This book belongs to

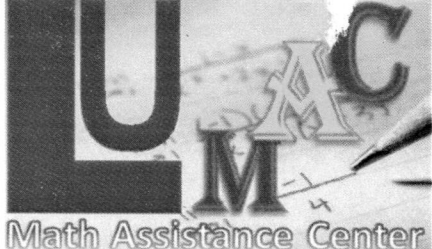

Please do not remove the book from this room.
Thank you.

SECOND CANADIAN EDITION

Elementary Statistics

A STEP-BY-STEP APPROACH

Allan G. Bluman

Community College of Allegheny County

John G. Mayer

SAIT Polytechnic

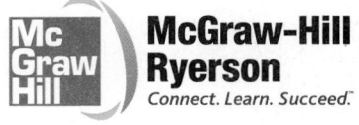
McGraw-Hill Ryerson

Connect. Learn. Succeed.

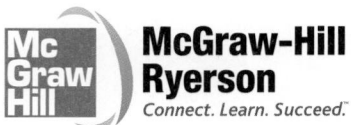

The McGraw-Hill Companies

McGraw-Hill
Ryerson
Connect. Learn. Succeed.

Elementary Statistics:
A Step-by-Step Approach
Second Canadian Edition

The Internet addresses listed in the text were accurate at the time of publication. The inclusion of a Web site
does not indicate an endorsement by the authors or McGraw-Hill Ryerson, nor does McGraw-Hill Ryerson
guarantee the accuracy of information presented at these sites.

ISBN-13: 978-0-07-000550-1
ISBN-10: 0-07-000550-8

1 2 3 4 5 6 7 8 9 10 TCP 1 9 8 7 6 5 4 3 2 1

Printed and bound in Canada.

Care has been taken to trace ownership of copyright material contained in this text; however, the publisher will
welcome any information that enables it to rectify any reference or credit for subsequent editions.

Vice-President and Editor-in-Chief: Joanna Cotton
Executive Sponsoring Editor: Leanna MacLean
Sponsoring Editor: James Booty
Developmental Editors: Sarah Fulton and Amy Rydzanicz
Marketing Manager: Cathie Lefebvre
Senior Editorial Associate: Stephanie Hess
Supervising Editor: Kara Stahl
Copy Editor: June Trusty
Production Coordinator: Sheryl MacAdam
Cover and Interior Design: Laserwords Private Limited
Cover Image Credit: Richard Glass, Getty Images (RM)
Page Layout: Aptara®, Inc.
Printer: Transcontinental Printing Group

Library and Archives Canada Cataloguing in Publication Bluman, Allan G.
     Elementary statistics: a step by step approach / Allan G. Bluman, John G.
Mayer. — 2nd Canadian ed.

Includes bibliographical references and index.
ISBN 978-0-07-000550-1

     1. Statistics—Textbooks. I. Mayer, John G., 1953-   II. Title.

QA276.12.B58 2011   519.5   C2010-905063-0

This text is dedicated to my wife, Janice, and our children, Tara, Jason, Christian, and Adam, and grandchild, Emily, who provided the inspiration and encouragement to promote our extraordinary Canadian heritage.

Brief Contents

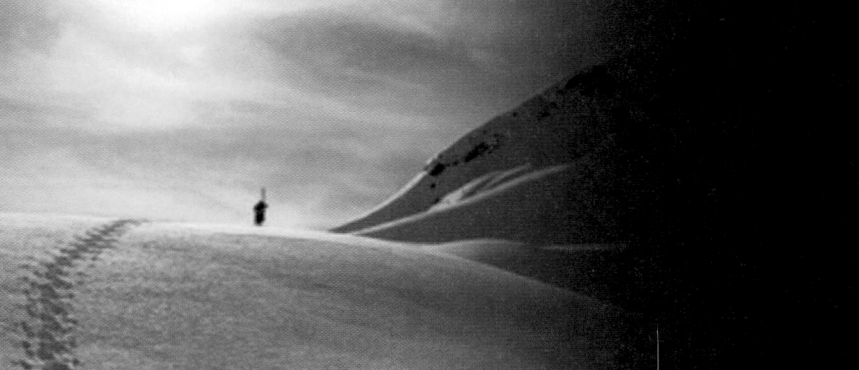

Contents

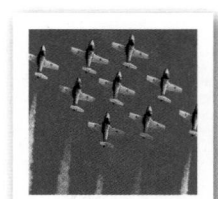
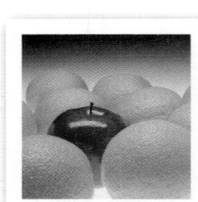

Chapter 4

Chapter 5

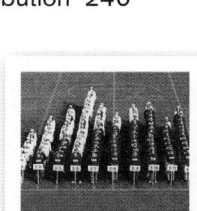

Chapter 6

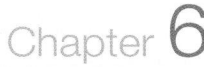

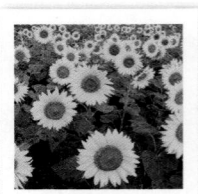
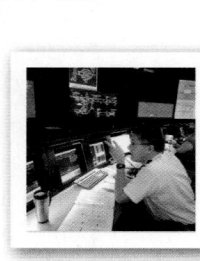

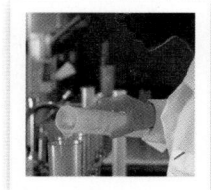

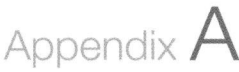

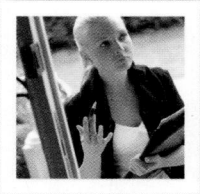

Preface

Approach

Elementary Statistics: A Step-by-Step Approach, Second Canadian Edition, was written to help students in the beginning statistics course whose mathematical background is limited to basic algebra. The book follows a nontheoretical approach without formal proofs, explaining concepts intuitively and supporting them with abundant examples. The applications span a broad range of topics certain to appeal to the interests of students of diverse backgrounds and include problems in business, sports, health, architecture, education, entertainment, political science, psychology, history, criminal justice, the environment, transportation, physical sciences, demographics, eating habits, and travel and leisure.

About This Book

The second Canadian edition of *Elementary Statistics: A Step-by-Step Approach* is for beginning statistics courses with a basic algebra prerequisite. The book follows a nontheoretical approach without formal proofs and teaches problem solving through worked examples and comprehensive step-by-step instructions.

Key features in this text include the following:

- **Over 1800** exercises with additional Canadian content are located at the end of major sections within each chapter.
- The **Applying the Concepts** feature is included in all sections of each chapter and gives students an opportunity to think about the new concepts they have studied and to apply them to hypothetical examples and scenarios similar to those found online, in newspapers and magazines, and on radio and television news programs.
- **Over 300** examples with detailed solutions serve as models to help students solve problems on their own.
- **Procedure Tables** summarize processes for students' quick reference and use the step-by-step method.
- **Hypothesis-Testing Summaries** are found at the end of Chapter 9 (z, t, χ^2, and F tests for testing means, proportions, and variances), Chapter 12 (correlation, chi-square, and ANOVA), and Chapter 13 (nonparametric tests) to show students the different types of hypotheses and the types of tests to use.
- A **databank** listing various attributes (educational level, cholesterol level, gender, etc.) for 100 people and 13 additional data sets using real data and SI units are included and referenced in various exercises and projects throughout the book, including the projects presented in Data Projects sections.
- The end-of-chapter **Summary, Important Terms,** and **Important Formulas** give students a concise summary of the chapter topics and provide a good source for quiz or test preparation.
- **Review Exercises** are found at the end of each chapter.
- Special sections called **Data Analysis** require students to work with a data set to perform various statistical tests or procedures and then summarize the results. The

data are included in the databank in Appendix D and can be downloaded from the book's website.

- **Chapter Quizzes**, found at the end of each chapter, include multiple-choice, true/false, and completion questions, along with exercises to test students' knowledge and comprehension of chapter content.

- The **appendices** provide students with an essential algebra review, an outline for report writing, Bayes' theorem, extensive reference tables, a technology review, a glossary, and answers to all quiz questions, all odd-numbered exercises, and selected even-numbered exercises. Alternative methods of solving for areas under the normal distribution curve from the centre, $z = 0$, are illustrated with examples and are available in Appendix B–3 for download from *Connect*.

Changes to the Canadian Edition

The second Canadian edition of *Elementary Statistics: A Step-by-Step Approach* features a substantial amount of new Canadian content, and improvements based on the feedback provided by expert statistics specialists throughout Canada.

- Hundreds of new and updated Canadian exercises and examples have been inserted, most using real data from verified Canadian sources, and many incorporating thought-provoking questions requiring students to interpret their results.

- The text is updated with an abundance of the most currently available Canadian content, including Unusual Stats, Interesting Facts, Statistics Today, Speaking of Statistics, Critical Thinking Challenges, chapter openers, worked examples, Data Analysis exercises, and Data Projects data sets in SI units.

- Six new Speaking of Statistics topics have been included.

- The Data Projects near the end of each chapter are all new and are specific to the areas of business and finance, sports and leisure, technology, health and wellness, politics and economics, and the students themselves.

- A reference card containing formulas and z, t, χ^2, and PPMC tables is included with the textbook.

- New and updated data sets have been added throughout the text.

- An explanation of bar graphs has been added to Chapter 2, since bar graphs are one of the most commonly used graphs in statistics and they are slightly different from Pareto charts.

- Based on Canadian reviewer comments, the following specific improvements have been made:

  - Improved figures illustrating usage of the z, t, and χ^2 distributions have been inserted.

  - Contemporary methods have been introduced, such as procedures for normality plots and P-value techniques for hypothesis testing.

  - Two graphs have been added to the explanation of the chi-square distribution in Chapter 7 to help clarify the nature of the distribution and how the distribution is related to the chi-square table.

  - The shortcut formula for the standard deviation has been changed. The formula used now is $s = \sqrt{\dfrac{n(\Sigma X^2) - (\Sigma X)^2}{n(n - 1)}}$, which is the one used in most other statistics books. It also avoids the complex fraction used in the other formula. Many reviewers have stated that they prefer the less-complicated formula.

  - When σ or σ_1 and σ_2 are known, the z tests are used in hypothesis testing. When σ or σ_1 and σ_2 are unknown, the t tests are used in hypothesis testing.

- The F test for two variances is no longer used before the t test for the difference between two means when σ_1 and σ_2 are unknown.

Also based on Canadian reviewer comments, the following improvements were made:

Technology Step by Step: Procedures for use of TI-83 Plus and TI-84 Plus programmable calculators are provided in Appendix E of the textbook. Minitab and Excel procedures were simplified and have been moved to a full version of Appendix E online in *Connect*. In addition, SPSS procedures are included in the online appendix.

Canadian Perspective: This edition includes examples drawn from Canadian business, industry, health-care, and other diverse fields. All changes to Canadian content utilize new data sets with source reference information.

Acknowledgements

It is important to acknowledge the many people whose contributions have gone into the second Canadian edition of *Elementary Statistics*. Very special thanks are due to developmental editors Sarah Fulton and Amy Rydzanicz, supervising editor Kara Stahl, sponsoring editor James Booty, copy editor June Trusty, and technical checker Rafal Kulik.

Special thanks for their advice and recommendations for revisions found in the second Canadian edition go to

Karen Buro, *Grant MacEwan College*

Paul Cabilio, *Acadia University*

Nancy Chibry, *University of Calgary*

Dennis Connolly, *University of Lethbridge*

Robert Connolly, *Algonquin College*

Paola Di Muro, *Brandon University*

M. Estabrooks, *Red Deer College*

Jimmie Graham, *Dawson College*

Andreas J. Guelzow, *Concordia University College of Alberta*

David Holloway, *British Columbia Institute of Technology*

Wendy Huang, *Lakehead University*

Sohail Khan, *University of Winnipeg*

Stephen Krizan, *SAIT Polytechnic*

Rafal Kulik, *University of Ottawa*

Dorothy Levay, *Brock University*

Eugene Li, *Langara College*

Amoel Lisecki, *SAIT Polytechnic*

Brian D. Macpherson, *University of Manitoba*

Gordon Robertson, *University of Ottawa*

Geoffrey Salloum, *Camosun College*

Gordon Sarty, *University of Saskatchewan*

Mina Singh, *York University*

Gary Sneddon, *Memorial University*

Jim Stallard, *University of Calgary*

Robert Steacy, *University of Victoria*

Dave Tomkins, *Thompson Rivers University*

Sheldon Ungar, *University of Toronto—Scarborough*

John G. Mayer

Guided Tour:
Features and Supplements

Each chapter begins with an **outline** and a list of **learning objectives.** The objectives are repeated at the beginning of each section to help students focus on the concepts presented within that section.

| Chapter **9**

Testing the Difference between Two Means, Two Proportions, and Two Variances

Objectives >

After completing this chapter, you should be able to

- **LO1** Test the difference between sample means, using the z test.
- **LO2** Test the difference between two means for independent samples, using the t test.
- **LO3** Test the difference between two means for dependent samples.
- **LO4** Test the difference between two proportions.
- **LO5** Test the difference between two variances or standard deviations.

Outline >

Introduction
9–1 Testing the Difference between Two Means: Using the z Test
9–2 Testing the Difference between Two Means of Independent Samples: Using the t Test
9–3 Testing the Difference between Two Means: Dependent Samples
9–4 Testing the Difference between Two Proportions
9–5 Testing the Difference between Two Variances
Summary

connect Practise and learn online with Connect with data sets and algorithmic questions related to concepts covered in this chapter. Throughout this chapter, questions and tables with online data sets are marked with.

 Statistics Today

Do You Live As Well As Other Canadians?

The United Nations ranked Canada fourth in the world on its *Human Development Index* for 2009, ahead of the United States and Japan but trailing Norway and Australia. Unfortunately, this reputation for outstanding living conditions merely represents the well-being of the average Canadian. Regional disparities abound. One measure of quality of life is economic well-being. In 2008, the average Canadian per capita income was $39,648. How did your province or territory compare to this average? See Statistics Today—Revisited on page 140.

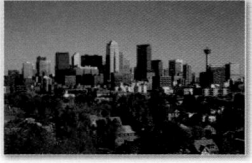

This chapter will show you how to obtain and interpret descriptive statistics as measures of average, measures of variation, and measures of position.

Source: United Nations, *Human Development Report, 2009.*

Introduction >

Chapter 2 showed how one can gain useful information from raw data by organizing them into a frequency distribution and then presenting the data by using various graphs. This chapter shows the statistical methods that can be used to summarize data. The most familiar of these methods is the finding of averages.

For example, an average NHL hockey player earned $2.21 million in the 2009–2010 season.[1] The average 2009 undergraduate student debt ranges between $21,000 to $28,000, depending on the province or program of study.[2] The life expectancy at birth for average Canadian males, based on 2010 estimates, is 79.2 years, whereas the average Canadian female will live 83.2 years.[3]

Canadian nationalist writer and humourist Pierre Berton once described a typical Canadian as "*Someone who knows how to make love in a canoe without tipping it.*"

Are you an average Canadian? Statistics Canada and market researchers collect descriptive statistics from all facets of Canadian life. Here are some findings about the typical Canadian.

Interesting Fact

A person has on average 1460 dreams in one year.

Canadian brides marry at an average age of 31.7 years and their grooms at 34.3 years.[4]
Typical Canadian households spend an average of $142.08 on food each week.[5]
An average Canadian consumes 23.4 kg of red meat, 13.4 kg of poultry, and 12.7 dozen eggs each year.[6]
Canadians consume an average of 63.2 litres of milk, 160.1 litres of coffee or tea, and 65.8 litres of beer per capita each year.[7]
Canadians view an average of 147 online videos for an average of 605 minutes each month.[8]

[1] National Hockey League Players' Association, Players, "Player Compensation."
[2] Canadian Federation of Students, Research and Policy, Submission to House of Commons Standing Committee on Finance, August 2009.
[3] Office of the Superintendent of Financial Institutions Canada, Office of the Chief Actuary, Canada Pension Plan Mortality Study: Actuarial Study No. 7, July 2009.
[4] Adapted from CBC News, "Marriage by the Numbers," March 9, 2005.
[5] Adapted from Statistics Canada, Spending Patterns in Canada, 2008, Catalogue No. 62-202-X.
[6] Adapted from Statistics Canada, Food Statistics, 2009, Catalogue No. 21-020-X.
[7] Adapted from Statistics Canada, The Daily, Catalogue No. 11-001, May 26, 2005.
[8] comScore, Canada Ranks as a Global Leader in Online Video Viewing, April 21, 2008.

The outline and learning objectives are followed by a feature entitled **Statistics Today,** in which a **real-life problem** shows students the relevance of the material in the chapter. This problem is subsequently solved near the end of the chapter by using the statistical techniques presented in the chapter.

34   Chapter 2   Frequency Distributions and Graphs

Example 2–1

Distribution of Blood Types

Twenty-five armed forces recruits were given a blood test to determine their blood type. The data set is

A	B	B	AB	O
O	O	B	AB	B
B	B	O	A	O
A	O	O	O	AB
AB	A	O	B	A

Construct a frequency distribution for the data.

Solution

Since the data are categorical, discrete classes can be used. There are four blood types: A, B, O, and AB. These types will be used as the classes for the distribution.

The procedure for constructing a frequency distribution for categorical data is given next.

Step 1   Make a table as shown.

A	B	C	D
Class	**Tally**	**Frequency**	**Percentage**
A			
B			
O			
AB			

Step 2   Tally the data and place the results in column B.

Step 3   Count the tallies and place the results in column C.

Step 4   Find the percentage of values in each class by using the formula

$$\% = \frac{f}{n} \cdot 100$$

where f = frequency of the class and n = total number of values in the data set. For example, in the class of type A blood, the percentage is

$$\% = \frac{5}{25} \cdot 100 = 20\%$$

Percentages are not normally part of a frequency distribution, but they can be added since they are used in certain types of graphs such as pie graphs. Also, the decimal equivalent of a percentage is called a *relative frequency*.

Step 5   Find the totals for columns C (frequency) and D (percentage). The completed table is shown.

A	B	C	D
Class	**Tally**	**Frequency**	**Percentage**
A	⁄⁄⁄⁄	5	20
B	⁄⁄⁄⁄ ⁄⁄	7	28
O	⁄⁄⁄⁄ ⁄⁄⁄⁄	9	36
AB	⁄⁄⁄⁄	4	16
		Total 25	100

For the sample, more people have type O blood than any other type.

Over 300 **examples** with detailed solutions serve as models to help students solve problems on their own. Examples are solved by using a step-by-step explanation, and illustrations provide a clear display of results for students.

Section 7–2   Confidence Intervals for the Mean When σ Is Unknown   **319**

Exercises 7–2

1. What are the properties of the t distribution?

2. What is meant by *degrees of freedom*?

3. When should the t distribution be used to find a confidence interval for the mean?

4. Find the values for each.

    a. $t_{\alpha/2}$ and $n = 18$ for the 99% confidence interval for the mean

    b. $t_{\alpha/2}$ and $n = 23$ for the 95% confidence interval for the mean

    c. $t_{\alpha/2}$ and $n = 15$ for the 98% confidence interval for the mean

    d. $t_{\alpha/2}$ and $n = 10$ for the 90% confidence interval for the mean

    e. $t_{\alpha/2}$ and $n = 20$ for the 95% confidence interval for the mean

For Exercises 5 through 20, assume that all variables are approximately normally distributed.

5. Blood Hemoglobin The average hemoglobin reading for a sample of 20 teachers was 16 grams per 100 millilitres, with a sample standard deviation of 2 grams. Find the 99% confidence interval of the true mean.

6. Professors' Salaries The following data represent annual salaries of a random selection of academics with the rank of professor (or full professor) in Ontario universities. Estimate the mean salary of all Ontario university professors at a 95% confidence level.

$119,843	$149,749	$152,311
$115,914	$132,184	$153,454
$159,845	$150,261	$178,068

Source: Ontario Ministry of Finance. Universities, "Disclosure for 2008 under the Public Sector Salary Disclosure Act, 1996."

7. Tuition Fees A sample of undergraduate university tuition fees across Canada is listed below. Estimate, with 98% confidence, the true population tuition fees for all undergraduate students.

$1968	$4673	$4988
$2550	$4920	$5101
$3108	$4872	$5630
$4638	$5004	$4989
$4719	$5008	$2911

Source: Macleans.ca, "On Campus: The Bottom Line." November 5, 2009.

8. Oil Production A random sample of oil-producing countries lists oil production measured in barrels of oil per day (bbl/day). Estimate the true population mean oil consumption for all oil-producing countries in the world at a 90% confidence level. Data shown are thousands of bbl/day.

33	2,422	3186	11	368
20	115	36	2466	305
2531	133	797	287	71
586	10,780	4174	30	12
18	51	1584	359	38

Source: Central Intelligence Agency, The World Factbook, "Country Comparison: Oil Production," (2009 est.).

9. College Wrestler Weights A sample of 6 university wrestlers had an average weight of 125 kg with a standard deviation of 5.5 kg. Find the 90% confidence interval of the true mean weight of all university wrestlers. If a coach claimed that the average weight of the wrestlers on his team was 141 kg, would the claim be believable?

10. Charitable Donations Different regions of Canada were sampled to determine per capita charitable donations. Results are listed below. At a 98% level of confidence, estimate the mean charitable donations for all Canadians.

$253	$333	$322	$299	$150
$415	$387	$367	$426	$397

Source: Human Resources and Skills Development Canada, Indicators of Well-Being in Canada, "Social Participation—Charitable Donations, 2004."

11. Distance Travelled to Work A recent study of 28 employees of XYZ company showed that the mean of the distance they travelled to work was 23 km. The standard deviation of the sample mean was 3 km. Find the 95% confidence interval of the true mean. If a manager wanted to be sure that most of his employees would not be late, how much time would he suggest they allow for the commute if the average speed was 48 km per hour?

12. Sunny Days A random selection of Canadian cities yielded the following annual number of sunny days. Estimate the average number of sunny days for all Canadian cities at a 99% confidence level.

272	299	320	324	275
300	277	294	287	323
292	293	307	274	312
286	292	306	300	277

Source: Environment Canada.

13. Student Gas Consumption A study of 25 students showed that they spent an average of $18.53 for gasoline per week. The standard deviation of the sample was $3.00. Find the 95% confidence interval of the true mean.

Numerous examples and exercises use **real data.** The icon shown here indicates that the data set for the exercise is available in a variety of file formats on the text's *Connect* site.

Numerous **Procedure Tables** summarize processes for students' quick reference. All use the step-by-step method.

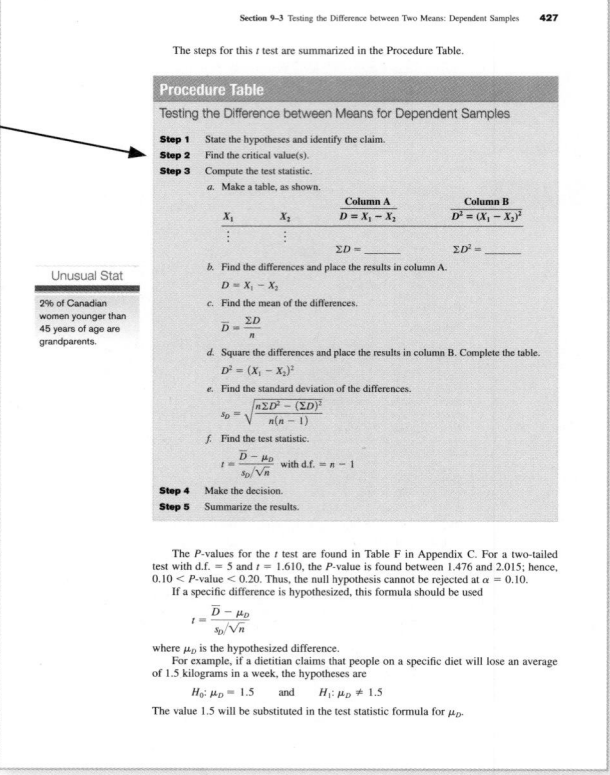

The steps for this t test are summarized in the Procedure Table.

Procedure Table

Testing the Difference between Means for Dependent Samples

Step 1 State the hypotheses and identify the claim.

Step 2 Find the critical value(s).

Step 3 Compute the test statistic.

  a. Make a table, as shown.

X_1	X_2	Column A $D = X_1 - X_2$	Column B $D^2 = (X_1 - X_2)^2$
⋮	⋮	$\Sigma D =$ _____	$\Sigma D^2 =$ _____

  b. Find the differences and place the results in column A.

  $$D = X_1 - X_2$$

  c. Find the mean of the differences.

  $$\overline{D} = \frac{\Sigma D}{n}$$

  d. Square the differences and place the results in column B. Complete the table.

  $$D^2 = (X_1 - X_2)^2$$

  e. Find the standard deviation of the differences.

  $$s_D = \sqrt{\frac{n\Sigma D^2 - (\Sigma D)^2}{n(n-1)}}$$

  f. Find the test statistic.

  $$t = \frac{\overline{D} - \mu_D}{s_D/\sqrt{n}} \quad \text{with d.f.} = n - 1$$

Step 4 Make the decision.

Step 5 Summarize the results.

Unusual Stat

2% of Canadian women younger than 45 years of age are grandparents.

The P-values for the t test are found in Table F in Appendix C. For a two-tailed test with d.f. = 5 and $t = 1.610$, the P-value is found between 1.476 and 2.015; hence, $0.10 < P\text{-value} < 0.20$. Thus, the null hypothesis cannot be rejected at $\alpha = 0.10$.

If a specific difference is hypothesized, this formula should be used

$$t = \frac{\overline{D} - \mu_D}{s_D/\sqrt{n}}$$

where μ_D is the hypothesized difference.

For example, if a dietitian claims that people on a specific diet will lose an average of 1.5 kilograms in a week, the hypotheses are

$$H_0: \mu_D = 1.5 \quad \text{and} \quad H_1: \mu_D \neq 1.5$$

The value 1.5 will be substituted in the test statistic formula for μ_D.

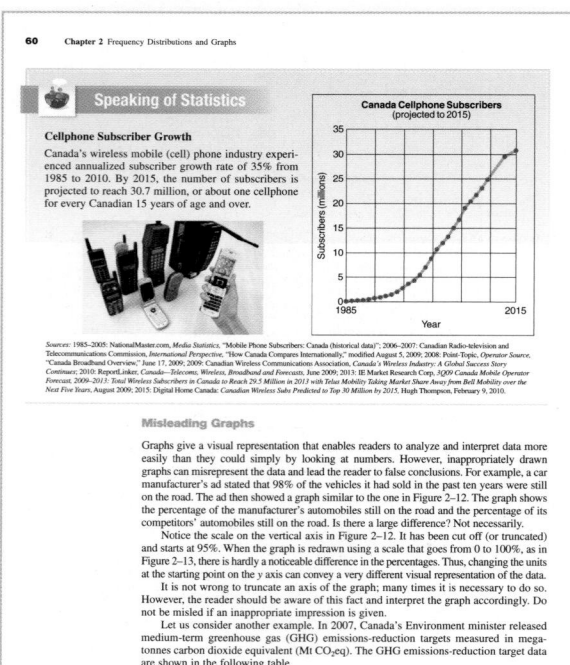

Speaking of Statistics

Cellphone Subscriber Growth

Canada's wireless mobile (cell) phone industry experienced annualized subscriber growth rate of 35% from 1985 to 2010. By 2015, the number of subscribers is projected to reach 30.7 million, or about one cellphone for every Canadian 15 years of age and over.

Canada Cellphone Subscribers (projected to 2015)

Sources: 1985–2005: NationalMaster.com, *Media Statistics,* "Mobile Phone Subscribers: Canada (historical data)"; 2006–2007: Canadian Radio-television and Telecommunications Commission, *International Perspective,* "How Canada Compares Internationally," modified August 5, 2009; 2008: Point-Topic, *Operator Source,* "Canada Broadband Overview," June 17, 2009; 2009: Canadian Wireless Communications Association, *Canada's Wireless Industry: A Global Success Story Continues;* 2010: ReportLinker, *Canada—Telecoms, Wireless, Broadband and Forecasts,* June 2009; 2013: IE Market Research Corp, 3Q09 *Canada Mobile Operator Forecast, 2009–2013: Total Wireless Subscribers in Canada to Reach 29.5 Million in 2013 with Telus Mobility Taking Market Share Away from Bell Mobility over the Next Five Years,* August 2009; 2015: Digital Home Canada: *Canadian Wireless Subs Predicted to Top 30 Million by 2015,* Hugh Thompson, February 9, 2010.

Misleading Graphs

Graphs give a visual representation that enables readers to analyze and interpret data more easily than they could simply by looking at numbers. However, inappropriately drawn graphs can misrepresent the data and lead the reader to false conclusions. For example, a car manufacturer's ad stated that 98% of the vehicles it had sold in the past ten years were still on the road. The ad then showed a graph similar to the one in Figure 2–12. The graph shows the percentage of the manufacturer's automobiles still on the road and the percentage of its competitors' automobiles still on the road. Is there a large difference? Not necessarily.

Notice the scale on the vertical axis in Figure 2–12. It has been cut off (or truncated) and starts at 95%. When the graph is redrawn using a scale that goes from 0 to 100%, as in Figure 2–13, there is hardly a noticeable difference in the percentages. Thus, changing the units at the starting point on the y axis can convey a very different visual representation of the data.

It is not wrong to truncate an axis of the graph; many times it is necessary to do so. However, the reader should be aware of this fact and interpret the graph accordingly. Do not be misled if an inappropriate impression is given.

Let us consider another example. In 2007, Canada's Environment minister released medium-term greenhouse gas (GHG) emissions-reduction targets measured in mega-tonnes carbon dioxide equivalent (Mt CO_2eq). The GHG emissions-reduction target data are shown in the following table.

Year	2010	2011	2012	2015	2020
Target reductions (Mt CO_2eq)	49	54	58	72	88

Source: Climate Action Network Canada: The Pembina Institute, *Analysis of the Government of Canada's April 2007 Greenhouse Gas Policy Announcement,* Matthew Bramley.

The **Speaking of Statistics** sections invite students to think about poll results and other statistics-related news stories in another connection between statistics and the real world.

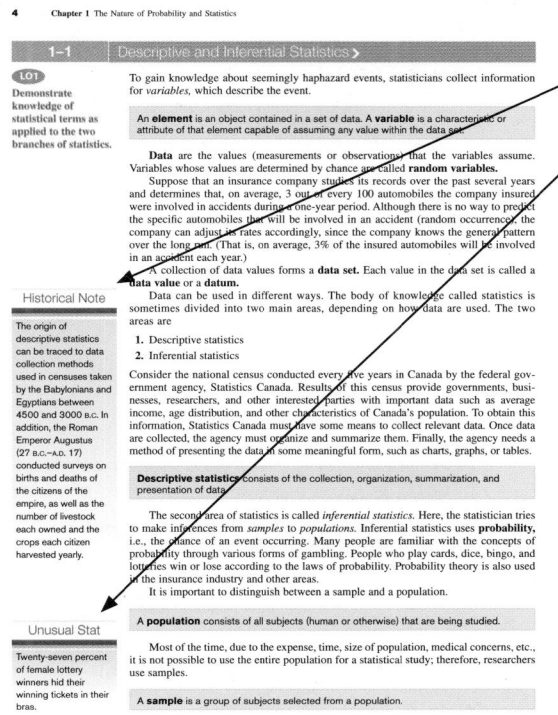

Historical Notes, Unusual Stats, and **Interesting Facts,** located in the margins, make statistics come alive for the reader.

Rules and definitions are set off for easy referencing by the student.

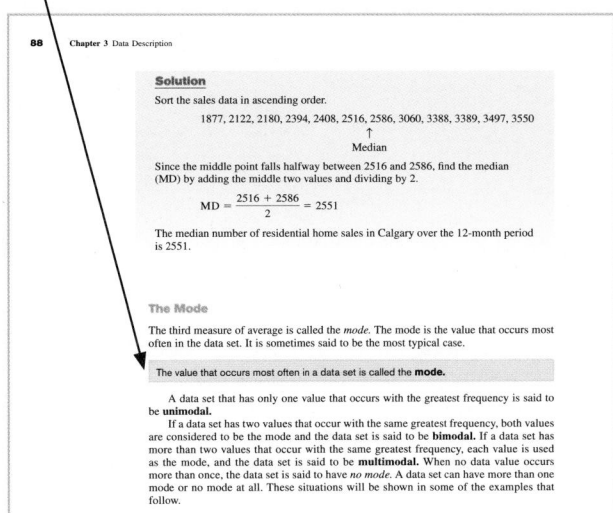

Critical Thinking sections at the end of each chapter challenge students to apply what they have learned to new situations. The problems presented are designed to deepen conceptual understanding and/or to extend topical coverage.

Applying the Concepts exercises are found at the end of each section, and their purpose is to reinforce the concepts explained in the section. They give the student an opportunity to think about the concepts and apply them to hypothetical examples similar to real-life ones found in newspapers, magazines, and professional journals. Most contain open-ended questions—questions that require interpretation and may have more than one correct answer. These exercises can also be used as classroom discussion topics for instructors who like to use this type of teaching technique.

Data Projects further challenge students' understanding and application of the material presented in the chapter. Many of these require the student to gather, analyze, and report on real data.

Step-by-step procedures for TI-83 Plus and TI-84 Plus calculators are included in Appendix E in the textbook for easy reference. A brief overview of each of the principal **statistics technologies, such as Minitab, SPSS, and Excel,** is included in the extended version of Appendix E, available on this text's *Connect* site.

5–4   Applying the Concepts

Rockets and Targets

During the latter days of World War II, the Germans developed flying rocket bombs. These bombs were used to attack London. Allied military intelligence didn't know whether these bombs were fired at random or had a sophisticated aiming device. To determine the answer, they used the Poisson distribution.

To assess the accuracy of these bombs, London was divided into 576 square regions. Each region was $\frac{1}{4}$ square kilometre in area. They then compared the number of actual hits with the theoretical number of hits by using the Poisson distribution. If the values in both distributions were close, then they would conclude that the rockets were fired at random. The actual distribution is as follows:

Hits	0	1	2	3	4	5
Regions	229	211	93	35	7	1

1. Using the Poisson distribution, find the theoretical values for each number of hits. In this case, the number of bombs was 535, and the number of regions was 576. So

$$\mu = \frac{535}{576} \approx 0.929$$

For 3 hits,

$$P(X) = \frac{\mu^x \cdot e^{-\mu}}{X!}$$

$$= \frac{(0.929)^3 (2.7183)^{-0.929}}{3!} \approx 0.0528$$

Hence the number of hits is $(0.0528)(576) = 30.4128$.

Complete the table for the other number of hits.

Hits	0	1	2	3	4	5
Regions				30.4		

2. Write a brief statement comparing the two distributions.
3. Based on your answer to question 2, can you conclude that the rockets were fired at random?

See page 251 for the answer.

Exercises 5–4

1. Use the multinomial formula and find the probabilities for each.
   a. $n = 6$, $X_1 = 3$, $X_2 = 2$, $X_3 = 1$, $p_1 = 0.5$, $p_2 = 0.3$, $p_3 = 0.2$
   b. $n = 5$, $X_1 = 1$, $X_2 = 2$, $X_3 = 2$, $p_1 = 0.3$, $p_2 = 0.6$, $p_3 = 0.1$
   c. $n = 4$, $X_1 = 1$, $X_2 = 1$, $X_3 = 2$, $p_1 = 0.8$, $p_2 = 0.1$, $p_3 = 0.1$
   d. $n = 3$, $X_1 = 1$, $X_2 = 1$, $X_3 = 1$, $p_1 = 0.5$, $p_2 = 0.3$, $p_3 = 0.2$
   e. $n = 5$, $X_1 = 1$, $X_2 = 3$, $X_3 = 1$, $p_1 = 0.7$, $p_2 = 0.2$, $p_3 = 0.1$

2. **Textbook Typographical Errors** The probabilities that a textbook page will have 0, 1, 2, or 3 typographical errors are 0.79, 0.12, 0.07, and 0.02, respectively. If eight pages are randomly selected, find the probability that four will contain no errors, two will contain 1 error, one will contain 2 errors, and one will contain 3 errors.

3. **Truck Safety Violations** The probabilities are 0.25, 0.40, and 0.35 that an 18-wheel truck will have 0 violations, 1 violation, or 2 or more violations when it is given a safety inspection. If eight trucks are inspected, find the probability that three will have 0 violations, two will have 1 violation, and three will have 2 or more violations.

Data Projects ≫

Where appropriate, use Minitab, SPSS, TI-83 Plus, TI-84 Plus, Excel, or a computer program of your choice to complete the following exercises.

1. **Business and Finance** A car salesperson has six automobiles on the car lot. Roll a die, using the numbers 1 through 6 to represent each car. If only one car can be sold on each day, how long will it take him to sell all the automobiles? In other words, see how many tosses of the die it will take to get the numbers 1 through 6.

2. **Sports and Leisure** Using the rules given in Figure 14–11 on page 634, play the simulated bowling game. Each game consists of 10 frames.

3. **Technology** In a carton of 12 iPods, three are defective. If four are sold on Saturday, find the probability that at least one will be defective. Use random numbers to simulate this exercise 50 times.

4. **Health and Wellness** Of people who go on a special diet, 25% will lose at least 5 kilograms in 10 weeks. A drug manufacturer says that if people take its special herbal pill, the number of people who lose at least 5 kilograms

in 10 weeks will increase. The company conducts an experiment, giving its pill to 20 people. Seven people lost at least 5 kilograms in 10 weeks. The drug manufacturer claims that the study "proves" the success of the herbal pill. Using random numbers, simulate the experiment 30 times, assuming the pill is ineffective. What can you conclude about the result that 7 out of 20 people lost at least 5 kilograms?

5. **Politics and Economics** Research the home provinces of all prime ministers of Canada since Confederation. Select two of the prime ministers at random. What is the probability that both prime ministers will be from the same province? Use random numbers to simulate the experiment and perform the experiment 50 times.

6. **Your Class** Simulate the classical birthday problem given in Critical Thinking Challenge 3 in Chapter 4. Select a sample size of 25 and generate random numbers between 1 and 365. Are any two random numbers the same? Select a sample of 50. Are any two random numbers the same? Repeat the experiments 10 times each and explain your answers.

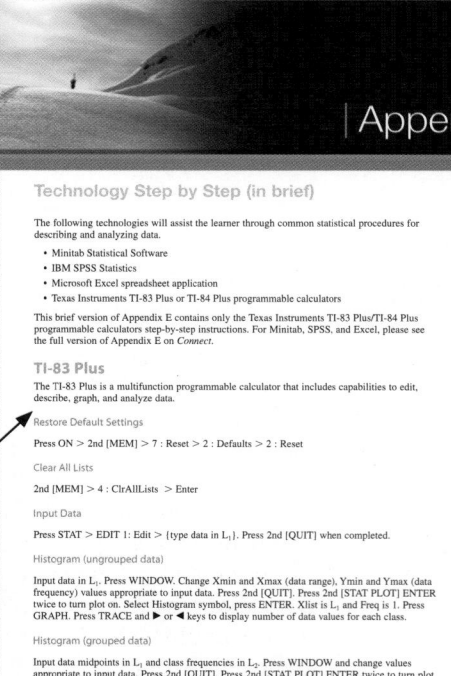

Appendix E

Technology Step by Step (in brief)

The following technologies will assist the learner through common statistical procedures for describing and analyzing data.

- Minitab Statistical Software
- IBM SPSS Statistics
- Microsoft Excel spreadsheet application
- Texas Instruments TI-83 Plus or TI-84 Plus programmable calculators

This brief version of Appendix E contains only the Texas Instruments TI-83 Plus/TI-84 Plus programmable calculators step-by-step instructions. For Minitab, SPSS, and Excel, please see the full version of Appendix E on *Connect*.

TI-83 Plus

The TI-83 Plus is a multifunction programmable calculator that includes capabilities to edit, describe, graph, and analyze data.

Restore Default Settings

Press ON > 2nd [MEM] > 7 : Reset > 2 : Defaults > 2 : Reset

Clear All Lists

2nd [MEM] > 4 : ClrAllLists > Enter

Input Data

Press STAT > EDIT 1: Edit > {type data in L_1}. Press 2nd [QUIT] when completed.

Histogram (ungrouped data)

Input data in L_1. Press WINDOW. Change Xmin and Xmax (data range), Ymin and Ymax (data frequency) values appropriate to input data. Press 2nd [QUIT]. Press 2nd [STAT PLOT] ENTER twice to turn plot on. Select Histogram symbol, press ENTER. Xlist is L_1 and Freq is 1. Press GRAPH. Press TRACE and ▶ or ◀ keys to display number of data values for each class.

Histogram (grouped data)

Input data midpoints in L_1 and class frequencies in L_2. Press WINDOW and change values appropriate to input data. Press 2nd [QUIT]. Press 2nd [STAT PLOT] ENTER twice to turn plot on. Select Histogram symbol, press ENTER. Xlist is L_1 and Freq is L_2. Press GRAPH. Press TRACE and ▶ or ◀ keys to display number of data values for each class.

Superior Service

Service takes on a whole new meaning with McGraw-Hill Ryerson and *Elementary Statistics*. More than just bringing you the textbook, we have consistently raised the bar in terms of innovation and educational research—both in operations management and in education in general. These investments in learning and the education community have helped us to understand the needs of students and educators across the country, and allowed us to foster the growth of truly innovative, integrated learning.

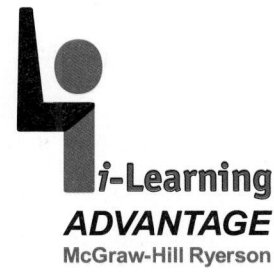

Integrated Learning

Your Integrated *i*Learning Sales Specialist is a McGraw-Hill Ryerson representative who has the experience, product knowledge, training, and support to help you assess and integrate any of our products, technology, and services into your course for optimal teaching and learning performance. Whether it's helping your students improve their grades, or putting your entire course online, your *i*Learning Sales Specialist is there to help you do it. Contact your *i*Learning Sales Specialist today to learn how to maximize all of McGraw-Hill Ryerson's resources!

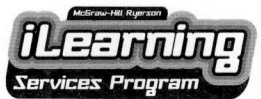

*i*Learning Services

McGraw-Hill Ryerson offers a unique *i*Services package designed for Canadian faculty. Our mission is to equip providers of higher education with superior tools and resources required for excellence in teaching. For additional information, visit www.mcgrawhill.ca/highereducation/iservices.

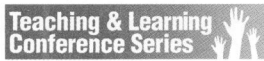

Teaching & Learning Conference Series

The educational environment has changed tremendously in recent years, and McGraw-Hill Ryerson continues to be committed to helping you acquire the skills you need to succeed in this new milieu. Our innovative Teaching & Learning Conference Series brings faculty together from across Canada with 3M Teaching Excellence award winners to share teaching and learning best practices in a collaborative and stimulating environment. Pre-conference workshops on general topics, such as teaching large classes and technology integration, will also be offered. We will also work with you at your own institution to customize workshops that best suit the needs of your faculty.

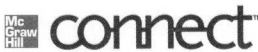

Connect™

Connect is a Web-based assignment and assessment platform that gives students the means to better connect with their course work, with their instructors, and with the important concepts that they will need to know for success now and in the future. *Connect* embraces diverse study behaviours and preferences with breakthrough features that help students master course content and achieve better results. The powerful course management tool in *Connect* also offers a wide range of exclusive features that help instructors spend less time managing and more time teaching.

With *Connect*, you can deliver assignments, quizzes, and tests online. A robust set of questions and problems are presented and tied to the textbook's learning objectives. Track individual student performance—by question, assignment, or in relation to the class overall—with detailed grade reports. Integrate grade reports easily with Learning Management Systems (LMS) such as WebCT and Blackboard. And much more.

Connect helps you teach for today's needs:

Unlimited Practice, Instant Feedback
Provide instant feedback to unlimited practice problems, acknowledging correct answers and pointing to areas that need more work.

Automatic Grading
Focus on teaching instead of administrating, with electronic access to the class roster and gradebook, which easily sync with your school's course management system.

Test Bank Questions
Assign students online homework, and test and quiz questions with multiple problem types, algorithmic variation, and randomized question order.

Integrated eBooks
Connect directly integrates the McGraw-Hill textbooks you already use into the engaging, easy-to-use interface.

Dedicated Canadian Support and Training
The *Connect* development team and customer service groups are located in our Canadian offices and work closely together to provide expert technical support and training for both instructors and students.

Connect™ for Students

Connect provides students with a powerful tool for improving academic performance and truly mastering course material, plus 24/7 online access to an interactive and searchable eBook. *Connect* allows students to practise important skills at their own pace and on their own schedule. Importantly, students' assessment results and instructors' feedback are all saved online—so students can continually review their progress and plot their course to success.

Instructor's Supplements

Instructor's Solutions Manual

Prepared by the author and adapted to reflect the second Canadian edition, this manual includes worked-out solutions to all the exercises in the text and answers to all quiz questions.

Computerized Test Bank

Prepared by Nancy Chibry, University of Calgary, the computerized test bank has been extensively revised and technically checked for accuracy. The computerized test bank contains a variety of questions, including true/false, multiple-choice, and short-answer, as well as short problems requiring analysis and written answers. The computerized test bank is available through EZ Test Online—a flexible and easy-to-use electronic testing program—that allows instructors to create tests from book-specific items. EZ Test accommodates a wide range of question types and allows instructors to add their own questions. Test items are also available in Word format (Rich Text Format). For secure online testing, exams created in EZ Test can be exported to WebCT and Blackboard. EZ Test Online is supported at www.mhhe.com/eztest, where users can download a Quick Start Guide, access FAQs, or log a ticket for help with specific issues.

Microsoft®PowerPoint® Lecture Slides

Prepared by Cristina Anton, Grant MacEwan University, the PowerPoint slides draw on the highlights of each chapter and provide an opportunity for the instructor to emphasize the most relevant visuals in class discussions.

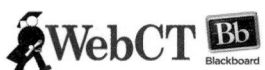

Course Management

McGraw-Hill Ryerson offers a range of flexible integration solutions for **WebCT** and **Blackboard** platforms. Please contact your local McGraw-Hill Ryerson *i*Learning Sales specialist for details.

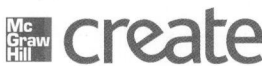

Create Online

McGraw-Hill's Create Online places the most abundant resource at your fingertips—literally. With a few mouse clicks, you can create customized learning tools simply and affordably. McGraw-Hill Ryerson has included many of its market-leading textbooks within Create Online for eBook and print customization as well as many licensed readings and cases. For more information, please visit www.mcgrawhillcreate.com.

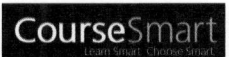

CourseSmart

CourseSmart brings together thousands of textbooks across hundreds of courses in an eTextbook format providing unique benefits to students and faculty. By purchasing an eTextbook, students can save up to 50 percent off the cost of a print textbook, reduce their impact on the environment, and gain access to powerful Web tools for learning, including full text search, notes and highlighting, and email tools for sharing notes among classmates. For faculty, CourseSmart provides instant access to review and compare textbooks and course materials in their discipline area without the time, cost, and environmental impact of mailing print examination copies. For further details, contact your *i*Learning Sales Specialist or visit www.coursesmart.com.

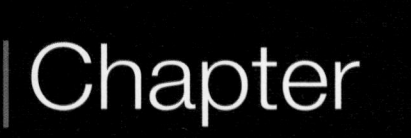

Chapter 1

The Nature of Probability and Statistics

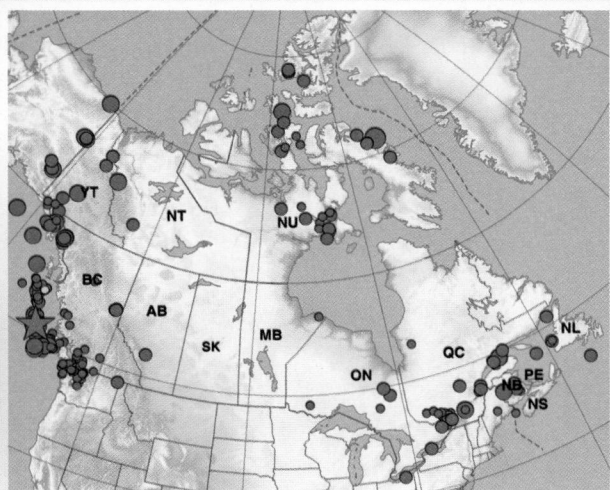

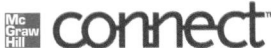 **Practise and learn online with *Connect* with data sets and algorithmic questions related to concepts covered in this chapter.**

Statistics Today

Are We Improving Our Diet?

Canada's Guide To Healthy Eating and Physical Activity suggests that the benefits of a healthy diet

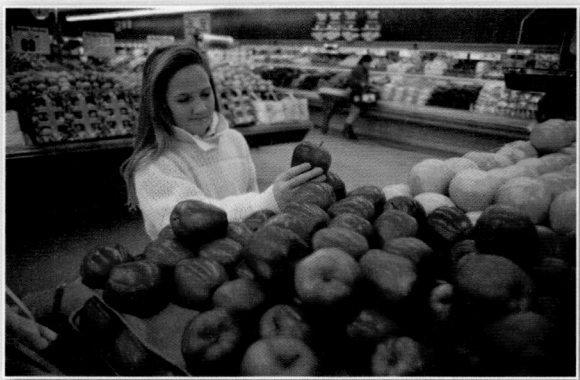

and an active lifestyle improve the quality of life and may prevent the onset of illnesses such as stroke, heart disease, and some types of cancer. Nutritionists recommend consumption of five or more servings of fruits and vegetables per day as part of a healthy diet. North American researchers from the Division of Nutrition, the National Center for Chronic Disease Control and Prevention, the National Cancer Institute, and the National Institute of Health decided to use statistical procedures to see how much progress is being made toward this goal.

The procedures they used and the results of the study will be explained in this chapter. See Statistics Today—Revisited, page 26, near the end of this chapter.

Source: Healthy Living: Canada's Guide to Healthy Eating and Physical Activity. Health Canada, 2004. Adapted and reproduced with the permission of the Minister of Public Works and Government Services Canada, 2007.

Introduction >

Most people become familiar with probability and statistics through radio, television, newspapers, magazines, and online resources. For example, the following statements were found in print and digital media.

Unusual Stat

Most Canadian women animal owners (82%) embrace or stroke their pets at least four times a day.

- On average, the Geological Survey of Canada (GSC) locates and records over 1500 earthquakes in Canada each year. *Source:* Reproduced with the permission of the Minister of Public Works and Government Services Canada, 2007, and courtesy of Natural Resources Canada, *Geological Survey of Canada.*

- Average undergraduate student debt at graduation in Canada is $26,680. *Source: The Price of Knowledge: Access and Student Finance in Canada,* Chapter 7, "Student Debt in Canada," Joseph Berger, 2009.

- Canadian police services reported approximately 2.2 million Criminal Code incidents (excluding traffic) in 2008. *Source:* Statistics Canada, *Juristat,* "Police-Reported Crime Statistics in Canada, 2008," July 2009.

- In 2008, the average Canadian family income was $90,678, with $40,667 (44.8%) paid in taxes. *Source: Canadian Capitalist,* "The Fraser Institute and 'Average Canadian Family.'" August 24, 2009.

- The Canadian median age is 40.4 years, compared to Japan at 44.2 years and Uganda at 15 years. *Source: CIA—The World Factbook, 2009.*

- Globally, the average ecological footprint is 2.2 hectares, with Canada ranking second-highest at 7.6 hectares per person. *Source: David Suzuki's Green Guide,* David Suzuki and David Boyd, 2008.

- Fifty-five percent of Canadians aged 18–34 have placed an online profile on a social network or community. *Source: MarketingCharts*: Ipsos-Reid, "37% of Canadians Have Visited a Social Network, 29% Have a Profile."
- More than 21 million Canadian viewers, or 88% of the total Canadian Internet population, watched an average of 147 videos per viewer in February 2009. *Source: ComScore,* "Canada Ranks as a Global Leader in Online Video Viewing," April 21, 2008.

Interesting Fact

Of the 20 hottest years on record, 19 occurred in the 1980s or later.

Statistics is used in almost all fields of human endeavour. In sports, for example, a statistician may keep records of the number of yards a running back gains during a football game, or the number of hits a baseball player gets in a season. In other areas, such as public health, an administrator might be concerned with the number of residents who contract a new strain of flu virus during a certain year. In education, a researcher might want to know if new methods of teaching are better than old ones. These are only a few examples of how statistics can be used in various occupations.

Furthermore, statistics is used to analyze the results of surveys and as a tool in scientific research to make decisions based on controlled experiments. Other uses of statistics include industrial operations research, quality engineering, manufacturing quality control, scientific estimation, and prediction.

Statistics is the science of conducting studies to collect, organize, summarize, analyze, and draw conclusions from data.

Students study statistics for several reasons:

1. Students, like professional people, must be able to read and understand the various statistical studies performed in their fields. To have this understanding, they must be knowledgeable about the vocabulary, symbols, concepts, and statistical procedures used in these studies.

2. Students and professional people may be called on to conduct research in their fields, since statistical procedures are basic to research. To accomplish this, they must be able to design experiments; collect, organize, summarize, and analyze data; and possibly make reliable predictions or forecasts for future use. They must also be able to communicate the results of the study in their own words.

3. Students and professional people can also use the knowledge gained from studying statistics to become better consumers and citizens. For example, they can make intelligent decisions about what products to purchase based on consumer studies, about government spending based on utilization studies, and so on.

These reasons can be considered the goals for students and professionals who study statistics.

It is the purpose of this chapter to introduce the student to the basic concepts of *probability* and *statistics* by answering questions such as the following:

What are the branches of statistics?

What are data?

How are samples selected?

It is important for the student to understand and apply statistical concepts but also to focus on the merits and limitations of each procedure. This approach will assist the student in evaluating the profusion of data presented in all forms of media and then apply that knowledge beyond this course into everyday life.

| 1–1 | Descriptive and Inferential Statistics > |

Demonstrate knowledge of statistical terms as applied to the two branches of statistics.

To gain knowledge about seemingly haphazard events, statisticians collect information for *variables,* which describe the event.

> An **element** is an object contained in a set of data. A **variable** is a characteristic or attribute of that element capable of assuming any value within the data set.

Data are the values (measurements or observations) that the variables assume. Variables whose values are determined by chance are called **random variables.**

Suppose that an insurance company studies its records over the past several years and determines that, on average, 3 out of every 100 automobiles the company insured were involved in accidents during a one-year period. Although there is no way to predict the specific automobiles that will be involved in an accident (random occurrence), the company can adjust its rates accordingly, since the company knows the general pattern over the long run. (That is, on average, 3% of the insured automobiles will be involved in an accident each year.)

A collection of data values forms a **data set.** Each value in the data set is called a **data value** or a **datum.**

Data can be used in different ways. The body of knowledge called statistics is sometimes divided into two main areas, depending on how data are used. The two areas are

1. Descriptive statistics
2. Inferential statistics

Consider the national census conducted every five years in Canada by the federal government agency, Statistics Canada. Results of this census provide governments, businesses, researchers, and other interested parties with important data such as average income, age distribution, and other characteristics of Canada's population. To obtain this information, Statistics Canada must have some means to collect relevant data. Once data are collected, the agency must organize and summarize them. Finally, the agency needs a method of presenting the data in some meaningful form, such as charts, graphs, or tables.

> **Descriptive statistics** consists of the collection, organization, summarization, and presentation of data.

The second area of statistics is called *inferential statistics.* Here, the statistician tries to make inferences from *samples* to *populations.* Inferential statistics uses **probability,** i.e., the chance of an event occurring. Many people are familiar with the concepts of probability through various forms of gambling. People who play cards, dice, bingo, and lotteries win or lose according to the laws of probability. Probability theory is also used in the insurance industry and other areas.

It is important to distinguish between a sample and a population.

> A **population** consists of all subjects (human or otherwise) that are being studied.

Most of the time, due to the expense, time, size of population, medical concerns, etc., it is not possible to use the entire population for a statistical study; therefore, researchers use samples.

> A **sample** is a group of subjects selected from a population.

Speaking of Statistics

Statistics and a New Celestial Object
Bound by the sun's gravity, orbiting celestial objects include planets and dwarf planets. Pluto was officially demoted from planet to dwarf planet status in 2006. Another dwarf planet, Eris, identified in 2005, has a mass 27% greater than Pluto. Eris, at its peak elliptical orbit, is approximately 14.5 million kilometres from the sun and takes nearly 557 years to complete the orbit. The diameter of Eris is approximately 2400 kilometres. Its surface temperature has been estimated at −230.7°C. How does Eris compare with other solar system celestial objects? Let's look at the statistics.

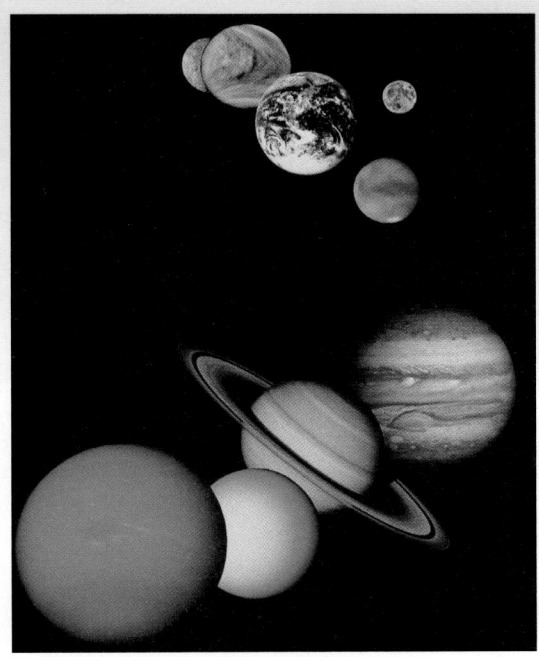

Planet / *Dwarf Planet*	Diameter (kilometres)	Mean Distance from the Sun (millions of kilometres)	Orbital Period (days)	Mean Temperature (°C)	Number of Moons
Mercury	4,880	57.9	88	167.2	0
Venus	12,104	108.1	224.7	463.9	0
Earth	12,756	149.7	365.2	15.0	1
Mars	6,795	227.9	687	−65.0	2
Jupiter	142,984	778.6	4,331	−110.0	63
Saturn	120,535	1,433.6	10,747	−140.0	47
Uranus	51,118	2,872.4	30,589	−195.6	27
Neptune	49,528	4,495.1	59,800	−201.1	13
Pluto	*2,306*	*5,869.6*	*90,588*	*−226.1*	*3*
Eris	*2,400*	*10,127.8*	*203,489*	*−230.7*	*1*

With these statistics, we can make some comparisons. For example, Eris is about one-quarter the size of Venus and Earth. Eris takes more than twice as long as Pluto to orbit the sun. What other comparisons can you make?

If the subjects of a sample are properly selected, most of the time they should possess the same or similar characteristics as the subjects in the population. The techniques used to properly select a sample will be explained in Section 1–3.

An area of inferential statistics called **hypothesis testing** is a decision-making process for evaluating claims about a population, based on information obtained from samples. For example, a researcher may wish to know if a new drug will reduce the number of heart attacks in men over 70 years of age. For this study, two groups of men over 70 would be selected. One group would be given the drug, and the other would be given a placebo (a substance with no medical benefits or harm). Later, the number of heart attacks occurring in each group of men would be counted, a statistical hypothesis test would be run, and a decision would be made about the effectiveness of the drug.

Unusual Stat

Only one-third of crimes committed are reported to the police.

Statisticians also use statistics to determine *relationships* among variables. For example, relationships were the focus of one of the most noted studies in the past few decades, *Smoking and Health,* published by the Surgeon General of the United States in 1964. He stated that after reviewing and evaluating the data, his group found a definite relationship between smoking and lung cancer. He did not say that cigarette smoking actually causes lung cancer, but that there is a relationship between smoking and lung cancer. This conclusion was based on a study done in 1958 by Hammond and Horn. In this study, 187,783 men were observed over a period of 45 months. The death rate from lung cancer in this group of volunteers was ten times as great for smokers as for nonsmokers.

Finally, by studying past and present data and conditions, statisticians try to make predictions based on this information. For example, a car dealer may look at past sales records for a specific month to decide what types of automobiles and how many of each type to order for that month next year.

> **Inferential statistics** consists of generalizing from samples to populations, performing estimations and hypothesis tests, determining relationships among variables, and making predictions.

1–1   Applying the Concepts

Attendance and Grades

Read the following on attendance and grades, and answer the questions.

A study conducted at Red Deer Community College revealed that students who attended class 95 to 100% of the time usually received an A in the class. Students who attended class 80 to 90% of the time usually received a B or C in the class. Students who attended class less than 80% of the time usually received a D or an F or eventually withdrew from the class.

Based on this information, attendance and grades are related. The more you attend class, the more likely you will receive a higher grade. If you improve your attendance, your grades will probably improve. Many factors affect your grade in a course. One factor that you have considerable control over is attendance. You can increase your opportunities for learning by attending class more often.

1. What are the variables under study?
2. What are the data in the study?
3. Are descriptive, inferential, or both types of statistics used?
4. What is the population under study?
5. Was a sample collected? If so, from where?
6. From the information given, comment on the relationship between the variables.

See page 30 for the answers.

1–2   Variables and Types of Data

Categorize data by type and level of measurement.

As stated in Section 1–1, statisticians gain information about a particular situation by collecting data for random variables. This section will explore in greater detail the nature of variables and types of data.

Variables can be classified as qualitative or quantitative. **Qualitative variables** are variables that can be placed into distinct categories, according to some characteristic or attribute. For example, if subjects are classified according to gender (male or female), then the variable *gender* is qualitative. Other examples of qualitative variables are religious preference and geographic locations. Letter grades (A, B, C, D, F) and race results (1st, 2nd, 3rd) are nonnumeric qualitative variables with the additional ranking attribute. This is discussed in the "Levels of Measurement" section on page 8.

Quantitative variables are numerical and can be ordered, ranked, or measured. For example, the variable *age* is numerical, and people can be ranked in order according to the value of their ages. Other examples of quantitative variables are heights, weights, and body temperatures.

Quantitative variables can be further classified into two groups: discrete and continuous. *Discrete variables* can be assigned values such as 0, 1, 2, 3 and are said to be countable. Examples of discrete variables are the number of children in a family, the number of students in a classroom, and the number of calls received by a switchboard operator each day for a month.

> **Discrete variables** assume values that can be counted.

Continuous variables, by comparison, can assume an infinite number of values in an interval between any two specific values. Temperature, for example, is a continuous variable, since the variable can assume an infinite number of values between any two given temperatures, such as 15.5°C low and 27.1°C high.

> **Continuous variables** can assume an infinite number of values between any two specific values. They are obtained by measuring. They often include fractions and decimals.

The classification of variables can be summarized as follows:

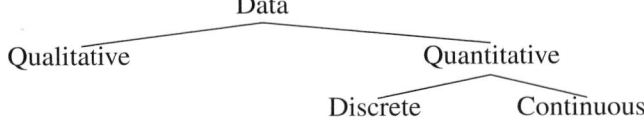

Data

Qualitative   Quantitative

Discrete   Continuous

Unusual Stat

Seventy-five percent of Canada's population lives within 160 kilometres of the United States border.

Since continuous data must be measured, answers must be rounded because of the limits of the measuring device. Usually, answers are rounded to the nearest given unit. For example, heights might be rounded to the nearest centimetre (cm), weights to the nearest gram (g), etc. Hence, a recorded height of 186 cm could mean any measure from 185.5 cm up to but not including 186.6 cm. Thus, the boundary of this measure is given as 185.5–186.5 cm. *Boundaries are written for convenience at 185.5–186.5 but are understood to mean all values up to but not including 186.5.* Actual data values of 186.5 would be rounded to 187 and would be included in a class with boundaries 186.5 up to but not including 187.5, written as 186.5–187.5. As another example, if a recorded weight is 39 kilograms (kg), the exact boundaries are 38.5 up to but not including 39.5 kg. Table 1–1 helps to clarify this concept. The boundaries of a continuous variable are given in one additional decimal place and always end with the digit 5.

Table 1–1 Recorded Values and Boundaries		
Variable	**Recorded value**	**Boundaries**
Length	15 centimetres (cm)	14.5–15.5 cm
Temperature	30 degrees Celsius (°C)	29.5–30.5°C
Time	0.43 seconds (sec)	0.425–0.435 sec
Mass	1.6 grams (g)	1.55–1.65 g

Levels of Measurement

In addition to being classified as qualitative or quantitative, variables can be classified by how they are categorized, counted, or measured. For example, can the data be organized into specific categories, such as area of residence (rural, suburban, or urban)? Can the data values be ranked, such as first place, second place, etc.? Or are the values obtained from measurement, such as heights, IQs, or temperature? This type of classification—i.e., how variables are categorized, counted, or measured—uses **measurement scales,** and four common types of scales are used: nominal, ordinal, interval, and ratio.

The first level of measurement is called the *nominal level* of measurement. A sample of college or university instructors classified according to subject taught (e.g., English, history, psychology, or mathematics) is an example of nominal-level measurement. Classifying residents according to telephone numbers is also an example of the nominal level of measurement. Even though numbers are assigned as phone numbers, there is no meaningful order of ranking. Other examples of nominal-level data are political party (Liberal, Conservative, Bloc Québécois, New Democratic Party, etc.), religious preference (Christian, Muslim, Jewish, nonreligious, etc.), and marital status (single, married, common-law, divorced, etc.).

> The **nominal level of measurement** classifies data into mutually exclusive (nonoverlapping), exhausting categories in which no order or ranking can be imposed on the data.

The next level of measurement is called the *ordinal level.* Data measured at this level can be placed into categories, and these categories can be ordered, or ranked. For example, from student evaluations, guest speakers might be ranked as superior, average, or poor. Floats in a homecoming parade might be ranked as first place, second place, etc. *Note that precise measurement of differences in the ordinal level of measurement* does not *exist.* For instance, when people are classified according to their build (small, medium, or large), a large variation exists among the individuals in each class.

Other examples of ordinal data are letter grades (A, B, C, D, F).

> The **ordinal level of measurement** classifies data into categories that can be ranked; however, precise differences between the ranks do not exist.

The third level of measurement is called the *interval level.* This level differs from the ordinal level in that precise differences do exist between units. For example, many standardized psychological tests yield values measured on an interval scale. IQ is an example of such a variable. There is a meaningful difference of 1 point between an IQ of 109 and an IQ of 110. Temperature is another example of interval measurement, since there is a meaningful difference of 1°C between each unit, such as 29°C and 30°C. *One property is lacking in the interval scale: There is no true zero.* For example, IQ tests do not measure people who have no intelligence. For temperature, 0°C does not mean no heat at all. There are few data types that satisfy the criteria for the interval measurement level.

> The **interval level of measurement** ranks data, and precise differences between units of measure do exist; however, there is no meaningful zero.

The final level of measurement is called the *ratio level.* Examples of ratio scales are those used to measure height, weight, area, and number of phone calls received. Ratio scales have differences between units (1 cm, 1 kg, etc.) and a true zero. In addition, the ratio scale contains a true ratio between values. For example, if one person can lift 100 kg and another can lift 50 kg, then the ratio between them is 2 to 1. Put another way, the first person can lift twice as much weight as the second person.

The **ratio level of measurement** possesses all the characteristics of interval measurement, and there exists a true zero. In addition, true ratios exist when the same variable is measured on two different members of the population.

There is not complete agreement among statisticians about the classification of data into one of the four categories. For example, some researchers classify IQ data as ratio data rather than interval. Also, data can be altered so that they fit into a different category. For instance, if the incomes of all professors of a college are classified into the three categories of low, average, and high, then a ratio variable becomes an ordinal variable. Table 1–2 gives some examples of each type of data.

Table 1–2	Examples of Measurement Scales		
Nominal-level data	**Ordinal-level data**	**Interval-level data**	**Ratio-level data**
Postal code	Grade (A, B, C, D, F)	Temperature (°C)	Height
Gender (male, female)	Rating scale (poor, good, excellent)	Calendar years	Weight
Eye colour (blue, brown, green, hazel)	Race results (1st, 2nd, 3rd)	SAT or GMAT score	Volume
Political preference	Ranking of universities	IQ	Age
Religious affiliation	Income level (low, middle, high)		Salary
Major field (business, medicine, law, etc.)			Time of Day
Nationality			Distance
			Precipitation

1–2 Applying the Concepts

Be Aware of Motor Vehicles

Read the following information about motor vehicle traffic injuries and answer the questions.

Major Injury Report—Motor Vehicle Traffic

The chart indicates the number of individuals injured in motor vehicle accidents by injury class.

Classification of injured	Number of injuries
Pedestrian	256
Pedal cyclist	56
Driver (nonmotorcycle)	752
Passenger (nonmotorcycle)	335
Motorcycle driver	181
Motorcycle passenger	14

Source: Canadian Institute for Health Information, *Ontario Trauma Registry Report: Major Injury in Ontario, 2007–2008.*

1. What are the variables under study?

2. Categorize each variable as quantitative or qualitative.

3. Categorize each quantitative variable as discrete or continuous.

4. Identify the level of measurement for each variable.

5. The motorcycle driver is shown as having fewer injuries than the nonmotorcycle driver. Does that mean that it is safer to drive a motorcycle? Explain.

6. List other factors that may affect the number of injuries reported.

7. From the information given, comment on the relationship between the variables.

See page 30 for the answers.

1–3   Data Collection and Sampling Techniques ❯

Identify the four basic sampling techniques.

In research, statisticians use data to describe or analyze situations or events. Examples of data usage are shown below:

- Manufacturer may collect consumer data in order to plan an effective marketing strategy.
- Management may survey the company's employees to assess their needs in order to negotiate a new contract with the employees' union.
- Administrators may collect student data to determine if the educational goals of a school district are being met.
- Analysts may collect market data to disseminate to clients to make intelligent investment decisions.

These examples illustrate a few situations where collecting data will help people decide on the appropriate course of action.

Data can be collected in a variety of ways. One of the most common methods is through the use of surveys. Surveys can be done by using a variety of methods. Three of the most common methods are the telephone survey, the mailed questionnaire, and the personal interview.

Telephone surveys have an advantage over personal interview surveys in that they are less costly. Also, people may be more candid in their opinions since there is no face-to-face contact. A major drawback to the telephone survey is that some people in the population will not have phones or will not answer when the calls are made; hence, not all people have a chance of being surveyed. Also, many people now have unlisted numbers and cellphones, so they cannot be surveyed. Finally, even the tone of the voice of the interviewer might influence the response of the person who is being interviewed.

Mailed questionnaire surveys can be used to cover a wider geographic area than telephone surveys or personal interviews since mailed questionnaire surveys are less expensive to conduct. Also, respondents can remain anonymous if they desire. Disadvantages of mailed questionnaire surveys include a low number of responses and inappropriate answers to questions. Another drawback is that some people may have difficulty reading or understanding the questions.

Interesting Fact

Market research organizations conducting polls or surveys are exempt from Canada's telemarketing *National Do Not Call List*.

Historical Note

A pioneer in census taking was Pierre-Simon de Laplace. In 1780, he developed the Laplace method of estimating the population of a country. The principle behind his method was to take a census of a few selected communities and to determine the ratio of the population to the number of births in these communities. (Good birth records were kept.) This ratio would be used to multiply the number of births in the entire country to estimate the number of citizens in the country.

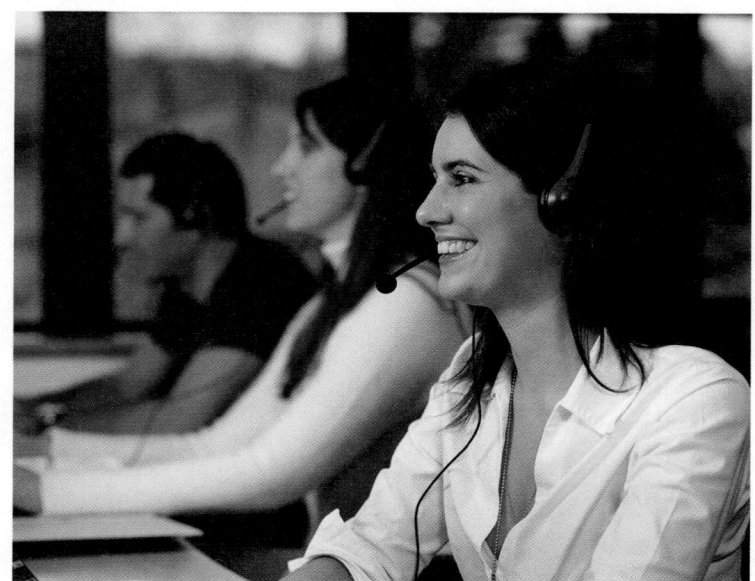

Internet surveys using techniques such as email, hyperlinks, and pop-up windows have been utilized by Web sites in order to collect data from a diverse population. A burgeoning industry has evolved for businesses that collect and then sell email addresses. Hyperlinks can trigger a survey request by visitors clicking on either text or graphics. Pop-up windows may be used to request random visitors to participate in surveys. One method is to display a pop-up window survey request after a few seconds have elapsed. Challenges for these data collection methods include technology such as email spam filters and pop-up blockers. Low response rates may require saturation techniques that are socially unacceptable. Concerns of reliability, validity and generalization of results must also be addressed.

Personal interview surveys have the advantage of obtaining in-depth responses to questions from the person being interviewed. One disadvantage is that interviewers must be trained in asking questions and recording responses, which makes the personal interview survey more costly than the other two survey methods. Another disadvantage is that the interviewer may be biased in his or her selection of respondents.

Data can also be collected in other ways, such as *surveying records* or *direct observation* of situations.

As stated in Section 1–1, researchers use samples to collect data and information about a particular variable from a large population. Using samples saves time and money and, in some cases, enables the researcher to get more detailed information about a particular subject. Samples cannot be selected in haphazard ways because the information obtained might be biased. For example, interviewing people on a street corner during the day would not include responses from people working in offices at that time or from people attending school; hence, not all subjects in a particular population would have a chance of being selected.

To obtain samples that are unbiased—i.e., give each subject in the population an equally likely chance of being selected—statisticians use four basic methods of sampling: random, systematic, stratified, and cluster sampling.

Speaking of Statistics

Canada's wireless projections to 2013 point to 29.7 million subscribers, with Rogers Wireless leading the competition with a 35.8% market share. What data types, measurement levels, and possible sampling methods were used in obtaining the market share information?

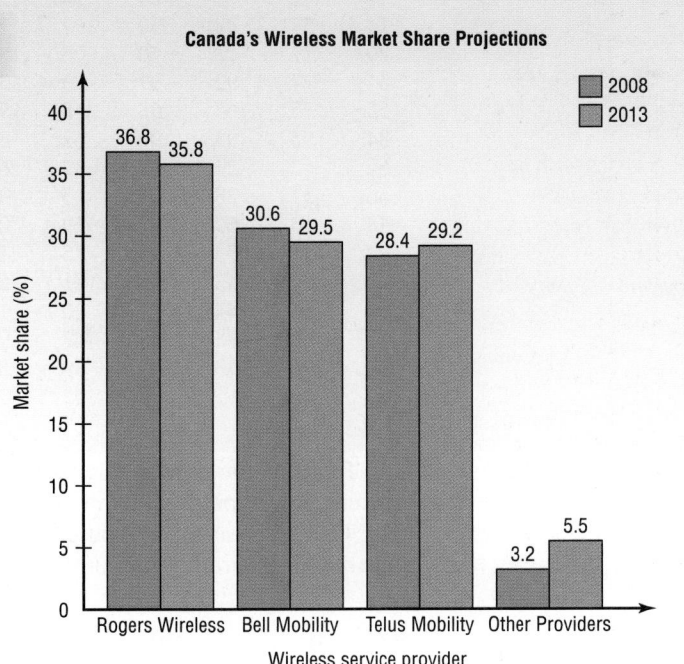

Canada's Wireless Market Share Projections

Source: IE Market Research Corp. (May 2009). *Research and Markets*, "2Q09 Canada Mobile Operator Forecast, 2008–2013."

Random Sampling

Random samples are selected by using chance methods or random numbers. One such method is to number each subject in the population. Then place numbered cards in a bowl, mix them thoroughly, and select as many cards as needed. The subjects whose numbers are selected constitute the sample. Since it is difficult to mix the cards thoroughly, there is a chance of obtaining a biased sample. For this reason, statisticians use another method of obtaining numbers. They generate random numbers with a computer or calculator. Before the invention of computers, random numbers were obtained from tables.

Some two-digit random numbers are shown in Table 1–3. To select a random sample of, say, 15 subjects out of 85 subjects, it is necessary to number each subject from 1 to 85. Then select a starting number by closing your eyes and placing your finger on a number in the table. (Although this may sound somewhat unusual, it enables us to find a starting number at random.) In this case suppose your finger landed on the number 12 in the second column. (It is the sixth number down from the top.) Then proceed downward until you have selected 15 different numbers between 01 and 85. When you reach the bottom of the column, go to the top of the next column. If you select a number greater than 85 or the number 00 or a duplicate number, just omit it. In our example, we will use the subjects numbered 12, 27, 75, 62, 57, 13, 31, 06, 16, 49, 46, 71, 53, 41, and 02. A more detailed procedure for selecting a random sample using a table of random numbers is given in Chapter 14, using Table D in Appendix C.

Table 1–3		Random Numbers										
79	41	71	93	60	35	04	67	96	04	79	10	86
26	52	53	13	43	50	92	09	87	21	83	75	17
18	13	41	30	56	20	37	74	49	56	45	46	83
19	82	02	69	34	27	77	34	24	93	16	77	00
14	57	44	30	93	76	32	13	55	29	49	30	77
29	12	18	50	06	33	15	79	50	28	50	45	45
01	27	92	67	93	31	97	55	29	21	64	27	29
55	75	65	68	65	73	07	95	66	43	43	92	16
84	95	95	96	62	30	91	64	74	83	47	89	71
62	62	21	37	82	62	19	44	08	64	34	50	11
66	57	28	69	13	99	74	31	58	19	47	66	89
48	13	69	97	29	01	75	58	05	40	40	18	29
94	31	73	19	75	76	33	18	05	53	04	51	41
00	06	53	98	01	55	08	38	49	42	10	44	38
46	16	44	27	80	15	28	01	64	27	89	03	27
77	49	85	95	62	93	25	39	63	74	54	82	85
81	96	43	27	39	53	85	61	12	90	67	96	02
40	46	15	73	23	75	96	68	13	99	49	64	11

Table methods of random numbers have been replaced by modern computational devices or computer software applications. Graphing calculators, such as the TI-83 Plus and TI-84 Plus, and computer applications, such as Excel, Minitab, or SPSS, are all capable of generating random numbers within a defined range of values.

Systematic Sampling

Researchers obtain **systematic samples** by numbering each subject of the population and then selecting every kth subject. For example, suppose there were 2000 subjects in the population and a sample of 50 subjects was needed. Since $2000 \div 50 = 40$, then $k = 40$, and every 40th subject would be selected; however, the first subject (numbered between 1 and 40) would be selected at random. Suppose subject 12 was the first subject selected; then the sample would consist of the subjects whose numbers were 12, 52, 92, etc., until 50 subjects were obtained. When using systematic sampling, one must be careful about how the subjects in the population are numbered. If subjects were arranged in a manner such as wife, husband, wife, husband, and every 40th subject was selected, the sample would consist of all husbands. Numbering is not always necessary. For example, a researcher may select every tenth item from an assembly line to test for defects.

Stratified Sampling

Researchers obtain **stratified samples** by dividing the population into groups (called *strata*) according to some characteristic that is important to the study, then sampling from each group. Samples within the strata should be randomly selected. For example, suppose the president of a two-year college wants to learn how students feel about a certain issue. Furthermore, the president wishes to see if the opinions of the first-year students differ from those of the second-year students. The president will select students from each group to use in the sample. Another example is that a polling organization would like to determine the popularity of political parties throughout Canada. To ensure representation from all regions in the country, random samples are drawn from western, central, and eastern provinces and territories.

Cluster Sampling

Researchers also use **cluster samples.** Here the population is divided into groups called clusters by some means, such as geographic area or schools in a large school district. Then the researcher randomly selects some of these clusters and uses all members of the selected clusters as the subjects of the samples. Suppose a researcher wishes to survey apartment dwellers in a large city. If there are ten apartment buildings in the city, the researcher can select at random two buildings from the ten and interview all the residents of these buildings. Cluster sampling is used when the population is large or when it involves subjects residing in a large geographic area. For example, if one wanted to do a study involving the patients in the hospitals in Montreal, it would be very costly and time-consuming to try to obtain a random sample of patients since they would be spread over a large area. Instead, a few hospitals could be selected at random, and the patients in these hospitals would be interviewed in a cluster.

The four basic sampling methods are summarized in Table 1–4.

Other Sampling Methods

In addition to the four basic sampling methods, researchers use other methods to obtain samples. One such method is called a **convenience sample.** Here a researcher uses subjects that are convenient. For example, the researcher may interview subjects entering a local mall to determine the nature of their visit or perhaps what stores they will be patronizing. This sample is probably not representative of the general customers for several reasons. For one thing, it was probably taken at a specific time of day, so not all customers entering the mall have an equal chance of being selected since they were not there when the survey was being conducted. But convenience samples can be representative of the population. If the researcher investigates the characteristics of the population and determines that the sample is representative, then it can be used.

Other sampling techniques, such as *sequential sampling, double sampling,* and *multistage sampling,* are explained in Chapter 14, along with a more detailed explanation of the four basic sampling techniques.

Table 1–4	Summary of Sampling Methods

Random Subjects are selected by random numbers.

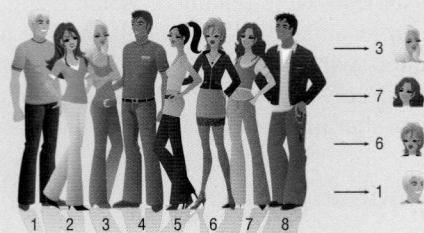

Systematic Subjects are selected by using every *k*th number after the first subject is randomly selected from 1 through *k*.

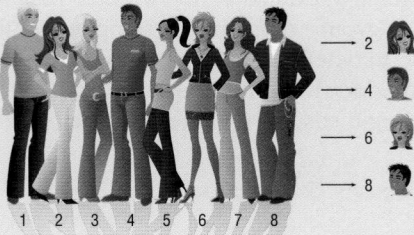

Stratified Subjects are selected by dividing up the population into groups (strata), and subjects within groups are randomly selected.

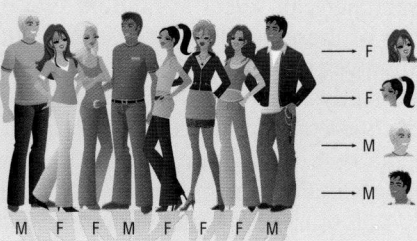

Cluster Subjects are selected by using an intact group that is representative of the population.

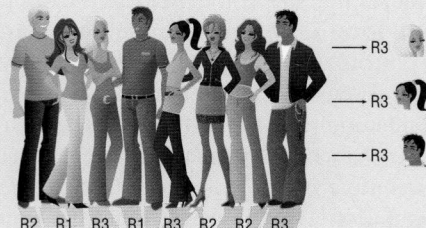

1–3 Applying the Concepts

Canadian Culture and Drug Abuse

Assume you are a member of the National Research Council and have become increasingly concerned about drug use by professional sports players. You set up a plan and conduct a survey on how people believe the Canadian culture (television, movies, magazines, and popular music) influences illegal drug use. Your survey consists of 2250 adults and adolescents from around the country. A consumer group petitions you for more information about your survey. Answer the following questions about your survey.

1. What type of survey did you use (phone, mail, or interview)?
2. What are the advantages and disadvantages of the surveying methods you did not use?
3. What type of scores did you use? Why?
4. Did you use a random method for deciding who would be in your sample?
5. Which of the methods (stratified, systematic, cluster, or convenience) did you use?
6. Why was that method more appropriate for this type of data collection?
7. If a convenience sample was obtained, consisting of only adolescents, how would the results of the study be affected?

See page 30 for the answers.

1–4 Observational and Experimental Studies

Explain the difference between an observational and an experimental study.

There are several different ways to classify statistical studies. This section explains two types of studies: *observational studies* and *experimental studies.*

> In an **observational study,** the researcher merely observes what is happening or what has happened in the past and tries to draw conclusions based on these observations.

For example, data from the *Canadian Social Trends Survey* (Statistics Canada) stated that "Participation in exercise, as well as walking and jogging, grew from 1992 to 2005." The survey also mentioned that "Groups more likely to participate in active leisure, while holding other factors constant, were women, university-educated people, married people, and those with incomes of $60,000 and over, those who reported their lives had a relatively low level of time stress, and those living in British Columbia or Quebec."

In this study, the researcher merely observed what had happened to the survey participants within the indicated time frame. There was no type of research intervention.

> In an **experimental study,** the researcher manipulates one of the variables and tries to determine how the manipulation influences other variables.

For example, a study conducted at Virginia Polytechnic Institute and presented in *Psychology Today* divided 56 female undergraduate students into two groups and had the students perform as many sit-ups as possible in 90 seconds. The first group was told only to "Do your best," while the second group was told to try to increase the actual number of sit-ups done each day by 10%. After four days, the subjects in the group who were given the vague instructions to "Do your best" averaged 43 sit-ups, while the group that was given the more specific instructions to increase the number of sit-ups by 10% averaged 56 sit-ups by the last day's session. The conclusion then

Interesting Fact

The average age of a Harley-Davidson motorcycle owner is 52 years.

was that athletes who were given specific goals performed better than those who were not given specific goals.

This study is an example of a statistical experiment since the researchers intervened in the study by manipulating one of the variables, namely, the type of instructions given to each group.

In a true experimental study, the subjects should be assigned to groups randomly. Also, the treatments should be assigned to the groups at random. In the sit-up study, the article did not mention whether the subjects were randomly assigned to the groups.

Sometimes when random assignment is not possible, researchers use intact groups. These types of studies are done quite often in education where already intact groups are available in the form of existing classrooms. When these groups are used, the study is said to be a **quasi-experimental study.** The treatments, though, should be assigned at random. Most articles do not state whether random assignment of subjects was used.

Statistical studies usually include one or more *independent variables* and one *dependent variable.*

> The **independent variable** in an experimental study is the one that is being manipulated by the researcher. The independent variable is also called the **explanatory variable.** The response variable is called the **dependent variable** or the **outcome variable.**

The outcome variable is the variable that is studied to see if it has changed significantly due to the manipulation of the independent variable. For example, in the sit-up study, the researchers gave the groups two different types of instructions, general and specific. Hence, the independent variable is the type of instruction. The dependent variable, then, is the response variable, that is, the number of sit-ups each group was able to perform after four days of exercise. If the differences in the dependent or outcome variable are large and other factors are equal, these differences can be attributed to the manipulation of the independent variable. In this case, specific instructions were shown to increase athletic performance.

In the sit-up study, there were two groups. The group that received the special instruction is called the **treatment group** while the other is called the **control group.** The treatment group receives a specific treatment (in this case, instructions for improvement) while the control group does not.

A common experimental study is the **double-blind study,** in which neither the doctor nor the patient knows whether a drug or placebo (i.e., no active drug) is delivered. For example, a researcher may want to determine the effect of a new weight-loss drug for obesity. Patients are randomly assigned to two groups. The treatment group is given the drug and the control group is given the placebo. After a period of time, the patients' weights are measured. Figure 1–1 identifies the two groups and variables in this study.

Figure 1–1

Example of Experimental Study

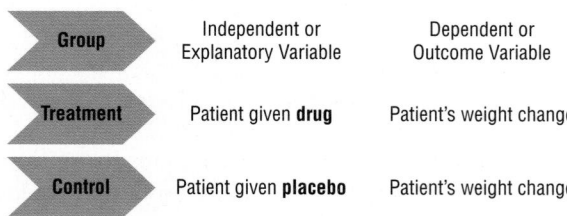

Both types of statistical studies have advantages and disadvantages. Experimental studies have the advantage that the researcher can decide how to select subjects and how to assign them to specific groups. The researcher can also control or manipulate the independent variable. For example, in studies that require the subjects to consume a certain amount of medicine each day, the researcher can determine the precise dosages and, if necessary, vary the dosage for the groups.

There are several disadvantages to experimental studies. First, they may occur in unnatural settings, such as laboratories and special classrooms. This can lead to several problems. One such problem is that the results might not apply to the natural setting. The age-old question then is "This mouthwash may kill 10,000 germs in a test tube, but how many germs will it kill in my mouth?"

Another disadvantage with an experimental study is the **Hawthorne effect.** This effect was discovered in 1924 in a study of workers at the Hawthorne plant of the Western Electric Company. In this study, researchers found that the subjects who knew they were participating in an experiment actually changed their behaviour in ways that affected the results of the study.

Another problem is called *confounding of variables.*

Two variables are **confounded** when their effects on a response variable cannot be distinguished from each other.

Researchers try to control most variables in a study, but this is not possible in some studies. For example, subjects who are put on an exercise program might also improve their diet unbeknownst to the researcher and perhaps improve their health in other ways not due to exercise alone. Then diet becomes a confounding variable.

Observational studies also have advantages and disadvantages. One advantage of an observational study is that it usually occurs in a natural setting. For example, researchers can observe people's driving patterns on streets and highways in large cities. Another advantage of an observational study is that it can be done in situations where it would be unethical or downright dangerous to conduct an experiment. Using observational studies, researchers can study suicides, rapes, murders, etc. In addition, observational studies can be done using variables that cannot be manipulated by the researcher, such as drug users versus nondrug users and right-handedness versus left-handedness.

Observational studies have disadvantages, too. As mentioned previously, since the variables are not controlled by the researcher, a definite cause-and-effect situation cannot be shown since other factors may have had an effect on the results. Observational studies can be expensive and time-consuming. For example, if one wanted to study the habitat of lions in Africa, one would need a lot of time and money, and there would be a certain amount of danger involved. Finally, since the researcher may not be using his or her own measurements, the results could be subject to the inaccuracies of those who collected the data. For example, if the researchers were doing a study of events that occurred in the 1800s, they would have to rely on information and records obtained by others from a previous era. There is no way to ensure the accuracy of these records.

When you read the results of statistical studies, decide if the study was observational or experimental. Then see if the conclusion follows logically, based on the nature of these studies.

No matter what type of study is conducted, two studies on the same subject sometimes have conflicting conclusions. Why might this occur? An article entitled "Bottom Line: Is It Good for You?" (*USA TODAY Weekend*) states that in the 1960s studies suggested that margarine was better for the heart than butter since margarine contains less saturated fat and users had lower cholesterol levels. In a 1980 study, researchers found that butter was better than margarine since margarine contained trans-fatty acids, which are worse for the heart than butter's saturated fat. Then in a 1998 study, researchers found that margarine was better for a person's health. Now, what is to be believed? Should one use butter or margarine?

The answer here is to take a closer look at these studies. Actually, it is not a choice between butter or margarine that counts, but the type of margarine used. In the 1980s, studies showed that solid margarine contains trans-fatty acids, and scientists believe that they are worse for the heart than butter's saturated fat. In the 1998 study, liquid margarine was used. It is very low in trans-fatty acids, and hence it is more healthful than butter because trans-fatty acids have been shown to raise cholesterol. Hence, the conclusion is to use liquid margarine instead of solid margarine or butter.

Before decisions based on research studies are made, it is important to get all the facts and examine them in light of the particular situation.

1–4 Applying the Concepts

Just a Pinch between Your Cheek and Gum

As the evidence on the adverse effects of cigarette smoke grew, people tried many different ways to quit smoking. Some people tried chewing tobacco or, as it was called, smokeless tobacco. A small amount of tobacco was placed between the cheek and gum. Certain chemicals from the tobacco were absorbed into the bloodstream and gave the sensation of smoking cigarettes. This prompted studies on the adverse effects of smokeless tobacco. One study in particular used 40 university students as subjects. Twenty were given smokeless tobacco to chew, and 20 given a substance that looked and tasted like smokeless tobacco, but did not contain any of the harmful substances. The students were randomly assigned to one of the groups. The students' blood pressure and heart rate were measured before they started chewing and 20 minutes after they had been chewing. A significant increase in heart rate occurred in the group that chewed the smokeless tobacco. Answer the following questions.

1. What type of study was this (observational, quasi-experimental, or experimental)?
2. What are the independent and dependent variables?
3. Which was the treatment group?
4. Could the students' blood pressures be affected by knowing that they are part of a study?
5. List some possible confounding variables.
6. Do you think this is a good way to study the effect of smokeless tobacco?

See page 30 for the answers.

1–5   Uses and Misuses of Statistics❯

Explain how statistics can be used and misused.

As explained previously, statistical techniques can be used to describe data, compare two or more data sets, determine if a relationship exists between variables, test hypotheses, and make estimates about population characteristics. However, there is another aspect of statistics, and that is the misuse of statistical techniques to sell products that don't work properly, to attempt to prove something true that is really not true, or to get our attention by using statistics to evoke fear, shock, and outrage.

There are two sayings that have been around for a long time that illustrate this point:

"There are three types of lies—lies, damn lies, and statistics."

"Figures don't lie, but liars figure."

Just because we read or hear the results of a research study or an opinion poll in the media, this does not mean that these results are reliable or that they can be applied to any and all situations. For example, reporters sometimes leave out critical details such as the size of the sample used or how the research subjects were selected. Without this information, one cannot properly evaluate the research and properly interpret the conclusions of the study or survey.

It is the purpose of this section to show some ways that statistics can be misused. One should not infer that all research studies and surveys are suspect, but that there are many factors to consider when making decisions based on the results of research studies and surveys. Here are some ways that statistics can be misrepresented.

Suspect Samples

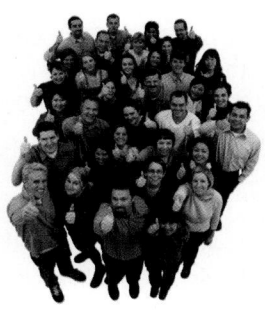

The first thing to consider is the sample that was used in the research study. Sometimes researchers use very small samples to obtain information. Several years ago, advertisements contained such statements as "Three out of four doctors surveyed recommend brand such and such." If only four doctors were surveyed, the results could have been obtained by chance alone; however, if 100 doctors were surveyed, the results might be quite different.

Not only is it important to have a sample size that is large enough, but also it is necessary to see how the subjects in the sample were selected. Studies using volunteers sometimes have a built-in bias. Volunteers generally do not represent the population at large. Sometimes they are recruited from a particular socioeconomic background, and sometimes unemployed people volunteer for research studies to get a stipend. Studies that require the subjects to spend several days or weeks in an environment other than their home or workplace automatically exclude people who are employed and cannot take time away from work. Sometimes only college students or retirees are used in studies. In the past, many studies have used only men, but have attempted to generalize the results to both men and women. Opinion polls that require a person to phone or mail in a response most often are not representative of the population in general, since only those with strong feelings for or against the issue usually call or respond by mail.

Another type of sample that may not be representative is the convenience sample. Educational studies sometimes use students in intact classrooms since it is convenient. Quite often, the students in these classrooms do not represent the student population of the entire school district.

When results are interpreted from studies using small samples, convenience samples, or volunteer samples, care should be used in generalizing the results to the entire population.

Ambiguous Averages

In Chapter 3, you will learn that there are four commonly used measures that are loosely called *averages.* They are the *mean, median, mode,* and *midrange.* For the same data set, these averages can differ markedly. People who know this can, without lying, select the one measure of average that lends the most evidence to support their position.

Changing the Subject

Another type of statistical distortion can occur when different values are used to represent the same data. For example, one political candidate who is running for reelection might say, "During my administration, expenditures increased a mere 3%." His opponent, who is trying to unseat him, might say, "During my opponent's administration, expenditures have increased a whopping $6,000,000." Here both figures are correct; however, expressing a 3% increase as $6,000,000 makes it sound like a very large increase. Here again, ask yourself, Which measure best represents the data?

Detached Statistics

A claim that uses a detached statistic is one in which no comparison is made. For example, you may hear a claim such as "Our brand of crackers has one-third fewer calories." Here, no comparison is made. One-third fewer calories than what? Another example is a claim that uses a detached statistic such as "Brand A painkiller works four times faster." Four times faster than what? When you see statements such as this, always ask yourself, Compared to what?

Implied Connections

Many claims attempt to imply connections between variables that may not actually exist. For example, consider the following statement: "Eating fish may help to reduce your cholesterol." Notice the words *may help*. There is no guarantee that eating fish will definitely help you reduce your cholesterol.

"Studies suggest that using our exercise machine will reduce your weight." Here the word *suggest* is used, and again, there is no guarantee that you will lose weight by using the exercise machine advertised.

Another claim might say, "Taking calcium will lower blood pressure in some people." Note the word *some* is used. You may not be included in the group of "some" people. Be careful when you draw conclusions from claims that use words such as *may, in some people,* and *might help.*

Misleading Graphs

Statistical graphs give a visual representation of data that enables viewers to analyze and interpret data more easily than by simply looking at numbers. In Chapter 2, you will see how some graphs are used to represent data. However, if graphs are drawn inappropriately, they can misrepresent the data and lead the reader to false conclusions. The misuse of graphs is also explained in Chapter 2, on pages 60–63.

Faulty Survey Questions

When analyzing the results of a survey using questionnaires, you should be sure that the questions are properly written since the way questions are phrased can often influence the way people answer them. For example, the responses to a question such as "Do you feel that the North Huntingdon School District should build a new football stadium?" might be answered differently than a question such as "Do you favour increasing school taxes so that the North Huntingdon School District can build a new football stadium?" Each question asks something a little different, and the responses could be radically different. When you read and interpret the results obtained from questionnaire surveys, watch out for some of these common mistakes made in the writing of the survey questions.

In Chapter 14, you will find some common ways that survey questions could be misinterpreted by those responding and could therefore result in incorrect conclusions.

To restate the premise of this section, statistics, when used properly, can be beneficial in obtaining much information, but when used improperly, can lead to much misinformation. It is like your automobile. If you use your automobile to get to school or work or to go on a vacation, that's good. But if you use it to run over your neighbour's dog because it barks all night long and tears up your flower garden, that's not so good!

1–6	Computers and Calculators >

Explain the importance of computers and calculators in statistics.

Statistical computing continues to evolve with the advent of more powerful computers and calculators. Modern statistical software takes advantage of this computing power, allowing for easy, fast, and accurate analysis on simple and complex data sets.

Affordable tools available to students to perform data analysis include portable hand-held graphing calculators with built-in or downloadable statistical software. One of the most widely used models is the Texas Instruments TI-83 Plus and TI-84 Plus series.

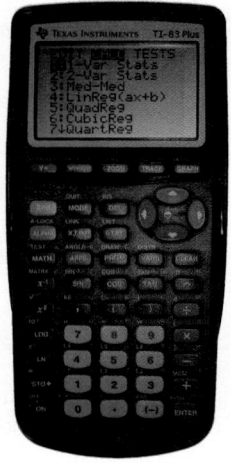

Figure 1–2

Texas Instruments TI-83 Plus graphing calculator with statistics menu displayed

Hewlett-Packard (HP 40gs or HP 50g), Sharp (EL-9900C), and Casio (FX-9750II) are also excellent models for both descriptive and inferential statistics. Be aware that many academic programs disallow the use of graphing calculators during examinations due to their storage and display capabilities.

Computer-based application software is an indispensable resource for statisticians. Statistical software is available on a variety of hardware platforms—notebook, personal computer, or network server, and operating systems—Windows, Mac OS, or UNIX. The Microsoft Excel spreadsheet application is one of the most widely used software for statistical data analysis and charting due to its ease of use and prevalence in the marketplace. Although not as versatile as dedicated statistical programs, Excel's built-in functions can be enhanced with a wide array of add-in programs, such as the Analysis ToolPak. Many third-party add-in programs are available that enhance Excel's already impressive statistical feature set. Other statistical solutions include mathematics programs, such as MATLAB, Mathematica, Maple, Mathcad, and open-source software, such as "R."

Dedicated statistical application software offers all, or at least most, of the required tools for statisticians without the need for optional add-in products. These programs can range from a nongraphical command line interface to the more intuitive menu-driven, spreadsheet-oriented graphical user interface. Popular dedicated programs incorporate both interfaces. Depending on the field of study, there are numerous choices for the statistician. Minitab uses a cross-discipline approach and targets entry-level scientists and business and industrial users. Experimental researchers may opt for the SAS System for Statistical Analysis. The SPSS software focuses on marketing, scientific, government, and education researchers. Many other statistical applications are prevalent in the marketplace.

The purpose of this elementary statistics textbook is to teach the student the concepts and methodologies required to make informed statistical decisions. Statistical software used on either calculators or computers represent tools that ease the burden of time-consuming computations. Learning procedures, formulas, and table-lookup will give the student a much better understanding of the underlying work performed by the chosen technology.

Figure 1–3

Microsoft Excel statistical data analysis output with chart

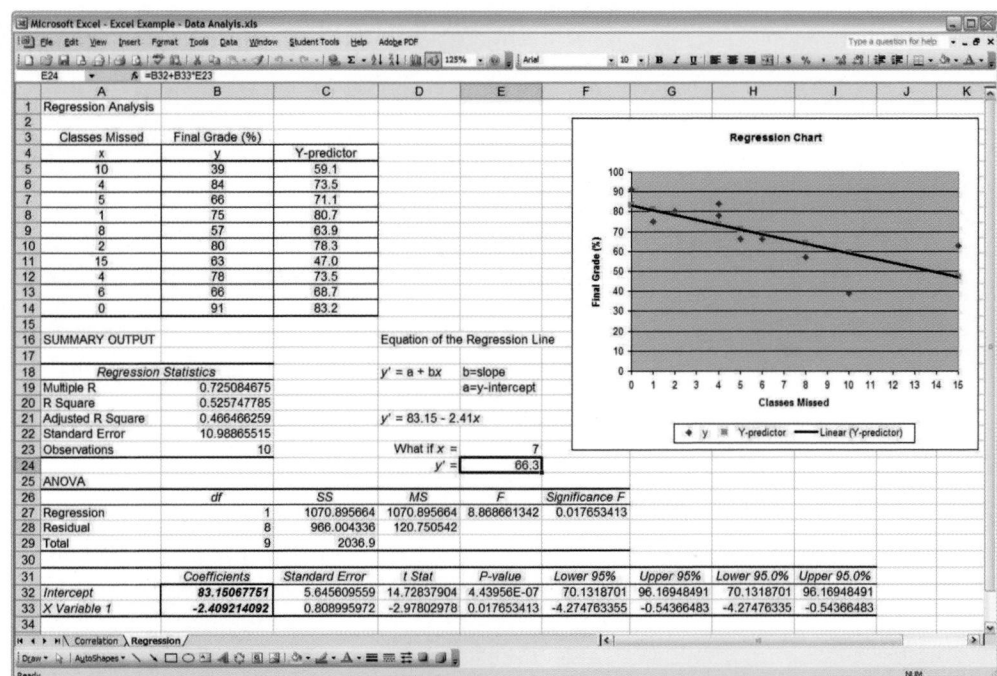

Figure 1–4

Minitab statistical
software with
command-line and
menu interface

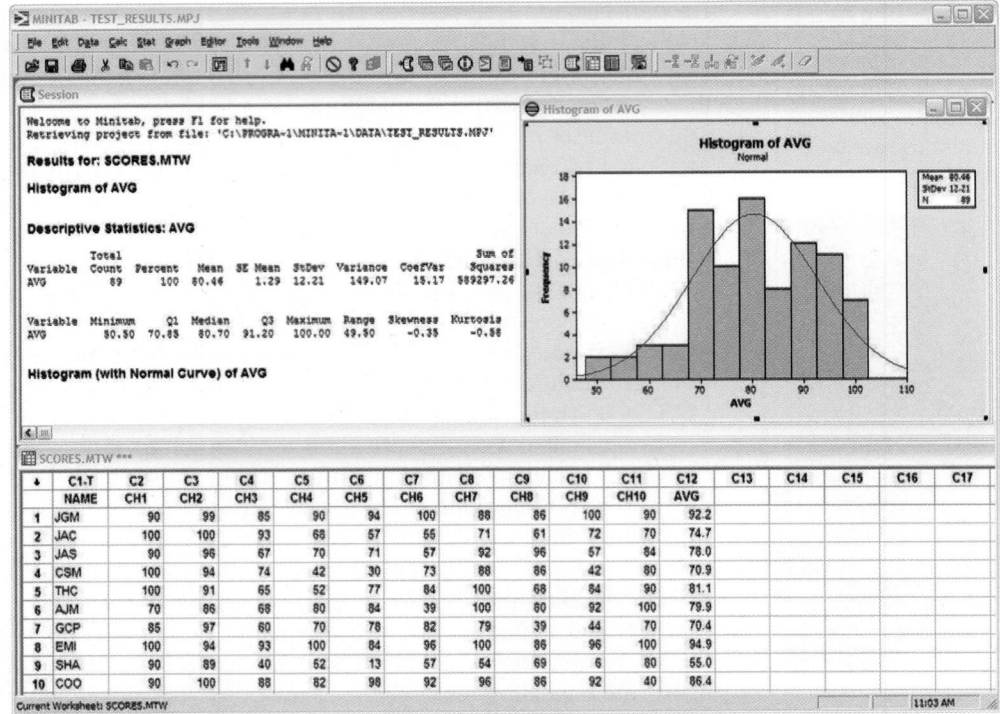

For step-by-step guidance on the use of Texas Instruments TI-83 Plus/TI-84 Plus programmable calculators, see Appendix E at the back of this book. For summary procedures for Minitab, SPSS, and Excel, please see the full version of Appendix E on *Connect*.

The author has left it up to each instructor to choose how much technology he or she will incorporate into the course.

Summary >

The two major areas of statistics are descriptive and inferential. Descriptive statistics includes the collection, organization, summarization, and presentation of data. Inferential statistics includes making inferences from samples to populations, estimations and hypothesis testing, determining relationships, and making predictions. Inferential statistics is based on *probability theory.*

Since in most cases the populations under study are large, statisticians use subgroups called *samples* to get the necessary data for their studies. There are four basic methods used to obtain samples: random, systematic, stratified, and cluster.

Data can be classified as qualitative or quantitative. Quantitative data can be either discrete or continuous, depending on the values they can assume. Data can also be measured by various scales. The four basic levels of measurement are nominal, ordinal, interval, and ratio.

There are two basic types of statistical studies: observational studies and experimental studies. When conducting observational studies, researchers observe what is happening or what has happened and then draw conclusions based on these observations. They do not attempt to manipulate the variables in any way.

When conducting an experimental study, researchers manipulate one or more of the independent or explanatory variables and see how this manipulation influences the dependent or outcome variable.

Finally, the applications of statistics are many and varied. People encounter them in everyday life, such as in reading newspapers or magazines, listening to the radio, or watching television. Since statistics is used in almost every field of endeavour, the educated individual should be knowledgeable about the vocabulary, concepts, and procedures of statistics.

Today, computers and calculators are used extensively in statistics to facilitate the computations.

Unusual Stat

Twenty percent of Canadians believe that extraterrestrials visit the earth on a regular basis.

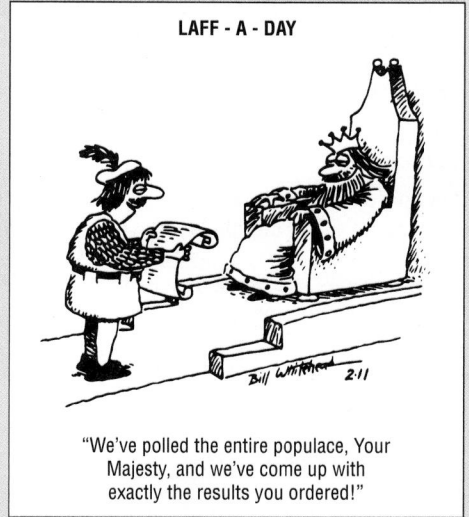

LAFF - A - DAY

"We've polled the entire populace, Your Majesty, and we've come up with exactly the results you ordered!"

Source: © 1993 King Features Syndicate, Inc. World Rights reserved. Reprinted with special permission of King Features Syndicate.

Important Terms »

cluster sample 13	double-blind study 16	nominal level of measurement 8	random sample 12
confounded variables 17	element 4		random variable 4
continuous variables 7	experimental study 15	observational study 15	ratio level of measurement 8
control group 16	explanatory variable 16	ordinal level of measurement 8	
convenience sample 13	Hawthorne effect 17		sample 4
data 4	hypothesis testing 5	outcome variable 16	statistics 3
data set 4	independent variable 16	population 4	stratified sample 13
data value or datum 4	inferential statistics 6	probability 4	systematic sample 12
dependent variable 16	interval level of measurement 8	qualitative variables 6	treatment group 16
descriptive statistics 4		quantitative variables 7	variable 4
discrete variables 7	measurement scales 8	quasi-experimental study 16	

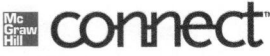 Practise and learn online with *Connect* with data sets and algorithmic questions related to concepts covered in this chapter.

Review Exercises »

Note: **All odd-numbered problems as well as the even-numbered problems marked with "(ans)" are included in Appendix J: Selected Answers at the back of the book.**

1. Name and define the two areas of statistics.

2. What is probability? Name two areas where probability is used.

3. Suggest some ways statistics can be used in everyday life.

4. Explain the differences between a sample and a population.

5. Why are samples used in statistics?

6. In each of these statements, tell whether descriptive or inferential statistics have been used.

   a. Projected numbers for space tourists by 2021 is 25,000 passengers per year in suborbital flights. (*Source:* Futron Corporation)
   b. Wireless (cell) phone subscribers in Canada reached 22.5 million in 2009. (*Source:* Canadian Wireless Telecommunications Association)
   c. The value of Canada's building permits in December 2005 set a new record at $6.5 billion. (*Source:* Statistics Canada)
   d. In 2008, police reported 611 homicide victims in Canada. (*Source:* Statistics Canada)
   e. Flu shots may also protect against heart disease and stroke. (*Source:* Heart and Stroke Foundation)
   f. By 2031, 25% of Canada's population will be 65 years of age or over. (*Source:* Statistics Canada)
   g. Total health-care spending per Canadian in 2009 was $5452. (*Source:* Canadian Institute for Health Information)
   h. Canada's finance minister revealed that the budget shortfall will swell to a record $55.9 billion in 2009

and pledged that the government will reduce the deficit to $5.2 billion by 2015. (*Source:* canada.com)

7. Classify each as nominal-level, ordinal-level, interval-level, or ratio-level measurement:

   a. Pages in the city of Winnipeg telephone book.
   b. Rankings of tennis players.
   c. Weights of air conditioners.
   d. Temperatures inside ten refrigerators.
   e. Salaries of the top five CEOs in Canada.
   f. Ratings of eight local plays (poor, fair, good, excellent).
   g. Times required for mechanics to do a tune-up.
   h. Ages of students in a classroom.
   i. Marital status of patients in a doctor's office.
   j. Horsepower of tractor engines.

8. **(ans)** Classify each variable as qualitative or quantitative.

   a. Number of bicycles sold in one year by a large sporting goods store.
   b. Colours of baseball caps in a store.
   c. Time it takes to cut a lawn.
   d. Capacity in cubic metres of six truck beds.
   e. Classification of children in a day-care centre (infant, toddler, preschool).
   f. Weights of fish caught in Lake Winnipeg.
   g. Marital status of faculty members in a large university.

9. Classify each variable as discrete or continuous.

   a. Number of doughnuts sold each day by Doughnut Heaven.
   b. Water temperatures of six swimming pools in Saskatoon on a given day.
   c. Weights of cats in a pet shelter.

d. Lifetime (in hours) of 12 flashlight batteries.

e. Number of cheeseburgers sold each day by a hamburger stand on a college campus.

f. Number of Blu-ray discs rented each day by a video store.

g. Daily volume of raw sewage and storm water (in litres) entering St. John's Harbour.

10. Give the boundaries of each value.

a. 42.8 kilometres   *d.* 18 kilograms
b. 1.6 millilitres   *e.* 13.8°C
c. 5.36 grams   *f.* 40 centimetres

11. Name and define the four basic sampling methods.

12. (ans) Classify each sample as random, systematic, stratified, or cluster.

a. In a large school district, all teachers from two buildings are interviewed to determine whether they believe the students have less homework to do now than in previous years.

b. Every seventh customer entering a shopping mall is asked to select her or his favourite store.

c. Nursing supervisors are selected using random numbers in order to determine annual salaries.

d. Every 100th hamburger manufactured is checked to determine its fat content.

e. Mail carriers of a large city are divided into four groups according to gender (male or female) and according to whether they walk or ride on their routes. Then ten are selected from each group and interviewed to determine whether they have been bitten by a dog in the last year.

13. Give three examples each of nominal, ordinal, interval, and ratio data.

14. For each of these statements, define a population and state how a sample might be obtained.

a. The average cost of an airline meal is $4.55. (*Source: Everything Has Its Price,* Richard E. Donley, Simon and Schuster)

b. Some 25% of Canadian children are obese today. (*Source: Reader's Digest Canada*)

c. Every ten minutes, two people die in car crashes and 170 are injured. (*Source:* National Safety Council estimates)

d. When older people with mild to moderate hypertension were given mineral salt for six months, the average blood pressure reading dropped by 8 points systolic and 3 points diastolic. (*Source: Prevention*)

e. The average amount spent per gift for Mom on Mother's Day is $25.95. (*Source:* The Gallup Organization)

15. Select a newspaper or magazine article that involves a statistical study, and write a paper answering these questions.

a. Is this study descriptive or inferential? Explain your answer.

b. What are the variables used in the study? In your opinion, what level of measurement was used to obtain the data from the variables?

c. Does the article define the population? If so, how is it defined? If not, how could it be defined?

d. Does the article state the sample size and how the sample was obtained? If so, determine the size of the sample and explain how it was selected. If not, suggest a way it could have been obtained.

e. Explain *in your own words* what procedure (survey, comparison of groups, etc.) might have been used to determine the study's conclusions.

f. Do you agree or disagree with the conclusions? State your reasons.

16. Information from research studies is sometimes taken out of context. Explain why the claims of these studies might be suspect.

a. The average university tuition for international students in 2010 was $31,081.

b. It is estimated that over 100,000 stray cats roam Toronto streets.

c. Only 3% of the men surveyed read *Cosmopolitan* magazine.

d. Based on a recent mail survey, 85% of the respondents favoured gun control.

e. A recent study showed that high school dropouts drink more coffee than students who graduated; therefore, coffee dulls the brain.

f. Since most automobile accidents occur within 24 km of a person's residence, it is safer to make long trips.

17. Identify each study as being either observational or experimental.

a. Subjects were randomly assigned to two groups, and one group was given an herb and the other group a placebo. After six months, the numbers of respiratory tract infections each group had were compared.

b. A researcher stood at a busy intersection to see if the colour of the automobile that a person drives is related to running red lights.

c. A researcher finds that people who are more hostile have higher total cholesterol levels than those who are less hostile.

d. Subjects are randomly assigned to four groups. Each group is placed on one of four special diets—a low-fat diet, a high-fish diet, a combination of low-fat diet and high-fish diet, and a regular diet. After six months, the blood pressures of the groups are compared to see if diet has any effect on blood pressure.

18. Identify the independent variable(s) and the dependent variable for each of the studies in Exercise 17.

19. For each of the studies in Exercise 17, suggest possible confounding variables.

20. Beneficial Bacteria According to a pilot study of 20 people conducted at the University of Minnesota, daily doses of a compound called arabinogalactan over a period of six months resulted in a significant increase in the beneficial lactobacillus species of bacteria. Why can't it be concluded that the compound is beneficial for the majority of people?

21. Comment on the following statement, taken from a magazine advertisement: "In a recent clinical study, Brand ABC [actual brand will not be named] was proved to be 1950% better than creatine!"

22. In an ad for women, the following statement was made: "For every 100 women, 91 have taken the road less travelled." Comment on this statement.

23. In many ads for weight-loss products, under the product claims and in small print, the following statement is made: "These results are not typical." What does this say about the product being advertised?

24. In an ad for moisturizing lotion, the following claim is made: " . . . it's the #1 dermatologist-recommended brand." What is misleading about this claim?

25. An ad for an exercise product stated: "Using this product will burn 74% more calories." What is misleading about this statement?

26. "Vitamin E is a proven antioxidant and may help in fighting cancer and heart disease." Is there anything ambiguous about this claim? Explain.

27. "Just 1 capsule of Brand X can provide 24 hours of acid control." [Actual brand will not be named.] What needs to be more clearly defined in this statement?

28. ". . . Male children born to women who smoke during pregnancy run a risk of violent and criminal behaviour that lasts well into adulthood." Can we infer that smoking during pregnancy is responsible for criminal behaviour in people?

29. Caffeine and Health In the 1980s, a study linked coffee to a higher risk of heart disease and pancreatic cancer. In the early 1990s, studies showed that drinking coffee posed minimal health threats. However, in 1994, a study showed that pregnant women who drank 3 or more cups of tea daily may be at risk for spontaneous abortion. In 1998, a study claimed that women who drank more than a half-cup of caffeinated tea every day may actually increase their fertility. In 1998, a study showed that over a lifetime, a few extra cups of coffee a day can raise blood pressure, heart rate, and stress. (*Source:* "Bottom Line: Is It Good for You? Or Bad?" by Monika Guttman, *USA TODAY Weekend*) Suggest some reasons why these studies appear to be conflicting.

Extending the Concepts

30. Find an article that describes a statistical study, and identify the study as observational or experimental.

31. For the article that you used in Exercise 30, identify the independent variable(s) and dependent variable for the study.

32. For the article that you selected in Exercise 30, suggest some confounding variables that may have an effect on the results of the study.

 Statistics Today

Are We Improving Our Diet?—Revisited

Researchers selected a *sample* of 23,699 adults in the United States, using phone numbers selected at *random,* and conducted a *telephone survey.* All respondents were asked six questions:

1. How often do you drink juices such as orange, grapefruit, or tomato?
2. Not counting juice, how often do you eat fruit?
3. How often do you eat green salad?
4. How often do you eat potatoes (not including french fries, fried potatoes, or potato chips)?
5. How often do you eat carrots?
6. Not counting carrots, potatoes, or salad, how many servings of vegetables do you usually eat?

Researchers found that men consumed fewer servings of fruits and vegetables per day (3.3) than women (3.7). Only 20% of the population consumed the recommended five or more daily servings. In addition, they found that youths and less-educated people consumed an even lower amount than the average.

Based on this study, they recommend that greater educational efforts are needed to improve fruit and vegetable consumption by North Americans and to provide environmental and institutional support to encourage increased consumption.

Source: Mary K. Serdula, M.D., et al., "Fruit and Vegetable Intake Among Adults in 16 States: Results of a Brief Telephone Survey," *American Journal of Public Health* 85, no. 2. Copyright by the American Public Health Association; Government of Canada.

Chapter Quiz »

Determine whether each statement is true or false. If the statement is false, explain why.

1. Probability is used as a basis for inferential statistics.

2. The height of Sir John A. Macdonald is an example of a variable.

3. The highest level of measurement is the interval level.

4. When the population of college professors is divided into groups according to their rank (instructor, assistant professor, etc.) and then several are selected from each group to make up a sample, the sample is called a *cluster sample*.

5. The variable *age* is an example of a qualitative variable.

6. The weight of pumpkins is considered to be a continuous variable.

7. The boundary of a value such as 6 centimetres would be 5.9–6.1 centimetres.

Select the best answer.

8. The number of absences per year that a worker has is an example of what type of data?

   a. Nominal   c. Discrete
   b. Qualitative   d. Continuous

9. What are the boundaries of 25.6 grams?

   a. 25–26 grams   c. 25.5–25.7 grams
   b. 25.55–25.65 grams   d. 20–39 grams

10. A researcher divided subjects into two groups according to gender and then selected members from each group for her sample. What sampling method was the researcher using?

    a. Cluster   c. Systematic
    b. Random   d. Stratified

11. Data that can be classified according to colour are measured on what scale?

    a. Nominal   c. Ordinal
    b. Ratio   d. Interval

12. A study that involves no researcher intervention is called

    a. An experimental study.
    b. A noninvolvement study.
    c. An observational study.
    d. A quasi-experimental study.

13. A variable that interferes with other variables in the study is called

    a. A confounding variable.
    b. An explanatory variable.
    c. An outcome variable.
    d. An interfering variable.

Use the best answer to complete these statements.

14. Two major branches of statistics are _____ and _____.

15. Two uses of probability are _____ and _____.

16. The group of all subjects under study is called a(n) _____.

17. A group of subjects selected from the group of all subjects under study is called a(n) _____.

18. Three reasons why samples are used in statistics are

    a. _____   b. _____   c. _____.

19. The four basic sampling methods are

    a. _____   b. _____   c. _____   d. _____.

20. A study that uses intact groups when it is not possible to randomly assign participants to the groups is called a(n) _____ study.

21. In a research study, participants should be assigned to groups using _____ methods, if possible.

22. For each statement, decide whether descriptive or inferential statistics is used.

    a. The average life expectancy for Canadian females is 83.91 years and 78.69 years for males. (*Source:* CIA, *The World Factbook, 2009*)
    b. The world population is projected to reach 8.9 billion by 2050. (*Source:* United Nations)
    c. In 2006, there were 140,040 artists in Canada, with combined earnings of $3.2 billion. (*Source:* Hill Strategies Research Inc.)
    d. Researchers stated that the shape of a person's ears is related to the person's aggression. (*Source: American Journal of Human Biology*)
    e. Federal health care funding to the provinces and territories will reach $30 billion by 2013. (*Source:* Health Canada)

23. Classify each as nominal-level, ordinal-level, interval-level, or ratio-level measurement.

    a. Rating of movies as G, PG, and R.
    b. Number of candy bars sold on a fund drive.
    c. Classification of automobiles as subcompact, compact, standard, and luxury.
    d. Temperatures of hair dryers.
    e. Weights of suitcases on a commercial airline.

24. Classify each variable as discrete or continuous.

    a. Ages of people working in a large factory.
    b. Number of cups of coffee served at a restaurant.
    c. The amount of a drug injected into a guinea pig.
    d. The time it takes a student to drive to school.
    e. The number of litres of milk sold each day at a grocery store.

25. Give the boundaries of each.

    a. 48 seconds
    b. 0.56 centimetre
    c. 9.1 litres
    d. 13.7 kilograms
    e. 7 metres

Critical Thinking Challenges »

1. **World's Busiest Airports** A study of the world's busiest airports was conducted by *Airports Council International*. Describe three variables that one could use to determine which airports are the busiest. What *units* would one use to measure these variables? Are these variables categorical, discrete, or continuous?

2. **Smoking and Criminal Behaviour** The results of a study published in *Archives of General Psychiatry* stated that male children born to women who smoke during pregnancy run a risk of violent and criminal behaviour that lasts into adulthood. The results of this study were challenged by some people in the media. Give several reasons why the results of this study would be challenged.

3. **Piano Lessons Improve Math Ability** The results of a study published in *Neurological Research* stated that second-graders who took piano lessons and played a computer math game more readily grasped math problems in fractions and proportions than a similar group who took an English class and played the same math game. What type of inferential study was this? Give several reasons why piano lessons could improve a student's math ability.

4. **ACL Tears in Collegiate Soccer Players** A study of 2958 collegiate soccer players (1565 male and 1393 female) showed that in 46 anterior cruciate ligament (ACL) tears, 36 were in women. Calculate the percentages of tears for each gender.

   a. Can it be concluded that female athletes tear their knees more often than male athletes?
   b. Comment on how this study's conclusion might have been reached.

5. **Anger and Snap Judgments** Read the article below entitled "Anger Can Cause Snap Judgments" and answer the following questions.

   a. Is the study experimental or observational?
   b. What is the independent variable?
   c. What is the dependent variable?
   d. Do you think the sample sizes are large enough to merit the conclusion?
   e. Based on the results of the study, what changes would you recommend to a normally unbiased person to help that person reduce his or her anger?

6. **Hostile Children Fight Unemployment** Read the article entitled "Hostile Children Fight Unemployment" and answer the following questions.

   a. Is the study experimental or observational?
   b. What is the independent variable?
   c. What is the dependent variable?
   d. Suggest some confounding variables that may have influenced the results of the study.
   e. Identify the three groups of subjects used in the study.

ANGER CAN CAUSE SNAP JUDGMENTS

Anger can make a normally unbiased person act with prejudice, according to a forthcoming study in the journal *Psychological Science*.

Assistant psychology professors David DeSteno at Northeastern University in Boston and Nilanjana Dasgupta at the University of Massachusetts, Amherst, randomly divided 81 study participants into two groups and assigned them a writing task designed to induce angry, sad or neutral feelings. In a subsequent test to uncover nonconscious associations, angry subjects were quicker to connect negatively charged words—like war, death and vomit—with members of the opposite group—even though the groupings were completely arbitrary.

"These automatic responses guide our behavior when we're not paying attention," says DeSteno, and they can lead to discriminatory acts when there is pressure to make a quick decision. "If you're aware that your emotions might be coloring these gut reactions," he says, "you should take time to consider that possibility and adjust your actions accordingly."

—*Eric Strand*

UNEMPLOYMENT

Hostile Children Fight Unemployment

Aggressive children may be destined for later long-term unemployment. In a study that began in 1968, researchers at the University of Jyvaskyla in Finland examined about 300 participants at ages 8, 14, 27, and 36. They looked for aggressive behaviors like hurting other children, kicking objects when angry, or attacking others without reason.

Their results, published recently in the *International Journal of Behavioral Development*, suggest that children with low self-control of emotion—especially aggression—were significantly more prone to long-term unemployment. Children with behavioral inhibitions—such as passive and anxious behaviors—were also indirectly linked to unemployment as they lacked the preliminary initiative needed for school success. And while unemployment rates were high in Finland during the last data collection, jobless participants who were aggressive as children were less likely to have a job two years later than their nonaggressive counterparts.

Ongoing unemployment can have serious psychological consequences, including depression, anxiety and stress. But lead researcher Lea Pulkkinen, Ph.D., a Jyvaskyla psychology professor, does have encouraging news for parents: Aggressive children with good social skills and child-centered parents were significantly less likely to be unemployed for more than two years as adults.

—Tanya Zimbardo

Source: Reprinted with permission from *Psychology Today.* Copyright © (2001) Sussex Publishers, Inc.

Data Projects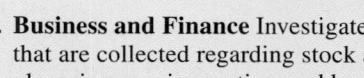

1. **Business and Finance** Investigate the types of data that are collected regarding stock and bonds; for example, price, earnings ratios, and bond ratings. Find as many types of data as possible. For each, identify the level of measure as nominal, ordinal, interval, or ratio. For any quantitative data, also note if they are discrete or continuous.

2. **Sports and Leisure** Select a professional sport. Investigate the types of data that are collected about that sport; for example, in hockey, the level of play (Midget A, AA, AAA; Junior A, B, or C; Semi-Pro League and National League), team records (wins, losses, ties) and individual records (goals, assists, points). For each, identify the level of measure as nominal, ordinal, interval, or ratio. For any quantitative data, also note if they are discrete or continuous.

3. **Technology** Music organization programs on computers and music players maintain information about a song, such as the writer, song length, genre, and your personal rating. Investigate the types of data collected about a song. For each, identify the level of measure as nominal, ordinal, interval, or ratio. For any quantitative data, also note if they are discrete or continuous.

4. **Health and Wellness** Think about the types of data that can be collected about your health and wellness, things such as blood type, cholesterol level, smoking status, and BMI. Find as many data items as you can. For each, identify the level of measure as nominal, ordinal, interval, or ratio. For any quantitative data, also note if they are discrete or continuous.

5. **Politics and Economics** Every five years, on the first and sixth year of each decade, Statistics Canada conducts a Canada-wide census of every resident in the country. Investigate the types of data that were collected in the 2006 census or, if available, the 2011 census. For each data type, identify the level of measure as nominal, ordinal, interval, or ratio. For any quantitative data, also note if they are discrete or continuous. Use the library or a government or genealogy Web site to find a census form or data from the early 1900s. What types of data were recollected? How do the types of data differ?

6. **Your Class** Your school probably has a database that contains information about each student, such as age, county of residence, credits earned, and ethnicity. Investigate the types of student data that your college or university collects and reports. For each, identify the level of measure as nominal, ordinal, interval, or ratio. For any quantitative data, also note if they are discrete or continuous.

Answers to Applying the Concepts »

Section 1–1 Attendance and Grades

1. The variables are grades and attendance.

2. The data consist of specific grades and attendance numbers.

3. These are descriptive statistics.

4. The population under study is students at Red Deer Community College (RDCC).

5. While not specified, we probably have data from a sample of RDCC students.

6. Based on the data, it appears that in general, the better your attendance the higher your grade.

Section 1–2 Be Aware of Motor Vehicles

1. The variables are "classification of injured" and "number of injuries" from motor vehicle traffic.

2. "Classification of injured" is a qualitative variable, while "number of injuries" is a quantitative variable.

3. The number of injuries from motor vehicle traffic is a discrete variable.

4. The classification of injured is classified in the nominal measurement level and the number of injuries is classified in the ratio level of measurement.

5. The motorcycle driver does show fewer injuries than the nonmotorcycle driver; however, there may be other factors to consider. For example, there are fewer motorcyclists on the road than nonmotorcyclists.

6. Answers will vary. Other factors to consider for the number of reported injuries may include severity of injury (minor injuries may not be reported; whereas injuries leading to death may be classified elsewhere). Location of accident (remote accident locations may not be reported). Private settlements, solo accident, alcohol or drug abuse (insurance ramifications or legal consequences may affect reporting).

7. Answers will vary. There are almost five times more reported injuries to pedestrians than pedal cyclists. The ratio of driver-to-passenger injuries is higher for nonmotorcycle vehicles (2.24:1) than for motorcycle vehicles (12.93:1).

Section 1–3 Canadian Culture and Drug Abuse

Answers will vary, so these are possible answers.

1. I used a telephone survey. The advantage to my survey method is that this was a relatively inexpensive survey method (although more expensive than using the mail) that could get a fairly sizable response. The disadvantage to my survey method is that I have not included anyone without a telephone. (*Note:* My survey used a random dialing method to include unlisted numbers and cellphone exchanges.)

2. A mail survey also would have been fairly inexpensive, but my response rate may have been much lower than what I got with my telephone survey. Interviewing would have allowed me to use follow-up questions and to clarify any questions of the respondents at the time of the interview. However, interviewing is very labour- and cost-intensive.

3. I used ordinal data on a scale of 1 to 5. The scores were 1 = strongly disagree, 2 = disagree, 3 = neutral, 4 = agree, 5 = strongly agree.

4. The random method that I used was a random dialing method.

5. To include people from each province, I used a stratified random sample, collecting data randomly from each of the area codes and telephone exchanges available.

6. This method allowed me to make sure that I had representation from each area of Canada.

7. Convenience samples may not be representative of the population, and a convenience sample of adolescents would probably differ greatly from the general population with regard to the influence of Canadian culture on illegal drug use.

Section 1–4 Just a Pinch between Your Cheek and Gum

1. This was an experiment, since the researchers imposed a treatment on each of the two groups involved in the study.

2. The independent variable is whether the participant chewed tobacco or not. The dependent variables are the students' blood pressures and heart rates.

3. The treatment group is the tobacco group—the other group was used as a control.

4. A student's blood pressure might not be affected by knowing that he or she was part of a study. However, if the student's blood pressure was affected by this knowledge, all the students (in both groups) would be affected similarly. This might be an example of the placebo effect.

5. Answers will vary. One possible answer is that confounding variables might include the way that the students chewed the tobacco, whether or not the students smoked (although this would hopefully have been evened out with the randomization), and that all the participants were university students.

6. Answers will vary. One possible answer is that the study design was fine, but that it cannot be generalized beyond the population of university students (or people around that age).

Chapter 2

Frequency Distributions and Graphs

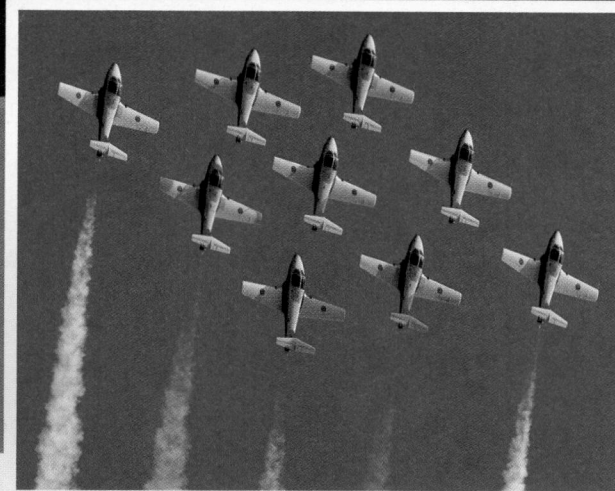

Objectives >

After completing this chapter, you should be able to

LO1 Organize data using frequency distributions.

LO2 Represent data in frequency distributions graphically using histograms, frequency polygons, and ogives.

LO3 Analyze data by constructing Pareto charts, time series graphs, pie graphs, and stem and leaf plots.

Outline >

McGraw Hill **connect**™ Practise and learn online with *Connect* with data sets and algorithmic questions related to concepts covered in this chapter. Throughout this chapter, questions and tables with online data sets are marked with 🖱 .

Statistics Today

Identity Theft, Identity Fraud, and You

Criminal Intelligence Services Canada defines the term *identity theft* as "the collection, possession, and trafficking in personal information, which typically takes place independent of, or in preparation for, the commission of identity fraud." Thieves may exploit your name; address; birth date; gender; Social Insurance, driver's licence, banking, phone, and credit card numbers; email address; passwords; employment and income data; and passport and personal health records

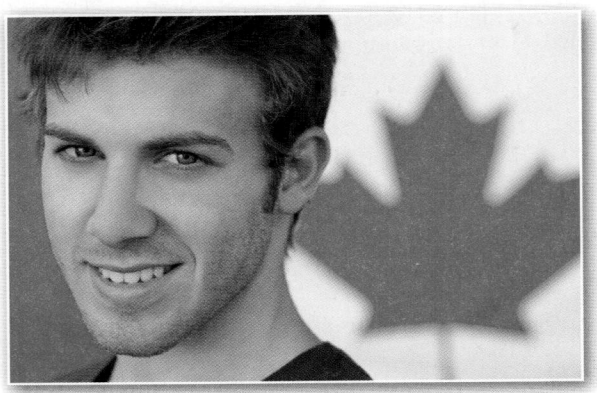

without your knowledge or consent. Could you be a victim of identity fraud?

Phonebusters, Canada's anti-fraud call centre, reported 11,370 identity theft victims in 2008, accounting for $9.5 million in losses, or an average of over $835 per victim. Reported losses increased almost 50% over the previous year. Benefits that thieves obtained with personal information were reported as follows.

Credit card usage	860	27%
Merchandise purchase	595	19%
Credit card application	395	12%
Cellphone lease	343	11%
Cash withdrawal	306	10%
Account access	128	4%
Other benefits	547	17%
	3174	100%

Although disturbing, the numbers presented in the table do not have the same impact as illustrating the figures in a well-drawn chart or graph. This chapter will demonstrate procedures to organize data and to construct appropriate charts and graphs that will help to emphasize key points in the data.

See Statistics Today—Revisited, page 75, for some suggestions on how to represent the data graphically.

Sources: Criminal Intelligence Services Canada, *2008 Annual Report;* Phonebusters, *2008 Annual Report.*

Introduction >

When conducting a statistical study, the researcher must gather data for the particular variable under study. For example, if a Parks Canada researcher wishes to study the number of people in a region who suffered swimmer's itch, in which parasites from freshwater snails and water fowl burrow under the skin, he or she needs to gather data from camper surveys, pharmacists, doctors, hospitals, or health agencies.

To describe situations, draw conclusions, or make inferences about events, the researcher must organize the data in some meaningful way. The most convenient method of organizing data is to construct a *frequency distribution.*

After organizing the data, the researcher must present them so they can be understood by those who will benefit from reading the study. The most useful method of presenting the data is by constructing *statistical charts* and *graphs.* There are many different types of charts and graphs, and each one has a specific purpose.

This chapter explains how to organize data by constructing frequency distributions and how to present the data by constructing charts and graphs. The charts and graphs illustrated here are histograms, frequency polygons, ogives, pie graphs, Pareto charts, and time series graphs. A graph that combines the characteristics of a frequency distribution and a histogram, called a *stem and leaf plot,* is also explained.

2–1	Organizing Data >

LO1

Organize data using frequency distributions.

Wealthy People   Suppose a researcher wished to do a study on the ages of the top 50 wealthiest people in the world. The researcher first would have to get the data on the ages of the people. In this case, these ages are listed in *Forbes* magazine. When the data are in original form, they are called **raw data,** which can look like the following.

53	89	61	80	86	76	78	66	86	81
78	51	59	67	54	35	56	83	63	77
69	58	54	61	65	36	49	85	89	69
64	87	65	73	51	53	47	82	73	72
83	73	60	68	44	57	46	43	66	42

Since little information can be obtained from looking at raw data, the researcher organizes the data into what is called a **frequency distribution.** A frequency distribution consists of *classes* and their corresponding *frequencies.* Each raw data value is placed into a quantitative or qualitative category called a **class.** The **frequency** of a class then is the number of data values contained in a specific class. A frequency distribution is shown for the preceding age data set.

Class limits	Tally	Frequency
31–40	//	2
41–50	///// /	6
51–60	///// ///// /	11
61–70	///// ///// //	12
71–80	///// ////	9
81–90	///// /////	10
	Total	50

Now some general observations can be made from looking at the frequency distribution. For example, it can be stated that the majority of the wealthy people in the study are over 60 years of age.

> A **frequency distribution** is the organization of raw data in table form, using classes and frequencies.

The classes in this distribution are 31–40, 41–50, etc. These values are called *class limits.* The data values 35 and 26 can be tallied in the first class; 42, 43, 44, 46, 47, and 49 in the second class; and so on.

Two types of frequency distributions that are most often used are the *categorical frequency distribution* and the *grouped frequency distribution.* The procedures for constructing these distributions are shown now.

Interesting Fact

Forbes magazine reported that the world's wealthiest people lost $1.4 trillion during the 2008 recession.

Categorical Frequency Distributions

The **categorical frequency distribution** is used for data that can be placed in specific categories, such as nominal- or ordinal-level data. For example, data such as political affiliation, religious affiliation, or major field of study would use categorical frequency distributions.

Example 2–1

Distribution of Blood Types

Twenty-five armed forces recruits were given a blood test to determine their blood type. The data set is

A	B	B	AB	O
O	O	B	AB	B
B	B	O	A	O
A	O	O	O	AB
AB	A	O	B	A

Construct a frequency distribution for the data.

Solution

Since the data are categorical, discrete classes can be used. There are four blood types: A, B, O, and AB. These types will be used as the classes for the distribution.

    The procedure for constructing a frequency distribution for categorical data is given next.

Step 1   Make a table as shown.

A Class	B Tally	C Frequency	D Percentage
A			
B			
O			
AB			

Step 2   Tally the data and place the results in column B.

Step 3   Count the tallies and place the results in column C.

Step 4   Find the percentage of values in each class by using the formula

$$\% = \frac{f}{n} \cdot 100$$

where f = frequency of the class and n = total number of values in the data set. For example, in the class of type A blood, the percentage is

$$\% = \frac{5}{25} \cdot 100 = 20\%$$

    Percentages are not normally part of a frequency distribution, but they can be added since they are used in certain types of graphs such as pie graphs. Also, the decimal equivalent of a percentage is called a *relative frequency*.

Step 5   Find the totals for columns C (frequency) and D (percentage). The completed table is shown.

A Class	B Tally	C Frequency	D Percentage
A	〥	5	20
B	〥 //	7	28
O	〥 ////	9	36
AB	////	4	16
		Total 25	100

For the sample, more people have type O blood than any other type.

Grouped Frequency Distributions

When the range of the data is large, the data must be grouped into classes that are more than one unit in width, in what is called a **grouped frequency distribution.** For example, a distribution of the number of hours that boat batteries lasted is the following.

Class limits	Class boundaries	Tally	Frequency	Cumulative frequency
24–30	23.5–30.5	///	3	3
31–37	30.5–37.5	/	1	4
38–44	37.5–44.5	7#L	5	9
45–51	44.5–51.5	7#L ////	9	18
52–58	51.5–58.5	7#L /	6	24
59–65	58.5–65.5	/	1	25
			$\overline{25}$	

The procedure for constructing a frequency distribution including cumulative frequencies is given in Example 2–2; however, several things should be noted. In this distribution, the values 24 and 30 of the first class are called *class limits.* The **lower class limit** is 24; it represents the smallest data value that can be included in the class. The **upper class limit** is 30; it represents the largest data value that can be included in the class. The numbers in the second column are called **class boundaries.** These numbers are used to separate the classes so that there are no gaps in the frequency distribution. The gaps are due to the limits; for example, there is a gap between 30 and 31.

Students sometimes have difficulty finding class boundaries when given the class limits. The basic rule of thumb is that *the class limits should have the same decimal place value as the data, but the class boundaries should have one additional place value and end in a 5.* For example, if the values in the data set are whole numbers, such as 24, 32, 18, the limits for a class might be 31–37, and the boundaries are 30.5–37.5. Find the boundaries by subtracting 0.5 from 31 (the lower class limit) and adding 0.5 to 37 (the upper class limit).

$$\text{Lower limit} - 0.5 = 31 - 0.5 = 30.5 = \text{lower boundary}$$
$$\text{Upper limit} + 0.5 = 37 + 0.5 = 37.5 = \text{upper boundary}$$

If the data are in tenths, such as 6.2, 7.8, and 12.6, the limits for a class hypothetically might be 7.8–8.8, and the boundaries for that class would be 7.75–8.85. Find these values by subtracting 0.05 from 7.8 and adding 0.05 to 8.8.

Finally, the **class width** for a class in a frequency distribution is found by subtracting the lower (or upper) class limit of one class from the lower (or upper) class limit of the next class. For example, the class width in the preceding distribution on the duration of boat batteries is 7, found from $31 - 24 = 7$.

The class width can also be found by subtracting the lower boundary from the upper boundary for any given class. In this case, $30.5 - 23.5 = 7$.

Note: Do not subtract the limits of a single class. It will result in an incorrect answer.

The researcher must decide how many classes to use and the width of each class. To construct a frequency distribution, follow these rules:

1. *There should be between 5 and 20 classes.* Although there is no hard-and-fast rule for the number of classes contained in a frequency distribution, it is of the utmost importance to have enough classes to present a clear description of the collected data.

2. *It is preferable but not absolutely necessary that the class width be an odd number.* This ensures that the midpoint of each class has the same place value as the data.

The **class midpoint** X_m is obtained by adding the lower and upper boundaries and dividing by 2, or adding the lower and upper limits and dividing by 2:

$$X_m = \frac{\text{Lower boundary} + \text{Upper boundary}}{2}$$

or

$$X_m = \frac{\text{Lower limit} + \text{Upper limit}}{2}$$

For example, the midpoint of the first class in the example with boat batteries is

$$\frac{24 + 30}{2} = 27 \qquad \text{or} \qquad \frac{23.5 + 30.5}{2} = 27$$

The midpoint is the numeric location of the centre of the class. Midpoints are necessary for graphing (see Section 2–2). If the class width is an even number, the midpoint is in tenths. For example, if the class width is 6 and the boundaries are 5.5 and 11.5, the midpoint is

$$\frac{5.5 + 11.5}{2} = \frac{17}{2} = 8.5$$

Rule 2 is only a suggestion and it is not rigorously followed, especially when a computer is used to group data.

3. *The classes must be mutually exclusive.* Mutually exclusive classes have nonoverlapping class limits so that data cannot be placed into two classes. Many times, frequency distributions such as

Age
10–20
20–30
30–40
40–50

are found in the literature or in surveys. If a person is 40 years old, into which class should she or he be placed? A better way to construct a frequency distribution is to use classes such as

Age
10–20
21–31
32–42
43–53

4. *The classes must be continuous.* Even if there are no values in a class, the class must be included in the frequency distribution. There should be no gaps in a frequency distribution. The only exception occurs when the class with a zero frequency is the first or last class. A class with a zero frequency at either end can be omitted without affecting the distribution.

5. *The classes must be exhaustive.* There should be enough classes to accommodate all the data.

6. *The classes must be equal in width.* This avoids a distorted view of the data.

One exception occurs when a distribution has a class that is open-ended. That is, the class has no specific beginning value or no specific ending value. A frequency distribution with an open-ended class is called an **open-ended distribution.** Here are two examples of distributions with open-ended classes.

Age	Frequency		Minutes	Frequency
10–20	3		Below 110	16
21–31	6		110–114	24
32–42	4		115–119	38
43–53	10		120–124	14
54 and above	8		125–129	5

The frequency distribution for age is open-ended for the last class, which means that anybody who is 54 years or older will be tallied in the last class. The distribution for minutes is open-ended for the first class, meaning that any minute values below 110 will be tallied in that class.

Example 2–2 shows the procedure for constructing a grouped frequency distribution, as well as cumulative frequencies of data values up to and including each class.

Example 2–2

Statistics Final Grades

The following data represent final grades for Professor Fisher's introductory statistics course. Construct a frequency distribution using 7 classes.

74	73	71	55	91	62	78	83	63	81
68	93	37	78	57	56	65	67	81	95
65	58	83	65	72	76	81	53	57	67
88	85	73	97	73	82	43	69	62	31
75	75	62	41	68	87	78	41	98	73

Solution

The procedure for constructing a grouped frequency distribution for numerical data follows.

Step 1 Determine the classes.

Find the highest value and lowest value: $H = 98$ and $L = 31$.

Find the range: $R = $ highest value $-$ lowest value $= H - L$, so $R = 98 - 31 = 67$

Select the number of classes desired (usually between 5 and 20). In this case, 7 is arbitrarily chosen.

Find the class width by dividing the range by the number of classes.

$$\text{Width} = \frac{R}{\text{Number of classes}} = \frac{67}{7} = 9.6$$

Round the answer up to the nearest whole number if there is a remainder: $9.6 \approx 10$. (Rounding *up* is different from rounding *off*. A number is rounded up if there is any decimal remainder when dividing. For example, $85 \div 6 = 14.167$ and is rounded up to 15. Also, $53 \div 4 = 13.25$ and is rounded up to 14. Also, after dividing, if there is no remainder, you will need to add an extra class to accommodate all the data.)

Select a starting point for the lowest class limit. This can be the smallest data value or any convenient number less than the smallest data value. (*Note:* A convenient starting point may require an additional class to accommodate all data.) In this case, 30 is used. Add the width to the lowest score taken as the starting point to get the lower limit of the next class. Keep adding until there are 7 classes, as shown, 30, 40, 50, etc.

Subtract one unit from the lower limit of the second class to get the upper limit of the first class. Then add the width to each upper limit to get all the upper limits.

$$40 - 1 = 39$$

The first class is 30–39, the second class is 40–49, etc.

Find the class boundaries by subtracting 0.5 from each lower class limit and adding 0.5 to each upper class limit:

29.5–39.5, 39.5–49.5, etc.

Step 2   Tally the data and place the tally for each data point in the appropriate class.

Step 3   Find the numerical frequencies (f) from the tallies for each class.

Step 4   Find the cumulative frequencies.

A cumulative frequency (*cf*) column can be added to the distribution by adding the frequency in each class to the total of the frequencies of the classes preceding that class, such as $0 + 2 = 2, 2 + 3 = 5, 5 + 6 = 11$, and $11 + 12 = 23$, etc. (*Note:* "Σf" is "sum of frequencies.")

The completed frequency distribution is

Class limits	Class boundaries	Tally	Frequency	Cumulative frequency
30–39	29.5–39.5	//	2	2
40–49	39.5–49.5	⊬	3	5
50–59	49.5–59.5	⊬⊢	6	11
60–69	59.5–69.5	⊬ ⊬ //	12	23
70–79	69.5–79.5	⊬ //// ///	13	36
80–89	79.5–89.5	⊬ ////	9	45
90–99	89.5–99.5	////	5	50

$$n = \Sigma f = 50$$

The frequency distributions shows that the class 69.5–79.5 contains the largest number of grades (13) followed by the class 59.5–69.5 with 12 grades. Hence, exactly one-half of the grades (25) fall between 59.5 and 79.5.

The cumulative frequency column indicates how many data values are less than a specific class. In Example 2–2, 11 of the final grades are less than 60. The number of grades less than 70 is 23, less than 80 is 36, and so on.

After the raw data have been organized into a frequency distribution, it will be analyzed by looking for peaks and extreme values. The peaks show which class or classes have the most data values compared to the other classes. Extreme values, called **outliers,** show large or small data values that are relative to other data values. Refer to Section 3–3 for a detailed explanation of outliers.

When the range of the data values is relatively small, a frequency distribution can be constructed using single data values for each class. This type of distribution is called an **ungrouped frequency distribution** and is shown next.

| Example 2–3 | **Fuel Economy SPVs** 🖊 |

The data shown here represent highway fuel economy ratings, L/100 km (rounded to the nearest whole number), for 30 selected special-purpose vehicles (sports utility vehicles, truck class hybrids, etc.) from various manufacturers with sales in Canada. Construct a frequency distribution and then analyze the distribution.

7	9	12	8	10	14
10	11	8	9	11	10
9	10	7	10	9	8
9	9	11	8	12	9
13	8	10	11	9	11

Source: Natural Resources Canada, *Fuel Consumption Guide, 2009.*

Solution

Step 1 Determine the classes. Since the range of the data set is small ($14 - 7 = 7$), classes consisting of a single data value can be used. They are 7, 8, 9, 10, 11, 12, 13, and 14.

Note: If the data are continuous, class boundaries can be used. Subtract 0.5 from each class value to get the lower class boundary, and add 0.5 to each class value to get the upper class boundary.

Step 2 Tally the data and place the tally in the appropriate class.

Step 3 Count and record the numerical frequencies from the tallies.

Step 4 Determine the cumulative frequencies, beginning with the lowest class.

Class limits	Class boundaries	Tally	Frequency	Cumulative frequency
7	6.5–7.5	//	2	2
8	7.5–8.5	////	5	7
9	8.5–9.5	//// ///	8	15
10	9.5–10.5	//// /	6	21
11	10.5–11.5	////	5	26
12	11.5–12.5	//	2	28
13	12.5–13.5	/	1	29
14	13.5–14.5	/	1	30

$$n = \Sigma f = 30$$

In this case, exactly one-half (15/30) of the special-purpose vehicles are fuel-efficient, with 9 or less L/100 km highway fuel consumption.

The steps for constructing a grouped frequency distribution are summarized in the following Procedure Table.

Procedure Table

Constructing a Grouped Frequency Distribution

Step 1   Determine the classes.

Find the highest and lowest value.

Find the range.

Select the number of classes desired.

Find the width by dividing the range by the number of classes and rounding up.

Select a starting point (usually the lowest value or any convenient number less than the lowest value); add the width to get the lower limits.

Find the upper class limits.

Find the boundaries.

Step 2   Tally the data.

Step 3   Find the numerical frequencies from the tallies.

Step 4   Find the cumulative frequencies.

When one is constructing a frequency distribution, the guidelines presented in this section should be followed. However, one can construct several different but correct frequency distributions for the same data by using a different class width, a different number of classes, or a different starting point.

Furthermore, the method shown here for constructing a frequency distribution is not unique, and there are other ways of constructing one. Slight variations exist, especially in computer packages. But regardless of what methods are used, classes should be mutually exclusive, continuous, exhaustive, and of equal width.

In summary, the different types of frequency distributions were shown in this section. The first type, shown in Example 2–1, is used when the data are categorical (nominal), such as blood type or political affiliation. This type is called a *categorical frequency distribution*. The second type of distribution is used when the range is large and classes several units in width are needed. This type is called a *grouped frequency distribution* and is shown in Example 2–2. Another type of distribution is used for numerical data and when the range of data is small, as shown in Example 2–3. Since each class is only one unit, this distribution is called an *ungrouped frequency distribution*.

All the different types of distributions are used in statistics and are helpful when one is organizing and presenting data.

The reasons for constructing a frequency distribution are as follows:

1. To organize the data in a meaningful, intelligible way.

2. To enable the reader to determine the nature or shape of the distribution.

3. To facilitate computational procedures for measures of average and spread (shown in Chapter 3, Sections 3–1 and 3–2).

4. To enable the researcher to draw charts and graphs for the presentation of data (shown in Section 2–2).

5. To enable the reader to make comparisons among different data sets.

The factors used to analyze a frequency distribution are essentially the same as those used to analyze histograms and frequency polygons, which are shown in Section 2–2.

2–1 Applying the Concepts

Prime Ministers' Ages at Swearing-In

The data represent the ages of Canada's prime ministers at their swearing-in ceremony.

52	51	70	47	69	74
54	57	46	47	60	66
61	66	48	39	55	45
46	59	65	46		

Source: Parliament of Canada.

1. Were the data obtained from a population or a sample? Explain your answer.
2. What was the age of the oldest prime minister?
3. What was the age of the youngest prime minister?
4. Construct a frequency distribution for the data. (Use your own judgment as to the number of classes and class size.)
5. Are there any peaks in the distribution?
6. Identify any possible outliers.
7. Write a brief summary of the nature of the data as shown in the frequency distribution.

See page 79 for the answers.

Exercises 2–1

1. List five reasons for organizing data into a frequency distribution.

2. Name the three types of frequency distributions, and explain when each should be used.

3. Find the class boundaries, midpoints, and widths for each class.

   a. 12–18
   b. 56–74
   c. 695–705
   d. 13.6–14.7
   e. 2.15–3.93

4. How many classes should frequency distributions have? Why should the class width be an odd number?

5. Shown here are four frequency distributions. Each is incorrectly constructed. State the reason why.

   a.
Class	Frequency
27–32	1
33–38	0
39–44	6
45–49	4
50–55	2

   b.
Class	Frequency
5–9	1
9–13	2
13–17	5
17–20	6
20–24	3

   c.
Class	Frequency
123–127	3
128–132	7
138–142	2
143–147	19

   d.
Class	Frequency
9–13	1
14–19	6
20–25	2
26–28	5
29–32	9

6. What are open-ended frequency distributions? Why are they necessary?

7. **Trust in Internet Information** A survey was taken on how much trust people place in the information they read on the Internet. Construct a categorical frequency distribution for the data, A = trust in everything they

read, M = trust in most of what they read, H = trust in about one-half of what they read, S = trust in a small portion of what they read. (Based on information from the *UCLA Internet Report.*)

M	M	M	A	H	M	S	M	H	M
S	M	M	M	M	A	M	M	A	M
M	M	H	M	M	M	H	M	H	M
A	M	M	M	H	M	M	M	M	M

8. Pumpkin Weights At a Prince Edward County, Ontario, pumpkinfest, the heaviest-pumpkin contest had the following entries. Weights are in kilograms. Construct a frequency distribution beginning at 30 with a class width of 50. (*Trivia:* The 2010 *Guinness World Records* listed the heaviest pumpkin grown at 821.23 kg.)

215	342	266	233	158	134	362
405	240	417	228	276	422	134
396	287	251	366	150	254	
34	113	245	215	147	94	
347	269	153	177	140	48	

Source: www.pec.on.ca/pumpkinfest.

9. NHL Point Totals The National Hockey League expanded from 6 to 12 teams in 1967. The data shown represent the NHL leading scorer point total since the expansion. Construct a frequency distribution for the data beginning at the minimum data value and use a class width of 20.

125	122	199	164	130
94	161	168	137	133
106	70	183	134	152
96	130	215	132	120
121	160	208	136	126
96	131	205	125	87
127	163	196	135	97
102	142	212	145	

Source: National Hockey League.

10. Global Warming Trends The Earth Policy Institute's study of global warming trends (1956–2005) published the following data. Temperatures shown are in °C. Construct a frequency distribution using 6 classes, starting at a minimum value, and analyze the nature of the data.

1956–1965	1966–1975	1976–1985	1986–1995	1996–2005
13.8	13.9	13.8	14.2	14.4
14.1	14.0	14.2	14.4	14.4
14.1	13.9	14.1	14.4	14.7
14.1	14.0	14.1	14.3	14.4
14.0	14.0	14.3	14.5	14.4
14.1	13.9	14.4	14.4	14.6
14.1	14.0	14.1	14.2	14.7
14.0	14.2	14.3	14.2	14.6
13.7	13.9	14.2	14.3	14.6
13.8	14.0	14.1	14.5	14.8

Source: Earth Policy Institute.

11. Engineering Schools GRE Scores The average quantitative Graduate Records Exam (GRE) scores for the top 30 graduate schools of engineering are listed. Construct a frequency distribution with 6 classes starting at the minimum data value.

767	770	761	760	771	768	776	771	756	770
763	760	747	766	754	771	771	778	766	762
780	750	746	764	769	759	757	753	758	746

Source: U.S. News & World Report Best Graduate Schools.

12. Masters Golf Scores In 2003, Canadian Mike Weir won golf's prestigious Masters Championship in an exciting playoff. Below are the final results for the tournament. Construct a frequency distribution with 7 classes beginning at 280. (The data in this exercise will be used in Exercise 22 in Section 3–1.)

281	288	290	292	294	295	297
281	288	290	293	294	296	298
283	288	290	293	294	296	301
284	288	290	293	294	297	301
286	288	290	293	295	297	302
287	289	290	293	295	297	304
287	289	291	294	295	297	305

Source: www.augusta.com.

13. Prime Ministers' Terms of Office The data below represent the term served (in months) of Canada's prime ministers since Confederation. Five prime ministers served multiple nonconsecutive terms. Construct a frequency distribution using 24-month intervals beginning at 1. (The data for this exercise will be used for Exercise 5 in Section 2–2 and Exercise 23 in Section 3–1.)

26	121	5	105	3	9
51	134	60	70	103	62
157	47	54	3	17	33
72	183	14	16	24	17
59	152	76			

Source: Parliament of Canada.

14. Automobile Fatalities The data below represent the number of automobile fatalities in Canada over the past 20 years. Construct a frequency distribution beginning at 2400 with a class width of 200. (The data for this exercise will be used for Exercise 6 in Section 2–2 and Exercise 24 in Section 3–1.)

3774	3651	3121	2646	2434
3510	3445	2869	2612	2593
3729	3228	2854	2636	2484
3610	3073	2708	2569	2434

Source: Transport Canada.

15. Exchange Rates The following data represent the quarterly exchange (in cents) for Canadian to United States dollars over a ten-year period. Construct a frequency distribution using 7 classes starting at the minimum value and class width rounded up to nearest cent. (The information in this exercise will be used for Exercise 9 in Section 2–2 and Exercise 25 in Section 3–1.)

90	82	76	63	66	68	66	72
86	82	73	65	64	68	68	72
86	78	74	63	66	68	68	73
85	74	68	63	67	68	71	73
81	75	64	64	68	66	71	73

Source: Bank of Canada.

16. Area of National Parks The area, in square kilometres, of Canada's national parks under 10,000 km^2 is shown here. Construct a frequency distribution for the data beginning at 1 with a class width of 1000. (The data in this exercise will be used in Exercise 11 in Section 2–2.)

6641	16	206	4766	3050
1349	1406	400	1943	1495
1313	3874	404	1878	4345
505	2973	239	907	1138
194	26	544	151	33
260	948	500	154	
9	22	240	112	

Source: Parks Canada.

17. World's Highest Mountains The heights (in metres above sea level) for the top 50 of the world's highest mountains are given here. Construct a frequency distribution for the data using 7 classes beginning at 7000 and class width rounded up to the nearest hundred. (The data in this exercise will be used in Exercise 9 in Section 3–1 and Exercise 17 in Section 3–2.)

8848	8068	7785	7654	7313
8611	8047	7756	7619	7291
8586	8035	7756	7555	7285
8511	8012	7756	7553	7273
8463	7885	7546	7546	7245
8201	7852	7742	7495	7150
8167	7820	7723	7485	7142
8163	7816	7720	7439	7135
8125	7815	7719	7406	7134
8091	7788	7690	7398	7129

Source: www.scaruffi.com/travel/tallest.html.

18. Home Run Record-Breakers During the 1998 baseball season, Mark McGwire and Sammy Sosa both broke Roger Maris's home run record of 61. The distances (in feet) for each home run follow. Construct a frequency distribution for each player, using 8 classes. (The information in this exercise will be used for Exercise 12 in Section 2–2, Exercise 10 in Section 3–1, and Exercise 14 in Section 3–2.)

McGwire				Sosa			
306	370	370	430	371	350	430	420
420	340	460	410	430	434	370	420
440	410	380	360	440	410	420	460
350	527	380	550	400	430	410	370
478	420	390	420	370	410	380	340
425	370	480	390	350	420	410	415
430	388	423	410	430	380	380	366
360	410	450	350	500	380	390	400
450	430	461	430	364	430	450	440
470	440	400	390	365	420	350	420
510	430	450	452	400	380	380	400
420	380	470	398	370	420	360	368
409	385	369	460	430	433	388	440
390	510	500	450	414	482	364	370
470	430	458	380	400	405	433	390
430	341	385	410	480	480	434	344
420	380	400	440	410	420		
377	370						

Source: USA TODAY.

Extending the Concepts »

19. JFK Assassination A researcher conducted a survey asking people if they believed more than one person was involved in the assassination of United States President John F. Kennedy in 1963. The results were as follows: 73% said yes, 19% said no, and 9% had no opinion. Is there anything suspicious about the results?

2–2 | Histograms, Frequency Polygons, and Ogives >

LO2

Represent data in frequency distributions graphically using histograms, frequency polygons, and ogives.

After the data have been organized into a frequency distribution, they can be presented in graphical form. The purpose of graphs in statistics is to convey the data to the viewers in pictorial form. It is easier for most people to comprehend the meaning of data presented graphically than data presented numerically in tables or frequency distributions. This is especially true if the users have little or no statistical knowledge.

Statistical graphs can be used to describe the data set or to analyze it. Graphs are also useful in getting the audience's attention in a publication or a speaking presentation. They can be used to discuss an issue, reinforce a critical point, or summarize a data set. They can also be used to discover a trend or pattern in a situation over a period of time.

The three most commonly used graphs in research are

1. The histogram
2. The frequency polygon
3. The cumulative frequency graph, or ogive (pronounced o-jive)

An example of each type of graph is shown in Figure 2–1. The data for each graph represent the distribution of record high temperatures, in °C, for each of the 50 states in the United States.

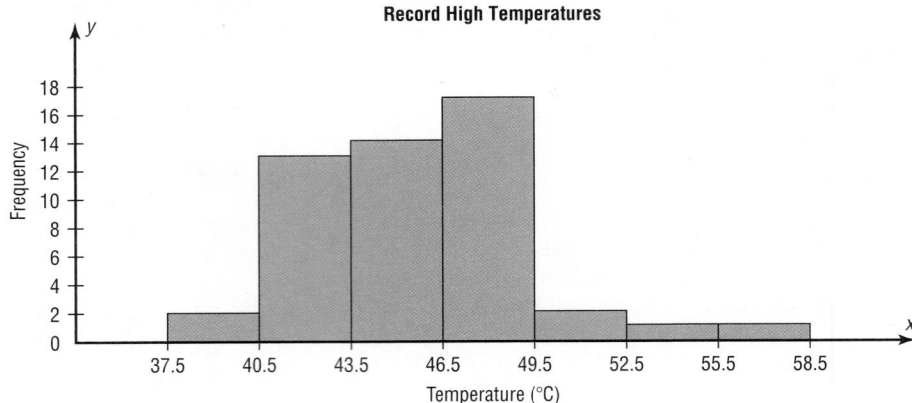

(a) Histogram

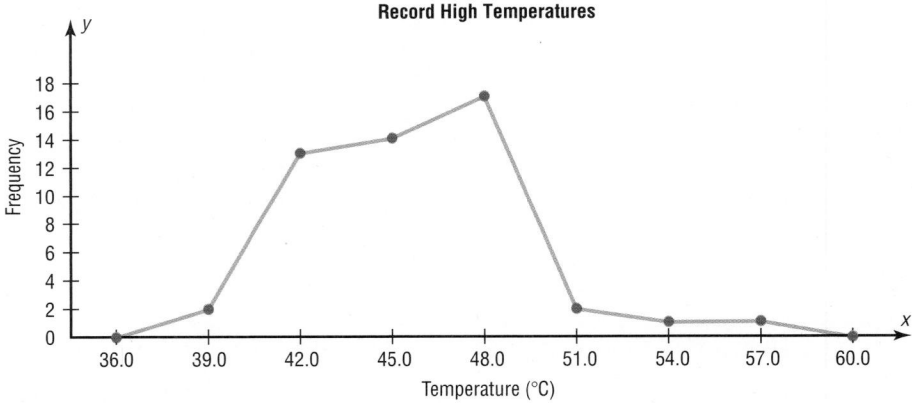

(b) Frequency polygon

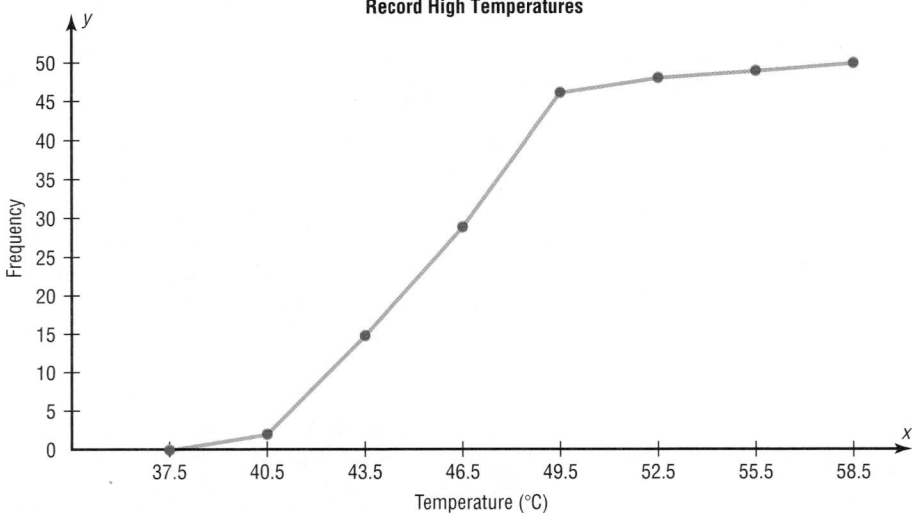

(c) Cumulative frequency graph—ogive

The Histogram

> The **histogram** is a graph of a frequency distribution in which the bar heights correspond to class frequencies and the bar widths represent class boundaries.

Note: The difference between a **histogram** and a **bar chart** is that the histogram plots frequencies for quantitative (numerical) data and the bar chart plots frequencies for qualitative (categorical) data.

Example 2–4

Historical Note

Graphs originated when ancient astronomers drew the position of the stars in the heavens. Roman surveyors also used coordinates to locate landmarks on their maps.

   The development of statistical graphs can be traced to William Playfair (1748–1819), an engineer and drafter who used graphs to present economic data pictorially.

Statistics Final Grades

Construct a histogram to represent the data shown for final grades in Professor Fisher's introductory statistics course.

Class boundaries	Frequency
29.5–39.5	2
39.5–49.5	3
49.5–59.5	6
59.5–69.5	12
69.5–79.5	13
79.5–89.5	9
89.5–99.5	5

Solution

Step 1 Draw and label the x and y axes. The x axis is always the horizontal axis, and the y axis is always the vertical axis.

Step 2 Represent the frequency on the y axis and the class boundaries on the x axis.

Step 3 Using the frequencies as the heights, draw vertical bars for each class. See Figure 2–2.

Figure 2–2

Histogram for Example 2–4

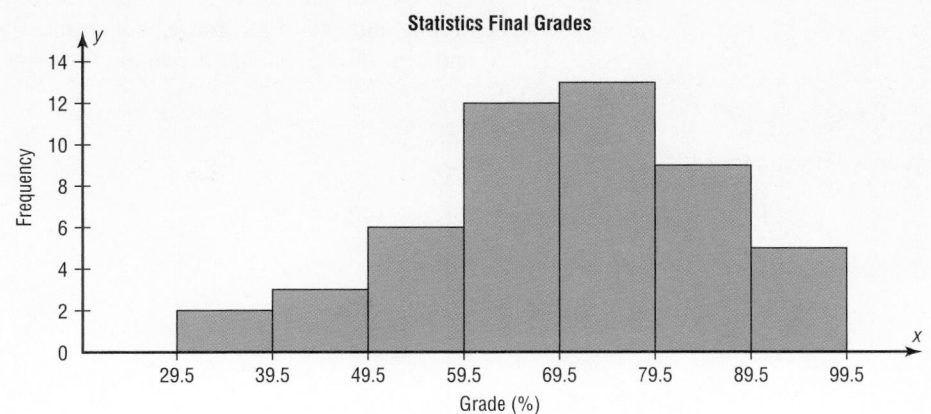

As the histogram shows, the class with the greatest number of data values (13) is 69.5–79.5, followed by 12 for 59.5–69.5. The graph also has one peak, with the data clustering around it.

The Frequency Polygon

Another way to represent the same data set is by using a frequency polygon.

> The **frequency polygon** is a graph that displays the data by using lines that connect points plotted for the frequencies at the midpoints of the classes. The frequencies are represented by the heights of the points.

Example 2–5 shows the procedure for constructing a frequency polygon.

Example 2–5

Statistics Final Grades

Using the frequency distribution given in Example 2–4, construct a frequency polygon.

Solution

Step 1   Find the midpoints of each class. Recall that midpoints are found by adding the upper and lower boundaries and dividing by 2:

$$\frac{29.5 + 39.5}{2} = 34.5 \qquad \frac{39.5 + 49.5}{2} = 44.5$$

and so on. The midpoints are

Class boundaries	Midpoints	Frequency
29.5–39.5	34.5	2
39.5–49.5	44.5	3
49.5–59.5	54.5	6
59.5–69.5	64.5	12
69.5–79.5	74.5	13
79.5–89.5	84.5	9
89.5–99.5	94.5	5

Step 2   Draw the x and y axes. Label the x axis with the midpoint of each class, and then use a suitable scale on the y axis for the frequencies.

Step 3   Using the midpoints for the x values and the frequencies as the y values, plot the points.

Step 4   Connect adjacent points with line segments. Draw a line back to the x axis at the beginning and end of the graph, at the same distance that the previous (24.5) and next (104.5) midpoints would be located, as shown in Figure 2–3.

Figure 2–3

Frequency Polygon for Example 2–5

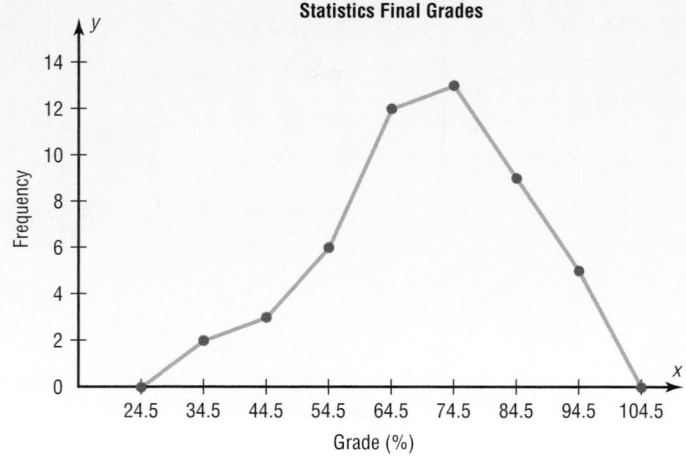

The frequency polygon and the histogram are two different ways to represent the same data set. The choice of which one to use is left to the discretion of the researcher.

The Ogive

The third type of graph that can be used represents the cumulative frequencies for the classes. This type of graph is called the *cumulative frequency graph* or *ogive*. The **cumulative frequency** is the sum of the frequencies accumulated up to the upper boundary of a class in the distribution.

> The **ogive** is a graph that represents the cumulative frequencies for the classes in a frequency distribution.

Example 2–6 shows the procedure for constructing an ogive.

| Example 2–6 | **Statistics Final Grades** |

Construct an ogive for the frequency distribution described in Example 2–4.

Solution

Step 1 Find the cumulative frequency for each class.

Class boundaries	Cumulative frequency
29.5–39.5	2
39.5–49.5	5
49.5–59.5	11
59.5–69.5	23
69.5–79.5	36
79.5–89.5	45
89.5–99.5	50

Step 2 Draw the x and y axes. Label the x axis with the class boundaries, beginning with the lower class boundary of the first class and ending with the upper class boundary of the last class. Use an appropriate scale for the y axis for the cumulative frequency column.

Step 3 Plot the cumulative frequencies at each upper class boundary as the cumulative frequency represents the number of data values below each upper class boundary.

Step 4 Starting with the first upper class boundary, 39.5, connect the adjacent points with line segments. Extend the graph to the first lower class boundary, 29.5, on the x axis. Refer to Figure 2–4.

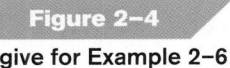

Figure 2–4

Ogive for Example 2–6

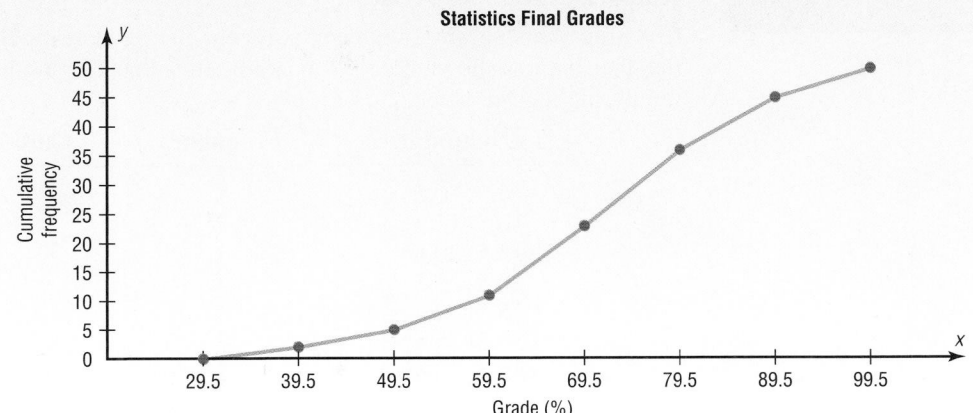

Cumulative frequency graphs are used to visually represent how many values are below a certain upper class boundary. For example, to find out how many grades are less then 79.5, locate 79.5 on the x axis, draw a vertical line up until it intersects the graph, and then draw a horizontal line at that point to the y axis. The y axis value is 36. Therefore, 36 grades are less than 79.5.

The steps for drawing these three types of graphs are shown in the following Procedure Table.

Unusual Stat

Thirty-seven percent of Canadian teens report talking to friends on their cellphones while in school.

Procedure Table

Constructing Statistical Graphs

Step 1 Draw and label the x and y axes.

Step 2 Choose a suitable scale for the frequencies or cumulative frequencies, and label it on the y axis.

Step 3 Represent the class boundaries for the histogram or ogive, or the midpoint for the frequency polygon, on the x axis.

Step 4 Plot the points and then draw the bars or lines.

Relative Frequency Graphs

The histogram, the frequency polygon, and the ogive shown previously were constructed by using frequencies in terms of the raw data. These distributions can be converted to distributions using *proportions* instead of raw data as frequencies. These types of graphs are called **relative frequency graphs.**

Graphs of relative frequencies instead of frequencies are used when the proportion of data values that fall into a given class is more important than the actual number of data values that fall into that class. For example, if one wanted to compare the age distribution of adults in Toronto, Ontario, with adults in Niagara Falls, Ontario, one would use relative frequency distributions. The reason is that since the population of the City of Toronto is 2,480,000 whereas the City of Niagara Falls (not including tourists) is 78,815, the bars using the actual data values for Toronto would be much taller than those for the same classes for Niagara Falls.

To convert a frequency into a proportion or relative frequency, divide the frequency for each class by the total of the frequencies. The sum of the relative frequencies will always be 1. These graphs are similar to the ones that use raw data as frequencies, but the values on the y axis are in terms of proportions. Example 2–7 shows the three types of relative frequency graphs.

Example 2–7

Kilometres Run per Week

Construct a histogram, frequency polygon, and ogive using relative frequencies for the distribution (shown here) of the kilometres that 20 randomly selected runners ran during a given week.

Class boundaries	Frequency	Cumulative frequency
5.5–10.5	1	1
10.5–15.5	2	3
15.5–20.5	3	6
20.5–25.5	5	11
25.5–30.5	4	15
30.5–35.5	3	18
35.5–40.5	2	20
	20	

Solution

Step 1 Convert each frequency to a proportion or relative frequency by dividing the frequency for each class by the total number of observations.

For class 5.5–10.5, the relative frequency is $\frac{1}{20} = 0.05$; for class 10.5–15.5, the relative frequency is $\frac{2}{20} = 0.10$; for class 15.5–20.5, the relative frequency is $\frac{3}{20} = 0.15$; and so on.

Place these values in the column labelled Relative frequency.

Step 2 Find the cumulative relative frequencies. To do this, add the frequency in each class to the total frequency of the preceding class. In this case, $0 + 0.05 = 0.05, 0.05 + 0.10 = 0.15, 0.15 + 0.15 = 0.30, 0.30 + 0.25 = 0.55$, etc. Place these values in the column labelled Cumulative relative frequency.

Using the same procedure, find the relative frequencies for the Cumulative frequency column. The relative frequencies are shown here.

Class boundaries	Midpoints	Relative frequency	Cumulative relative frequency
5.5–10.5	8	0.05	0.05
10.5–15.5	13	0.10	0.15
15.5–20.5	18	0.15	0.30
20.5–25.5	23	0.25	0.55
25.5–30.5	28	0.20	0.75
30.5–35.5	33	0.15	0.90
35.5–40.5	38	0.10	1.00
		$\overline{1.00}$	

Step 3 Draw each graph as shown in Figure 2–5. For the histogram and ogive, use the class boundaries along the x axis. For the frequency polygon, use the midpoints on the x axis. The scale on the y axis uses proportions.

Figure 2–5

Graphs for Example 2–7

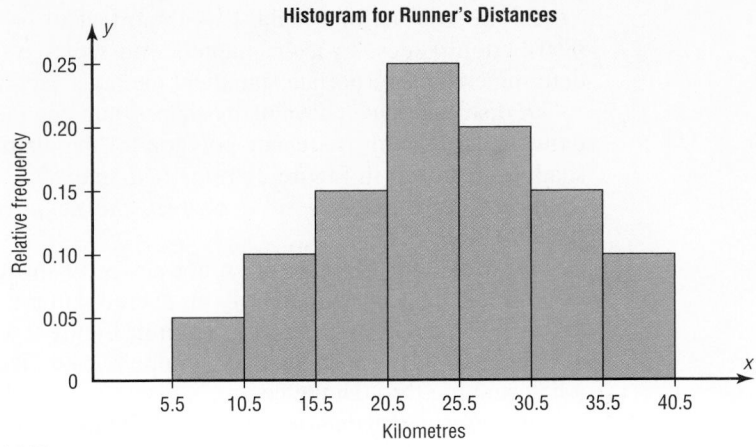

(a) Histogram

(Continued)

Figure 2–5

(Continued)

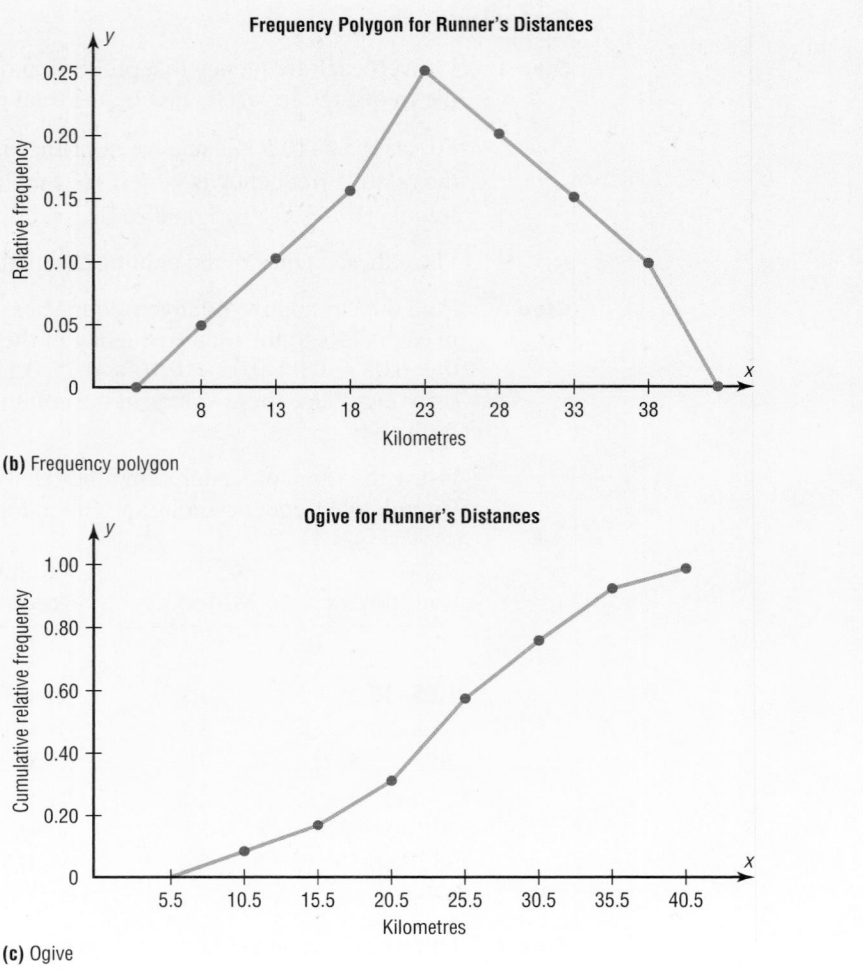

(b) Frequency polygon

(c) Ogive

Distribution Shapes

When one is describing data, it is important to be able to recognize the shapes of the distribution values. In later chapters you will see that the shape of a distribution also determines the appropriate statistical methods used to analyze the data.

A distribution can have many shapes, and one method of analyzing a distribution is to draw a histogram or frequency polygon for the distribution. Several of the most common shapes are shown in Figure 2–6: *the bell-shaped or mound-shaped, the uniform-shaped, the positively or right-skewed shaped, the negatively or left-skewed shaped, and the bimodal-shaped.*

Distributions are most often not perfectly shaped, so it is not necessary to have an exact shape but rather to identify an overall pattern.

A *bell-shaped distribution* shown in Figure 2–6(a) has a single peak and tapers off at either end. It is approximately symmetric; i.e., it is roughly the same on both sides of a line running through the centre.

A *uniform distribution* is basically flat or rectangular. See Figure 2–6(b).

When the peak of a distribution is to the left and the data values taper off to the right, a distribution is said to be *positively or right-skewed*. See Figure 2–6(c). When the data values

Figure 2–6

Distribution Shapes

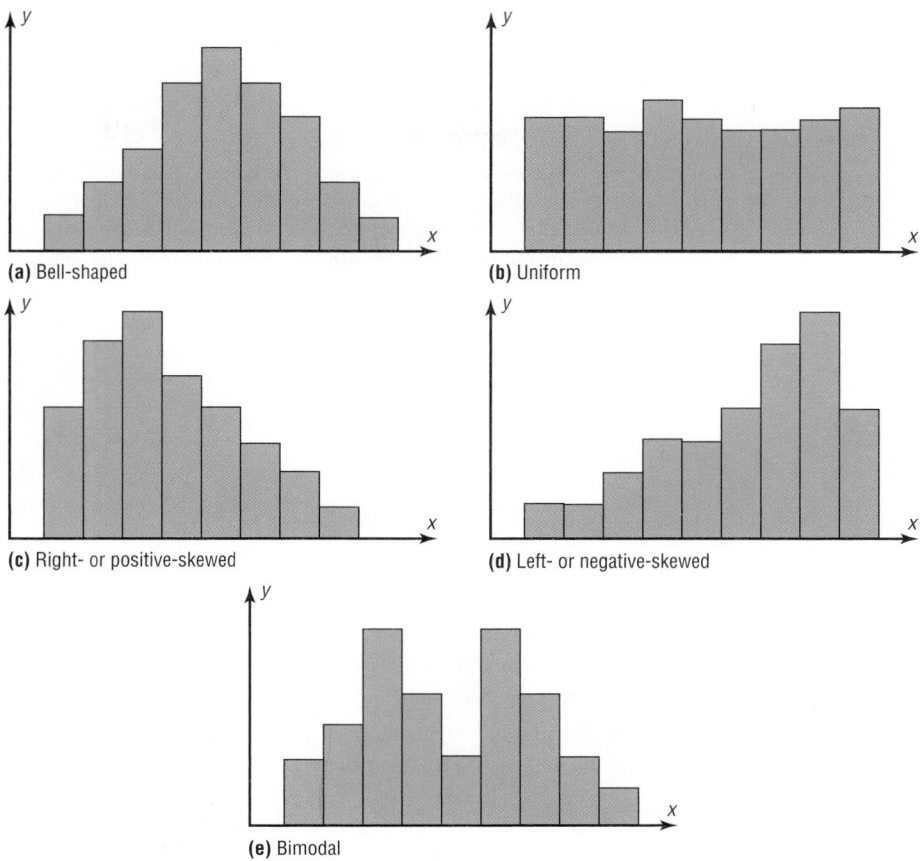

(a) Bell-shaped

(b) Uniform

(c) Right- or positive-skewed

(d) Left- or negative-skewed

(e) Bimodal

are clustered to the right and taper off to the left, a distribution is said to be *negatively or left-skewed*. See Figure 2–6(d). Skewness will be explained in detail in Chapter 3, pages 93–94. Distributions with one peak, such as those shown in Figure 2–6(a), (c), and (d), are said to be *unimodal*. (The highest peak of a distribution indicates where the mode of the data values is. The mode is the data value that occurs more often than any other data value. Modes are explained in Chapter 3.) When a distribution has two peaks of the same height, it is said to be *bimodal*. See Figure 2–6(e).

Distributions can have other shapes in addition to the ones shown here; however, these are some of the more common ones that you will encounter in analyzing data.

When you are analyzing histograms and frequency polygons, look at the shape of the curve. For example, does it have one peak or two peaks? Is it relatively flat, or is it bimodal? Are the data values spread out on the graph, or are they clustered around the centre? Are there data values in the extreme ends? These may be *outliers*. (See Section 3–3 for an explanation of outliers.) Are there any gaps in the histogram, or does the frequency polygon touch the *x* axis somewhere other than the ends? Finally, are the data clustered at one end or the other, indicating a *skewed distribution*?

For example, the histogram for the statistics final grades shown in Figure 2–2 shows a single peaked distribution, with the class 69.5–79.5 containing the largest number of grades. The distribution has no gaps, and there are fewer grades in the lowest class than in the highest class.

2-2   Applying the Concepts

Selling Real Estate

Assume you are a realtor in St. John's, Newfoundland and Labrador. You have recently obtained a listing of the selling prices of the homes that have sold in that area in the last six months. You wish to organize that data so you will be able to provide potential buyers with useful information. Use the following data to create a histogram, frequency polygon, and cumulative frequency polygon.

142,000	127,000	99,600	162,000	89,000	93,000	99,500
73,800	135,000	119,500	67,900	156,300	104,500	108,650
123,000	91,000	205,000	110,000	156,300	104,000	133,900
179,000	112,000	147,000	321,550	87,900	88,400	180,000
159,400	205,300	144,400	163,000	96,000	81,000	131,000
114,000	119,600	93,000	123,000	187,000	96,000	80,000
231,000	189,500	177,600	83,400	77,000	132,300	166,000

1. What questions could be answered more easily by looking at the histogram rather than the listing of home prices?

2. What different questions could be answered more easily by looking at the frequency polygon rather than the listing of home prices?

3. What different questions could be answered more easily by looking at the cumulative frequency polygon rather than the listing of home prices?

4. Are there any extremely large or extremely small data values compared to the other data values?

5. Which graph displays these extremes the best?

6. Is the distribution skewed?

See page 79 for the answers.

Exercises 2-2

1. **Student Summer Development Needs** For 108 randomly selected college applicants, the following frequency distribution for entrance exam scores was obtained. Construct a histogram, frequency polygon, and ogive for the data. (The data for this exercise will be used for Exercise 13 in this section.)

Class limits	Frequency
90–98	6
99–107	22
108–116	43
117–125	28
126–134	9

Applicants who score above 107 need not enroll in a summer developmental program. In this group, how many students do not have to enroll in the developmental program?

2. **Employee Years of Service** For 75 employees of a large department store, the following distribution for years of service was obtained. Construct a histogram, frequency polygon, and ogive for the data. (The data for this exercise will be used for Exercise 14 in this section.)

Class limits	Frequency
1–5	21
6–10	25
11–15	15
16–20	0
21–25	8
26–30	6

A majority of the employees have worked fewer than how many years?

3. **PGA Tournament Scores** Calgarian Stephen Ames won The Players Championship in 2006. This victory earned the Canadian golfer US$1.44 million or C$1,682,928. The final results represent player scores after four completed rounds of golf and are shown as a frequency distribution.

Class limits	Frequency
280–283	5
284–287	13
288–291	16
292–295	20
296–299	13
300–303	4
304–307	2

Source: www.pgatour.com.

Construct a histogram, frequency polygon, and ogive for the distribution. Comment on the skewness of the distribution.

4. **NFL Player Salaries** The salaries (in millions of dollars) for 31 NFL teams for a specific season are given in this frequency distribution.

Class limits	Frequency
39.9–42.8	2
42.9–45.8	2
45.9–48.8	5
48.9–51.8	5
51.9–54.8	12
54.9–57.8	5

Source: NFL.com.

Construct a histogram, frequency polygon, and ogive for the data; and comment on the shape of the distribution.

5. **Prime Ministers' Terms of Office** Federal elections in Canada are not held at fixed dates, so prime ministers serve for terms of variable lengths. The following distribution illustrates the number of months served by prime ministers since Confederation. Construct a histogram, frequency polygon, and ogive for the data Comment on the distribution's shape.

Term (months)	Class boundaries	Frequency
1–24	0.5–24.5	9
25–48	24.5–48.5	3
49–72	48.5–72.5	7
73–96	72.5–96.5	1
97–120	96.5–120.5	2
121–144	120.5–144.5	2
145–168	144.5–168.5	2
169–192	168.5–192.5	1

Source: Parliament of Canada.

6. **Masters Golf Scores** Construct a histogram, frequency polygon, and ogive for the data in Exercise 14 in Section 2–1, and analyze the results.

7. **Air Quality Index** The Air Quality Index (AQI) is measured by ground-level ozone (O_3), where a high AQI reading is bad for your health. The following data represent a random selection of AQI daily readings for Canada's mining capital, Sudbury, Ontario, in 2009. Use the data to construct a grouped frequency distribution with 7 classes, a histogram, a frequency polygon, and an ogive. (The distribution in this exercise will be used for Exercise 17 in this section.)

13	11	17	27	31	24
19	16	18	32	25	23
21	18	8	35	28	14
11	28	22	49	33	19
20	18	24	42	20	17
13	25	25	15	16	18

8. **Dog Reaction Times** In a study of reaction times of dogs to a specific stimulus, an animal trainer obtained the following data, given in seconds. Construct a histogram, frequency polygon, and ogive for the data, and analyze the results. (The histogram in this exercise will be used for Exercise 18 in this section, Exercise 16 in Section 3–1, and Exercise 26 in Section 3–2.)

Class limits	Frequency
2.3–2.9	10
3.0–3.6	12
3.7–4.3	6
4.4–5.0	8
5.1–5.7	4
5.8–6.4	2

9. **Exchange Rates** Construct a histogram, frequency polygon, and ogive for the data in Exercise 15 in Section 2–1, and analyze the results.

10. **Driver and Passenger Fatalities** The following data show the percentage of drivers and passenger fatalities in Canada by age group. Draw histograms for each category using age groups as x axis labels. Decide if there is any difference in age group fatalities.

Age group	Drivers	Passengers
0–4	0	1.4
5–14	0.2	7.7
15–19	8.8	19.0
20–24	14.6	15.5
25–34	17.5	12.0
35–44	17.0	9.5
45–54	14.9	9.6
55–64	11.1	7.7
65+	15.4	16.6

Source: Transport Canada.

11. **Area of National Parks** Construct a histogram, frequency polygon, and ogive for the data in Exercise 16 in Section 2–1, and analyze the results.

12. **Home Run Record Breakers** For the data in Exercise 18 in Section 2–1, construct a histogram for the home run distances for each player and compare them. Are they basically the same, or are there any noticeable differences? Explain your answer.

13. **Student Summer Development Needs** For the data in Exercise 1 in this section, construct a histogram, frequency polygon, and ogive, using relative frequencies. What proportion of the applicants need to enroll in the summer developmental program?

14. **Employee Years of Service** For the data in Exercise 2 in this section, construct a histogram, frequency polygon, and ogive, using relative frequencies. What proportion of the employees have been with the store for more than 20 years?

15. **Cereal Calories** The number of calories per serving for selected ready-to-eat cereals is listed here. Construct

a frequency distribution using 7 classes. Draw a histogram, frequency polygon, and ogive for the data, using relative frequencies. Describe the shape of the histogram.

130	190	140	80	100	120	220	220	110	100
210	130	100	90	210	120	200	120	180	120
190	210	120	200	130	180	260	270	100	160
190	240	80	120	90	190	200	210	190	180
115	210	110	225	190	130				

Source: The Doctor's Pocket Calorie, Fat, and Carbohydrate Counter.

16. Protein Grams in Fast Food The amount of protein (in grams) for a variety of fast-food sandwiches is reported here. Construct a frequency distribution using 6 classes. Draw a histogram, frequency polygon, and ogive for the data, using relative frequencies. Describe the shape of the histogram.

23	30	20	27	44	26	35	20	29	29
25	15	18	27	19	22	12	26	34	15
27	35	26	43	35	14	24	12	23	31
40	35	38	57	22	42	24	21	27	33

Source: The Doctor's Pocket Calorie, Fat, and Carbohydrate Counter.

17. Air Quality Index For the 2009 Sudbury AQI data in Exercise 7 in this section, construct a relative frequency histogram and relative frequency polygon.

18. Dog Reaction Times The animal trainer in Exercise 8 in this section selected another group of dogs that were much older than the first group and measured their reaction times to the same stimulus. Construct a histogram, frequency polygon, and ogive for the data.

Class limits	Frequency
2.3–2.9	1
3.0–3.6	3
3.7–4.3	4
4.4–5.0	16
5.1–5.7	14
5.8–6.4	4

Analyze the results and compare the histogram for this group with the one obtained in Exercise 8 in this section. Are there any differences in the histograms? (The data in this exercise will be used for Exercise 16 in Section 3–1 and Exercise 26 in Section 3–2.)

Extending the Concepts »

19. Using the histogram shown here, do the following.

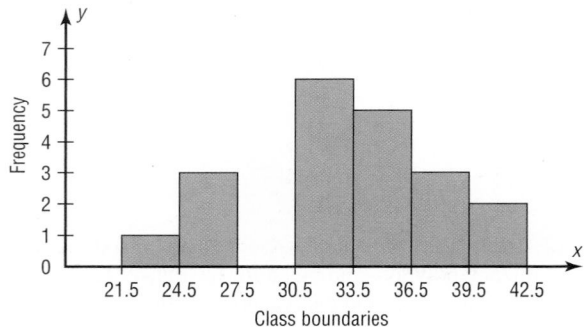

Class boundaries

a. Construct a frequency distribution; include class limits, class frequencies, midpoints, and cumulative frequencies.

b. Construct a frequency polygon.

c. Construct an ogive.

20. Using the results from Exercise 19, answer these questions.

a. How many values are in the class 27.5–30.5?

b. How many values fall between 24.5 and 36.5?

c. How many values are below 33.5?

d. How many values are above 30.5?

2–3 | Other Types of Graphs ›

Analyze data by constructing Pareto charts, time series graphs, pie graphs, and stem and leaf plots.

In addition to the histogram, the frequency polygon, and the ogive, several other types of graphs are often used in statistics. They are the Pareto chart, the time series graph, and the pie graph. Figure 2–7 shows an example of each type of graph.

Pareto Charts

In Section 2–2, graphs such as the histogram, frequency polygon, and ogive showed how data can be represented when the variable displayed on the horizontal axis is quantitative, such as heights and weights.

On the other hand, when the variable displayed on the horizontal axis is qualitative or categorical data, a **bar chart** or **Pareto chart** can be used. The Pareto chart is simply a bar chart in which the plotted data are sorted in descending order (high to low frequencies). Bars on a Pareto chart can be displayed with or without a space between bars.

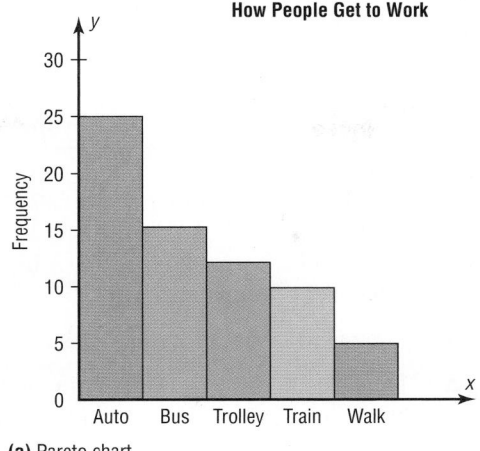

(a) Pareto chart

Figure 2–7

**Other Types of Graphs
Used in Statistics**

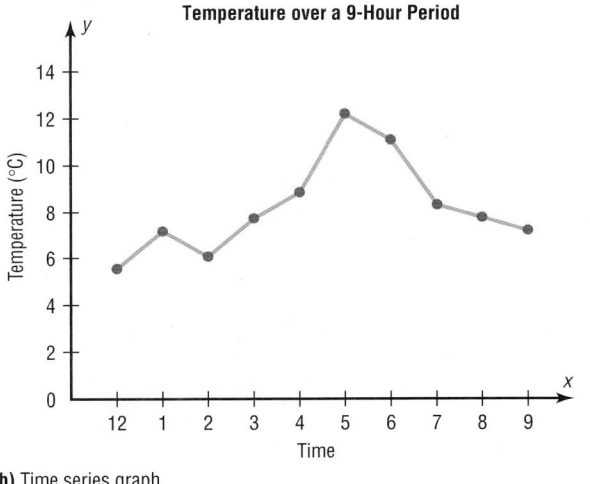

(b) Time series graph

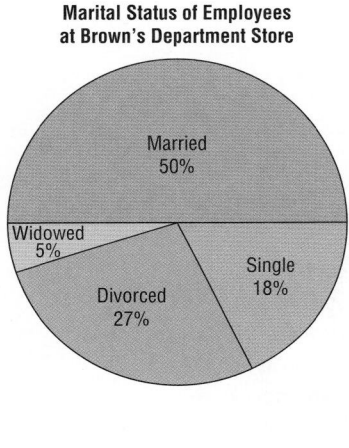

(c) Pie graph

A **Pareto chart** is used to represent a frequency distribution for a categorical variable, and the frequencies are displayed by the heights of vertical bars, which are arranged in order from highest to lowest.

Example 2–8

How Young Smokers Obtain Cigarettes

The table shown represents the usual source from which student smokers, Grades 5 to 9, obtain their cigarettes. Construct and analyze a Pareto chart for the data.

Source	Number
Take from family	9
Friend gives	30
Family gives	14
Buy from friends/other	25
Store	22

Source: Youth Smoking Survey, Technical Report, Health Canada, 2002. Adapted and reproduced with the permission of the Minister of Public Works and Government Services Canada, 2007.

Solution

Step 1 Arrange the data from the largest to the smallest according to frequency.

Source	Number
Friend gives	30
Buy from friends/other	25
Store	22
Family gives	14
Take from family	9

Step 2 Draw and label the *x* and *y* axes.

Step 3 Draw the bars corresponding to the frequencies. See Figure 2–8. The Pareto chart shows that the usual source from which student smokers, Grades 5 to 9, obtain cigarettes is from friends. This source is more than triple the source of taking cigarettes from family.

Figure 2–8

Pareto Chart for Example 2–8

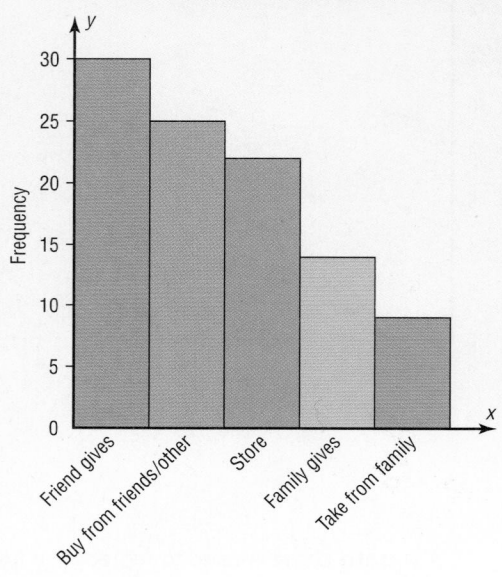

Usual Source of Cigarettes for Smokers (Grades 5 to 9)

Source: Health Canada.

Historical Note

Vilfredo Pareto (1848–1923) was an Italian scholar who developed theories in economics, statistics, and the social sciences. His contributions to statistics include the development of a mathematical function used in economics. This function has many statistical applications and is called the *Pareto distribution*. In addition, he researched income distribution, and his findings became known as Pareto's law.

Suggestions for Drawing Pareto Charts

1. Make the bars the same width.
2. Arrange the data from largest to smallest according to frequency.
3. Make the units that are used for the frequency equal in size.

When you analyze a Pareto chart, make comparisons by looking at the heights of the bars.

The Time Series Graph

When data are collected over a period of time, they can be represented by a time series graph.

A **time series graph** represents data that occur over a specific period of time.

Example 2–9 shows the procedure for constructing a time series graph.

Example 2–9

Rapid Population Growth

Fuelled by high oil prices and Alberta's booming economy, Calgary's population is rising sharply. The following data (in thousands) illustrate Calgary's rapid growth. Construct and analyze a time series graph for the data.

Year	Population
1980	560.6
1985	625.1
1990	692.9
1995	749.1
2000	860.7
2005	956.1
2010	1065.5

Source: CMHC and City of Calgary.

Historical Note

Time series graphs are over 1000 years old. The first ones were used to chart the movements of the planets and the sun.

Solution

Step 1   Draw and label the *x* and *y* axes.

Step 2   Label the *x* axis for years and the *y* axis for the number of vehicles.

Step 3   Plot each point according to the table.

Step 4   Draw line segments connecting adjacent points. Do not try to fit a smooth curve through the data points. See Figure 2–9. The graph shows a steady increase over the 30-year period.

Figure 2–9

Time Series Graph for Example 2–9

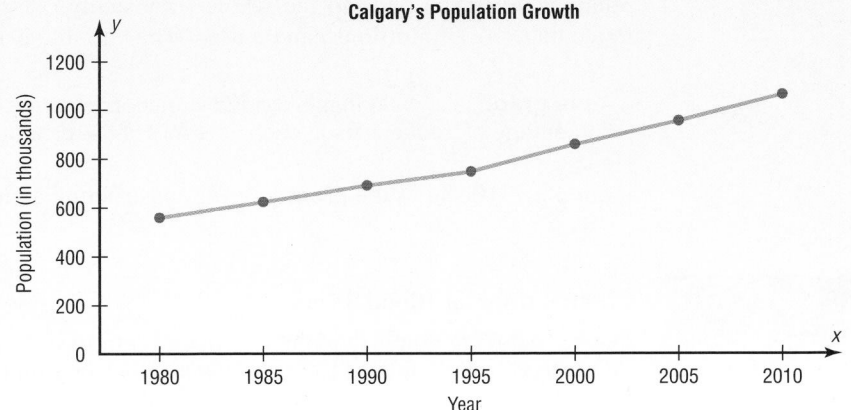

When you analyze a time series graph, look for a trend or pattern that occurs over the time period. For example, is the line ascending (indicating an increase over time) or descending (indicating a decrease over time)? Another thing to look for is the slope, or steepness, of the line. A line that is steep over a specific time period indicates a rapid increase or decrease over that period.

Two data sets can be compared on the same graph (called a *compound time series graph*) if two lines are used, as shown in Figure 2–10. This graph shows the population trend for India and China over a 100-year period.

Figure 2–10

Two Time Series Graphs for Comparison

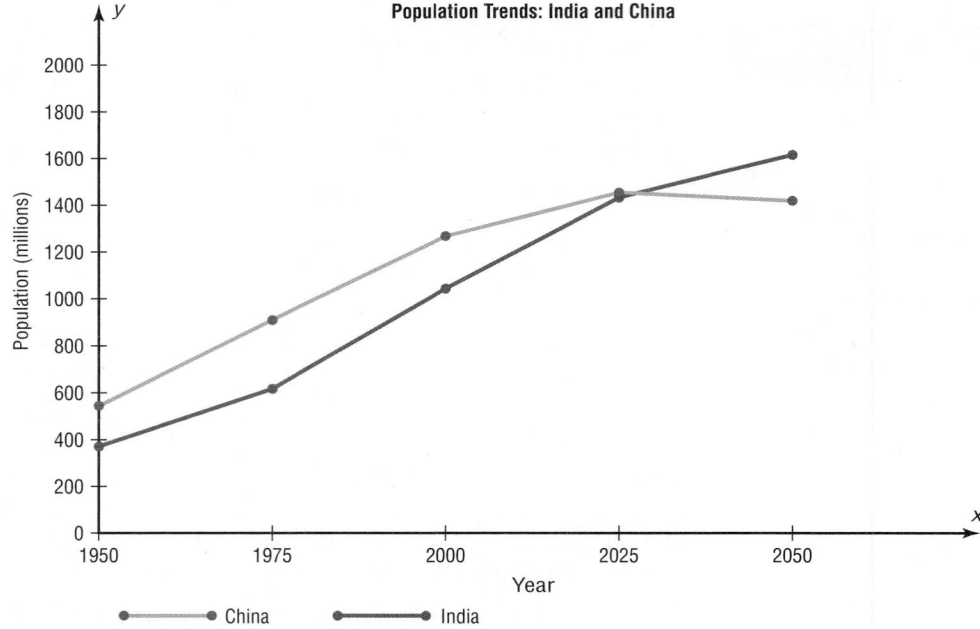

Source: United Nations Department of Economic and Social Affairs, Population Division.

The Pie Graph

Pie graphs are used extensively in statistics. The purpose of the pie graph is to show the relationship of the parts to the whole by visually comparing the sizes of the sections. Percentages or proportions can be used. The variable is nominal or categorical.

A **pie graph** is a circle that is divided into sections or wedges according to the percentage of frequencies in each category of the distribution.

Example 2–10 shows the procedure for constructing a pie graph.

Example 2–10

Distribution of Blood Types

Construct a pie graph showing the blood types of the armed forces recruits described in Example 2–1. The frequency distribution is repeated here.

Class	Frequency	Percent
A	5	20
B	7	28
O	9	36
AB	4	16
	25	100

Solution

Step 1   Find the number of degrees for each class, using the formula

$$\text{Degree} = \frac{f}{n} \cdot 360°$$

For each class, then, the following results are obtained.

A $\frac{5}{25} \cdot 360° = 72°$

B $\frac{7}{25} \cdot 360° = 100.8°$

O $\frac{9}{25} \cdot 360° = 129.6°$

AB $\frac{4}{25} \cdot 360° = 57.6°$

Step 2   Find the percentages. (This was already done in Example 2–1.)

Step 3   Using a protractor, graph each section and write its name and corresponding percentage, as shown in Figure 2–11.

Figure 2–11

Pie Graph for
Example 2–10

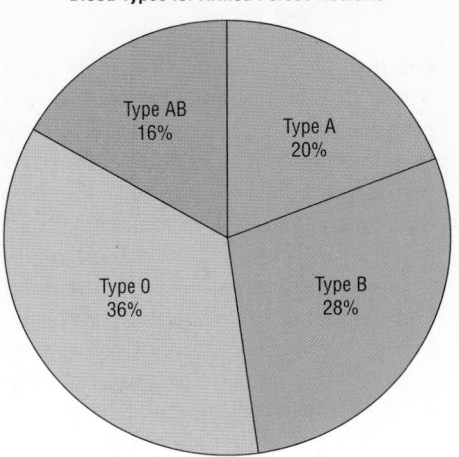

Blood Types for Armed Forces Recruits

To analyze the nature of the data shown in the pie graph, compare the sections. For example, are any sections relatively large compared to the rest?

Figure 2–11 shows that among the recruits, type O blood is more prevalent than any other type. People who have type AB blood are in the minority. More than twice as many people have type O blood as type AB.

Speaking of Statistics

Cellphone Subscriber Growth

Canada's wireless mobile (cell) phone industry experienced annualized subscriber growth rate of 35% from 1985 to 2010. By 2015, the number of subscribers is projected to reach 30.7 million, or about one cellphone for every Canadian 15 years of age and over.

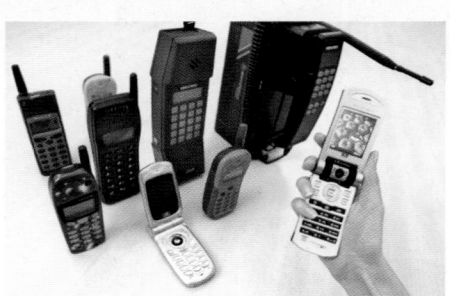

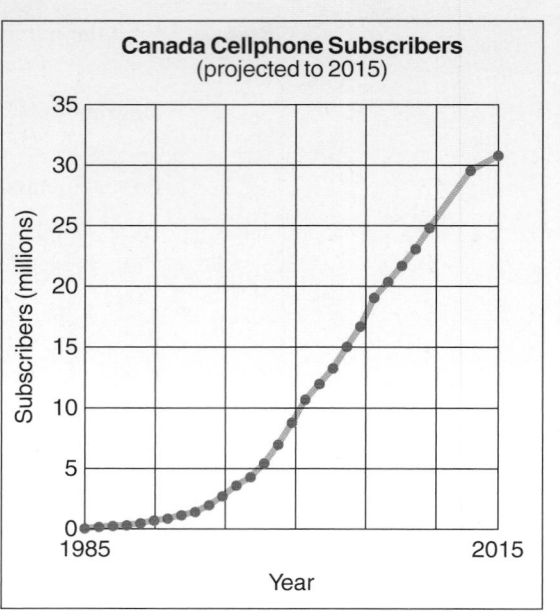

Canada Cellphone Subscribers
(projected to 2015)

Sources: 1985–2005: NationalMaster.com, *Media Statistics,* "Mobile Phone Subscribers: Canada (historical data)"; 2006–2007: Canadian Radio-television and Telecommunications Commission, *International Perspective,* "How Canada Compares Internationally," modified August 5, 2009; 2008: Point-Topic, *Operator Source,* "Canada Broadband Overview," June 17, 2009; 2009: Canadian Wireless Communications Association, *Canada's Wireless Industry: A Global Success Story Continues*; 2010: ReportLinker, *Canada—Telecoms, Wireless, Broadband and Forecasts,* June 2009; 2013: IE Market Research Corp, *3Q09 Canada Mobile Operator Forecast, 2009–2013: Total Wireless Subscribers in Canada to Reach 29.5 Million in 2013 with Telus Mobility Taking Market Share Away from Bell Mobility over the Next Five Years,* August 2009; 2015: Digital Home Canada: *Canadian Wireless Subs Predicted to Top 30 Million by 2015,* Hugh Thompson, February 9, 2010.

Misleading Graphs

Graphs give a visual representation that enables readers to analyze and interpret data more easily than they could simply by looking at numbers. However, inappropriately drawn graphs can misrepresent the data and lead the reader to false conclusions. For example, a car manufacturer's ad stated that 98% of the vehicles it had sold in the past ten years were still on the road. The ad then showed a graph similar to the one in Figure 2–12. The graph shows the percentage of the manufacturer's automobiles still on the road and the percentage of its competitors' automobiles still on the road. Is there a large difference? Not necessarily.

Notice the scale on the vertical axis in Figure 2–12. It has been cut off (or truncated) and starts at 95%. When the graph is redrawn using a scale that goes from 0 to 100%, as in Figure 2–13, there is hardly a noticeable difference in the percentages. Thus, changing the units at the starting point on the *y* axis can convey a very different visual representation of the data.

It is not wrong to truncate an axis of the graph; many times it is necessary to do so. However, the reader should be aware of this fact and interpret the graph accordingly. Do not be misled if an inappropriate impression is given.

Let us consider another example. In 2007, Canada's Environment minister released medium-term greenhouse gas (GHG) emissions-reduction targets measured in megatonnes carbon dioxide equivalent (Mt CO_2eq). The GHG emissions-reduction target data are shown in the following table.

Year	2010	2011	2012	2015	2020
Target reductions (Mt CO_2eq))	49	54	58	72	88

Source: Climate Action Network Canada: The Pembina Institute, *Analysis of the Government of Canada's April 2007 Greenhouse Gas Policy Announcement,* Matthew Bramley.

Graph of Automaker's Claim Using a Scale from 95 to 100%

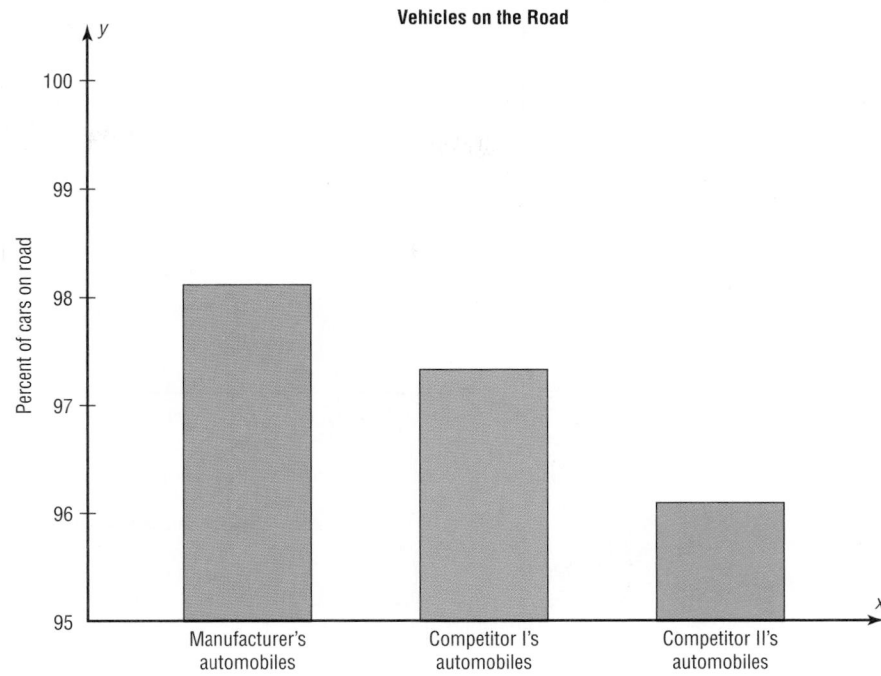

Graph in Figure 2–12 Redrawn Using a Scale from 0 to 100%

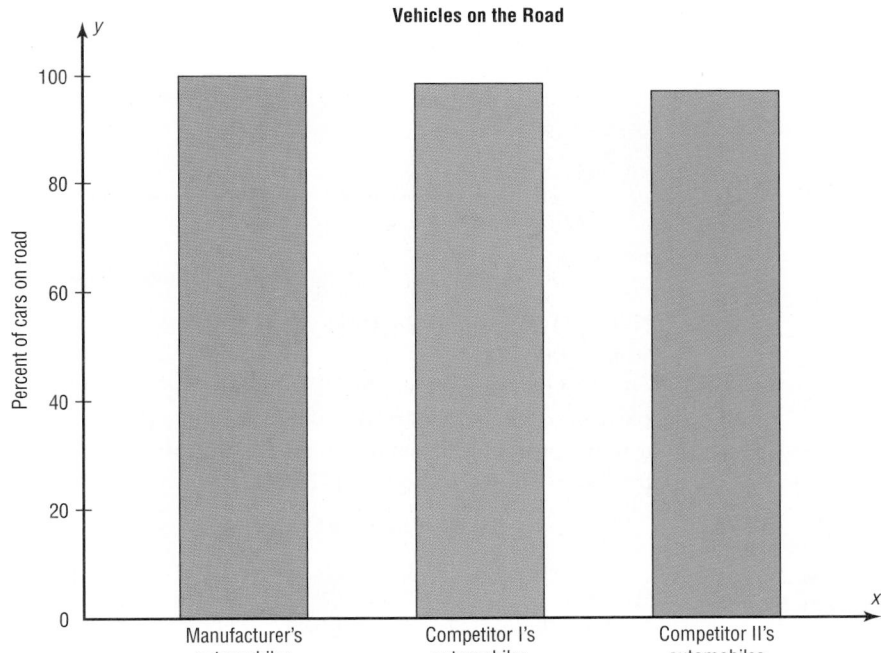

Interesting Fact

The most popular flavour of ice cream is vanilla, and about one-third of the ice cream sold is vanilla.

When Figure 2–14(a) is examined, the GHG emissions-reduction targets appear to be extreme and short-termed. This effect is achieved by narrowing the scale (40 to 90) and evenly spacing the years, even though the dates are inconsistent.

In Figure 2–14(b), the units begin at a zero starting point and the scaling of the dates is fixed. These corrections offer a more realistic representation of the data, making the GHG emission-reduction targets appear more attainable.

Another misleading graphing technique sometimes used involves exaggerating a one-dimensional increase by showing it in two dimensions. For example, the average

Figure 2–14

**Misrepresenting Data
by Changing the Scale:
(a) Incorrect Scale,
(b) Correct Scale**

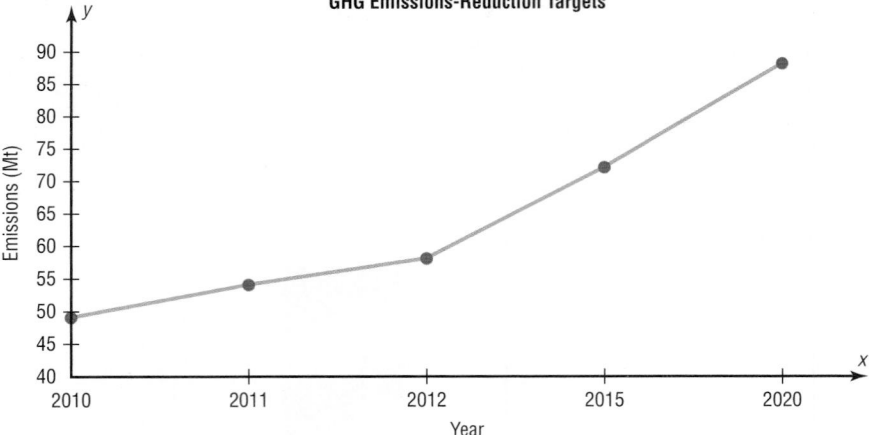

(a) Graph Misrepresenting GHG Emissions-Reduction Targets

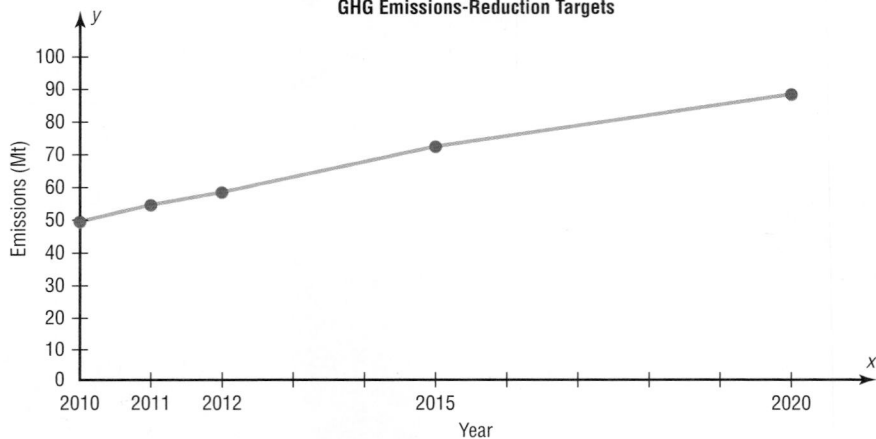

(b) Graph Correctly Illustrating GHG Emissions-Reduction Targets

NHL player's salary in 1990 was $271,000, whereas the estimated average 2010 salary was $2,000,000.[1]

The increase shown by the graph in Figure 2–15(a) represents the change by a comparison of the heights of the two bars in one dimension. The same data visually illustrate a more pronounced salary change when utilizing two-dimensional shapes (i.e., hockey pucks) as shown in Figure 2–15(b).

Figure 2–15

**Time Comparison of
NHL Average Salaries**

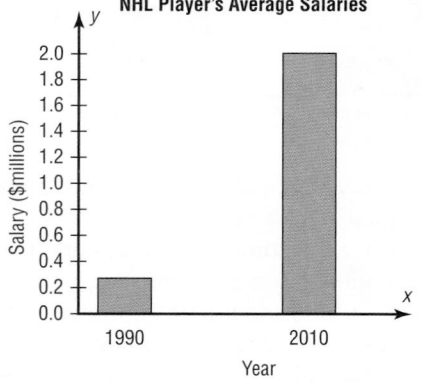

(a) One-dimensional column chart

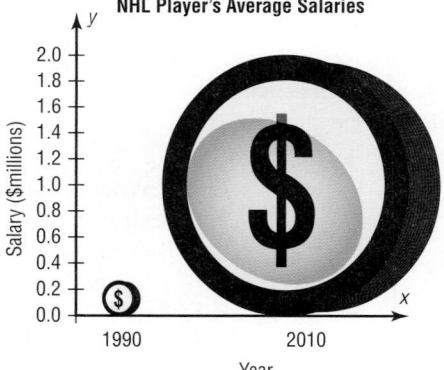

(b) Two-dimensional chart using shapes

[1]*Source:* www.proicehockey.about.com.

Note that it is not wrong to use the graphing techniques of truncating the scales or representing data by two-dimensional pictures. But when these techniques are used, the reader should be cautious of the conclusion drawn on the basis of the graphs.

Another way to misrepresent data on a graph is by omitting labels or units on the axes of the graph. The graph shown in Figure 2–16 compares the cost of living, economic growth, population growth, and crime rate of four main geographic areas in the United States. However, since there are no numbers on the *y* axis, very little information can be gained from this graph, except a crude ranking of each factor. There is no way to decide the actual magnitude of the differences.

Figure 2–16

A Graph with No Units on the *y* Axis

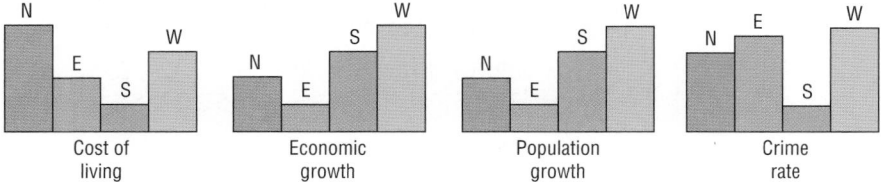

Finally, all graphs should contain a source for the information presented. The inclusion of a source for the data will enable you to check the reliability of the organization presenting the data. A summary of the types of graphs and their uses is shown in Figure 2–17.

Figure 2–17

Summary of Graphs and Uses of Each

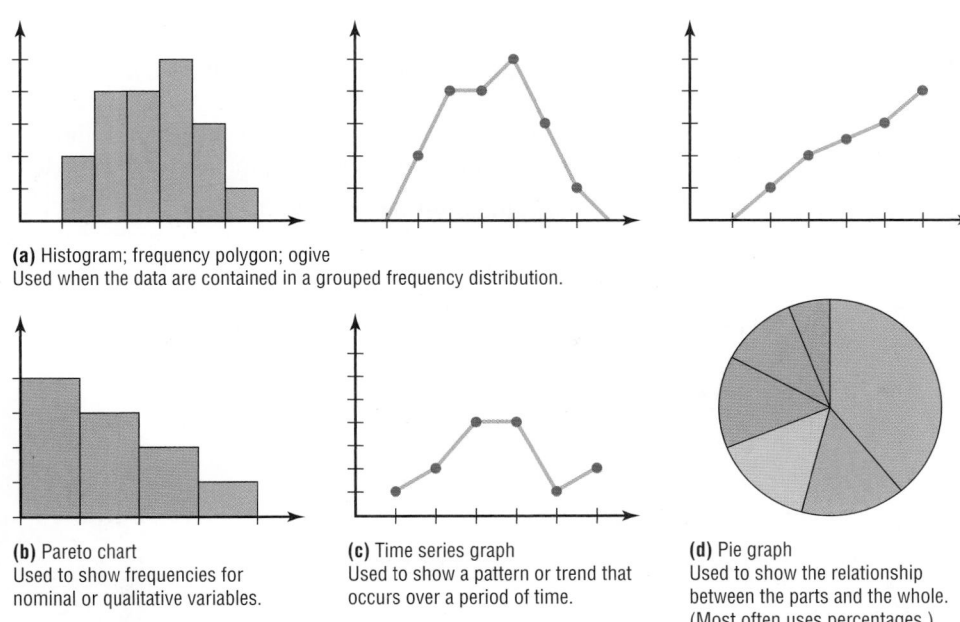

(a) Histogram; frequency polygon; ogive
Used when the data are contained in a grouped frequency distribution.

(b) Pareto chart
Used to show frequencies for nominal or qualitative variables.

(c) Time series graph
Used to show a pattern or trend that occurs over a period of time.

(d) Pie graph
Used to show the relationship between the parts and the whole. (Most often uses percentages.)

Stem and Leaf Plots

The stem and leaf plot is a method of organizing data and is a combination of sorting and graphing. It has the advantage over a grouped frequency distribution of retaining the actual data while showing them in graphical form.

A **stem and leaf plot** is a data plot that uses the stem as the leading part of the data value with the leaf as the remaining part of the data value to form groups or classes.

Example 2–11 shows the procedure for constructing a stem and leaf plot.

Example 2–11

Outpatient Cardiograms

At an outpatient testing centre, the number of cardiograms performed each day for 20 days is shown. Construct a stem and leaf plot for the data.

25	31	20	32	13
14	43	02	57	23
36	32	33	32	44
32	52	44	51	45

Solution

Step 1   Arrange the data in order:

02, 13, 14, 20, 23, 25, 31, 32, 32, 32,
32, 33, 36, 43, 44, 44, 45, 51, 52, 57

Note: Arranging the data in order is not essential and can be cumbersome when the data set is large; however, it is helpful in constructing a stem and leaf plot. The leaves in the final stem and leaf plot should be arranged in order.

Step 2   Separate the data according to the first digit, as shown.

02   13, 14   20, 23, 25   31, 32, 32, 32, 32, 33, 36
43, 44, 44, 45   51, 52, 57

Figure 2–18

Stem and Leaf Plot for Example 2–11

```
0 | 2
1 | 3 4
2 | 0 3 5
3 | 1 2 2 2 2 3 6
4 | 3 4 4 5
5 | 1 2 7
```

Step 3   A display can be made by using the leading digit as the *stem* and the trailing digit as the *leaf*. For example, for the value 32, the leading digit, 3, is the stem and the trailing digit, 2, is the leaf. For the value 14, the 1 is the stem and the 4 is the leaf. Now a plot can be constructed as shown in Figure 2–18.

Leading digit (stem)	Trailing digit (leaf)
0	2
1	3 4
2	0 3 5
3	1 2 2 2 2 3 6
4	3 4 4 5
5	1 2 7

Speaking of Statistics

How much money is held at the Bank of Canada as unclaimed balances?

At the end of December 2008, approximately 1,023,000 unclaimed balances, worth some $351 million, were on the Bank of Canada's books. Over 93.5% of these were under $1000, representing 31.7% of the total value outstanding. The oldest balance dates back to 1900.

Source: Bank of Canada, *Services,* "Unclaimed Balances."

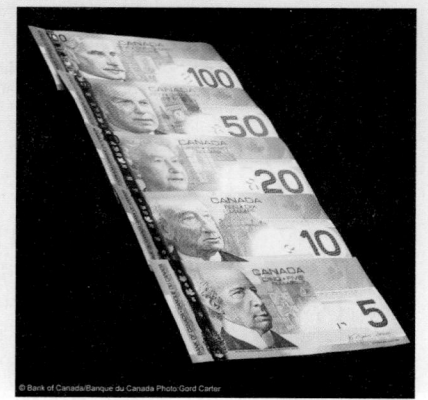

Figure 2–18 shows that the distribution peaks in the centre and that there are no gaps in the data. For 7 of the 20 days, the number of patients receiving cardiograms was between 31 and 36. The plot also shows that the testing centre treated from a minimum of 2 patients to a maximum of 57 patients in any one day.

If there are no data values in a class, you should write the stem number and leave the leaf row blank. Do not put a zero in the leaf row.

Example 2–12	**Car Thefts** 🖱

An insurance company researcher conducted a survey on the number of car thefts in a large city for a period of 30 days last summer. The raw data are shown. Construct a stem and leaf plot by using classes 50–54, 55–59, 60–64, 65–69, 70–74, and 75–79.

52	62	51	50	69
58	77	66	53	57
75	56	55	67	73
79	59	68	65	72
57	51	63	69	75
65	53	78	66	55

Solution

Step 1   Arrange the data in order.

50, 51, 51, 52, 53, 53, 55, 55, 56, 57, 57, 58, 59, 62, 63, 65, 65, 66, 66, 67, 68, 69, 69, 72, 73, 75, 75, 77, 78, 79

Step 2   Separate the data according to the classes.

50, 51, 51, 52, 53, 53   55, 55, 56, 57, 57, 58, 59
62, 63   65, 65, 66, 66, 67, 68, 69, 69   72, 73
75, 75, 77, 78, 79

Step 3   Plot the data as shown here.

Leading digit (stem)	Trailing digit (leaf)
5	0 1 1 2 3 3
5	5 5 6 7 7 8 9
6	2 3
6	5 5 6 6 7 8 9 9
7	2 3
7	5 5 7 8 9

The graph for this plot is shown in Figure 2–19.

Figure 2–19

Stem and Leaf Plot for Example 2–12

5	0 1 1 2 3 3
5	5 5 6 7 7 8 9
6	2 3
6	5 5 6 6 7 8 9 9
7	2 3
7	5 5 7 8 9

When the data values are in the hundreds, such as 325, the stem is 32 and the leaf is 5. For example, the stem and leaf plot for the data values 325, 327, 330, 332, 335, 341, 345, and 347 looks like this.

32	5 7
33	0 2 5
34	1 5 7

Interesting Fact

The average number of pencils and index cards David Letterman tosses over his shoulder during one show is four.

When you analyze a stem and leaf plot, look for peaks and gaps in the distribution. See if the distribution is symmetric or skewed. Check the variability of the data by looking at the spread.

Related distributions can be compared by using a back-to-back stem and leaf plot. The back-to-back stem and leaf plot uses the same digits for the stems of both distributions, but the digits that are used for the leaves are arranged in order out from the stems on both sides. Example 2–13 shows a back-to-back stem and leaf plot.

Example 2–13	**Comparison of Skyscraper Storeys**

The number of storeys in two selected samples of skyscrapers in North America and Asia are shown. Construct a back-to-back stem and leaf plot, and compare the distributions.

North America			Asia		
108	72	65	105	78	70
102	72	64	101	75	69
100	72	64	88	75	69
83	71	64	88	73	68
77	70	64	88	73	68
76	69	62	88	73	68
75	68	61	85	72	66
75	67	60	85	72	66
74	66	60	80	70	66
73	66	60	80	70	66

Source: www.emporis.com.

Solution

Step 1 Arrange the data for both data sets in order.

Step 2 Construct a stem and leaf plot using the same digits as stems. Place the digits for the leaves for North America on the left side of the stem and the digits for the leaves for Asia on the right side, as shown. See Figure 2–20.

Figure 2–20
Back-to-Back Stem and Leaf Plot for Example 2–13

North America		Asia
9 8 7 6 6 5 4 4 4 4 2 1 0 0 0	**6**	6 6 6 6 8 8 8 8 9
7 6 5 5 4 3 2 2 2 1 0	**7**	0 0 2 2 3 3 3 5 5 8
3	**8**	0 0 5 5 8 8 8 8
	9	
8 2 0	**10**	1 5

Step 3 Compare the distributions. Both the buildings in North America and Asia have a large variation in the number of storeys per building. The North American buildings are congested in the 60- to 79-storey class, whereas the Asian buildings are more evenly distributed in the 60- to 89-storey class.

Stem and leaf plots are part of the techniques called *exploratory data analysis,* discussed in Section 3–4. This section also introduces *boxplots,* a chart type that requires understanding of the data description techniques presented in Chapter 3.

Another graph, *scatter plots,* is explained in Section 10–1. This type of chart illustrates trends derived from paired data sets or two variable data (*x, y*). Applications and procedures utilizing scatter plots are explained in detail in Chapter 10.

Sections 2–2 and 2–3 demonstrated the most commonly used statistical chart types but variations of these graphs may be used to represent, explore, and interpret data sets. Depending on the field of study, a researcher may employ dotplots, cluster charts, candlestick charts, hi-lo-close charts, radar charts, area charts, and pictograms, to list but a few. A Web search will find and give details of these and many other chart types.

2–3 Applying the Concepts

Trends in Cancer Deaths

The following graph shows mortality rates for selected cancer sites for Canadian females from 1977 to 2006. The rates are per 100,000 females. Answer the following questions about the graph.

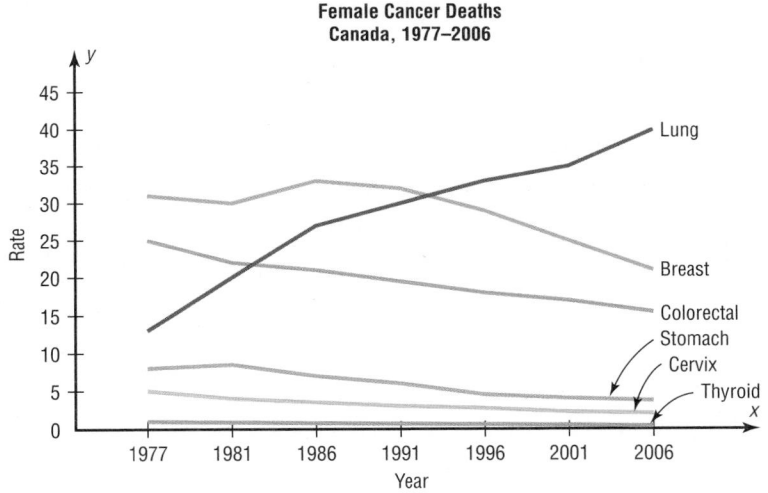

Source: Canadian Cancer Statistics, 2006.

1. What are the variables in the graph?
2. Are the variables qualitative or quantitative?
3. Are the variables discrete or continuous?
4. What type of graph was used to display the data?
5. Could a Pareto chart be used to display the data?
6. Could a pie chart be used to display the data?
7. List some typical uses for the Pareto chart.
8. List some typical uses for the time series chart.

See page 79 for the answers.

Exercises 2–3

1. **Criminal Offences** Police in Canada reported the following nonviolent criminal offences (excluding non-Criminal Code traffic violations). Construct a Pareto chart. Based on the Pareto chart, where should police activity and public education be focused?

Type of violation	Number
Violent offences	441,782
Nonviolent offences	1,752,923
Criminal Code traffic violations	143,169
Federal statute (drug) offences	101,965
Federal statute (other) offences	33,248

Source: Statistics Canada, *The Daily,* "Police-Reported Crime Statistics," Table 2, July 21, 2009.

2. **Homicide Rates** Construct a Pareto chart illustrating the overall homicide rate (per 100,000 population) reported for the following Canadian cities in 2005. Rates are based on incidents reported to the police in each of Canada's census metropolitan areas (CMA).

City	Homicide rate
Vancouver	2.9
Winnipeg	3.7
Edmonton	4.3
Montreal	1.3
Calgary	2.4
Ottawa	1.3
Hamilton	1.6
Toronto	2.0
Quebec City	0.7

Source: Statistics Canada, *The Daily,* July 20, 2006.

3. **Internet Connections** The following data represent the estimated number (in millions) of computers connected to the Internet worldwide. Construct a Pareto chart for the data. Based on the data, suggest the best place to market appropriate Internet products.

Location	Number of computers
Homes	240
Small companies	102
Large companies	148
Government agencies	33
Schools	47

Source: IDC.

4. **Roller Coaster Census** The *Roller Coaster Census Report* lists the following number of roller coasters on each continent. Represent the data graphically, using a Pareto chart.

Africa	17
Asia	315
Australia	22
Europe	413
North America	643
South America	45

Source: Roller Coaster DataBase: www.rcdb.com.

5. **World Energy Use** The following percentages indicate the source of energy used worldwide. Construct a Pareto chart for the energy used.

Petroleum	39.8%
Coal	23.2
Dry natural gas	22.4
Hydroelectric	7.0
Nuclear	6.4
Other (wind, solar, etc.)	1.2

Source: N.Y. Times Almanac.

6. **Airport Passenger Volume** Canada's busiest airport is Toronto's Lester B. Pearson International Airport. The following data represent total domestic and international passenger volume (in millions) from 2000 to 2008. Construct a time series chart for the data. Give a possible reason for less airport traffic for the two years following 2001.

Year	2000	2001	2002	2003	2004
Total	28.9	28.0	25.9	24.7	28.6

Year	2005	2006	2007	2008
Total	29.9	30.8	31.4	32.3

Source: Greater Toronto Airport Authority, *GTAA Corporate, Statistics,* "Passenger Traffic."

7. **Global Warming** The data represent average global temperature for each decade since the beginning of the 20th century. Plot a time series graph. Interpret the trend.

Year	1900s	1910s	1920s	1930s	1940s	1950s
Temperature (°C)	13.6	13.7	13.7	13.9	13.9	13.9

Year	1960s	1970s	1980s	1990s	2000s
Temperature (°C)	13.9	13.9	14.1	14.2	14.4

Sources: World Almanac; 2000s data estimate: *BBC News,* "This Decade Warmest on Record," December 8, 2009, Richard Black.

8. **University Graduate Trends** The following data (in thousands) represent trends in Canadian university graduates, by gender. Construct a time series plot for both female and male graduates on the same chart. Compare the results.

Year	1993	1995	1997	1999	2001	2003	2005	2007
Female	98.5	102.0	100.9	101.4	105.2	118.9	129.0	146.7
Male	75.4	76.0	73.0	72.2	72.9	80.3	86.8	94.8

Source: Statistics Canada, *Trends in University Graduation, 1992 to 2007,* and *Description for Chart 1, Number of university graduates, by sex, Canada, 1992 to 2007,* Catalogue no. 81-004-X.

9. Voter Apathy The percentage of eligible voters who turned out for Canada's federal elections from 1972–2008 is shown below. Construct a time series graph and analyze the results.

Election year	Voter turnout (%)
1972	76.7
1974	71.0
1980	69.3
1984	75.3
1988	75.3
1993	69.9
1997	67.0
2000	61.3
2004	60.9
2006	64.7
2008	59.8

Source: Elections Canada.

10. How Do You Spend Your Day? Statistics Canada's *General Social Survey* published the following results on a typical day for 15- to 24-year-olds. Construct a pie chart for the data.

Activity	Hours
Paid work and commuting	3.1
Household work and shopping	1.4
Civic and voluntary activities	0.2
Education, including studying	2.6
Sleep, meals, and personal time	10.7
Socializing, including eating out	2.4
Television, reading, and relaxing	1.9
Sports, movies, and entertainment	0.2
Active leisure and sports	1.5

Source: Statistics Canada, *General Social Survey 2005, Table 2.*

11. Mortality by Cancer Type Each year, the Canadian Cancer Society publishes estimates of cancer-related deaths. The following table indicates deaths by type of cancer for 2009. Construct a pie chart for the data.

Lung	20,500
Colorectal	9,100
Breast	5,400
Prostate	4,400
Pancreas	3,900
All other cancers	32,000

Source: Canadian Cancer Society.

12. Components of the Earth's Crust The following elements comprise the earth's crust, the outermost solid layer. Illustrate the composition of the earth's crust with a pie graph.

Oxygen	45.6%
Silicon	27.3
Aluminum	8.4
Iron	6.2
Calcium	4.7
Other	7.8

Source: The New York Times Almanac.

13. Workers Switch Jobs In a recent survey, 3 in 10 people indicated that they are likely to leave their jobs when the economy improves. Of those surveyed, 34% indicated that they would make a career change, 29% want a new job in the same industry, 21% are going to start a business, and 16% are going to retire. Make a pie chart and a Pareto chart for the data. Which chart do you think better represents the data?
Source: National Survey Institute.

14. State which graph (Pareto chart, time series graph, or pie graph) would most appropriately represent the given situation.

  a. The number of students enrolled at a local college for each year during the last five years.

  b. The budget for the student activities department at a certain college for each year during the last five years.

  c. The means of transportation the students use to get to school.

  d. The percentage of votes each of the four candidates received in the last election.

  e. The record temperatures of a city for the last 30 years.

  f. The frequency of each type of crime committed in a city during the year.

15. Prime Ministers' Ages The age at the swearing-in ceremony of each Canadian prime minister is shown. Construct a stem and leaf plot and analyze the data.

52	74	60	39	65
51	54	66	55	46
70	57	61	45	
47	46	66	46	
69	47	48	59	

Source: www.canadainfolink.ca.

16. Calories in Salad Dressings A listing of calories per 28 grams of selected salad dressings (not fat-free) is given below. Construct a stem and leaf plot for the data.

100	130	130	130	110	110	120	130	140	100
140	170	160	130	160	120	150	100	145	145
145	115	120	100	120	160	140	120	180	100
160	120	140	150	190	150	180	160		

17. Plant Growth The growth (in centimetres) of two varieties of plants after 20 days is shown in this table. Construct a back-to-back stem and leaf plot for the data, and compare the distributions.

Variety 1				Variety 2			
20	12	39	38	18	45	62	59
41	43	51	52	53	25	13	57
59	55	53	59	42	55	56	38
50	58	35	38	41	36	50	62
23	32	43	53	45	55		

18. NHL Conferences Team Scoring The data shown indicate the number of goals scored by teams in the Eastern and Western Conferences of the National Hockey League for the 2008–2009 season. Construct a back-to-back stem and leaf plot comparing the two conferences.

Eastern Conference			Western Conference		
274	239	217	257	233	234
272	210	250	295	226	230
244	249	257	246	245	208
264	234	210	264	219	207
264	250	201	254	213	199

Source: National Hockey League, *Standings.*

19. Music Sales by Genre The North American music industry's 2007 market share by genre is shown in the table below. Create an appropriate graph to represent the data.

Genre	%
Alternative	14.4
Christian/gospel	5.5
Classical	2.9
Country	10.2
Jazz	2.3
Latin	5.2
Metal	8.6
New Age	0.5
R&B	15.5
Rap	6.8
Rock	24.2
Soundtrack	3.9

Source: Nielsen SoundScan.

Extending the Concepts »

20. Recording Artists The Canadian Recording Industry Association awarded gold album status (50,000 units sold), platinum status (100,000 units), or diamond (1,000,000 units) to Canadian artists as shown. Construct a compound time series graph for the data. Comment on the state of Canada's music industry.

	1999	2000	2001	2002	2003	2004	2005
Gold	27	29	24	35	27	40	38
Platinum	41	29	24	35	14	35	26
Diamond	3	2	1	1	1	1	0

Source: Canadian Heritage, *The Music Market,* "Music Sales."

21. Meat Production Meat production for veal and lamb for the years 1960–2000 is shown here. (Data are in millions of pounds.) Construct a compound time series graph for the data. What comparison can be made regarding meat production?

Year	1960	1970	1980	1990	2000
Veal	1109	588	400	327	225
Lamb	769	551	318	358	234

Source: The World Almanac and Book of Facts.

22. Top 10 Airlines The top ten airlines based on fleet size are listed. Represent these data with an appropriate graph.

United–Continental	708	China Southern	354
Delta	690	US Airways	339
FedEx Express	619	Lufthansa	334
American	619	SkyWest	294
Southwest	544	Air China	265

Source: ITP Business Publishing Ltd., *Arabian Supply Chain.com,* "Top 10: Largest Airline Fleets," David Ingham, November 3, 2010.

23. Nobel Prizes in Physiology or Medicine The top prize-winning countries for Nobel Prizes in Physiology or Medicine are listed here. Represent the data with an appropriate graph.

United States	80	Denmark	5
United Kingdom	24	Austria	4
Germany	16	Belgium	4
Sweden	8	Italy	3
France	7	Australia	3
Switzerland	6		

Source: Top 10 of Everything.

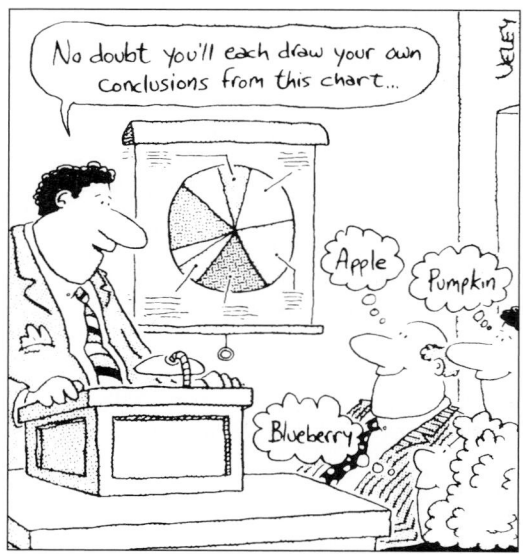

Source: Cartoon by Bradford Veley, Marquette, Michigan. Used with permission.

24. Cost of Milk The graph shows the increase in the price of a litre of milk. Why might the increase appear to be larger than it really is?

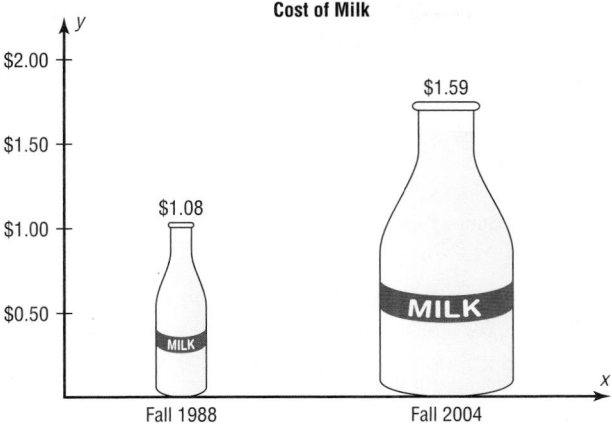

25. Boom in Number of Births The graph shows the projected boom (in millions) in the number of births. Cite several reasons why the graph might be misleading.

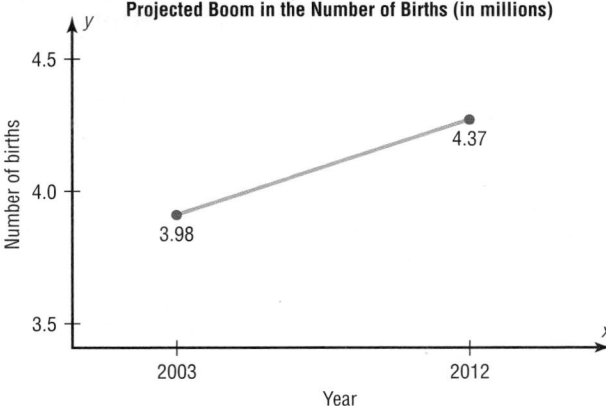

Summary >

When data are collected, they are called *raw data*. Since very little knowledge can be obtained from raw data, they must be organized in some meaningful way. A frequency distribution using classes is the solution. Once a frequency distribution is constructed, the representation of the data by graphs is a simple task. The most commonly used graphs in research statistics are the histogram, frequency polygon, and ogive. Other graphs, such as the Pareto chart, time series graph, and pie graph, can also be used. Some of these graphs are seen frequently in newspapers, magazines, and various statistical reports.

Finally, a stem and leaf plot uses part of the data values as stems and part of the data values as leaves. This graph has the advantages of a frequency distribution and a histogram.

For step-by-step guidance on the use of Texas Instruments TI-83 Plus/TI-84 Plus programmable calculators, see Appendix E at the back of this book. For summary procedures for Minitab, SPSS, and Excel, please see the full version of Appendix E on *Connect*.

Important Terms »

bar chart 45, 54

categorical frequency distribution 33

class 33

class boundaries 35

class midpoint 36

class width 35

cumulative frequency 47

frequency 33

frequency distribution 33

frequency polygon 46

grouped frequency distribution 35

histogram 45

lower class limit 35

ogive 47

open-ended distribution 37

outliers 38

Pareto chart 54

pie graph 58

raw data 33

relative frequency graph 48

stem and leaf plot 63

time series graph 57

ungrouped frequency distribution 39

upper class limit 35

Important Formulas »

Formula for the percentage of values in each class:

$$\% = \frac{f}{n} \cdot 100$$

where

f = **frequency of the class**

n = **total number of values**

Formula for the range:

R = **highest value − lowest value**

Formula for the class width:

Class width = upper boundary − lower boundary

Formula for the class midpoint:

$$X_m = \frac{\text{lower boundary + upper boundary}}{2}$$

or

$$X_m = \frac{\text{lower limit + upper limit}}{2}$$

Formula for the degrees for each section of a pie graph:

$$\text{Degrees} = \frac{f}{n} \cdot 360°$$

McGraw Hill **connect**™ Practise and learn online with *Connect* with data sets and algorithmic questions related to concepts covered in this chapter. Questions and tables with online data sets are marked with ✈.

Review Exercises »

1. **How People Get Their News** The Brunswick Research Organization surveyed 50 randomly selected individuals and asked them the primary way they received the daily news. Their choices were via newspaper (N), television (T), radio (R), or Internet (I). Construct a categorical frequency distribution for the data and interpret the results. The data in this exercise will be used for Exercise 2 in this section.

N	N	T	T	T	I	R	R	I	T
I	N	R	R	I	N	N	I	T	N
I	R	T	T	T	T	N	R	R	I
R	R	I	N	T	R	T	I	I	T
T	I	N	T	T	I	R	N	R	T

2. Construct a pie graph for the data in Exercise 1, and analyze the results.

3. **Ball Sales** A sporting goods store kept a record of sales of five items for one randomly selected hour during a recent sale. Construct a frequency distribution for the data (B = baseballs, G = golf balls, T = tennis balls, S = soccer balls, F = footballs). (The data for this exercise will be used for Exercise 4 in this section.)

F	B	B	B	G	T	F
G	G	F	S	G	T	
F	T	T	T	S	T	
F	S	S	G	S	B	

4. Draw a pie graph for the data in Exercise 3 showing the sales of each item, and analyze the results.

5. **BUN Count** The blood urea nitrogen (BUN) count of 20 randomly selected patients is given here in milligrams per decilitre (mg/dL). Construct an ungrouped frequency distribution for the data. (The data for this exercise will be used for Exercise 6.)

17	18	13	14
12	17	11	20
13	18	19	17
14	16	17	12
16	15	19	22

6. Construct a histogram, frequency polygon, and ogive for the data in Exercise 5 in this section, and analyze the results.

7. **Road Maintenance and Vehicle Costs** The data show the estimated added cost per vehicle use due to bad roads. Construct a frequency distribution using 6 classes. (The data for this exercise will be used for Exercises 8 and 11 in this section.)

165	186	122	172	140	153	208	169
156	114	113	135	131	125	177	136
136	127	112	188	171	179	152	155
116	90	187	136	159	97	141	85
91	170	111	147	165	163	159	150

Source: Federal Highway Administration.

8. Construct a histogram, frequency polygon, and ogive for the data in Exercise 7 in this section, and analyze the results.

9. **NFL Franchise Values** The data shown (in millions of dollars) are the values of the 30 National Football League franchises. Construct a frequency distribution for the data using 8 classes. (The data for this exercise will be used for Exercises 10 and 12 in this section.)

170	191	171	235	173	187	181	191
200	218	243	200	182	320	184	239
186	199	186	210	209	240	204	193
211	186	197	204	188	242		

Source: Pittsburgh Post-Gazette.

10. Construct a histogram, frequency polygon, and ogive for the data in Exercise 9 in this section, and analyze the results.

11. Construct a histogram, frequency polygon, and ogive by using relative frequencies for the data in Exercise 7 in this section.

12. Construct a histogram, frequency polygon, and ogive by using relative frequencies for the data in Exercise 9 in this section.

13. **City Homicides** Construct a Pareto chart for the number of homicides reported for the following cities.

City	Number of homicides
Winnipeg	34
Edmonton	34
Vancouver	56
Calgary	20
Toronto	94
Montreal	63

Source: Statistics Canada.

14. **Bankruptcy Debt Source** The Office of the Superintendent of Bankruptcy Canada reports the primary sources of debt for Canadians, 55 years and older, as follows. Construct a Pareto chart.

Debt source	Total
Credit cards	71,220
Mortgages	289,033
Bank loans	49,077
Finance companies	40,181
Individuals	30,165

Source: Office of the Superintendent of Bankruptcy Canada, *Resources for Academics,* "Growing Old Gracefully: An Investigation into the Growing Number of Bankrupt Canadians over Age 55."

15. **Minimum Wage** The given data represent the federal minimum hourly wage in the years shown. Draw a time series graph to represent the data and analyze the results.

Year	Wage
1960	$1.00
1965	1.25
1970	1.60
1975	2.10
1980	3.10
1985	3.35
1990	3.80
1995	4.25
2000	5.15
2005	5.15

Source: The World Almanac and Book of Facts.

16. **World Oil Prices** The following data represent average annual world oil prices, adjusted for inflation, over a ten-year period. Construct a time series chart for the data. Analyze the results.

Year	Price per barrel (US$)
1999	$21.39
2000	$34.29
2001	$28.03
2002	$27.33
2003	$32.47
2004	$42.97
2005	$55.21
2006	$62.36
2007	$66.66
2008	$91.35
2009	$43.56

Source: InflationData.com, *Historical Oil Prices*, "Historical Crude Oil Prices (Table)."

17. **Consumer Bankruptcies** The data show the number of consumer bankruptcies in Ontario and Quebec from 2003 to 2009. Illustrate a compound time series graph (i.e., two sets of data on the same chart) and compare the results.

Year	Quebec	Ontario
2003	26,341	38,531
2004	26,840	39,341
2005	27,351	40,687
2006	28,997	39,936
2007	32,457	46,454
2008	36,987	53,294
2009	44,114	69,494

18. **Women at Work** In a study of 100 women, the numbers shown here indicate the major reason why each woman surveyed worked outside the home. Construct a pie graph for the data and analyze the results.

Reason	Number of women
To support self/family	62
For extra money	18
For something different to do	12
Other	8

19. **Career Changes** A survey asked if people would like to spend the rest of their careers with their present employers. The results are shown. Construct a pie graph for the data and analyze the results.

Answer	Number of people
Yes	660
No	260
Undecided	80

20. **Museum Visitors** The number of visitors to the Railroad Museum during 24 randomly selected hours is shown here. Construct a stem and leaf plot for the data.

67	62	38	73	34	43	72	35
53	55	58	63	47	42	51	62
32	29	47	62	29	38	36	41

21. **Employee Work Hours** The data set shown here represents the number of hours that 25 part-time employees worked at the Sea Side Amusement Park during a randomly selected week in June. Construct a stem and leaf plot for the data and summarize the results.

16	25	18	39	25	17	29	14	37
22	18	12	23	32	35	24	26	
20	19	25	26	38	38	33	29	

22. **Job Aptitude Test** A special aptitude test is given to job applicants. The data shown here represent the scores of 30 applicants. Construct a stem and leaf plot for the data and summarize the results.

204	210	227	218	254
256	238	242	253	227
251	243	233	251	241
237	247	211	222	231
218	212	217	227	209
260	230	228	242	200

Data Analysis ≫

The databanks for these questions can be found in Appendix D at the back of the text and are also available on ▓ **connect**.

1. From the databank, choose one of the following variables: age, weight, cholesterol level, systolic pressure, IQ, or sodium level. Select at least 30 values. For these values, construct a grouped frequency distribution. Draw a histogram, frequency polygon, and ogive for the distribution. Describe briefly the shape of the distribution.

2. From the databank, choose one of the following variables: educational level, smoking status, or exercise. Select at least 20 values. Construct an ungrouped frequency distribution for the data. For the distribution, draw a Pareto chart and describe briefly the nature of the chart.

Statistics Today

Identity Theft, Identity Fraud, and You–Revisited

Data presented in numerical form do not convey an easy-to-interpret conclusion; however, when data are presented in graphical form, readers can see the visual impact of the numbers. In the case of identify fraud, the reader can see that the most common mechanism is through improper usage of the victim's credit card, whereas fewer criminals access the victim's personal account. Both the Pareto chart and pie chart clearly illustrate these points.

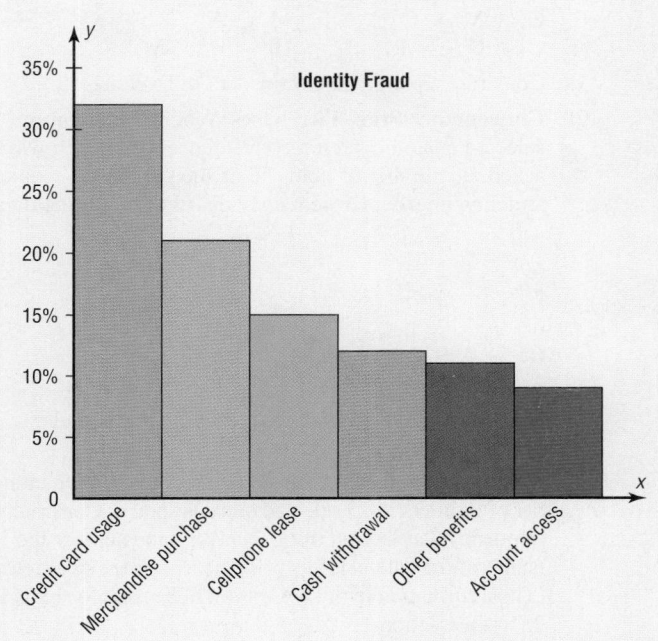

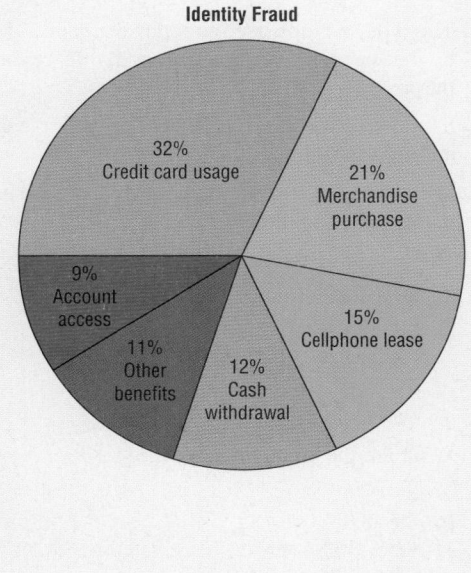

3. From the databank, select at least 30 subjects and construct a categorical distribution for their marital status. Draw a pie graph and describe briefly the findings.

4. Using the data from Data Set IV in Appendix D, construct a frequency distribution and draw a histogram. Describe briefly the shape of the distribution of the tallest buildings in Calgary.

5. Using the data from Data Set XI in Appendix D, construct a frequency distribution and draw a frequency polygon. Describe briefly the shape of the distribution for the number of pages in statistics books.

6. Using the data from Data Set XIV in Appendix D, divide Canada into three provincial regions, as follows:

East	NL NB NS PE
Central	QC ON
West	MB SK AB BC

Find the total population for each region, and draw a Pareto chart and a pie graph for the data. Analyze the results. Explain which chart might be a better representation of the data.

7. Using the data from Data Set I in Appendix D, make a stem and leaf plot for the record high temperatures in Canada. Describe the nature of the plot.

Chapter Quiz   »

Determine whether each statement is true or false. If the statement is false, explain why.

1. In the construction of a frequency distribution, it is a good idea to have overlapping class limits, such as 10–20, 20–30, 30–40.

2. Histograms can be drawn by using vertical or horizontal bars.

3. It is not important to keep the width of each class the same in a frequency distribution.

4. Frequency distributions can aid the researcher in drawing charts and graphs.

5. The type of graph used to represent data is determined by the type of data collected and by the researcher's purpose.

6. In construction of a frequency polygon, the class limits are used for the *x* axis.

7. Data collected over a period of time can be graphed by using a pie graph.

Select the best answer.

8. What is another name for the ogive?
   a. Histogram
   b. Frequency polygon
   c. Cumulative frequency graph
   d. Pareto chart

9. What are the boundaries for 8.6–8.8?
   a. 8–9
   b. 8.5–8.9
   c. 8.55–8.85
   d. 8.65–8.75

10. What graph should be used to show the relationship between the parts and the whole?
    a. Histogram
    b. Pie graph
    c. Pareto chart
    d. Ogive

11. Except for rounding errors, relative frequencies should add up to what sum?
    a. 0   *c.* 50
    b. 1   *d.* 100

Complete these statements with the best answers.

12. The three types of frequency distributions are _____, _____, and _____.

13. In a frequency distribution, the number of classes should be between _____ and _____.

14. Data such as blood types (A, B, AB, O) can be organized into a(n) _____ frequency distribution.

15. Data collected over a period of time can be graphed using a(n) _____ graph.

16. A statistical device used in exploratory data analysis that is a combination of a frequency distribution and a histogram is called a(n) _____.

17. On a Pareto chart, the frequencies should be represented on the _____ axis.

18. **Housing Arrangements** A questionnaire on housing arrangements showed this information obtained from 25 respondents. Construct a frequency distribution for the data (H = house, A = apartment, M = mobile home, C = condominium).

H	C	H	M	H	A	C	A	M
C	M	C	A	M	A	C	C	M
C	C	H	A	H	H	M		

19. Construct a pie graph for the data in Exercise 18.

20. **Convenience Store Purchases** When 30 randomly selected customers left a convenience store, each was asked the number of items he or she purchased. Construct an ungrouped frequency distribution for the data.

2	9	4	3	6
6	2	8	6	5
7	5	3	8	6
6	2	3	2	4
6	9	9	8	9
4	2	1	7	4

21. Construct a histogram, a frequency polygon, and an ogive for the data in Exercise 20.

22. **Murders in Selected Cities** For a recent year, the number of murders in 25 selected cities is shown. Construct a frequency distribution using 9 classes, and analyze the nature of the data in terms of shape, extreme values, etc. (The information in this exercise will be used for Exercise 23 in this section.

248	348	74	514	597
270	71	226	41	39
366	73	241	46	34
149	68	73	63	65
109	598	278	69	27

Source: Pittsburgh Tribune Review.

23. Construct a histogram, frequency polygon, and ogive for the data in Exercise 22. Analyze the histogram.

24. **Recycled Trash** Construct a Pareto chart for the number of tonnes (in millions) of trash recycled per year by Americans based on an Environmental Protection Agency study.

Type	Amount
Paper	320.0
Iron/steel	292.0
Aluminum	276.0
Yard waste	242.4
Glass	196.0
Plastics	41.6

Source: USA TODAY.

25. Internet Growth Worldwide Internet users, in millions, have grown significantly, as illustrated in the following table. Construct a time series chart for the data.

Year	1999	2000	2001	2002	2003
World users	279	393	494	680	790
Year	2004	2005	2006	2007	2008
World users	935	1048	1217	1402	1542

Source: Encyclopaedia Almanac 2010.

26. Museum Visitors The number of visitors to the Historic Museum for 25 randomly selected hours is shown. Construct a stem and leaf plot for the data.

15	53	48	19	38
86	63	98	79	38
62	89	67	39	26
28	35	54	88	76
31	47	53	41	68

Critical Thinking Challenges »

1. Greenhouse Tomatoes The chart shows Canada's greenhouse tomato production by leading province. Can you see anything misleading about the graph as drawn?

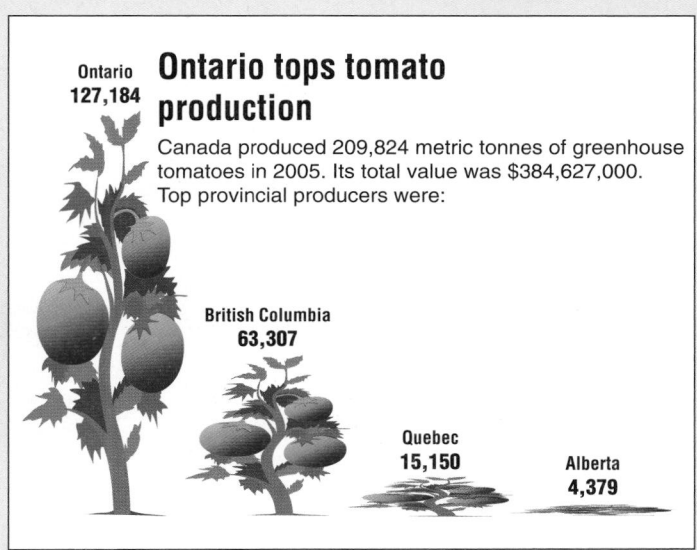

Ontario tops tomato production

Ontario 127,184

Canada produced 209,824 metric tonnes of greenhouse tomatoes in 2005. Its total value was $384,627,000. Top provincial producers were:

British Columbia 63,307

Quebec 15,150

Alberta 4,379

Source: Adapted from Statistics Canada website, www.statcan.ca/cgi-bin/downpub/listpub.cgi?catno=22-003-XIB2006001. Accessed, March 19, 2007.

2. The Great Lakes Shown are various statistics about the Great Lakes. Using appropriate graphs (your choice) and summary statements, write a report analyzing the data.

	Superior	Michigan	Huron	Erie	Ontario
Length (kilometres)	563	494	332	388	311
Breadth (kilometres)	257	190	295	92	85
Depth (metres)	405	281	229	64	244
Volume (cubic kilometres)	12,088	4,918	3,543	484	1,638
Area (square kilometres)	82,103	57,757	59,570	25,667	19,554
Shoreline (U.S., kilometres)	1,389	2,253	933	694	483

Source: The World Almanac and Book of Facts.

3. **Vehicle Longevity** A hot topic in the Canadian automotive industry is the survival rates of domestic versus import branded vehicles. The following chart illustrates the longevity of vehicles from a 2006 study compared with the results from a 2000 study. Refer to the chart to answer the following questions.

    a. Which year has the biggest gap between domestic and import longevity?
    b. Which brand shows the greatest improvement in longevity between 2000 and 2006? Give a possible explanation.

    c. In what year(s) does the import branded vehicle longevity decline begin to escalate? The domestic brand?
    d. For 2006 data, estimate the percentage of both brands on the road after (i) 5 years, (ii) 10 years, and (iii) 15 years.
    e. What other observations can be made from this chart? Is there an environmental impact?

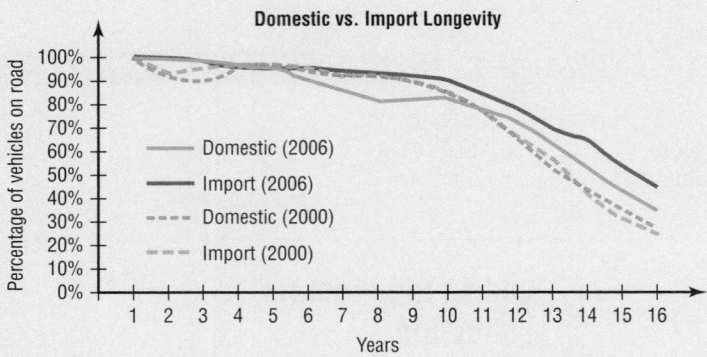

Source: DesRosiers Automotive Consultants Inc.

Data Projects

Where appropriate, use Minitab, SPSS, the TI-83 Plus, the TI-84 Plus, Excel, or a computer program of your choice to complete the following exercises.

1. **Business and Finance** Consider the 30 stocks listed as the "Dow Jones Industrials." Look up each stock's earnings per share. Randomly select 30 stocks traded on the Toronto Stock Exchange (TSX). Look up their earnings per share for each selected stock. Create a frequency table with 5 categories for each data set. Sketch a histogram for each. How do the two data sets compare?

2. **Sports and Leisure** Use systematic sampling to create a sample of 25 National League and 25 American League baseball players from the most recently completed season. Find the number of home runs for each player. Create a frequency table with 5 categories for each data set. Sketch a histogram for each. How do the two leagues compare?

3. **Technology** Randomly select 50 songs from your music player or music organization program. Find the length (in seconds) for each song. Use these data to create a frequency table with 6 categories. Sketch a frequency polygon for the frequency table. Is the shape of the distribution of times uniform, skewed, or bell-shaped? Also

note the genre of each song. Create a Pareto chart showing the frequencies of the various categories. Finally, note the year each song was released. Create a pie chart organized by decade to show the percentage of songs from various time periods.

4. **Health and Wellness** Use information from Canadian Blood Services to create a pie chart depicting the percentages of Canadians with various blood types. Search for information about blood donations and the percentage of each blood type donated. How do the charts compare? Why is the collection of type O blood so important?

5. **Politics** Search the Elections Canada website and construct appropriate charts comparing the previous two federal election results illustrating (i) federal party gains and losses, (ii) distribution by region, (iii) distribution of seats by gender and political affiliation, and (iv) voter turnout.

6. **Your Class** Have each person in class take his or her pulse and determine the heart rate (beats in one minute). Use the data to create a frequency table with 6 classes. Then have everyone in the class do 25 jumping jacks and immediately take the pulse again after the activity. Create a frequency table for those data as well. Compare the two results. Are they similarly distributed? How does the range of scores compare?

Answers to Applying the Concepts »

Section 2–1 Prime Ministers' Ages at Swearing-In

1. The data were obtained from the population of all prime ministers at the time this text was written.

2. The oldest swearing-in age was 74 years old.

3. The youngest swearing-in age was 39 years old.

4. Answers will vary. One possible answer is

Age at Swearing-In	Frequency
36–40	1
41–45	1
46–50	6
51–55	4
56–60	3
61–65	2
66–70	4
71–75	1

5. Answers will vary. For the frequency distribution given in Exercise 4, there is a peak for the 46–50 class.

6. Answers will vary. Two possible outliers are indicated in class 36–40 (age 39) and class 71–75 (age 74) from raw data.

7. Answers will vary. Data appear to be bimodal with peaks around the 46–55 and 66–70 age groups. (Refer to Section 2–2 for a discussion of distribution shapes.)

Section 2–2 Selling Real Estate

1. A histogram of the data gives price ranges and the counts of homes in each price range. We can also talk about how the data are distributed by looking at a histogram.

2. A frequency polygon shows increases or decreases in the number of home prices around values.

3. A cumulative frequency polygon shows the number of homes sold at or below a given price.

4. The house that sold for $321,550 is an extreme value in this data set.

5. Answers will vary. One possible answer is that the histogram displays the outlier well since there is a gap in the prices of the homes sold.

6. The distribution of the data is skewed to the right.

Section 2–3 Trends in Cancer Deaths

1. The variables in the graph are the year, cause of death, and rate of death per 100,000 women.

2. The cause of death is qualitative, while the year and death rates are quantitative.

3. Year is a discrete variable, and death rate is continuous. Since cause of death is qualitative, it is neither discrete nor continuous.

4. A time series plot was used to display the data.

5. No, a Pareto chart could not be used to display the data, since we can have only one quantitative variable and one categorical variable in a Pareto chart.

6. We cannot use a pie chart for the same reasons as given for the Pareto chart.

7. A Pareto chart is typically used to show a categorical variable listed from the highest-frequency category to the category with the lowest frequency.

8. A time series chart is used to see trends in the data. It can also be used for forecasting and predicting.

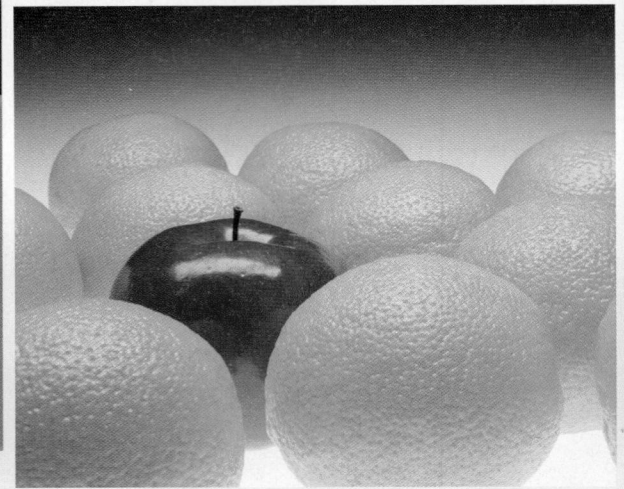

| Chapter 3

Data Description

Objectives >

After completing this chapter, you should be able to

LO1 Summarize data using measures of central tendency, such as the mean, median, mode, and midrange.

LO2 Describe data using measures of variation, such as the range, variance, and standard deviation.

LO3 Identify the position of a data value in a data set, using various measures of position, such as percentiles, deciles, and quartiles.

LO4 Use the techniques of exploratory data analysis, including boxplots and five-number summaries, to discover various aspects of data.

Outline >

Mc Graw Hill connect™ Practise and learn online with *Connect* with data sets and algorithmic questions related to concepts covered in this chapter. Throughout this chapter, questions and tables with online data sets are marked with .

Statistics Today

Do You Live As Well As Other Canadians?

The United Nations ranked Canada fourth in the world on its *Human Development Index* for 2009, ahead of the United States and Japan but trailing Norway and Australia. Unfortunately, this reputation for outstanding living conditions merely represents the well-being of the average Canadian. Regional disparities abound. One measure of quality of life is economic well-being. In 2008, the average Canadian per capita income was $39,648. How did your province or territory compare to this average? See Statistics Today—Revisited on page 140.

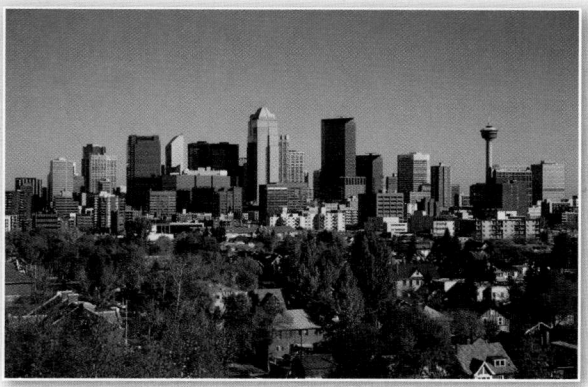

This chapter will show you how to obtain and interpret descriptive statistics as measures of average, measures of variation, and measures of position.

Source: United Nations, *Human Development Report, 2009.*

Introduction ›

Chapter 2 showed how one can gain useful information from raw data by organizing them into a frequency distribution and then presenting the data by using various graphs. This chapter shows the statistical methods that can be used to summarize data. The most familiar of these methods is the finding of averages.

For example, an average NHL hockey player earned $2.21 million in the 2009–2010 season.[1] The average 2009 undergraduate student debt ranges between $21,000 to $28,000, depending on the province or program of study.[2] The life expectancy at birth for average Canadian males, based on 2010 estimates, is 79.2 years, whereas the average Canadian female will live 83.2 years.[3]

Canadian nationalist writer and humourist Pierre Berton once described a typical Canadian as "*Someone who knows how to make love in a canoe without tipping it.*"

Are you an average Canadian? Statistics Canada and market researchers collect descriptive statistics from all facets of Canadian life. Here are some findings about the typical Canadian.

Interesting Fact

A person has on average 1460 dreams in one year.

Canadian brides marry at an average age of 31.7 years and their grooms at 34.3 years.[4]

Typical Canadian households spend an average of $142.08 on food each week.[5]

An average Canadian consumes 23.4 kg of red meat, 13.4 kg of poultry, and 12.7 dozen eggs each year.[6]

Canadians consume an average of 63.2 litres of milk, 160.1 litres of coffee or tea, and 65.8 litres of beer per capita each year.[7]

Canadians view an average of 147 online videos for an average of 605 minutes each month.[8]

[1]National Hockey League Players' Association, *Players,* "Player Compensation."
[2]Canadian Federation of Students, Research and Policy, *Submission to House of Commons Standing Committee on Finance,* August 2009.
[3]Office of the Superintendent of Financial Institutions Canada, Office of the Chief Actuary, *Canada Pension Plan Mortality Study: Actuarial Study No. 7,* July 2009.
[4]Adapted from *CBC News,* "Marriage by the Numbers," March 9, 2005.
[5]Adapted from Statistics Canada, *Spending Patterns in Canada, 2008,* Catalogue No. 62-202-X.
[6]Adapted from Statistics Canada, *Food Statistics, 2009,* Catalogue No. 21-020-X.
[7]Adapted from Statistics Canada, *The Daily,* Catalogue No. 11-001, May 26, 2005.
[8]comScore, *Canada Ranks as a Global Leader in Online Video Viewing,* April 21, 2008.

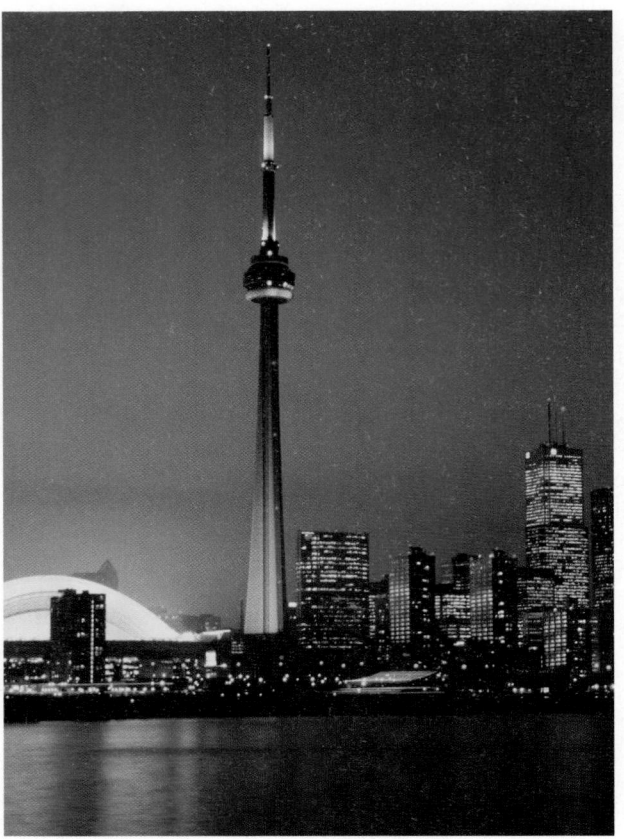

In these examples, the word *average* is ambiguous, since several different methods can be used to obtain an average. Loosely stated, the average means the centre of the distribution or the most typical case. Measures of average are also called *measures of central tendency* and include the *mean, median, mode,* and *midrange.*

Knowing the average of a data set is not enough to describe the data set entirely. Even though a shoe store owner knows that the average size of a man's shoe is size 10, she would not be in business very long if she ordered only size 10 shoes.

As this example shows, in addition to knowing the average, one must know how the data values are dispersed. That is, do the data values cluster around the mean, or are they spread more evenly throughout the distribution? The measures that determine the spread of the data values are called *measures of variation* or *measures of dispersion.* These measures include the *range, variance,* and *standard deviation.*

Finally, another set of measures is necessary to describe data. These measures are called *measures of position.* They tell where a specific data value falls within the data set or its relative position in comparison with other data values. Common position measures are *percentiles, deciles, quartiles,* and standard scores or *z* scores. These measures are used extensively in psychology and education. Sometimes they are referred to as *norms.*

The measures of central tendency, variation, and position explained in this chapter are part of what is called *traditional statistics.*

Section 3–4 shows the techniques of what is called *exploratory data analysis.* These techniques include the *boxplot* and the *five-number summary.* They can be used to explore data to see what they show (as opposed to the traditional techniques, which are used to confirm conjectures about the data).

3–1   Measures of Central Tendency >

Summarize data using measures of central tendency, such as the mean, median, mode, and midrange.

Historical Note

In 1796, Adolphe Quetelet investigated the characteristics (heights, weights, etc.) of French conscripts to determine the "average man." Florence Nightingale was so influenced by Quetelet's work that she began collecting and analyzing medical records in the military hospitals during the Crimean War. Based on her work, hospitals began keeping accurate records on their patients.

Chapter 1 stated that statisticians use samples taken from populations; however, when populations are small, it is not necessary to use samples since the entire population can be used to gain information. For example, suppose an insurance manager wanted to know the average weekly sales of all the company's representatives. If the company employed a large number of salespeople, say, nationwide, he would have to use a sample and make an inference to the entire sales force. But if the company had only a few salespeople, say, only 87 agents, he would be able to use all representatives' sales for a randomly chosen week and thus use the entire population.

Measures found by using all the data values in the population are called *parameters.* Measures obtained by using the data values from samples are called *statistics;* hence, the average of the sales from a sample of representatives is called a *statistic,* and the average of sales obtained from the entire population is called a *parameter.*

> A **statistic** is a characteristic or measure obtained by using the data values from a sample.
>
> A **parameter** is a characteristic or measure obtained by using all the data values from a specific population.

These concepts as well as the symbols used to represent them will be explained in detail in this chapter.

General Rounding Rule   In statistics the basic rounding rule is that when computations are done in the calculation, rounding should not be done until the final answer is calculated. When rounding is done in the intermediate steps, it tends to increase the difference between that answer and the exact one. But in the textbook and solutions manual, it is not practical to show long decimals in the intermediate calculations; hence, the values in the examples are carried out to enough places (usually three or four) to obtain the same answer that a calculator would give after rounding on the last step. Detailed examples in this chapter will illustrate proper rounding techniques.

The Mean

The *mean,* also known as the *arithmetic average,* is found by adding the values of the data and dividing by the total number of values. For example, the mean of 3, 2, 6, 5, and 4 is found by adding $3 + 2 + 6 + 5 + 4 = 20$ and dividing by 5; hence, the mean of the data is $20 \div 5 = 4$. The values of the data are represented by Xs. In this data set, $X_1 = 3$, $X_2 = 2$, $X_3 = 6$, $X_4 = 5$, and $X_5 = 4$. To show a sum of the total X values, the symbol Σ (the capital Greek letter sigma) is used, and ΣX means to find the sum of the X values in the data set. The summation notation is explained in Appendix A.

> The **mean** is the sum of the values, divided by the total number of values. The symbol $\overline{X}$ represents the sample mean.
>
> $$\overline{X} = \frac{X_1 + X_2 + X_3 + \cdots + X_n}{n} = \frac{\Sigma X}{n}$$
>
> where n represents the total number of values in the sample.

For a population, the Greek letter μ (mu) is used for the mean.

$$\mu = \frac{X_1 + X_2 + X_3 + \cdots + X_N}{N} = \frac{\Sigma X}{N}$$

where N represents the total number of values in the population.

In statistics, Greek letters are often used to denote parameters, and Roman letters are often used to denote statistics. Assume that the data are obtained from samples unless otherwise specified.

Example 3–1

Annual Holidays

The data represent the total number of paid days off (vacation and statutory holidays) for a sample of individuals selected from nine different countries. Find the mean.

$$20, 26, 40, 36, 23, 42, 35, 24, 30$$

Source: World Tourism Organization.

Solution

$$\overline{X} = \frac{\Sigma X}{n} = \frac{20 + 26 + 40 + 36 + 23 + 42 + 35 + 24 + 30}{9}$$

$$= \frac{276}{9} \approx 30.7 \text{ days (rounded)}$$

Therefore, the mean of the number of paid days off is 30.7 days.

Example 3–2

Monthly Water Consumption

A sample of monthly residential utility bills measuring water consumption, in cubic metres (m^3), for the past year is selected. The following readings were observed.

(*Note:* 1 m^3 = 1000 litres)

23.7   31.2   24.3   33.0   29.1   29.9   25.9   30.8   32.1   27.6   21.3   25.4

Source: Enmax Corporation utilities statements.

Solution

$$\overline{X} = \frac{\Sigma X}{n} = \frac{23.7 + 31.2 + 24.3 + 33.0 + 29.1 + 29.9 + 25.9 + 30.8 + 32.1 + 27.6 + 21.3 + 25.4}{12}$$

$$= \frac{334.3}{12} \approx 27.86 \text{ m}^3 \text{ (rounded)}$$

The mean water consumption for the past year was 27.86 m^3 or 27,860 litres per month.

The mean, in most cases, is not an actual data value.

Rounding Rule for the Mean   The mean should be rounded to one more decimal place than occurs in the raw data. For example, if the raw data are given in whole numbers, the mean should be rounded to the nearest tenth. If the data are given in tenths, the mean should be rounded to the nearest hundredth, and so on.

The procedure for finding the mean for grouped data uses the midpoints of the classes. This procedure is shown next.

| Example 3–3 | **Kilometres Run per Week** |

Kilometres Run per Week

Using the frequency distribution for Example 2–7 on page 48, find the mean. The data represent the number of kilometres run during one week for a sample of 20 runners.

Solution

The procedure for finding the mean for grouped data is given here.

Step 1   Make a table as shown.

A Class	B Frequency (f)	C Midpoint (X_m)	D $f \cdot X_m$
5.5–10.5	1		
10.5–15.5	2		
15.5–20.5	3		
20.5–25.5	5		
25.5–30.5	4		
30.5–35.5	3		
35.5–40.5	2		
	$n = 20$		

Step 2   Find the midpoints of each class and enter them in column C.

$$X_m = \frac{5.5 + 10.5}{2} = 8 \qquad \frac{10.5 + 15.5}{2} = 13 \qquad \text{etc.}$$

Step 3   For each class, multiply the frequency by the midpoint, as shown, and place the product in column D.

$$1 \cdot 8 = 8 \qquad 2 \cdot 13 = 26 \qquad \text{etc.}$$

The completed table is shown here.

A Class	B Frequency (f)	C Midpoint (X_m)	D $f \cdot X_m$
5.5–10.5	1	8	8
10.5–15.5	2	13	26
15.5–20.5	3	18	54
20.5–25.5	5	23	115
25.5–30.5	4	28	112
30.5–35.5	3	33	99
35.5–40.5	2	38	76
	$n = 20$		$\Sigma f \cdot X_m = 490$

Step 4   Find the sum of column D.

Step 5   Divide the sum by n to get the mean.

$$\overline{X} = \frac{\Sigma f \cdot X_m}{n} = \frac{490}{20} = 24.5 \text{ kilometres}$$

The procedure for finding the mean for grouped data assumes that the mean of all the raw data values in each class is equal to the midpoint of the class. In reality, this is not true, since the average of the raw data values in each class usually will not be exactly equal to the midpoint. However, using this procedure will give an acceptable approximation of the mean, since some values fall above the midpoint and other values fall below the midpoint for each class, and the midpoint represents an estimate of all values in the class.

The steps for finding the mean for grouped data are summarized in the next Procedure Table.

Procedure Table

Finding the Mean for Grouped Data

Step 1 Make a table as shown.

A Class	B Frequency (f)	C Midpoint (X_m)	D $f \cdot X_m$

Step 2 Find the midpoints of each class and place them in column C.

Step 3 Multiply the frequency by the midpoint for each class, and place the product in column D.

Step 4 Find the sum of column D.

Step 5 Divide the sum obtained in column D by the sum of the frequencies obtained in column B.

The formula for the mean is

$$\overline{X} = \frac{\Sigma f \cdot X_m}{n}$$

(*Note:* The symbols $\Sigma f \cdot X_m$ mean to find the sum of the product of the frequency (f) and the midpoint (X_m) for each class.)

 Speaking of Statistics

All things are not equal! Only wealthy Canadian families can afford to purchase a house in parts of Canada. This Snapshot illustrates the average house prices in select Canadian cities in May 2007. Which type of average (mean, median, mode) do you think was used?

Snapshot

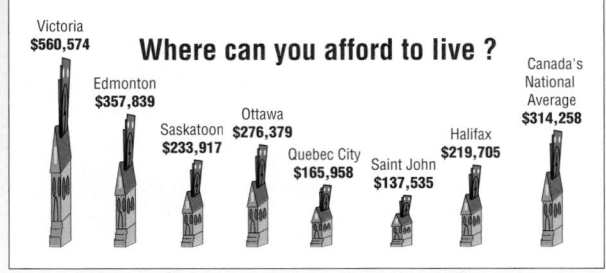

Source: CREA—Canadian Real Estate Association (May 2007).

Unusual Stat

A person looks, on average, at about 14 homes before buying one.

The Median

An article recently reported that the median income for college and university professors was \$81,104. This measure of central tendency means that one-half of all the professors surveyed earned more than \$81,104, and one-half earned less than \$81,104.[9]

The *median* is the halfway point in a data set. Before one can find this point, the data must be arranged in order. When the data set is ordered, it is called a **data array.** The median either will be a specific value in the data set or will fall between two values, as shown in Examples 3–4 and 3–5.

> The **median** is the midpoint of the data array. The symbol for the median is MD.

Steps in computing the median of a data array

Step 1 Arrange the data in order.

Step 2 Select the middle point.

Example 3–4

Hotel Rates

Whistler, British Columbia, hosted the downhill ski events in the 2010 Winter Olympic Games. The data represent pre-Olympic hotel rates (per night) in select hotels. Find the median.

$$\$134, \$149, \$179, \$330, \$170, \$208, \$170, \$99, \$159$$

Source: www.expedia.com.

Solution

Step 1 Arrange the data in order.

99, 134, 149, 159, 170, 170, 179, 208, 330

Step 2 Select the middle value.

99, 134, 149, 159, 170, 170, 179, 208, 330

↑

Median

Hence, the median hotel price is \$170.

Example 3–4 had an odd number of values in the data set; hence, the median was an actual data value. When there are an even number of values in the data set, the median will fall between two given values, as illustrated in Example 3–5.

Example 3–5

Residential Home Sales

The number of residential home sales per month in Calgary over a 12-month period is listed below. Find the median.

1877, 2408, 3060, 3497, 3389, 3550, 3388, 2586, 2516, 2180, 2122, 2394

Source: Calgary Real Estate Board.

---

[9]*University of Toronto Faculty Association Comparative Study.*

Solution

Sort the sales data in ascending order.

1877, 2122, 2180, 2394, 2408, 2516, 2586, 3060, 3388, 3389, 3497, 3550

↑

Median

Since the middle point falls halfway between 2516 and 2586, find the median (MD) by adding the middle two values and dividing by 2.

$$MD = \frac{2516 + 2586}{2} = 2551$$

The median number of residential home sales in Calgary over the 12-month period is 2551.

The Mode

The third measure of average is called the *mode.* The mode is the value that occurs most often in the data set. It is sometimes said to be the most typical case.

> The value that occurs most often in a data set is called the **mode.**

   A data set that has only one value that occurs with the greatest frequency is said to be **unimodal.**
   If a data set has two values that occur with the same greatest frequency, both values are considered to be the mode and the data set is said to be **bimodal.** If a data set has more than two values that occur with the same greatest frequency, each value is used as the mode, and the data set is said to be **multimodal.** When no data value occurs more than once, the data set is said to have *no mode.* A data set can have more than one mode or no mode at all. These situations will be shown in some of the examples that follow.

Example 3–6

Space Shuttle Flight Missions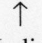

NASA's space shuttle robotic arm, Canadarm, has been in service since 1981. The following data represent the number of NASA shuttle flight missions each year that utilized one of the five Canadian-built Canadarms. Find the mode.

1, 2, 2, 4, 7, 1, 0, 1, 0, 3, 3, 4, 4, 6, 4, 3, 3, 3, 2, 4, 6, 5, 0, 0, 1, 3, 3, 4, 5

Source: Canadian Space Agency, *Flight History of Canadarm.*

Solution

It is helpful to arrange the data in order, although it is not necessary.

0, 0, 0, 0, 1, 1, 1, 1, 2, 2, 2, 3, 3, 3, 3, 3, 3, 3, 4, 4, 4, 4, 4, 4, 5, 5, 6, 6, 7

Since 3 space shuttle missions occurred in 7 different years—a frequency larger than any other number—the mode for the data is 3.

| Example 3-7 | **World Nuclear Reactors** |

The number of operable nuclear reactors for the top 12 countries in the world is shown. Canada ranks seventh, with 16 nuclear reactors. Find the mode.

| 104 | 59 | 53 | 30 | 27 | 19 | 16 | 14 | 13 | 11 | 9 | 7 |

Source: NationMaster.com, *Energy Statistics,* "Nuclear Reactors Operable (most recent) by Country."

Solution

Since each value occurs only once, there is no mode.

Note: Do not state that the mode is zero. That would be incorrect because in some data, such as temperature, zero can be an actual value. No mode would also occur if all data values occurred with equal frequency (i.e., 2 or 3 times).

| Example 3-8 | **Air Quality Index** |

The number of moderate to poor Air Quality Index (AQI) days for select Ontario cities in 2009 is shown below. Find the mode.

| 23 | 12 | 26 | 57 | 38 | 26 | 25 | 34 |
| 30 | 28 | 22 | 15 | 32 | 28 | 49 | 42 |

Solution

Since the AQI readings of 26 and 28 both occur two times, the modes are 26 and 28. Data sets with two modes are bimodal.

The mode for grouped data is the modal class. The **modal class** is the class with the largest frequency.

| Example 3-9 | **Kilometres Run per Week** |

Find the modal class for the frequency distribution of kilometres that 20 runners ran in one week, used in Example 2-7 on page 48.

Class	Frequency
5.5–10.5	1
10.5–15.5	2
15.5–20.5	3
20.5–25.5	5 ← Modal class
25.5–30.5	4
30.5–35.5	3
35.5–40.5	2

Solution

The modal class is 20.5–25.5, since it has the largest frequency. Sometimes the midpoint of the class is used rather than the boundaries; hence, the mode could also be given as 23 kilometres per week.

The mode is the only measure of central tendency that can be used in finding the most typical case when the data are nominal or categorical.

Example 3–10

International Student Enrollment

In 2009, McGill University registered the following number of full-time and part-time international students, based on country of citizenship. Find the mode.

United States	2305
France	695
China	413
India	291
Saudi Arabia	248

Source: McGill University, *Enrolment Reports: International Students.*

Solution

The category with the highest frequency is the mode, which is the United States.

An extremely high or extremely low data value in a data set can have a striking effect on the mean of the data set. These extreme values are called *outliers*. This is one reason why when analyzing a frequency distribution, you should be aware of any of these values. For the data set shown in Example 3–11, the mean, median, and mode can be quite different because of extreme values. A method for identifying outliers is given in Section 3–3.

Example 3–11

Graduate Student Funding

Graduate students in an environmental studies research program each received funding from different sources as shown. (Assume that this represents the entire population under study.) Find the mean, median and mode.

$14,750 $15,900 $17,500 $17,500 $18,000 $21,750 $23,250 $39,900

Solution

$$\mu = \frac{\Sigma X}{N} = \frac{\$168,550}{8} = \$21,069$$

$$MD = \frac{\$17,500 + \$18,000}{2} = \$17,750$$

Hence, the mean is $21,069, the median is the $17,750, and the mode—$17,500—occurs two times.

In Example 3–11, the mean is much higher than the median or the mode. This is so because the extremely high scholarship awarded to one graduate student tends to raise the value of the mean. In this and similar situations, the median should be used as the measure of central tendency.

The Midrange

The *midrange* is a rough estimate of the middle. It is found by adding the lowest and highest values in the data set and dividing by 2. It is a very rough estimate of the average and can be affected by one extremely high or low value.

> The **midrange** is defined as the sum of the lowest and highest values in the data set, divided by 2. The symbol MR is used for the midrange.
>
> $$MR = \frac{\text{Lowest value } + \text{ Highest value}}{2}$$

Example 3–12

Deli Luncheon Sales

A Montreal delicatessen had the following daily luncheon sales (rounded to the nearest dollar) over a one-week period. Find the midrange.

$$\$230 \quad \$390 \quad \$377 \quad \$410 \quad \$383 \quad \$398 \quad \$265$$

Solution

$$MR = \frac{\$230 + \$410}{2} = \frac{\$640}{2} = \$320$$

Hence, the midrange is $320.

If the data set contains one extremely large value or one extremely small value, a higher or lower midrange value will result and may not be a typical description of the middle.

Example 3–13

Deli Luncheon Sales

Assume the Montreal deli's luncheon sales for the following week were affected by a major storm. Listed below, rounded to the nearest dollar, are the deli's luncheon sales for the following week. Find the midrange.

$$\$255 \quad \$425 \quad \$333 \quad \$395 \quad \$361 \quad \$328 \quad \$45$$

Solution

$$MR = \frac{\$425 + \$45}{2} = \frac{\$470}{2} = \$235$$

Hence, the midrange is $235. The value $235 is not typical of the average luncheon sales at the deli as the outlier value $45 is not typical of the sales.

In statistics, several measures can be used for an average. The most common measures are the mean, median, mode, and midrange. Each has its own specific purpose and use. Exercises 39 through 41 at the end of this section show examples of other averages, such as the harmonic mean, the geometric mean, and the quadratic mean. Their applications are limited to specific areas, as shown in the exercises.

The Weighted Mean

Sometimes, one must find the mean of a data set in which not all values are equally represented. Consider the case of finding the average cost of a litre of gasoline for three taxis. Suppose the drivers buy gasoline at three different service stations at a cost of $0.99, $1.07, and $1.21 per litre. One might try to find the average by using the formula

$$\overline{X} = \frac{\Sigma X}{n}$$

$$= \frac{0.99 + 1.07 + 1.21}{3} = \frac{3.27}{3} = \$1.09$$

But not all of the drivers purchased the same number of litres. Hence, to find the true average cost per litre, one must take into consideration the number of litres each driver purchased.

The type of mean that considers an additional factor is called the *weighted mean,* and it is used when the values are not all equally represented.

Find the **weighted mean** of a variable X by multiplying each value by its corresponding weight and dividing the sum of the products by the sum of the weights.

$$\overline{X} = \frac{w_1 X_1 + w_2 X_2 + \cdots + w_n X_n}{w_1 + w_2 + \cdots + w_n} = \frac{\Sigma wX}{\Sigma w}$$

where $w_1, w_2, \ldots, w_n$ are the weights and $X_1, X_2, \ldots, X_n$ are the values.

Example 3–14 shows how the weighted mean is used to compute a grade point average. Since courses vary in their credit value, the number of credits must be used as weights.

| Example 3–14 | **Grade Point Average** |

A student received an A in English Composition I (3 credits), a C in Introduction to Psychology (3 credits), a B in Biology I (4 credits), and a D in Physical Education (2 credits). Assuming A = 4 grade points, B = 3 grade points, C = 2 grade points, D = 1 grade point, and F = 0 grade points, find the student's grade point average.

Solution

Course	Credits (w)	Grade (X)
English Composition I	3	A (4 points)
Introduction to Psychology	3	C (2 points)
Biology I	4	B (3 points)
Physical Education	2	D (1 point)

$$\overline{X} = \frac{\Sigma wX}{\Sigma w} = \frac{3 \cdot 4 + 3 \cdot 2 + 4 \cdot 3 + 2 \cdot 1}{3 + 3 + 4 + 2} = \frac{32}{12} = 2.7$$

The grade point average is 2.7.

Table 3–1 summarizes the measures of central tendency.

Table 3–1	**Summary of Measures of Central Tendency**	
Measure	**Definition**	**Symbol(s)**
Mean	Sum of values, divided by total number of values	$\mu, \overline{X}$
Median	Middle point in data set that has been ordered	MD
Mode	Most frequent data value	None
Midrange	Lowest value plus highest value, divided by 2	MR

Researchers and statisticians must know which measure of central tendency is being used and when to use each measure of central tendency. The properties and uses of the four measures of central tendency are summarized next.

Properties and Uses of Central Tendency

The Mean

1. One computes the mean by using all the values of the data.
2. The mean usually varies less than the median or mode when samples are taken from the same population and all three measures are computed for these samples.
3. The mean is used in computing other statistics, such as the variance.
4. The mean for the data set is unique and not necessarily one of the data values.
5. The mean cannot be computed for the data in a frequency distribution that has an open-ended class.
6. The mean is affected by unusual and extreme high or low values, called *outliers,* and may not be the appropriate average to use in these situations.

The Median

1. The median is used when one must find the centre or middle value of a data set.
2. The median is used when one must determine whether the data values fall into the upper half or lower half of the distribution.
3. The median is used for an open-ended distribution.
4. The median is affected less than the mean by extremely high or extremely low values.

The Mode

1. The mode is used when the most typical case is desired.
2. The mode is the easiest average to compute.
3. The mode can be used when the data are nominal, such as religious preference, gender, or political affiliation.
4. The mode is not always unique. A data set can have more than one mode, or the mode may not exist for a data set.

The Midrange

1. The midrange is easy to compute.
2. The midrange gives the midpoint.
3. The midrange is affected by extremely high or low values in a data set.

Distribution Shapes

In the previous chapter, data were organized into classes in tables and graphed. These data organization and presentation methods are essential to understanding the structure of a data set.

Frequency distributions can assume many shapes. The three most important shapes are positively skewed, symmetric, and negatively skewed. Figure 3–1 shows histograms of each.

In a **positively skewed** or **right-skewed distribution,** the majority of the data values fall to the left of the mean and cluster at the lower end of the distribution; the "tail" is to the right. Typically, the mean is to the right of the median, and the mode is to the left of the median.

For example, if an instructor gave an examination and most of the students did poorly, their scores would tend to cluster on the left side of the distribution. A few high scores would constitute the tail of the distribution, which would be on the right side. Another example of a positively skewed distribution is the incomes of the population of Canada. Most of the incomes cluster about the low end of the distribution; those with high incomes are in the minority and are in the tail at the right of the distribution.

In a **symmetric distribution,** the data values are evenly distributed on both sides of the mean. In addition, when the distribution is unimodal, the mean, median, and mode are the same and are at the centre of the distribution. Examples of symmetric distributions are IQ scores and heights of adult males.

Figure 3–1

Types of Distributions

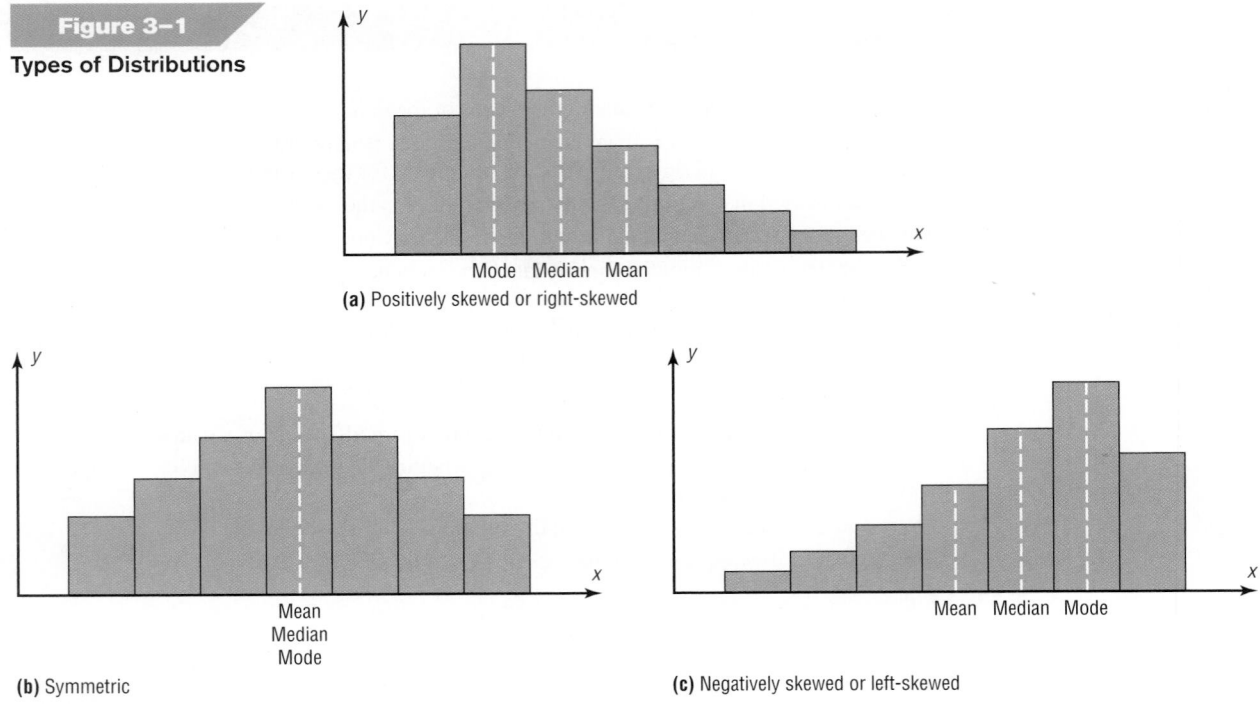

(a) Positively skewed or right-skewed

(b) Symmetric

(c) Negatively skewed or left-skewed

When the majority of the data values fall to the right of the mean and cluster at the upper end of the distribution, with the tail to the left, the distribution is said to be **negatively skewed** or **left-skewed.** Typically, the mean is to the left of the median, and the mode is to the right of the median. As an example, a negatively skewed distribution results if the majority of students score very high on an instructor's examination. These scores will tend to cluster to the right of the distribution.

When a distribution is extremely skewed, the value of the mean will be pulled toward the tail, but the majority of the data values will be greater than the mean or less than the mean (depending on which way the data are skewed); hence, the median rather than the mean is a more appropriate measure of central tendency. An extremely skewed distribution can also affect other statistics.

A measure of skewness for a distribution is discussed in Exercise 48 in Section 3–2.

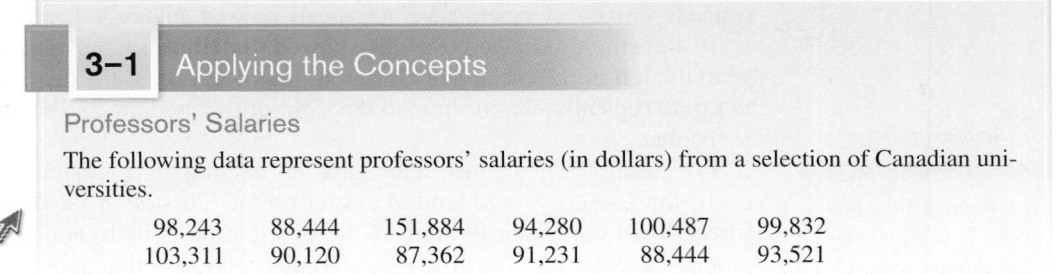

3–1   Applying the Concepts

Professors' Salaries

The following data represent professors' salaries (in dollars) from a selection of Canadian universities.

| 98,243 | 88,444 | 151,884 | 94,280 | 100,487 | 99,832 |
| 103,311 | 90,120 | 87,362 | 91,231 | 88,444 | 93,521 |

Source: Adapted from Statistics Canada, excerpts from salaries and salary scales of full-time teaching staff at Canadian universities, 2001–2002; www.statcan.ca/bsolc/english/bsolc?catno=81-595-M2004013, February 28, 2007.

1. First, assume that you are employed as a researcher for an association of university administrators and do not wish to raise tuition fees to increase salaries. Compute the mean, median, midrange, and mode and decide which one would best support your position to not raise salaries.

2. Second, assume you work for a university faculty association and want to provide the rationale for a faculty salary increase. Use the best measure of central tendency to support your position.

3. Explain how outliers can be used to support one or the other position.

4. If the salaries represented every professor in Canada, would the averages be parameters or statistics?

5. Which measure of central tendency can be misleading when a data set contains outliers?

6. When one is comparing the measures of central tendency, does the distribution display any skewness? Explain.

See page 145 for the answers.

Exercises 3–1

For Exercises 1 through 8, find (a) the mean, (b) the median, (c) the mode, and (d) the midrange.

1. **Grade Point Averages** The average undergraduate grade point average (GPA) for the 25 top-ranked medical schools is listed below

3.80	3.77	3.70	3.74	3.70
3.86	3.76	3.68	3.67	3.57
3.83	3.70	3.80	3.74	3.67
3.78	3.74	3.73	3.65	3.66
3.75	3.64	3.78	3.73	3.64

Source: U.S. News & World Report Best Graduate Schools.

2. **World Waterfall Heights** The heights (in metres) of 20 of the world's tallest waterfalls are shown here. (*Note: The height of Niagara Falls is 50.9 metres!*)

979	948	914	900	860	850	840	836	820	818
792	788	773	771	762	755	751	739	725	720

Source: World Waterfall Database.

3. **Number of Burglaries** The following data are the number of burglaries reported for a 12-month period in select Calgary communities. Which measure of average might be the best in this case? Explain your answer.

13	8	22	73	13	2	24	7	13	4	33
7	4	3	6	8	4	16	8	17	9	72

Source: Calgary Police Service.

4. **Earnings of Dead Celebrities** *Forbes* magazine prints an annual "Top-Earning Dead Celebrities" list (based on royalties and estate earnings). Find the measures of central tendency for these data and comment on the skewness. Figures represent millions of dollars.

Kurt Cobain	50	Ray Charles	10
Elvis Presley	42	Marilyn Monroe	8
Charles M. Schulz	35	Johnny Cash	8
John Lennon	24	J. R. R. Tolkien	7
Albert Einstein	20	George Harrison	7
Andy Warhol	19	Bob Marley	7
Theodor Geisel			
(Dr. Seuss)	10		

Source: Lacey Rose, Louis Hau, and Amanda Schupak, "Top-Earning Dead Celebrities," Forbes.com, October 24, 2006.

5. **Identity Theft Victims** A researcher claims that each year, there is an average of 300 victims of identity theft in major cities. Twelve were randomly selected, and the number of victims of identity theft in each city is shown. Can you conclude that the researcher was correct?

574	229	663	372	102	88
117	239	465	136	189	75

6. **World's Wealthiest People** For a recent year, the worth (in billions of dollars) of a sample of the 10 wealthiest people under the age of 60 is shown:

14, 12, 48, 20, 18, 18, 12.6, 10.4, 7.3, 5.3

The worth of a sample of 10 of the wealthiest people age 60 and over is shown:

41.0, 13.7, 10.0, 18.0, 11.3, 7.6, 7, 18, 20, 60

Based on the averages, can you conclude that those 60 years old and over have a higher net worth?

Source: Forbes magazine.

7. **Earthquake Magnitude** Twelve major earthquakes had Richter magnitudes shown here.

7.0, 6.2, 7.7, 8.0, 6.4, 6.2,
7.2, 5.4, 6.4, 6.5, 7.2, 5.4

Which would you consider the best measure of average?

Source: The Universal Almanac.

8. **CEO Salaries** The data shown are the total compensation (in millions of dollars) for the 50 top-paid CEOs for a recent year. Compare the averages, and state which one you think is the best measure.

17.5	18.0	36.8	31.7	31.7
17.3	24.3	47.7	38.5	17.0
23.7	16.5	25.1	17.4	18.0
37.6	19.7	21.4	28.6	21.6
19.3	20.0	16.9	25.2	19.8
25.0	17.2	20.4	20.1	29.1
19.1	25.2	23.2	25.9	24.0
41.7	24.0	16.8	26.8	31.4
16.9	17.2	24.1	35.2	19.1
22.9	18.2	25.4	35.4	25.5

Source: USA TODAY.

9. **World's Highest Mountains** Find the (a) mean, (b) median, (c) mode, and (d) midrange for the data in Exercise 17 in Section 2–1 on page 43. Is the distribution symmetric or skewed? Use the individual data values.

10. **Home Run Record Breakers** Find the (a) mean, (b) median, (c) mode, and (d) midrange for the distances of the home runs for McGwire and Sosa, using the data in Exercise 18 in Section 2–1 on page 43.

     Compare the means. Decide if the means are approximately equal or if one of the players is hitting longer home runs. Use the individual data values.

11. **City Population Census** Population data, in thousands, for Canada's largest cities are compared for the 2001 and 2006 census years. Find the mean, median, mode, and midrange for each data set. What do your findings suggest?

2001			2006		
4683	414	148	5113	451	177
3451	377	148	3636	390	162
1987	359	147	2117	373	159
1064	296	156	1131	330	158
951	312	147	1079	330	152
938	308	155	1035	323	152
687	226	138	716	234	142
677	193	117	695	195	127
662	176	119	693	187	126
436	173	118	458	181	125

Source: Statistics Canada.

For Exercises 12 through 21, find the (a) mean and (b) modal class.

12. **Exam Scores** For 108 randomly selected college students, this exam score frequency distribution was obtained.

Exam score	Frequency
90–98	6
99–107	22
108–116	43
117–125	28
126–134	9

13. **Golf Scores** The final golf scores for The Players Championship in 2006 were

Score	Frequency
280–283	5
284–287	13
288–291	16
292–295	20
296–299	13
300–303	4
304–307	2

Source: PGA.com.

14. **Automobile Fuel Efficiency** Thirty-five different vehicle manufacturers are listed in *Canada's Fuel Consumption Guide, 2006*. The following distribution indicates the most fuel-efficient vehicle reported from each manufacturer. Data shown indicate highway fuel consumption in L/100 km. (This data will be used in Exercise 20 in Section 3–2.)

Fuel consumption	Frequency
3.5–6.5	5
6.5–9.5	15
9.5–12.5	8
12.5–15.5	4
15.5–18.5	0
18.5–21.5	2
21.5–24.5	1

Source: Natural Resources Canada, *Fuel Consumption Guide, 2006.*

15. **Police Crime Index** The *Police-Reported Crime Series Index* (PRCSI) measures crimes based on a factor weighted by judicial criminal sentences, with more serious offences receiving a higher index weighting. The base year for comparison was 2006, with an index weighting of 100. The following distribution represents the PRCSI for metropolitan areas in Canada for 2008.

PRCSI	Frequency
40–59	2
60–79	14
80–99	6
100–119	5
120–139	4
140–159	1
160–179	1

Do you think that the mean is the best measure of average for these data? Explain.

Source: Statistics Canada, *Juristat,* "Police-Reported Crime Statistics in Canada, 2008," July 2009, Vol. 29, No. 3

16. **Dog Reaction Times** Find the mean and modal class for the two frequency distributions in Exercises 8 and 18 in Section 2–2. Are the "average" reactions the same? Explain your answer.

17. **Light Bulb Life Span** Eighty randomly selected light bulbs were tested to determine their lifetimes (in hours). This frequency distribution was obtained. (The data in this exercise will be used in Exercise 23 in Section 3–2.)

Bulb lifetime	Frequency
52.5–63.5	6
63.5–74.5	12
74.5–85.5	25
85.5–96.5	18
96.5–107.5	14
107.5–118.5	5

18. Net Worth of Corporations These data represent the net worth (in millions of dollars) of 45 national corporations.

Net worth	Frequency
10–20	2
21–31	8
32–42	15
43–53	7
54–64	10
65–75	3

19. Laundry Detergent Cost per Load The cost per load (in cents) of 35 laundry detergents tested by a consumer organization is shown. (The data in this exercise will be used for Exercise 19 in Section 3–2.)

Cost per load	Frequency
13–19	2
20–26	7
27–33	12
34–40	5
41–47	6
48–54	1
55–61	0
62–68	2

20. Commissions Earned This frequency distribution represents the commission earned (in dollars) by 100 salespeople employed at several branches of a large chain store.

Commissions	Frequency
150–158	5
159–167	16
168–176	20
177–185	21
186–194	20
195–203	15
204–212	3

21. Copying Machine Service Calls This frequency distribution represents the data obtained from a sample of 75 copying machine service technicians. The values represent the days between service calls for various copying machines.

Days between calls	Frequency
15.5–18.5	14
18.5–21.5	12
21.5–24.5	18
24.5–27.5	10
27.5–30.5	15
30.5–33.5	6

22. Masters Golf Scores Find the mean and modal class for the data in Exercise 12 in Section 2–1.

23. Prime Ministers' Terms of Office Find the mean and modal class for the data in Exercise 13 in Section 2–1.

24. Automobile Fatalities Find the mean and modal class for the data in Exercise 14 in Section 2–1.

25. Exchange Rates Find the mean and modal class for the data in Exercise 15 in Section 2–1.

26. Automobile Sales Find the weighted mean price of three models of automobiles sold. The number and price of each model sold are shown in this list.

Model	Number	Price
A	8	$10,000
B	10	12,000
C	12	8,000

27. Fat Grams Using the weighted mean, find the average number of grams of fat per 100 grams of meat or fish that a person would consume over a one-week period if that person ate the following.

Meat or fish	Fat (g/100 g)
84 g fried shrimp	11.9
84 g veal cutlet (broiled)	10.7
56 g fried chicken drumstick	8.9
70 g fried chicken drumstick	15.7
112 g tuna (canned in oil)	6.3

28. Diet Cola Preference A recent survey of a new diet cola reported the following percentages of people who liked the taste. Find the weighted mean of the percentages.

Area	% Favoured	Number surveyed
1	40	1000
2	30	3000
3	50	800

29. Helicopter Costs The costs of three models of helicopters are shown here. Find the weighted mean of the costs of the models.

Model	Number sold	Cost
Sunscraper	9	$427,000
Skycoaster	6	365,000
High-Flyer	12	725,000

30. Final Grade An instructor grades exams, 20%; term paper, 30%; final exam, 50%. A student had grades of 83, 72, and 90, respectively, for exams, term paper, and final exam. Find the student's final average. Use the weighted mean.

31. Final Grade Another instructor gives four 1-hour exams and one final exam, which counts as two 1-hour exams. Find a student's grade if she received 62, 83, 97, and 90 on the 1-hour exams and 82 on the final exam.

32. For these situations, state which measure of central tendency—mean, median, or mode—should be used.

  a. The most typical case is desired.

  b. The distribution is open-ended.

c. There is an extreme value in the data set.

d. The data are categorical.

e. Further statistical computations will be needed.

f. The values are to be divided into two approximately equal groups, one group containing the larger values and one containing the smaller values.

33. Describe which measure of central tendency—mean, median, or mode—was probably used in each situation.

a. One-half of the factory workers make more than $5.37 per hour, and one-half make less than $5.37 per hour.

b. The average number of children per family in the Plaza Heights Complex is 1.8.

c. Most people prefer red convertibles over any other colour.

d. The average person cuts the lawn once a week.

e. The most common fear today is fear of speaking in public.

f. The average age of college and university professors is 42.3 years.

34. 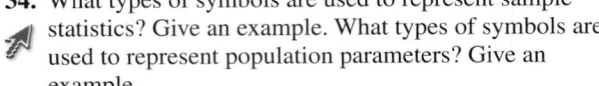 What types of symbols are used to represent sample statistics? Give an example. What types of symbols are used to represent population parameters? Give an example.

35. **Fast-Food Earnings** A local fast-food company claims that the average salary of its employees is $13.23 per hour. An employee states that most employees make minimum wage. If both are being truthful, how could both be correct?

Extending the Concepts ≫

36. If the mean of five values is 64, find the sum of the values.

37. If the mean of five values is 8.2 and four of the values are 6, 10, 7, and 12, find the fifth value.

38. Find the mean of 10, 20, 30, 40, and 50.

a. Add 10 to each value and find the mean.

b. Subtract 10 from each value and find the mean.

c. Multiply each value by 10 and find the mean.

d. Divide each value by 10 and find the mean.

e. Make a general statement about each situation.

39. The *harmonic mean* (HM) is defined as the number of values, divided by the sum of the reciprocals of each value. The formula is

$$HM = \frac{n}{\Sigma(1/X)}$$

For example, the harmonic mean of 1, 4, 5, and 2 is

$$HM = \frac{4}{1/1 + 1/4 + 1/5 + 1/2} = 2.05$$

This mean is useful for finding the average speed. Suppose a person drove 180 kilometres at 60 kilometres per hour and returned, driving 80 kilometres per hour. The average speed is not 70 kilometres per hour, which is found by adding 60 and 80 and dividing by 2. The average speed is found as shown.

Since

Time = distance ÷ rate

then

$$\text{Time 1} = \frac{180}{60} = 3.0 \text{ hours to the destination}$$

$$\text{Time 2} = \frac{180}{80} = 2.25 \text{ hours to make the return trip}$$

Hence, the total time is 5.25 hours, and the total kilometres driven are 360. Now, the average speed is

$$\text{Rate} = \frac{\text{Distance}}{\text{Time}} = \frac{360}{5.25} = 68.57 \begin{array}{l}\text{kilometres per}\\\text{hour (rounded)}\end{array}$$

This value can be found by using the harmonic mean formula

$$HM = \frac{2}{1/60 + 1/80} = 68.57 \text{ (rounded)}$$

a. A salesperson drives 300 kilometres round trip at 60 kilometres per hour going to Ottawa and 50 kilometres per hour returning home. Find the average kilometres per hour.

b. A bus driver drives 450 kilometres to Vancouver at 90 kilometres per hour and returns, driving 100 kilometres per hour. Find the average speed.

c. A carpenter buys $500 worth of nails at $25 per kilogram and $500 worth of nails at $5 per kilogram. Find the average cost of 1 kilogram of nails.

40. The *geometric mean* (GM) is defined as the *n*th root of the product of *n* values. The formula is

$$GM = \sqrt[n]{(X_1)(X_2)(X_3)\cdots(X_n)}$$

The geometric mean of 4 and 16 is

$$GM = \sqrt{(4)(16)} = \sqrt{64} = 8$$

The geometric mean of 1, 3, and 9 is

$$GM = \sqrt[3]{(1)(3)(9)} = \sqrt[3]{27} = 3$$

The geometric mean is useful in finding the average of percentages, ratios, indexes, or growth rates. For example, if a person receives a 20% raise after one year of service and a 10% raise after the second year of service, the average percentage raise per year is not 15 but 14.89%, as shown.

$$GM = \sqrt{(1.2)(1.1)} = 1.1489$$

or

$$GM = \sqrt{(120)(110)} = 114.89\%$$

His salary is 120% at the end of the first year and 110% at the end of the second year. This is equivalent to an average of 14.89%, since 114.89% − 100% = 14.89%.

This answer can also be shown by assuming that the person makes $10,000 to start and receives two raises of 20% and 10%.

Raise 1 = 10,000 · 20% = $2000
Raise 2 = 12,000 · 10% = $1200

His total salary raise is $3200. This total is equivalent to

$10,000 · 14.89% = $1489.00
$11,489 · 14.89% = _1710.71_
$3199.71 ≈ $3200

Find the geometric mean of each of these.

a. The growth rates of the Living Life Insurance Corporation for the past 3 years were 35, 24, and 18%.

b. A person received these percentage raises in salary over a 4-year period: 8, 6, 4, and 5%.

c. A stock increased each year for 5 years at these percentages: 10, 8, 12, 9, and 3%.

d. The price increases, in percentages, for the cost of food in a specific geographic region for the past 3 years were 1, 3, and 5.5%.

41. A useful mean in the physical sciences (such as voltage) is the *quadratic mean* (QM), which is found by taking the square root of the average of the squares of each value. The formula is

$$QM = \sqrt{\frac{\Sigma X^2}{n}}$$

The quadratic mean of 3, 5, 6, and 10 is

$$QM = \sqrt{\frac{3^2 + 5^2 + 6^2 + 10^2}{4}}$$
$$= \sqrt{42.5} = 6.52$$

Find the quadratic mean of 8, 6, 3, 5, and 4.

42. An approximate median can be found for data that have been grouped into a frequency distribution. First it is necessary to find the median class. This is the class that contains the median value. That is the $n/2$ data value. Then it is assumed that the data values are evenly distributed throughout the median class. The formula is

$$MD = \frac{(n/2) - cf}{f}(w) + L_m$$

where

n = sum of frequencies
cf = cumulative frequency of class immediately preceding the median class
w = width of median class
f = frequency of median class
L_m = lower boundary of median class

Using this formula, find the median for data in the frequency distribution in Exercise 15.

3–2	Measures of Variation ❯

In statistics, to describe the data set accurately, statisticians must know more than the measures of central tendency. Consider Example 3–15.

| Example 3–15 | **Comparison of Outdoor Paints** |

LO2

Describe data using measures of variation, such as the range, variance, and standard deviation.

A testing lab wishes to test two experimental brands of outdoor paint to see how long each will last before fading. The testing lab makes six 3.78-L pails of each paint to test. Since different chemical agents are added to each group and only six cans are involved, these two groups constitute two small populations. The results (in months) are shown. Find the mean and median of each group.

Brand A	Brand B
10	35
60	45
50	30
30	35
40	40
20	25

Solution

The mean for brand A is

$$\mu = \frac{\Sigma X}{N} = \frac{210}{6} = 35 \text{ months}$$

The mean for brand B is

$$\mu = \frac{\Sigma X}{N} = \frac{210}{6} = 35 \text{ months}$$

The median for brand A is

$$\text{MD} = \frac{30 + 40}{2} = 35 \text{ months}$$

The median for brand B is

$$\text{MD} = \frac{35 + 35}{2} = 35 \text{ months}$$

Since both the means and the medians are equal in Example 3–15, one might conclude that both brands of paint last equally well. However, when the data sets are examined graphically, a somewhat different conclusion might be drawn. See Figure 3–2.

Figure 3–2

Examining Data Sets Graphically

Variation of paint (in months)

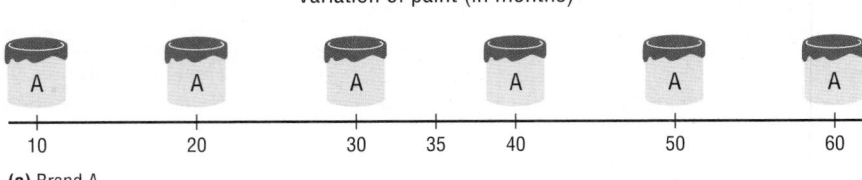

(a) Brand A

Variation of paint (in months)

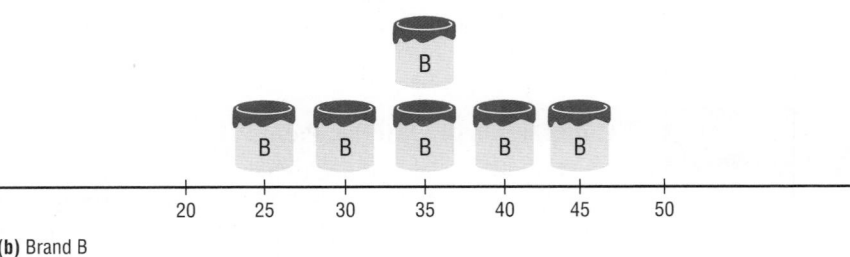

(b) Brand B

As Figure 3–2 shows, even though both the means and medians are the same for each brand, the spread, or variation, is quite different. Figure 3–2 shows that brand B performs more consistently; it is less variable. For the spread or variability of a data set, three measures are commonly used: *range, variance,* and *standard deviation.* Each measure will be discussed in this section.

Range

The range is the simplest of the three measures.

The **range** is the highest value minus the lowest value. The symbol R is used for the range.

$$R = \text{highest value} - \text{lowest value}$$

Example 3–16

Comparison of Outdoor Paints

Find the ranges for the paints in Example 3–15.

Solution

For brand A, the range is

$$R = 60 - 10 = 50 \text{ months}$$

For brand B, the range is

$$R = 45 - 25 = 20 \text{ months}$$

Make sure the range is given as a single number.

The range for brand A shows that 50 months separate the largest data value from the smallest data value. For brand B, 20 months separate the largest data value from the smallest data value, which is less than one-half of brand A's range.

One extremely high or one extremely low data value can affect the range markedly, as shown in Example 3–17.

Example 3–17

Employee Salaries

The salaries for the staff of the XYZ Manufacturing Co. are shown here. Find the range.

Staff	Salary
Owner	$100,000
Manager	40,000
Sales representative	30,000
Workers	25,000
	15,000
	18,000

Solution

The range is $R = \$100,000 - \$15,000 = \$85,000$.

Since the owner's salary is included in the data for Example 3–17, the range is a large number. To have a more meaningful statistic to measure the variability, statisticians use measures called the *variance* and *standard deviation.*

Population Variance and Standard Deviation

Before the variance and standard deviation are defined formally, the computational procedure will be shown, since the definition is derived from the procedure.

Rounding Rule for the Standard Deviation   The rounding rule for the standard deviation is the same as that for the mean. The final answer should be rounded to one more decimal place than that of the original data.

Example 3–18

Comparison of Outdoor Paints

Find the variance and standard deviation for the data set for brand A paint in Example 3–15.

10, 60, 50, 30, 40, 20

Solution

Step 1 Find the mean for the data.

$$\mu = \frac{\Sigma X}{N} = \frac{10 + 60 + 50 + 30 + 40 + 20}{6} = \frac{210}{6} = 35$$

Step 2 Subtract the mean from each data value.

$$10 - 35 = -25 \quad 50 - 35 = +15 \quad 40 - 35 = +5$$
$$60 - 35 = +25 \quad 30 - 35 = -5 \quad 20 - 35 = -15$$

Step 3 Square each result.

$$(-25)^2 = 625 \quad (+15)^2 = 225 \quad (+5)^2 = 25$$
$$(+25)^2 = 625 \quad (-5)^2 = 25 \quad (-15)^2 = 225$$

Step 4 Find the sum of the squares.

$$625 + 625 + 225 + 25 + 25 + 225 = 1750$$

Step 5 Divide the sum by N to get the variance.

Variance $= 1750 \div 6 = 291.7$ (rounded)

Step 6 Take the square root of the variance to get the standard deviation. Hence, the standard deviation equals $\sqrt{291.7}$, or approximately 17.1. It is helpful to make a table.

A Values (X)	B $X - \mu$	C $(X - \mu)^2$
10	−25	625
60	+25	625
50	+15	225
30	−5	25
40	+5	25
20	−15	225
		1750

Column A contains the raw data X. Column B contains the differences $X - \mu$ obtained in step 2. Column C contains the squares of the differences obtained in step 3.

The preceding computational procedure reveals several things. First, the square root of the variance gives the standard deviation, and vice versa, squaring the standard deviation gives the variance. Second, the variance is actually the average of the square of the distance that each value is from the mean. Therefore, if the values are near the mean, the variance will be small. In contrast, if the values are far from the mean, the variance will be large.

One might wonder why the squared distances are used instead of the actual distances. One reason is that the sum of the distances will always be zero. To verify this result for a specific case, add the values in column B of the table in Example 3–18. When each value is squared, the negative signs are eliminated.

Finally, why is it necessary to take the square root? The reason is that since the distances were squared, the units of the resultant numbers are the squares of the units of the original raw data. Finding the square root of the variance puts the standard deviation in the same units as the raw data.

When you are finding the square root, always use its positive or principal value, since the variance and standard deviation of a data set can never be negative.

The **variance** is the average of the squares of the distance each value is from the mean. The symbol for the population variance is σ^2 (σ is the Greek lower-case letter sigma). The formula for the population variance is

$$\sigma^2 = \frac{\Sigma(X - \mu)^2}{N}$$

where
  X = individual value
  μ = population mean
  N = population size

The **standard deviation** is the square root of the variance. The symbol for the population standard deviation is σ.
    The corresponding formula for the population standard deviation is

$$\sigma = \sqrt{\sigma^2} = \sqrt{\frac{\Sigma(X - \mu)^2}{N}}$$

Example 3–19

Comparison of Outdoor Paints

Find the variance and standard deviation for brand B paint data in Example 3–15. The months were

35, 45, 30, 35, 40, 25

Solution

Step 1 Find the mean.

$$\mu = \frac{\Sigma X}{N} = \frac{35 + 45 + 30 + 35 + 40 + 25}{6} = \frac{210}{6} = 35$$

Step 2 Subtract the mean from each value, and place the result in column B of the table.

Step 3 Square each result and place the squares in column C of the table.

A	B	C
X	$X - \mu$	$(X - \mu)^2$
35	0	0
45	10	100
30	−5	25
35	0	0
40	5	25
25	−10	100

Step 4   Find the sum of the squares in column C.

$$\Sigma(X - \mu)^2 = 0 + 100 + 25 + 0 + 25 + 100 = 250$$

Step 5   Divide the sum by N to get the variance.

$$\sigma^2 = \frac{\Sigma(X - \mu)^2}{N} = \frac{250}{6} = 41.7$$

Step 6   Take the square root to get the standard deviation.

$$\sigma = \sqrt{\frac{\Sigma(X - \mu)^2}{N}} = \sqrt{41.7} = 6.5 \text{ (rounded)}$$

Hence, the standard deviation is 6.5.

Since the standard deviation of brand A is 17.1 (see Example 3–18) and the standard deviation of brand B is 6.5, the data are more variable for brand A. *In summary, when the means are equal, the larger the variance or standard deviation is, the more variable the data are.*

Sample Variance and Standard Deviation

When computing the variance for a sample, one might expect the following expression to be used:

$$\frac{\Sigma(X - \overline{X})^2}{n}$$

where $\overline{X}$ is the sample mean and n is the sample size. *This formula is not usually used, however, since in most cases the purpose of calculating the statistic is to estimate the corresponding parameter.* For example, the sample mean $\overline{X}$ is used to estimate the population mean μ. The expression

$$\frac{\Sigma(X - \overline{X})^2}{n}$$

does not give the best estimate of the population variance because when the population is large and the sample is small (usually less than 30), the variance computed by this formula usually underestimates the population variance, resulting in a biased estimate. Therefore, instead of dividing by n, find the variance of the sample by dividing by $n - 1$, giving a slightly larger value and an *unbiased* estimate of the population variance.

The formula for the sample variance, denoted by s^2, is

$$s^2 = \frac{\Sigma(X - \overline{X})^2}{n - 1}$$

where
$\overline{X}$ = sample mean
n = sample size

To find the standard deviation of a sample, one must take the square root of the sample variance, which was found by using the preceding formula.

Formula for the Sample Standard Deviation

The standard deviation of a sample (denoted by s) is

$$s = \sqrt{s^2} = \sqrt{\frac{\Sigma(X - \overline{X})^2}{n - 1}}$$

where

$$
\begin{aligned}
X &= \text{individual value} \\
\overline{X} &= \text{sample mean} \\
n &= \text{sample size}
\end{aligned}
$$

Shortcut formulas for computing the variance and standard deviation are presented next and will be used in the remainder of the chapter and in the exercises. These formulas are mathematically equivalent to the preceding formulas and do not involve using the mean. They save time when repeated subtracting and squaring occur in the original formulas. They are also more accurate when the mean has been rounded.

Shortcut or Computational Formulas for s^2 and s

The shortcut formulas for computing the variance and standard deviation for data obtained from samples are as follows.

Variance

$$s^2 = \frac{n(\Sigma X^2) - (\Sigma X)^2}{n(n - 1)}$$

Standard deviation

$$s = \sqrt{\frac{n(\Sigma X^2) - (\Sigma X)^2}{n(n - 1)}}$$

Examples 3–20 and 3–21 explain how to use the shortcut formulas.

Example 3–20

European Auto Sales

Find the sample variance and standard deviation for the amount of European auto sales for a sample of 6 years shown. The data are in millions of dollars.

11.2, 11.9, 12.0, 12.8, 13.4, 14.3

Source: USA TODAY.

Solution

Step 1 Find the sum of the values.

$$\Sigma X = 11.2 + 11.9 + 12.0 + 12.8 + 13.4 + 14.3 = 75.6$$

Step 2 Square each value and find the sum.

$$\Sigma X^2 = 11.2^2 + 11.9^2 + 12.0^2 + 12.8^2 + 13.4^2 + 14.3^2 = 958.94$$

Step 3 Substitute in the formulas and solve.

$$s^2 = \frac{n(\Sigma X^2) - (\Sigma X)^2}{n(n-1)}$$

$$= \frac{6(958.94) - 75.6^2}{6(6-1)}$$

$$= \frac{5753.64 - 5715.36}{6(5)}$$

$$= \frac{38.28}{30}$$

$$= 1.276$$

The variance is 1.28 (rounded).

$$s = \sqrt{1.28} \approx 1.13$$

Hence, the sample standard deviation is 1.13.

Note that ΣX^2 is not the same as $(\Sigma X)^2$. The notation ΣX^2 means to square the values first, then sum; $(\Sigma X)^2$ means to sum the values first, then square the sum.

Variance and Standard Deviation for Grouped Data

The procedure for finding the variance and standard deviation for grouped data is similar to that for finding the mean for grouped data, and it uses the midpoints of each class.

Example 3–21

Kilometres Run per Week

Find the variance and the standard deviation for the frequency distribution of the data in Example 2–7 on page 48. The data represent the number of kilometres that 20 runners ran during one week.

Class	Frequency	Midpoint
5.5–10.5	1	8
10.5–15.5	2	13
15.5–20.5	3	18
20.5–25.5	5	23
25.5–30.5	4	28
30.5–35.5	3	33
35.5–40.5	2	38

Solution

Step 1 Make a table as shown, and find the midpoint of each class.

A Class	B Frequency (f)	C Midpoint (X_m)	D $f \cdot X_m$	E $f \cdot X_m^2$
5.5–10.5	1	8		
10.5–15.5	2	13		
15.5–20.5	3	18		
20.5–25.5	5	23		
25.5–30.5	4	28		
30.5–35.5	3	33		
35.5–40.5	2	38		

Step 2   Multiply the frequency by the midpoint for each class, and place the products in column D.

$$1 \cdot 8 = 8 \qquad 2 \cdot 13 = 26 \qquad \ldots \qquad 2 \cdot 38 = 76$$

Step 3   Multiply the frequency by the square of the midpoint, and place the products in column E.

$$1 \cdot 8^2 = 64 \qquad 2 \cdot 13^2 = 338 \qquad \ldots \qquad 2 \cdot 38^2 = 2888$$

Step 4   Find the sums of columns B, D, and E. The sum of column B is n, the sum of column D is $\Sigma f \cdot X_m$, and the sum of column E is $\Sigma f \cdot X_m^2$. The completed table is shown.

A Class	B Frequency	C Midpoint	D $f \cdot X_m$	E $f \cdot X_m^2$
5.5–10.5	1	8	8	64
10.5–15.5	2	13	26	338
15.5–20.5	3	18	54	972
20.5–25.5	5	23	115	2,645
25.5–30.5	4	28	112	3,136
30.5–35.5	3	33	99	3,267
35.5–40.5	2	38	76	2,888
	$n = 20$		$\Sigma f \cdot X_m = 490$	$\Sigma f \cdot X_m^2 = 13{,}310$

Step 5   Substitute in the formula and solve for s^2 to get the variance.

$$s^2 = \frac{n(\Sigma f \cdot X_m^2) - (\Sigma f \cdot X_m)^2}{n(n-1)}$$

$$= \frac{20(13{,}310) - 490^2}{20(20-1)}$$

$$= \frac{266{,}200 - 240{,}100}{20(19)}$$

$$= \frac{26{,}100}{380}$$

$$\approx 68.7$$

Step 6   Take the square root of the variance to get the standard deviation.

$$s = \sqrt{68.7} \approx 8.3$$

Be sure to use the number found in the sum of column B (i.e., the sum of the frequencies) for n. Do not use the number of classes.

The steps for finding the variance and standard deviation for grouped data are summarized in this Procedure Table.

Procedure Table

Finding the Sample Variance and Standard Deviation for Grouped Data

Step 1   Make a table as shown, and find the midpoint of each class.

A Class	B Frequency	C Midpoint	D $f \cdot X_m$	E $f \cdot X_m^2$

Step 2   Multiply the frequency by the midpoint for each class, and place the products in column D.

Step 3   Multiply the frequency by the square of the midpoint, and place the products in column E.

Step 4   Find the sums of columns B, D, and E. (The sum of column B is n. The sum of column D is $\Sigma f \cdot X_m$. The sum of column E is $\Sigma f \cdot X_m^2$.)

Step 5   Substitute in the formula and solve for s^2 to get the variance.

$$s^2 = \frac{n(\Sigma f \cdot X_m^2) - (\Sigma f \cdot X_m)^2}{n(n-1)}$$

Step 6   Take the square root of the variance to get the standard deviation.

$$s = \sqrt{s^2}$$

The three measures of variation are summarized in Table 3–2.

Table 3–2	Summary of Measures of Variation	
Measure	**Definition**	**Symbol(s)**
Range	Distance between highest value and lowest value	R
Variance	Average of the squares of the distance that each value is from the mean	σ^2, s^2
Standard deviation	Square root of the variance	σ, s

Uses of the Variance and Standard Deviation

1. As previously stated, variances and standard deviations can be used to determine the spread of the data. If the variance or standard deviation is large, the data are more dispersed. This information is useful in comparing two (or more) data sets to determine which is more (most) variable.

2. The measures of variance and standard deviation are used to determine the consistency of a variable. For example, in the manufacture of fittings, such as nuts and bolts, the variation in the diameters must be small, or the parts will not fit together.

3. The variance and standard deviation are used to determine the number of data values that fall within a specified interval in a distribution. For example, Chebyshev's theorem (explained later) shows that, for any distribution, at least 75% of the data values will fall within 2 standard deviations of the mean.

4. Finally, the variance and standard deviation are used quite often in inferential statistics. These uses will be shown in later chapters of this textbook.

Coefficient of Variation

Whenever two samples have the same units of measure, the variance and standard deviation for each can be compared directly. For example, suppose an automobile dealer wanted to compare the standard deviation of kilometres driven for the cars she received as trade-ins on new cars. She found that for a specific year, the standard deviation for Buicks was 679 kilometres and the standard deviation for Cadillacs was 563 kilometres. She could say that the variation in kilometres was greater in the Buicks. But what if a manager wanted to compare the standard deviations of two different variables, such as the number of sales per salesperson over a three-month period and the commissions made by these salespeople?

A statistic that allows one to compare standard deviations when the units are different, as in this example, is called the *coefficient of variation.*

> The **coefficient of variation,** denoted by CVar, is the standard deviation divided by the mean. The result is expressed as a percentage.
>
>   **For samples,**   **For populations,**
>
> $$\text{CVar} = \frac{s}{\overline{X}} \cdot 100\% \qquad \text{CVar} = \frac{\sigma}{\mu} \cdot 100\%$$

Example 3–22

Sales of Cars

The mean of the number of sales of cars over a 3-month period is 87, and the standard deviation is 5. The mean of the commissions is \$5225, and the standard deviation is \$773. Compare the variations of the two.

Solution

The coefficients of variation are

$$\text{CVar} = \frac{s}{\overline{X}} = \frac{5}{87} \cdot 100\% \approx 5.7\% \qquad\qquad \text{sales}$$

$$\text{CVar} = \frac{773}{5225} \cdot 100\% \approx 14.8\% \qquad\qquad \text{commissions}$$

Since the coefficient of variation is larger for commissions, the commissions are more variable than the sales.

Example 3–23

Nurses' Work Experience and Wages

The mean of emergency room registered nurses' work experience at a British Columbia regional hospital was 18.5 years, with a variance of 58.5. The mean hourly wage of the registered nurses was \$33.22, with a variance of 45.29. Compare the variations.

Solution

The coefficients of variation are

$$\text{CVar} = \frac{\sqrt{s^2}}{\overline{X}} = \frac{\sqrt{58.5}}{18.5} \cdot 100\% \approx 41.3\% \qquad\qquad \text{work experience}$$

$$\text{CVar} = \frac{\sqrt{s^2}}{\overline{X}} = \frac{\sqrt{45.29}}{33.22} \cdot 100\% \approx 20.3\% \qquad\qquad \text{hourly wage}$$

The registered nurses' work experience is more variable than the hourly wage since the coefficient of variation is higher.

Range Rule of Thumb

The range can be used to approximate the standard deviation. The approximation is called the **range rule of thumb.**

The Range Rule of Thumb

A rough estimate of the standard deviation is

$$s \approx \frac{\text{range}}{4}$$

In other words, if the range is divided by 4, an approximate value for the standard deviation is obtained. For example, the standard deviation for the data set 5, 8, 8, 9, 10, 12, and 13 is 2.7, and the range is $13 - 5 = 8$. The range rule of thumb is $s \approx 2$. The range rule of thumb in this case underestimates the standard deviation somewhat; however, it is in the ballpark.

A note of caution should be mentioned here. The range rule of thumb is only an *approximation* and should be used when the distribution of data values is unimodal and roughly symmetric.

The range rule of thumb can be used to estimate the largest and smallest data values of a data set. The smallest data value will be approximately 2 standard deviations below the mean, and the largest data value will be approximately 2 standard deviations above the mean of the data set. The mean for the previous data set is 9.3; hence,

$$\text{Smallest data value} = \overline{X} - 2s = 9.3 - 2(2.8) = 3.7$$
$$\text{Largest data value} = \overline{X} + 2s = 9.3 + 2(2.8) = 14.9$$

Notice that the smallest data value was 5, and the largest data value was 13. Again, these are rough approximations. For many data sets, almost all data values will fall within 2 standard deviations of the mean. Better approximations can be obtained by using Chebyshev's theorem and the empirical rule. These are explained next.

Chebyshev's Theorem

As stated previously, the variance and standard deviation of a variable can be used to determine the spread, or dispersion, of a variable. That is, the larger the variance or standard deviation, the more the data values are dispersed. For example, if two variables measured in the same units have the same mean, say, 70, and variable 1 has a standard deviation of 1.5 while variable 2 has a standard deviation of 10, then the data for variable 2 will be more spread out than the data for variable 1. *Chebyshev's theorem,* developed by the Russian mathematician Pafnuty L. Chebyshev (1821–1894), specifies the proportions of the spread in terms of the standard deviation.

> **Chebyshev's theorem** The proportion of values from a data set that will fall within k standard deviations of the mean will be at least $1 - 1/k^2$, where k is a number greater than 1 (k is not necessarily an integer).

This theorem states that at least three-fourths, or 75%, of the data values will fall within 2 standard deviations of the mean of the data set. This result is found by substituting $k = 2$ in the expression.

$$1 - \frac{1}{k^2} \qquad \text{or} \qquad 1 - \frac{1}{2^2} = 1 - \frac{1}{4} = \frac{3}{4} = 75\%$$

For the example in which variable 1 has a mean of 70 and a standard deviation of 1.5, at least three-fourths, or 75%, of the data values fall between 67 and 73. These values are found by adding 2 standard deviations to the mean and subtracting 2 standard deviations from the mean, as shown:

$$70 + 2(1.5) = 70 + 3 = 73$$

and

$$70 - 2(1.5) = 70 - 3 = 67$$

For variable 2, at least three-fourths, or 75%, of the data values fall between 50 and 90. Again, these values are found by adding and subtracting, respectively, 2 standard deviations to and from the mean.

$$70 + 2(10) = 70 + 20 = 90$$

and

$$70 - 2(10) = 70 - 20 = 50$$

Furthermore, the theorem states that at least eight-ninths, or 88.89%, of the data values will fall within 3 standard deviations of the mean. This result is found by letting $k = 3$ and substituting in the expression.

$$1 - \frac{1}{k^2} \quad \text{or} \quad 1 - \frac{1}{3^2} = 1 - \frac{1}{9} = \frac{8}{9} = 88.89\% \,(\text{rounded})$$

For variable 1, at least eight-ninths, or approximately 88.89%, of the data values fall between 65.5 and 74.5, since

$$70 + 3(1.5) = 70 + 4.5 = 74.5$$

and

$$70 - 3(1.5) = 70 - 4.5 = 65.5$$

For variable 2, at least eight-ninths, or approximately 88.89%, of the data values fall between 40 and 100.

This theorem can be applied to any distribution regardless of its shape (see Figure 3–3).

Examples 3–24 and 3–25 illustrate the application of Chebyshev's theorem.

Figure 3–3

Chebyshev's Theorem

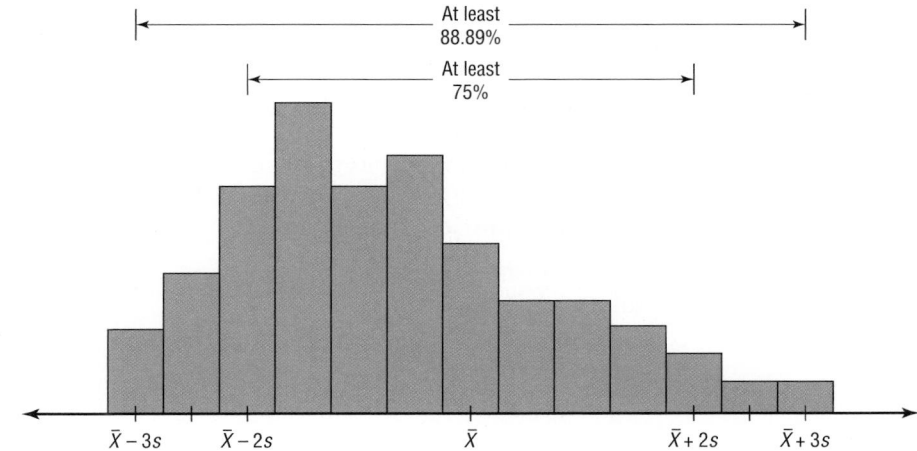

| Example 3–24 | **House Prices** |

The mean price of houses in a certain neighbourhood is $360,000, and the standard deviation is $45,000. Find the price range for which at least 75% of the houses will sell.

Solution

Chebyshev's theorem states that three-fourths, or 75%, of the data values will fall within 2 standard deviations of the mean. Thus,

$$\$360{,}000 + 2(\$45{,}000) = \$360{,}000 + \$90{,}000 = \$450{,}000$$

and

$$\$360{,}000 - 2(\$45{,}000) = \$360{,}000 - \$90{,}000 = \$270{,}000$$

Therefore, at least 75% of all homes sold in the area will have a price range from $270,000 and $450,000.

Chebyshev's theorem can be used to find the minimum percentage of data values that will fall between any two given values. The procedure is shown in Example 3–25.

| Example 3–25 | **Travel Allowances** |

A survey of local companies found that the mean amount of travel allowance for executives was $0.25 per kilometre. The standard deviation was $0.02. Using Chebyshev's theorem, find the minimum percentage of the data values that will fall between $0.20 and $0.30.

Solution

Step 1 Subtract the mean from the larger value.

$$\$0.30 - \$0.25 = \$0.05$$

Step 2 Divide the difference by the standard deviation to get k.

$$k = \frac{0.05}{0.02} = 2.5$$

Step 3 Use Chebyshev's theorem to find the percentage.

$$1 - \frac{1}{k^2} = 1 - \frac{1}{2.5^2} = 1 - \frac{1}{6.25} = 1 - 0.16 = 0.84 \qquad \text{or} \qquad 84\%$$

Hence, at least 84% of the data values will fall between $0.20 and $0.30.

The Empirical (Normal) Rule

Chebyshev's theorem applies to any distribution regardless of its shape. However, when a distribution is *bell-shaped* (or what is called *normal*), the following statements, which make up the **empirical rule,** are true.

Approximately 68% of the data values will fall within 1 standard deviation of the mean.

Approximately 95% of the data values will fall within 2 standard deviations of the mean.

Approximately 99.7% of the data values will fall within 3 standard deviations of the mean.

For example, suppose that the scores on a national achievement exam have a mean of 480 and a standard deviation of 90. If these scores are normally distributed, then approximately 68% will fall between 390 and 570 ($480 + 90 = 570$ and $480 - 90 = 390$). Approximately 95% of the scores will fall between 300 and 660 ($480 + 2 \cdot 90 = 660$ and $480 - 2 \cdot 90 = 300$). Approximately 99.7% will fall between 210 and 750 ($480 + 3 \cdot 90 = 750$ and $480 - 3 \cdot 90 = 210$). See Figure 3–4. (The empirical rule is explained in greater detail in Chapter 7.)

Figure 3–4

The Empirical Rule

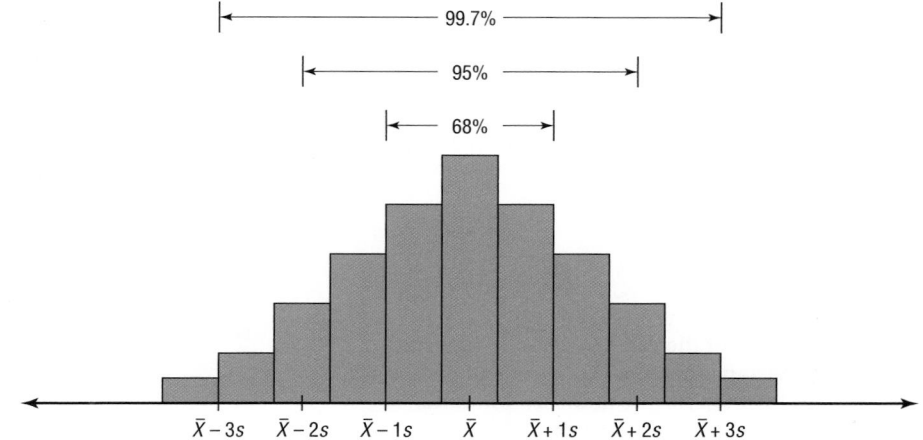

3–2   Applying the Concepts

Blood Pressure

The table lists means and standard deviations. The mean is the number before the plus/minus, and the standard deviation is the number after the plus/minus. The results are from a study attempting to find the average blood pressure of older adults. Use the results to answer the questions.

	Normotensive		**Hypertensive**	
	Men ($n = 1200$)	**Women** ($n = 1400$)	**Men** ($n = 1100$)	**Women** ($n = 1300$)
Age	55 ± 10	55 ± 10	60 ± 10	64 ± 10
Blood pressure (mm Hg)				
Systolic	123 ± 9	121 ± 11	153 ± 17	156 ± 20
Diastolic	78 ± 7	76 ± 7	91 ± 10	88 ± 10

1. Apply Chebyshev's theorem to the systolic blood pressure of normotensive men. At least how many of the men in the study fall within 1 standard deviation of the mean?

2. At least how many of those men in the study fall within 2 standard deviations of the mean?

Assume that blood pressure is normally distributed among older adults. Answer the following questions, using the empirical rule instead of Chebyshev's theorem.

3. Give ranges for the diastolic blood pressure (normotensive and hypertensive) of older women.

4. Do the normotensive, male, systolic blood pressure ranges overlap with the hypertensive, male, systolic, blood pressure ranges?

See page 145 for the answers.

Exercises 3–2

1. What is the relationship between the variance and the standard deviation?

2. Why might the range *not* be the best estimate of variability?

3. What are the symbols used to represent the population variance and standard deviation?

4. What are the symbols used to represent the sample variance and standard deviation?

5. Why is the unbiased estimator of variance used?

6. The three data sets have the same mean and range, but is the variation the same? Prove your answer by computing the standard deviation. Assume the data were obtained from samples.

   a. 5, 7, 9, 11, 13, 15, 17
   b. 5, 6, 7, 11, 15, 16, 17
   c. 5, 5, 5, 11, 17, 17, 17

For Exercises 7–13, find the range, variance, and standard deviation. Assume the data represent samples, and use the shortcut formula for the unbiased estimator to compute the variance and standard deviation.

7. **City Homicide Rates** The homicide rates per 100,000 population for Canada's largest cities with population over 500,000 are shown for a recent year. Are the data consistent or do they vary? Explain your answer.

   2.0, 1.3, 2.9, 2.5, 4.3, 1.3, 0.7, 3.7, 1.6
   Source: Statistics Canada, *Canada Year Book 2008.*

8. **Cigarette Cost** The following data represent the cost of one cigarette (in cents), out of a carton of 200, in each of Canada's provinces and territories.

   38, 40, 42, 36, 42, 40, 34, 39, 32, 42, 43, 37, 35

   Use the range rule of thumb to estimate the standard deviation. Compare the estimate to the actual standard deviation.
   Source: Smoking and Health Action Foundation.

9. **Country Life Expectancies** The countries with the highest life expectancy, in years, and the lowest life expectancies, in years, are shown below. Which data set is more variable?

High life expectancy		Low life expectancy	
Macau	84.4	Chad	47.7
Andorra	82.5	Nigeria	46.9
Japan	82.1	Zimbabwe	45.8
Singapore	82.0	Central African Republic	44.5
Hong Kong	81.9	Afghanistan	44.4
Australia	81.6	Liberia	41.8
Canada	81.2	Mozambique	41.2
France	81.0	Lesotho	40.4
Sweden	80.9	Zambia	38.6
Switzerland	80.9	Angola	38.2

Source: Central Intelligence Agency, *The World Factbook,* "Country Comparison: Life Expectancy at Birth."

10. **Areas of Provinces** The total land area (rounded to 1000 square kilometres or 1000 km²) for the five largest Canadian provinces is listed here.

QC	1,365,128	AB	642,317
BC	925,186	SK	591,670
ON	917,741		

The total land area (rounded to 1000 square kilometres or 1000 km²) for the five smallest Canadian provinces is listed here.

MB	553,556	NS	53,338
NL	373,872	PE	5,660
NB	71,450		

Which data set is more variable?
Source: Natural Resources Canada, *The Atlas of Canada.*

11. **Storeys in the Tallest Buildings** Shown here are the numbers of storeys in the 11 tallest buildings in Hong Kong, People's Republic of China.

   88, 78, 72, 73, 80, 62, 75, 59, 75, 72, 52

   Shown here are the numbers of storeys in the 11 tallest buildings in New York City.

   102, 77, 66, 70, 59, 72, 69, 75, 60, 48, 60

   Which data set is more variable?
   Source: www.emporis.com.

12. **Cost of Gasoline** The following data are the prices per litre of premium gasoline in Canadian dollars in eight foreign countries.

   $1.85, $1.76, $1.69, $1.64, $1.59, $1.34, $0.98, $0.70

   Do you think the standard deviation of these data is representative of the population standard deviation of gasoline prices in all foreign countries? Explain your answer.
   Source: Reuters News Service.

13. **Student–Teacher Ratios** The average (mean) student-to-educator ratio in Canada for elementary and secondary schools was 15.9 in a recent year. The number of students per educator ranged provincially 11.5 to 17.5. Use the range rule of thumb to estimate the standard deviation of student-to-educator ratio.
   Source: Statistics Canada, *Canada Yearbook 2008.*

14. **Home Runs** Find the range, variance, and standard deviation for the distances of the home runs for McGwire and Sosa, using the data in Exercise 18 in Section 2–1. Compare the ranges and standard deviations. Decide which is more variable or if the variability is about the same. (Use individual data.)

15. **City Population Census** Find the range, variance, and standard deviation for each data set in Exercise 11 of Section 3–1. Based on the results, which data set is more variable?

16. Unemployed Work Force The number of unemployed workers, in thousands, for each of Canada's provinces was reported during the 2009 recession. Find the range, variance and standard deviation.

40.6	9.4	47.5	35.5	341
674	34.3	28.5	158.5	204.9

Source: Statistics Canada, *The Daily,* "Latest Release from the Labour Force Survey," July 9, 2010.

17. World's Highest Mountains Find the range, variance, and standard deviation for the data in Exercise 17 of Section 2–1.

18. NHL Team Scoring The number of goals that each team scored (goals for) and the number of goals that were scored on the team (goals against) are represented below for the National Hockey League 2008–2009 regular season. Find the variance and standard deviation for each frequency distribution. Compare the results.

Goals for	Frequency	Goals against	Frequency
180–199	1	180–199	1
200–219	8	200–219	5
220–239	6	220–239	12
240–259	9	240–259	8
260–279	5	260–279	2
280–299	1	280–299	2

Source: NHL.com, *Standings, 2008–2009 Regular Season.*

For Exercises 19 through 27, find the variance and standard deviation.

19. Detergent Cost per Load of Laundry The costs per load (in cents) of 35 laundry detergents tested by a consumer organization are shown here.

Cost per load	Frequency
13–19	2
20–26	7
27–33	12
34–40	5
41–47	6
48–54	1
55–61	0
62–68	2

20. Automobile Fuel Efficiency Thirty-five automobiles were tested for fuel efficiency (in L/100 km). This frequency distribution was obtained.

Fuel consumption	Frequency
3.5–6.5	5
6.5–9.5	15
9.5–12.5	8
12.5–15.5	4
15.5–18.5	0
18.5–21.5	2
21.5–24.5	1

21. Aboriginal Age Distribution The data show the age group distribution, in years, of Prince Edward Island's under–25 Aboriginal population by identity.

Age	Frequency
0–4	230
5–9	210
10–14	160
15–19	170
20–25	100

Source: Statistics Canada, *Canada Yearbook 2008.*

22. Reaction to Stimulus In a study of reaction times to a specific stimulus, a psychologist recorded these data (in seconds).

Reaction time	Frequency
2.1–2.7	12
2.8–3.4	13
3.5–4.1	7
4.2–4.8	5
4.9–5.5	2
5.6–6.2	1

23. Light Bulb Life Span Eighty randomly selected light bulbs were tested to determine their lifetimes (in hours). This frequency distribution was obtained.

Bulb life span	Frequency
52.5–63.5	6
63.5–74.5	12
74.5–85.5	25
85.5–96.5	18
96.5–107.5	14
107.5–118.5	5

24. Homicide Rates The data represent the homicide rate per 100,000 population in selected Canadian cities.

Homicide rate	Frequency
0–0.9	7
1–1.9	13
2–2.9	3
3–3.9	3
4–4.9	2

Source: Statistics Canada, *Crime and Justice,* "Homicides, by Census Metropolitan Area."

25. Battery Lives Eighty randomly selected batteries were tested to determine their lifetimes (in hours). The following frequency distribution was obtained.

Battery life	Frequency
62.5–73.5	5
73.5–84.5	14
84.5–95.5	18
95.5–106.5	25
106.5–117.5	12
117.5–128.5	6

Can it be concluded that the lifetimes of these brands of batteries are consistent?

26. Dog Reaction Times Find the variance and standard deviation for the two distributions in Exercise 8 in Section 2–2 and Exercise 18 in Section 2–2. Compare the variation of the data sets. Decide if one data set is more variable than the other.

27. Photocopier Service Calls This frequency distribution represents the data obtained from a sample of photocopier service technicians. The values are the days between service calls on 80 photocopy machines.

Days between calls	Frequency
25.5–28.5	5
28.5–31.5	9
31.5–34.5	32
34.5–37.5	20
37.5–40.5	12
40.5–43.5	2

28. Exam Scores The average score of the students in one calculus class is 110, with a standard deviation of 5; the average score of students in a statistics class is 106, with a standard deviation of 4. Which class is more variable in terms of scores?

29. Suspension Bridges The data show the lengths (in metres) of suspension bridges in the eastern part of North America and western part of North America. Compare the variability of the two samples.

East: 1298, 1067, 375, 655, 610, 533
West: 1250, 853, 704, 472, 457, 368

Source: World Almanac and Book of Facts.

30. Exam Scores The average score on an English final examination was 85, with a standard deviation of 5; the average score on a history final exam was 110, with a standard deviation of 8. Which class was more variable?

31. Accountants' Ages The average age of the accountants at Three Rivers Corp. is 26 years, with a standard deviation of 6 years; the average salary of the accountants is $31,000, with a standard deviation of $4000. Compare the variations of age and income.

32. Using Chebyshev's theorem, solve these problems for a distribution with a mean of 80 and a standard deviation of 10.

a. At least what percentage of values will fall between 60 and 100?

b. At least what percentage of values will fall between 65 and 95?

33. The mean of a distribution is 20 and the standard deviation is 2. Use Chebyshev's theorem.

a. At least what percentage of the values will fall between 10 and 30?

b. At least what percentage of the values will fall between 12 and 28?

34. In a distribution of 200 values, the mean is 50 and the standard deviation is 5. Use Chebyshev's theorem.

a. At least how many values will fall between 30 and 70?

b. At most how many values will be less than 40 or more than 60?

35. Fast-Food Industry Wages A sample of hourly wages of employees in the fast-food industry has a mean of $8.26 and a standard deviation of $0.33. Using Chebyshev's theorem, find the range in which at least 75% of the data values will fall.

36. Time Spent Online Adult Canadians spend an average of 2.7 hours per day online. Assuming a standard deviation of 30 minutes, find the range in which at least 88.89% of adult Canadian users spend online. Use Chebyshev's theorem.

Source: Ipsos, *News and Polls,* "Canadian Teenagers Are Leading the Online Revolution? Maybe Not...," February 27, 2008.

37. Cereal Potassium per Serving A survey of a number of the leading brands of cereal shows that the mean content of potassium per serving is 95 milligrams, and the standard deviation is 2 milligrams. Find the range in which at least 88.89% of the data will fall. Use Chebyshev's theorem.

38. Solid Waste Production The average college student produces 290 kilograms of solid waste each year, including 500 disposable cups and 140 kilograms of paper. If the standard deviation is approximately 36 kilograms, within what weight limits will at least 75% of all students' garbage lie?

Source: Environmental Sustainability Committee, www.esc.mtu.edu.

39. Trials to Learn a Maze The average of the number of trials it took a sample of mice to learn to traverse a maze was 12. The standard deviation was 3. Using Chebyshev's theorem, find the minimum percentage of data values that will fall in the range of 4 to 20 trials.

40. Farm Size The average farm in Canada in 2005 contained 295 hectares. Assume a standard deviation of 16 hectares. Use Chebyshev's theorem to find the minimum percentage of farms that fell in the range of 255 to 335 hectares.

Source: Agriculture and Agri-Food Canada, *Special Features: Census of Agriculture Summary.*

41. Fresh Food Consumption The average yearly per capita consumption of fresh fruit in Canada is 68.8 kilograms. Suppose that the distribution of fruit amounts consumed is bell-shaped with a standard deviation equal to 3.1 kilograms. What percentage of Canadians would you expect to consume more than 75 kilograms of fresh fruit per year?

Source: Statistics Canada.

42. Faculty Work Hours The average full-time faculty member in a post-secondary degree-granting institution works an average of 53 hours per week.

a. If we assume the standard deviation is 2.8 hours, what percentage of faculty members work more than 58.6 hours a week?

b. If we assume a bell-shaped distribution, what percentage of faculty members work more than 58.6 hours a week?

Source: National Center for Education Statistics.

Extending the Concepts »

43. Serum Cholesterol Levels For this data set, find the
mean and standard deviation of the variable. The data
represent the serum cholesterol levels of 30 individuals.
Count the number of data values that fall within 2 standard deviations of the mean. Compare this with the
number obtained from Chebyshev's theorem. Comment
on the answer.

211	240	255	219	204
200	212	193	187	205
256	203	210	221	249
231	212	236	204	187
201	247	206	187	200
237	227	221	192	196

44. Ages of Consumers For this data set, find the mean
and standard deviation of the variable. The data
represent the ages of 30 customers who ordered a
product advertised on television. Count the number
of data values that fall within 2 standard deviations
of the mean. Compare this with the number obtained
from Chebyshev's theorem. Comment on the
answer.

42	44	62	35	20
30	56	20	23	41
55	22	31	27	66
21	18	24	42	25
32	50	31	26	36
39	40	18	36	22

45. Using Chebyshev's theorem, complete the table to find
the minimum percentage of data values that fall within k
standard deviations of the mean.

k	1.5	2	2.5	3	3.5
Percentage					

46. Use this data set: 10, 20, 30, 40, 50.

  a. Find the standard deviation.
  b. Add 5 to each value, and then find the standard
    deviation.
  c. Subtract 5 from each value and find the standard
    deviation.

  d. Multiply each value by 5 and find the standard
    deviation.
  e. Divide each value by 5 and find the standard
    deviation.
  f. Generalize the results of parts *b* through *e*.
  g. Compare these results with those in Exercise 38.

47. The mean deviation is found by using this formula:

$$\text{Mean deviation} = \frac{\Sigma|X - \overline{X}|}{n}$$

where
  X = value
  $\overline{X}$ = mean
  n = number of values
  $||$ = absolute value

Find the mean deviation for these data.

5, 9, 10, 11, 11, 12, 15, 18, 20, 22

48. A measure to determine the skewness of a distribution is
called the *Pearson coefficient of skewness.* The formula is

$$\text{Skewness} = \frac{3(\overline{X} - \text{MD})}{s}$$

The values of the coefficient usually range from -3 to
$+3$. When the distribution is symmetric, the coefficient
is zero; when the distribution is positively skewed, it is
positive; and when the distribution is negatively skewed,
it is negative.

  Using the formula, find the coefficient of skewness for each distribution, and describe the shape of
the distribution.

  a. Mean = 10, median = 8, standard deviation = 3.
  b. Mean = 42, median = 45, standard deviation = 4.
  c. Mean = 18.6, median = 18.6, standard
    deviation = 1.5.
  d. Mean = 98, median = 97.6, standard deviation = 4.

49. All values of a data set must be within $s\sqrt{n-1}$ of the
mean. If a person collected 25 data values that had a
mean of 50 and a standard deviation of 3 and you saw
that one data value was 67, what would you conclude?

3–3	Measures of Position ›

 LO3

**Identify the position
of a data value in a
data set, using various
measures of position,
such as percentiles,
deciles, and quartiles.**

In addition to measures of central tendency and measures of variation, there are measures
of position or location. These measures include standard scores, percentiles, deciles, and
quartiles. They are used to locate the relative position of a data value in the data set. For
example, if a value is located at the 80th percentile, it means that 80% of the values fall
below it in the distribution and 20% of the values fall above it. The *median* is the value
that corresponds to the 50th percentile, since one-half of the values fall below it and one-
half of the values fall above it. This section discusses these measures of position.

Standard Scores

There is an old saying, "You can't compare apples and oranges." But with the use of statistics, it can be done to some extent. Suppose that a student scored 90 on a music test and 45 on an English exam. Direct comparison of raw scores is impossible, since the exams might not be equivalent in terms of number of questions, value of each question, and so on. However, a comparison of both scores' positions relative to their respective evaluations' average scores and dispersion can be made. This comparison uses the mean and standard deviation and is called a *standard score* or *z score*. (We also use *z* scores in later chapters.)

A **z score** or **standard score** for a value is obtained by subtracting the mean from the value and dividing the result by the standard deviation. The symbol for a standard score is *z*. The formula is

$$z = \frac{\text{Value} - \text{Mean}}{\text{Standard deviation}}$$

For samples, the formula is

$$z = \frac{X - \overline{X}}{s}$$

For populations, the formula is

$$z = \frac{X - \mu}{\sigma}$$

The *z* score represents the number of standard deviations that a data value falls above or below the mean.

For the purpose of this book, it will be assumed that when we find *z* scores, the data were obtained from samples.

Example 3–26

Test Scores

A student scored 65 on a calculus test that had a mean of 50 and a standard deviation of 10; she scored 30 on a history test with a mean of 25 and a standard deviation of 5. Compare her relative positions on the two tests.

Solution

First, find the *z* scores. For calculus the *z* score is

$$z = \frac{X - \overline{X}}{s} = \frac{65 - 50}{10} = 1.5$$

For history the *z* score is

$$z = \frac{30 - 25}{5} = 1.0$$

Since the *z* score for calculus is larger, her relative position in the calculus class is higher than her relative position in the history class.

Note that if the *z* score is positive, the score is above the mean. If the *z* score is 0, the score is the same as the mean. And if the *z* score is negative, the score is below the mean.

Example 3–27	**Test Scores**

Find the z score for each test, and state which is higher.

Test A	$X = 38$	$\overline{X} = 40$	$s = 5$
Test B	$X = 94$	$\overline{X} = 100$	$s = 10$

Solution

For test A,

$$z = \frac{X - \overline{X}}{s} = \frac{38 - 40}{5} = -0.4$$

For test B,

$$z = \frac{94 - 100}{10} = -0.6$$

The score for test A is relatively higher than the score for test B.

When all data for a variable are transformed into z scores, the resulting distribution will have a mean of 0 and a standard deviation of 1. A z score, then, is actually the number of standard deviations each value is from the mean for a specific distribution. In Example 3–26, the calculus score of 65 was actually 1.5 standard deviations above the mean of 50. This will be explained in greater detail in Chapter 7.

Percentiles

Percentiles are position measures used in educational and health-related fields to indicate the position of an individual in a group.

Percentiles divide a data set into 100 equal parts in which the *p*th percentile is a value that at most *p*% of the observations in the data set are less than this value and the remainder are greater.

In many situations, the graphs and tables showing the percentiles for various measures such as test scores, heights, weights, and body mass index have already been completed. Table 3–3 shows the percentile ranks for scaled scores on the *Test of English as a Foreign Language* (TOEFL). For example, if a student had a scaled score of 60 for Section 1 (listening comprehension), that student would have a percentile rank of 79. Hence, that student did better than 79% of the students who took section 1 of the exam.

Figure 3–5 shows percentiles in graphical form of the body mass index (BMI) of girls from ages 5 to 19. The BMI is the ratio of a person's weight in kilograms (kg) to the square of their height in metres (m), or kg/m^2. To find the percentile rank of an 18-year-old girl whose BMI score is 25, start at the 25 BMI score on the left axis and move horizontally to the right. Find 18 on the horizontal axis and move up vertically. The two lines meet at the 85th percentile curved line; hence, an 18-year-old girl with a 25 BMI score is in the 85th percentile for her age group. If the lines do not meet exactly on one of the curved percentile lines, then the percentile rank must be approximated.

Percentiles are also used to compare an individual's test score with the national norm. For example, the *Canadian Achievement Test* (CAT), offered by the Canadian Test Centre (CTC) Educational Assessment Services, measures outcomes of skill sets in reading, language, spelling, and mathematics. Parents receive a report indicating a student's nationalized percentile ranking compared to students at the same grade level.

Table 3–3	Percentile Ranks for Paper-Based TOEFL Scores (2009)– Applicants for a Professional Licence*				
Scale Score	Section 1 Listening Comprehension	Section 2 Structure and Written Expression	Section 3 Reading Comprehension	Total Scale Score	Percentile Rank
68	99	96			
66	97	95	99	660	99
64	93	90	96	640	96
62	87	86	91	620	91
→ 60	79	80	85	600	85
58	71	71	77	580	77
56	61	63	67	560	67
54	50	54	55	540	55
52	39	45	43	520	43
50	28	34	33	500	32
48	19	26	23	480	22
46	11	19	16	460	14
44	6	12	11	440	8
42	3	8	7	420	5
40	2	5	4	400	2
38	1	2	3	380	1
36	1	1	2	360	
34		1	1	340	
32			1	320	
Mean.	53.6	52.7	52.3	Mean S.D.	529 64
S.D.	6.6	6.8	6.9		

*Based on examinees who indicated that they were taking TOEFL to become licensed to practise their professions in the United States or Canada.

Source: Educational Testing Service, *Test and Score Data Summary for TOEFL Internet-Based and Paper-Based Tests,* January 2009–December 2009 Test Data.

Percentiles are not the same as percentages. That is, if a student gets 72 correct answers out of a possible 100, she obtains a percentage score of 72. There is no indication of her position with respect to the rest of the class. She could have scored the highest, the lowest, or somewhere in between. On the other hand, if a raw score of 72 corresponds to the 64th percentile, then she did better than 64% of the students in her class.

Percentiles are symbolized by

$$P_0, P_1, P_2, P_3, \ldots, P_{99}, P_{100}$$

and divide the distribution into 100 groups.

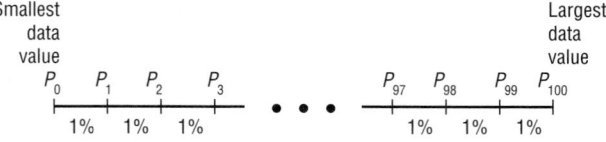

Percentile graphs can be constructed as shown in Example 3–28. Percentile graphs use the same values as the cumulative relative frequency graphs described in Section 2–2, except that the proportions have been converted to percents.

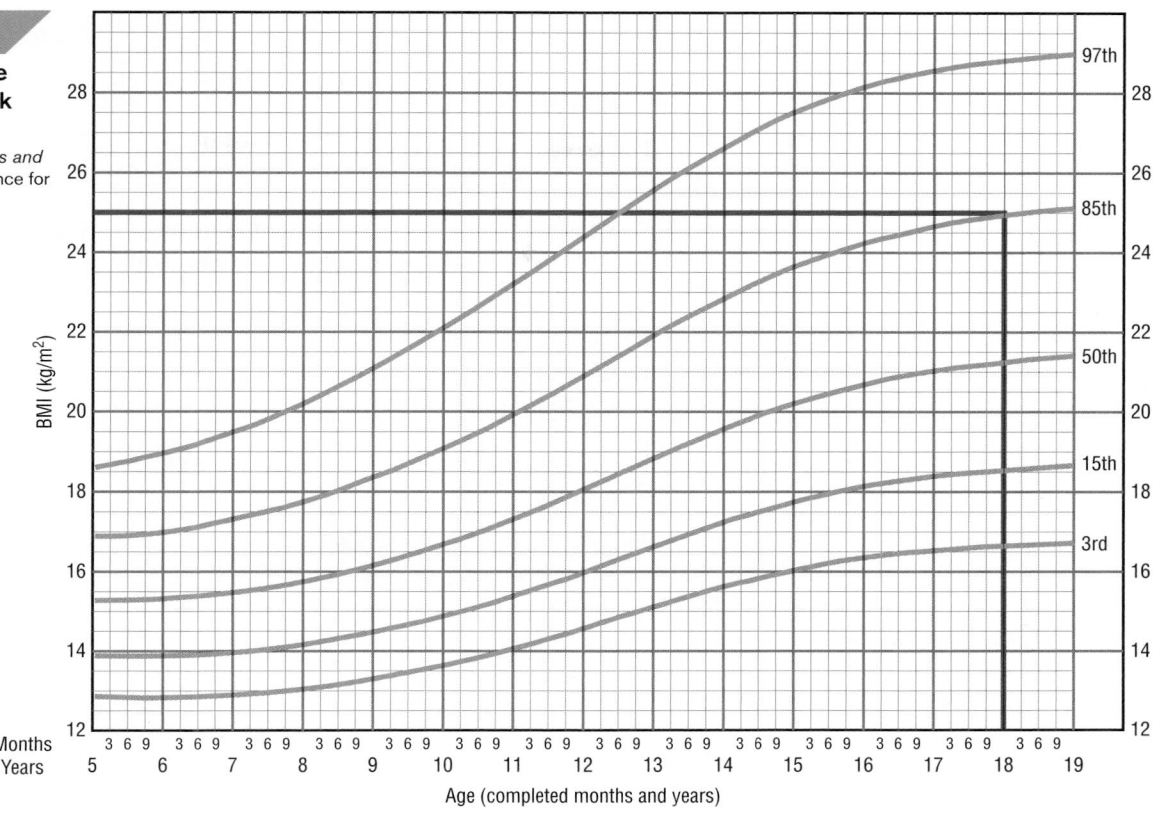

Figure 3–5

BMI of Girls by Age and Percentile Rank

Source: World Health Organization, *Programmes and Projects,* "Growth Reference for 5–19 Years."

Example 3–28

Systolic Blood Pressure

The frequency distribution for the systolic blood pressure readings (in millimetres of mercury, mm Hg) of 200 randomly selected college students is shown here. Construct a percentile graph.

A Class boundaries	B Frequency	C Cumulative frequency	D Cumulative percentage
89.5–104.5	24		
104.5–119.5	62		
119.5–134.5	72		
134.5–149.5	26		
149.5–164.5	12		
164.5–179.5	4		
	200		

Solution

Step 1   Find the cumulative frequencies and place them in column C.

Step 2   Find the cumulative percentages and place them in column D. To do this step, use the formula

$$\text{Cumulative \%} = \frac{\text{Cumulative frequency}}{n} \cdot 100\%$$

For the first class,

$$\text{Cumulative \%} = \frac{24}{200} \cdot 100\% = 12\%$$

The completed table is shown here.

A Class boundaries	B Frequency	C Cumulative frequency	D Cumulative percentage
89.5–104.5	24	24	12
104.5–119.5	62	86	43
119.5–134.5	72	158	79
134.5–149.5	26	184	92
149.5–164.5	12	196	98
164.5–179.5	4	200	100
	200		

Step 3 Graph the data, using class boundaries for the x axis and the percentages for the y axis, as shown in Figure 3–6.

Figure 3–6

Percentile Graph for
Example 3–28

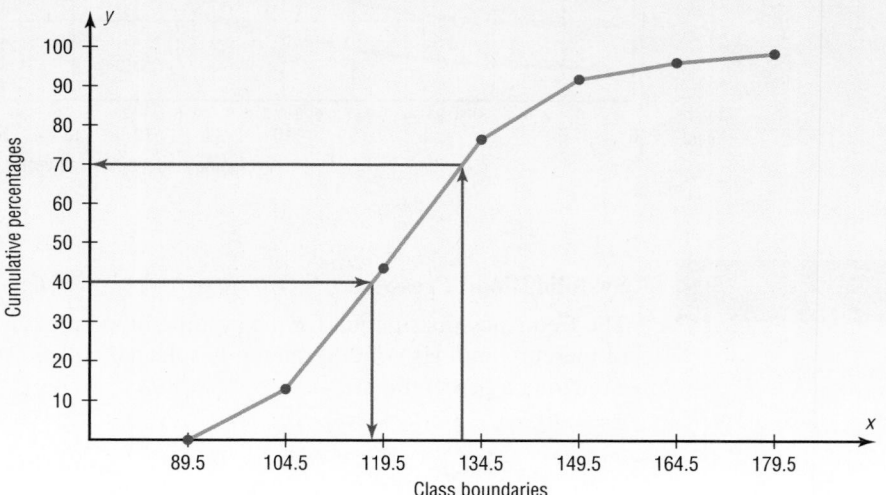

Once a percentile graph has been constructed, one can find the approximate corresponding percentile ranks for given blood pressure values and find approximate blood pressure values for given percentile ranks.

For example, to find the percentile rank of a blood pressure reading of 130, find 130 on the x axis of Figure 3–6, and draw a vertical line to the graph. Then move horizontally to the value on the y axis. Note that a blood pressure of 130 corresponds to approximately the 70th percentile.

If the value that corresponds to the 40th percentile is desired, start on the y axis at 40 and draw a horizontal line to the graph. Then draw a vertical line to the x axis and read the value. In Figure 3–6, the 40th percentile corresponds to a value of approximately 118. Thus, if a person has a blood pressure of 118, he or she is at the 40th percentile.

Estimating Percentile with Linear Interpolation The data value for a percentile rank from a frequency distribution can be approximated using linear interpolation. The following example demonstrates this procedure.

Example 3–29	**Systolic Blood Pressure**

Referring to Example 3–28, find the systolic blood pressure reading corresponding to the 70th percentile.

Step 1: Set up the cumulative frequency distribution, as previously outlined, then find the location of the 70th percentile.

$$c = \frac{n \cdot p}{100} = \frac{200 \cdot 70}{100} = 140$$

Therefore, 140 data values are below P_{70}.

Step 2: Using the cumulative frequency column (C), find the class containing the 140th cumulative data value. Alternatively, use the cumulative percentage column (D) to find the class containing P_{70}. The desired class is the 3rd class, 119.5 to 134.5.

Step 3: Use the linear interpolation method to approximate the data value corresponding to P_{70}.

$$P_k = LCB_2 + \frac{c_1 - cf_L}{f_2}(w_2) \quad where$$

$$P_{70} = 119.5 + \frac{140 - 86}{72}(15)$$

$$= 119.5 + 11.25$$

$$= 130.75$$

where

$P_k = percentile\ rank$
$LCB_2 = lower\ class\ boundary$ (step 2)
$c_1 = location\ (count)$ (step 1)
$cf_L = cumulative\ frequency$ of previous (lower) class
$f_2 = class\ frequency$ (step 2)
$w_2 = class\ width$ (step 2)

Therefore, a systolic blood pressure reading of 130.75 mm Hg corresponds to the 70th percentile, or 70% of college students have a systolic blood pressure of less than 130.75 mm Hg. Compare this value to the percentile graph in Figure 3–6.

Finding values and the corresponding percentile ranks by using a graph yields only approximate answers. Several mathematical methods exist for computing percentiles for data. These methods can be used to find the approximate percentile rank of a data value or to find a data value corresponding to a given percentile. When the data set is large (100 or more), these methods yield better results. Examples 3–30 through 3–33 show these methods.

Percentile Formula

The percentile corresponding to a given value X is computed by using the following formula:

$$Percentile = \frac{(Number\ of\ values\ below\ X) + 0.5}{Total\ number\ of\ values} \cdot 100\%$$

Example 3–30	**Test Scores**

A teacher gives a 20-point test to 10 students. The scores are shown here. Find the percentile rank of a score of 12.

18, 15, 12, 6, 8, 2, 3, 5, 20, 10

Solution

Arrange the data in order from lowest to highest.

$$2, 3, 5, 6, 8, 10, 12, 15, 18, 20$$

Then substitute into the formula.

$$\text{Percentile} = \frac{(\text{Number of values below } X) + 0.5}{\text{Total number of values}} \cdot 100\%$$

Since there are six values below a score of 12, the solution is

$$\text{Percentile} = \frac{6 + 0.5}{10} \cdot 100\% = 65\text{th percentile}$$

Thus, a student whose score was 12 did better than 65% of the class.

Note: One assumes that a score of 12 in Example 3–30, for instance, means theoretically any value between 11.5 and 12.5.

Example 3–31

Test Scores

Using the data in Example 3–30, find the percentile rank for a score of 6.

Solution

There are three values below 6. Thus

$$\text{Percentile} = \frac{3 + 0.5}{10} \cdot 100\% = 35\text{th percentile}$$

A student who scored 6 did better than 35% of the class.

Examples 3–32 and 3–33 show a procedure for finding a value corresponding to a given percentile.

Example 3–32

Test Scores

Using the test scores in Example 3–30, find the value corresponding to the 25th percentile.

Solution

Step 1   Arrange the data in order from lowest to highest.

$$2, 3, 5, 6, 8, 10, 12, 15, 18, 20$$

Step 2   Compute

$$c = \frac{n \cdot p}{100}$$

where

n = total number of values
p = percentile

Thus,

$$c = \frac{10 \cdot 25}{100} = 2.5$$

Step 3 If c is not a whole number, round it up to the next whole number; in this case, $c = 3$. (If c is a whole number, see Example 3–33.) Start at the lowest value and count over to the third value, which is 5. Hence, the value 5 corresponds to the 25th percentile.

Example 3–33

Test Scores

Using the data set in Example 3–30, find the value that corresponds to the 60th percentile.

Solution

Step 1 Arrange the data in order from smallest to largest.

2, 3, 5, 6, 8, 10, 12, 15, 18, 20

Step 2 Substitute in the formula.

$$c = \frac{n \cdot p}{100} = \frac{10 \cdot 60}{100} = 6$$

Step 3 If c is a whole number, use the value halfway between the c and $c + 1$ values when counting up from the lowest value—in this case, the 6th and 7th values.

2, 3, 5, 6, 8, 10, 12, 15, 18, 20

           ↗   ↖

    6th value   7th value

The value halfway between 10 and 12 is 11. Find it by adding the two values and dividing by 2.

$$\frac{10 + 12}{2} = 11$$

Hence, 11 corresponds to the 60th percentile. Anyone scoring 11 would have done better than 60% of the class.

The steps for finding a value corresponding to a given percentile are summarized in this Procedure Table.

Procedure Table

Finding a Data Value Corresponding to a Given Percentile

Step 1 Arrange the data in order from lowest to highest.

Step 2 Substitute into the formula

$$c = \frac{n \cdot p}{100}$$

where
    n = total number of values
    p = percentile

Step 3A If c is not a whole number, round up to the next whole number. Starting at the lowest value, count over to the number that corresponds to the rounded-up value.

Step 3B If c is a whole number, use the value halfway between the c and $c + 1$ values when counting up from the lowest value.

Quartiles and Deciles

Quartiles divide the distribution into four groups, separated by Q_1, Q_2, Q_3.

Note that Q_1 is the same as the 25th percentile; Q_2 is the same as the 50th percentile, or the median; Q_3 corresponds to the 75th percentile, as shown:

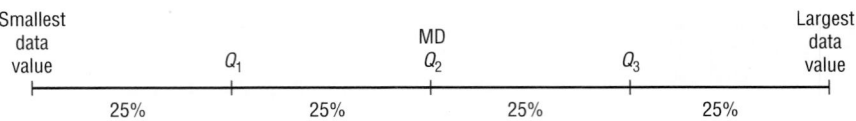

Unusual Stat

85% of Canadian banknotes in circulation contain traces of cocaine.

Quartiles can be computed by using the formula given for computing percentiles on page 123. For Q_1 use $p = 25$. For Q_2 use $p = 50$. For Q_3 use $p = 75$.

In addition to dividing the data set into four groups, quartiles can be used as a rough measurement of variability. The **interquartile range (IQR)** is defined as the difference between Q_1 and Q_3 and is the range of the middle 50% of the data.

The interquartile range is used to identify outliers, and it is also used as a measure of variability in exploratory data analysis, as shown in Section 3–4.

Example 3–34

Test Scores

Using the test scores in Example 3–30, find the interquartile range (IQR) for the data.

Solution

Example 3–32 solved for P_{25} which represents the first quartile, Q_1. Therefore, $Q_1 = 5$. Now solve for P_{75}, which represents the third quartile, Q_3, as follows.

Step 1 Arrange the data in order from lowest to highest.

2, 3, 5, 6, 8, 10, 12, 15, 18, 20

Step 2 Compute $c = \dfrac{n \cdot p}{100} = \dfrac{10 \cdot 75}{100} = 7.5$

Step 3 Since c is not a whole number, round it up to the next whole number; in this case, $c = 8$. Therefore $P_{75} = Q_3 = 15$.

Step 4 To obtain the IQR, subtract Q_3 from Q_1.

$$\text{IQR} = Q_3 - Q_1 = 15 - 5 = 10$$

Hence, the range for the middle 50% of scores, the interquartile range, is 10.

Deciles divide the distribution into 10 groups, as shown. They are denoted by D_1, D_2, etc.

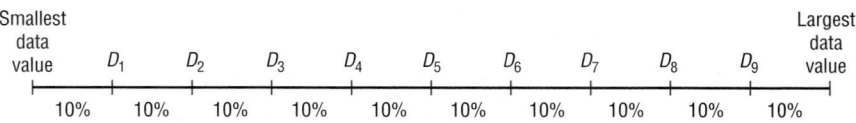

Note that D_1 corresponds to P_{10}; D_2 corresponds to P_{20}; etc. Deciles can be found by using the formulas given for percentiles. Taken altogether then, these are the relationships among percentiles, deciles, and quartiles.

Deciles are denoted by D_1, D_2, D_3, . . . , D_9, and they correspond to P_{10}, P_{20}, P_{30}, . . . , P_{90}.

Quartiles are denoted by Q_1, Q_2, Q_3 and they correspond to P_{25}, P_{50}, P_{75}.

The median is the same as P_{50} or Q_2 or D_5.

The position measures are summarized in Table 3–4.

Table 3–4	Summary of Position Measures	
Measure	**Definition**	**Symbol(s)**
Standard score or z score	Number of standard deviations that a data value is above or below the mean	z
Percentile	Position in hundredths that a data value holds in the distribution	P_n
Decile	Position in tenths that a data value holds in the distribution	D_n
Quartile	Position in fourths that a data value holds in the distribution	Q_n

Outliers

A data set should be checked for extremely high or extremely low values. These values are called *outliers.*

> An **outlier** is an extremely high or an extremely low data value when compared with the rest of the data values.

An outlier can strongly affect the mean and standard deviation of a variable. For example, suppose a researcher mistakenly recorded an extremely high data value. This value would then make the mean and standard deviation of the variable much larger than they really were. Outliers can have an effect on other statistics as well.

There are several ways to check a data set for outliers. One method is shown in this Procedure Table.

Procedure Table

Procedure for Identifying Outliers

Step 1   Arrange the data in order and find Q_1 and Q_3.

Step 2   Find the interquartile range: IQR = $Q_3 - Q_1$.

Step 3   Multiply the IQR by 1.5.

Step 4   Subtract the value obtained in step 3 from Q_1 and add the value to Q_3.

Step 5   Check the data set for any data value that is smaller than $Q_1 - 1.5(\text{IQR})$ or larger than $Q_3 + 1.5(\text{IQR})$.

This procedure is shown in Example 3–35.

Example 3–35

Check the following data set for outliers.

$$5, 6, 12, 13, 15, 18, 22, 50$$

Solution

The data value 50 is extremely suspect. These are the steps in checking for an outlier.

Step 1   Find Q_1 and Q_3 by solving for P_{25} and P_{75}, respectively, as previously shown. Q_1 is 9 and Q_3 is 20.

Step 2   Find the interquartile range (IQR).

$$\text{IQR} = Q_3 - Q_1 = 20 - 9 = 11$$

Step 3   Multiply this value by 1.5.

$$1.5(11) = 16.5$$

Step 4   Subtract the value obtained in step 3 from Q_1, and add the value obtained in step 3 to Q_3.

$$9 - 16.5 = -7.5 \quad \text{and} \quad 20 + 16.5 = 36.5$$

Step 5   Check the data set for any data values that fall outside the interval from -7.5 to 36.5. The value 50 is outside this interval; hence, it can be considered an outlier.

There are several reasons why outliers may occur. First, the data value may have resulted from a measurement or observational error. Perhaps the researcher measured the variable incorrectly. Second, the data value may have resulted from a recording error. That is, it may have been written or typed incorrectly. Third, the data value may have been obtained from a subject that is not in the defined population. For example, suppose test scores were obtained from a Grade 7 class, but a student in that class was actually in Grade 6 and had special permission to attend the class. This student might have scored extremely low on that particular exam on that day. Fourth, the data value might be a legitimate value that occurred by chance (although the probability is extremely small).

There are no hard-and-fast rules on what to do with outliers, nor is there complete agreement among statisticians on ways to identify them. Obviously, if they occurred as a result of an error, an attempt should be made to correct the error or else the data value should be omitted entirely. When they occur naturally by chance, the statistician must make a decision about whether to include them in the data set.

When a distribution is normal or bell-shaped, data values that are beyond 3 standard deviations of the mean can be considered suspected outliers.

3–3   Applying the Concepts

Determining Dosages

In an attempt to determine necessary dosages of a new drug (HDL) used to control sepsis, assume you administer varying amounts of HDL to 40 mice. You create four groups and label them *low dosage, moderate dosage, large dosage,* and *very large dosage.* The dosages also vary within each group. After the mice are injected with the HDL and the sepsis bacteria, the time until the onset of sepsis is recorded. Your job as a statistician is to effectively communicate the results of the study.

1. Which measures of position could be used to help describe the data results?
2. If 40% of the mice in the top quartile survived after the injection, how many mice would that be?
3. What information can be given from using percentiles?
4. What information can be given from using quartiles?
5. What information can be given from using standard scores?

See page 145 for the answers.

Exercises 3–3

1. What is a *z* score?

2. Define *percentile rank.*

3. What is the difference between a percentage and a percentile?

4. Define *quartile.*

5. What is the relationship between quartiles and percentiles?

6. What is a decile?

7. How are deciles related to percentiles?

8. To which percentile, quartile, and decile does the median correspond?

9. Vacation Days If the average number of vacation days for a selection of various countries has a mean of 29.4 days and a standard deviation of 8.6, find the *z* scores for the average number of vacation days in each of these countries.

Canada	26 days
Italy	42 days
United States	13 days

Source: Infoplease: www.infoplease.com.

10. Reaction Time of Sprinters The mean reaction time to the starting pistol for world-class sprinters is 153 milliseconds (ms) with a standard deviation of 28 ms. Find the corresponding *z* score for each sprinter's reaction time (in ms).

a. 195   *d.* 241.2

b. 90   *e.* 88.6

c. 139

Source: Kevin Duffy's Home Page, "Reaction Times and Sprint False Starts."

11. Exam Scores A final examination for a psychology course has a mean of 84 and a standard deviation of 4. Find the corresponding *z* score for each raw score.

a. 87   *d.* 76

b. 79   *e.* 82

c. 93

12. Temperature of the Human Body The healthy human body has a mean temperature of 36.8°C, with a standard deviation of 0.7°C. Find the corresponding *z* score for the following body temperatures (°C).

a. 37.5

b. 36.1

c. 34.77

d. 37.85

e. 38.41

Source: NationMaster.com, Normal Human Body Temperature.

13. Exam Scores A student scored 61 on the chemistry final exam, which had a mean of 54 and a standard deviation of 3.5, and she scored 85 on the biology final with a mean of 79 and a standard deviation of 2.5. On which exam did she perform relatively better?

14. Marathon Run An amateur male ran a marathon in 3 hours and 51 minutes; the mean time of the male runners was 4 hours and 30 minutes with a standard deviation of 39 minutes. An amateur female ran the same marathon in 4 hours and 40 minutes; the mean time of the female runners was 5 hours and 10 minutes with a standard deviation of 50 minutes. Which marathon runner did relatively better with respect to their gender? *Note:* A lower relative position is better in a marathon run.

Source: Marathon Training Expert.com, What Is the Average Marathon Time?

15. Graduate Record Exam A Canadian student applying to an American college wrote the three-part Graduate Record Exam (GRE). The student scores were as follows. In which part of the GRE did the student do relatively better?

Verbal reasoning	Quantitative reasoning	Analytical writing
$X = 593$	$X = 811$	$X = 5.2$
$\overline{X} = 462$	$\overline{X} = 584$	$\overline{X} = 4.0$
$s = 119$	$s = 151$	$s = 0.9$

Source: Educational Testing Services, GRE and Interpreting Your GRE Scores, 2008–2009.

16. College Room and Board Costs Room and board costs for selected schools are summarized in this distribution. Find the approximate cost of room and board corresponding to each of the following percentiles.

Costs (in dollars)	Frequency
3000.5–4000.5	5
4000.5–5000.5	6
5000.5–6000.5	18
6000.5–7000.5	24
7000.5–8000.5	19
8000.5–9000.5	8
9000.5–10,000.5	5

a. 30th percentile

b. 50th percentile

c. 75th percentile

d. 90th percentile

Source: World Almanac.

17. Using the data in Exercise 16, find the approximate percentile rank of each of the following costs.

a. 5500   *c.* 6500

b. 7200   *d.* 8300

18. (ans) Achievement Test Scores The data shown represent the scores on a national achievement test for a group of Grade 10 students. Find the approximate percentile ranks of these scores by constructing a percentile graph.

a. 220

b. 245

c. 276

d. 280

e. 300

Score	Frequency
196.5–217.5	5
217.5–238.5	17
238.5–259.5	22
259.5–280.5	48
280.5–301.5	22
301.5–322.5	6

19. For the data in Exercise 18, find the approximate scores that correspond to these percentiles.

a. 15th

b. 29th

c. 43rd

d. 65th

e. 80th

20. (ans) Aircraft Speeds The airborne speeds in kilometres per hour of 21 aircraft are shown. Find the approximate values that correspond to the given percentiles by constructing a percentile graph.

Speed (km/h)	Frequency
588–621	4
622–655	2
656–689	3
690–723	2
724–757	1
758–791	2
792–825	3
826–859	4
	21

a. 9th

b. 20th

c. 45th

d. 60th

e. 75th

Source: The World Almanac and Book of Facts.

21. Using the data in Exercise 20, estimate the percentile ranks of the following speeds.

a. 571 km/h

b. 604 km/h

c. 670 km/h

d. 736 km/h

e. 845 km/h

22. Weightlifting Results The final results of the men's super-heavyweight (+105 kg class) at the 77th Men's World Championships includes the total weight lifted (kg) for the snatch and the clean and jerk.

445   445   427   415   415   413   411   388   388
386   381   381   380   378   378   368   325

Find the percentile ranks for the following total weights.

a. 427

b. 413

c. 381

d. 368

Source: International Weightlifting Federation.

23. In Exercise 22, what weight corresponds to the following percentile ranks?

a. 60th percentile or P_{60}

b. 3rd quartile or Q_3

c. 4th decile or D_4

d. 85th percentile or P_{85}

24. Average Weekly Earnings Industry Canada reports the following weekly average earnings (in dollars) for sectors in the Information and Communication Technologies (ICT) industry. Find the percentile rank of each weekly wage.

978   1088   1094   1155   1121   1192   1310

Source: Industry Canada, Canadian ICT Sector Profile, August 2009.

25. In Exercise 24, find the weekly wage corresponding to the 70th percentile.

26. Hurricane Damage Find the percentile rank for each value in the data set. The data represent the values in billions of dollars of the damage of 10 hurricanes.

1.1, 1.7, 1.9, 2.1, 2.2, 2.5, 3.3, 6.2, 6.8, 20.3

Source: Insurance Services Office.

27. What value in Exercise 26 corresponds to the 40th percentile?

28. Employee Ages The following data represent the ages of employees in a law firm. Find the percentile rank of each employee age.

25   26   31   35   43   46   52   58   61

29. In Exercise 28, what age corresponds to the 33rd percentile?

30. Using the procedure shown in Example 3–35, check each data set for outliers.

a. 16, 18, 22, 19, 3, 21, 17, 20

b. 24, 32, 54, 31, 16, 18, 19, 14, 17, 20

c. 321, 343, 350, 327, 200

d. 88, 72, 97, 84, 86, 85, 100

e. 145, 119, 122, 118, 125, 116

f. 14, 16, 27, 18, 13, 19, 36, 15, 20

31. Another measure of average is called the *midquartile;* it is the numerical value halfway between Q_1 and Q_3, and the formula is

$$\text{Midquartile} = \frac{Q_1 + Q_3}{2}$$

Using this formula and other formulas, find Q_1, Q_2, Q_3, the midquartile, and the interquartile range for each data set.

a. 5, 12, 16, 25, 32, 38

b. 53, 62, 78, 94, 96, 99, 103

3–4   Exploratory Data Analysis ›

LO4

Use the techniques of exploratory data analysis, including boxplots and five-number summaries, to discover various aspects of data.

In traditional statistics, data are organized by using a frequency distribution. From this distribution, various graphs such as the histogram, frequency polygon, and ogive can be constructed to determine the shape or nature of the distribution. In addition, various statistics such as the mean and standard deviation can be computed to summarize the data.

The purpose of traditional analysis is to confirm various conjectures about the nature of the data. For example, from a carefully designed study, a researcher might want to know if the proportion of Canadians who are exercising today has increased from ten years ago. This study would contain various assumptions about the population, various definitions of terms such as *exercise,* and so on.

In **exploratory data analysis (EDA),** data can be organized using a *stem and leaf plot.* (See Chapter 2.) The measure of central tendency used in EDA is the *median.* The measure of variation used in EDA is the *interquartile range* $(Q_3 - Q_1)$. In EDA the data are represented graphically using a **boxplot** (sometimes called a *box-and-whisker plot*). The purpose of exploratory data analysis is to examine data in order to identify patterns, trends, or relationships. These observations can be simple descriptions such as central measures or dispersions that help in making decisions or suggest further actions. Exploratory data analysis was developed by John Tukey and presented in his book *Exploratory Data Analysis* (Addison-Wesley, 1977).

The Five-Number Summary and Boxplots

A boxplot can be used to graphically represent the data set. These plots involve five specific values:

1. The lowest value of the data set (i.e., minimum)
2. Q_1
3. The median
4. Q_3
5. The highest value of the data set (i.e., maximum)

These values are called a **five-number summary** of the data set.

A **boxplot** is a graph of a data set obtained by drawing a horizontal line from the minimum data value to Q_1, drawing a horizontal line from Q_3 to the maximum data value, and drawing a box whose vertical sides pass through Q_1 and Q_3 with a vertical line inside the box passing through the median or Q_2.

Example 3–36

Stockbroker Clients

A stockbroker recorded the number of clients she saw each day over an 11-day period. The data are shown. Construct a boxplot for the data.

33, 38, 43, 30, 29, 40, 51, 27, 42, 23, 31

Solution

Step 1   Arrange the data in order.

23, 27, 29, 30, 31, 33, 38, 40, 42, 43, 51

Step 2   Find the median.

$$23, 27, 29, 30, 31, 33, 38, 40, 42, 43, 51$$

$$\uparrow$$

Median

Step 3   Find Q_1 or P_{25}.

$$c = \frac{n \cdot p}{100} = \frac{11 \cdot 25}{100} = 2.75 \text{ (round up to 3)} \therefore Q_1 = 29$$

Step 4   Find Q_3 or P_{75}.

$$c = \frac{n \cdot p}{100} = \frac{11 \cdot 75}{100} = 8.25 \text{ (round up to 9)} \therefore Q_3 = 42$$

Step 5   Draw a scale for the data on the x axis.

Step 6   Locate the lowest value, Q_1, the median, Q_3, and the highest value on the scale.

Step 7   Draw a box around Q_1 and Q_3, draw a vertical line through the median, and connect the upper and lower values, as shown in Figure 3–7.

Figure 3–7

Boxplot for Example 3–36

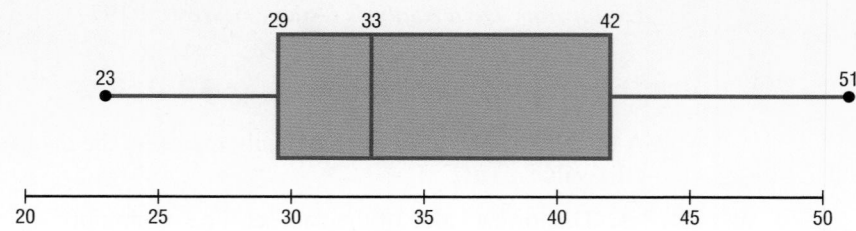

The box in Figure 3–7 represents the middle 50% of the data, and the lines represent the lower and upper ends of the data.

Information Obtained from a Boxplot

1. *a.* If the median is near the centre of the box, the distribution is approximately symmetric.
    b. If the median falls to the left of the centre of the box, the distribution is positively skewed.
    c. If the median falls to the right of the centre, the distribution is negatively skewed.
2. *a.* If the lines are about the same length, the distribution is approximately symmetric.
    b. If the right line is larger than the left line, the distribution is positively skewed.
    c. If the left line is larger than the right line, the distribution is negatively skewed.

The boxplot in Figure 3–7 indicates that the distribution is slightly positively skewed.

If the boxplots for two or more data sets are graphed on the same axis, the distributions can be compared. To compare the averages, use the location of the medians. To compare the variability, use the interquartile range, i.e., the length of the boxes. Example 3–37 shows this procedure.

Example 3–37

Sodium Content of Cheese

A dietitian is interested in comparing the sodium content of real cheese with the sodium content of a cheese substitute. The data for two random samples are shown. Compare the distributions, using boxplots.

Real cheese				Cheese substitute			
310	420	45	40	270	180	250	290
220	240	180	90	130	260	340	310

Source: The Complete Book of Food Counts.

Solution

Step 1 Find Q_1, MD, and Q_3 for the real cheese data.

$$c = \frac{n \cdot p}{100} = \frac{8 \cdot 25}{100} = 2 \therefore Q_1 = \frac{45 + 90}{2} = 67.5$$

$$\text{MD} = \frac{180 + 220}{2} = 200$$

$$c = \frac{n \cdot p}{100} = \frac{8 \cdot 75}{100} = 6 \therefore Q_3 = \frac{240 + 310}{2} = 275$$

Step 2 Find Q_1, MD, and Q_3 for the substitute cheese data.

$$c = \frac{n \cdot p}{100} = \frac{8 \cdot 25}{100} = 2 \therefore Q_1 = \frac{180 + 250}{2} = 215$$

$$\text{MD} = \frac{260 + 270}{2} = 265$$

$$c = \frac{n \cdot p}{100} = \frac{8 \cdot 75}{100} = 6 \therefore Q_3 = \frac{290 + 310}{2} = 300$$

Step 3 Draw the boxplots for each distribution on the same graph. See Figure 3–8.

Figure 3–8

Boxplots for
Example 3–37

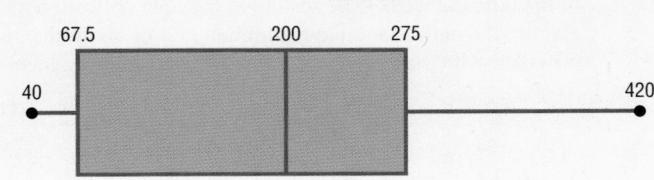

Real cheese

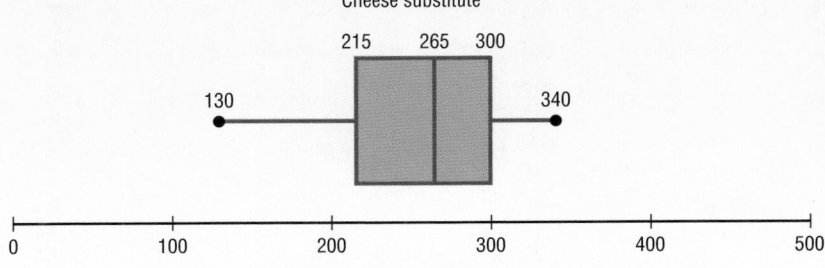

Cheese substitute

Step 4 Compare the plots. It is quite apparent that the distribution for the cheese substitute data has a higher median than the median for the distribution for the real cheese data. The variation or spread for the distribution of the real cheese data is larger than the variation for the distribution of the cheese substitute data.

In exploratory data analysis, *hinges* are used instead of quartiles to construct boxplots. When the data set consists of an even number of values, hinges are the same as quartiles. Hinges for a data set with an odd number of values differ somewhat from quartiles. However, since most calculators and computer programs use quartiles, they will be used in this textbook.

Another important point to remember is that the summary statistics (median and interquartile range) used in exploratory data analysis are said to be *resistant statistics*. A **resistant statistic** is relatively less affected by outliers than a *nonresistant statistic*. The mean and standard deviation are nonresistant statistics. Sometimes when a distribution is skewed or contains outliers, the median and interquartile range may more accurately summarize the data than the mean and standard deviation, since the mean and standard deviation are more affected in this case.

Table 3–5 compares the traditional versus the exploratory data analysis approach.

Table 3–5	Traditional versus EDA Techniques
Traditional	**Exploratory data analysis**
Frequency distribution	Stem and leaf plot
Histogram	Boxplot
Mean	Median
Standard deviation	Interquartile range

3–4   Applying the Concepts

The Noisy Workplace

Assume you work for CCOHS (Canadian Centre for Occupational Health and Safety) and have complaints about noise levels from some of the workers at a provincial power plant. You charge the power plant with taking decibel readings at six different areas of the plant at different times of the day and week. The results of the data collection are listed. Use boxplots to initially explore the data and make recommendations about the plant areas where the workers must be provided with protective ear wear. The safe hearing level is at approximately 120 decibels.

Area 1	Area 2	Area 3	Area 4	Area 5	Area 6
30	64	100	25	59	67
12	99	59	15	63	80
35	87	78	30	81	99
65	59	97	20	110	49
24	23	84	61	65	67
59	16	64	56	112	56
68	94	53	34	132	80
57	78	59	22	145	125
100	57	89	24	163	100
61	32	88	21	120	93
32	52	94	32	84	56
45	78	66	52	99	45
92	59	57	14	105	80
56	55	62	10	68	34
44	55	64	33	75	21

See page 146 for the answers.

Exercises 3–4

For Exercises 1–6, identify the five-number summary and find the interquartile range.

1. 8, 12, 32, 6, 27, 19, 54

2. 19, 16, 48, 22, 7

3. 362, 589, 437, 316, 192, 188

4. 147, 243, 156, 632, 543, 303

5. 14.6, 19.8, 16.3, 15.5, 18.2

6. 9.7, 4.6, 2.2, 3.7, 6.2, 9.4, 3.8

For Exercises 7–10, use each boxplot to identify the maximum value, minimum value, median, first quartile, third quartile, and interquartile range.

7.

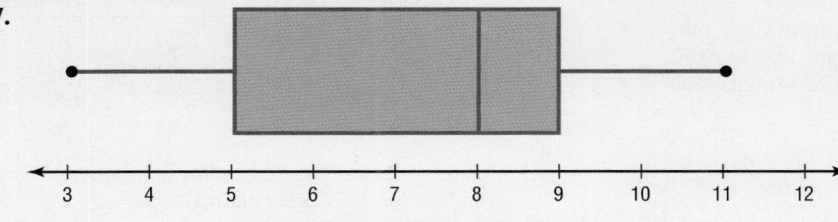

8.

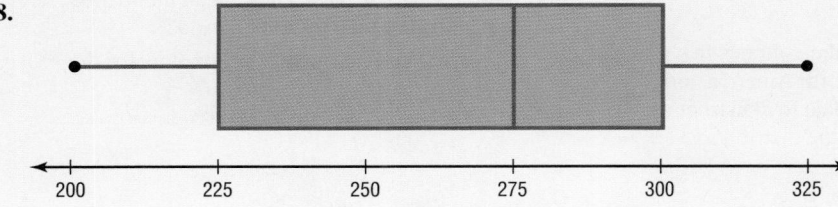

9.

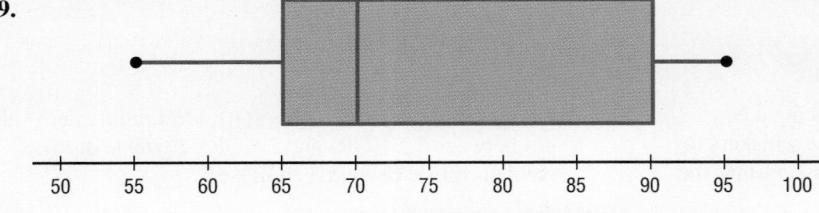

10.

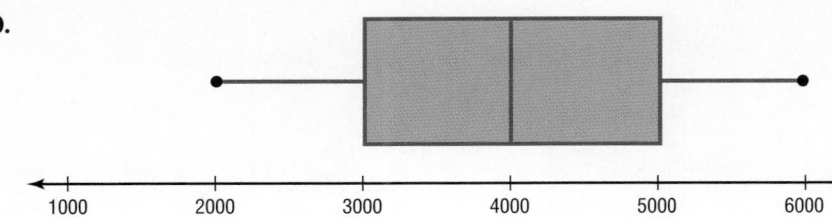

11. City Police Force Size Shown here are the sizes of the police forces in Canada's 10 largest cities in 2005 (the numbers represent hundreds). Construct a boxplot for the data and comment on the shape of the distribution.

89.4, 64.9, 16.0, 12.0, 12.4, 16.3, 31.7, 3.6, 10.0, 5.8

Source: Statistics Canada.

12. Parliamentary Bills Passed Construct a boxplot for the number of bills passed by the Canadian Parliament for the past 8 completed sessions. Comment on the shape of the distribution.

46, 21, 28, 47, 25, 58, 50, 82

Source: Parliament of Canada.

13. Vacation Days of Selected Countries Construct a box-plot for the following average number of vacation days in selected countries.

42	37	35
34	28	26
13	25	25

Source: World Tourism Organization.

14. Broadway Theatre Productions Shown here is the number of new theatre productions that appeared on NYC's Broadway for the past several years. Construct a boxplot for the data and comment on the shape of the distribution.

30	28	33	29	37	39
35	37	37	38	34	

Source: The League of American Theaters and Producers Inc.

15. April Showers These data represent the average rainfall (in millimetres) for select Canadian cities in April. Construct a boxplot and comment on the skewness of the data.

41.9	75.4	25.1	21.8	20.4	25.7
35.9	64.0	69.0	74.8	75.5	83.4
124.4	81.6	110.4	28.4	10.3	8.3

Source: Environment Canada.

16. Dam Volumes These data represent the volumes in cubic metres of the largest dams in North America and Central and South America. Use the data to construct a boxplot for each region and compare the distributions.

Data is in cubic metres (m³). *Note*: Canada's Syncrude Tailings Dam in Fort McMurray, Alberta, ranks second in the world at 0.54 million m³, compared to China's 39.3 million-m³ Three Gorges dam.

North America	Central/South America
540,000	296,200
209,500	238,180
96,049	81,000
70,339	78,000
65,440	43,000
59,639	35,600

Source: Infoplease, "World's Largest Dams."

17. Number of Tornadoes A four-month record for the number of tornadoes in 2007–2010 is given here.

	2007	2008	2009	2010
April	129	226	189	167
May	290	293	201	461
June	325	270	294	128
July	129	118	93	69

a. Which month had the highest mean number of tornadoes for this 4-year period?

b. Which year has the highest mean number of tornadoes for this 4-month period?

c. Construct and interpret four boxplots for the 4-year period.

Source: U.S. National Weather Service, Storm Prediction Center.

Extending the Concepts »

18. A *modified boxplot* can be drawn by placing a box around Q_1 and Q_3 and then extending the whiskers to the largest and/or smallest values within 1.5 times the interquartile range (i.e., $Q_3 - Q_1$). *Mild outliers* are values between 1.5 (IQR) and 3 (IQR). *Extreme outliers* are data values beyond 3 (IQR).

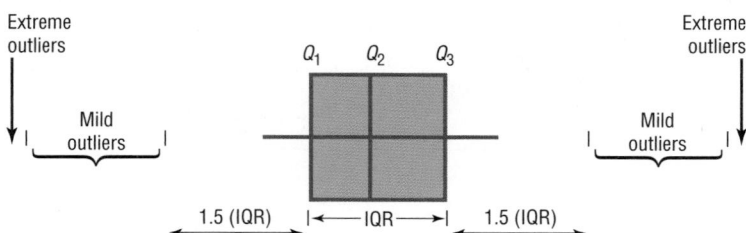

For the data shown here, draw a modified boxplot and identify any mild or extreme outliers. The data represent the number of unhealthful smog days for a specific year for the highest 10 locations.

97	39	43	66	91
43	54	42	53	39

Source: U.S. Public Interest Research Group and Clean Air Network.

Summary >

This chapter explains the basic ways to summarize data. These include measures of central tendency, measures of variation or dispersion, and measures of position. The three most commonly used measures of central tendency are the mean, median, and mode. The midrange is also used occasionally to represent an average. The three most commonly used measurements of variation are the range, variance, and standard deviation.

The most common measures of position are percentiles, quartiles, deciles, and standard scores or *z* scores. This chapter explains how data values are distributed according to Chebyshev's theorem and the empirical rule. The coefficient of variation is used to describe the standard deviation in relationship to the mean. These methods are commonly called *traditional statistical methods* and are primarily used to confirm various conjectures about the nature of the data.

Other methods, such as the boxplot and five-number summaries, are part of exploratory data analysis; they are used to examine data to see what they reveal.

After learning the techniques presented in Chapter 2 and this chapter, you will have a substantial knowledge of descriptive statistics. That is, you will be able to collect, organize, summarize, and present data.

For step-by-step guidance on the use of Texas Instruments TI-83 Plus/TI-84 Plus programmable calculators, see Appendix E at the back of this book. For summary procedures for Minitab, SPSS, and Excel, please see the full version of Appendix E on *Connect*.

Important Terms »

bimodal 88

boxplot 131

Chebyshev's theorem 110

coefficient of variation 109

data array 87

decile 126

empirical rule 112

exploratory data analysis 131

five-number summary 131

interquartile range 126

mean 83

median 87

midrange 91

modal class 89

mode 88

multimodal 88

negatively skewed or left-skewed distribution 94

outlier 127

parameter 83

percentile 119

positively skewed or right-skewed distribution 93

quartile 126

range 101

range rule of thumb 110

resistant statistic 134

standard deviation 103

statistic 83

symmetric distribution 93

unimodal 88

variance 103

weighted mean 92

z score or standard score 118

Important Formulas »

Formula for the mean for individual data:

$$\bar{X} = \frac{\Sigma X}{n} \text{ (sample data)} \qquad \mu = \frac{\Sigma X}{N} \text{ (population data)}$$

Formula for the mean for grouped data:

$$\bar{X} = \frac{\Sigma f \cdot X_m}{n}$$

Formula for the weighted mean:

$$\bar{X} = \frac{\Sigma wX}{\Sigma w}$$

Formula for the midrange:

$$\text{MR} = \frac{\textbf{lowest value} + \textbf{highest value}}{2}$$

Formula for the range:

$$R = \textbf{highest value} - \textbf{lowest value}$$

Formula for the variance for population data:

$$\sigma^2 = \frac{\Sigma(X - \mu)^2}{N}$$

Formula for the variance for sample data (shortcut formula for the unbiased estimator):

$$s^2 = \frac{n(\Sigma X^2) - (\Sigma X)^2}{n(n - 1)}$$

Formula for the variance for grouped data:

$$s^2 = \frac{n(\Sigma f \cdot X_m^2) - (\Sigma f \cdot X_m)^2}{n(n - 1)}$$

Formula for the standard deviation for population data:

$$\sigma = \sqrt{\frac{\Sigma(X - \mu)^2}{N}}$$

Formula for the standard deviation for sample data (shortcut formula):

$$s = \sqrt{\frac{n(\Sigma X^2) - (\Sigma X)^2}{n(n - 1)}}$$

Formula for the standard deviation for grouped data:

$$s = \sqrt{\frac{n(\Sigma f \cdot X_m^2) - (\Sigma f \cdot X_m)^2}{n(n - 1)}}$$

Formula for the coefficient of variation:

$$\text{CVar} = \frac{s}{\overline{X}} \cdot 100\% \quad \text{or} \quad \text{CVar} = \frac{\sigma}{\mu} \cdot 100\%$$

Range rule of thumb:

$$s \approx \frac{\text{range}}{4}$$

Expression for Chebyshev's theorem: The proportion of values from a data set that will fall within k standard deviations of the mean will be at least

$$1 - \frac{1}{k^2}$$

where k is a number greater than 1.

Formula for the z score (standard score):

$$z = \frac{X - \mu}{\sigma} \quad \text{or} \quad z = \frac{X - \overline{X}}{s}$$

Formula for the cumulative percentage:

$$\text{Cumulative \%} = \frac{\text{Cumulative frequency}}{n} \cdot 100\%$$

Formula for the percentile rank of a value X:

$$\text{Percentile} = \frac{(\text{Number of values below } X + 0.5)}{\text{Total number of values}} \cdot 100\%$$

Formula for finding a value corresponding to a given percentile:

$$c = \frac{n \cdot p}{100}$$

Formula for interquartile range:

$$\text{IQR} = Q_3 - Q_1$$

Mc Graw Hill **CONNECT**™ Practise and learn online with *Connect* with data sets and algorithmic questions related to concepts covered in this chapter. Questions and tables with online data sets are marked with 🖊.

Review Exercises ›

1. **Radio Listening Hours** The following data represent the reported number of hours of radio listening per week for each of Canada's provinces for young adults in the 18 to 24 age group.

12.9	19.0	13.5	13.4	14.6
15.7	17.4	19.4	18.3	13.3

   Source: Statistics Canada.

   Find each of these.
   a. Mean
   b. Median
   c. Mode
   d. Midrange
   e. Range
   f. Variance
   g. Standard deviation

2. **Island Areas** These data represent the area in square kilometres of major islands in the Caribbean Sea and the Mediterranean Sea.

Caribbean Sea			Mediterranean Sea	
280	2,398	1,129	4,991	3,654
194	259	8,648	593	246
13,939	443	300	8,259	1,399
5,957	751	4,828	9,251	24,089
430	1,779	153	223	25,708
110,862	10,992	347		
76,117				

   Source: The World Almanac and Book of Facts.

   For each data set, find the following descriptive measures.
   a. Mean
   b. Median
   c. Mode
   d. Midrange
   e. Range
   f. Variance
   g. Standard deviation
   h. Coefficient of variation

   Which data set is more variable?

3. **Battery Lives** Twelve batteries were tested to see how many hours they would last. The frequency distribution is shown here.

Hours	Frequency
1–3	1
4–6	4
7–9	5
10–12	1
13–15	1

   Find each of these.
   a. Mean
   b. Modal class
   c. Variance
   d. Standard deviation

4. **Student Internet Search Times** The following data represent the number of seconds it took 20 students to find information from the Internet on a personal computer.

Search time	Frequency
34–38	4
39–43	6
44–48	3
49–53	4
54–58	3

Find each of these.

a. Mean
b. Modal class
c. Variance
d. Standard deviation

5. **Tidal Changes** Shown here is a frequency distribution for the extreme tidal ranges (high tide to low tide) at selected locations in Canada. (*Note:* Canada's Bay of Fundy has the greatest tidal range in the world at 16.1 metres.)

Tidal change (m)	Frequency
0–2.95	4
2.95–5.95	7
5.95–8.95	5
8.95–11.95	1
11.95–14.95	1
14.95–17.95	1

Source: The Atlas of Canada.

Find each of the following.

a. Mean
b. Modal class
c. Variance
d. Standard deviation

6. **Truck Fuel Costs** The following distribution illustrates the fuel cost per year to operate various pickup trucks in Canada. *Note: The data assume a fuel price of 70¢/litre and 20,000 kilometres driving distance.*

Fuel cost ($/Year)	Frequency
1200–1499	9
1500–1799	48
1800–2099	47
2100–2399	8
2400–2699	0
2700–2999	3
3000–3299	1
3300–3599	1
	117

Source: Natural Resources Canada, Fuel Consumption Guide 2005.

Find the following descriptive measures.

a. Mean
b. Modal class
c. Variance
d. Standard deviation

7. **Number of Cavities** In a dental survey of Grade 3 students, this distribution was obtained for the number of cavities found. Find the average number of cavities for the class. Use the weighted mean.

Number of students	Number of cavities
12	0
8	1
5	2
5	3

8. **Investment Earnings** An investor calculated these percentages of each of three stock investments with payoffs as shown. Find the average payoff. Use the weighted mean.

Stock	Percent	Payoff
A	30	$10,000
B	50	3,000
C	20	1,000

9. **Employee Years of Service** In an advertisement, a transmission service centre stated that the average years of service of its employees were 13. The distribution is shown here. Using the weighted mean, calculate the correct average.

Number of employees	Years of service
8	3
1	6
1	30

10. **Textbooks in Professors' Offices** If the average number of textbooks in professors' offices is 16, the standard deviation is 5, and the average age of the professors is 43, with a standard deviation of 8, which data set is more variable?

11. **Bookstore Survey** A survey of bookstores showed that the average number of magazines carried is 56, with a standard deviation of 12. The same survey showed that the average length of time each store had been in business was 6 years, with a standard deviation of 2.5 years. Which is more variable, the number of magazines or the number of years?

12. **Supreme Court Judges' Years of Service** The number of years served, as of 2010, by members of the Canada's Supreme Court is listed below.

21   10   12   10   8   7   6   6   4   2

a. Find the percentile rank for each value.
b. Which value corresponds to the 3rd quartile or 75th percentile?
c. Construct a boxplot for the data and comment on the shape of the distribution.

Source: Supreme Court of Canada, About the Court, "Current Judges."

13. **NFL Salaries** The salary payroll (in millions of dollars) for 32 NFL teams for the 2009–2010 season are given in the following frequency distribution.

Payroll	Frequency
60–74	1
75–89	3
90–104	11
105–119	11
120–134	5
135–149	1

Source: USA Today, "Salaries Databases."

a. Construct a percentile graph.

b. Find the values that correspond to the 25th percentile, the median or 5th decile (P_{50}), and the 3rd quartile (P_{75}).

c. Estimate the percentile rank for payroll salaries of 85, 105, and 125.

14. Check each data set for outliers.

 a. 506, 511, 517, 514, 400, 521

 b. 3, 7, 9, 6, 8, 10, 14, 16, 20, 12

 c. 14, 18, 27, 26, 19, 13, 5, 25

 d. 112, 157, 192, 116, 153, 129, 131

15. Car Rental Costs A survey of car rental agencies shows that the average cost of a car rental is $0.32 per kilometre. The standard deviation is $0.03. Using Chebyshev's theorem, find the range in which at least 75% of the data values will fall.

16. Seed Costs The average cost of a certain type of seed per hectare is $42. The standard deviation is $3. Using Chebyshev's theorem, find the range in which at least 88.89% of the data values will fall.

17. Labour Charges The average labour charge for automobile mechanics is $54 per hour. The standard deviation is $4. Find the minimum percentage of data values that will fall within the range of $48 to $60. Use Chebyshev's theorem.

18. Cost to Train Employees For a certain type of job, it costs a company an average of $231 to train an employee to perform the task. The standard deviation is $5.

Find the minimum percentage of data values that will fall in the range of $219 to $243. Use Chebyshev's theorem.

19. Delivery Charges The average delivery charge for a refrigerator is $32. The standard deviation is $4. Find the minimum percentage of data values that will fall in the range of $20 to $44. Use Chebyshev's theorem.

20. Exam Grades Which of these exam grades has a better relative position?

a. A grade of 82 on a test with $X = 85$ and $s = 6$.

b. A grade of 56 on a test with $X = 60$ and $s = 5$.

21. Hours Worked The data shown here represent the number of hours that 12 part-time employees at a toy store worked during the weeks before and after Christmas. Construct two boxplots and compare the distributions.

Before	38	16	18	24	12	30	35	32	31	30	24	35
After	26	15	12	18	24	32	14	18	16	18	22	12

22. Commute Times to Work A lifestyles study indicated that 11.4 million Canadians, or 47% of the adult population, commute to work on weekdays. The average commute time was 62 minutes. If the standard deviation was 11 minutes, within what limits would you expect approximately 68% of adult commuters' times to fall? Assume the distribution is approximately bell-shaped.

Source: The Fraser Institute.

![Statistics Today logo] **Statistics Today**

Do You Live as Well as Other Canadians?–Revisited.

The nominal gross domestic product (GDP) per capita or average income for all Canadians was $39,648 but regional disparities exist. Provincial and territorial comparative average GDP for 2008 is shown here.

By making comparison using averages, you can see that the Northwest Territories leads the country in economic well-being, well above the Canadian average and more than double the averages of all provinces/territories except Alberta, Yukon, and Ontario.

Northwest Territories	$82,128
Alberta	$51,664
Yukon	$45,181
Ontario	$41,141
Saskatchewan	$41,025
Newfoundland and Labrador	$39,402
Canada	**$39,648**
Nunavut	$39,019
British Columbia	$37,529
Manitoba	$35,160
Quebec	$34,780
New Brunswick	$31,256
Nova Scotia	$31,193
Prince Edward Island	$29,735

Sources: Statistics Canada, *Summary Tables*, "Gross Domestic Product, Expenditure-Based, by Province and Territory, 2004–2008," and "Population by Year, by Province and Territory, 2005–2009."

Data Analysis »

The databanks for these questions can be found in Appendix D at the back of the text and on 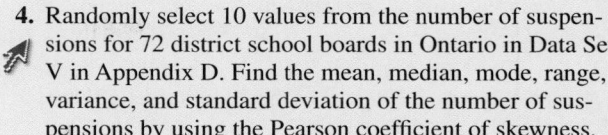 **connect**.

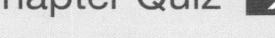 **1.** From the databank, choose one of the following variables: age, weight, cholesterol level, systolic pressure, IQ, or sodium level. Select at least 30 values, and find the mean, median, mode, and midrange. State which measurement of central tendency best describes the average and why.

2. Find the range, variance, and standard deviation for the data selected in Exercise 1.

3. From the databank, choose 10 values from any variable, construct a boxplot, and interpret the results.

4. Randomly select 10 values from the number of suspensions for 72 district school boards in Ontario in Data Set V in Appendix D. Find the mean, median, mode, range, variance, and standard deviation of the number of suspensions by using the Pearson coefficient of skewness.

5. Using the data from Data Set VII in Appendix D, find the mean, median, mode, range, variance, and standard deviation of the area of Canada's 30 most populated cities. Comment on the skewness of the data, using the Pearson coefficient of skewness.

Chapter Quiz »

Determine whether each statement is true or false. If the statement is false, explain why.

1. When the mean is computed for individual data, all values in the data set are used.

2. The mean cannot be found for grouped data when there is an open class.

3. A single, extremely large value can affect the median more than the mean.

4. One-half of all the data values will fall above the mode, and one-half will fall below the mode.

5. In a data set, the mode will always be unique.

6. The range and midrange are both measures of variation.

7. One disadvantage of the median is that it is not unique.

8. The mode and midrange are both measures of variation.

9. If a person's score on an exam corresponds to the 75th percentile, then that person obtained 75 correct answers out of 100 questions.

Select the best answer.

10. What is the value of the mode when all values in the data set are different?

   a. 0
   b. 1
   c. There is no mode.
   d. It cannot be determined unless the data values are given.

11. When data are categorized as, for example, places of residence (rural, suburban, urban), the most appropriate measure of central tendency is the

   a. Mean
   b. Median
   c. Mode
   d. Midrange

12. P_{50} corresponds to

   a. Q_2 *c.* IQR
   b. D_5 *d.* Midrange

13. Which is not part of the five-number summary used for boxplots?

   a. Q_1 and Q_3
   b. The mean
   c. The median
   d. The smallest and the largest data values

14. A statistic that tells the number of standard deviations a data value is above or below the mean is called

   a. A quartile
   b. A percentile
   c. A coefficient of variation
   d. A z score

15. When a distribution is bell-shaped, approximately what percentage of data values will fall within 1 standard deviation of the mean?

   a. 50%
   b. 68%
   c. 95%
   d. 99.7%

Complete these statements with the best answer.

16. A measure obtained from sample data is called a(n) _____.

17. Generally, Greek letters are used to represent _____, and Roman letters are used to represent _____.

18. The positive square root of the variance is called the _____.

19. The symbol for the population standard deviation is _____.

20. When the sum of the lowest data value and the highest data value is divided by 2, the measure is called _____.

21. If the mode is to the left of the median and the mean is to the right of the median, then typically the distribution is _____ skewed.

22. An extremely high or extremely low data value is called a(n) _____.

23. **Car Fuel Consumption** These data highlight the fuel consumption (L/100 km) of the 10 least fuel-efficient cars with Canadian sales.

    24.7 23.2 22.9 22.9 22.9 22.7 22.4 22.1 22.0 20.8

    Source: Natural Resources Canada—*Fuel Consumption Guide 2006.*

    Find each of the descriptive measures.

    a. Mean
    b. Median
    c. Mode
    d. Midrange
    e. Range
    f. Variance
    g. Standard deviation

24. **Typing Test Errors** The distribution of the number of errors that 10 students made on a typing test is shown.

Errors	Frequency
0–2	1
3–5	3
6–8	4
9–11	1
12–14	1

    Find each of these.

    a. Mean
    b. Modal class
    c. Variance
    d. Standard deviation

25. **Rainfall in October** Shown here is a frequency distribution for the number of selected Canadian cities with October precipitation (millimetres) in the indicated intervals.

Precipitation (mm)	Frequency
0.5–25.5	5
25.5–50.5	3
50.5–75.5	3
75.5–100.5	3
100.5–125.5	2
125.5–150.5	1
150.5–175.5	1

    Source: Environment Canada.

    Find each of the descriptive measures.

    a. Mean
    b. Modal class
    c. Variance
    d. Standard deviation

26. **Shipment Times** A survey of 36 selected recording companies showed these numbers of days that it took to receive a shipment from the day it was ordered.

Days	Frequency
1–3	6
4–6	8
7–9	10
10–12	7
13–15	0
16–18	5

    Find each of these.

    a. Mean
    b. Modal class
    c. Variance
    d. Standard deviation

27. **Student Best Friends** In a survey of Grade 3 students, this distribution was obtained for the number of "best friends" each had.

Number of students	Number of best friends
3	0
8	1
6	2
5	3

    Find the average number of best friends for the class. Use the weighted mean.

28. **Employee Years of Service** In an advertisement, a retail store stated that its employees averaged 9 years of service. The distribution is shown here.

Number of employees	Years of service
8	2
2	6
3	10

    Using the weighted mean, calculate the correct average.

29. **Newspapers for Sale** The average number of newspapers for sale in an airport newsstand is 12, and the standard deviation is 4. The average age of the pilots is 37 years, with a standard deviation of 6 years. Which data set is more variable?

30. **Toothpaste Brands** A survey of grocery stores showed that the average number of brands of toothpaste carried was 16, with a standard deviation of 5. The same survey showed the average length of time each store was in business was 7 years, with a standard deviation of 1.6 years. Which is more variable, the number of brands or the number of years?

31. **Test Scores** A student scored 76 on a general science test where the class mean and standard deviation were 82 and 8, respectively; he also scored 53 on a psychology test where the class mean and standard deviation were 58 and 3, respectively. In which class was his relative position higher?

32. **Graduate Record Exam** An American student applying to a Canadian university obtained the following scores on the three-part Graduate Record Exam (GRE). In which part of the GRE did the student do relatively better?

Verbal reasoning	Quantitative reasoning	Analytical writing
$X = 402$	$X = 471$	$X = 3.7$
$\overline{X} = 462$	$\overline{X} = 584$	$\overline{X} = 4.0$
$s = 119$	$s = 151$	$s = 0.9$

33. **Shopping Mall Areas** The number of square metres (in 1000s) of 10 of the largest shopping malls in the world is shown below.

    660, 557, 353, 297, 297, 279, 260, 232, 223, 214

a. Find the percentile rank for each value.
b. What value corresponds to the 40th percentile?
c. Construct a boxplot and comment on the nature of the distribution.

Source: East Connecticut State University, *Shopping Mall Studies.*

34. **Exam Results** On a philosophy comprehensive exam, this distribution was obtained from 25 students.

Score	Frequency
40.5–45.5	3
45.5–50.5	8
50.5–55.5	10
55.5–60.5	3
60.5–65.5	1

a. Construct a percentile graph.
b. Find the values that correspond to the 22nd, 78th, and 99th percentiles.
c. Find the percentiles of the values 52, 43, and 64.

35. **Rental Car Gas Prices** The first column of these data represents the prebuy gas price (in US$ per gallon) of a rental car, and the second column represents the price charged if the car is returned without refilling the gas tank for a selected car rental company. Draw two box-plots for the data and compare the distributions.

Prebuy cost	No prebuy cost
$1.55	$3.80
1.54	3.99
1.62	3.99
1.65	3.85
1.72	3.99
1.63	3.95
1.65	3.94
1.72	4.19
1.45	3.84
1.52	3.94

Source: USA TODAY.

36. **Body Mass Index** The mean body mass index (BMI) for Canadian males is 26.1, with a standard deviation of 5.1. Canadian females have a mean BMI of 24.7, with a standard deviation of 4.7. Assume the BMI data form a bell-shaped (normal) distribution. Apply the empirical rule to determine the BMI range that includes (a) 68%, (b) 95%, and (c) 99.7% of BMI readings for both genders.

Source: Nancy A. Ross, Stephane Treamblay, Saeeda Khan, Daniel Crouse, Mark Trembly, and Jean-Marie Berthelot, "Body Mass Index in Urban Canada: Neighborhood and Metropolitan Area Effects," *American Journal of Public Health,* January 31, 2007–March 31, 2007, Vol. 97, No. 3.

Critical Thinking Challenges »

1. **Average Cost of Weddings** Averages give us information to help us to see where we stand and enable us to make comparisons. Here is a study on the average cost of a wedding. What type of average—mean, median, mode or midrange—might have been used for each category?

Wedding Budget Woes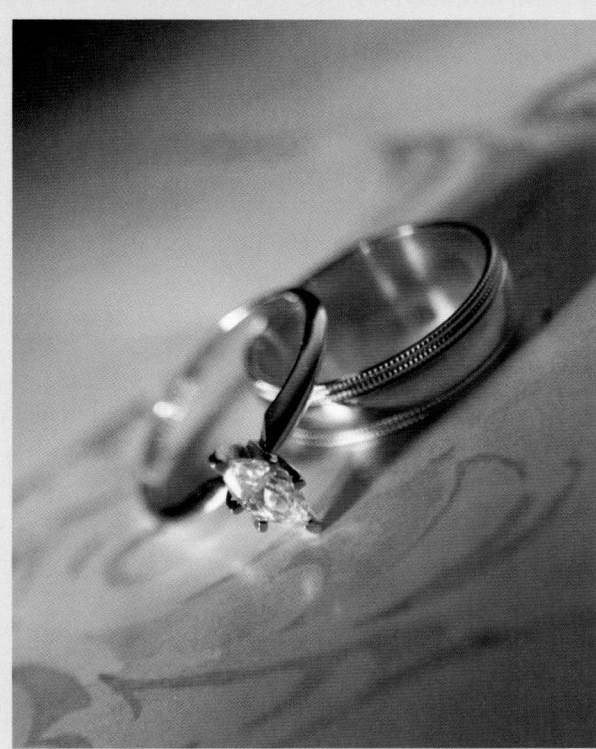

A 2009 survey of Canadian weddings showed that the average age of engaged women was 29 years, with the average engagement lasting 18 months. The most popular month for engagements was December, with 52% of weddings planned between July and September. The average wedding had 140 guests. Wedding costs increased more than 10% from 2007 to 2009. Here is a typical wedding budget. Yikes!

Reception venue	$7,782
Bridal gown	1,083
Wedding bands	1,557
Photographer	1,682
Wedding cake	335
Florist/decor	881
Transportation/limo	569
DJ/musicians	805
Honeymoon	3,632
Average wedding cost	**$18,326**

Source: www.weddingbells.ca, *Wedding Trends in Canada.*

2. **Average Cost of Smoking** This article states that the average yearly cost of smoking a pack of cigarettes a day is $3276. Find the average cost of a pack of cigarettes in your area, and compute the cost per day for one year. Compare your answer with the one in the article.

Save Your Cigarette Money
Bank on your health

On the face of it, it's an easy calculation—you spend so many dollars a day on cigarettes, there are 365 days in a year, a few clicks on the calculator and you can work out how much smoking will cost you in your lifetime. But money doesn't stay the same over time; the price of cigarettes goes up, and so does the cost of living. And your life expectancy doesn't decrease a year for every year you live—the longer you live, the older the age you'll probably live to. So what seems a simple calculation becomes a little trickier—and the numbers can be more than you would expect.

If you smoked a pack a day, your annual savings if you quit smoking could be $3276. Visit the following website to calculate the cost of cigarettes: www. quit4life.com/calc_e.asp.

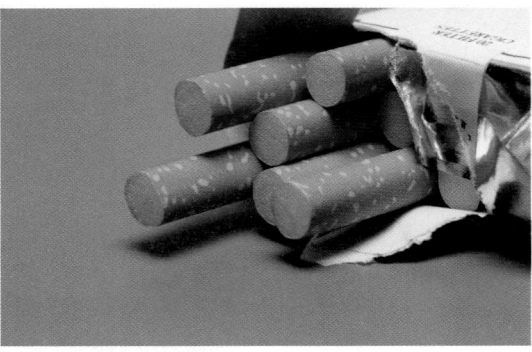

Source: Health Canada, *Quit 4 Life,* "How Much Money Will You Save?"

3. **Age of Canadians by Province** The table shows the median ages of Canadian males and females by province and territory based on data from the 2001 Census. Explain why the median is used instead of the mean.

| | Median Age | |
Name	Males	Females
Canada	36.8	38.4
Newfoundland and Labrador	37.9	38.8
Prince Edward Island	36.8	38.5
Nova Scotia	38.0	39.5
New Brunswick	37.7	39.4
Quebec	37.8	39.8
Ontario	36.4	38.0
Manitoba	35.8	37.8
Saskatchewan	35.8	37.6
Alberta	34.4	35.6
British Columbia	37.8	39.0
Yukon Territory	36.4	35.8
Northwest Territories	30.4	29.8
Nunavut	22.3	21.9

Source: Adapted from Statistics Canada website, www.statcan.ca/bsolc/english/ bsolc?catno=97F0024X2001001. Accessed March 19, 2007.

Data Projects »

Where appropriate, use Minitab, SPSS, the TI-83 Plus, the TI-84 Plus, Excel, or a computer program of your choice to complete the following exercises.

1. **Business and Finance** Use the data collected in Data Project 1 in Chapter 2 regarding stock earnings per share. Determine the mean, mode, median, and midrange for the two data sets. Is one measure of centre more appropriate than the other for these data? Do the measures of centre appear similar? What does this say about the symmetry of the distribution?

2. **Sports and Leisure** Use the data collected in Data Project 2 in Chapter 2 regarding baseball home runs. Determine the mean, mode, median, and midrange for the two data sets. Is one measure of centre more appropriate than the other for these data? Do the measures of centre appear similar? What does this say about the symmetry of the distribution?

3. **Technology** Use the data collected in Data Project 3 in Chapter 2. Determine the mean for the frequency table of song lengths created in that project. Find the actual mean length of all 50 songs. How does the grouped mean compare to the actual mean?

4. **Health and Wellness** Use the data collected in Data Project 6 in Chapter 2 regarding heart rates. Determine the mean and standard deviation for each set of data. Do the means seem very different from one another? Do the standard deviations appear very different from one another?

5. **Politics** Use the data collected in Data Project 5 in Chapter 2 regarding federal election results. Use the formulas for population mean and standard deviation to compute the parameters for all provinces and territories. What is the z score associated with Newfoundland and Labrador? Manitoba? British Columbia? Which provinces are more than 2 standard deviations from the mean?

6. **Your Class** Use your class as a sample. Determine the mean, median, and standard deviation for the age of students in your class. What z score would a 40-year-old have? Would it be unusual to have a 40-year-old in your sample? Determine the skew of the data using the Pearson coefficient of skewness. (See Exercise 48, page 117.)

Answers to Applying the Concepts »

Solution 3–1 Professors' Salaries

1. The sample mean is $98,929.92, the sample median is $93,900.50, the sample midrange is $119,623, and the sample mode is $88,444. If you work for the administrators and do not want to increase salaries, you would say that the average salary is $119,623.

2. If you work for the faculty association and want a salary increase for professors, the sample mode of $88,444 is the best indicator of low salaries followed by the sample median of $93,900.50.

3. The outlier is $151,884. With the outlier removed, the sample mean is $94,115.91, the sample median is $93,521, the sample midrange is $95,336.50, and the sample mode is $88,444. The outlier greatly affected the mean, allowing the administrators to report an average salary that is not representative of the "typical" faculty salary.

4. If the salaries represented every professor at all universities in Canada, the averages would be parameters, since we would have data from the entire population.

5. The mean can be misleading in the presence of outliers, since it is greatly affected by these extreme values.

6. Since the mean is greater than both the median and the mode, the distribution is typically skewed to the right (positively skewed). A sketch of the histogram verifies this distribution shape.

Section 3–2 Blood Pressure

1. Chebyshev's theorem does not work for scores within 1 standard deviation of the mean.

2. At least 75% (900) of the normotensive men will fall in the interval 105–141 mm Hg.

3. About 95% (1330) of the normotensive women have diastolic blood pressures between 62 and 90 mm Hg. About 95% (1235) of the hypertensive women have diastolic blood pressures between 68 and 108 mm Hg.

4. About 95% (1140) of the normotensive men have systolic blood pressures between 105 and 141 mm Hg. About 95% (1045) of the hypertensive men have systolic blood pressures between 119 and 187 mm Hg. These two ranges do overlap.

Section 3–3 Determining Dosages

1. The quartiles could be used to describe the data results.

2. Since there are 10 mice in the upper quartile, this would mean that 4 of them survived.

3. The percentiles would give us the position of a single mouse with respect to all other mice.

4. The quartiles divide the data into four groups of equal size.

5. Standard scores would give us the position of a single mouse with respect to the mean time until the onset of sepsis.

Section 3–4 The Noisy Workplace

From this boxplot, we see that about 25% of the readings in area 5 are above the safe hearing level of 120 decibels. Those workers in area 5 should definitely have protective ear wear. One of the readings in area 6 is above the safe hearing level. It might be a good idea to provide protective ear wear to those workers in area 6 as well. Areas 1–4 appear to be "safe" with respect to hearing level, with area 4 being the safest.

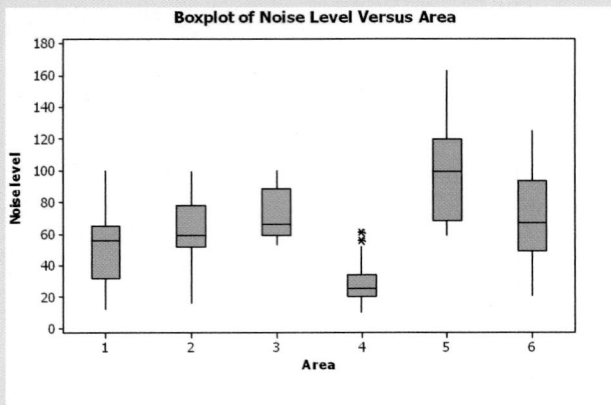

Chapter 4

Probability and Counting Rules

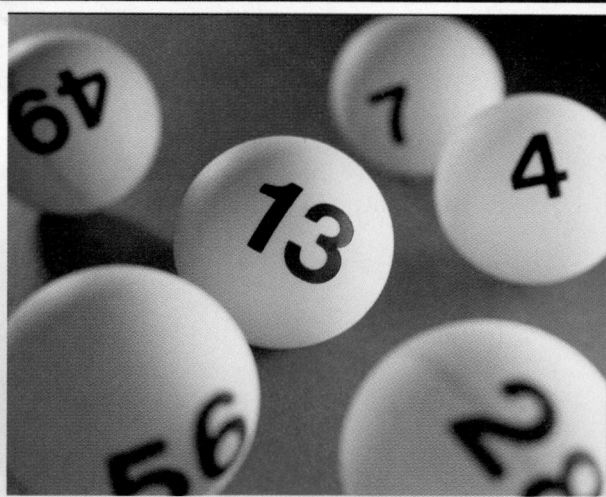

Objectives >

After completing this chapter, you should be able to

LO1 Determine sample spaces and find the probability of an event, using classical probability or empirical probability.

LO2 Use the addition rules to find the probability of simultaneous compound events.

LO3 Use the multiplication rules and conditional probability to find the probability of sequential compound events.

LO4 Use the fundamental counting rule, permutation rule, and combination rule to determine the number of ways that events can occur.

LO5 Combine probability and counting rules to determine outcomes of experiments.

Outline >

McGraw Hill **connect**™ Practise and learn online with *Connect* with data sets and algorithmic questions related to concepts covered in this chapter. Throughout this chapter, questions and tables with online data sets are marked with ✈.

Statistics Today

Would You Bet Your Life?

Humans not only bet money when they gamble, but also bet their lives by engaging in unhealthy activities such as smoking, drinking, using drugs, and exceeding the speed limit when driving. Many people don't care about the risks involved in these activities since they do not understand the concepts of probability. On the other hand, people may fear

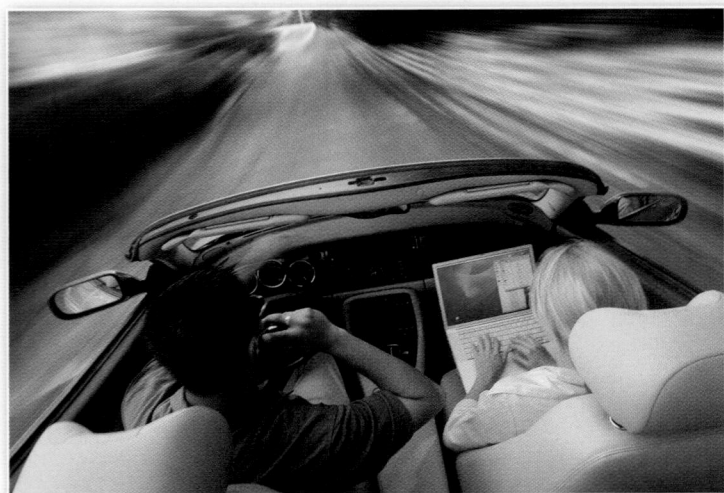

activities that involve little risk to health or life because these activities have been sensationalized by the press and media.

In his book *Probabilities in Everyday Life* (Ivy Books, p. 191), John D. McGervey states

When people have been asked to estimate the frequency of death from various causes, the most overestimated categories are those involving pregnancy, tornadoes, floods, fire, and homicide. The most underestimated categories include deaths from diseases such as diabetes, strokes, tuberculosis, asthma, and stomach cancer (although cancer in general is overestimated).

The question then is, would you feel safer if you flew across Canada on a commercial airline or if you drove? How much greater is the risk of one way to travel over the other? See Statistics Today—Revisited, page 203, near the end of the chapter for the answer.

In this chapter, you will learn about probability—its meaning, how it is computed, and how to evaluate it in terms of the likelihood of an event actually happening.

Introduction >

A cynical person once said, "The only two sure things are death and taxes." This philosophy no doubt arose because so much in people's lives is affected by chance. From the time a person awakes until he or she goes to bed, that person makes decisions regarding the possible events that are governed at least in part by chance. For example, should I carry an umbrella to work today? Will my car battery last until spring? Should I accept that new job?

Probability as a general concept can be defined as the chance of an event occurring. Many people are familiar with probability from observing or playing games of chance, such as card games, slot machines, or lotteries. In addition to being used in games of chance, probability theory is used in the fields of insurance, investment, weather forecasting, and in various other areas. Finally, as stated in Chapter 1, probability is the basis of inferential statistics. For example, predictions are based on probability, and hypotheses are tested by using probability.

The basic concepts of probability are explained in this chapter. These concepts include *probability experiments, sample spaces,* the *addition* and *multiplication rules,* and the *probabilities of complementary events.* Also in this chapter, you will learn the rule for counting, the differences between permutations and combinations, and how to figure out how many different combinations for specific situations exist. Finally, Section 4–5 explains how the counting rules and the probability rules can be used together to solve a wide variety of problems.

4–1 | Sample Spaces and Probability >

Determine sample spaces and find the probability of an event, using classical probability or empirical probability.

The theory of probability grew out of the study of various games of chance using coins, dice, and cards. Since these devices lend themselves well to the application of concepts of probability, they will be used in this chapter as examples. This section begins by explaining some basic concepts of probability. Then the types of probability and probability rules are discussed.

Basic Concepts

Processes such as flipping a coin, rolling a die, or drawing a card from a deck are called *probability experiments.*

> A **probability experiment** is a chance process that leads to well-defined results called *outcomes.*
>
> An **outcome** is the result of a single trial of a probability experiment.

A trial means flipping a coin once, rolling one die once, or the like. When a coin is tossed, there are two possible outcomes: head or tail. (*Note:* We exclude the possibility of a coin landing on its edge.) In the roll of a single die, there are six possible outcomes: 1, 2, 3, 4, 5, or 6. In any experiment, the set of all possible outcomes is called the *sample space.*

> A **sample space** is the set of all possible outcomes of a probability experiment.

Some sample spaces for various probability experiments are shown here.

Experiment	Sample space
Toss one coin	Head, tail
Roll a die	1, 2, 3, 4, 5, 6
Answer a true/false question	True, false
Toss two coins	Head-head, tail-tail, head-tail, tail-head

It is important to realize that when two coins are tossed, there are *four* possible outcomes, as shown in the fourth experiment above. Both coins could fall heads up. Both coins could fall tails up. Coin 1 could fall heads up and coin 2 tails up. Or coin 1 could fall tails up and coin 2 heads up. Heads and tails will be abbreviated as H and T throughout this chapter.

Example 4–1

Rolling Dice

Find the sample space for rolling two dice.

Solution

Since each die can land in six different ways, and two dice are rolled, the sample space can be presented by a rectangular array, as shown in Figure 4–1. The sample space is the list of pairs of numbers in the chart.

Figure 4–1

Figure 4–1

Sample Space for
Rolling Two Dice
(Example 4–1)

	Die 2					
Die 1	1	2	3	4	5	6
1	(1, 1)	(1, 2)	(1, 3)	(1, 4)	(1, 5)	(1, 6)
2	(2, 1)	(2, 2)	(2, 3)	(2, 4)	(2, 5)	(2, 6)
3	(3, 1)	(3, 2)	(3, 3)	(3, 4)	(3, 5)	(3, 6)
4	(4, 1)	(4, 2)	(4, 3)	(4, 4)	(4, 5)	(4, 6)
5	(5, 1)	(5, 2)	(5, 3)	(5, 4)	(5, 5)	(5, 6)
6	(6, 1)	(6, 2)	(6, 3)	(6, 4)	(6, 5)	(6, 6)

Example 4–2

Drawing Cards

Find the sample space for drawing one card from an ordinary deck of cards.

Solution

Since there are 4 suits (hearts, clubs, diamonds, and spades) and 13 cards for each suit (ace, numbers 2 through 10, jack, queen, king), there are 52 outcomes in the sample space. See Figure 4–2.

Figure 4–2

Sample Space for
Drawing a Card
(Example 4–2)

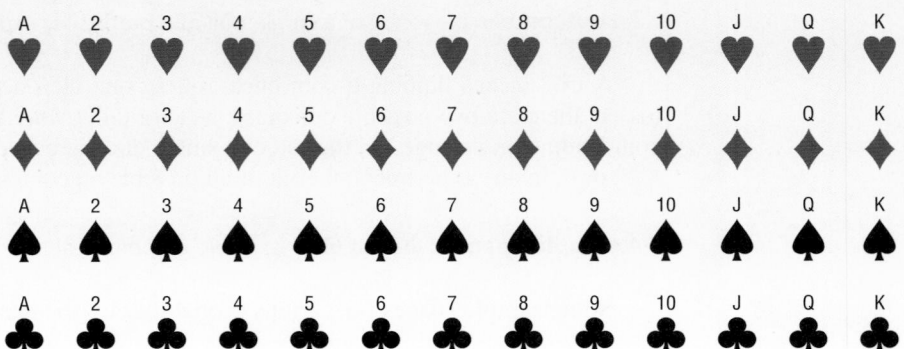

Example 4–3

Gender of Children

Find the sample space for the gender of the children if a family has three children. Use B for boy and G for girl.

Solution

There are two genders, male and female, and each child could be either gender. Hence, there are eight possibilities, as shown here.

BBB   BBG   BGB   GBB   GGG   GGB   GBG   BGG

In Examples 4–1 through 4–3, the sample spaces were found by observation and reasoning; however, another way to find all possible outcomes of a probability experiment is to use a *tree diagram*.

A **tree diagram** is a schematic with branches emanating from a starting point showing all possible outcomes of a probability experiment.

Example 4–4

Gender of Children

Use a tree diagram to find the sample space for the gender of three children in a family, as in Example 4–3.

Solution

Since there are two possibilities (boy or girl) for the first child, draw two branches from a starting point and label one B and the other G. Then if the first child is a boy, there are two possibilities for the second child (boy or girl), so draw two branches from B and label one B and the other G. Do the same if the first child is a girl. Follow the same procedure for the third child. The completed tree diagram is shown in Figure 4–3. To find the outcomes for the sample space, trace through all the possible branches, beginning at the starting point for each one.

Figure 4–3

Tree Diagram for Example 4–4

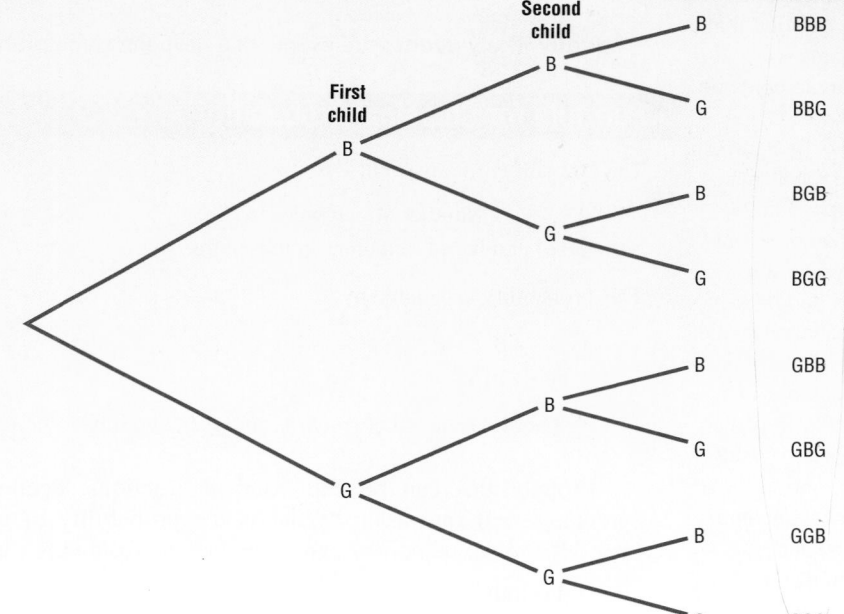

An outcome was defined previously as the result of a single trial of a probability experiment. In many problems, one must find the probability of two or more outcomes. For this reason, it is necessary to distinguish between an outcome and an event.

An **event** consists of a set of outcomes of a probability experiment.

An event can be one outcome or more than one outcome. For example, if a die is rolled and a 6 shows, this result is called an *outcome,* since it is a result of a single trial. An event with one outcome is called a **simple event.** The event of getting an odd number when a die is rolled is called a **compound event,** since it consists of three outcomes or three simple events. In general, a compound event consists of two or more outcomes or simple events.

There are three basic interpretations of probability:

1. Classical probability
2. Empirical or relative frequency probability
3. Subjective probability

Classical Probability

Classical probability uses sample spaces to determine the numerical probability that an event will happen. One does not actually have to perform the experiment to determine that probability. Classical probability is so named because it was the first type of probability studied formally by mathematicians in the seventeenth and eighteenth centuries.

Classical probability assumes that all outcomes in the sample space are equally likely to occur. For example, when a single die is rolled, each outcome has the same probability of occurring. Since there are six outcomes, each outcome has a probability of $\frac{1}{6}$. When a card is selected from an ordinary deck of 52 cards, one assumes that the deck has been shuffled, and each card has the same probability of being selected. In this case, it is $\frac{1}{52}$.

Equally likely events are events that have the same probability of occurring.

Formula for Classical Probability

The probability of any event E is

$$\frac{\text{Number of outcomes in } E}{\text{Total number of outcomes in the sample space}}$$

This probability is denoted by

$$P(E) = \frac{n(E)}{n(S)}$$

This probability is called *classical probability,* and it uses the sample space S.

Probabilities can be expressed as fractions, decimals, or—where appropriate—percentages. If one asks, "What is the probability of getting a head when a coin is tossed?" typical responses can be any of the following three.

"One-half."

"Point five."

"Fifty percent."[1]

These answers are all equivalent. In most cases, the answers to examples and exercises given in this chapter are expressed as fractions or decimals, but percentages are used where appropriate.

Rounding Rule for Probabilities Probabilities should be expressed as reduced fractions or rounded to two or three decimal places. When the probability of an event is an extremely small decimal, it is permissible to round the decimal to the first nonzero digit after the point. For example, 0.0000587 would be 0.00006. When obtaining probabilities from one of the tables in Appendix C, use the number of decimal places given in the table. If decimals are converted to percentages to express probabilities, move the decimal point two places to the right and add a percent sign.

---

[1]Strictly speaking, a percentage is not a probability. However, in everyday language, probabilities are often expressed as percentages (i.e., there is a 60% chance of rain tomorrow). For this reason, some probabilities will be expressed as percentages throughout this book.

Example 4–5

Drawing Cards

Find the probability of getting a red ace when a card is drawn at random from an ordinary deck of cards.

Solution

Since there are 52 card cards in a deck and there are 2 red aces, namely the ace of hearts and the ace of diamonds, $P(\text{red ace}) = \frac{2}{52} = \frac{1}{26}$.

Example 4–6

Gender of Children

If a family has three children, find the probability that all the children are girls.

Solution

The sample space for the gender of children for a family that has three children is BBB, BBG, BGB, GBB, GGG, GGB, GBG, and BGG (see Examples 4–3 and 4–4). Since there is one way in eight possibilities for all three children to be girls,

$$P(\text{GGG}) = \tfrac{1}{8}$$

Historical Note

Ancient Greeks and Romans made crude dice from animal bones, various stones, minerals, and ivory. When the dice were tested, some were found to be quite accurate and fair.

In probability theory, it is important to understand the meaning of the words *and* and *or*. For example, if you were asked to find the probability of getting a queen *and* a heart when you are drawing a single card from a deck, you would be looking for the queen of hearts. Here the word *and* means "at the same time." The word *or* has two meanings. For example, if you were asked to find the probability of selecting a queen *or* a heart when one card is selected from a deck, you would be looking for one of the 4 queens or one of the 13 hearts. In this case, the queen of hearts would be included in both cases and counted twice. So there would be $4 + 13 - 1 = 16$ possibilities.

On the other hand, if you were asked to find the probability of getting a queen *or* a king, you would be looking for one of the 4 queens or one of the 4 kings. In this case, there would be $4 + 4 = 8$ possibilities. In the first case, both events can occur at the same time; we say that this is an example of the *inclusive or*. In the second case, both events cannot occur at the same time, and we say that this is an example of the *exclusive or*.

Example 4–7

Drawing Cards

A card is drawn from an ordinary deck. Find these probabilities.

  a. Of getting a jack
  b. Of getting the 6 of clubs (i.e., a 6 and a club)
  c. Of getting a 3 or a diamond
  d. Of getting a 3 or a 6

Solution

  a. Refer to the sample space in Figure 4–2. There are 4 jacks so there are 4 outcomes in event E and 52 possible outcomes in the sample space. Hence,

  $$P(\text{jack}) = \tfrac{4}{52} = \tfrac{1}{13}$$

  b. Since there is only one 6 of clubs in event E, the probability of getting a 6 of clubs is

  $$P(\text{6 of clubs}) = \tfrac{1}{52}$$

c. There are four 3s and 13 diamonds, but the 3 of diamonds is counted twice in this listing. Hence, there are 16 possibilities of drawing a 3 or a diamond, so

$$P(3 \text{ or diamond}) = \frac{16}{52} = \frac{4}{13}$$

This is an example of the inclusive or.

d. Since there are four 3s and four 6s,

$$P(3 \text{ or } 6) = \frac{8}{52} = \frac{2}{13}$$

This is an example of the exclusive or.

There are four basic probability rules. These rules are helpful in solving probability problems, in understanding the nature of probability, and in deciding if your answers to the problems are correct.

Probability Rule 1

The probability of any event E is a number (either a fraction or decimal) between and including 0 and 1. This is denoted by $0 \le P(E) \le 1$.

Rule 1 states that probabilities cannot be negative or greater than 1.

Probability Rule 2

If an event E cannot occur (i.e., the event contains no members in the sample space), its probability is 0.

Example 4–8

Rolling a Die

When a single die is rolled, find the probability of getting a 9.

Solution

Since the sample space is 1, 2, 3, 4, 5, and 6, it is impossible to get a 9. Hence, the probability is $P(9) = \frac{0}{6} = 0$.

Probability Rule 3

If an event E is certain, then the probability of E is 1.

In other words, if $P(E) = 1$, then the event E is certain to occur. This rule is illustrated in Example 4–9.

Example 4–9

Rolling a Die

When a single die is rolled, what is the probability of getting a number less than 7?

Solution

Since all outcomes—1, 2, 3, 4, 5, and 6—are less than 7, the probability is

$$P(\text{number less than } 7) = \frac{6}{6} = 1$$

The event of getting a number less than 7 is certain.

In other words, probability values range from 0 to 1. When the probability of an event is close to 0, its occurrence is highly unlikely. When the probability of an event is near 0.5, there is about a 50–50 chance that the event will occur; and when the probability of an event is close to 1, the event is highly likely to occur.

Probability Rule 4

The sum of the probabilities of all the outcomes in the sample space is 1.

For example, in the roll of a fair die, each outcome in the sample space has a probability of $\frac{1}{6}$. Hence, the sum of the probabilities of the outcomes is as shown.

Outcome	1	2	3	4	5	6
Probability	$\frac{1}{6}$	$\frac{1}{6}$	$\frac{1}{6}$	$\frac{1}{6}$	$\frac{1}{6}$	$\frac{1}{6}$
Sum	\multicolumn{6}{l}{$\frac{1}{6} + \frac{1}{6} + \frac{1}{6} + \frac{1}{6} + \frac{1}{6} + \frac{1}{6} = \frac{6}{6} = 1$}

Complementary Events

Another important concept in probability theory is that of *complementary events.* When a die is rolled, for instance, the sample space consists of the outcomes 1, 2, 3, 4, 5, and 6. The event E of getting odd numbers consists of the outcomes 1, 3, and 5. The event of not getting an odd number is called the *complement* of event E, and it consists of the outcomes 2, 4, and 6.

> The **complement of an event** E is the set of outcomes in the sample space that are not included in the outcomes of event E. The complement of E is denoted by $\overline{E}$ (read "E bar").

Example 4–10 further illustrates the concept of complementary events.

Example 4–10

Finding Complements

Find the complement of each event.

    a. Rolling a die and getting a 4

    b. Selecting a letter of the alphabet and getting a vowel

    c. Selecting a month and getting a month that begins with a J

    d. Selecting a day of the week and getting a weekday

Solution

    a. Getting a 1, 2, 3, 5, or 6

    b. Getting a consonant (assume *y* is a consonant)

    c. Getting February, March, April, May, August, September, October, November, or December

    d. Getting Saturday or Sunday

The outcomes of an event and the outcomes of the complement make up the entire sample space. For example, if two coins are tossed, the sample space is HH, HT, TH, and TT. The complement of "getting all heads" is not "getting all tails," since the event "all heads" is HH, and the complement of HH is HT, TH, and TT. Hence, the complement of the event "all heads" is the event "getting at least one tail."

Since the event and its complement make up the entire sample space, it follows that the sum of the probability of the event and the probability of its complement will equal 1. That is, $P(E) + P(\overline{E}) = 1$. In Example 4–10, let E = all heads, or HH, and let $\overline{E}$ = at least one tail, or HT, TH, TT. Then $P(E) = \frac{1}{4}$ and $P(\overline{E}) = \frac{3}{4}$; hence, $P(E) + P(\overline{E}) = \frac{1}{4} + \frac{3}{4} = 1$.

The rule for complementary events can be stated algebraically in three ways.

Rule for Complementary Events

$$P(\overline{E}) = 1 - P(E) \quad \text{or} \quad P(E) = 1 - P(\overline{E}) \quad \text{or} \quad P(E) + P(\overline{E}) = 1$$

Stated in words, the rule is: *If the probability of an event or the probability of its complement is known, then the other can be found by subtracting the probability from 1.* This rule is important in probability theory because at times the best solution to a problem is to find the probability of the complement of an event and then subtract from 1 to get the probability of the event itself.

Example 4–11

Residence in Industrialized Country

If the probability that a person lives in an industrialized country of the world is $\frac{1}{5}$, find the probability that a person does not live in an industrialized country.

Source: Harper's Index.

Solution

$P(\text{not living in an industrialized country}) = 1 - P(\text{living in an industrialized country})$
$$= 1 - \frac{1}{5} = \frac{4}{5}$$

Probabilities can be represented pictorially by **Venn diagrams.** Figure 4–4(a) shows the probability of a simple event E. The area inside the circle represents the probability of event E, that is, $P(E)$. The area inside the rectangle represents the probability of all the events in the sample space $P(S)$.

The Venn diagram that represents the probability of the complement of an event $P(\overline{E})$ is shown in Figure 4–4(b). In this case, $P(\overline{E}) = 1 - P(E)$, which is the area inside the rectangle but outside the circle representing $P(E)$. Recall that $P(S) = 1$ and $P(E) = 1 - P(\overline{E})$, The reasoning is that $P(E)$ is represented by the area of the circle and $P(\overline{E})$ is the probability of the events that are outside the circle.

Figure 4–4

Venn Diagram for the Probability and Complement

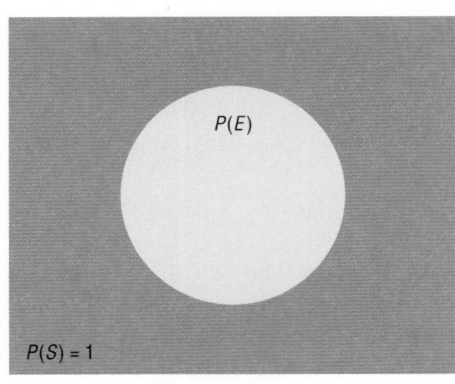

$P(E)$

$P(S) = 1$

(a) Simple probability

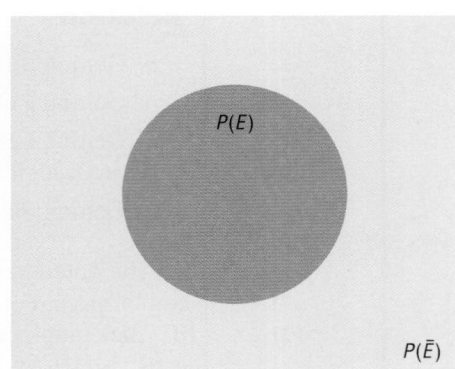

$P(E)$

$P(\overline{E})$

(b) $P(\overline{E}) = 1 - P(E)$

Empirical Probability

The difference between classical and **empirical probability** is that classical probability assumes that certain outcomes are equally likely (such as the outcomes when a die is rolled), while empirical probability relies on actual experience to determine the likelihood of outcomes. In empirical probability, one might actually roll a given die 6000 times, observe the various frequencies, and use these frequencies to determine the probability of an outcome.

Suppose, for example, that a researcher for the Canadian Automobile Association asked 50 people who plan to travel over the Labour Day long weekend how they will get to their destinations. The results can be categorized in a frequency distribution as shown.

Method	Frequency
Drive	41
Fly	6
Train or bus	3
	50

Now probabilities can be computed for various categories. For example, the probability of selecting a person who is driving is $\frac{41}{50}$, since 41 out of the 50 people said that they were driving.

Formula for Empirical Probability

Given a frequency distribution, the probability of an event being in a given class is

$$P(E) = \frac{\text{Frequency for the class}}{\text{Total frequencies in the distribution}} = \frac{f}{n}$$

This probability is called *empirical probability* and is based on observation.

Example 4–12

Travel Survey

In the travel survey just described, find the probability that a person will travel by airplane over the Labour Day long weekend.

Solution

$$P(E) = \frac{f}{n} = \frac{6}{50} = \frac{3}{25}$$

Example 4–13

Distribution of Blood Types

In a random sample of 50 people, 21 had type O blood, 22 had type A blood, 5 had type B blood, and 2 had type AB blood. Set up a frequency distribution and find the following probabilities.

  a. A person has type O blood.

  b. A person has type A or type B blood.

  c. A person has neither type A nor type O blood.

  d. A person does not have type AB blood.

Source: The American Red Cross.

Solution

Type	Frequency
A	22
B	5
AB	2
O	21
	Total 50

a. $P(\text{O}) = \dfrac{f}{n} = \dfrac{21}{50}$

b. $P(\text{A or B}) = \dfrac{22}{50} + \dfrac{5}{50} = \dfrac{27}{50}$

(Add the frequencies of the two classes.)

c. $P(\text{neither A nor O}) = \dfrac{5}{50} + \dfrac{2}{50} = \dfrac{7}{50}$

(Neither A nor O means that a person has either type B or type AB blood.)

d. $P(\text{not AB}) = 1 - P(\text{AB}) = 1 - \dfrac{2}{50} = \dfrac{48}{50} = \dfrac{24}{25}$

(Find the probability of not AB by subtracting the probability of type AB from 1.)

Example 4–14

Hospital Stays for Maternity Patients

Hospital records indicated that maternity patients stayed in the hospital for the number of days shown in the distribution.

Number of days stayed	Frequency
3	15
4	32
5	56
6	19
7	5
	127

Find the probabilities that a randomly sampled patient stayed

a. exactly 5 days.   c. at most 4 days.

b. less than 6 days.   d. at least 5 days.

Solution

a. $P(5) = \dfrac{56}{127}$

b. $P(\text{less than 6 days}) = \dfrac{15}{127} + \dfrac{32}{127} + \dfrac{56}{127} = \dfrac{103}{127}$

(Less than 6 days means 3, 4, or 5 days.)

c. $P(\text{at most 4 days}) = \dfrac{15}{127} + \dfrac{32}{127} = \dfrac{47}{127}$

(At most 4 days means 3 or 4 days.)

d. $P(\text{at least 5 days}) = \dfrac{56}{127} + \dfrac{19}{127} + \dfrac{5}{127} = \dfrac{80}{127}$

(At least 5 days means 5, 6, or 7 days.)

Empirical probabilities can also be found by using a relative frequency distribution, as shown in Section 2–2.

For example, the relative frequency distribution of the travel survey shown previously is

Method	Frequency	Relative frequency
Drive	41	0.82
Fly	6	0.12
Train or bus	3	0.06
	50	1.00

Therefore, the probability that a person's method of travel was to drive is 0.82, which is equal to $\frac{41}{50}$. These frequencies are the same as the relative frequencies explained in Chapter 2.

Law of Large Numbers

When a coin is tossed one time, it is common knowledge that the probability of getting a head is $\frac{1}{2}$. But what happens when the coin is tossed 50 times? Will it come up heads 25 times? Not all the time. One should expect about 25 heads if the coin is fair. But due to chance variation, 25 heads will not occur most of the time.

If the empirical probability of getting a head is computed by using a small number of trials, it is usually not exactly $\frac{1}{2}$. However, as the number of trials increases, the empirical probability of getting a head will approach the theoretical probability of $\frac{1}{2}$, if in fact the coin is fair (i.e., balanced). This phenomenon is an example of the **law of large numbers.**

One should be careful to not think that the number of heads and number of tails tend to "even out." As the number of trials increases, the proportion of heads to the total number of trials will approach $\frac{1}{2}$. This law holds for any type of gambling game—tossing dice, playing roulette, and so on.

It should be pointed out that the probabilities that the proportions steadily approach may or may not agree with those theorized in the classical model. If not, it can have important implications, such as "the die is not fair." Pit bosses in Las Vegas watch for empirical trends that do not agree with classical theories, and they will sometimes take a set of dice out of play if observed frequencies are too far out of line with classical expected frequencies.

Subjective Probability

The third type of probability is called *subjective probability*. **Subjective probability** uses a probability value based on an educated guess or estimate, employing opinions and inexact information.

In subjective probability, a person or group makes an educated guess at the chance that an event will occur. This guess is based on the person's experience and evaluation of a solution. For example, a sportswriter may say that there is a 70% probability that the Toronto Blue Jays will win the pennant next year. A physician might say that, on the basis of her diagnosis, there is a 30% chance the patient will need an operation. A seismologist might say there is an 80% probability that an earthquake will occur in a certain area. These are only a few examples of how subjective probability is used in everyday life.

All three types of probability (classical, empirical, and subjective) are used to solve a variety of problems in business, engineering, and other fields.

Probability and Risk Taking

An area in which people fail to understand probability is risk taking. Actually, people fear situations or events that have a relatively small probability of happening rather than those events that have a greater likelihood of occurring. For example, many people think that the crime rate is increasing every year. However, a published report from the Canadian Centre for Justice Statistics indicates that nationally both property and violent crimes have been steadily decreasing since their peak in 1992.[2]

In his book *How Risk Affects Your Everyday Life,* author James Walsh states, "Today most media coverage of risk to health and well-being focuses on shock and outrage." Shock and outrage make good stories and can scare us about the wrong dangers. For example, the author states that if a person is 20% overweight, the loss of life expectancy is 900 days (about three years), but loss of life expectancy from exposure to radiation emitted by nuclear power plants is 0.02 day. As you can see, being overweight is much more of a threat than being exposed to radioactive emission.

Many people gamble daily with their lives, for example, by using tobacco, drinking and driving, and riding motorcycles. When people are asked to estimate the probabilities or frequencies of death from various causes, they tend to overestimate causes such as accidents, fires, and floods and to underestimate the probabilities of death from diseases (other than cancer), strokes, etc. For example, most people think that their chances of dying of a heart attack are 1 in 20, when in fact they are almost 1 in 3; the chances of dying by pesticide poisoning are 1 in 200,000 (*True Odds* by James Walsh). The reason people think this way is that the news media sensationalize deaths resulting from catastrophic events and rarely mention deaths from disease.

When you are dealing with life-threatening catastrophes such as hurricanes, floods, automobile accidents, or smoking, it is important to get the facts. That is, get the actual numbers from accredited statistical agencies or reliable statistical studies, and then compute the probabilities and make decisions based on your knowledge of probability and statistics.

In summary, then, when you make a decision or plan a course of action based on probability, make sure that you understand the true probability of the event occurring. Also, find out how the information was obtained (i.e., from a reliable source). Weigh the cost of the action and decide if it is worth it. Finally, look for other alternatives or courses of action with less risk involved.

Historical Note

The first book on probability, *The Book of Chance and Games,* was written by Jerome Cardan (1501–1576). Cardan was an astrologer, philosopher, physician, mathematician, and gambler. This book contained techniques on how to cheat and how to catch others at cheating.

4–1 Applying the Concepts

Tossing a Coin

Assume you are at a carnival and decide to play one of the games. You spot a table where a person is flipping a coin, and since you have an understanding of basic probability, you believe that the odds of winning are in your favour. When you get to the table, you find out that all you have to do is guess which side of the coin will be facing up after it is tossed. You are assured that the coin is fair, meaning that each of the two sides has an equally likely chance of occurring. You think back about what you learned in your statistics class about probability before you decide what to bet on. Answer the following questions about the coin-tossing game.

1. What is the sample space?
2. What are the possible outcomes?
3. What does the classical approach to probability say about computing probabilities for this type of problem?

---

[2]Adapted from Statistics Canada, "Table: Uniform Crime Reporting Survey, CCJS," *Juristat,* Crime statistics in Canada, 2004, Catalogue 85-002, Vol. 25, No. 5, page 5.

You decide to bet on heads, believing that it has a 50% chance of coming up. A friend of yours, who had been playing the game for awhile before you got there, tells you that heads has come up the last 9 times in a row. You remember the law of large numbers.

4. What is the law of large numbers, and does it change your thoughts about what will occur on the next toss?

5. What does the empirical approach to probability say about this problem, and could you use it to solve this problem?

6. Can subjective probabilities be used to help solve this problem? Explain.

7. Assume you could win $1 million if you could guess what the results of the next toss will be. What would you bet on? Why?

See page 207 for the answers.

Exercises 4–1

1. What is a probability experiment?

2. Define *sample space*.

3. What is the difference between an outcome and an event?

4. What are equally likely events?

5. What is the range of the values of the probability of an event?

6. When an event is certain to occur, what is its probability?

7. If an event cannot happen, what value is assigned to its probability?

8. What is the sum of the probabilities of all the outcomes in a sample space?

9. If the probability that it will rain tomorrow is 0.20, what is the probability that it won't rain tomorrow? Would you recommend taking an umbrella?

10. A probability experiment is conducted. Which of these cannot be considered a probability of an outcome?

   a. $\frac{1}{3}$ d. -0.59 g. 1

   b. $-\frac{1}{5}$ e. 0   h. 33%

   c. 0.80   f. 1.45   i. 112%

11. Classify each statement as an example of classical probability, empirical probability, or subjective probability.

   a. The probability that a person will watch the 6 o'clock evening news is 0.15.

   b. The probability of winning at Chuck-a-Luck, a three-dice game, is $\frac{75}{216}$.

   c. The probability that a bus will be in an accident on a specific run is about 6%.

   d. The probability of getting a royal flush when five cards are selected at random is $\frac{1}{649,740}$.

   e. The probability that a student will get a C or better in a statistics course is about 70%.

   f. The probability that a new fast-food restaurant will be a success in Regina is 35%.

   g. The probability that interest rates will rise in the next 6 months is 0.50.

12. (ans) **Rolling a Die** If a die is rolled one time, find these probabilities.

   a. Of getting a 4

   b. Of getting an even number

   c. Of getting a number greater than 4

   d. Of getting a number less than 7

   e. Of getting a number greater than 0

   f. Of getting a number greater than 3 or an odd number

   g. Of getting a number greater than 3 and an odd number

13. **Rolling Two Dice** If two dice are rolled one time, find the probability of getting these results.

   a. A sum of 6

   b. Doubles

   c. A sum of 7 or 11

   d. A sum greater than 9

   e. A sum less than or equal to 4

14. (ans) **Drawing a Card** If one card is drawn from a deck, find the probability of getting these results.

   a. An ace

   b. A diamond

   c. An ace of diamonds

   d. A 4 or a 6

e. A 4 or a club

f. A 6 or a spade

g. A heart or a club

h. A red queen

i. A red card or a 7

j. A black card and a 10

15. **Shopping Mall Promotion** A shopping mall has set up a promotion as follows. With any mall purchase of $50 or more, the customer gets to spin the wheel shown here. If a number 1 comes up, the customer wins $10. If the number 2 comes up, the customer wins $5, and if the number 3 or 4 comes up, the customer wins a discount coupon. Find the following probabilities.

a. The customer wins $10.

b. The customer wins money.

c. The customer wins a coupon.

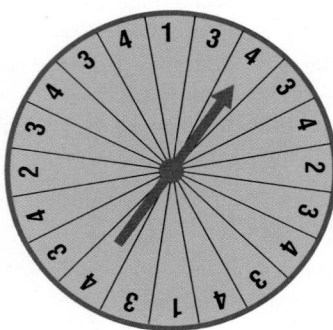

16. **Selecting a Province/Territory** Choose one of Canada's 13 provinces or territories at random.

a. What is the probability that it begins with an N?

b. What is the probability that it doesn't begin with a vowel? (*Note:* Assume that "Y" is a vowel.)

17. **Human Blood Types** Human blood is grouped into four types. The percentage of Canadians with each type is listed below.

O 46%   A 42%   B 9%   AB 3%

Choose one Canadian at random. Find the probability that this person

a. Has type O blood

b. Has type A or B

c. Does not have type O

Source: Canadian Blood Services, *Blood,* "Types & Rh System."

18. **Firearms Registry Support** Seventy-six percent of Canadians of voting age support a national firearms registry. Choose one Canadian voter at random. What is the

probability that the selected voter will be opposed to the firearms registry?

Source: The Gallup Poll Organization.

19. **Children Living at Home** In the 2006 census, Statistics Canada reported that 38.5% of Canadian families had no children living at home, 27.3% had one child, 23.9% had two children, and 10.3% had three or more children living at home. If a family is selected at random, find the probability that living at home included

a. Either one or two children

b. More than one child

c. Less than three children

d. Based on the answers to parts *a, b,* and *c,* which is most likely to occur?

Source: Statistics Canada, *Summary Tables,* "Census Families by Number of Children at Home, by Province and Territory (2006 Census)."

20. **Prime Numbers** A prime number is a number that is evenly divisible by 1 and itself. The prime numbers less than 100 are listed below.

2	3	4	7	11	13	17	19	23	29	31
37	41	43	47	53	59	61	67	71	73	79
83	89	97								

Choose one of these numbers at random. Find the probability that

a. The number is even.

b. The sum of the number's digits is even.

c. The number is greater than 50.

21. **Gender of Children** A couple has three children. Find each probability.

a. All boys

b. All girls or all boys

c. Exactly two boys or two girls

d. At least one child of each gender

22. **Craps Game** In the game of craps using two dice, a person wins on the first roll if a 7 or an 11 is rolled. Find the probability of winning on the first roll.

23. **Craps Game** In a game of craps, a player loses on the roll if a 2, 3, or 12 is tossed on the first roll. Find the probability of losing on the first roll.

24. **Workplace Fatalities** The Association of Workers' Compensation Boards of Canada (AWCBC) publishes statistics on injuries in the workplace. In 2008, the AWCBC reported the following workplace fatalities by province.

NL	23	ON	396
PEI	3	MB	24
NS	23	SK	26
NB	14	AB	166
QC	195	BC	160

If one workplace fatality is selected at random, what is the probability that the worker was

a. From Ontario (ON)

b. From an Atlantic province (NL or PEI or NS or NB)

c. Not from a Prairie province (MB or SK or AB)

Source: Association of Workers' Compensation Boards of Canada, *National Work Injury Statistics Program.*

25. **Roulette** A roulette wheel has 38 spaces numbered 1 through 36, 0, and 00. Find the probability of getting these results.

a. An odd number (Do not count 0 or 00 as odd.)

b. A number greater than 27

c. A space that contains the digit 0

d. Based on the answers to parts *a*, *b*, and *c*, which is most likely to occur? Explain why.

26. **Federal Prison Sentences** The following data represents the federal prison sentences for Canadian males convicted of various criminal offences in a recent year.

Sentence	Number
Under three years	1848
Three to six years	1548
Six to ten years	341
Ten years or more	96
Life or indeterminate	155
	3988

Source: Correctional Services Canada.

If one male prisoner is selected at random, find the probability that the sentence was

a. Under three years

b. Between three and ten years

c. At least ten years (including life or indeterminate)

27. **Counterfeit Bills** The Bank of Canada reported the following number of counterfeit bills in circulation in 2008.

$5	$10	$20
5337	8454	38,445

If one of these bills is randomly selected, find the probability that the bill is

a. A $20 bill

b. A $5 or $10 bill

c. Not a $10 bill

Source: Bank of Canada, *Bank of Canada Banking and Financial Statistics,* December 2009.

28. **Equal Treatment of People** A *Reader's Digest* survey indicated that 85% of Canadian teens said "it was absolutely essential" to treat "all people equally, regardless of race or ethnic background." If a Canadian teen is selected at random, find the probability that the teen disagrees with this viewpoint on equality of treatment.

Source: www.readersdigest.ca.

29. **Rolling Dice** Roll two dice and multiply the numbers together.

a. Write out the sample space.

b. What is the probability that the product is a multiple of 6?

c. What is the probability that the product is less than 10?

30. **Distribution of Tax Dollars** The Canadian government's Department of Finance publishes a pamphlet entitled *Where Your Tax Dollar Goes*. A 2005 publication breaks down the tax burden as follows:

45.2% from personal income tax

15.0% from goods and services tax (GST)

15.1% from corporate income tax

8.7% from Employment Insurance premiums

8.4% from other taxes

7.5% from other revenues

If a revenue source is selected at random, what is the probability that it does not come from either personal income tax or corporate income tax?

Source: Finance Canada.

31. **Coin Selection** A box contains one of each coin: 1¢, 5¢, 10¢, and 25¢. A coin is selected at random, and it is not replaced; then a second coin is selected at random. Draw a tree diagram and determine the sample space.

32. **Coin Toss** Draw a tree diagram and determine the sample space for tossing four coins.

33. **Numbered Ball Selection** Four balls numbered 1 through 4 are placed in a box. A ball is selected at random, and its number is noted; then it is replaced. A second ball is selected at random, and its number is noted. Draw a tree diagram and determine the sample space.

34. **Digital TV Purchase** Fred and Robin decide to replace their old CRT analogue television with a modern flat panel digital television. They are offered the following options.

Manufacturer	Screen size	Display type
LG Electronics	46″	LCD
Samsung	52″	Plasma
Sony		

Draw a tree diagram for all possible types of digital televisions.

35. **Required First-Year College Courses** First-year students at a particular college must take 1 English class, 1 class in mathematics, a first-year seminar, and an elective. There are 2 English classes to choose from, 3 mathematics classes, 5 electives, and everyone takes the same first-year seminar. Represent the possible schedules using a tree diagram

36. **Tossing a Coin and Rolling a Die** A coin is tossed; if it falls heads up, it is tossed again. If it falls tails up, a die is rolled. Draw a tree diagram and determine the outcomes.

Extending the Concepts »

37. CEO Age Distribution The distribution of ages of CEOs is as follows:

Age	Frequency
21–30	1
31–40	8
41–50	27
51–60	29
61–70	24
71–up	11

Source: Information based on *USA TODAY* Snapshot.

If a CEO is selected at random, find the probability that his or her age is

a. Between 31 and 40

b. Under 31

c. Over 30 and under 51

d. Under 31 or over 60

38. Coin Toss A person flipped a coin 100 times and obtained 73 heads. Can the person conclude that the coin was unbalanced?

39. Medical Treatment A medical doctor stated that with a certain treatment, a patient has a 50% chance of recovering without surgery. That is, "Either he will get well or he won't get well." Comment on this statement.

40. Wheel Spinner The wheel spinner shown here is spun twice. Find the sample space, and then determine the probability of the following events.

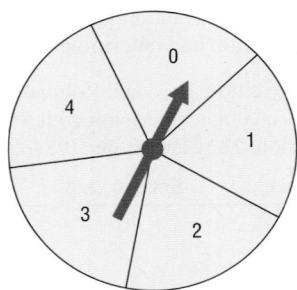

a. An odd number on the first spin and an even number on the second spin (*Note:* 0 is considered even.)

b. A sum greater than 4

c. Even numbers on both spins

d. A sum that is odd

e. The same number on both spins

41. Tossing Coins Toss three coins 128 times and record the number of heads (0, 1, 2, or 3); then record your results with the theoretical probabilities. Compute the empirical probabilities of each.

42. Tossing Coins Toss two coins 100 times and record the number of heads (0, 1, 2). Compute the probabilities of each outcome, and compare these probabilities with the theoretical results.

43. Gambling Odds Odds are used in gambling games to make them fair. For example, if a person rolled a die and won every time he or she rolled a 6, then the person would win on average once every 6 times. So that the game is fair, the odds of 5 to 1 are given. This means that if the person bet $1 and won, he or she could win $5. On average, the player would win $5 once in 6 rolls and lose $1 on the other 5 rolls—hence the term *fair game.*

In most gambling games, the odds given are not fair. For example, if the odds of winning are really 20 to 1, the house might offer 15 to 1 in order to make a profit.

Odds can be expressed as a fraction or as a ratio, such as $\frac{5}{1}$, 5:1, or 5 to 1. Odds are computed in favour of the event or against the event. The formulas for odds are

$$\text{Odds in favour} = \frac{P(E)}{1 - P(E)}$$

$$\text{Odds against} = \frac{P(\overline{E})}{1 - P(\overline{E})}$$

In the die example,

$$\text{Odds in favour of a 6} = \frac{\frac{1}{6}}{\frac{5}{6}} = \frac{1}{5} \text{ or } 1{:}5$$

$$\text{Odds against a 6} = \frac{\frac{5}{6}}{\frac{1}{6}} = \frac{5}{1} \text{ or } 5{:}1$$

Find the odds in favour of and against each event.

a. Rolling a die and getting a 2

b. Rolling a die and getting an even number

c. Drawing a card from a deck and getting a spade

d. Drawing a card and getting a red card

e. Drawing a card and getting a queen

f. Tossing two coins and getting two tails

g. Tossing two coins and getting one tail

| 4–2 | The Addition Rules for Probability > |

Use the addition rules to find the probability of simultaneous compound events.

Many problems involve finding the probability of two or more events. For example, at a large political gathering, one might wish to know, for a person selected at random, the probability that the person is a female or is a Conservative. In this case, there are three possibilities to consider:

1. The person is a female.
2. The person is a Conservative.
3. The person is both a female and a Conservative.

Consider another example. At the same gathering there are Conservatives, Liberals, and New Democrats. If a person is selected at random, what is the probability that the person is a Liberal or a New Democrat? In this case, there are only two possibilities:

1. The person is a Liberal.
2. The person is a New Democrat.

The difference between the two examples is that in the first case, the person selected can be a female and a Conservative at the same time. In the second case, the person selected cannot be both a Liberal and a New Democrat at the same time. In the second case, the two events are said to be *mutually exclusive;* in the first case, they are not mutually exclusive.

> Two events are **mutually exclusive events** if they cannot occur at the same time (i.e., they have no outcomes in common).

In another situation, the events of getting a 4 and getting a 6 when a single card is drawn from a deck are mutually exclusive events, since a single card cannot be both a 4 and a 6. On the other hand, the events of getting a 4 and getting a heart on a single draw are not mutually exclusive, since one can select the 4 of hearts when drawing a single card from an ordinary deck.

Historical Note

Paintings in tombs excavated in Egypt show that the Egyptians played games of chance. One game called *Hounds and Jackals* played in 1800 B.C. is similar to the present-day game of *Snakes and Ladders.*

Example 4–15

Rolling a Die

Determine which events are mutually exclusive and which are not, when a single die is rolled.

  a. Getting an odd number and getting an even number
  b. Getting a 3 and getting an odd number
  c. Getting an odd number and getting a number less than 4
  d. Getting a number greater than 4 and getting a number less than 4

Solution

  a. The events are mutually exclusive, since the first event can be 1, 3, or 5 and the second event can be 2, 4, or 6.
  b. The events are not mutually exclusive, since the first event is a 3 and the second can be 1, 3, or 5. Hence, 3 is contained in both events.
  c. The events are not mutually exclusive, since the first event can be 1, 3, or 5 and the second can be 1, 2, or 3. Hence, 1 and 3 are contained in both events.
  d. The events are mutually exclusive, since the first event can be 5 or 6 and the second event can be 1, 2, or 3.

Example 4–16	**Drawing a Card**

Determine which events are mutually exclusive, and which are not, when a single card is drawn from a deck.

    a. Getting a 7 and getting a jack

    b. Getting a club and getting a king

    c. Getting a face card and getting an ace

    d. Getting a face card and getting a spade

Solution

Only the events in parts *a* and *c* are mutually exclusive.

The probability of two or more events can be determined by the *addition rules*. The first addition rule is used when the events are mutually exclusive.

Addition Rule 1

When two events *A* and *B* are mutually exclusive, the probability that *A* or *B* will occur is

$$P(A \text{ or } B) = P(A) + P(B)$$

Example 4–17	**Selecting a Doughnut**

A box contains 3 glazed doughnuts, 4 jelly doughnuts, and 5 chocolate doughnuts. If a person selects a doughnut at random, find the probability that it is either a glazed doughnut or a chocolate doughnut.

Solution

Since the box contains 3 glazed doughnuts, 5 chocolate doughnuts, and a total of 12 doughnuts, $P(\text{glazed or chocolate}) = P(\text{glazed}) + P(\text{chocolate}) = \frac{3}{12} + \frac{5}{12} = \frac{8}{12} = \frac{2}{3}$. The events are mutually exclusive.

Example 4–18	**Political Affiliation at a Rally**

At a political rally, there are 20 Conservatives, 13 Liberals, and 6 New Democrats. If a person is selected at random, find the probability that person is either a Liberal or a New Democrat.

Solution

$$P(\text{Liberal or New Democrat}) = P(\text{Liberal}) + P(\text{New Democrat})$$
$$= \tfrac{13}{39} + \tfrac{6}{39} = \tfrac{19}{39}$$

Example 4–19	**Selecting a Day of the Week**

A day of the week is selected at random. Find the probability that it is a weekend day.

Solution

$$P(\text{Saturday or Sunday}) = P(\text{Saturday}) + P(\text{Sunday}) = \tfrac{1}{7} + \tfrac{1}{7} = \tfrac{2}{7}$$

When two events are not mutually exclusive, then the probability of the common elements of the two events must be subtracted from the combined probabilities. Refer to the Venn diagram, Figure 4–5(b) on the next page. This technique is illustrated in Example 4–20.

Example 4–20

Drawing a Card

A single card is drawn from a deck. Find the probability that it is a king or a club.

Solution

Since the king of clubs means a king and a club, it has been counted twice—once as a king and once as a club; therefore, one of the outcomes must be subtracted, as shown.

$$P(\text{king or club}) = P(\text{king}) + P(\text{club}) - P(\text{king of clubs})$$

$$= \frac{4}{52} + \frac{13}{52} - \frac{1}{52} = \frac{16}{52} = \frac{4}{13}$$

When events are not mutually exclusive, Addition Rule 2 can be used to find the probability of the events.

Addition Rule 2

If A and B are *not* mutually exclusive, then

$$P(A \text{ or } B) = P(A) + P(B) - P(A \text{ and } B)$$

Note: This rule can also be used when the events are mutually exclusive, since $P(A$ and $B)$ will always equal 0. However, it is important to make a distinction between the two situations.

Example 4–21

Selecting Medical Personnel

In a hospital unit there are 8 nurses and 5 physicians; 7 nurses and 3 physicians are females. If a staff person is randomly selected, find the probability that the subject is a nurse or a male.

Solution

The sample space is shown here.

Staff	Females	Males	Total
Nurses	7	1	8
Physicians	3	2	5
Total	10	3	13

The probability is

$$P(\text{nurse or male}) = P(\text{nurse}) + P(\text{male}) - P(\text{male nurse})$$

$$= \frac{8}{13} + \frac{3}{13} - \frac{1}{13} = \frac{10}{13}$$

Example 4–22

Driving While Intoxicated

On New Year's Eve, the probability of a person driving while intoxicated is 0.32, the probability of a person having a driving accident is 0.09, and the probability of a person having a driving accident while intoxicated is 0.06. What is the probability of a person driving while intoxicated or having a driving accident?

Solution

$$P(\text{intoxicated or accident}) = P(\text{intoxicated}) + P(\text{accident})$$
$$- P(\text{intoxicated and accident})$$
$$= 0.32 + 0.09 - 0.06 = 0.35$$

In summary, then, when the two events are mutually exclusive, use Addition Rule 1. When the events are not mutually exclusive, use Addition Rule 2.

The probability rules can be extended to three or more events. For three mutually exclusive events A, B, and C,

$$P(A \text{ or } B \text{ or } C) = P(A) + P(B) + P(C)$$

For three events that are *not* mutually exclusive,

$$P(A \text{ or } B \text{ or } C) = P(A) + P(B) + P(C) - P(A \text{ and } B) - P(A \text{ and } C)$$
$$- P(B \text{ and } C) + P(A \text{ and } B \text{ and } C)$$

See Exercises 23, 24, and 25 in this section.

Figure 4–5(a) shows a Venn diagram that represents two mutually exclusive events A and B. In this case, $P(A \text{ or } B) = P(A) + P(B)$, since these events are mutually exclusive and do not overlap. In other words, the probability of occurrence of event A or event B is the sum of the areas of the two circles.

Figure 4–5(b) represents the probability of two events that are *not* mutually exclusive. In this case, $P(A \text{ or } B) = P(A) + P(B) - P(A \text{ and } B)$. The area in the intersection or overlapping part of both circles corresponds to $P(A \text{ and } B)$; and when the area of circle A is added to the area of circle B, the overlapping part is counted twice. It must therefore be subtracted once to get the correct area or probability.

Figure 4–5

Venn Diagrams for the Addition Rules

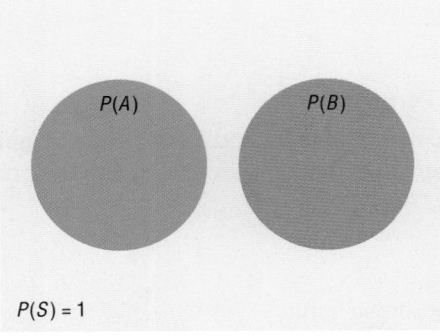

$P(S) = 1$

(a) Mutually exclusive events
$P(A \text{ or } B) = P(A) + P(B)$

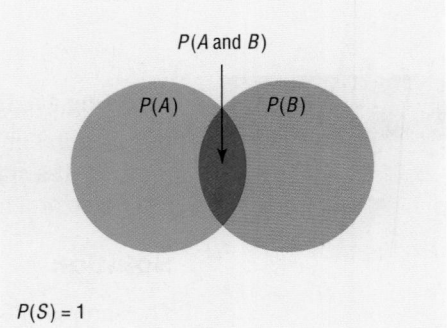

$P(S) = 1$

(b) Non-mutually exclusive events
$P(A \text{ or } B) = P(A) + P(B) - P(A \text{ and } B)$

Note: Venn diagrams were developed by mathematician John Venn (1834–1923) and are used in set theory and symbolic logic. They have been adapted to probability theory also. In set theory, the symbol $\cup$ represents the *union* of two sets, and $A \cup B$ corresponds to A or B. The symbol $\cap$ represents the *intersection* of two sets, and $A \cap B$ corresponds to A and B. Venn diagrams show only a general picture of the probability rules and do not portray all situations, such as $P(A) = 0$, accurately.

4–2 Applying the Concepts

Which Pain Reliever Is Best?

Assume that following an injury you received from playing your favourite sport, you obtain and read information on new pain medications. In that information you read of a study that was conducted to test the side effects of two new pain medications. Use the following table to answer the questions and decide which, if any, of the two new pain medications you will use.

Side effect	Number of side effects in 12-week clinical trial		
	Placebo $n = 192$	Drug A $n = 186$	Drug B $n = 188$
Upper respiratory congestion	10	32	19
Sinus headache	11	25	32
Stomach ache	2	46	12
Neurological headache	34	55	72
Cough	22	18	31
Lower respiratory congestion	2	5	1

1. How many subjects were in the study?

2. How long was the study?

3. What were the variables under study?

4. What type of variables are they and what level of measurement are they on?

5. Are the numbers in the table exact figures?

6. What is the probability that a randomly selected person was receiving a placebo?

7. What is the probability that a person was receiving a placebo or drug A? Are these mutually exclusive events? What is the complement to this event?

8. What is the probability that a randomly selected person was receiving a placebo or experienced a neurological headache?

9. What is the probability that a randomly selected person was not receiving a placebo or experienced a sinus headache?

See page 207 for the answers.

Exercises 4–2

1. Define mutually exclusive events, and give an example of two events that are mutually exclusive and two events that are not mutually exclusive.

2. Determine whether these events are mutually exclusive.

   a. Roll a die: Get an even number, and get a number less than 3.

   b. Roll a die: Get a prime number (2, 3, 5), and get an odd number.

   c. Roll a die: Get a number greater than 3, and get a number less than 3.

   d. Select a student in your class: The student has blond hair, and the student has blue eyes.

   e. Select a student in your college or university: The student is in second year, and the student is a business major.

   f. Select any course: It is a calculus course, and it is an English course.

   g. Select a registered voter: The voter is a Conservative, and the voter is a Liberal.

3. **University Degrees Awarded** The table below represents Canadian university degrees awarded in a recent year by gender.

	Bachelor's	Master's	Doctorate
Male	66,669	16,035	2,676
Female	108,696	23,880	2,151

Choose a degree at random. Find the probability that it is

   a. A bachelor's degree

   b. A doctorate or a degree awarded to a female

c. A doctorate degree awarded to a male

d. Not a master's degree

Source: Statistics Canada, *The Daily*, "Table 1: University qualifications awarded by program level and gender," July 13, 2009.

4. Staff Person Selection At a community swimming pool there are 2 managers, 8 lifeguards, 3 concession stand clerks, and 2 maintenance people. If a person is selected at random, find the probability that the person is either a lifeguard or a manager.

5. Instructor Selection At a convention there are 7 mathematics instructors, 5 computer science instructors, 3 statistics instructors, and 4 science instructors. If an instructor is selected, find the probability of getting a science instructor or a math instructor.

6. Movie Selection A media rental store rented the following number of movie titles in each of these categories: 170 horror, 230 drama, 120 mystery, 310 romance, and 150 comedy. If a person selects a movie to rent, find the probability that it is a romance or a comedy. Is this event likely or unlikely to occur? Explain your answer.

7. Nurse Selection A recent study of 200 nurses found that of 125 female nurses, 56 had bachelor's degrees; and of 75 male nurses, 34 had bachelor's degrees. If a nurse is selected at random, find the probability that the nurse is

a. A female nurse with a bachelor's degree

b. A male nurse

c. A male nurse with a bachelor's degree

d. Based on your answers to parts *a*, *b*, and *c*, explain which is most likely to occur. Explain why.

8. Online Bookings The probability that a travel Web site booking is for a flight is 0.47, and the probability that the booking is for a hotel is 0.58. If the probability that the booking is for either a hotel or a flight is 0.95, what is the probability that both a flight and hotel are booked together?

9. Sports Participation At a particular school with 200 male students, 58 play football, 40 play basketball, and 8 play both. What is the probability that a randomly selected male student plays neither sport?

10. Card Selection A single card is drawn from a deck. Find the probability of selecting the following.

a. A 4 or a diamond

b. A club or a diamond

c. A jack or a black card

11. Student Selection In a statistics class there are 18 juniors and 10 seniors; 6 of the seniors are females, and 12 of the juniors are males. If a student is selected at random, find the probability of selecting the following.

a. A junior or a female

b. A senior or a female

c. A junior or a senior

12. Book Selection At a used-book sale, 100 books are adult books and 160 are children's books. Of the adult books, 70 are nonfiction while 60 of the children's books are nonfiction. If a book is selected at random, find the probability that it is

a. Fiction

b. Not a children's nonfiction book

c. An adult book or a children's nonfiction book

13. Age Groups and Gender The population distribution by age and gender for Halifax, Nova Scotia, following the 2006 census was as follows.

	Age (years)		
	24 and under	**25 to 49**	**50 and older**
Male	56,575	68,900	53,420
Female	56,110	74,720	63,135

If one person from Halifax is selected at random, find the probability that the person is

a. A female and age 24 and under

b. A male or age 50 and older

c. Age 25 to 49 and not male

Source: Statistics Canada, *2006 Census: Data Products*, "Profile of Labour Market Activity, Industry, Occupation, Education, Language of Work, Place of Work and Mode of Transportation for Census Metropolitan Areas and Census Agglomerations."

14. Endangered Species The number of North American endangered species for several groups are listed here.

	Mammals	**Birds**	**Reptiles**	**Amphibians**
Canada	18	21	3	1
United States	41	79	27	53

If one endangered species is selected at random, find the probability that it is

a. Found in Canada and is a bird

b. Is a reptile or found in the United States

c. Warm-blooded

Source: IUCN—The World Conservation Union.

15. Graduates by Field of Study The table below represents the number of Canadian university undergraduates receiving degrees in various disciplines in a recent year by gender.

	Education	**Humanities**	**Science**
Female	20,943	17,613	2,553
Male	6,468	9,606	5,988

Find the probability that a randomly selected student

a. Received an Education degree

b. Was male or was awarded a Science degree

c. Was a female Humanities graduate

d. Was not male

Source: Statistics Canada, http://www.statcan.gc.ca/daily-quotidien/090713/t090713b2-eng.htm

16. Vehicle Collisions The following data illustrate vehicle collisions by time of day and age group.

	16–24	25–54	55+
Morning	29	31	30
Afternoon	42	46	54
Evening	29	23	16

What is the probability that a randomly selected driver was involved in a collision

a. In the evening, from the age group 16–24 years?

b. Was not in the 55+ age group?

c. In the afternoon or was in the age group 25–54 years?

Source: Statistics Canada, *Research Paper: Driving Characteristics of the Young and Aging Population,* John Nicoletta, Transportation Division.

17. Cable Channel Programming Three cable channels (6, 8, and 10) have quiz shows, comedies, and dramas. The number of each is shown here.

Type of show	Channel 6	Channel 8	Channel 10
Quiz show	5	2	1
Comedy	3	2	8
Drama	4	4	2

If a show is selected at random, find these probabilities.

a. The show is a quiz show, or it is shown on Channel 8.

b. The show is a drama or a comedy.

c. The show is shown on Channel 10, or it is a drama.

18. Mail Delivery A local postal carrier distributes first-class letters, advertisements, and magazines. For a certain day, she distributed the following numbers of each type of item.

Delivered to	First-class letters	Ads	Magazines
Home	325	406	203
Business	732	1021	97

If an item of mail is selected at random, find these probabilities.

a. The item went to a home.

b. The item was an ad, or it went to a business.

c. The item was a first-class letter, or it went to a home.

19. Medical Tests on Emergency Patients The frequency distribution shown here illustrates the number of medical tests conducted on 30 randomly selected emergency patients.

Number of tests performed	Number of patients
0	12
1	8
2	2
3	3
4 or more	5

If a patient is selected at random, find these probabilities.

a. The patient had exactly 2 tests done.

b. The patient had at least 2 tests done.

c. The patient had at most 3 tests done.

d. The patient had 3 or fewer tests done.

e. The patient had 1 or 2 tests done.

20. Patient Recovery Time This distribution represents the length of time a patient spends in a hospital.

Days	Frequency
0–3	2
4–7	15
8–11	8
12–15	6
16+	9

If a patient is randomly selected, find these probabilities.

a. The patient spends 3 days or fewer in the hospital.

b. The patient spends fewer than 8 days in the hospital.

c. The patient spends 16 or more days in the hospital.

d. The patient spends a maximum of 11 days in the hospital.

21. Door-to-Door Sales A sales representative who visits customers at home finds she sells 0, 1, 2, 3, or 4 items according to the following frequency distribution.

Items sold	Frequency
0	8
1	10
2	3
3	2
4	1

Find the probability that she sells the following.

a. Exactly 1 item   c. At least 1 item

b. More than 2 items   d. At most 3 items

22. Alcoholic Cholesterol Levels A recent study of 300 patients found that of 100 alcoholic patients, 87 had elevated cholesterol levels, and of 200 nonalcoholic patients, 43 had elevated cholesterol levels. If a patient is selected at random, find the probability that the patient is the following.

a. An alcoholic with elevated cholesterol level

b. A nonalcoholic

c. A nonalcoholic with nonelevated cholesterol level

23. Drawing a Card If one card is drawn from an ordinary deck of cards, find the probability of getting the following.

a. A king or a queen or a jack

b. A club or a heart or a spade

c. A king or a queen or a diamond

d. An ace or a diamond or a heart

e. A 9 or a 10 or a spade or a club

24. Rolling Dice Two dice are rolled. Find the probability of getting

   a. A sum of 5, 6, or 7

   b. Doubles or a sum of 6 or 8

   c. A sum greater than 8 or less than 3

   d. Based on the answers to parts *a*, *b*, and *c*, which is least likely to occur? Explain why.

25. Selecting Coloured Balls An urn contains 6 red balls, 2 green balls, 1 blue ball, and 1 white ball. If a ball is drawn, find the probability of getting a red or a white ball.

26. Rolling Dice Three dice are rolled. Find the probability of getting

   a. Triples

   b. A sum of 5

Extending the Concepts »

27. Purchasing a Pizza The probability that a customer selects a pizza with mushrooms or pepperoni is 0.43, and the probability that the customer selects only mushrooms is 0.32. If the probability that he or she selects only pepperoni is 0.17, find the probability of the customer selecting both items.

28. Building a New Home In building new homes, a contractor finds that the probability of a home buyer selecting a two-car garage is 0.70 and of selecting a one-car garage is 0.20. Find the probability that the buyer will select no garage. The builder does not build houses with three-car or more garages.

29. In Exercise 28, find the probability that the buyer will not want a two-car garage.

30. Suppose that $P(A) = 0.42$, $P(B) = 0.38$, and $P(A \cup B) = 0.70$. Are *A* and *B* mutually exclusive? Explain.

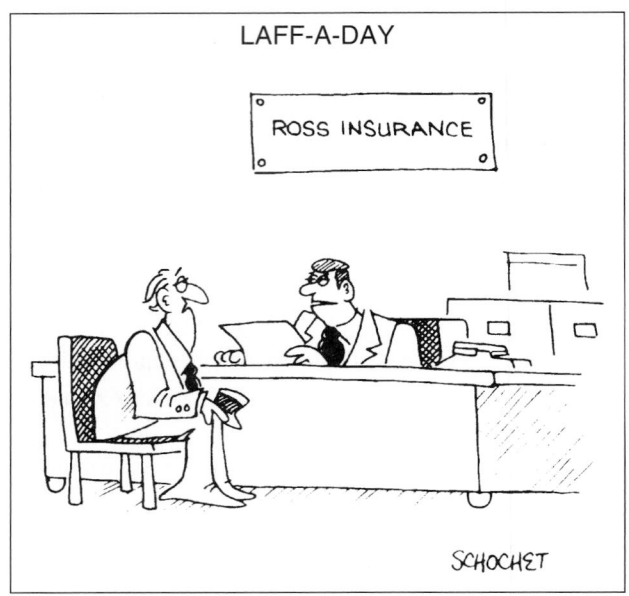

LAFF-A-DAY

ROSS INSURANCE

"I know you haven't had an accident in thirteen years. We're raising your rates because you're about due one."

Source: Reprinted with special permission of King Features Syndicate.

| 4–3 | The Multiplication Rules and Conditional Probability > |

 LO3

Use the multiplication rules and conditional probability to find the probability of sequential compound events.

Section 4–2 showed that the addition rules are used to compute probabilities for mutually exclusive and non-mutually exclusive events. This section introduces the multiplication rules.

The Multiplication Rules

The *multiplication rules* can be used to find the probability of two or more events that occur in sequence. For example, if a coin is tossed and then a die is rolled, one can find the probability of getting a head on the coin *and* a 4 on the die. These two events are said to be *independent* since the outcome of the first event (tossing a coin) does not affect the probability outcome of the second event (rolling a die).

> Two events *A* and *B* are **independent events** if the fact that *A* occurs does not affect the probability of *B* occurring.

Here are other examples of independent events:

Rolling a die and getting a 6, and then rolling a second die and getting a 3.

Drawing a card from a deck and getting a queen, replacing it, and drawing a second card and getting a queen.

To find the probability of two independent events that occur in sequence, one must find the probability of each event occurring separately and then multiply the answers. For example, if a coin is tossed twice, the probability of getting two heads is $\frac{1}{2} \cdot \frac{1}{2} = \frac{1}{4}$. This result can be verified by looking at the sample space HH, HT, TH, TT. Then $P(\text{HH}) = \frac{1}{4}$.

Multiplication Rule 1

When two events are independent, the probability of both occurring is

$$P(A \text{ and } B) = P(A) \cdot P(B)$$

Example 4–23

Tossing a Coin

A coin is flipped and a die is rolled. Find the probability of getting a head on the coin and a 4 on the die.

Solution

$$P(\text{head and } 4) = P(\text{head}) \cdot P(4) = \frac{1}{2} \cdot \frac{1}{6} = \frac{1}{12}$$

Note that the sample space for the coin is H, T and for the die it is 1, 2, 3, 4, 5, 6.

The problem in Example 4–23 can also be solved by using the sample space

H1   H2   H3   H4   H5   H6   T1   T2   T3   T4   T5   T6

The solution is $\frac{1}{12}$, since there is only one way to get the head–4 outcome.

Example 4–24

Drawing a Card

A card is drawn from a deck and replaced; then a second card is drawn. Find the probability of getting a queen and then an ace.

Solution

The probability of getting a queen is $\frac{4}{52}$, and since the card is replaced, the probability of getting an ace is $\frac{4}{52}$ Hence, the probability of getting a queen and an ace is

$$P(\text{queen and ace}) = P(\text{queen}) \cdot P(\text{ace}) = \frac{4}{52} \cdot \frac{4}{52} = \frac{16}{2704} = \frac{1}{169}$$

Example 4–25

Selecting a Coloured Ball

An urn contains 3 red balls, 2 green balls, and 5 white balls. A ball is selected and its colour noted. Then it is replaced. A second ball is selected and its colour noted. Find the probability of each of these.

  a. Selecting 2 green balls

  b. Selecting 1 green ball and then 1 white ball

  c. Selecting 1 red ball and then 1 green ball

Solution

a. $P(\text{green and green}) = P(\text{green}) \cdot P(\text{green}) = \dfrac{2}{10} \cdot \dfrac{2}{10} = \dfrac{4}{100} = \dfrac{1}{25}$

b. $P(\text{green and white}) = P(\text{green}) \cdot P(\text{white}) = \dfrac{2}{10} \cdot \dfrac{5}{10} = \dfrac{10}{100} = \dfrac{1}{10}$

c. $P(\text{red and green}) = P(\text{red}) \cdot P(\text{green}) = \dfrac{3}{10} \cdot \dfrac{2}{10} = \dfrac{6}{100} = \dfrac{3}{50}$

Multiplication Rule 1 can be extended to three or more independent events by using the formula

$$P(A \text{ and } B \text{ and } C \text{ and } \cdots \text{ and } K) = P(A) \cdot P(B) \cdot P(C) \cdots P(K)$$

When a small sample is selected from a large population and the subjects are not replaced, the probability of the event occurring changes so slightly that for the most part, it is considered to remain the same. Examples 4–26 and 4–27 illustrate this concept.

Example 4–26

Stress Factors

A Statistics Canada health report found that adult Canadians 18 or older experienced five or more sources of stress, with time pressure particularly common. The report indicated that 44% of Canadians acknowledged that they were trying to do too many things at once. If three adult Canadians are selected, find the probability that all three will suffer stress due to time pressure.

Source: Adapted from Statistics Canada, Excerpt of health reports: stress and chronic conditions, excess weight, and arthritis, www.statcan.ca/Daily/English/040121/d040121b.htm. February 28, 2007.

Solution

Let S denote stress. Then

$$
\begin{aligned}
P(S \text{ and } S \text{ and } S) &= P(S) \cdot P(S) \cdot P(S) \\
&= (0.44)(0.44)(0.44) \approx 0.085
\end{aligned}
$$

Example 4–27

Male Colour Blindness

Approximately 9% of men have a type of colour blindness that prevents them from distinguishing between red and green. If 3 men are selected at random, find the probability that all of them will have this type of red–green colour blindness.

Source: USA TODAY.

Solution

Let C denote red–green colour blindness. Then

$$
\begin{aligned}
P(C \text{ and } C \text{ and } C) &= P(C) \cdot P(C) \cdot P(C) \\
&= (0.09)(0.09)(0.09) \\
&= 0.000729
\end{aligned}
$$

Hence, the rounded probability is 0.0007.

In Examples 4–23 through 4–27, the events were independent of one another, since the occurrence of the first event in no way affected the outcome of the second event. On the other hand, when the occurrence of the first event changes the probability of the occurrence of the second event, the two events are said to be *dependent.* For example, suppose a card is drawn from a deck and *not* replaced, and then a second card is drawn. What is the probability of selecting an ace on the first card and a king on the second card?

Before an answer to the question can be given, one must realize that the events are dependent. The probability of selecting an ace on the first draw is $\frac{4}{52}$. If that card is *not* replaced, the probability of selecting a king on the second card after selecting an ace on the first draw is $\frac{4}{51}$, since there are 4 kings and 51 cards remaining. The outcome of the first draw has affected the outcome of the second draw.

Dependent events are formally defined now.

> When the outcome or occurrence of the first event affects the outcome or occurrence of the second event in such a way that the probability is changed, the events are said to be **dependent events.**

Here are some examples of dependent events:

Drawing a card from a deck, not replacing it, and then drawing a second card.

Selecting a ball from an urn, not replacing it, and then selecting a second ball.

Being a lifeguard and getting a suntan.

Having high grades and getting a scholarship.

Parking in a no-parking zone and getting a parking ticket.

To find probabilities when events are dependent, use the multiplication rule with a modification in notation. For the problem just discussed, the probability of getting an ace on the first draw is $\frac{4}{52}$, and the probability of getting a king on the second draw is $\frac{4}{51}$. By the multiplication rule, the probability of both events occurring is

$$\frac{4}{52} \cdot \frac{4}{51} = \frac{16}{2652} = \frac{4}{663}$$

The event of getting a king on the second draw *given* that an ace was drawn the first time is called a *conditional probability.*

The **conditional probability** of an event B in relationship to an event A is the probability that event B occurs after event A has already occurred. The notation for conditional probability is $P(B|A)$. This notation does not mean that B is divided by A; rather, it means the probability that event B occurs given that event A has already occurred. In the card example, $P(B|A)$ is the probability that the second card is a king given that the first card is an ace, and it is equal to $\frac{4}{51}$ since the first card was *not* replaced.

Multiplication Rule 2

When two events are dependent, the probability of both occurring is

$$P(A \text{ and } B) = P(A) \cdot P(B|A)$$

Example 4–28

Selecting Music CDs

A person owns a collection of 30 CDs, of which 5 are country music. If 2 CDs are selected at random, find the probability that both are country music.

Solution

Since the events are dependent,

$$P(C_1 \text{ and } C_2) = P(C_1) \cdot P(C_2|C_1) = \frac{5}{30} \cdot \frac{4}{29} = \frac{20}{870} = \frac{2}{87}$$

| Example 4–29 | **Homeowner's and Automobile Insurance** |

The World Wide Insurance Company found that 53% of the residents of a city had homeowner's insurance (H) with the company. Of these clients, 27% also had automobile insurance (A) with the company. If a resident is selected at random, find the probability that the resident has both homeowner's and automobile insurance with the World Wide Insurance Company.

Solution

$$P(\text{H and A}) = P(\text{H}) \cdot P(\text{A}|\text{H}) = (0.53)(0.27) = 0.1431$$

This multiplication rule can be extended to three or more events, as shown in Example 4–30.

| Example 4–30 | **Drawing Cards** |

Three cards are drawn from an ordinary deck and not replaced. Find the probability of these.

    a. Getting 3 jacks

    b. Getting an ace, a king, and a queen in order

    c. Getting a club, a spade, and a heart in order

    d. Getting 3 clubs

Solution

  a. $P(3 \text{ jacks}) = \dfrac{4}{52} \cdot \dfrac{3}{51} \cdot \dfrac{2}{50} = \dfrac{24}{132,600} = \dfrac{1}{5525}$

  b. $P(\text{ace and king and queen}) = \dfrac{4}{52} \cdot \dfrac{4}{51} \cdot \dfrac{4}{50} = \dfrac{64}{132,600} = \dfrac{8}{16,575}$

  c. $P(\text{club and spade and heart}) = \dfrac{13}{52} \cdot \dfrac{13}{51} \cdot \dfrac{13}{50} = \dfrac{2197}{132,600} = \dfrac{169}{10,200}$

  d. $P(3 \text{ clubs}) = \dfrac{13}{52} \cdot \dfrac{12}{51} \cdot \dfrac{11}{50} = \dfrac{1716}{132,600} = \dfrac{11}{850}$

Tree diagrams can be used as an aid to finding the solution to probability problems when the events are sequential. Example 4–31 illustrates the use of tree diagrams.

| Example 4–31 | **Selecting Coloured Balls** |

Box 1 contains 2 red balls and 1 blue ball. Box 2 contains 3 blue balls and 1 red ball. A coin is tossed. If it falls heads up, box 1 is selected and a ball is drawn. If it falls tails up, box 2 is selected and a ball is drawn. Find the probability of selecting a red ball.

Solution

With the use of a tree diagram, the sample space can be determined as shown in Figure 4–6. First, assign probabilities to each branch. Next, using the multiplication rule, multiply the probabilities for each branch.

    Finally, use the addition rule, since a red ball can be obtained from box 1 or box 2.

$$P(\text{red}) = \tfrac{2}{6} + \tfrac{1}{8} = \tfrac{8}{24} + \tfrac{3}{24} = \tfrac{11}{24}$$

(*Note:* The sum of all final probabilities will always be equal to 1.)

Figure 4–6

Tree Diagram for Example 4–31

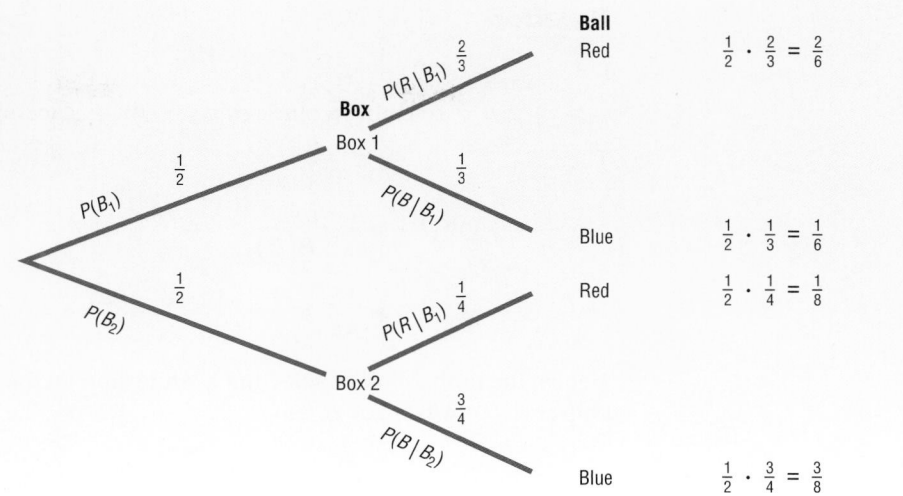

Tree diagrams can be used when the events are independent or dependent, and they can also be used for sequences of three or more events.

Conditional Probability

The conditional probability of an event B in relationship to an event A was defined as the probability that event B occurs after event A has already occurred.

The conditional probability of an event can be found by dividing both sides of the equation for Multiplication Rule 2 by $P(A)$, as shown:

$$P(A \text{ and } B) = P(A) \cdot P(B|A)$$

$$\frac{P(A \text{ and } B)}{P(A)} = \frac{\cancel{P(A)} \cdot P(B|A)}{\cancel{P(A)}}$$

$$\frac{P(A \text{ and } B)}{P(A)} = P(B|A)$$

Formula for Conditional Probability

The probability that the second event B occurs given that the first event A has occurred can be found by dividing the probability that both events occurred by the probability that the first event has occurred. The $P(A)$ cannot equal 0. The formula is

$$P(B|A) = \frac{P(A \text{ and } B)}{P(A)}$$

Examples 4–32, 4–33, and 4–34 illustrate the use of this rule.

Example 4–32

Selecting Coloured Chips

A box contains black chips and white chips. A person selects two chips without replacement. If the probability of selecting a black chip *and* a white chip is $\frac{15}{56}$, and the probability of selecting a black chip on the first draw is $\frac{3}{8}$, find the probability of selecting the white chip on the second draw, *given* that the first chip selected was a black chip.

Solution

Let

B = selecting a black chip W = selecting a white chip

Then

$$P(W|B) = \frac{P(B \text{ and } W)}{P(B)} = \frac{\frac{15}{56}}{\frac{3}{8}}$$

$$= \frac{15}{56} \div \frac{3}{8} = \frac{15}{56} \cdot \frac{8}{3} = \frac{\overset{5}{\cancel{15}}}{\underset{7}{\cancel{56}}} \cdot \frac{\overset{1}{\cancel{8}}}{\underset{1}{\cancel{3}}} = \frac{5}{7}$$

Hence, the probability of selecting a white chip on the second draw given that the first chip selected was black is $\frac{5}{7}$.

Example 4–33

Parking Tickets

The probability that Sam parks in a no-parking zone *and* gets a parking ticket is 0.06, and the probability that Sam cannot find a legal parking space and has to park in the no-parking zone is 0.20. On Tuesday, Sam arrives at school and has to park in a no-parking zone. Find the probability that he will get a parking ticket.

Solution

Let

N = parking in a no-parking zone T = getting a ticket

Then

$$P(T|N) = \frac{P(N \text{ and } T)}{P(N)} = \frac{0.06}{0.20} = 0.30$$

Hence, Sam has a 0.30 probability of getting a parking ticket, given that he parked in a no-parking zone.

The conditional probability of events occurring can also be computed when the data are given in table form, as shown in Example 4–34.

Example 4–34

Survey of Women in the Armed Forces

A recent survey asked 100 people if they thought women in the armed forces should be permitted to participate in combat. The results of the survey are shown.

Gender	Yes	No	Total
Male	32	18	50
Female	8	42	50
Total	40	60	100

Find these probabilities.

a. The respondent answered yes, given that the respondent was a female.

b. The respondent was a male, given that the respondent answered no.

Solution

Let

M = respondent was a male	Y = respondent answered yes
F = respondent was a female	N = respondent answered no

a. The problem is to find $P(Y|F)$. The rule states

$$P(Y|F) = \frac{P(F \text{ and } Y)}{P(F)}$$

The probability $P(F \text{ and } Y)$ is the number of females who responded yes, divided by the total number of respondents:

$$P(F \text{ and } Y) = \frac{8}{100}$$

The probability $P(F)$ is the probability of selecting a female:

$$P(F) = \frac{50}{100}$$

Then

$$P(Y|F) = \frac{P(F \text{ and } Y)}{P(F)} = \frac{8/100}{50/100}$$

$$= \frac{8}{100} \div \frac{50}{100} = \frac{\overset{4}{\cancel{8}}}{\underset{1}{\cancel{100}}} \cdot \frac{\overset{1}{\cancel{100}}}{\underset{25}{\cancel{50}}} = \frac{4}{25}$$

b. The problem is to find $P(M|N)$.

$$P(M|N) = \frac{P(N \text{ and } M)}{P(N)} = \frac{18/100}{60/100}$$

$$= \frac{18}{100} \div \frac{60}{100} = \frac{\overset{3}{\cancel{18}}}{\underset{1}{\cancel{100}}} \cdot \frac{\overset{1}{\cancel{100}}}{\underset{10}{\cancel{60}}} = \frac{3}{10}$$

The Venn diagram for conditional probability is shown in Figure 4–7. In this case,

$$P(B|A) = \frac{P(A \text{ and } B)}{P(A)}$$

Figure 4–7

Venn Diagram for Conditional Probability

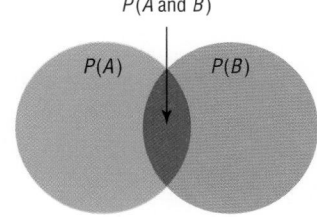

$P(A \text{ and } B)$

$P(A)$ $P(B)$

$P(S)$

$$P(B|A) = \frac{P(A \text{ and } B)}{P(A)}$$

which is represented by the area in the intersection or overlapping part of the circles A and B, divided by the area of circle A. The reasoning here is that if one assumes

A has occurred, then A becomes the sample space for the next calculation and is the denominator of the probability fraction $\dfrac{P(A \text{ and } B)}{P(A)}$. The numerator $P(A \text{ and } B)$ represents the probability of the part of B that is contained in A. Hence, $P(A \text{ and } B)$ becomes the numerator of the probability fraction $\dfrac{P(A \text{ and } B)}{P(A)}$. Imposing a condition reduces the sample space.

Bayes' Theorem (Optional)

The procedure of revising the probability of an event occurring based on knowledge of the occurrence of a prior event is known as *Bayes' theorem* (or *Bayes' rule*). For example when calculating the probability of drawing two cards from a deck of playing cards without replacement, the conditional probability of the 2nd drawn card may be revised after the 1st card is revealed. Refer to Appendix B–2 for a detailed explanation of Bayes' theorem with tree diagrams, formulas, solved problems, and exercises using this procedure.

Probabilities for "At Least"

The multiplication rules can be used with the complementary event rule (Section 4–1) to simplify solving probability problems involving "at least." Examples 4–35, 4–36, and 4–37 illustrate how this is done.

| Example 4–35 | **Drawing Cards** |

A game is played by drawing four cards from an ordinary deck and replacing each card after it is drawn. Find the probability of winning if at least one ace is drawn.

Solution

It is much easier to find the probability that no aces are drawn (i.e., losing) and then subtract that value from 1 than to find the solution directly, because that would involve finding the probability of getting one ace, two aces, three aces, and four aces and then adding the results.

Let E = at least one ace is drawn and $\overline{E}$ = no aces drawn. Then

$$P(\overline{E}) = \frac{48}{52} \cdot \frac{48}{52} \cdot \frac{48}{52} \cdot \frac{48}{52}$$

$$= \frac{12}{13} \cdot \frac{12}{13} \cdot \frac{12}{13} \cdot \frac{12}{13} = \frac{20{,}736}{28{,}561}$$

Hence,

$$P(E) = 1 - P(\overline{E})$$

$$P(\text{winning}) = 1 - P(\text{losing}) = 1 - \frac{20{,}736}{28{,}561} = \frac{7{,}825}{28{,}561} \approx 0.27$$

or a hand with at least one ace will win about 27% of the time.

| Example 4–36 | **Tossing Coins** |

A coin is tossed 5 times. Find the probability of getting at least one tail.

Solution

It is easier to find the probability of the complement of the event, which is "all heads," and then subtract the probability from 1 to get the probability of at least one tail.

$$P(E) = 1 - P(\overline{E})$$
$$P(\text{at least 1 tail}) = 1 - P(\text{all heads})$$
$$P(\text{all heads}) = \left(\tfrac{1}{2}\right)^5 = \tfrac{1}{32}$$

Hence,

$$P(\text{at least 1 tail}) = 1 - \tfrac{1}{32} = \tfrac{31}{32}$$

Example 4–37

Food Bank Recipients

The Canadian Association of Food Banks publishes a national report on hunger in Canada. A 2007 survey indicated that 38% of Canadian food bank recipients are from Ontario. If 4 Canadian food bank recipients are randomly selected, find the probability that at least one is from Ontario.

Source: The Canadian Association of Food Banks, *HungerCount 2007.*

Solution

Let E = at least one Ontario food bank recipient and $\overline{E}$ = no Ontario food bank recipients.
Then

$$P(E) = 0.38 \quad \text{and} \quad P(\overline{E}) = 1 - 0.38 = 0.62$$

$P(\text{no Ontario food bank recipients}) = (0.62)(0.62)(0.62)(0.62) \approx 0.148$; hence,
$P(\text{at least one Ontario food bank recipient}) = 1 - 0.148 = 0.852.$

Similar methods can be used for problems involving "at most."

4–3 Applying the Concepts

Guilty or Innocent?

In July 1964, an elderly woman was mugged in Costa Mesa, California. In the vicinity of the crime a tall, bearded man sat waiting in a yellow car. Shortly after the crime was committed, a young, tall woman, wearing her blond hair in a ponytail, was seen running from the scene of the crime and getting into the car, which sped off. The police broadcast a description of the suspected muggers. Soon afterward, a couple fitting the description was arrested. Although the evidence in the case was largely circumstantial, the two people arrested were nonetheless convicted of the crime. The prosecutor based his entire case on basic probability theory, showing the unlikelihood of another couple being in that area while having all the same characteristics that the elderly woman described. The following probabilities were used.

Characteristic	Assumed probability
Drives yellow car	1 out of 12
Man over 6 feet tall	1 out of 10
Man wearing tennis shoes	1 out of 4
Man with beard	1 out of 11
Woman with blond hair	1 out of 3
Woman with hair in a ponytail	1 out of 13
Woman over 6 feet tall	1 out of 100

1. Compute the probability of another couple being in that area with the same characteristics.

2. Would you use the addition or multiplication rule? Why?

3. Are the characteristics independent or dependent?

4. How are the computations affected by the assumption of independence or dependence?

5. Should any court case be based solely on probabilities?

6. Would you convict the couple who was arrested even if there were no eyewitnesses?

7. Comment on why in today's justice system no person can be convicted solely on the results of probabilities.

8. In actuality, aren't most court cases based on uncalculated probabilities?

See page 207 for the answers.

Exercises 4–3

1. State which events are independent and which are dependent.

   a. Tossing a coin and drawing a card from a deck

   b. Drawing a ball from an urn, not replacing it, and then drawing a second ball

   c. Getting a raise in salary and purchasing a new car

   d. Driving on ice and having an accident

   e. Having a large shoe size and having a high IQ

   f. A father being left-handed and a daughter being left-handed

   g. Smoking excessively and having lung cancer

   h. Eating an excessive amount of ice cream and smoking an excessive number of cigarettes

2. **Exercise** If 37% of high school students said that they exercise regularly, find the probability that 5 randomly selected high school students will say that they exercise regularly. Would you consider this event likely or unlikely to occur? Explain your answer.

3. **Aerobics** If 84% of all people who do aerobics are women, find the probability that if 2 people who do aerobics are randomly selected, both are women. Would you consider this event likely or unlikely to occur? Explain your answer.

4. **Seat Belt Use** Transport Canada reports that 87.1% of Canadian drivers and passengers buckle up for safety. If 4 people are selected at random, find the probability that they all used a seat belt while driving.
   Source: Transport Canada.

5. **Clerical and Administrative Roles** Statistics Canada reports that 24.1% of clerical and administrative roles are performed by men. If 3 women are randomly selected, find the probability that they all perform clerical and administrative duties. Would you consider this event likely or unlikely to occur? Explain your answer.
   Source: Statistics Canada.

6. **Prison Inmates** If 18% of Canada's federal prison inmates are Aboriginal, find the probability that 2 randomly selected federal prison inmates are Aboriginal.
   Source: Statistics Canada.

7. **Teen Usage of Wireless Devices** A Harris Interactive poll stated that four out of five teens carry a wireless device,

primarily for cellphone and text messaging usage. If 3 teens are randomly selected, find the following probabilities.

   a. None of the teens have a wireless device.

   b. At least one has a wireless device.

   c. All three have wireless devices.

   Source: MarketingCharts: Harris Interactive, *Cell Phones Key to Teens' Social Lives, 47% Can Text with Eyes Closed,* July 2008 survey.

8. **Drawing Cards** If 2 cards are selected from a standard deck of 52 cards without replacement, find these probabilities.

   a. Both are spades.

   b. Both are the same suit.

   c. Both are kings.

9. **NHL Players** Of 714 players in the National Hockey League (NHL), 383 or 53.6% are Canadian citizens. If 3 NHL players are randomly selected, what is the probability that all are Canadian citizens?
   Source: NHL.com.

10. **Death Penalty Survey** A *Reader's Digest* survey reported that one-half of Canadian teens favoured the death penalty for persons convicted of murder. If 3 Canadian teens are randomly selected, find the probability that all 3 teens favour the death penalty for convicted murderers.
    Source: www.readersdigest.ca.

11. **NFL Licensed Apparel** Of fans who own sports league-licensed apparel, 31% have National Football League (NFL) apparel. If 3 of these fans are selected at random, what is the probability that all have NFL apparel?
    Source: ESPN Chilton Sports Poll.

12. **Flashlight Batteries** A flashlight has 6 batteries, 2 of which are defective. If 2 are selected at random without replacement, find the probability that both are defective.

13. **Child Poverty** According to the Campaign 2000—End Child Poverty in Canada Web site, 16% of Ontario children live in poverty. If 4 Ontario children are randomly selected, what is the probability that none of the children live in poverty?
    Source: www.campaign2000.ca.

14. **Firearm Ownership** Alberta ranks first among Canada's provinces, with 39% of Alberta households owning firearms. If 3 Alberta households are randomly

selected, what is the probability that none of the households own a firearm?

Source: Alberta Centre for Injury Control & Research.

15. **Customer Purchases** In a department store there are 120 customers, 90 of whom will buy at least one item. If 5 customers are selected at random, one by one, find the probability that all will buy at least one item.

16. **Drawing Cards** Three cards are drawn from a deck *without* replacement. Find these probabilities.

    a. All are jacks.

    b. All are clubs.

    c. All are red cards.

17. **Scientific Study** In a scientific study there are 8 guinea pigs, 5 of which are pregnant. If 3 are selected at random without replacement, find the probability that all are pregnant.

18. For Exercise 17, find the probability that none are pregnant.

19. **Civic Organization Members** In a civic organization, there are 38 members; 15 are men and 23 are women. If 3 members are selected to plan the Canada Day parade, find the probability that all 3 are women. Would you consider this event likely or unlikely to occur? Explain your answer.

20. In Exercise 19, find the probability that all 3 members are men.

21. **Item Sales** A manufacturer makes two models of an item: Model I, which accounts for 80% of unit sales, and Model II, which accounts for 20% of unit sales. Because of defects, the manufacturer has to replace (or exchange) 10% of its Model I and 18% of its Model II. If a model is selected at random, find the probability that it will be defective.

22. **Student Loans** Statistics Canada reported that 41% of college graduates and 45% of university graduates with bachelor's degrees had government student loans. Of these, 18% of the college graduates and 22% of the university graduates with bachelor's degrees paid off their loans within two years of graduation. Select one student at random. (*Hint:* Draw a tree diagram.) Find the probability that the student is a

    a. College graduate who did not pay back the student loan within two years.

    b. University graduate with a bachelor's degree, given that the student did pay back the loan within two years.

    c. University graduate with a bachelor's degree or a graduate student who did not pay back the student loan within two years.

    Source: Statistics Canada, *The Daily,* "National Graduates Survey: Student Debt," April 26, 2004.

23. **Automobile Insurance** An insurance company classifies drivers as low-risk, medium-risk, and high-risk. Of those insured, 60% are low-risk, 30% are medium-risk, and 10% are high-risk. After a study, the company finds that during a one-year period, 1% of the low-risk drivers had an accident, 5% of the medium-risk drivers had an accident, and 9% of the high-risk drivers had an accident. If a driver is selected at random, find the probability that the driver will have had an accident during the year.

24. **Defective Parts** A production process produces a part. On average, 15% of all parts produced are defective. Each part is inspected before being shipped, and the inspector misclassifies a part 10% of the time. What proportion of the parts will be "classified as good"? What is the probability that a part is defective, given that it was classified as good?

25. **Selecting Coloured Balls** Urn 1 contains 5 red balls and 3 black balls. Urn 2 contains 3 red balls and 1 black ball. Urn 3 contains 4 red balls and 2 black balls. If an urn is selected at random and a ball is drawn, find the probability it will be red.

26. **Women in Prison** For a recent year, 6.1% of persons transferred to federal prison jurisdiction were women. Of these women, 3.3% were under the age of 20. If a federal jurisdiction prisoner is selected at random, find the probability that the person is under the age of 20, given that the person is a woman.

    Source: Public Safety Canada, *Corrections and Conditional Release Statistical Overview 2008.*

27. **Rolling Dice** Roll two standard dice and add the numbers. What is the probability of getting a number larger than 9 for the first time on the third roll?

28. **Model Railroad Circuit** A circuit to run a model railroad has 8 switches. Two are defective. If a person selects 2 switches at random and tests them, find the probability that the second one is defective, given that the first one is defective.

29. **Country Club Activities** At the Avonlea Country Club, 73% of the members play bridge and swim, and 82% play bridge. If a member is selected at random, find the probability that the member swims, given that the member plays bridge.

30. **College Courses** At a large college, the probability that a student takes calculus and is on the Dean's List is 0.042. The probability that a student is on the Dean's List is 0.21. Find the probability that the student is taking calculus, given that he or she is on the Dean's List.

31. **House Types** In Rolling Acres, 42% of the houses have a deck and a garage; 60% have a deck. Find the probability that a home has a garage, given that it has a deck.

32. **Pizza and Salad** In a pizza restaurant, 95% of the customers order pizza. If 65% of the customers order pizza and a salad, find the probability that a customer who orders pizza will also order a salad.

33. **Gift Baskets** The Gift Basket Store had the following premade gift baskets containing the following combinations in stock.

	Cookies	Mugs	Candy
Coffee	20	13	10
Tea	12	10	12

Choose 1 basket at random. Find the probability that it contains

a. Coffee or candy

b. Tea, given that it contains mugs

c. Tea and cookies

Source: Infoplease: www.infoplease.com

34. **Blood Types and Rh Factors** In addition to being grouped into four types, human blood is grouped by its Rhesus (Rh) factor. Consider the figures below, which show the distributions of these groups for Canadians.

	O	A	B	AB
Rh+	39%	36%	7.6%	2.5%
Rh−	7%	6%	1.4%	0.5%

Choose 1 Canadian at random. Find the probability that the person

a. Is a universal donor, i.e., has O negative blood

b. Has type O blood given that the person is Rh+

c. Has A+ or AB− blood

d. Has Rh− given that the person has type B

Source: Canadian Blood Services, What Can I Donate? "Blood: Types & Rh System."

35. **Intellectual Property Protection** The following table represents intellectual property protection granted and/or registered in Canada for a specific year, organized by product output (type) and nationality of applicant.

	Patents	Trademarks	Copyrights
Canada	1,461	14,273	6,862
Foreign	12,092	15,507	788

Select one product output at random.

a. What is the probability that it was granted to a Canadian, given that it was a patent product type?

b. What is the probability that it was a copyright product type, given that it was registered to a foreign applicant?

Source: Canadian Intellectual Property Office.

36. **2010 Winter Olympics** The medal distribution for the 2010 Winter Olympic Games in Vancouver, British Columbia, is shown in the table.

Country	Gold	Silver	Bronze
United States	9	15	13
Germany	10	13	7
Canada	14	7	5
Norway	9	8	6
Austria	4	6	6
Russian Federation	3	5	7
Other	37	33	41

Choose one medal winner at random.

a. Find the probability that the winner won a gold medal, given that the winner was from Canada.

b. Find the probability that the winner was from Canada, given that the medal was gold.

c. Are the events "medal winner from Canada" and "gold medal won" independent? Explain.

Source: The Vancouver Organizing Committee for the 2010 Olympic and Paralympic Winter Games, Medal Count: www.vancouver2010.com.

37. **Wedding Day** Statistics Canada reports that 71% of marriages occur on a Saturday. If 5 Canadian marriages were randomly selected, find the probability that

a. None of the marriages occurred on a Saturday.

b. At least one of the marriages occurred on a Saturday.

Source: Statistics Canada.

38. **Fatal Accidents** Transport Canada reports that 7.4% of road fatalities involve motorcyclists. If 3 road fatality reports are randomly selected, what is the probability that

a. All involve a motorcyclist?

b. None involve a motorcyclist?

c. At least 1 involves a motorcyclist?

Source: Transport Canada.

39. **Toddler Immunization** Eighty percent of toddlers are immunized against the major childhood killer diseases—measles, tetanus, whooping cough, polio, diphtheria, and tuberculosis. Suppose that 6 toddlers are selected at random. What is the probability that at least one has not received the recommended immunizations?

Source: Canadian International Development Agency, Global Citizenship in Action, Special Edition on Global Health, "The Facts on Health."

40. **Online Electronic Games** Fifty-six percent of electronic gamers play games online, and sixty-four percent of those gamers are female. What is the probability that a randomly selected gamer plays games online and is male?

Source: msnbc.com, Technology & Science.

41. **University Degrees** Statistics Canada reports that 17.2% of Canadians have a university degree. Suppose that 5 Canadians are randomly selected. What is the probability that at least one of the selected has a university degree?

Source: Statistics Canada.

42. **Teacher Performance** The Canadian Education Association reports that 70% of Canadians feel that teachers are doing a good job educating their youth. If 3 Canadians are selected at random, find the probabilities that

a. All 3 feel that teachers are doing a good job

b. None of the respondents believe that teachers are doing a good job

c. At least one agrees that teachers are doing a good job

Source: Canadian Education Association, Public Education in Canada: Facts, Trends and Attitudes.

43. Drawing Cards If 4 cards are drawn from a deck of 52 and not replaced, find the probability of getting at least one club.

44. Clinic Patients At a local clinic there are 8 men, 5 women, and 3 children in the waiting room. If 3 patients are randomly selected, find the probability that there is at least one child among them.

45. Defective Brakes It has been found that 6% of all automobiles on the road have defective brakes. If 5 automobiles are stopped and checked by the police, find the probability that at least one will have defective brakes.

46. Medication Effectiveness A medication is 75% effective against a bacterial infection. Find the probability that if 12 people take the medication, at least one person's infection will not improve.

47. Tossing a Coin A coin is tossed 5 times; find the probability of getting at least one tail. Would you consider this event likely to happen? Explain your answer.

48. Selecting a Letter of the Alphabet If 3 letters of the alphabet are selected at random, find the probability of getting at least one letter x. Letters can be used more than once. Would you consider this event likely to happen? Explain your answer.

49. Rolling a Die A die is rolled 7 times. Find the probability of getting at least one 3. Would you consider this event likely to occur? Explain your answer.

50. Teachers' Conference At a teachers' conference, there were 4 English teachers, 3 mathematics teachers, and 5 science teachers. If 4 teachers are selected for a committee, find the probability that at least one is a science teacher.

51. Rolling a Die If a die is rolled 3 times, find the probability of getting at least one even number.

52. Selecting a Flower In a large vase, there are 8 roses, 5 daisies, 12 lilies, and 9 orchids. If 4 flowers are selected at random, find the probability that at least one of the flowers is a rose. Would you consider this event likely to occur? Explain your answer.

Extending the Concepts »

53. Let A and B be two mutually exclusive events. Are A and B independent events? Explain your answer.

54. Types of Vehicles The Bargain Auto Mall has the following cars in stock.

	SUV	Compact	Mid-sized
Foreign	20	50	20
Domestic	65	100	45

Are the events "compact" and "domestic" independent? Explain.

55. College Enrollment An admissions director knows that the probability a student will enroll after a campus visit is 0.55, or $P(E) = 0.55$. While students are on campus visits, interviews with professors are arranged. The admissions director computes these conditional probabilities for students enrolling after visiting three professors, DW, LP, and MH.

$$P(E|DW) = 0.95 \qquad P(E|LP) = 0.55 \qquad P(E|MH) = 0.15$$

Is there something wrong with the numbers? Explain.

56. Commercials Event A is the event that a person remembers a certain product commercial. Event B is the event that a person buys the product. If $P(B) = 0.35$, comment on each of these conditional probabilities if you were vice president for sales.

a. $P(B|A) = 0.20$
b. $P(B|A) = 0.35$
c. $P(B|A) = 0.55$

4–4   Counting Rules ›

Use the fundamental counting rule, permutation rule, and combination rule to determine the number of ways that events can occur.

Many times one wishes to know the number of all possible outcomes for a sequence of events. To determine this number, three rules can be used: the *fundamental counting rule,* the *permutation rule,* and the *combination rule.* These rules are explained here, and they will be used in Section 4–5 to find probabilities of events.

The first rule is called the **fundamental counting rule.**

The Fundamental Counting Rule

Fundamental Counting Rule

In a sequence of n events in which the first one has k_1 possibilities and the second event has k_2 and the third has k_3, and so forth, the total number of possibilities of the sequence will be

$$k_1 \cdot k_2 \cdot k_3 \cdots k_n$$

Note: In this case *and* means to multiply.

Examples 4–38 through 4–41 illustrate the fundamental counting rule.

| Example 4–38 | **Tossing a Coin and Rolling a Die** |

A coin is tossed and a die is rolled. Find the number of outcomes for the sequence of events.

Solution

Since the coin can land either heads up or tails up and since the die can land with any one of six numbers showing face up, there are $2 \cdot 6 = 12$ possibilities. A tree diagram can also be drawn for the sequence of events. See Figure 4–8.

Figure 4–8

Complete Tree Diagram for Example 4–38

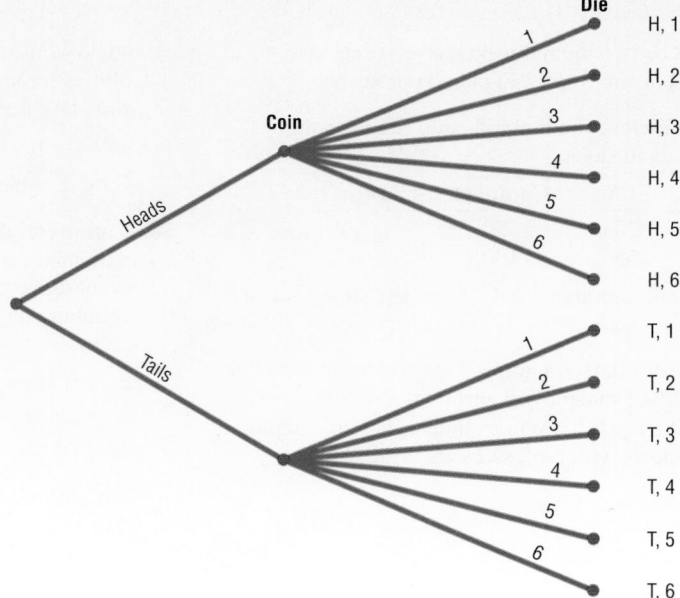

| Example 4–39 | **Types of Paint** |

A paint manufacturer wishes to manufacture several different paints. The categories include

Colour	Red, blue, white, black, green, brown, yellow
Type	Latex, oil
Texture	Flat, semigloss, high gloss
Use	Outdoor, indoor

How many different kinds of paint can be made if a person can select one colour, one type, one texture, and one use?

Solution

A person can choose one colour and one type and one texture and one use. Since there are 7 colour choices, 2 type choices, 3 texture choices, and 2 use choices, the total number of possible different paints is

Colour		Type		Texture		Use	
7	$\cdot$	2	$\cdot$	3	$\cdot$	2	= 84

Example 4–40

Blood Type Distribution

There are four blood types, A, B, AB, and O, Blood can also be Rh+ and Rh−. Finally, a blood donor can be classified as either male or female. How many different ways can a donor have his or her blood labelled?

Solution

Since there are 4 possibilities for blood type, 2 possibilities for Rh factor, and 2 possibilities for the gender of the donor, there are $4 \cdot 2 \cdot 2$, or 16, different classification categories, as shown.

Blood type		Rh		Gender	
4	$\cdot$	2	$\cdot$	2	= 16

A tree diagram for the events is shown in Figure 4–9.

Figure 4–9

Complete Tree Diagram for Example 4–40

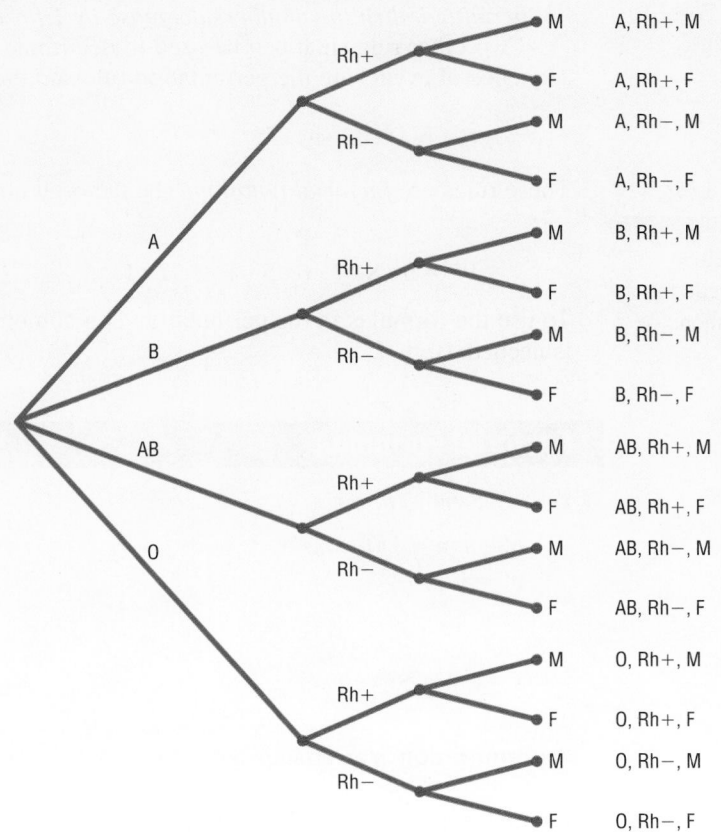

When determining the number of different possibilities of a sequence of events, one must know whether repetitions are permissible.

Example 4–41

Identification Cards

The digits 0, 1, 2, 3, and 4 are to be used in a four-digit ID card. How many different cards are possible if repetitions are permitted?

Solution

Since there are 4 spaces to fill and 5 choices for each space, the solution is

$$5 \cdot 5 \cdot 5 \cdot 5 = 5^4 = 625$$

Now, what if repetitions are not permitted? For Example 4–41, the first digit can be chosen in 5 ways. But the second digit can be chosen in only 4 ways, since there are only four digits left, etc. Thus, the solution is

$$5 \cdot 4 \cdot 3 \cdot 2 = 120$$

The same situation occurs when one is drawing balls from an urn or cards from a deck. If the ball or card is replaced before the next one is selected, then repetitions are permitted, since the same one can be selected again. But if the selected ball or card is not replaced, then repetitions are not permitted, since the same ball or card cannot be selected the second time.

These examples illustrate the fundamental counting rule. In summary: *If repetitions are permitted, then the numbers stay the same going from left to right. If repetitions are not permitted, then the numbers decrease by 1 for each place left to right.*

Two other rules that can be used to determine the total number of possibilities of a sequence of events are the permutation rule and the combination rule.

Factorial Notation

Historical Note

In 1808 Christian Kramp first used the factorial notation.

These rules use *factorial notation*. The factorial notation uses the exclamation point.

$$5! = 5 \cdot 4 \cdot 3 \cdot 2 \cdot 1$$
$$9! = 9 \cdot 8 \cdot 7 \cdot 6 \cdot 5 \cdot 4 \cdot 3 \cdot 2 \cdot 1$$

To use the formulas in the permutation and combination rules, a special definition of 0! is needed. $0! = 1$.

Factorial Formulas

For any counting n

$$n! = n(n - 1)(n - 2) \cdots 1$$
$$0! = 1$$

Permutations

A **permutation** is an arrangement of n objects in a specific order.

Examples 4–42 and 4–43 illustrate permutations.

Example 4–42

Business Locations

Suppose a business owner has a choice of five locations in which to establish her business. She decides to rank each location according to certain criteria, such as price of the store and parking facilities. How many different ways can she rank the five locations?

Solution

There are

$$5! = 5 \cdot 4 \cdot 3 \cdot 2 \cdot 1 = 120$$

different possible rankings. The reason is that she has 5 choices for the first location, 4 choices for the second location, 3 choices for the third location, etc.

In Example 4–42 all objects were used up. But what happens when not all objects are used up? The answer to this question is given in Example 4–43.

Example 4–43

Business Locations

Suppose the business owner in Example 4–42 wishes to rank only the top three of the five locations. How many different ways can she rank them?

Solution

Using the fundamental counting rule, she can select any one of the five for first choice, then any one of the remaining four locations for her second choice, and finally, any one of the remaining locations for her third choice, as shown.

First choice		Second choice		Third choice
$\boxed{5}$	$\cdot$	$\boxed{4}$	$\cdot$	$\boxed{3}$ = 60

The solutions in Examples 4–42 and 4–43 are permutations.

Permutation Rule

The arrangement of n objects in a specific order using r objects at a time is called a *permutation of n objects taking r objects at a time*. It is written as $_nP_r$, and the formula is

$$_nP_r = \frac{n!}{(n - r)!}$$

The notation $_nP_r$ is used for permutations.

$$_6P_4 \text{ means } \frac{6!}{(6 - 4)!} \qquad \text{or} \qquad \frac{6!}{2!} = \frac{6 \cdot 5 \cdot 4 \cdot 3 \cdot \cancel{2} \cdot \cancel{1}}{\cancel{2} \cdot \cancel{1}} = 360$$

Although Examples 4–42 and 4–43 were solved by the multiplication rule, they can now be solved by the permutation rule.

In Example 4–42, five locations were taken and then arranged in order; hence,

$$_5P_5 = \frac{5!}{(5 - 5)!} = \frac{5!}{0!} = \frac{5 \cdot 4 \cdot 3 \cdot 2 \cdot 1}{1} = 120$$

(Recall that $0! = 1$.)

In Example 4–43, three locations were selected from five locations, so $n = 5$ and $r = 3$; hence

$$_5P_3 = \frac{5!}{(5-3)!} = \frac{5!}{2!} = \frac{5 \cdot 4 \cdot 3 \cdot \cancel{2} \cdot \cancel{1}}{\cancel{2} \cdot \cancel{1}} = 60$$

Examples 4–44 and 4–45 illustrate the permutation rule.

Example 4–44

Television News Stories

A television news director wishes to use 3 news stories on an evening show. One story will be the lead story, one will be the second story, and the last will be a closing story. If the director has a total of 8 stories to choose from, how many possible ways can the program be set up?

Solution

Since order is important, the solution is

$$_8P_3 = \frac{8!}{(8-3)!} = \frac{8!}{5!} = 336$$

Hence, there would be 336 ways to set up the program.

Example 4–45

School Musical Plays

A school musical director can select 2 musical plays to present next year. One will be presented in the fall, and one will be presented in the spring. If she has 9 to pick from, how many different possibilities are there?

Solution

Order is important since one play can be presented in the fall and the other play in the spring.

$$_9P_2 = \frac{9!}{(9-2)!} = \frac{9!}{7!} = \frac{9 \cdot 8 \cdot 7!}{7!} = 72$$

There are 72 different possibilities.

Combinations

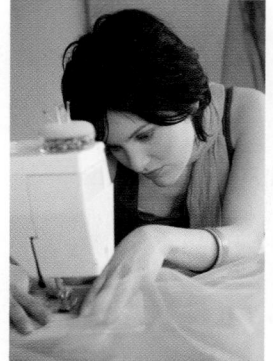

Suppose a dress designer wishes to select two colours of material to design a new dress, and she has on hand four colours. How many different possibilities can there be in this situation?

This type of problem differs from previous ones in that the order of selection is not important. That is, if the designer selects yellow and red, this selection is the same as the selection red and yellow. This type of selection is called a *combination*. The difference between a permutation and a combination is that in a combination, the order or arrangement of the objects is not important; by contrast, order *is* important in a permutation. Example 4–46 illustrates this difference.

A selection of distinct objects without regard to order is called a **combination.**

Example 4–46

Letters

Given the letters A, B, C, and D, list the permutations and combinations for selecting two letters.

Solution

The permutations are

AB	BA	CA	DA
AC	BC	CB	DB
AD	BD	CD	DC

In permutations, AB is different from BA. But in combinations, AB is the same as BA since the order of the objects does not matter in combinations. Therefore, if duplicates are removed from a list of permutations, what is left is a list of combinations, as shown.

AB	~~BA~~	~~CA~~	~~DA~~
AC	BC	~~CB~~	~~DB~~
AD	BD	CD	~~DC~~

Hence the combinations of A, B, C, and D are AB, AC, AD, BC, BD, and CD. (Alternatively, BA could be listed and AB crossed out, etc.) The combinations have been listed alphabetically for convenience, but this is not a requirement.

Combinations are used when the order or arrangement is not important, as in the selecting process. Suppose a committee of 5 students is to be selected from 25 students. The 5 selected students represent a combination, since it does not matter who is selected first, second, etc.

Interesting Fact

Excluding traffic offences, 2,194,705 Criminal Code offences were reported in Canada in 2008.

Combination Rule

The number of combinations of r objects selected from n objects is denoted by $_nC_r$ and is given by the formula

$$_nC_r = \frac{n!}{(n-r)!r!}$$

Example 4–47

Combinations

How many combinations of 4 objects are there, taken 2 at a time?

Solution

Since this is a combination problem, the answer is

$$_4C_2 = \frac{4!}{(4-2)!2!} = \frac{4!}{2!2!} = \frac{\overset{2}{\cancel{4}} \cdot 3 \cdot \cancel{2!}}{\cancel{2} \cdot 1 \cdot \cancel{2!}} = 6$$

This is the same result shown in Example 4–46.

Notice that the expression for $_nC_r$ is

$$\frac{n!}{(n-r)!r!}$$

which is the formula for permutations with $r!$ in the denominator. In other words,

$$_nC_r = \frac{_nP_r}{r!}$$

This $r!$ divides out the duplicates from the number of permutations, as shown in Example 4–46. For each 2 letters, there are 2 permutations but only one combination. Hence, dividing the number of permutations by $r!$ eliminates the duplicates. This result can be verified for other values of n and r. Note: $_nC_n = 1$.

| Example 4–48 | **Mountain Bikes** |

A bicycle shop owner has 12 mountain bicycles in the showroom. The owner wishes to select 5 of them to display at a bicycle show. How many different ways can a group of 5 be selected?

Solution

$$_{12}C_5 = \frac{12!}{(12-5)!5!} = \frac{12!}{7!5!} = \frac{12 \cdot 11 \cdot \overset{2}{\cancel{10}} \cdot \overset{3}{\cancel{9}} \cdot \overset{2}{\cancel{8}} \cdot \cancel{7!}}{\cancel{7!} \cdot \cancel{5} \cdot \cancel{4} \cdot \cancel{3} \cdot 2 \cdot 1} = 792$$

| Example 4–49 | **Committee Selection** |

In a club there are 7 women and 5 men. A committee of 3 women and 2 men is to be chosen. How many different possibilities are there?

Solution

Here, one must select 3 women from 7 women, which can be done in $_7C_3$, or 35, ways. Next, 2 men must be selected from 5 men, which can be done in $_5C_2$, or 10, ways. Finally, by the fundamental counting rule, the total number of different ways is $35 \cdot 10 = 350$, since one is choosing both men and women. Using the formula gives

$$_7C_3 \cdot {_5C_2} = \frac{7!}{(7-3)!3!} \cdot \frac{5!}{(5-2)!2!} = 350$$

Table 4–1 Summarizes the counting rules.

Table 4–1	**Summary of counting rules**	
Rule	**Definition**	**Formula**
Fundamental counting rule	The number of ways a sequence of n events can occur if the first event can occur in k_1 ways, the second event can occur in k_2 ways, etc.	$k_1 \cdot k_2 \cdot k_3 \cdots k_n$
Permutation rule	The number of permutations of n objects taking r objects at a time (order is important)	$_nP_r = \dfrac{n!}{(n-r)!}$
Combination rule	The number of combinations of r objects taken from n objects (order is not important)	$_nC_r = \dfrac{n!}{(n-r)!r!}$

4–4 Applying the Concepts

Garage Door Openers

Garage door openers originally had a series of 4 on/off switches so that homeowners could personalize the frequencies that opened their garage doors. If all garage door openers were set at the same frequency, anyone with a garage door opener could open anyone else's garage door.

1. Use a tree diagram to show how many different positions 4 consecutive on/off switches could be in.

After garage door openers became more popular, another set of 4 on/off switches was added to the systems.

2. Find a pattern of how many different positions are possible with the addition of each on/off switch.

3. How many different positions are possible with 8 consecutive on/off switches?

4. Is it reasonable to assume, if you owned a garage door opener with 8 switches, that someone could use his or her garage door opener to open your garage door by trying all the different possible positions?

In 1989 it was reported that the ignition keys for 1988 Dodge Caravans were made from a single blank that had 5 cuts on it. Each cut was made at one out of 5 possible levels. In 1988, assume there was 420,000 Dodge Caravans sold in Canada.

5. How many different possible keys can be made from the same key blank?

6. How many different 1988 Dodge Caravans could any one key start?

Look at the ignition key for your car and count the number of cuts on it. Assume that the cuts are made at one of five possible levels. Most car companies use one key blank for all their makes and models of cars.

7. Conjecture how many cars your car company sold over recent years, and then figure out how many other cars your car key could start. What would you do to decrease the odds of someone being able to open another vehicle with his or her key?

See page 208 for the answers.

Exercises 4–4

1. **U.S. Zip Codes** How many 5-digit United States numeric postal (zip) codes are possible if the same 5 digits can be repeated? If the 5 digits cannot be repeated?

2. **Batting Order** How many ways can a baseball manager arrange a batting order of 9 players?

3. **Video Games** How many different ways can 7 different video game discs be arranged on a shelf?

4. **Seating Arrangements** In how many ways can 5 speakers be seated in a row on a stage?

5. **Shampoo Display** A store manager wishes to display 8 different brands of shampoo in a row. How many ways can this be done?

6. **Show Programs** Three bands and two comics are performing for a student talent show. How many different programs (in terms of order) can be arranged? How many different programs can be arranged if the comics must perform between bands?

7. **Campus Tours** Student volunteers take visitors on a tour of 7 campus buildings. How many different tours are possible? (Assume order is important.)

8. **Radio Station Call Letters** Assume a radio station must have 4 call letters for identification. If the call letters for a radio station must begin with C or V, how many different call letters can be made if repetitions are not allowed? If repetitions are allowed?

9. **Identification Tags** How many different 3-digit identification tags can be made if the digits can be used more than once? If the first digit must be a 5 and repetitions are not permitted?

10. **Book Arrangements** How many different ways can 9 trophies be arranged on a shelf?

11. **Selection of Officers** Six students are running for the positions of president and vice-president, and five students are running for secretary and treasurer. If the two highest vote-getters in each of the two contests are elected, how many winning combinations can there be?

12. **Auto Trips** There are 2 major roads from city X to city Y and 4 major roads from city Y to city Z. How many different trips can be made from city X to city Z passing through city Y?

13. Evaluate each of these.

    a. $8!$ e. $_7P_5$ i. $_5C_5$

    b. $10!$ f. $_{12}P_4$ j. $_6P_2$

    c. $0!$ g. $_5P_3$

    d. $1!$ h. $_6P_0$

14. **County Assessments** The County Assessment Bureau decides to reassess homes in 8 different areas. How many different ways can this be accomplished?

15. **Sports Car Stripes** How many different 4-colour code stripes can be made on a sports car if each code consists of the colours green, red, blue, and white? All colours are used only once.

16. **Manufacturing Tests** An inspector must select 3 tests to perform in a certain order on a manufactured part. He has a choice of 7 tests. How many ways can he perform 3 different tests?

17. **Threatened Species of Reptiles** There are 22 threatened species of reptiles in the United States. In how many ways can you choose 4 to write about? (Order is not important.)
    Source: Infoplease: www.infoplease.com.

18. **Restaurant Inspections** How many different ways can a city health department inspector visit 5 restaurants in a city with 10 restaurants?

19. **Permutations** How many different 4-letter permutations can be formed from the letters in the word *decagon*?

20. **Cellphone Models** A particular cellphone company offers 4 models of phones, each in 6 different colours and each available with any one of 5 calling plans. How many combinations are possible?

21. **Identification Cards** How many different ID cards can be made if there are 6 digits on a card and no digit can be used more than once?

22. **Free-Sample Requests** An online coupon service has 13 offers for free samples. How many different requests

are possible if a customer must request exactly 3 free samples? How many are possible if the customer may request up to 3 free samples?

23. **Ticket Selection** How many different ways can 4 tickets be selected from 50 tickets if each ticket wins a different prize?

24. **Research Rat Tests** How many different ways can a researcher select 5 rats from 20 rats and assign each to a different test?

25. **Task Assignments** How many ways can an adviser choose 4 students from a class of 12 if they are all assigned the same task? How many ways can the students be chosen if they are each given a different task?

26. **Agency Cases** An investigative agency has 7 cases and 5 agents. How many different ways can the cases be assigned if only 1 case is assigned to each agent?

27. **(ans)** Evaluate each expression.

    a. $_5C_2$ d. $_6C_2$ g. $_3C_3$ j. $_4C_3$

    b. $_8C_3$ e. $_6C_4$ h. $_9C_7$

    c. $_7C_4$ f. $_3C_0$ i. $_{12}P_2$

28. **Selecting Cards** How many ways can 3 cards be selected from a standard deck of 52 cards, disregarding the order of selection?

29. **Selecting Bracelets** How many ways are there to select 3 bracelets from a box of 10 bracelets, disregarding the order of selection?

30. **Selecting Players** How many ways can 4 baseball players and 3 basketball players be selected from 12 baseball players and 9 basketball players?

31. **Selecting a Committee** How many ways can a committee of 4 people be selected from a group of 10 people?

32. **Selecting Christmas Presents** If a person can select 3 presents from 10 presents under a Christmas tree, how many different combinations are there?

33. **Test Questions** How many different tests can be made from a test bank of 20 questions if the test consists of 5 questions?

34. **Promotional Programs** The general manager of a fast-food restaurant chain must select 6 restaurants from 11 for a promotional program. How many different possible ways can this selection be done?

35. **Music Program Selections** A jazz band has prepared 18 selections for a concert tour. At each stop, the band will perform 10. How many different programs are possible? How many programs are possible if the band always begins with the same song and ends with the same song?

36. Freight Train Cars In a train yard there are 4 tank cars, 12 boxcars, and 7 flatcars. How many ways can a train be made up consisting of 2 tank cars, 5 boxcars, and 3 flatcars? (In this case, order is not important.)

37. Selecting a Committee There are 7 women and 5 men in a department. How many ways can a committee of 4 people be selected? How many ways can this committee be selected if there must be 2 men and 2 women on the committee? How many ways can this committee be selected if there must be at least 2 women on the committee?

38. Selecting Cereal Boxes Wake Up cereal comes in 2 types, crispy and crunchy. If a researcher has 10 boxes of each, how many ways can she select 3 boxes of each for a quality control test?

39. Hawaiian Words The Hawaiian alphabet consists of 7 consonants and 5 vowels. How many three-letter "words" are possible if there are never two consonants together and if a word must always end in a vowel?

40. Selecting a Jury How many ways can a jury of 6 women and 6 men be selected from 10 women and 12 men?

41. Selecting a Golf Foursome How many ways can a foursome of 2 men and 2 women be selected from 10 men and 12 women in a golf club?

42. Investigative Team The RCMP Drug Enforcement Branch must form a 5-member investigative team. If it has 25 agents from which to choose, how many different possible teams can be formed?

43. Dominoes A domino is a flat rectangular block, the face of which is divided into two square parts, each part showing from zero to six pips (or dots). Playing a game consists of playing dominoes with a matching number of pips. Explain why there are 28 dominoes in a complete set.

44. Charity Event Participants There are 16 seniors and 15 juniors in a particular social organization. In how many ways can 4 seniors and 2 juniors be chosen to participate in a charity event?

45. Selecting Commercials How many ways can a person select 7 television commercials from 11 television commercials?

46. DVD Selection How many ways can a person select 8 DVDs from a display of 13 DVDs?

47. Candy Bar Selection How many ways can a person select 6 candy bars from a list of 10 and 6 salty snacks from a list of 12 to put in a vending machine?

48. Selecting a Location An advertising manager decides to have an ad campaign in which 8 special calculators will be hidden at various locations in a shopping mall: If she has 17 locations from which to pick, how many different possible combinations can she choose?

Extending the Concepts   »

49. Coin Selections How many different ways can a person select one or more coins if she has 2 nickels, 1 dime, and 1 quarter?

50. Farm Animals In a barnyard there is an assortment of chickens and cows. Counting heads, one gets 15; counting legs, one gets 46. How many of each are there?

51. Movie Seat Arrangement How many different ways can five people—A, B, C, D, and E—sit in a row at a movie theatre if (*a*) A and B must sit together; (*b*) C must sit to the right of, but not necessarily next to, B; (*c*) D and E will not sit next to each other?

52. Poker Hands Using combinations, calculate the number of each poker hand in a deck of cards. (A poker hand consists of 5 cards dealt in any order.)

a. Royal flush   *c.* Four of a kind

b. Straight flush   *d.* Full house

4–5   Probability and Counting Rules (Optional) >

Combine probability and counting rules to determine outcomes of experiments.

The counting rules can be combined with the probability rules in this chapter to solve many types of probability problems. By using the fundamental counting rule, the permutation rules, and the combination rule, one can compute the probability of outcomes of many experiments, such as getting a full house when 5 cards are dealt or selecting a committee of 3 women and 2 men from a club consisting of 10 women and 10 men.

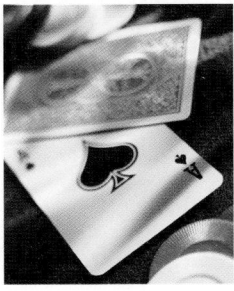

Example 4–50

Four Aces

Find the probability of getting 4 aces when 5 cards are drawn from an ordinary deck of cards.

Solution

There are $_{52}C_5$ ways to draw 5 cards from a deck. There is only one way to get 4 aces (i.e., $_4C_4$), but there are 48 possibilities to get the fifth card. Therefore, there are 48 ways to get 4 aces and 1 other card. Hence,

$$P(4 \text{ aces}) = \frac{_4C_4 \cdot 48}{_{52}C_5} = \frac{1 \cdot 48}{2{,}598{,}960} = \frac{48}{2{,}598{,}960} = \frac{1}{54{,}145}$$

Example 4–51

Defective Transistors

A box contains 24 transistors, 4 of which are defective. If 4 are sold at random, find the following probabilities.

   a. Exactly 2 are defective.   *c.* All are defective.

   b. None is defective.   *d.* At least 1 is defective.

Solution

There are $_{24}C_4$ ways to sell 4 transistors, so the denominator in each case will be 10,626.

   a. Two defective transistors can be selected as $_4C_2$ and 2 nondefective ones as $_{20}C_2$. Hence,

$$P(\text{exactly 2 defectives}) = \frac{_4C_2 \cdot {_{20}C_2}}{_{24}C_4} = \frac{1{,}140}{10{,}626} = \frac{190}{1{,}771}$$

   b. The number of ways to choose no defectives is $_{20}C_4$. Hence,

$$P(\text{no defectives}) = \frac{_{20}C_4}{_{24}C_4} = \frac{4{,}845}{10{,}626} = \frac{1{,}615}{3{,}542}$$

   c. The number of ways to choose 4 defectives from 4 is $_4C_4$, or 1. Hence,

$$P(\text{all defectives}) = \frac{1}{_{24}C_4} = \frac{1}{10{,}626}$$

   d. To find the probability of at least 1 defective transistor, find the probability that there are no defective transistors, and then subtract that probability from 1.

$$P(\text{at least 1 defective}) = 1 - P(\text{no defectives})$$
$$= 1 - \frac{_{20}C_4}{_{24}C_4} = 1 - \frac{1{,}615}{3{,}542} = \frac{1{,}927}{3{,}542}$$

Example 4–52

Magazines

A store has 6 *TV Graphic* magazines and 8 *Newstime* magazines on the counter. If two customers purchased a magazine, find the probability that one of each magazine was purchased.

Solution

$$P(1 \text{ } TV \text{ } Graphic \text{ and } 1 \text{ } Newstime) = \frac{_6C_1 \cdot {_8C_1}}{_{14}C_2} = \frac{6 \cdot 8}{91} = \frac{48}{91}$$

| Example 4–53 | **Combination Lock** |

A combination lock consists of the 26 letters of the alphabet. If a 3-letter combination is needed, find the probability that the combination will consist of the letters ABC in that order. The same letter can be used more than once. (*Note:* A combination lock is really a permutation lock.)

Solution

Since repetitions are permitted, there are $26 \cdot 26 \cdot 26 = 17{,}576$ different possible combinations. And since there is only one ABC combination, the probability is $P(\text{ABC}) = 1/26^3 = 1/17{,}576$.

| Example 4–54 | **Tennis Tournament** |

There are 8 married couples in a tennis club. If 1 man and 1 woman are selected at random to plan the summer tournament, find the probability that they are married to each other.

Solution

Since there are 8 ways to select the man and 8 ways to select the woman, there are $8 \cdot 8$, or 64, ways to select 1 man and 1 woman. Since there are 8 married couples, the solution is $\frac{8}{64} = \frac{1}{8}$.

As indicated at the beginning of this section, the counting rules and the probability rules can be used to solve a large variety of probability problems found in business, gambling, economics, biology, and other fields.

4–5 Applying the Concepts

Counting Rules and Probability

One of the biggest problems for students when doing probability problems is to decide which formula or formulas to use. Another problem is to decide whether two events are independent or dependent. Use the following problem to help develop a better understanding of these concepts.

Assume you are given a 5-question multiple-choice quiz. Each question has 5 possible answers: A, B, C, D, and E.

1. How many events are there?
2. Are the events independent or dependent?
3. If you guess at each question, what is the probability that you will get all of them correct?
4. What is the probability that a person would guess answer A for each question?

Assume that you are given a test in which you are to match the correct answers in the right column with the questions in the left column. You can use each answer only once.

5. How many events are there?
6. Are the events independent or dependent?
7. What is the probability of getting them all correct if you are guessing?
8. What is the difference between the two problems?

See page 208 for the answers.

Speaking of Statistics

The Mathematics of Gambling

Gambling is big business. There are provincial lotteries, casinos, sports betting, and church bingos. It seems that today, everybody is either watching or playing Texas Hold 'em Poker.

Using permutations, combinations, and the probability rules, mathematicians can find the probabilities of various gambling games. Here are the probabilities of the various 5-card poker hands.

Hand	Number of ways	Probability
Straight flush	40	0.000015
Four of a kind	624	0.000240
Full house	3,744	0.001441
Flush	5,108	0.001965
Straight	10,200	0.003925
Three of a kind	54,912	0.021129
Two pairs	123,552	0.047539
One pair	1,098,240	0.422569
Less than one pair	1,302,540	0.501177
Total	2,598,960	1.000000

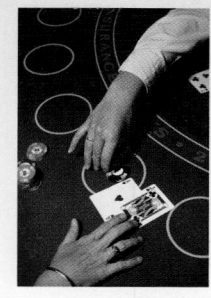

The chance of winning at gambling games can be compared by using what is called the *house advantage, house edge,* or *house percentage.* For example, the house advantage for roulette is about 5.26%, which means that in the long run, the house wins 5.26 cents on every $1 bet, or that you will lose, on average, 5.26 cents on every $1 you bet. The lower the house advantage, the more favourable the game is to you.

For the game of craps, the house advantage is anywhere between 1.4 and 15%, depending on what you bet on. For keno, the house advantage is 29.5%. The house advantage for Chuck-a-Luck is 7.87%, and for baccarat, it is either 1.36 or 1.17%, depending on your bet.

Slot machines have a house advantage anywhere from about 4 to 10%, depending on the geographic location, such as Atlantic City, Las Vegas, and Windsor, and the amount put into the machine, such as 5¢, 25¢, and $1.

Actually, gamblers found winning strategies for the game blackjack or 21 such as card counting. However, the casinos retaliated by using multiple decks and by banning card counters.

Exercises 4–5

1. **Selecting Cards** Find the probability of getting 2 face cards (king, queen, or jack) when 2 cards are drawn from a deck without replacement.

2. **Selecting a Committee** A parent–teacher committee consisting of 4 people is to be formed from 20 parents and 5 teachers. Find the probability that the committee will consist of these people. (Assume that the selection will be random.)

   a. All teachers

   b. 2 teachers and 2 parents

   c. All parents

   d. 1 teacher and 3 parents

3. **Management Seminar** In a company there are 7 executives: 4 women and 3 men. Three are selected to attend a management seminar. Find these probabilities.

   a. All 3 selected will be women.

   b. All 3 selected will be men.

   c. 2 men and 1 woman will be selected.

   d. 1 man and 2 women will be selected.

4. **Senate Party Affiliation** The composition of Canada's Senate, based on party affiliation as of January 2010, is

   53 Conservative   49 Liberals   3 Others

   A new committee is being formed to study ways to benefit the arts in education. If 3 senators are selected at random to head the committee, what is the probability that they will all be Liberals? What is the probability that they will all be Conservatives? What is the probability that there will be one from each designated party affiliation, including "Other" parties? Note: *Conservative senators include Progressive Conservatives.*
   Source: The Senate of Canada.

5. **Provincial/Territorial Premiers** Since each jurisdiction joined Canada's confederation, there have been

255 elected provincial and territorial premiers, as of 2007, as shown.

Alberta	13	Nunavut	1
British Columbia	34	Ontario	24
Manitoba	21	Prince Edward Island	32
New Brunswick	31	Quebec	34
Nova Scotia	26	Saskatchewan	14
Newfoundland/Labrador	9	Yukon	7
Northwest Territories	9		

Suppose that 4 premiers are chosen at random to be the subject of a documentary. Find the probability that

a. All 4 hail from British Columbia.

b. 2 are from the Northwest Territories and 2 are from Yukon.

Source: Canada Info Link: www.canadainfolink.ca.

6. **Defective Pixels** A package contains 12 LCD panels, 3 of which have defective pixels. If 4 LCD panels are selected, find the probability of getting

a. No defective LCD panels

b. 1 defective LCD panel

c. 3 defective LCD panels

7. **Winning Tickets** If 50 tickets are sold and 2 prizes are to be awarded, find the probability that one person will win 2 prizes if that person buys 2 tickets.

8. **Drawing a Full House** Find the probability of getting a full house (3 cards of one denomination and 2 of another) when 5 cards are dealt from an ordinary deck.

9. **Medical Committee** A committee of 4 people is to be formed from 6 doctors and 8 dentists. Find the probability that the committee will consist of

a. All dentists

b. 2 dentists and 2 doctors

c. All doctors

d. 3 doctors and 1 dentist

e. 1 doctor and 3 dentists

10. **Insurance Policies** An insurance sales representative selects 3 policies to review. The group of policies she can select from contains 8 life policies, 5 automobile policies, and 2 homeowner policies. Find the probability of selecting

a. All life policies

b. Both homeowner policies

c. All automobile policies

d. 1 of each policy

e. 2 life policies and 1 automobile policy

11. **Socks in a Drawer** A drawer contains 11 identical red socks and 8 identical black socks. Suppose that you choose 2 socks at random in the dark

a. What is the probability that you get a pair of red socks?

b. What is the probability that you get a pair of black socks?

c. What is the probability that you get 2 unmatched socks?

d. Where did the other red sock go?

12. **Selecting Books** Find the probability of selecting 3 science books and 4 math books from 8 science books and 9 math books. The books are selected at random.

13. **Rolling Three Dice** When 3 dice are rolled, find the probability of getting a sum of 7.

14. **Football Team Selection** A football team consists of 20 each freshmen and sophomores, 15 juniors, and 10 seniors. Four players are selected at random to serve as captains. Find the probability that

a. All 4 are seniors.

b. There is 1 each: freshman, sophomore, junior, and senior.

c. There are 2 sophomores and 2 freshmen.

d. At least 1 of the students is a senior.

15. **Arrangement of Washers** Find the probability that if 5 different-sized washers are arranged in a row, they will be arranged in order of size.

16. **Poker Hands** Using the information in Exercise 52 in Section 4–4, find the probability of each poker hand.

a. Royal flush

b. Straight flush

c. 4 of a kind

17. **Plant Selection** All holly plants are dioecious; that is, a male plant must be planted within 9 to 12 metres of the female plants in order to yield berries. A home improvement store has 12 unmarked holly plants for sale, 8 of which are female. If a homeowner buys 3 plants at random, what is the probability that berries will be produced?

Summary ›

In this chapter, the basic concepts and rules of probability are explained. The three types of probability are classical, empirical, and subjective. Classical probability uses sample spaces. Empirical probability uses frequency distributions and is based on observation. In subjective probability, the researcher makes an educated guess about the chance of an event occurring.

A probability event consists of one or more outcomes of a probability experiment. Two events are said to be mutually exclusive if they cannot occur at the same time. Events can also be classified as independent or dependent. If events are independent, whether or not the first event occurs does not affect the probability of the next event occurring. If the probability of the second event occurring is changed by the occurrence of the first event, then the events are dependent. The complement of an event is the set of outcomes in the sample space that are not included in the outcomes of the event itself. Complementary events are mutually exclusive.

Probability problems can be solved by using the addition rules, the multiplication rules, and the complementary event rules.

Finally, the fundamental counting rule, the permutation rule, and the combination rule can be used to determine the number of outcomes of events; then these numbers can be used to determine the probabilities of events.

For step-by-step guidance on the use of Texas Instruments TI-83 Plus/TI-84 Plus programmable calculators, see Appendix E at the back of this book. For summary procedures for Minitab, SPSS, and Excel, please see the full version of Appendix E on *Connect*.

Important Terms »

classical probability 152

combination 190

complement of an event 155

compound event 151

conditional probability 175

dependent events 175

empirical probability 157

equally likely events 152

event 151

fundamental counting rule 185

independent events 172

law of large numbers 159

mutually exclusive events 165

outcome 149

permutation 188

probability 148

probability experiment 149

sample space 149

simple event 151

subjective probability 159

tree diagram 150

Venn diagrams 156

Important Formulas »

Formula for classical probability:

$$P(E) = \frac{\text{Number of outcomes in } E}{\text{Total number of outcomes in sample space}} = \frac{n(E)}{n(S)}$$

Formula for empirical probability:

$$P(E) = \frac{\text{Frequency for class}}{\text{Total frequencies in distribution}} = \frac{f}{n}$$

Addition Rule 1, for two mutually exclusive events:

$$P(A \text{ or } B) = P(A) + P(B)$$

Addition Rule 2, for events that are not mutually exclusive:

$$P(A \text{ or } B) = P(A) + P(B) - P(A \text{ and } B)$$

Multiplication Rule 1, for independent events:

$$P(A \text{ and } B) = P(A) \cdot P(B)$$

Multiplication Rule 2, for dependent events:

$$P(A \text{ and } B) = P(A) \cdot P(B|A)$$

Formula for conditional probability:

$$P(B|A) = \frac{P(A \text{ and } B)}{P(A)}$$

Formula for complementary events:

$$P(\overline{E}) = 1 - P(E) \quad \text{or} \quad P(E) = 1 - P(\overline{E})$$
$$\text{or} \quad P(E) + P(\overline{E}) = 1$$

Fundamental counting rule: In a sequence of n events in which the first one has k_1 possibilities, the second event has k_2 possibilities, the third has k_3 possibilities, etc., the total number possibilities of the sequence will be

$$k_1 \cdot k_2 \cdot k_3 \cdots k_n$$

Permutation rule: The number of permutations of n objects taking r objects at a time when order is important is

$$_nP_r = \frac{n!}{(n-r)!}$$

Combination rule: The number of combinations of r objects selected from n objects when order is not important is

$$_nC_r = \frac{n!}{(n-r)!r!}$$

Mc Graw Hill Connect™ Practise and learn online with *Connect* with data sets and algorithmic questions related to concepts covered in this chapter. Questions and tables with online data sets are marked with .

Review Exercises »

1. **Rolling a Die** When a die is rolled, find the probability of getting a
   a. 5
   b. 6
   c. Number less than 5

2. **Selecting a Card** When a card is selected from a deck, find the probability of getting
   a. A club
   b. A face card or a heart
   c. A 6 and a spade
   d. A king
   e. A red card

3. **Software Selection** The top-ten-selling computer software titles last year consisted of 3 for doing taxes, 5 antivirus or security programs, and 2 "other" programs. Choose one title at random.
   a. What is the probability that it is not used for doing taxes?
   b. What is the probability that it is used for taxes or is one of the "other" programs?
   Source: Infoplease: www.infoplease.com.

4. **Renumbered Die** A six-sided die is printed with the numbers 1, 2, 3, 5, 8, and 13. Roll the die once. What is the probability of getting an even number? Roll the die twice and add the numbers on each rolled die. What is the probability of getting an odd sum on two rolled dice?

5. **Cordless Phone Survey** A recent survey indicated that in a town of 1500 households, 850 had cordless telephones. If a household is randomly selected, find the probability that it has a cordless telephone.

6. **Sweater Selection** During a sale at a men's store, 16 white sweaters, 3 red sweaters, 9 blue sweaters, and 7 yellow sweaters were purchased. If a customer is selected at random, find the probability that he bought
   a. A blue sweater
   b. A yellow or a white sweater

   c. A red, a blue, or a yellow sweater
   d. A sweater that was not white

7. **Budget Rental Cars** Cheap Rentals has nothing but budget cars for rental. The probability that a car has air conditioning is 0.5, and the probability that a car has a CD player is 0.37. The probability that a car has both air conditioning and a CD player is 0.06. What is the probability that a randomly selected car has neither air conditioning nor a CD player?

8. **Rolling Two Dice** When two dice are rolled, find the probability of getting
   a. A sum of 5 or 6
   b. A sum greater than 9
   c. A sum less than 4 or greater than 9
   d. A sum that is divisible by 4
   e. A sum of 14
   f. A sum less than 13

9. **Car and Boat Ownership** The probability that a person owns a car is 0.80, that a person owns a boat is 0.30, and that a person owns both a car and a boat is 0.12. Find the probability that a person owns either a boat or a car.

10. **Purchasing a New Car** There is a 0.39 probability that John will purchase a new car, a 0.73 probability that Mary will purchase a new car, and a 0.36 probability that both will purchase a new car. Find the probability that neither will purchase a new car.

11. **Avian Flu Risk** A *CTV Newsnet* poll indicates that 36% of Canadians believe that authorities are exaggerating the level of risk of the avian flu in order to encourage people to take precautions. If 5 Canadians are randomly selected, find the probability that all 5 feel the avian flu risk is exaggerated.
    Source: CTV Newsnet, March 2005.

12. **Public Library Usage** A study entitled "Canadians, Public Libraries and the Information Highway" examined Canadians' usage of public libraries. On a basic

level, 63% of survey respondents reported having a public library card. Find the probability that 5 randomly selected Canadians have a public library card.

Source: Canadian Library Association.

13. **Drawing Cards** Three cards are drawn from an ordinary deck *without* replacement. Find the probability of getting

   a. All black cards
   b. All spades
   c. All queens

14. **Coin Toss and Card Selection** A coin is tossed and a card is drawn from a deck. Find the probability of getting

   a. A head and a 6
   b. A tail and a red card
   c. A head and a club

15. **Movie Releases** The top five countries for movie releases so far this year are the United States with 471 releases, the United Kingdom with 386, Japan with 79, Germany with 316, and France with 132. Choose one new movie release at random. Find the probability that it is

   a. European
   b. From the United States
   c. German or French
   d. German, given that it is European

   Source: ShowBIZ Data: www.showbizdata.com.

16. **Factory Output** A manufacturing company has three factories: X, Y, and Z. The daily output of each is shown here.

Product	Factory X	Factory Y	Factory Z
TVs	18	32	15
Stereos	6	20	13

   If one item is selected at random, find these probabilities.

   a. It was manufactured at factory X or is a stereo.
   b. It was manufactured at factory Y or factory Z.
   c. It is a TV or was manufactured at factory Z.

17. **Vaccine Effectiveness** A vaccine has a 90% probability of being effective in preventing a certain disease. The probability of getting the disease if a person is not vaccinated is 50%. In a certain geographic region, 25% of the people get vaccinated. If a person is selected at random, find the probability that he or she will contract the disease.

18. **Television Models** A manufacturer makes three models of a television set, Models A, B, and C. A store sells 40% of Model A sets, 40% of Model B sets, and 20% of Model C sets. Of Model A sets, 3% have stereo sound; of Model B sets, 7% have stereo sound; and of Model C sets, 9% have stereo sound. If a set is sold at random, find the probability that it has stereo sound.

19. **Car Purchase** The probability that Sue will live on campus and buy a new car is 0.37. If the probability that she will live on campus is 0.73, find the probability that she will buy a new car, given that she lives on campus.

20. **Applying Shipping Labels** Four unmarked packages lost their shipping labels, and you must reapply them. What is the probability that you will apply the labels and get

   a. All four of them correct?
   b. Exactly three correct?
   c. At least two correct?
   d. At most one correct?

21. **Health Club Membership** Of the members of the Blue River Health Club, 43% have a lifetime membership and exercise regularly (three or more times a week). If 75% of the club members exercise regularly, find the probability that a randomly selected member is a life member, given that he or she exercises regularly.

22. **Bad Weather** The probability that it snows and the bus arrives late is 0.023. José hears the weather forecast, and there is a 40% chance of snow tomorrow. Find the probability that the bus will be late, given that it snows.

23. **Education Level and Smoking** At a large factory, the employees were surveyed and classified according to their level of education and whether they smoked. The data are shown in the table.

Smoking habit	Educational level		
	Not high school graduate	High school graduate	College/ university graduate
Smoke	6	14	19
Do not smoke	18	7	25

   If an employee is selected at random, find these probabilities.

   a. The employee smokes, given that he or she graduated from college or university.
   b. Given that the employee did not graduate from high school, he or she is a smoker.

24. **Bike Helmet Usage** A survey found that 77% of bike riders sometimes ride without a helmet. If 4 bike riders are randomly selected, find the probability that at least one of the riders does not wear a helmet all the time.

   Source: USA TODAY.

25. **Meteor Strikes** Canada's territory contains approximately 2 million lakes covering about 7.6% of the Canadian landmass. Of the next 5 meteor strikes hitting Canada, find the probability that

   a. None strike a lake.
   b. At most, one strikes a lake.
   c. At least three do not strike a lake.

   Source: Canada Info Link: www.canadainfolink.ca

26. **Asthma Sufferers** Health Canada reports that an estimated 2.7 million or 8.2% of Canadians suffer from asthma, a chronic lung disease. If 5 Canadians are randomly selected, find the probability that at least one has asthma.

   Source: Health Canada.

27. Licence Plates Most Canadian provincial automobile licence plates contain 6 digits—3 letters followed by 3 numbers. How many different licence plates can be made if repetitions are allowed? If repetitions are not allowed? If repetitions are allowed in the letters but not the digits?

28. Types of Copy Paper White copy paper is offered in 5 different strengths and 11 different degrees of brightness, recycled or not, and acid-free or not. How many different types of paper are available for order?

29. Baseball Players How many ways can 3 outfielders and 4 infielders be chosen from 5 outfielders and 7 infielders?

30. Selection of Board Members In a board of directors composed of 8 people, how many ways can one chief executive officer, one director, and one treasurer be selected?

31. Student Electives How many ways can a student select 2 electives from a possible choice of 10 electives?

32. Government Committee There are 6 Conservative, 5 Liberal, and 4 New Democrat MPs who have volunteered to serve on a House of Commons committee. If the committee must contain 3 Conservatives, 2 Liberals, and 1 New Democrat, how many ways can the committee be selected?

33. Song Selections A promotional MP3 player is available with the capacity to store 100 songs that can be reordered at the push of a button. How many different arrangements of these songs are possible? (*Note*: Factorials get very big, very fast! How large a factorial will your calculator calculate?)

34. Employee Benefit Plans A new employee has a choice of 5 health care plans, 3 retirement plans, and 2 different expense accounts. If a person selects one of each option, how many different options does he or she have?

35. Course Enrollment There are 12 students who wish to enroll in a particular course. There are only 4 seats left in the classroom. How many different ways can 4 students be selected to attend the class?

36. Candy Selection A candy store allows customers to select 3 different types of candies to be packaged and mailed. If there are 13 varieties available, how many possible selections can be made?

37. Book Selection If a student can select 5 novels from a reading list of 20 for a course in literature, how many different possible ways can this selection be done?

38. Course Selection If a student can select one of 3 language courses, one of 5 mathematics courses, and one of 4 history courses, how many different schedules can be made?

39. Licence Plates New Ontario licence plates are being issued in the form of ABCD-123—4 letters followed by 3 digits. How many such licence plates are possible? If the plates are issued at random, what is the probability of the issuing of licence plate LUCK-777?

40. Leisure Activities A newspaper advertises 5 different movies, 3 plays, and 2 baseball games for the weekend. If a couple selects 3 activities, find the probability that they attend 2 plays and 1 movie.

41. Territorial Selection Several territories and colonies today are still under the jurisdiction of another country. France holds the most, with 16 territories; the United Kingdom has 15; the United States has 14; and several other countries have territories as well. Choose 3 territories at random from those held by France, the United Kingdom, and the United States. What is the probability that all 3 belong to the same country?

Source: Infoplease: www.infoplease.com.

42. Yahtzee Yahtzee is a game played with 5 dice. Players attempt to score points by rolling various combinations. When all 5 dice show the same number, it is called a *Yahtzee* and scores 50 points for the first one and 100 points for each subsequent Yahtzee in the same game. Find the probability that a person throws

a. A Yahtzee on the very first roll
b. Two Yahtzees on two successive turns

43. Personnel Classification For a survey, a subject can be classified as follows:

Gender: male or female

Marital status: single, married, widowed, divorced

Occupation: administration, faculty, staff

Draw a tree diagram for the different ways a person can be classified.

Statistics Today

Would You Bet Your Life?–Revisited

In his book *Probabilities in Everyday Life,* John D. McGervey states that the chance of being killed on any given commercial airline flight is almost 1 in 1 million and that the chance of being killed during a transcontinental auto trip is about 1 in 8000. The corresponding probabilities are $1/1{,}000{,}000 = 0.000001$ as compared to $1/8000 = 0.000125$. Since the second number is 125 times greater than the first number, you have a much higher risk driving than flying across Canada.

Chapter Quiz »

Determine whether each statement is true or false. If the statement is false, explain why.

1. Subjective probability has little use in the real world.

2. Classical probability uses a frequency distribution to compute probabilities.

3. In classical probability, all outcomes in the sample space are equally likely.

4. When two events are not mutually exclusive,
   $P(A \text{ or } B) = P(A) + P(B)$.

5. If two events are dependent, they must have the same probability of occurring.

6. An event and its complement can occur at the same time.

7. The arrangement ABC is the same as BAC for combinations.

8. When objects are arranged in a specific order, the arrangement is called a *combination*.

Select the best answer.

9. The probability that an event happens is 0.42. What is the probability that the event won't happen?

   a. -0.42 c. 0
   b. 0.58   d. 1

10. When a meteorologist says that there is a 30% chance of showers, what type of probability is the person using?

    a. Classical
    b. Empirical
    c. Relative
    d. Subjective

11. The sample space for tossing 3 coins consists of how many outcomes?

    a. 2   c. 6
    b. 4   d. 8

12. The complement of guessing 5 correct answers on a 5-question true/false exam is

    a. Guessing 5 incorrect answers
    b. Guessing at least 1 incorrect answer
    c. Guessing at least 1 correct answer
    d. Guessing no incorrect answers

13. When two dice are rolled, the sample space consists of how many events?

    a. 6   c. 36
    b. 12   d. 54

14. What is $_nP_0$?

    a. 0
    b. 1
    c. n
    d. It cannot be determined.

15. What is the number of permutations of 6 different objects taken all together?

    a. 0   c. 36
    b. 1   d. 720

16. What is 0!?

    a. 0   c. Undefined
    b. 1   d. 10

17. What is $_nC_n$?

    a. 0   c. n
    b. 1   d. It cannot be determined.

Complete the following statements with the best answer.

18. The set of all possible outcomes of a probability experiment is called the _____.

19. The probability of an event can be any number between and including _____ and _____.

20. If an event cannot occur, its probability is _____.

21. The sum of the probabilities of the events in the sample space is _____.

22. When two events cannot occur at the same time, they are said to be _____.

23. **Card Selection** When a card is drawn, find the probability of getting

    a. A jack
    b. A 4
    c. A card less than 6 (an ace is considered above 6)

24. **Card Selection** When a card is drawn from a deck, find the probability of getting

    a. A diamond
    b. A 5 or a heart
    c. A 5 and a heart
    d. A king
    e. A red card

25. **Sweater Selection** At a men's clothing store, 12 men purchased blue golf sweaters, 8 purchased green sweaters, 4 purchased grey sweaters, and 7 bought black sweaters. If a customer is selected at random, find the probability that he purchased

    a. A blue sweater
    b. A green or grey sweater
    c. A green or black or blue sweater
    d. A sweater that was not black

26. **Rolling Dice** When 2 dice are rolled, find the probability of getting

    a. A sum of 6 or 7
    b. A sum greater than 8
    c. A sum less than 3 or greater than 8
    d. A sum that is divisible by 3
    e. A sum of 16
    f. A sum less than 11

27. **Appliance Ownership** The probability that a person owns a microwave oven is 0.75, that a person owns a CD player is 0.25, and that a person owns both a microwave and a CD player is 0.16. Find the probability that a person owns either a microwave or a CD player, but not both.

28. **Starting Salaries** Of the physics graduates of a university, 30% received a starting salary of $30,000 or more. If 5 of the graduates are selected at random, find the probability that all had a starting salary of $30,000 or more.

29. **Card Selection** Five cards are drawn from an ordinary deck *without* replacement. Find the probability of getting

    a. All red cards
    b. All diamonds
    c. All aces

30. **Scholarship Probability** The probability that Samantha will be accepted by the college or university of her choice and obtain a scholarship is 0.35. If the probability that she is accepted by the college or university is 0.65, find the probability that she will obtain a scholarship given that she is accepted by the college or university.

31. **New-Car Warranty** The probability that a customer will buy a car and an extended warranty is 0.16. If the probability that a customer will purchase a car is 0.30, find the probability that the customer will also purchase the extended warranty.

32. **Bowling and Club Membership** Of the members of the Spring Lake Bowling Lanes, 57% have a lifetime membership and bowl regularly (three or more times a week). If 70% of the club members bowl regularly, find the probability that a randomly selected member is a lifetime member, given that he or she bowls regularly.

33. **Work and Weather** The probability that Mike has to work overtime and it rains is 0.028. Mike hears the weather forecast, and there is a 50% chance of rain. Find the probability that he will have to work overtime, given that it rains.

34. **Education Level and Sports** At a large factory, the employees were surveyed and classified according to their level of education and whether they attend a sports event at least once a month. The data are shown in the table.

| | Educational level | | |
	High school graduate	Two-year college degree	Four-year college degree
Sports event			
Attend	16	20	24
Do not attend	12	19	25

If an employee is selected at random, find the probability that

a. The employee attends sports events regularly, given that he or she graduated from college (2- or 4-year degree)

b. Given that the employee is a high school graduate, he or she does not attend sports events regularly

35. **Heart Attacks** In a certain high-risk group, the chances of a person having suffered a heart attack are 55%. If 6 people are chosen, find the probability that at least 1 will have had a heart attack.

36. **Rolling a Die** A single die is rolled 4 times. Find the probability of getting at least one 5.

37. **Eye Colour** If 85% of all people have brown eyes and 6 people are selected at random, find the probability that at least 1 of them has brown eyes.

38. **Singer Selection** How many ways can 5 sopranos and 4 altos be selected from 7 sopranos and 9 altos?

39. **Speaker Seating** How many different ways can 8 speakers be seated on a stage?

40. **Soda Machine Service** A soda machine servicer must restock and collect money from 15 machines, each one at a different location. How many ways can she select 4 machines to service in 1 day?

41. **ID Cards** One company's ID cards consist of 5 letters followed by 2 digits. How many cards can be made if repetitions are allowed? If repetitions are not allowed?

42. **Letter Arrangement** How many different arrangements of the letters in the word *number* can be made?

43. **Physics Test** A physics test consists of 25 true/false questions. How many different possible answer keys can be made?

44. **Cellular Telephones** How many different ways can 5 cellphones be selected from 8 cellphones?

45. **Food Selection** On a lunch counter, there are 3 oranges, 5 apples, and 2 bananas. If 3 pieces of fruit are selected, find the probability that 1 orange, 1 apple, and 1 banana are selected.

46. **Cruise Ship Activities** A cruise director schedules 4 different movies, 2 bridge games, and 3 tennis games for a 2-day period. If a couple selects 3 activities, find the probability that they attend 2 movies and 1 tennis game.

47. **Committee Selection** At a sorority meeting, there are 6 third-year students, 4 second-year students, and 2 first-year students. If a committee of 3 is to be formed, find the probability that 1 of each will be selected.

48. **Banquet Meal Choices** For a banquet, a committee can select beef, pork, chicken, or veal; baked potatoes or mashed potatoes; and peas or green beans for a vegetable. Draw a tree diagram for all possible choices of a meat, a potato, and a vegetable.

Critical Thinking Challenges »

1. **Con Man Game** Consider this problem: A con man has 3 coins. One coin has been specially made and has a head on each side. A second coin has been specially made, and on each side it has a tail. Finally, a third coin has a head and a tail on it. All coins are of the same denomination. The con man places the 3 coins in his pocket, selects one, and shows you one side. It is heads. He is willing to bet you even money that it is the two-headed coin. His reasoning is that it can't be the two-tailed coin since a head is showing; therefore, there is a 50–50 chance of it being the two-headed coin. Would you take the bet?

2. **de Méré Dice Game** Chevalier de Méré won money when he bet unsuspecting patrons that in 4 rolls of 1 die, he could get at least one 6, but he lost money when he bet that in 24 rolls of 2 dice, he could get at least a double 6. Using the probability rules, find the probability of each event and explain why he won the majority of the time on the first game but lost the majority of the time when playing the second game. (*Hint:* Find the probabilities of losing each game and subtract from 1.)

3. **Classical Birthday Problem** How many people do you think need to be in a room so that 2 people will have the same birthday (month and day)? You might think it is 366. This would, of course, guarantee it (excluding leap year), but how many people would need to be in a room so that there would be a 90% probability that 2 people would be born on the same day? What about a 50% probability?

   Actually, the number is much smaller than you may think. For example, if you have 50 people in a room, the probability that 2 people will have the same birthday is 97%. If you have 23 people in a room, there is a 50% probability that 2 people were born on the same day!

   The problem can be solved by using the probability rules. It must be assumed that all birthdays are equally likely, but this assumption will have little effect on the answers. The way to find the answer is by using the complementary event rule as P (2 people having the same birthday) $= 1 - P$ (all have different birthdays).

For example, suppose there were 3 people in the room. The probability that each had a different birthday would be

$$\frac{365}{365} \cdot \frac{364}{365} \cdot \frac{363}{365} = \frac{{}_{365}P_3}{365^3} = 0.992$$

Hence, the probability that at least 2 of the 3 people will have the same birthday will be

$$1 - 0.992 = 0.008$$

Hence, for k people, the formula is

$$P(\text{at least 2 people have the same birthday})$$

$$= 1 - \frac{{}_{365}P_k}{365^k}$$

Using your calculator, complete the table and verify that for at least a 50% chance of 2 people having the same birthday, 23 or more people will be needed.

Number of people	Probability that at least 2 have the same birthday
1	0.000
2	0.003
5	0.027
10	
15	
20	
21	
22	
23	

4. **Contracting Diseases** We know that if the probability of an event happening is 100%, then the event is a certainty. Can it be concluded that if there is a 50% chance of contracting a communicable disease through contact with an infected person, there would be a 100% chance of contracting the disease if 2 contacts were made with the infected person? Explain your answer.

Data Projects »

1. **Business and Finance** Select a pizza restaurant and a sandwich shop. For the pizza restaurant, look at the menu to determine how many sizes, crust types, and toppings are available. How many different pizza types are possible? For the sandwich shop, determine how many breads, meats, veggies, cheeses, sauces, and condiments are available. How many different sandwich choices are possible?

2. **Sports and Leisure** When poker games are shown on television, there are often percentages displayed that

show how likely it is that a certain hand will win. Investigate how these percentages are determined. Show an example with two competing hands in a Texas Hold 'em game. Include the percentages that each hand will win after the deal, the flop, the turn, and the river.

3. **Technology** A music player or music organization program can keep track of how many different artists are in a library. First note how many different artists are in your music library. Then find the probability that if 25 songs are selected at random, none will have the same artist.

4. **Health and Wellness** Assume that the gender distribution of babies is such that one-half of the time females are born and one-half of the time males are born. In a family of 3 children, what is the probability that all are girls? In a family of 4? Is it unusual that in a family with 4 children, all would be girls? In a family of 5?

5. **Politics and Economics** Consider the Senate of Canada. For the most recent parliamentary session, find out about the composition of any three of the Senate's standing or special committees. How many

different committees of senators are possible, knowing the party composition of the Senate and the number of committee members from each party for each committee?

6. **Your Class** Research the famous Monty Hall probability problem. Conduct a simulation of the Monty Hall problem online using a simulation program or in class using live "contestants." After 50 simulations compare your results to those stated in the research you did. Did your simulation support the conclusions?

Answers to Applying the Concepts »

Section 4–1 Tossing a Coin

1. The sample space is the listing of all possible outcomes of the coin toss.

2. The possible outcomes are heads or tails.

3. Classical probability says that a fair coin has a 50–50 chance of coming up heads or tails.

4. The law of large numbers says that as you increase the number of trials, the overall results will approach the theoretical probability. However, since the coin has no "memory," it still has a 50–50 chance of coming up heads or tails on the next toss. Knowing what has already happened should not change your opinion on what will happen on the next toss.

5. The empirical approach to probability is based on running an experiment and looking at the results. You cannot do that at this time.

6. Subjective probabilities could be used if you believe the coin is biased.

7. Answers will vary; however, they should address that a fair coin has a 50–50 chance of coming up heads or tails on the next flip.

Section 4–2 Which Pain Reliever Is Best?

1. There were $192 + 186 + 188 = 566$ subjects in the study.

2. The study lasted for 12 weeks.

3. The variables are the type of pain reliever and the side effects.

4. Both variables are qualitative and nominal.

5. The numbers in the table are exact figures.

6. The probability that a randomly selected person was receiving a placebo is $192/566 = 0.3392$ (about 34%).

7. The probability that a randomly selected person was receiving a placebo or drug A is $(192 + 186)/566 = 378/566 = 0.6678$ (about 67%). These are mutually exclusive events. The complement is that a randomly selected person was receiving drug B.

8. The probability that a randomly selected person was receiving a placebo or experienced a neurological headache is $(192 + 55 + 72)/566 = 319/566 = 0.5636$ (about 56%).

9. The probability that a randomly selected person was not receiving a placebo or experienced a sinus headache is $(186 + 188)/566 + 11/566 = 385/566 = 0.6802$ (about 68%).

Section 4–3 Guilty or Innocent?

1. The probability of another couple with the same characteristics being in that area is $\frac{1}{12} \cdot \frac{1}{10} \cdot \frac{1}{4} \cdot \frac{1}{11} \cdot \frac{1}{3} \cdot \frac{1}{13} \cdot \frac{1}{100} = \frac{1}{20,592,000}$, assuming the characteristics are independent of one another.

2. You would use the multiplication rule, since we are looking for the probability of multiple events happening together.

3. We do not know if the characteristics are dependent or independent, but we assumed independence for the calculation in question 1.

4. The probabilities would change if there was dependence among two or more events.

5. Answers will vary. One possible answer is that probabilities can be used to explain how unlikely it is to have a set of events occur at the same time (in this case, how unlikely it is to have another couple with the same characteristics in that area).

6. Answers will vary. One possible answer is that if the only eyewitness was the woman who was mugged and the probabilities are accurate, it seems very unlikely that a couple matching these characteristics would be in that area at that time. This might cause you to convict the couple.

7. Answers will vary. One possible answer is that our probabilities are theoretical and serve a purpose when appropriate, but that court cases are based on much more than impersonal chance.

8. Answers will vary. One possible answer is that juries decide whether or not to convict a defendant if they find evidence "beyond a reasonable doubt" that the person is guilty. In

probability terms, this means that if the defendant was actually innocent, then the chance of seeing the events that occurred are so unlikely as to have occurred by chance. Therefore, the jury concludes that the defendant is guilty.

Section 4–4 Garage Door Openers

1. Four on/off switches lead to 16 different settings.

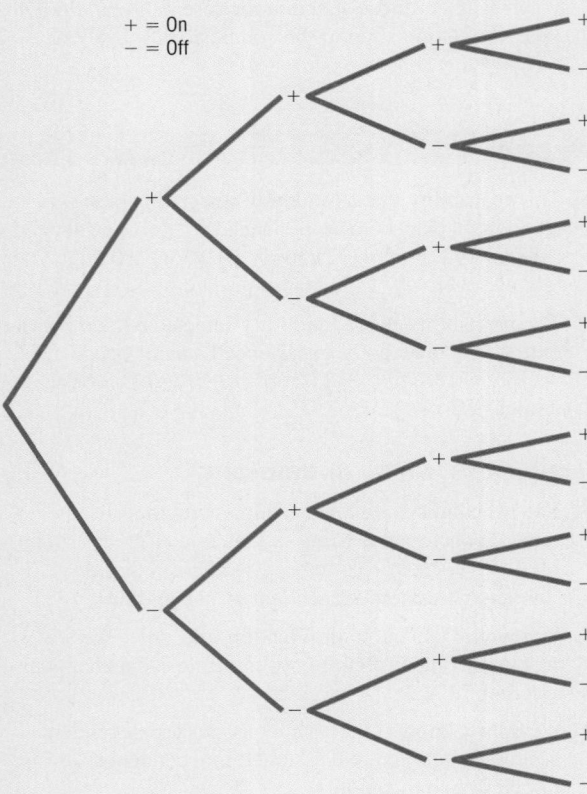

$+ =$ On
$- =$ Off

2. With 5 on/off switches, there are $2^5 = 32$ different settings. With 6 on/off switches, there are $2^6 = 64$ different settings. In general, if there are k on/off switches, there are 2^k different settings.

3. With 8 consecutive on/off switches, there are $2^8 = 256$ different settings.

4. It is less likely for someone to be able to open your garage door if you have 8 on/off settings (probability about 0.4%) than if you have 4 on/off switches (probability about 6.0%). Having 8 on/off switches in the opener seems pretty safe.

5. Each key blank could be made into $5^5 = 3{,}125$ possible keys.

6. If there were 420,000 Dodge Caravans sold in Canada, then any one key could start about $420{,}000/3{,}125 = 134.4$, or about 134, different Caravans.

7. Answers will vary.

Section 4–5 Counting Rules and Probability

1. There are five different events: each multiple-choice question is an event.

2. These events are independent.

3. If you guess on 1 question, the probability of getting it correct is 0.20. Thus, if you guess on all 5 questions, the probability of getting all of them correct is $(0.20)^5 = 0.00032$.

4. The probability that a person would guess answer A for a question is 0.20, so the probability that a person would guess answer A for each question is $(0.20)^5 = 0.00032$.

5. There are five different events: each matching question is an event.

6. These are dependent events.

7. The probability of getting them all correct if you are guessing is $\frac{1}{5} \cdot \frac{1}{4} \cdot \frac{1}{3} \cdot \frac{1}{2} \cdot \frac{1}{1} = \frac{1}{120} = 0.0083$.

8. The difference between the two problems is that we are sampling without replacement in the second problem, so the denominator changes in the event probabilities.

Chapter 5

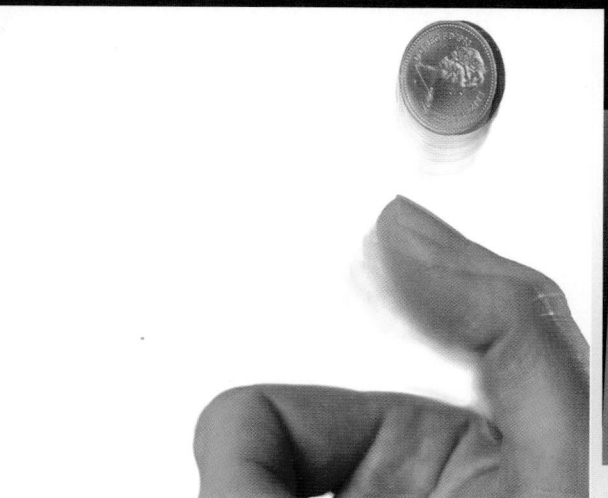

Discrete Probability Distributions

Objectives >

After completing this chapter, you should be able to

LO1 Construct a probability distribution for a random variable.

LO2 Find the mean, variance, standard deviation, and expected value for a discrete random variable.

LO3 Calculate exact probabilities for a binomial experiment and determine the mean, standard deviation, and variance for the variable of a binomial distribution.

LO4 Find probabilities for outcomes of variables, using the Poisson, hypergeometric, and multinomial distributions.

Outline >

Statistics Today

Is Pooling Worthwhile?

Blood samples are used to screen people for certain diseases. When the disease is rare, health-care workers sometimes combine or pool the blood samples of a group of individuals into one batch and then test it. If the test result of the batch is negative, no further testing is needed since none of the individuals in the group has the disease. However, if the test result of the batch is positive, each individual in the group must be tested.

Consider this hypothetical example: Suppose the probability of a person having the disease is 0.05, and a pooled sample of 15 individuals is tested. What is the probability that no further testing will be needed for the individuals in the sample? The answer to this question can be found by using what is called the

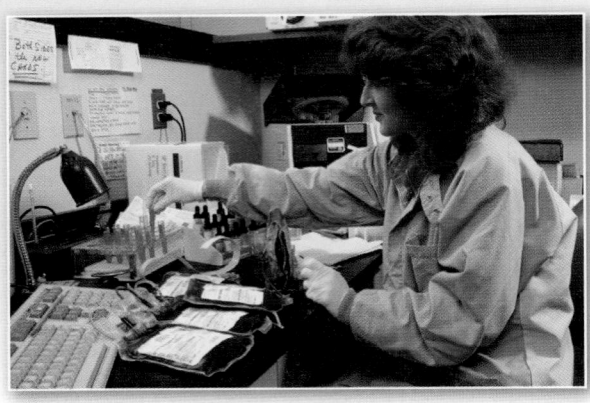

binomial distribution. See Statistics Today—Revisited, page 247, near the end of the chapter.

This chapter explains probability distributions in general and a specific, often-used distribution called the *binomial distribution.* The Poisson, hypergeometric, and multinomial distributions are also explained.

Introduction >

Many decisions in business, insurance, and other real-life situations are made by assigning probabilities to all possible outcomes pertaining to the situation and then evaluating the results. For example, a saleswoman can compute the probability that she will make 0, 1, 2, or 3 or more sales in a single day. An insurance company might be able to assign probabilities to the number of vehicles a family owns. A self-employed speaker might be able to compute the probabilities for giving 0, 1, 2, 3, or 4 or more speeches each week. Once these probabilities are assigned, statistics such as the mean, variance, and standard deviation can be computed for these events. With these statistics, various decisions can be made. The saleswoman will be able to compute the average number of sales she makes per week, and if she is working on commission, she will be able to approximate her weekly income over a period of time, say, monthly. The public speaker will be able to plan ahead and approximate his average income and expenses. The insurance company can use its information to design special computer forms and programs to accommodate its customers' future needs.

This chapter explains the concepts and applications of what is called a *probability distribution.* In addition, special probability distributions, such as the *binomial, multinomial, Poisson,* and *hypergeometric* distributions, are explained.

5–1	Probability Distributions >

Construct a probability distribution for a random variable.

Before probability distribution is defined formally, the definition of a variable is reviewed. In Chapter 1, a *variable* was defined as a characteristic or attribute that can assume different values. Various letters of the alphabet, such as *X*, *Y*, or *Z*, are used to represent variables. Since the variables in this chapter form a probability distribution, they are called *random variables.*

For example, if a die is rolled, a letter such as *X* can be used to represent the outcomes. Then the value that *X* can assume is 1, 2, 3, 4, 5, or 6, corresponding to the outcomes of rolling a single die. If two coins are tossed, a letter, say Y, can be used to represent the number of heads, in this case 0, 1, or 2. As another example, if the temperature at 8:00 A.M. is 6°C and at noon it is 12°C, then the values T that the temperature assumes are said to be random, since they are due to varying atmospheric conditions at the time the temperature was taken.

> A **random variable** is a function that assigns a unique numerical value, determined by chance, to each outcome of an experiment.

Also recall from Chapter 1 that one can classify variables as discrete or continuous by observing the values the variable can assume. If a variable can assume only a specific number of values, such as the outcomes for the roll of a die or the outcomes for the toss of a coin, then the variable is called a *discrete variable*.

Discrete variables have a finite number of possible values or an infinite number of values that can be counted. The word *counted* means that they can be enumerated using the numbers 1, 2, 3, etc. For example, the number of joggers in Riverview Park each day and the number of phone calls received after a TV commercial airs are examples of discrete variables, since they can be counted.

Variables that can assume all values in the interval between any two given values are called *continuous variables*. For example, if the temperature goes from 17°C to 26°C in a 24-hour period, it has passed through every possible number from 17°C to 26°C. *Continuous random variables are obtained from data that can be measured rather than counted.* Continuous random variables can assume an infinite number of values and can be decimal and fractional values. On a continuous scale, a person's weight might be exactly 83.201 kilograms if a scale could measure weight to the thousandth place; however, on a digital scale that measures only to tenths of kilograms, the weight would be 83.2 kilograms. Examples of continuous variables are heights, weights, temperatures, and time. In this chapter only discrete random variables are used; Chapter 6 explains continuous random variables.

The procedure shown here for constructing a probability distribution for a discrete random variable uses the probability experiment of tossing three coins. Recall that when three coins are tossed, the sample space is represented as TTT, TTH, THT, HTT, HHT, HTH, THH, HHH; and if X is the random variable for the number of heads, then X assumes the value 0, 1, 2, or 3.

Probabilities for the values of X can be determined as follows:

No heads	One head			Two heads			Three heads
TTT	TTH	THT	HTT	HHT	HTH	THH	HHH
$\frac{1}{8}$	$\frac{1}{8}$	$\frac{1}{8}$	$\frac{1}{8}$	$\frac{1}{8}$	$\frac{1}{8}$	$\frac{1}{8}$	$\frac{1}{8}$
$\frac{1}{8}$	$\frac{3}{8}$			$\frac{3}{8}$			$\frac{1}{8}$

Hence, the probability of getting no heads is $\frac{1}{8}$, one head is $\frac{3}{8}$, two heads is $\frac{3}{8}$, and three heads is $\frac{1}{8}$. From these values, a probability distribution can be constructed by listing the outcomes and assigning the probability of each outcome, as shown here.

Number of heads X	0	1	2	3
Probability $P(X)$	$\frac{1}{8}$	$\frac{3}{8}$	$\frac{3}{8}$	$\frac{1}{8}$

> A **discrete probability distribution** consists of the values a discrete random variable can assume and the corresponding probabilities of the values. The probabilities are determined theoretically or by observation.

Discrete probability distributions can be shown by using a graph or a table. Probability distributions can also be represented by a formula. See Exercises 31–36 at the end of this section for examples.

Probability examples in this section utilize discrete data procedures whereas Chapter 6 makes use of methods for solving problems relating to continuous data.

Example 5–1

Rolling a Die

Construct a probability distribution for rolling a single die.

Solution

Since the sample space is 1, 2, 3, 4, 5, 6 and each outcome has a probability of $\frac{1}{6}$, the distribution is as shown.

Outcome X	1	2	3	4	5	6
Probability $P(X)$	$\frac{1}{6}$	$\frac{1}{6}$	$\frac{1}{6}$	$\frac{1}{6}$	$\frac{1}{6}$	$\frac{1}{6}$

Probability distributions can be shown graphically by representing the values of X on the x axis and the probabilities $P(X)$ on the y axis.

Example 5–2

Tossing a Coin

Represent graphically the probability distribution for the sample space for tossing three coins.

Number of heads X	0	1	2	3
Probability $P(X)$	$\frac{1}{8}$	$\frac{3}{8}$	$\frac{3}{8}$	$\frac{1}{8}$

Solution

The values that X assumes are located on the x axis, and the values for $P(X)$ are located on the y axis. The graph in Figure 5–1 illustrates a single point column chart of the $P(X)$, using a vertical line for each X value.

Figure 5–1

Probability Distribution for Example 5–2

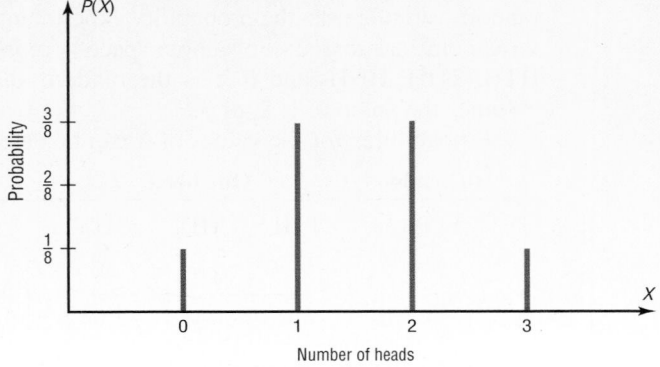

Note that for visual appearances, it is not necessary to start with 0 at the origin.

Examples 5–1 and 5–2 are illustrations of *theoretical* probability distributions. One did not need to actually perform the experiments to compute the probabilities. In contrast, to construct actual probability distributions, one must observe the variable over a period of time. They are empirical, as shown in Example 5–3.

Example 5–3

Hockey Final Series

The National Hockey League (NHL) championship final involves two teams vying for the coveted Stanley Cup trophy, the oldest professional sports trophy in North America. The final two remaining teams play a "best of seven" series, with the first team to win four games crowned the champion. The final series could be won in 4, 5, 6, or 7 games. The data shown consist of the number of games played in the

Stanley Cup finals from 1959 through 2009, with the exception of the 2005 NHL lockout. The number of games played is represented by the variable X. Find the probability $P(X)$ for each X value, construct a probability distribution, and draw graphs for the data using a single point column chart and histogram chart for $P(X)$.

X	Frequency
4	14
5	11
6	15
7	10
	50

Source: TSN.ca: *NHL*, "Stanley Cup Playoffs."

Solution

The probability $P(X)$ can be computed for each X by calculating the relative frequency for each occurrence of the random variable X; that is, dividing the frequency by the total.

For 4 games, $\frac{14}{50} = 0.28$ For 5 games, $\frac{11}{50} = 0.22$

For 6 games, $\frac{15}{50} = 0.30$ For 7 games, $\frac{10}{50} = 0.20$

The probability distribution is

Number of games X	4	5	6	7
Probability $P(X)$	0.28	0.22	0.3	0.2

The graph is shown in Figure 5–2.

Figure 5–2

Probability Distributions for Example 5–3

(a) Point Column Chart of $P(X)$

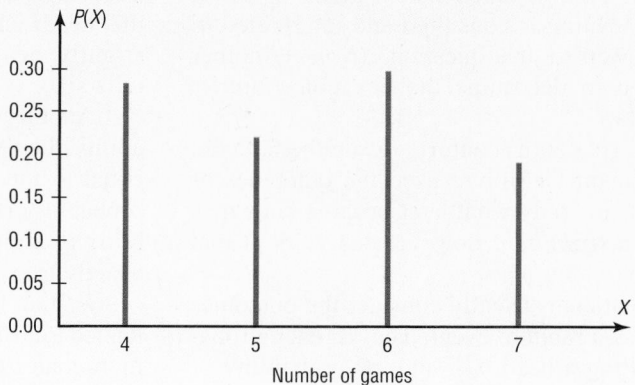

(b) Histogram Chart of $P(X)$

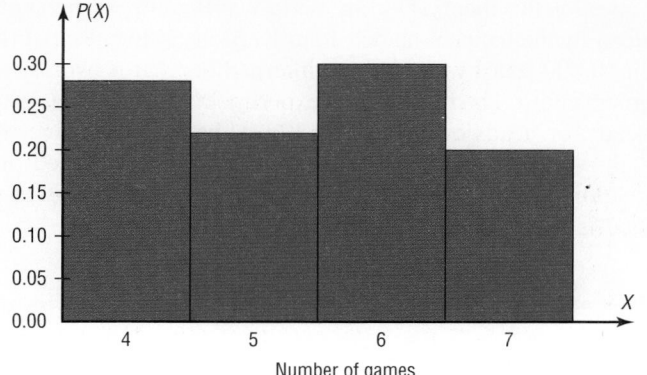

Speaking of Statistics

Coins, Births, and Other Random (?) Events

Examples of random events such as tossing coins are used in almost all books on probability. But is flipping a coin really a random event?

Tossing coins dates back to ancient Roman times when the coins usually consisted of the emperor's head on one side (i.e., heads) and another icon such as a ship on the other side. Tossing coins was used in both fortune telling and ancient Roman games.

A Chinese form of divination called the *I-Ching* (pronounced E-Ching) is thought to be at least 4000 years old. It consists of 64 hexagrams made up of six horizontal lines. Each line is either broken or unbroken, representing the yin and the yang. These 64 hexagrams are supposed to represent all possible situations in life. To consult the I-Ching, a question is asked and then three coins are tossed six times. The way the coins fall, either heads up or heads down, determines whether the line is broken (yin) or unbroken (yang). Once the hexagon is determined, its meaning is consulted and interpreted to get the answer to the question. (*Note:* Another method used to determine the hexagon employs yarrow sticks.)

In the sixteenth century, a mathematician named Abraham DeMoivre used the outcomes of tossing coins to study what later became known as the *normal distribution;* however, his work at that time was not widely known.

Mathematicians usually consider the outcomes of a coin toss a random event. That is, each probability of getting a head is $\frac{1}{2}$, and the probability of getting a tail is $\frac{1}{2}$. Also, it is not possible to predict with 100% certainty which outcome will occur. But new studies question this theory. During World War II a South African mathematician named John Kerrich tossed a coin 10,000 times while he was interned in a German prison camp. The result of his experiment was 5067 heads, or heads occurred 50.67% of the time.*

Several studies have shown that when a coin-tossing device is used, the probability that a coin

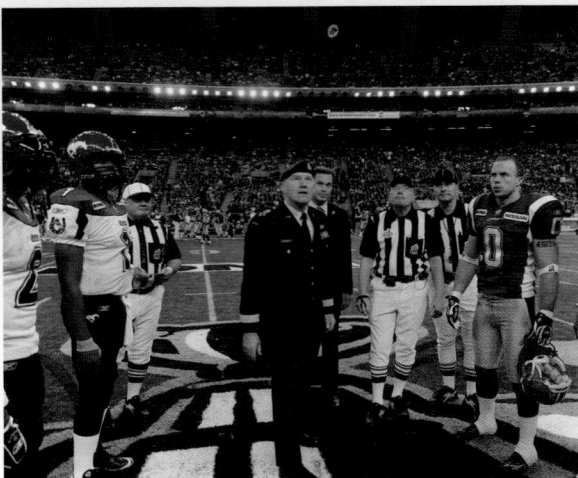

will land on the same side on which it is placed on the coin-tossing device is about 51%. It would take about 10,000 tosses to become aware of this bias. Furthermore, researchers showed that when a coin is spun on its edge, the coin would fall tails up about 80% of the time since there is more metal on the heads side of a coin. This makes the coin slightly heavier on the heads side than on the tails side.

Another assumption commonly made in probability theory is that the number of male births is equal to the number of female births and that the probability of a boy being born is $\frac{1}{2}$ and the probability of a girl being born is $\frac{1}{2}$. We know this is not exactly true.

In the later 1700s, a French mathematician named Pierre Simon Laplace attempted to prove that more males than females are born. He used records from 1745 to 1770 in Paris and showed that the percentage of females born was about 49%. Although these percentages vary somewhat from location to location, further surveys show they are generally true worldwide. Even though there are discrepancies, we generally consider the outcomes to be 50–50 since these discrepancies are relatively small.

Based on this article, would you consider the coin toss at the beginning of a football game to be fair?

*Source: Journal of Statistics Education, "Topics for Discussion from Current Newspapers and Journals," William P. Peterson, Vol. 10, No. 1, 2002.

Two Requirements for a Probability Distribution

1. The sum of the probabilities of all the events in the sample space must equal 1; that is, $\Sigma P(X) = 1$.
2. The probability of each event in the sample space must be between or equal to 0 and 1. That is, $0 \leq P(X) \leq 1$.

The first requirement states that the sum of the probabilities of all the events must be equal to 1. This sum cannot be less than 1 or greater than 1 since the sample space includes *all* possible outcomes of the probability experiment. The second requirement states that the probability of any individual event must be a value from 0 to 1. The reason (as stated in Chapter 4) is that the range of the probability of any individual value can be 0, 1, or any value between 0 and 1. A probability cannot be a negative number or greater than 1.

Example 5–4

Determine whether each distribution is a probability distribution.

a.

X	0	5	10	15	20
P(X)	$\frac{1}{5}$	$\frac{1}{5}$	$\frac{1}{5}$	$\frac{1}{5}$	$\frac{1}{5}$

c.

X	1	2	3	4
P(X)	$\frac{1}{4}$	$\frac{1}{8}$	$\frac{1}{16}$	$\frac{9}{16}$

b.

X	0	2	4	6
P(X)	-1.0	1.5	0.3	0.2

d.

X	2	3	7
P(X)	0.5	0.3	0.4

Solution

a. Yes, it is a probability distribution.

b. No, it is not a probability distribution, since $P(X)$ cannot be 1.5 or -1.0.

c. Yes, it is a probability distribution.

d. No, it is not, since $\Sigma P(X) = 1.2$.

Many variables in business, education, engineering, and other areas can be analyzed by using probability distributions. Section 5–2 shows methods for finding the mean and standard deviation for a probability distribution.

5–1 Applying the Concepts

Dropping College/University Courses

Use the following table to answer the questions.

Reason for Dropping a College/University Course	Frequency	Percentage
Too difficult	45	
Illness	40	
Change in work schedule	20	
Change of major	14	
Family-related problems	9	
Money	7	
Miscellaneous	6	
No meaningful reason	3	

1. What is the variable under study? Is it a random variable?
2. How many people were in the study?
3. Complete the table.
4. From the information given, what is the probability that a student will drop a class because of illness? Money? Change of major?
5. Would you consider the information in the table to be a probability distribution?
6. Are the categories mutually exclusive?
7. Are the categories independent?
8. Are the categories exhaustive?
9. Are the two requirements for a discrete probability distribution met?

See page 250 for the answers.

Exercises 5–1

1. Define and give three examples of a random variable.
2. Explain the difference between a discrete and a continuous random variable.
3. Give three examples of a discrete random variable.
4. Give three examples of a continuous random variable.
5. What is a probability distribution? Give an example.

For Exercises 6 through 11, determine whether the distribution represents a probability distribution. If it does not, state why.

6.

X	1	6	11	16	21
P(X)	$\frac{1}{7}$	$\frac{1}{7}$	$\frac{3}{7}$	$\frac{2}{7}$	$\frac{1}{7}$

7.

X	3	6	8	12
P(X)	0.3	0.5	0.7	−0.8

8.

X	3	6	8
P(X)	−0.3	0.6	0.7

9.

X	1	2	3	4	5
P(X)	$\frac{3}{10}$	$\frac{1}{10}$	$\frac{1}{10}$	$\frac{2}{10}$	$\frac{3}{10}$

10.

X	20	30	40	50
P(X)	0.05	0.35	0.4	0.2

11.

X	5	10	15
P(X)	1.2	0.3	0.5

For Exercises 12 through 18, state whether the variable is discrete or continuous.

12. The speed of a jet airplane
13. The number of cheeseburgers a fast-food restaurant serves each day
14. The number of people who play the national Lotto 6/49 lottery each day
15. The weight of a Siberian tiger
16. The time it takes to complete a marathon
17. The number of mathematics majors in your school
18. The blood pressures of all patients admitted to a hospital on a specific day

For Exercises 19 through 26, construct a probability distribution for the data and draw a graph for the distribution.

19. **Medical Tests** The probabilities that a patient will have 0, 1, 2, or 3 medical tests performed on entering a hospital are $\frac{6}{15}$, $\frac{5}{15}$, $\frac{3}{15}$, and $\frac{1}{15}$, respectively.

20. **Student Volunteers** The probabilities that a student volunteer will host 1, 2, 3, or 4 prospective first-year students are 0.4, 0.3, 0.2, and 0.1, respectively.

21. **Defective Parts** The probabilities of a machine manufacturing 0, 1, 2, 3, 4, or 5 defective parts in one day are 0.75, 0.17, 0.04, 0.025, 0.01, and 0.005, respectively.

22. **Book Purchase** The probabilities that a customer will purchase 0, 1, 2, or 3 books are 0.45, 0.30, 0.15, and 0.10, respectively.

23. **Loaded Die** A die is loaded in such a way that the probabilities of getting 1, 2, 3, 4, 5, and 6 are $\frac{1}{2}$, $\frac{1}{6}$, $\frac{1}{12}$, $\frac{1}{12}$, $\frac{1}{12}$, and $\frac{1}{12}$, respectively.

24. **Item Selection** The probabilities that a customer selects 1, 2, 3, 4, and 5 items at a convenience store are 0.32, 0.12, 0.23, 0.18, and 0.15, respectively.

25. **Surgeon Operations** The probabilities that a surgeon operates on 3, 4, 5, 6, or 7 patients in any one day are 0.15, 0.20, 0.25, 0.20, and 0.20, respectively.

26. **Headache Relief** Three patients are given a headache relief tablet. The probabilities for 0, 1, 2, or 3 successes are 0.18, 0.52, 0.21, and 0.09, respectively.

27. **Monetary Bill Selection** A box contains two $5 bills, three $10 bills, one $20 bill, and three $50 bills. Construct a probability distribution for the data if X represents the value of a single bill drawn at random and then replaced.

28. **Family with Children** Construct a probability distribution for a family of 3 children. Let X represent the number of boys.

29. **Drawing a Card** Construct a probability distribution for drawing a card from a deck of 40 cards consisting of 10 cards numbered 1, 10 cards numbered 2, 15 cards numbered 3, and 5 cards numbered 4.

30. **Rolling Two Dice** Using the sample space for tossing 2 dice, construct a probability distribution for the sums 2 through 12.

Extending the Concepts »

A probability distribution can be written in formula notation such as $P(X) = 1/X$, where $X = 2, 3, 6$. The distribution is shown as follows:

X	2	3	6
$P(X)$	$\frac{1}{2}$	$\frac{1}{3}$	$\frac{1}{6}$

For Exercises 31 through 36, write the distribution for the formula and determine whether it is a probability distribution.

31. $P(X) = X/6$ for $X = 1, 2, 3$

32. $P(X) = X$ for $X = 0.2, 0.3, 0.5$

33. $P(X) = X/6$ for $X = 3, 4, 7$

34. $P(X) = X + 0.1$ for $X = 0.1, 0.02, 0.04$

35. $P(X) = X/7$ for $X = 1, 2, 4$

36. $P(X) = X/(X + 2)$ for $X = 0, 1, 2$

5–2   Mean, Variance, Standard Deviation, and Expectation ›

Find the mean, variance, standard deviation, and expected value for a discrete random variable.

The mean, variance, and standard deviation for a probability distribution are computed differently from the mean, variance, and standard deviation for samples. This section explains how these measures—as well as a new measure called the *expectation*—are calculated for probability distributions.

Mean

In Chapter 3, the mean for a sample or population was computed by adding the values and dividing by the total number of values, as shown in the formulas

$$\overline{X} = \frac{\Sigma X}{n} \qquad \mu = \frac{\Sigma X}{N}$$

Historical Note

A professor, Augustin Louis Cauchy (1789–1857), wrote a book on probability. While he was teaching at the Military School of Paris, one of his students was Napoleon Bonaparte.

But how would one compute the mean of the number of spots that show on top when a die is rolled? One could try rolling the die, say, 10 times, recording the number of spots, and finding the mean; however, this answer would only approximate the true mean. What about 50 rolls or 100 rolls? Actually, the more times the die is rolled, the better the approximation. One might ask, then, How many times must the die be rolled to get the exact answer? *It must be rolled an infinite number of times.* Since this task is impossible, the previous formulas cannot be used because the denominators would be infinity. Hence, a new method of computing the mean is necessary. This method gives the exact theoretical value of the mean as if it were possible to roll the die an infinite number of times.

Before the formula is stated, an example will be used to explain the concept. Suppose two coins are tossed repeatedly, and the number of heads that occurred is recorded. What will be the mean of the number of heads? The sample space is

HH, HT, TH, TT

and each outcome has a probability of $\frac{1}{4}$. Now, in the long run, one would *expect* two heads (HH) to occur approximately $\frac{1}{4}$ of the time, one head to occur approximately $\frac{1}{2}$ of the time (HT or TH), and no heads (TT) to occur approximately $\frac{1}{4}$ of the time. Hence, on average, one would expect the number of heads to be

$$\tfrac{1}{4} \cdot 2 + \tfrac{1}{2} \cdot 1 + \tfrac{1}{4} \cdot 0 = 1$$

That is, if it were possible to toss the coins many times or an infinite number of times, the *average* of the number of heads would be 1.

Hence, to find the mean for a probability distribution, one must multiply each possible outcome by its corresponding probability and find the sum of the products.

Formula for the Mean of a Probability Distribution

The mean of a random variable with a discrete probability distribution is

$$\mu = X_1 \cdot P(X_1) + X_2 \cdot P(X_2) + X_3 \cdot P(X_3) + \cdots + X_n \cdot P(X_n)$$
$$= \Sigma X \cdot P(X)$$

where $X_1, X_2, X_3, \ldots, X_n$ are the outcomes and $P(X_1), P(X_2), P(X_3), \ldots, P(X_n)$ are the corresponding probabilities.

Note: $\Sigma X \cdot P(X)$ means to sum the products.

Rounding Rule for the Mean, Variance, and Standard Deviation for a Probability Distribution The rounding rule for the mean, variance, and standard deviation for variables of a probability distribution is this: The mean, variance, and standard deviation should be rounded to one more decimal place than the outcome X. When fractions are used, they should be reduced to lowest terms.

Examples 5–5 through 5–8 illustrate the use of the formula.

Example 5–5

Rolling a Die

Find the mean of the number of spots that appear when a die is tossed.

Solution

In the toss of a die, the mean can be computed thus.

Outcome X	1	2	3	4	5	6
Probability $P(X)$	$\frac{1}{6}$	$\frac{1}{6}$	$\frac{1}{6}$	$\frac{1}{6}$	$\frac{1}{6}$	$\frac{1}{6}$

$$\mu = \Sigma X \cdot P(X) = 1 \cdot \tfrac{1}{6} + 2 \cdot \tfrac{1}{6} + 3 \cdot \tfrac{1}{6} + 4 \cdot \tfrac{1}{6} + 5 \cdot \tfrac{1}{6} + 6 \cdot \tfrac{1}{6}$$
$$= \tfrac{21}{6} = 3\tfrac{1}{2} \text{ or } 3.5$$

That is, when a die is tossed many times, the theoretical mean will be 3.5. Note that even though the die cannot show a 3.5, the theoretical average is 3.5.

The reason why this formula gives the theoretical mean is that in the long run, each outcome would occur approximately $\frac{1}{6}$ of the time. Hence, multiplying the outcome by its corresponding probability and finding the sum would yield the theoretical mean. In other words, outcome 1 would occur approximately $\frac{1}{6}$ of the time, outcome 2 would occur approximately $\frac{1}{6}$ of the time, etc.

Example 5–6

Children in a Family

In a family with 2 children, find the mean of the number of children who will be girls.

Solution

The probability distribution is as follows:

Number of girls X	0	1	2
Probability $P(X)$	$\frac{1}{4}$	$\frac{1}{2}$	$\frac{1}{4}$

Hence, the mean is

$$\mu = \Sigma X \cdot P(X) = 0 \cdot \tfrac{1}{4} + 1 \cdot \tfrac{1}{2} + 2 \cdot \tfrac{1}{4} = 1$$

Example 5–7

Tossing Coins

If 3 coins are tossed, find the mean of the number of heads that occur. (See the table preceding Example 5–1.)

Solution

The probability distribution is

Number of heads X	0	1	2	3
Probability $P(X)$	$\frac{1}{8}$	$\frac{3}{8}$	$\frac{3}{8}$	$\frac{1}{8}$

The mean is

$$\mu = \Sigma X \cdot P(X) = 0 \cdot \tfrac{1}{8} + 1 \cdot \tfrac{3}{8} + 2 \cdot \tfrac{3}{8} + 3 \cdot \tfrac{1}{8} = \tfrac{12}{8} = 1\tfrac{1}{2} \text{ or } 1.5$$

The value 1.5 cannot occur as an outcome. Nevertheless, it is the long-run or theoretical average.

Example 5–8

Number of Extended Trips

The probability distribution shown represents the number of extended trips (i.e., trips of five nights or more) that Canadian adults take per year. (That is, 6% do not take any extended trips per year, 70% take one extended trip per year, etc.) Find the mean.

Number of trips X	0	1	2	3	4
Probability $P(X)$	0.06	0.70	0.20	0.03	0.01

Solution

$$\mu = \Sigma X \cdot P(X)$$
$$= (0)(0.06) + (1)(0.70) + (2)(0.20) + (3)(0.03) + (4)(0.01)$$
$$= 0 + 0.70 + 0.40 + 0.09 + 0.04$$
$$= 1.23 \approx 1.2$$

Hence, the mean of the number of extended trips taken by Canadians adults is 1.2.

Historical Note

In 1892, the Canadian Criminal Code declared a complete ban on all gambling activities.

Variance and Standard Deviation

For a probability distribution, the mean of the random variable describes the measure of the so-called long-run or theoretical average, but it does not tell anything about the spread of the distribution. Recall from Chapter 3 that in order to measure this spread or variability, statisticians use the variance and standard deviation. These formulas were used:

$$\sigma^2 = \frac{\Sigma(X - \mu)^2}{N} \qquad \text{or} \qquad \sigma = \sqrt{\frac{\Sigma(X - \mu)^2}{N}}$$

These formulas cannot be used for a random variable of a probability distribution since N is infinite, so the variance and standard deviation must be computed differently.

To find the variance for the random variable of a probability distribution, subtract the theoretical mean of the random variable from each outcome and square the difference. Then multiply each difference by its corresponding probability and add the products. The formula is

$$\sigma^2 = \Sigma[(X - \mu)^2 \cdot P(X)]$$

Finding the variance by using this formula is somewhat tedious. So for simplified computations, a shortcut formula can be used. This formula is algebraically equivalent to the longer one and is used in the examples that follow.

Formula for the Variance of a Probability Distribution

Find the variance of a probability distribution by multiplying the square of each outcome by its corresponding probability, summing those products, and subtracting the square of the mean. The formula for the variance of a probability distribution is

$$\sigma^2 = \Sigma[X^2 \cdot P(X)] - \mu^2$$

The standard deviation of a probability distribution is

$$\sigma = \sqrt{\sigma^2} \qquad \text{or} \qquad \sqrt{\Sigma[X^2 \cdot P(X)] - \mu^2}$$

Remember that the variance and standard deviation cannot be negative.

| Example 5–9 | **Rolling a Die** |

Compute the variance and standard deviation for the probability distribution in Example 5–5.

Solution

Recall that the mean is $\mu = 3.5$, as computed in Example 5–5. Square each outcome and multiply by the corresponding probability, sum those products, and then subtract the square of the mean.

$$\sigma^2 = \left(1^2 \cdot \tfrac{1}{6} + 2^2 \cdot \tfrac{1}{6} + 3^2 \cdot \tfrac{1}{6} + 4^2 \cdot \tfrac{1}{6} + 5^2 \cdot \tfrac{1}{6} + 6^2 \cdot \tfrac{1}{6}\right) - (3.5)^2 \approx 2.9$$

To get the standard deviation, find the square root of the variance.

$$\sigma = \sqrt{2.9} \approx 1.7$$

Example 5–10

Selecting Numbered Balls

A box contains 5 balls. Two are numbered 3, one is numbered 4, and two are numbered 5. The balls are mixed, and one is selected at random. After a ball is selected, its number is recorded. Then it is replaced. If the experiment is repeated many times, find the variance and standard deviation of the numbers on the balls.

Solution

Let X be the number on each ball. The probability distribution is

Number on ball X	3	4	5
Probability $P(X)$	$\tfrac{2}{5}$	$\tfrac{1}{5}$	$\tfrac{2}{5}$

The mean is

$$\mu = \Sigma X \cdot P(X) = 3 \cdot \tfrac{2}{5} \cdot 4 \cdot \tfrac{1}{5} \cdot 5 \cdot \tfrac{2}{5} = 4$$

The variance is

$$\begin{aligned}
\sigma^2 &= \Sigma[X^2 \cdot P(X)] - \mu^2 \\
&= \left[3^2 \cdot \tfrac{2}{5} + 4^2 \cdot \tfrac{1}{5} + 5^2 \cdot \tfrac{2}{5}\right] - 4^2 \\
&= 16\tfrac{4}{5} - 16 \\
&= \tfrac{4}{5}
\end{aligned}$$

The standard deviation is

$$\sigma = \sqrt{\frac{4}{5}} = \sqrt{0.8} \approx 0.894$$

The mean, variance, and standard deviation can also be found by using vertical columns, as shown.

X	$P(X)$	$X \cdot P(X)$	$X^2 \cdot P(X)$
3	0.4	1.2	3.6
4	0.2	0.8	3.2
5	0.4	2.0	10.0
		4.0	16.8

Find the mean by summing the $X \cdot P(X)$ column, and find the variance by summing the $X^2 \cdot P(X)$ column and subtracting the square of the mean.

$$\sigma^2 = 16.8 - 4^2 = 16.8 - 16 = 0.8$$

and

$$\sigma = \sqrt{0.8} \approx 0.894$$

Example 5–11

On Hold for Talk Radio

A talk radio station has 4 telephone lines. If the host is unable to talk (i.e., during a commercial) or is talking to a person, the other callers are placed on hold. When all lines are in use, others who are trying to call in get a busy signal. The probability that 0, 1, 2, 3, or 4 people will get through is shown in the distribution. Find the variance and standard deviation for the distribution.

X	0	1	2	3	4
$P(X)$	0.18	0.34	0.23	0.21	0.04

Should the station consider getting more phone lines installed?

Solution

The mean is

$$\mu = \Sigma X \cdot P(X)$$
$$= 0 \cdot (0.18) + 1 \cdot (0.34) + 2 \cdot (0.23) + 3 \cdot (0.21) + 4 \cdot (0.04)$$
$$= 1.6 \text{ (rounded)}$$

The variance is

$$\sigma^2 = \Sigma[X^2 \cdot P(X)] - \mu^2$$
$$= [0^2 \cdot (0.18) + 1^2 \cdot (0.34) + 2^2 \cdot (0.23) + 3^2 \cdot (0.21) + 4^2 \cdot (0.04)] - 1.6^2$$
$$= [0 + 0.34 + 0.92 + 1.89 + 0.64] - 2.56$$
$$= 3.79 - 2.56 = 1.23$$
$$= 1.2 \text{ (rounded)}$$

The standard deviation is $\sigma = \sqrt{\sigma^2}$, or $\sigma = \sqrt{1.2} = 1.1$ (rounded)

No. The mean number of people calling at any one time is 1.6. Since the standard deviation is 1.1, most callers are accommodated by having 4 phone lines because $\mu + 2\sigma$ is $1.6 + 2(1.1) = 1.6 + 2.2 = 3.8$. Very few callers get a busy signal since at least 75% of the callers either get through or are put on hold. (See Chebyshev's theorem in Section 3–2.)

Expectation

Another concept related to the mean for a probability distribution is the concept of expected value or expectation. Expected value is used in various types of games of chance, in insurance, and in other areas, such as decision theory.

> The **expected value** of a discrete random variable of a probability distribution is the theoretical average of the variable. The formula is
>
> $$\mu = E(X) = \Sigma X \cdot P(X)$$
>
> The symbol $E(X)$ is used for the expected value.

The formula for the expected value is the same as the formula for the theoretical mean. The expected value, then, is the theoretical mean of the probability distribution. That is, $E(X) = \mu$.

When expected value problems involve money, it is customary to round the answer to the nearest cent.

| Example 5–12 | **Winning Tickets** |

One thousand tickets are sold at $1 each for a colour television valued at $350. What is the expected value of the gain if a person purchases one ticket?

Solution

The problem can be set up as follows:

	Win	Lose
Gain X	$349	−$1
Probability $P(X)$	$\dfrac{1}{1000}$	$\dfrac{999}{1000}$

Two things should be noted. First, for a win, the net gain is $349, since the person does not get the cost of the ticket ($1) back. Second, for a loss, the gain is represented by a negative number, in this case −$1. The solution, then, is

$$E(X) = \$349 \cdot \frac{1}{1000} + (-\$1) \cdot \frac{999}{1000} = -\$0.65$$

Historical Note

In 1657 a Dutch mathematician, Christian Huygens, wrote a treatise on the Pascal–Fermat correspondence and introduced the idea of *mathematical expectation.*

Expected value problems of this type can also be solved by finding the overall gain (i.e., the value of the prize won or the amount of money won, not considering the cost of the ticket for the prize or the cost to play the game) and subtracting the cost of the tickets or the cost to play the game, as shown:

$$E(X) = \$350 \cdot \frac{1}{1000} - \$1 = -\$0.65$$

Here, the overall gain ($350) must be used.

Note that the expectation is −$0.65. This does not mean that a person loses $0.65, since the person can only win a television set valued at $350 or lose $1 on the ticket. What this expectation means is that the average of the losses is $0.65 for each of the 1000 ticket holders. Here is another way of looking at this situation: If a person purchased one ticket each week over a long time, the average loss would be $0.65 per ticket, since theoretically, on average, that person would win the set once for each 1000 tickets purchased.

| Example 5–13 | **Winning Tickets** |

One thousand tickets are sold at $1 each for 4 prizes of $100, $50, $25, and $10. After each prize drawing, the winning ticket is then returned to the pool of tickets. What is the expected value if a person purchases 2 tickets?

Gain X	$98	$48	$23	$8	−$2
Probability $P(X)$	$\dfrac{2}{1000}$	$\dfrac{2}{1000}$	$\dfrac{2}{1000}$	$\dfrac{2}{1000}$	$\dfrac{992}{1000}$

Solution

$$E(X) = \$98 \cdot \frac{2}{1000} + \$48 \cdot \frac{2}{1000} + \$23 \cdot \frac{2}{1000} + \$8 \cdot \frac{2}{1000} + (-\$2) \cdot \frac{992}{1000}$$

$$= -\$1.63$$

An alternative solution is

$$E(X) = \$100 \cdot \frac{2}{1000} + \$50 \cdot \frac{2}{1000} + \$25 \cdot \frac{2}{1000} + \$10 \cdot \frac{2}{1000} - \$2$$

$$= -\$1.63$$

Example 5–14

Bond Investment

A financial adviser suggests that his client select one of two types of bonds in which to invest \$5000. Bond X pays a return of 4% and has a default rate of 2%. Bond Y has a $2\frac{1}{2}$% return and a default rate of 1%. Find the expected rate of return and decide which bond would be a better investment. When the bond defaults, the investor loses all the investment.

Solution

The return on bond X is \$5000 · 4% = \$200. The expected return then is

$$E(X) = \$200(0.98) - \$5000(0.02) = \$96$$

The return on bond Y is \$5000 · $2\frac{1}{2}$% = \$125. The expected return then is

$$E(X) = \$125(0.99) - \$5000(0.01) = \$73.75$$

Hence, bond X would be a better investment since the expected return is higher.

In gambling games, if the expected value of the game is zero, the game is said to be fair. If the expected value of a game is positive, then the game is in favour of the player. That is, the player has a better-than-even chance of winning. If the expected value of the game is negative, then the game is said to be in favour of the house. That is, in the long run, the players will lose money.

In their book *The Complete Idiot's Guide to Gambling Like a Pro* (Alpha Books, 2002), authors Stanford Wong and Susan Spector give the expectations for various gambling games. The expected earnings game from a \$100 keno bet is \$73, roulette is \$94.70, and baccarat is \$98.80. That means that the house wins \$27 on keno, \$5.30 on roulette, and \$1.20 on baccarat for every \$100 bet. The bottom line here is that if you gamble long enough, sooner or later you will end up losing money.

5–2 Applying the Concepts

Expected Value

On March 28, 1979, the nuclear generating facility at Three Mile Island, Pennsylvania, began discharging radiation into the atmosphere. People exposed to even low levels of radiation can experience health problems ranging from very mild to severe, even death. A local newspaper reported that 11 babies were born with kidney problems in the three-county area surrounding the Three Mile Island nuclear power plant. The expected value for that problem in infants in that area was 3. Answer the following questions.

1. What does *expected value* mean?

2. Would you expect the exact value of 3 all the time?

3. If a news reporter stated that the number of cases of kidney problems in newborns was nearly four times as much as was usually expected, do you think pregnant mothers living in that area would be overly concerned?

4. Is it unlikely that 11 occurred by chance?

5. Are there any other statistics that could better inform the public?

6. Assume that 3 out of 2500 babies were born with kidney problems in that three-county area the year before the accident. Also assume that 11 out of 2500 babies were born with kidney problems in that three-county area the year after the accident. What is the real percentage of increase in that abnormality?

7. Do you think that pregnant mothers living in that area should be overly concerned after looking at the results in terms of rates?

See page 250 for the answers.

Exercises 5–2

1. Defective Transistors From past experience, a company has found that in cartons of transistors, 92% contain no defective transistors, 3% contain one defective transistor, 3% contain two defective transistors, and 2% contain three defective transistors. Find the mean, variance, and standard deviation for the defective transistors. About how many extra transistors per day would the company need to replace the defective ones if it used 10 cartons per day?

2. Suit Sales The number of suits sold per day at a retail store is shown in the table, with the corresponding probabilities. Find the mean, variance, and standard deviation of the distribution.

Number of suits sold X	19	20	21	22	23
Probability P(X)	0.2	0.2	0.3	0.2	0.1

If the manager of the retail store wants to be sure that he has enough suits for the next 5 days, how many should the manager purchase?

3. Number of Credit Cards A bank vice-president feels that each savings account customer has, on average, three credit cards. The following distribution represents the number of credit cards people own. Find the mean, variance, and standard deviation. Is the vice-president correct?

Number of cards X	0	1	2	3	4
Probability P(X)	0.18	0.44	0.27	0.08	0.03

4. Trivia Questions The probabilities that a player will get 5 to 10 questions right on a trivia quiz are shown below. Find the mean, variance, and standard deviation for the distribution.

X	5	6	7	8	9	10
P(X)	0.05	0.2	0.4	0.1	0.15	0.1

5. Cellphone Sales The probability that a cellphone company kiosk sells X number of new phone contracts per day is shown. Find the mean, variance, and standard deviation for this probability distribution.

X	4	5	6	8	10
P(X)	0.4	0.3	0.1	0.15	0.05

What is the probability that the kiosk will sell 6 or more contracts three days in a row?

6. Animal Shelter Adoptions The local animal shelter adopts out cats and dogs each week with the following probabilities.

X	3	4	5	6	7	8
P(X)	0.15	0.3	0.25	0.18	0.1	0.02

Find the mean, variance, and standard deviation for the number of animals adopted each week. What is the probability that the shelter finds homes for more than 5 animals in a given week?

7. Children's TV Program Commercials A concerned parents group determined the number of commercials shown in each of 5 children's programs over a period of time. Find the mean, variance, and standard deviation for the distribution shown.

Number of commercials X	5	6	7	8	9
Probability P(X)	0.2	0.25	0.38	0.10	0.07

8. Televisions per Household A study conducted by a TV station showed the number of televisions per household and the corresponding probabilities for each. Find the mean, variance, and standard deviation.

Number of televisions X	1	2	3	4
Probability P(X)	0.32	0.51	0.12	0.05

If you were taking a survey on the programs that were watched on each television set, how many program diaries would you send to each household in the survey?

9. CPR Class Enrollment The following distribution shows the number of students enrolled in CPR classes offered by the local fire department. Find the mean, variance, and standard deviation for the distribution.

Number of students X	12	13	14	15	16
Probability $P(X)$	0.15	0.20	0.38	0.18	0.09

10. Pizza Deliveries A pizza shop owner determines the number of pizzas that are delivered each day. Find the mean, variance, and standard deviation for the distribution shown. If the manager stated that 45 pizzas were delivered on one day, do you think that this is a believable claim?

Number of deliveries X	35	36	37	38	39
Probability $P(X)$	0.1	0.2	0.3	0.3	0.1

11. Insurance An insurance company insures a person's antique coin collection worth $20,000 for an annual premium of $300. If the company figures that the probability of the collection being stolen is 0.002, what will be the company's expected profit?

12. Job Bids A landscape contractor bids on jobs where he can make $3000 profit. The probabilities of getting 1, 2, 3, or 4 jobs per month are shown.

Number of jobs	1	2	3	4
Probability	0.2	0.3	0.4	0.1

Find the contractor's expected profit per month.

13. Rolling Dice If a person rolls doubles when he tosses two dice, he wins $5. For the game to be fair, how much should the person pay to play the game?

14. Dice Game A person pays $2 to play a certain game by rolling a single die once. If a 1 or a 2 comes up, the person wins nothing. If, however, the player rolls a 3, 4, 5, or 6, the player wins the difference between the number rolled and $2. Find the expectation for this game. Is the game fair?

15. Lottery Prizes A lottery offers one $1000 prize, one $500 prize, and five $100 prizes. One thousand tickets are sold at $3 each. Find the expectation of winning a prize if a person buys one ticket.

16. Lottery Prizes In Exercise 15, find the expectation of winning if a person buys two tickets. Assume that the player's ticket is replaced after each draw and that the same ticket can win more than one prize.

17. Winning the Lottery For a daily lottery, a person selects a three-digit number. If the person plays for $1, she can win $500. Find the expectation. In the same daily lottery, if a person boxes a number, she will win $80. Find the expectation if the number 123 is played for $1 and boxed. (When a number is "boxed," it can win when the digits occur in any order.)

18. Life Insurance A 35-year-old woman purchases a $100,000 term life insurance policy for an annual payment of $360. Based on a period life table the probability that she will survive the year is 0.999057. Find the expected value of the policy for the insurance company.

19. Raffle Ticket Sales A civic group sells 1000 raffle tickets to raise $2500 for its charity. First prize is $1000, second prize is $300, and third prize is $200. How much should the group charge for each ticket?

Extending the Concepts »

20. Rolling Dice Construct a probability distribution for the sum shown on the faces when two dice are rolled. Find the mean, variance, and standard deviation of the distribution.

21. Rolling a Die When one die is rolled, the expected value of the number of spots is 3.5. In Exercise 20, the mean number of spots was found for rolling two dice. What is the mean number of spots if three dice are rolled?

22. The formula for finding the variance for a probability distribution is

$$\sigma^2 = \Sigma[(X - \mu)^2 \cdot P(X)]$$

Verify algebraically that this formula gives the same result as the shortcut formula shown in this section.

23. Rolling a Die Roll a die 100 times. Compute the mean and standard deviation. How does the result compare with the theoretical results of Example 5–5?

24. Rolling Two Dice Roll two dice 100 times and find the mean, variance, and standard deviation of the sum of the spots. Compare the result with the theoretical results obtained in Exercise 20.

25. Extracurricular Activities Conduct a survey of the number of extracurricular activities your classmates are enrolled in. Construct a probability distribution and find the mean, variance, and standard deviation.

26. Promotional Campaign In a recent promotional campaign, a company offered these prizes and the corresponding probabilities. Find the expected value of winning. The tickets are free.

Number of prizes	Amount	Probability
1	$100,000	$\frac{1}{1,000,000}$
2	10,000	$\frac{1}{50,000}$
5	1,000	$\frac{1}{10,000}$
10	100	$\frac{1}{1000}$

If the winner has to mail in the winning ticket to claim the prize, what will be the expectation if the cost of the stamp is considered? Use the current cost of a stamp for a first-class letter.

Speaking of Statistics

This study shows that a part of the brain reacts to the impact of losing, and it might explain why people tend to increase their bets after losing when gambling. Explain how this type of decision making may influence fighter pilots, firefighters, or police officers, as the article states.

THE GAMBLER'S FALLACY

WHY WE EXPECT TO STRIKE IT RICH AFTER A LOSING STREAK

A GAMBLER USUALLY WAGERS more after taking a loss, in the misguided belief that a run of bad luck increases the probability of a win. We tend to cling to the misconception that past events can skew future odds. "On some level, you're thinking, 'If I just lost, it's going to even out.' The extent to which you're disturbed by a loss seems to go along with risky behaviour," says University of Michigan psychologist William Gehring, Ph.D., co-author of a new study linking dicey decision-making to neurological activity originating in the medial frontal cortex, long thought to be an area of the brain used in error detection.

Because people are so driven to up the ante after a loss, Gehring believes that the medial frontal cortex unconsciously influences future decisions based on the impact of the loss, in addition to registering the loss itself.

Gehring drew this conclusion by asking 12 subjects fitted with electrode caps to choose either the number 5 or 25, with the larger number representing the riskier bet.

On any given round, both numbers could amount to a loss, both could amount to a gain or the results could split, one number signifying a loss, the other a gain.

The medial frontal cortex responded to the outcome of a gamble within a quarter of a second, registering sharp electrical impulses only after a loss. Gehring points out that if the medial frontal cortex simply detected errors it would have reacted after participants chose the lesser of two possible gains. In other words, choosing "5" during a round in which both numbers paid off and betting on "25" would have yielded a larger profit.

After the study appeared in *Science*, Gehring received several emails from stock traders likening the "gambler's fallacy" to impulsive trading decisions made directly after off-loading a losing security. Researchers speculate that such risky, split-second decision-making could extend to fighter pilots, firefighters, and police officers—professions in which rapid-fire decisions are crucial and frequent.

—Dan Schulman

Source: Psychology Today, August 2002, p. 22. Used with permission.

5–3 The Binomial Distribution >

 LO3

Calculate exact probabilities for a binomial experiment and determine the mean, standard deviation, and variance for the variable of a binomial distribution.

Many types of probability problems have only two outcomes or can be reduced to two outcomes. For example, when a coin is tossed, it can land heads or tails. When a baby is born, it will be either male or female. In a basketball game, a team either wins or loses. A true/false item can be answered in only two ways, true or false. Other situations can be reduced to two outcomes. For example, a medical treatment can be classified as effective or ineffective, depending on the results. A person can be classified as having normal or abnormal blood pressure, depending on the measure of the blood pressure gauge.

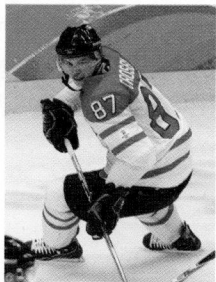

A multiple-choice question, even though there are four or five answer choices, can be classified as correct or incorrect. Situations like these are called *binomial experiments*.

Historical Note

In 1653, Blaise Pascal created a triangle of numbers called *Pascal's triangle* that can be used in the binomial distribution.

A **binomial experiment,** also known as *Bernoulli trials,* is a probability experiment that satisfies the following four requirements:

1. There must be a fixed number of trials.
2. Each trial can have only two outcomes or outcomes that can be reduced to two outcomes. These outcomes can be considered as either *success* or *failure.*
3. The outcomes of each trial must be independent of each other.
4. The probability of a success must remain the same for each trial.

A binomial experiment and its results give rise to a special probability distribution called the *binomial distribution.*

The **binomial distribution** is a discrete probability distribution of the number of successes in a series of *n* independent trials, with each trial having two possible outcomes and a constant probability of success.

In binomial experiments, the outcomes are usually classified as successes or failures. For example, the correct answer to a multiple-choice item can be classified as a success, but any of the other choices would be incorrect and hence classified as a failure. The notation that is commonly used for binomial experiments and the binomial distribution is defined now.

Notation for the Binomial Distribution

$P(S)$	The symbol for the probability of success
$P(F)$	The symbol for the probability of failure
p	The numerical probability of a success
q	The numerical probability of a failure

$$P(S) = p \quad \text{and} \quad P(F) = 1 - p = q$$

n	The number of trials
X	The number of successes in n trials

Note that $0 \leq X \leq n$ and $X = 0, 1, 2, 3, \ldots, n$

The probability of a success in a binomial experiment can be computed with this formula.

Binomial Probability Formula

In a binomial experiment, the probability of exactly X successes in n trials is

$$P(X) = \frac{n!}{(n - X)!X!} \cdot p^X \cdot q^{n-X}$$

An explanation of why the formula works is given following Example 5–15.

Example 5–15

Tossing Coins

A coin is tossed 3 times. Find the probability of getting exactly 2 heads.

Solution

This problem can be solved by looking at the sample space. There are 3 ways to get 2 heads.

HHH, <u>HHT,</u> <u>HTH,</u> <u>THH,</u> TTH, THT, HTT, TTT

The answer is $\frac{3}{8}$, or 0.375.

Looking at the problem in Example 5–15 from the standpoint of a binomial experiment, one can show that it meets the four requirements.

1. There are a fixed number of trials (three).

2. There are only two outcomes for each trial, heads or tails.

3. The outcomes are independent of one another (the outcome of one toss in no way affects the outcome of another toss).

4. The probability of a success (heads) is $\frac{1}{2}$ in each case.

In this case, $n = 3$, $X = 2$, $p = \frac{1}{2}$, and $q = \frac{1}{2}$. Hence, substituting in the formula gives

$$P(2 \text{ heads}) = \frac{3!}{(3-2)!2!} \cdot \left(\tfrac{1}{2}\right)^2 \left(\tfrac{1}{2}\right)^1 = \tfrac{3}{8} = 0.375$$

which is the same answer obtained by using the sample space.

The same example can be used to explain the formula. First, note that there are three ways to get exactly two heads and one tail from a possible eight ways. They are HHT, HTH, and THH. In this case, then, the number of ways of obtaining two heads from three coin tosses is $_3C_2$, or 3, as shown in Chapter 4. In general, the number of ways to get X successes from n trials without regard to order is

$$_nC_X = \frac{n!}{(n-X)!X!}$$

This is the first part of the binomial formula. (Some calculators can be used for this.)

Next, each success has a probability of $\frac{1}{2}$ and can occur twice. Likewise, each failure has a probability of $\frac{1}{2}$ and can occur once, giving the $\left(\frac{1}{2}\right)^2\left(\frac{1}{2}\right)^1$ part of the formula. To generalize, then, each success has a probability of p and can occur X times, and each failure has a probability of q and can occur $n - X$ times. Putting it all together yields the binomial probability formula.

Example 5–16

Doctor Visits

A publication entitled *Statistical Report on the Health of Canadians* indicated that 3 out of 5 Canadians aged 12 years and over visited a physician one or more times in the previous year. If 10 Canadians aged 12+ years are randomly selected, find the probability that exactly 3 people visited a physician at least once last year.

Source: Public Health Agency of Canada.

Solution

In this case, $n = 10$, $X = 3$, $p = 3/5$, and $q = 2/5$. Hence,

$$P(3) = \frac{10!}{(10-3)!3!}\left(\tfrac{3}{5}\right)^3\left(\tfrac{2}{5}\right)^7 \approx 0.042$$

Source: Statistics Canada.

Example 5–17

Youth Employment

A recent study on youth and the labour market reports that the employment rate for young Canadians aged 15 to 24 was 86.6%. If 5 Canadian youths are selected at random, find the probability that at least 3 of them are employed.

Source: Statistics Canada.

Solution

To find the probability that at least 3 youths are employed, it is necessary to find the individual probabilities for 3, 4, or 5, and then add them to get the total probability.

$$P(3) = \frac{5!}{(5-3)!3!}(0.866)^3(0.134)^2 \approx 0.117$$

$$P(4) = \frac{5!}{(5-4)!4!}(0.866)^4(0.134)^1 \approx 0.377$$

$$P(5) = \frac{5!}{(5-5)!5!}(0.866)^5(0.134)^0 \approx 0.487$$

Hence,

$$P(\text{at least 3 youths are employed})$$

$$= 0.117 + 0.377 + 0.487 = 0.981$$

Source: Adapted from Statistics Canada, *The Daily,* "Study: Youth and the Labour Market," November 23, 2005.

Computing probabilities by using the binomial probability formula can be quite tedious at times, so tables have been developed for selected values of n and p. Table B in Appendix C gives the probabilities for individual events. Example 5–18 shows how to use Table B to compute probabilities for binomial experiments.

Example 5–18

Tossing Coins

Solve the problem in Example 5–15 by using Table B, Binomial Distribution, in Appendix C.

Solution

Since $n = 3$, $X = 2$, and $p = 0.5$, the value 0.375 is found as shown in Figure 5–3.

Figure 5–3

Using Table B for Example 5–18

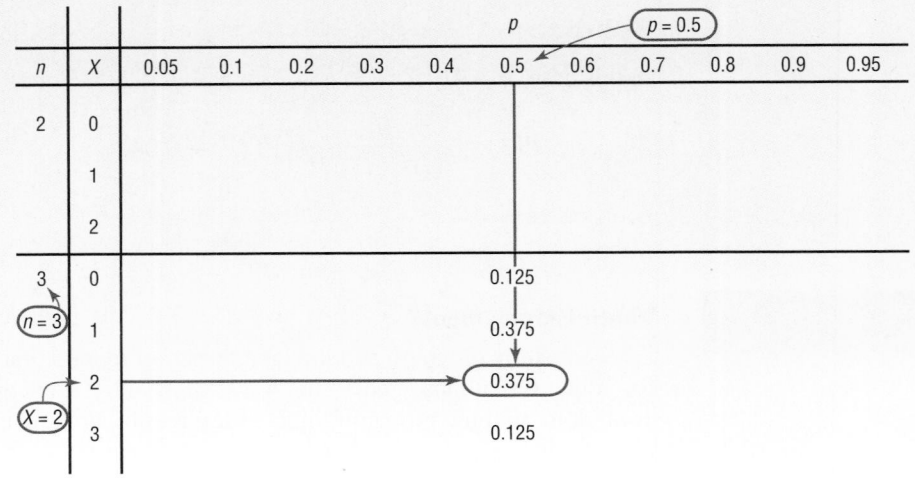

Example 5–19	**Fear of Crime Study**

Results of a study on fear of crime finds that 22% of young Canadians (15 to 24 years old) feel worried when home alone at night. If a random sample of 20 young Canadians is selected, find these probabilities by using the binomial table.

    a. There are exactly 5 people in the sample who are worried when home alone at night.

    b. There are at most 3 people in the sample who are worried when home alone at night.

    c. There are at least 3 people in the sample who are worried when home alone at night.

Source: Statistics Canada.

Solution

    a. $n = 20$, $p = 0.22$, and $X = 5$. From the table, one gets 0.192.

    b. $n = 20$ and $p = 0.22$, "At most 3 people" means 0, or 1, or 2, or 3.

    Hence, the solution is

$$P(0) + P(1) + P(2) + P(3) = 0.007 + 0.039 + 0.105 + 0.178$$
$$= 0.329$$

    c. $n = 20$ and $p = 0.22$. "At least 3 people" means 3, 4, 5, . . . , 20. This problem can best be solved by finding $P(0) + P(1) + P(2)$ and subtracting from 1.

$$P(0) + P(1) + P(2) = 0.007 + 0.039 + 0.105 = 0.151$$
$$1 - 0.151 = 0.849$$

Source: Adapted from Statistics Canada, *A Profile of Criminal Victimization: Results of the 1999 General Social Survey,* page 54, Catalogue 85-553. Release date: August 8, 2001.

Example 5–20	**Drinking Driver Fatalities**

Transport Canada reports that in a recent year 40% of fatally injured drivers tested had been drinking, based on tests of blood alcohol content. If a random sample of 15 driver traffic fatalities is selected, find the probability that at least 12 involved a driver who had been drinking.

Source: Transport Canada.

Solution

Now, $n = 15$, $P = 0.40$, and $X = \{12, 13, 14, 15\}$. From Table B in Appendix C, $P(12) = 0.002$. Since $P(13)$, $P(14)$, and $P(15)$ are not indicated in the table, use the rounded value 0.000 as the respective probabilities are less than 0.0005. Hence, the probability of at least 12 is 0.002 or 0.2%.

Source: Adapted from Transport Canada, *Canadian Motor Vehicle Traffic Collision Statistics: 2004.* Reprinted with the permission of the Minister of Public Works and Government Services Canada, 2007.

Remember that in the use of the binomial distribution, the outcomes must be independent. For example, in the selection of components from a batch to be tested, each component must be replaced before the next one is selected. Otherwise, the outcomes are not independent. However, a dilemma arises because there is a chance that the same component could be selected again. This situation can be avoided by not replacing the component and using a distribution called the *hypergeometric distribution* to calculate the probabilities. The hypergeometric distribution is presented later in this chapter. Note that when the population is large and the sample is small, the binomial probabilities can be shown to be nearly the same as the corresponding hypergeometric probabilities.

Mean, Variance, and Standard Deviation for the Binomial Distribution

The mean, variance, and standard deviation of a variable that has the *binomial distribution* can be found by using the following formulas.

$$\text{Mean } \mu = n \cdot p \qquad \text{Variance } \sigma^2 = n \cdot p \cdot q \qquad \text{Standard deviation } \sigma = \sqrt{n \cdot p \cdot q}$$

These formulas are algebraically equivalent to the formulas for the mean, variance, and standard deviation of the variables for probability distributions, but because they are for variables of the binomial distribution, they have been simplified by using algebra. The algebraic derivation is omitted here, but their equivalence is shown in Example 5–21.

Example 5–21

Tossing a Coin

A coin is tossed 4 times. Find the mean, variance, and standard deviation of the number of heads that will be obtained.

Solution

With the formulas for the binomial distribution and $n = 4$, $p = \frac{1}{2}$, and $q = \frac{1}{2}$, the results are

$$\mu = n \cdot p = 4 \cdot \tfrac{1}{2} = 2$$
$$\sigma^2 = n \cdot p \cdot q = 4 \cdot \tfrac{1}{2} \cdot \tfrac{1}{2} = 1$$
$$\sigma = \sqrt{1} = 1$$

From Example 5–21, when four coins are tossed many, many times, the average of the number of heads that appear is 2, and the standard deviation of the number of heads is 1. Note that these are theoretical values.

As stated previously, this problem can be solved by using the formulas for expected value. The distribution is shown.

No. of heads X	0	1	2	3	4
Probability $P(X)$	$\frac{1}{16}$	$\frac{4}{16}$	$\frac{6}{16}$	$\frac{4}{16}$	$\frac{1}{16}$

$$\mu = E(X) = \Sigma X \cdot P(X) = 0 \cdot \tfrac{1}{16} + 1 \cdot \tfrac{4}{16} + 2 \cdot \tfrac{6}{16} + 3 \cdot \tfrac{4}{16} + 4 \cdot \tfrac{1}{16} = \tfrac{32}{16} = 2$$
$$\sigma^2 = \Sigma X^2 \cdot P(X) - \mu^2$$
$$= 0^2 \cdot \tfrac{1}{16} + 1^2 \cdot \tfrac{4}{16} + 2^2 \cdot \tfrac{6}{16} + 3^2 \cdot \tfrac{4}{16} + 4^2 \cdot \tfrac{1}{16} - 2^2 = \tfrac{80}{16} - 4 = 1$$
$$\sigma = \sqrt{1} = 1$$

Hence, the simplified binomial formulas give the same results.

Example 5–22

Rolling a Die

A die is rolled 480 times. Find the mean, variance, and standard deviation of the number of 2s that will be rolled.

Solution

This is a binomial situation, where getting a 2 is a success and not getting a 2 is a failure; hence, $n = 480$, $p = \frac{1}{6}$, and $q = \frac{5}{6}$.

$$\mu = n \cdot p = 480 \cdot \frac{1}{6} = 80$$
$$\sigma^2 = n \cdot p \cdot q = 480 \cdot \left(\frac{1}{6}\right)\left(\frac{5}{6}\right) \approx 66.7$$
$$\sigma = \sqrt{n \cdot p \cdot q} = \sqrt{66.7} \approx 8.2$$

On average, there will be eighty 2s. The standard deviation is 8.2.

Example 5–23

Multiple Births

A Statistics Canada publication reported that 3% of Canadian mothers experience multiple births, primarily twins. If a random sample of 5000 births is taken, find the mean, variance, and standard deviation of the number of mothers delivering twins or more.

Source: Statistics Canada.

Solution

This is a binomial situation, since a birth can result in multiple births or not multiple births (i.e., two outcomes):

$$\mu = n \cdot p = (5000)(0.03) = 150$$
$$\sigma^2 = n \cdot p \cdot q = (5000)(0.03)(0.97) = 145.5$$
$$\sigma = \sqrt{n \cdot p \cdot q} = \sqrt{145.5} \approx 12.1$$

For the sample, the average number of multiple births is 150, the variance is 145.5, or 146, and the standard deviation is 12.1 or 12 (if rounded).

Source: Adapted from Statistics Canada, *Births, 2003,* Catalogue 84F0210X. Release date: July 12, 2005.

5–3 Applying the Concepts

Unsanitary Restaurants

Health officials routinely check sanitary conditions of restaurants. Assume you visit a popular tourist spot and read in the newspaper that in 3 out of every 7 restaurants checked, unsatisfactory health conditions were found. Assuming you are planning to eat out 10 times while you are there on vacation, answer the following questions.

1. How likely is it that you will eat at 3 restaurants with unsanitary conditions?
2. How likely is it that you will eat at 4 or 5 restaurants with unsanitary conditions?
3. Explain how you would compute the probability of eating in at least 1 restaurant with unsanitary conditions. Could you use the complement to solve this problem?
4. What is the most likely number to occur in this experiment?
5. How variable will the data be around the most likely number?
6. Is this a binomial distribution?
7. If it is a binomial distribution, does that mean that the likelihood of a success is always 50% since there are only two possible outcomes?

Check your answers by using the following computer-generated table.

Mean = 4.3   **Std. dev. = 1.56492**

X	P(X)	Cum. Prob.
0	0.00371	0.00371
1	0.02784	0.03155
2	0.09396	0.12552
3	0.18792	0.31344
4	0.24665	0.56009
5	0.22199	0.78208
6	0.13874	0.92082
7	0.05946	0.98028
8	0.01672	0.99700
9	0.00279	0.99979
10	0.00021	1.00000

See page 250 for the answers.

Exercises 5–3

1. Which of the following are binomial experiments or can be reduced to binomial experiments?

   a. Surveying 100 people to determine if they like Sudsy Soap

   b. Tossing a coin 100 times to see how many heads occur

   c. Drawing a card with replacement from a deck and getting a heart

   d. Asking 1000 people which brand of cigarettes they smoke

   e. Testing 4 different brands of painkillers to see which brands are effective

   f. Testing one brand of painkiller by using 10 people to determine whether it is effective

   g. Asking 100 people if they smoke

   h. Checking 1000 applicants to see whether they were admitted to White Oak College

   i. Surveying 300 prisoners to see how many different crimes they were convicted of

   j. Surveying 300 prisoners to see whether this is a first offence

2. **(ans)** Compute the probability of X successes, using Table B in Appendix C.

   a. $n = 2, p = 0.30, X = 1$
   b. $n = 4, p = 0.60, X = 3$
   c. $n = 5, p = 0.10, X = 0$
   d. $n = 10, p = 0.40, X = 4$
   e. $n = 12, p = 0.90, X = 2$
   f. $n = 15, p = 0.80, X = 12$
   g. $n = 17, p = 0.05, X = 0$
   h. $n = 20, p = 0.50, X = 10$
   i. $n = 16, p = 0.20, X = 3$

3. Compute the probability of X successes, using the binomial formula.

   a. $n = 6, X = 3, p = 0.03$
   b. $n = 4, X = 2, p = 0.18$
   c. $n = 5, X = 3, p = 0.63$
   d. $n = 9, X = 0, p = 0.42$
   e. $n = 10, X = 5, p = 0.37$

For Exercises 4 through 13, assume all variables are binomial. (*Note:* If values are not found in Table B of Appendix C, use the binomial formula.)

4. **Burglar Alarm** A burglar alarm system has 6 fail-safe components. The probability of each failing is 0.05. Find these probabilities.

   a. Exactly 3 will fail.
   b. Fewer than 2 will fail.
   c. None will fail.
   d. Compare the answers for parts *a*, *b*, and *c*, and explain why the results are reasonable.

5. **True/False Exam** A student takes a 20-question, true/false exam and guesses on each question. Find the probability of passing if the lowest passing grade is 15 correct out of 20. Would you consider this event likely to occur? Explain your answer.

6. **Multiple-Choice Exam** A student takes a 20-question, multiple-choice exam with 5 choices for each question and guesses on each question. Find the probability of guessing at least 15 out of 20 correctly. Would you consider this event likely or unlikely to occur? Explain your answer.

7. **Teens and Smoking** The Canadian Lung Association reports that 20% of Canadian teens (aged 12–19)

currently smoke (daily or occasionally). In a random sample of seven Canadian teens, find the probability that

a. Exactly two smoke.

b. At least two smoke.

c. At most two smoke.

d. Between one and three, inclusive, smoke.

Source: Canadian Lung Association, *Facts about Smoking,* "Teens and Smoking," September 28, 2006.

8. Cellphone Usage A recent study cautions that brain cancer may be linked to youngsters using cellphones. In Canada, 71% of youth between the ages of 12 and 19 have a cellphone. If 7 Canadian youths, aged 12 to 19 years, are randomly selected, find the probability that

a. Exactly 5 have a cellphone.

b. More than 5 have a cellphone.

c. Fewer than 5 have a cellphone.

Source: Brain Injury Association of Canada, *Brain Cancer Linked to Youngsters Using Cellphones,* Sarah Schmidt, Canwest News Service.

9. Survey on Concern for Criminals In a survey, 3 of 4 students said the courts show "too much concern" for criminals. Find the probability that at most 3 out of 7 randomly selected students will agree with this statement.
Source: Harper's Index.

10. Victimization of Aboriginal People *Juristat,* a Statistics Canada publication concerning Canada's criminal justice system, reported that 31.9% of Aboriginal people have been involved in some form of violent victimization. If 10 Aboriginals were selected at random, find the probability that at least 5 have been victimized.
Source: Statistics Canada.

11. Attitudes toward Seal Hunt The Environics Research Group conducted a poll for the Department of Fisheries and Oceans (DFO) on Canadian attitudes toward the east coast seal hunt. A majority, 53%, of informed respondents offered conditional support for the seal hunt. If a random sample of 5 Canadians were given the same arguments for and against the seal hunt, find these probabilities.

a. Exactly 2 respondents will support the seal hunt.

b. At most 3 respondents will support the seal hunt.

c. At least 2 respondents will support the seal hunt.

d. Fewer than 3 respondents will support the seal hunt.

Source: Fisheries and Oceans Canada.

12. Destination Weddings Twenty-six percent of couples who plan to marry this year are planning destination weddings. In a random sample of 12 couples who plan to marry, find the probability that

a. Exactly 6 couples will have a destination wedding.

b. At least 6 couples will have a destination wedding.

c. Fewer than 5 couples will have a destination wedding.

Source: Time Magazine

13. Internet Access If 84.3% of Canadian homes have Internet access, find the probability that in a random sample of 15 Canadians that

a. Exactly 13 have Internet access.

b. Between 12 and 14, inclusive, have Internet access.

c. At least 13 have Internet access.

d. At most 13 have Internet access.

Source: Miniwatts Marketing Group, *Internet World Stats.*

14. (ans) Find the mean, variance, and standard deviation for each of the values of n and p when the requirements for a binomial distribution are satisfied.

a. $n = 100, p = 0.75$

b. $n = 300, p = 0.3$

c. $n = 20, p = 0.5$

d. $n = 10, p = 0.8$

e. $n = 1000, p = 0.1$

f. $n = 500, p = 0.25$

g. $n = 50, p = \frac{2}{5}$

h. $n = 36, p = \frac{1}{6}$

15. Earned Doctorate Degree According to the 2006 census of Canada, approximately 0.7% of Canadian adults, 15 years and older, had earned a doctorate degree. If 500 Canadian adults are selected at random, find the mean, variance, and standard deviation of the number who earned a doctorate degree.
Source: Statistics Canada, Culture, Tourism, and the Centre for Education Statistics, *Doctorate Education in Canada: Findings from the Survey of Earned Doctorates, 2005/2006.*

16. Coin Tosses Find the mean, variance, and standard deviation for the number of heads when 20 coins are tossed.

17. Defective Calculators If 3% of calculators are defective, find the mean, variance, and standard deviation of a lot of 300 calculators.

18. Distracted Drivers A survey of Canadian attitudes toward controlling distractions while driving indicated that 37.7% favour banning certain devices while driving. If a random sample of 250 Canadians is selected, find the mean, variance, and standard deviation of the number who favour the banning of certain devices by drivers.
Source: Traffic Injury Research Foundation, *The Road Safety Monitor, 2006,* "Distracted Driving."

19. Teen TV Viewing Hours The average Canadian teen views 14.1 hours of TV per week, with approximately 8% of the week devoted to TV. If 1000 Canadian teens are randomly selected, find the mean, variance, and standard deviation of the number of teens who watch TV each week.
Source: Statistics Canada.

20. Climate Change Taxes A recent survey showed that 80% of Canadians support higher taxes on condition that the revenues would be devoted to promoting energy efficiency and developing alternative energy sources. If 900 Canadians are selected at random, find the mean, variance, and standard deviation of the number who support higher taxes on the conditions indicated.

21. Survey on Bathing Pets A survey found that 25% of pet owners had their pets bathed professionally rather than do it themselves. If 18 pet owners are randomly selected, find the probability that exactly 5 people have their pets bathed professionally.
Source: USA Snapshot, *USA TODAY.*

22. Household Cellphones The proportion of Canadian households that rely only on cellphones for communications instead of land-line phones was estimated at 4.8% by a Statistics Canada residential telephone service survey. If 15 Canadian households are randomly selected, find the probability that exactly 2 use only cellphones at home.
Source: Statistics Canada

23. Condominium Purchase A TD Bank-sponsored Ipsos Reid survey reported that 35% of Canada's urban-dwelling adults are likely to consider purchasing a condominium as their primary residence. If 10 urbanites are randomly selected, find the probability that at least 3 of the adults are likely to consider a condominium purchase.
Source: Ipos Reid Survey.

24. Recession Youth Unemployment During the 2009 recession, the unemployment rate for Canadian youths, aged 15 to 24 years, peaked at 16.0%. If 15 Canadian youths were randomly surveyed during the recession's peak, find the probability that at least 10 youths were employed.
Source: Statistics Canada, *The Daily,* "*Labour Force Survey,* July 2010," August 6, 2010.

25. Legalization of Marijuana An Angus Reid poll suggested that 55% of Canadians support the legalization of marijuana. If 20 Canadians are randomly surveyed, find the probability that at most 10 support marijuana's legalization.
Source: The Globe and Mail, "The True North, Stoned and Free," Rebecca Dube, July 16, 2007.

26. RRSP Contributions According to a recent survey, 23% of Canadian taxpayers do not plan to contribute to their registered retirement savings plans (RRSPs) for the current taxation year. If 30 Canadian taxpayers are randomly selected, find the probability that between 18 and 22 will contribute to their RRSPs for the current taxation year.
Source: Financial Post, "One in Four Don't Contribute to RRSPs At All, 28% Will Contribute Less, ING Finds," Jonathan Chevreau, January 20, 2010.

27. Youth Crime The Canadian Centre for Justice Statistics reported that 7% of Canada's youth, aged 12 to 17, were charged with Criminal Code offences (excluding traffic). If 13 Canadian youths are randomly selected, find the probability that 2 have been charged with a Criminal Code offence.
Source: Statistics Canada.

Extending the Concepts »

28. Children in a Family The graph shown here represents the probability distribution for the number of girls in a family of 3 children. From this graph, construct a probability distribution.

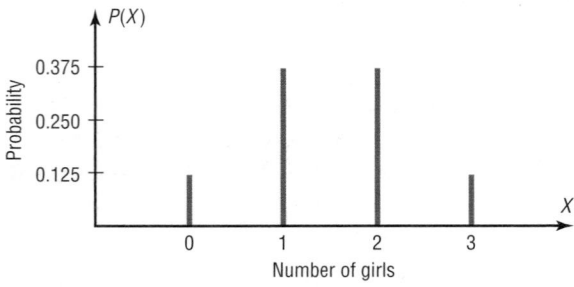

29. Defective Chips Construct a binomial distribution graph for the number of defective computer chips in a lot of four if $p = 0.3$.

5–4   Other Types of Distributions (Optional) ›

Find probabilities for outcomes of variables, using the Poisson, hypergeometric, and multinomial distributions.

In addition to the binomial distribution, other types of distributions are used in statistics. Three of the most commonly used distributions are the multinomial distribution, the Poisson distribution, and the hypergeometric distribution. They are described next.

The Multinomial Distribution

Recall that in order for an experiment to be binomial, two outcomes are required for each trial. But if each trial in an experiment has more than two outcomes, a distribution called the **multinomial distribution** must be used. For example, a survey might require the responses of "approve," "disapprove," or "no opinion." In another situation, a person may have a choice of one of five activities for Friday night, such as a movie, dinner, baseball game, play, or party. Since these situations have more than two possible outcomes for each trial, the binomial distribution cannot be used to compute probabilities.

The multinomial distribution can be used for such situations if the probabilities for each trial remain constant and the outcomes are independent for a fixed number of trials. The events must also be mutually exclusive.

Formula for the Multinomial Distribution

If X consists of events $E_1, E_2, \ldots, E_k$, which have corresponding probabilities $p_1, p_2, \ldots, p_k$ of occurring, and X_1 is the number of times E_1 will occur, X_2 is the number of times E_2 will occur, etc., then the probability that X will occur is

$$P(X) = \frac{n!}{X_1! \cdot X_2! \cdots X_k!} \cdot p_1^{X_1} \cdot p_2^{X_2} \cdots p_k^{X_k}$$

where $X_1 + X_2 + \cdots + X_k = n$ and $p_1 + p_2 + \cdots + p_k = 1$.

Example 5–24

Leisure Activities

In a large city, 50% of the people choose a movie, 30% choose dinner and a play, and 20% choose shopping as a leisure activity. If a sample of 5 people is randomly selected, find the probability that 3 are planning to go to a movie, one to dinner and a play, and one to a shopping mall.

Solution

We know that $n = 5$, $X_1 = 3$, $X_2 = 1$, $X_3 = 1$, $p_1 = 0.50$, $p_2 = 0.30$, and $p_3 = 0.20$. Substituting in the formula gives

$$P(X) = \frac{5!}{3! \cdot 1! \cdot 1!} \cdot (0.50)^3 (0.30)^1 (0.20)^1 = 0.15$$

Again, note that the multinomial distribution can be used even though replacement is not done, provided that the sample is small in comparison with the population.

Example 5–25

CD Purchases

In a music store, a manager found that the probabilities that a person buys 0, 1, or 2 or more CDs are 0.3, 0.6, and 0.1, respectively. If six customers enter the store, find the probability that one won't buy any CDs, three will buy 1 CD, and two will buy 2 or more CDs.

Solution

It is given that $n = 6$, $X_1 = 1$, $X_2 = 3$, $X_3 = 2$, $p_1 = 0.3$, $p_2 = 0.6$, and $p_3 = 0.1$. Then

$$P(X) = \frac{6!}{1!3!2!} \cdot (0.3)^1 (0.6)^3 (0.1)^2$$

$$= 60 \cdot (0.3)(0.216)(0.01) = 0.03888$$

Example 5–26

Selecting Coloured Balls

A box contains 4 white balls, 3 red balls, and 3 blue balls. A ball is selected at random, and its colour is written down. It is replaced each time. Find the probability that if 5 balls are selected, 2 are white, 2 are red, and 1 is blue.

Solution

We know that $n = 5$, $X_1 = 2$, $X_2 = 2$, $X_3 = 1$; $p_1 = \frac{4}{10}$, $p_2 = \frac{3}{10}$, and $p_3 = \frac{3}{10}$; hence,

$$P(X) = \frac{5!}{2!2!1!} \cdot \left(\frac{4}{10}\right)^2\left(\frac{3}{10}\right)^2\left(\frac{3}{10}\right)^1 = \frac{81}{625}$$

Thus, the multinomial distribution is similar to the binomial distribution but has the advantage of allowing one to compute probabilities when there are more than two outcomes for each trial in the experiment. That is, the multinomial distribution is a general distribution, and the binomial distribution is a special case of the multinomial distribution.

The Poisson Distribution

A discrete probability distribution that is useful when n is large and p is small and when the independent variables occur over a period of time is called the **Poisson distribution.** In addition to being used for the stated conditions (i.e., n is large, p is small, and the variables occur over a period of time), the Poisson distribution can be used when a density of items is distributed over a given area or volume, such as the number of plants growing per hectare or the number of defects in a given length of videotape.

Formula for the Poisson Distribution

The probability of X occurrences in an interval of time, volume, area, etc., for a variable where λ (Greek letter lambda) is the mean number of occurrences per unit (time, volume, area, etc.) is

$$P(X; \lambda) = \frac{e^{-\lambda}\lambda^X}{X!} \qquad \text{where } X = 0, 1, 2, \ldots$$

The letter e is a constant approximately equal to 2.7183.

Round the probabilities to four decimal places.

Example 5–27

Typographical Errors

If there are 200 typographical errors randomly distributed in a 500-page manuscript, find the probability that a given page contains exactly 3 errors.

Solution

First, find the mean number λ of errors. Since there are 200 errors distributed over 500 pages, each page has an average of

$$\lambda = \frac{200}{500} = \frac{2}{5} = 0.4$$

or 0.4 error per page. Since $X = 3$, substituting into the formula yields

$$P(X; \lambda) = \frac{e^{-\lambda}\lambda^X}{X!} = \frac{(2.7183)^{-0.4}(0.4)^3}{3!} \approx 0.0072$$

Thus, there is less than a 1% probability that any given page will contain exactly 3 errors.

Since the mathematics involved in computing Poisson probabilities is somewhat complicated, tables have been compiled for these probabilities. Table C in Appendix C gives P for various values for λ and X.

In Example 5–27, where X is 3 and λ is 0.4, the table gives the value 0.0072 for the probability. See Figure 5–4.

Figure 5–4

Using Table C in Appendix C

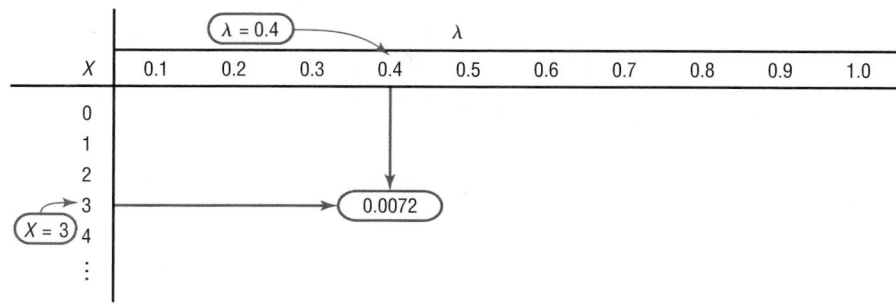

Example 5–28

Toll-Free Telephone Calls

A sales firm receives, on the average, 3 calls per hour on its toll-free number. For any given hour, find the probability that it will receive the following.

    a. At most 3 calls   *b.* At least 3 calls   *c.* 5 or more calls

Solution

    a. "At most 3 calls" means 0, 1, 2, or 3 calls. Hence,

$$P(0; 3) + P(1; 3) + P(2; 3) + P(3; 3)$$
$$= 0.0498 + 0.1494 + 0.2240 + 0.2240$$
$$= 0.6472$$

    b. "At least 3 calls" means 3 or more calls. It is easier to find the probability of 0, 1, and 2 calls and then subtract this answer from 1 to get the probability of at least 3 calls.

$$P(0; 3) + P(1; 3) + P(2; 3) = 0.0498 + 0.1494 + 0.2240 = 0.4232$$

    and

$$1 - 0.4232 = 0.5768$$

    c. For the probability of 5 or more calls, it is easier to find the probability of getting 0, 1, 2, 3, or 4 calls and subtract this answer from 1. Hence,

$$P(0; 3) + P(1; 3) + P(2; 3) + P(3; 3) + P(4; 3)$$
$$= 0.0498 + 0.1494 + 0.2240 + 0.2240 + 0.1680$$
$$= 0.8152$$

    and

$$1 - 0.8152 = 0.1848$$

Thus, for the events described, the part *a* event is most likely to occur and the part *c* event is least likely to occur.

The Poisson distribution can also be used to approximate the binomial distribution when the expected value $\lambda = n \cdot p$ is less than 5, as shown in Example 5–29. (The same is true when $n \cdot q < 5$.)

Example 5–29

Left-Handed People

If approximately 2% of the people in a room of 200 people are left-handed, find the probability that exactly 5 people there are left-handed.

Solution

Since $\lambda = n \cdot p$, then $\lambda = (200)(0.02) = 4$. Hence,

$$P(X; \lambda) = \frac{(2.7183)^{-4}(4)^5}{5!} \approx 0.1563$$

which is verified by the formula $_{200}C_5(0.02)^5(0.98)^{195} \approx 0.1579$. The difference between the two answers is based on the fact that the Poisson distribution is an approximation and rounding has been used.

The Hypergeometric Distribution

When sampling is done *without* replacement, the binomial distribution does not give exact probabilities, since the trials are not independent. The smaller the size of the population, the less accurate the binomial probabilities will be.

For example, suppose a committee of four people is to be selected from seven women and five men. What is the probability that the committee will consist of three women and one man?

To solve this problem, one must find the number of ways a committee of three women and one man can be selected from seven women and five men. This answer can be found by using combinations; it is

$$_7C_3 \cdot {}_5C_1 = 35 \cdot 5 = 175$$

Next, find the total number of ways a committee of four people can be selected from 12 people. Again, by the use of combinations, the answer is

$$_{12}C_4 = 495$$

Finally, the probability of getting a committee of three women and one man from seven women and five men is

$$P(X) = \frac{175}{495} = \frac{35}{99}$$

The results of the problem can be generalized by using a special probability distribution called the *hypergeometric distribution*. The **hypergeometric distribution** is a distribution of a variable that has two outcomes when sampling is done without replacement.

The probabilities for the hypergeometric distribution can be calculated by using the formula given next.

Formula for the Hypergeometric Distribution

Given a population with only two types of objects (females and males, defective and nondefective, successes or failures, etc.), such that there are a items of one kind and b items of another kind and $a + b$ equals the total population, the probability $P(X)$ of selecting without replacement a sample of size n with X items of type a and $n - X$ items of type b is

$$P(X) = \frac{{}_aC_X \cdot {}_bC_{n-X}}{{}_{a+b}C_n}$$

The basis of the formula is that there are $_aC_X$ ways of selecting the first type of items, $_bC_{n-X}$ ways of selecting the second type of items, and $_{a+b}C_n$ ways of selecting n items from the entire population.

Example 5–30

Assistant Manager Applicants

Ten people apply for a job as assistant manager of a restaurant. Five have completed college and 5 have not. If the manager selects 3 applicants at random, find the probability that all 3 are college graduates.

Solution

Assigning the values to the variables gives

$$a = 5 \text{ college graduates} \qquad n = 3$$
$$b = 5 \text{ nongraduates} \qquad X = 3$$

and $n - X = 0$. Substituting in the formula gives

$$P(X) = \frac{_5C_3 \cdot {}_5C_0}{_{10}C_3} = \frac{10}{120} = \frac{1}{12}$$

Example 5–31

House Insurance

A recent study found that 4 out of 9 houses were underinsured. If 5 houses are selected from the 9 houses, find the probability that exactly 2 are underinsured.

Solution

In this problem

$$a = 4 \qquad b = 5 \qquad n = 5 \qquad X = 2 \qquad n - X = 3$$

Then

$$P(X) = \frac{_4C_2 \cdot {}_5C_3}{_9C_5} = \frac{60}{126} = \frac{10}{21}$$

In many situations where objects are manufactured and shipped to a company, the company selects a few items and tests them to see whether they are satisfactory or defective. If a certain percentage is defective, the company then can refuse the whole shipment. This procedure saves the time and cost of testing every single item. To make the judgment about whether to accept or reject the whole shipment based on a small sample of tests, the company must know the probability of getting a specific number of defective items. To calculate the probability, the company uses the hypergeometric distribution.

Example 5–32

Defective Compressor Tanks

A lot of 12 compressor tanks is checked to see whether there are any defective tanks. Three tanks are checked for leaks. If 1 or more of the 3 is defective, the lot is rejected. Find the probability that the lot will be rejected if there are actually 3 defective tanks in the lot.

Solution

Since the lot is rejected if at least 1 tank is found to be defective, it is necessary to find the probability that none are defective and subtract this probability from 1.

Here, $a = 3$, $b = 9$, $n = 3$, $X = 0$; so

$$P(X) = \frac{{}_3C_0 \cdot {}_9C_3}{{}_{12}C_3} = \frac{1 \cdot 84}{220} = 0.38$$

Hence,

$$P(\text{at least one defective}) = 1 - P(\text{no defectives}) = 1 - 0.38 = 0.62$$

There is a 0.62, or 62%, probability that the lot will be rejected when 3 of the 12 tanks are defective.

A summary of the discrete distributions used in this chapter is shown in Table 5–1.

Table 5–1	**Summary of Discrete Distributions**

1. Binomial distribution

$$P(X) = \frac{n!}{(n - X)!X!} \cdot p^X \cdot q^{n - X}$$

$$\mu = n \cdot p \qquad \sigma = \sqrt{n \cdot p \cdot q}$$

Used when there are only two independent outcomes for a fixed number of independent trials and the probability for each success remains the same for each trial.

2. Multinomial distribution

$$P(X) = \frac{n!}{X_1! \cdot X_2! \cdots X_k!} \cdot p_1^{X_1} \cdot p_2^{X_2} \cdots p_k^{X_k}$$

where

$$X_1 + X_2 + \cdots + X_k = n \quad \text{and} \quad p_1 + p_2 + \cdots + p_k = 1$$

Used when the distribution has more than two outcomes, the probabilities for each trial remain constant, trials are independent, and there are a fixed number of trials.

3. Poisson distribution

$$P(X; \lambda) = \frac{e^{-\lambda}\lambda^X}{X!} \qquad \text{where } X = 0, 1, 2, \ldots$$

Used when n is large and p is small, the independent variable occurs over a period of time, or a density of items is distributed over a given area or volume.

4. Hypergeometric distribution

$$P(X) = \frac{{}_aC_X \cdot {}_bC_{n-X}}{{}_{a+b}C_n}$$

Used when there are two outcomes and sampling is done without replacement.

5–4   Applying the Concepts

Rockets and Targets

During the latter days of World War II, the Germans developed flying rocket bombs. These bombs were used to attack London. Allied military intelligence didn't know whether these bombs were fired at random or had a sophisticated aiming device. To determine the answer, they used the Poisson distribution.

To assess the accuracy of these bombs, London was divided into 576 square regions. Each region was $\frac{1}{4}$ square kilometre in area. They then compared the number of actual hits with the theoretical number of hits by using the Poisson distribution. If the values in both distributions were close, then they would conclude that the rockets were fired at random. The actual distribution is as follows:

Hits	0	1	2	3	4	5
Regions	229	211	93	35	7	1

1. Using the Poisson distribution, find the theoretical values for each number of hits. In this case, the number of bombs was 535, and the number of regions was 576. So

$$\mu = \frac{535}{576} \approx 0.929$$

For 3 hits,

$$P(X) = \frac{\mu^X \cdot e^{-\mu}}{X!}$$

$$= \frac{(0.929)^3 (2.7183)^{-0.929}}{3!} \approx 0.0528$$

Hence the number of hits is $(0.0528)(576) = 30.4128$.

Complete the table for the other number of hits.

Hits	0	1	2	3	4	5
Regions				30.4		

2. Write a brief statement comparing the two distributions.

3. Based on your answer to question 2, can you conclude that the rockets were fired at random?

See page 251 for the answer.

Exercises 5–4

1. Use the multinomial formula and find the probabilities for each.

   a. $n = 6, X_1 = 3, X_2 = 2, X_3 = 1, p_1 = 0.5, p_2 = 0.3,$ $p_3 = 0.2$

   b. $n = 5, X_1 = 1, X_2 = 2, X_3 = 2, p_1 = 0.3, p_2 = 0.6,$ $p_3 = 0.1$

   c. $n = 4, X_1 = 1, X_2 = 1, X_3 = 2, p_1 = 0.8, p_2 = 0.1,$ $p_3 = 0.1$

   d. $n = 3, X_1 = 1, X_2 = 1, X_3 = 1, p_1 = 0.5, p_2 = 0.3,$ $p_3 = 0.2$

   e. $n = 5, X_1 = 1, X_2 = 3, X_3 = 1, p_1 = 0.7, p_2 = 0.2,$ $p_3 = 0.1$

2. **Textbook Typographical Errors** The probabilities that a textbook page will have 0, 1, 2, or 3 typographical errors are 0.79, 0.12, 0.07, and 0.02, respectively. If eight pages are randomly selected, find the probability that four will contain no errors, two will contain 1 error, one will contain 2 errors, and one will contain 3 errors.

3. **Truck Safety Violations** The probabilities are 0.25, 0.40, and 0.35 that an 18-wheel truck will have 0 violations, 1 violation, or 2 or more violations when it is given a safety inspection. If eight trucks are inspected, find the probability that three will have 0 violations, two will have 1 violation, and three will have 2 or more violations.

4. **Number of Prescriptions** When a customer enters a pharmacy, the probabilities that he or she will have 0, 1, 2, or 3 prescriptions filled are 0.60, 0.25, 0.10, and 0.05, respectively. For a sample of six people who enter the pharmacy, find the probability that two will have 0 prescriptions, two will have 1 prescription, one will have 2 prescriptions, and one will have 3 prescriptions.

5. **Rolling a Die** A die is rolled 6 times. Find the probability of getting a 1, 2, 3, 4, 5, 6 exactly one time each.

6. **Mendel's Theory** According to Mendel's theory, if tall and colourful plants are crossed with short and colourless plants, the corresponding probabilities are $\frac{9}{16}$, $\frac{3}{16}$, $\frac{3}{16}$, and $\frac{1}{16}$ for tall and colourful, tall and colourless, short and colourful, and short and colourless, respectively. If eight plants are selected, find the probability that one will be tall and colourful, three will be tall and colourless, three will be short and colourful, and one will be short and colourless.

7. Find each probability $P(X; \lambda)$, using Table C, Poisson Distribution, in Appendix C.

   a. $P(5; 4)$

   b. $P(2; 4)$

   c. $P(6; 3)$

   d. $P(10; 7)$

   e. $P(9; 8)$

8. **Copy Machine Output** A copy machine randomly puts out 10 blank sheets per 500 copies processed. Find the probability that in a run of 300 copies, 5 sheets of paper will be blank.

9. **Study of Robberies** A recent study of robberies for a certain geographic region showed an average of one robbery per 20,000 people. In a city of 80,000 people, find the probability of the following.

   a. No robberies

   b. One robbery

   c. Two robberies

   d. Three or more robberies

10. **Misprints on Manuscript Pages** In a 400-page manuscript, there are 200 randomly distributed misprints. If a page is selected, find the probability that it has one misprint.

11. **Telephone Soliciting** A telephone soliciting company obtains an average of 5 orders per 1000 solicitations. If the company reaches 250 potential customers, find the probability of obtaining at least 2 orders.

12. **Mail Ordering** A mail-order company receives an average of 5 orders per 500 solicitations. If it sends out 100 advertisements, find the probability of receiving at least 2 orders.

13. **Company Mailing** Of a company's mailings, 1.5% are returned because of incorrect or incomplete addresses. In a mailing of 200 pieces, find the probability that none will be returned.

14. **Emission Inspection Failures** If 3% of all cars fail the emissions inspection, find the probability that in a sample of 90 cars, 3 will fail. Use the Poisson approximation.

15. **Phone Inquiries** The average number of phone inquiries per day at a poison control centre is 4. Find the probability it will receive 5 calls on a given day. Use the Poisson approximation.

16. **Defective Calculators** In a batch of 2000 calculators, there are, on average, 8 defective ones. If a random sample of 150 is selected, find the probability of 5 defective ones.

17. **School Newspaper Staff** A school newspaper staff is composed of 5 seniors, 4 juniors, 5 sophomores, and 7 freshmen. If four staff members are chosen at random for a publicity photo, what is the probability that there will be 1 student from each class?

18. **Missing Pages from Books** A bookstore owner examines 5 books from each lot of 25 to check for missing pages. If he finds at least 2 books with missing pages, the entire lot is returned. If, indeed, there are 5 books with missing pages, find the probability that the lot will be returned.

19. **Types of CDs** A CD case contains 10 jazz albums, 4 classical music albums, and 2 soundtracks. Choose 3 at random to put into a CD changer. What is the probability of selecting 2 jazz albums and 1 classical music album?

20. **Defective Computer Keyboards** A shipment of 24 computer keyboards is rejected if 4 are checked for defects and at least 1 is found to be defective. Find the probability that the shipment will be returned if there are actually 6 defective keyboards.

21. **Defective Devices** A shipment of 24 hand-held global positioning system (GPS) devices is rejected if 3 are checked for defects and at least 1 is found to be defective. Find the probability that the shipment will be returned if 6 GPS devices are defective.

Summary ›

Many variables have special probability distributions. This chapter presented several of the most common probability distributions, including the binomial distribution, the multinomial distribution, the Poisson distribution, and the hypergeometric distribution.

　　The binomial distribution is used when there are only two outcomes for an experiment, there are a fixed number of trials, the probability is the same for each trial, and the outcomes are independent of one another. The multinomial distribution is an extension of the binomial distribution and is used when there are three or more outcomes for an experiment. The hypergeometric distribution is used when sampling is done without replacement. Finally, the Poisson distribution is used in special cases when independent events occur over a period of time, area, or volume.

　　A probability distribution can be graphed, and the mean, variance, and standard deviation can be found. The mathematical expectation can also be calculated for a probability distribution. Expectation is used in insurance and games of chance.

For step-by-step guidance on the use of Texas Instruments TI-83 Plus/TI-84 Plus programmable calculators, see Appendix E. For summary procedures for Minitab, SPSS, and Excel, please see the full version of Appendix E on *Connect*.

Important Terms »

binomial distribution 228

binomial experiment 228

discrete probability distribution 211

expected value 222

hypergeometric distribution 240

multinomial distribution 236

Poisson distribution 238

random variable 211

Important Formulas »

Formula for the mean of a probability distribution:

$$\mu = \Sigma X \cdot P(X)$$

Formulas for the variance and standard deviation of a probability distribution:

$$\sigma^2 = \Sigma[X^2 \cdot P(X)] - \mu^2$$
$$\sigma = \sqrt{\Sigma[X^2 \cdot P(X)] - \mu^2}$$

Formula for expected value:

$$E(X) = \Sigma X \cdot P(X)$$

Binomial probability formula:

$$P(X) = \frac{n!}{(n - X)!X!} \cdot p^X \cdot q^{n-X}$$

Formula for the mean of the binomial distribution:

$$\mu = n \cdot p$$

Formulas for the variance and standard deviation of the binomial distribution:

$$\sigma^2 = n \cdot p \cdot q \qquad \sigma = \sqrt{n \cdot p \cdot q}$$

Formula for the multinomial distribution:

$$P(X) = \frac{n!}{X_1! \cdot X_2! \cdots X_k!} \cdot p_1^{X_1} \cdot p_2^{X_2} \cdots p_k^{X_k}$$

Formula for the Poisson distribution:

$$P(X; \lambda) = \frac{e^{-\lambda}\lambda^x}{X!} \quad \text{where } X = 0, 1, 2, \cdots$$

Formula for the hypergeometric distribution:

$$P(X) = \frac{{}_aC_X \cdot {}_bC_{n-X}}{{}_{a+b}C_n}$$

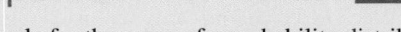

Review Exercises »

For Exercises 1 through 3, determine whether the distribution represents a probability distribution. If it does not, state why.

1.

X	1	2	3	4	5
P(X)	$\frac{1}{10}$	$\frac{3}{10}$	$\frac{1}{10}$	$\frac{2}{10}$	$\frac{3}{10}$

2.

X	10	20	30
P(X)	0.1	0.4	0.3

3.

X	8	12	16	20
P(X)	$\frac{5}{6}$	$\frac{1}{12}$	$\frac{1}{12}$	$\frac{1}{12}$

4. Emergency Calls The number of emergency calls a local police department receives per 24-hour period is distributed as shown here. Construct a graph for the data.

Number of calls X	10	11	12	13	14
Probability P(X)	0.02	0.12	0.40	0.31	0.15

5. Credit Cards A large retail company encourages its employees to get customers to apply for the store credit card. Below is the distribution for the number of credit card applications received per employee for an 8-hour shift.

X	0	1	2	3	4	5
P(X)	0.27	0.28	0.20	0.15	0.08	0.02

a. What is the probability that an employee will get 2 or 3 applications during any given shift?
b. Find the mean, variance, and standard deviation for this probability distribution.

6. Coins in a Box A box contains 5 pennies, 3 dimes, 1 quarter, and 1 loonie. Construct a probability distribution and draw a graph for the data.

7. Tie Purchases At Tyler's Tie Shop, Tyler found the probabilities that a customer will buy 0, 1, 2, 3, or 4 ties, as shown. Construct a graph for the distribution.

Number of ties X	0	1	2	3	4
Probability P(X)	0.30	0.50	0.10	0.08	0.02

8. Bank Customers A bank has a drive-through service. The number of customers arriving during a 15-minute period is distributed as shown. Find the mean, variance, and standard deviation for the distribution.

Number of customers X	0	1	2	3	4
Probability P(X)	0.12	0.20	0.31	0.25	0.12

9. Museum Visitors At a small community museum, the number of visitors per hour during the day has the distribution shown here. Find the mean, variance, and standard deviation for the data.

Number of visitors X	13	14	15	16	17
Probability P(X)	0.12	0.15	0.29	0.25	0.19

10. Cans of Paint Purchased During a recent paint sale at Corner Hardware, the number of cans of paint purchased was distributed as shown. Find the mean, variance, and standard deviation of the distribution.

Number of cans X	1	2	3	4	5
Probability P(X)	0.42	0.27	0.15	0.10	0.06

11. Inquiries Received The number of inquiries received per day for a university catalogue is distributed as shown. Find the mean, variance, and standard deviation for the data.

Number of inquiries X	22	23	24	25	26	27
Probability P(X)	0.08	0.19	0.36	0.25	0.07	0.05

12. Outdoor Regatta A producer plans an outdoor regatta for May 3. The cost of the regatta is $8000. This includes advertising, security, printing tickets, entertainment, etc. The producer plans to make $15,000 profit if all goes well. However, if it rains, the regatta will have to be cancelled. According to the weather report, the probability of rain is 0.3. Find the producer's expected profit.

13. Card Game A game is set up as follows: All the diamonds are removed from a deck of cards, and these 13 cards are placed in a bag. The cards are mixed up, and then one card is chosen at random (and then replaced). The player wins according to the following rules.

If the ace is drawn, the player loses $20.
If a face card is drawn, the player wins $10.
If any other card (2–10) is drawn, the player wins $2.

How much should be charged to play this game in order for it to be fair?

14. Commuter Train Rides If 30% of all commuters ride the train to work, find the probability that if 10 workers are selected, 5 will ride the train.

15. Car Drivers If 90% of all people between the ages of 30 and 50 drive a car, find these probabilities for a sample of 20 people in that age group.

a. Exactly 20 drive a car.
b. At least 15 drive a car.
c. At most 15 drive a car.

16. Internet Access via Cellphone Fourteen percent of cellphone users use their cellphones to access the Internet. In a random sample of 10 cellphone users, what is the probability that exactly 2 have used their phones to access the Internet? More than 2?

Source: Infoplease: www.infoplease.com.

17. **Drug Calculation Test** If 75% of nursing students are able to pass a drug calculation test, find the mean, variance, and standard deviation of the number of students who pass the test in a sample of 180 nursing students.

18. **Attendance at Meetings** A club has 225 members. If there is a 70% attendance rate per meeting, find the mean, variance, and standard deviation of the number of people who will be present at each meeting.

19. **Death Penalty** Amnesty International reports that 69% of Canadians moderately or strongly support the return of the death penalty, abolished by Parliament in 1976. If 7 Canadians are selected at random, what is the probability that at least 3 will support the return of capital punishment?
    Source: www.amnesty.ca.

20. **Home Heating Fuel** A Statistics Canada article on home heating and the environment estimates that 50% of Canadian households rely on natural gas heating, 33% use electricity, 13% heat with oil furnaces, and about 4% use wood-burning heaters. If a random sample of 500 Canadian households was selected, find the mean, variance, and standard deviation for each category of heating fuel.
    Source: Statistics Canada.

21. **Cigarette Smokers** Health Canada reports that 1 in 5 Canadians, aged 15 years of age and older, smokes cigarettes. If a random sample of 20 Canadians aged 15 years and older is selected, find the probability that exactly 5 are current smokers.
    Source: Health Canada.

22. **Youth Sex Survey** A survey on youth sexual attitudes points to abstinence as being preferential to sex. The report indicates that 56% of Canadian youths have never had sex. If 10 Canadian youths are selected at random, find the probability that exactly 5 have never had sex.
    Source: Macleans.ca, "Youth Survey: Teen Girls in Charge," Cathy Gulli, April 10, 2009.

23. **(Opt.) Insurance Claim Errors** The probabilities that a person will make 0, 1, 2, and 3 errors on an insurance claim are 0.70, 0.20, 0.08, and 0.02, respectively. If 20 claims are selected, find the probability that 12 will contain no errors, 4 will contain 1 error, 3 will contain 2 errors, and 1 will contain 3 errors.

24. **(Opt.) DVD Player Defects** Before a DVD player leaves the factory, it is given a quality-control check. The probabilities that a DVD player contains 0, 1, or 2 defects are 0.90, 0.06, and 0.04, respectively. In a sample of 12 players, find the probability that 8 have 0 defects, 3 have 1 defect, and 1 has 2 defects.

25. **(Opt.) Christmas Light Display** In a Christmas display, the probability that all lights are the same colour is 0.50; that 2 colours are used is 0.40; and that 3 or more colours are used is 0.10. If a sample of 10 displays is selected, find the probability that 5 have only 1 colour of light, 3 have 2 colours, and 2 have 3 or more colours.

26. **(Opt.) Genetic Trait** If 4% of the population carries a certain genetic trait, find the probability that in a sample of 100 people, there are exactly 8 people who have the trait. Assume the distribution is approximately Poisson.

27. **(Opt.) Computer Help Line** Computer Help Line receives, on the average, 6 calls per hour asking for assistance. The distribution is Poisson. For any randomly selected hour, find the probability that the company will receive

    a. At least 6 calls.
    b. 4 or more calls.
    c. At most 5 calls.

28. **(Opt.) Boating Accidents** The number of boating accidents on Lake Emilie follows a Poisson distribution. The probability of an accident is 0.003. If there are 1000 boats on the lake during a summer month, find the probability that there will be 6 accidents.

29. **(Opt.) Selecting Cards** If 5 cards are drawn from a deck, find the probability that 2 will be hearts.

30. **(Opt.) Used-Car Sales** Of the 50 automobiles in a used-car lot, 10 are white. If 5 automobiles are selected to be sold at an auction, find the probability that exactly 2 will be white.

31. **(Opt.) Food Bank Donations** At a food bank, a case of donated items contains 10 cans of soup, 8 cans of vegetables, and 8 cans of fruit. If 3 cans are selected at random to distribute, find the probability of getting 1 can of vegetables and 2 cans of fruit.

Statistics Today

Is Pooling Worthwhile?–Revisited

In the case of the pooled sample, the probability that only one test will be needed can be determined by using the binomial distribution. The question being asked is: In a sample of 15 individuals, what is the probability that no individual will have the disease? Hence, $n = 15$, $p = 0.05$, and $X = 0$. From Table B in Appendix C, the probability is that 0.463, or 46%, of the time, only one test will be needed. For screening purposes, then, pooling samples in this case would save considerable time, money, and effort as opposed to testing every individual in the population.

Chapter Quiz

Determine whether each statement is true or false. If the statement is false, explain why.

1. The expected value of a random variable can be thought of as a long-run average.

2. The number of courses a student is taking this semester is an example of a continuous random variable.

3. When the multinomial distribution is used, the outcomes must be dependent.

4. A binomial experiment has a fixed number of trials.

Complete these statements with the best answer.

5. Random variable values are determined by _____.

6. The mean for a binomial variable can be found by using the formula _____.

7. One requirement for a probability distribution is that the sum of all the events in the sample space must equal _____.

Select the best answer.

8. What is the sum of the probabilities of all outcomes in a probability distribution?

   a. 0
   b. $\frac{1}{2}$
   c. 1
   d. It cannot be determined.

9. How many outcomes are there in a binomial experiment?

   a. 0   *c.* 2
   b. 1   *d.* It varies.

10. The number of plants growing in a specific area can be approximated by what distribution?

   a. Binomial
   b. Multinomial
   c. Hypergeometric
   d. Poisson

For questions 11 through 14, determine if the distribution represents a probability distribution. If not, state why.

11.

X	1	2	3	4	5
P(X)	$\frac{1}{7}$	$\frac{2}{7}$	$\frac{2}{7}$	$\frac{3}{7}$	$\frac{2}{7}$

12.

X	3	6	9	12	15
P(X)	0.3	0.5	0.1	0.08	0.02

13.

X	50	75	100
P(X)	0.5	0.2	0.3

14.

X	4	8	12	16
P(X)	$\frac{1}{6}$	$\frac{3}{12}$	$\frac{1}{2}$	$\frac{1}{12}$

15. **Fire Department Calls** The number of fire calls the Conestoga Valley Fire Department receives per day is distributed as follows:

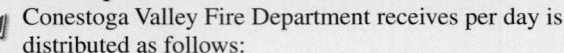

Number X	5	6	7	8	9
Probability P(X)	0.28	0.32	0.09	0.21	0.10

Construct a graph for the data.

16. **Telephones per Household** A study was conducted to determine the number of telephones each household has. The data are shown here.

Number of telephones	0	1	2	3	4
Frequency	2	30	48	13	7

Construct a probability distribution and draw a graph for the data.

17. **CD Purchases** During a recent CD sale at Matt's Music Store, the number of CDs customers purchased was distributed as follows:

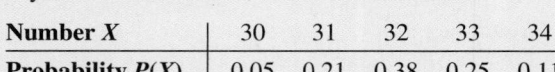

Number X	0	1	2	3	4
Probability P(X)	0.10	0.23	0.31	0.27	0.09

Find the mean, variance, and standard deviation of the distribution.

18. **Crisis Hot Line Calls** The number of calls received per day at a crisis hot line is distributed as follows:

Number X	30	31	32	33	34
Probability P(X)	0.05	0.21	0.38	0.25	0.11

Find the mean, variance, and standard deviation of the distribution.

19. **Selecting a Card** There are 6 playing cards placed face down in a box. They are the 4 of diamonds, the 5 of hearts, the 2 of clubs, the 10 of spades, the 3 of diamonds, and the 7 of hearts. A person selects a card. Find the expected value of the draw.

20. **Selecting a Card** A person selects a card from an ordinary deck of cards. If it is a black card, she wins $2. If it is a red card between or including 3 and 7, she wins $10. If it is a red face card, she wins $25; and if it is a black jack, she wins an extra $100. Find the expectation of the game.

21. **Carpooling** If 40% of all commuters ride to work in carpools, find the probability that if 8 workers are selected, 5 will ride in carpools.

22. **Employed Women** If 60% of all women are employed outside the home, find the probability that in a sample of 20 women,

   a. Exactly 15 are employed outside the home.
   b. At least 10 are employed outside the home.
   c. At most 5 are not employed outside the home.

23. **Driver's Exam** If 80% of the applicants are able to pass a driver's proficiency road test, find the mean, variance, and standard deviation of the number of people who pass the test in a sample of 300 applicants.

24. **Class Attendance** A history class has 75 members. If there is a 12% absentee rate per class meeting, find the mean, variance, and standard deviation of the number of students who will be absent from each class.

25. **Income Tax Errors** The probability that a person will make 0, 1, 2, or 3 errors on his or her income tax return is 0.50, 0.30, 0.15, and 0.05, respectively. If 30 claims are selected, find the probability that 15 will contain zero errors, 8 will contain one error, 5 will contain two errors, and 2 will contain three errors.

26. **Quality-Control Check** Before a television set leaves the factory, it is given a quality-control check. The probability that a television contains zero, one, or two defects is 0.88, 0.08, and 0.04, respectively. In a sample of 16 televisions, find the probability that 9 will have no defects, 4 will have one defect, and 3 will have two defects.

27. **Bowling Team Uniforms** Among the teams in a bowling league, the probability that the uniforms are all one colour is 0.45, that two colours are used is 0.35, and that three or more colours are used is 0.20. If a sample of 12 uniforms is selected, find the probability that 5 contain only one colour, 4 contain two colours, and 3 contain three or more colours.

28. **Elm Trees** If 8% of the population of trees are elm trees, find the probability that in a sample of 100 trees, there are exactly 6 elm trees. Assume the distribution is approximately Poisson.

29. **Sports Scores Hot Line Calls** A sports scores hot line receives, on the average, 8 calls per hour requesting the latest sports scores. The distribution is Poisson in nature. For any randomly selected hour, find the probability that the company will receive

    a. At least 8 calls
    b. 3 or more calls
    c. At most 7 calls

30. **Raincoat Colours** There are 48 raincoats for sale at a local men's clothing store. Twelve are black. If 6 raincoats are selected to be marked down, find the probability that exactly 3 will be black.

31. **Youth Group Officers** A youth group has 8 boys and 6 girls. If a slate of 4 officers is selected, find the probability that exactly

    a. 3 are girls.
    b. 2 are girls.
    c. 4 are boys.

Critical Thinking Challenges

1. **Lottery Numbers** The Ontario Lottery Corporation sells Pick 4, a game of chance in which 4 numbers are selected from a field of 0 to 9, with replacement. The top prize is awarded if the 4 digits on the ticket match the 4 digits randomly selected, in the same order. If one ticket is purchased, find the probability of winning the top prize.
   Source: Ontario Lottery Corporation.

2. **Lottery Numbers** In the Pick 4 game, a $1 ticket will earn a top prize of $5000 if the 4 digits on the ticket match the winning selection in the order drawn. What is the expected value of winning? Is it worth it?
   Source: Ontario Lottery Corporation.

3. **Lottery Numbers** If you play the same 4 numbers in the Pick 4 daily game, in how many years and days would you expect your first win, assuming that you have average luck?
   Source: Ontario Lottery Corporation.

4. **Chuck-A-Luck Game** In the game Chuck-a-Luck, three dice are rolled. A player bets a certain amount (say $1.00) on a number from 1 to 6. If the number appears on one die, the person wins $1.00. If it appears on two dice, the person wins $2.00, and if it appears on all three dice, the person wins $3.00. What are the chances of winning $1.00? $2.00? $3.00?

5. **Chuck-A-Luck Game** What is the expected value of the game of Chuck-a-Luck if a player bets $1.00 on one number?

Data Projects

Where appropriate, use Minitab, SPSS, TI-83 Plus, TI-84 Plus, Excel, or a computer program of your choice to complete the following exercises.

1. **Business and Finance** Assume that a life insurance company would like to make a profit of $250 on a $100,000 policy sold to a person whose probability of surviving the year is 0.9985. What premium should the company charge the customer? If the company would like to make a $250 profit on a $100,000 policy at a premium of $500, what is the lowest life expectancy it should accept for a customer?

2. **Sports and Leisure** Baseball, hockey, and basketball all use a seven-game series to determine the championship winners. Find the probability that with two evenly matched teams, a champion will be found in 4 games. Repeat for 5, 6, and 7 games. Look at the historical

results for the three sports. How do the actual results compare to the theoretical?

3. **Technology** Use your most recent itemized phone bill for the data in this problem. Assume that incoming and outgoing calls are equal in the population. (Why is this a reasonable assumption?) This means assume $p = 0.5$. For the number of calls you made last month, what would be the mean number of outgoing calls in a random selection of calls? Also, compute the standard deviation. Was the number of outgoing calls you made an unusual amount, given the above? In a selection of 12 calls, what is the probability that less than 3 were outgoing?

4. **Health and Wellness** Use Canadian Blood Services data to determine the percentage of the population with an Rh factor that is positive (A+, B+, AB+, or O+ blood types). Use that value for p. How many students

in your class have a positive Rh factor? Is this an unusual amount?

5. **Politics and Economics** Find out what percentage of citizens in your province or territory is registered to vote. Assuming that this is a binomial variable, what would be the mean number of registered voters in a random group of citizens with a sample size equal to the number of students in your class? Also determine the standard deviation. How many students in your class are registered to vote? Is this an unusual number, given the above?

6. **Your Class** Have each student in class toss 4 coins on a desk, and note how many heads are showing. Create a frequency table displaying the results. Compare the frequency table to the theoretical probability distribution for the outcome when 4 coins are tossed. Find the mean for the frequency table. How does it compare with the mean for the probability distribution?

Answers to Applying the Concepts »

Section 5–1 Dropping College/University Courses

1. The random variable under study is the reason for dropping a college/university course.

2. A total of 144 people were in the study.

3. The complete table is as follows:

Reason for dropping a college/university course	Frequency	Percentage
Too difficult	45	31.25
Illness	40	27.78
Change in work schedule	20	13.89
Change of major	14	9.72
Family-related problems	9	6.25
Money	7	4.86
Miscellaneous	6	4.17
No meaningful reason	3	2.08

4. The probability that a student will drop a class because of illness is about 28%. The probability that a student will drop a class because of money is about 5%. The probability that a student will drop a class because of a change of major is about 10%.

5. The information is not itself a probability distribution, but it can be used as one.

6. The categories are not necessarily mutually exclusive, but we treated them as such in computing the probabilities.

7. The categories are not independent.

8. The categories are exhaustive.

9. Since all the probabilities are between 0 and 1, inclusive, and the probabilities sum to 1, the requirements for a discrete probability distribution are met.

Section 5–2 Expected Value

1. The expected value is the mean in a discrete probability distribution.

2. We would expect variation from the expected value of 3.

3. Answers will vary. One possible answer is that pregnant mothers in that area might be overly concerned upon hearing that the number of cases of kidney problems in newborns was nearly 4 times what was usually expected. Other mothers (particularly those who had taken a statistics course!) might ask for more information about the claim.

4. Answers will vary. One possible answer is that it does seem unlikely to have 11 newborns with kidney problems when we expect only 3 newborns to have kidney problems.

5. The public might better be informed by percentages or rates (e.g., rate per 1000 newborns).

6. The increase of eight babies born with kidney problems represents a 0.32% increase (less than $\frac{1}{2}$ of 1%).

7. Answers will vary. One possible answer is that the percentage increase does not seem to be something to be overly concerned about.

Section 5–3 Unsanitary Restaurants

1. The probability of eating at 3 restaurants with unsanitary conditions out of the 10 restaurants is 0.18792.

2. The probability of eating at 4 or 5 restaurants with unsanitary conditions out of the 10 restaurants is $0.24665 + 0.22199 = 0.46864$.

3. To find this probability, you could add the probabilities for eating at 1, 2, ... , 10 unsanitary restaurants. An easier

way to compute the probability is to subtract the probability of eating at no unsanitary restaurants from 1 (using the complement rule).

4. The highest probability for this distribution is 4, but the expected number of unsanitary restaurants that you would eat at is $10 \cdot \frac{3}{7} = 4.3$.

5. The standard deviation for this distribution is

$$\sqrt{10\left(\tfrac{3}{7}\right)\left(\tfrac{4}{7}\right)} = 1.56$$

6. This is a binomial distribution. We have two possible outcomes: "success" is eating in an unsanitary restaurant; "failure" is eating in a sanitary restaurant. The probability that one restaurant is unsanitary is independent of the probability that any other restaurant is unsanitary. The probability that a restaurant is unsanitary remains constant at $\frac{3}{7}$. And we are looking at the number of unsanitary restaurants that we eat at out of 10 "trials."

7. The likelihood of success will vary from situation to situation. Just because we have two possible outcomes, this does not mean that each outcome occurs with probability 0.50.

Section 5–4 Rockets and Targets

1. The theoretical values for the number of hits are

Hits	0	1	2	3	4	5
Regions	227.5	211.3	98.2	30.4	7.1	1.3

2. The actual values are very close to the theoretical values.

3. Since the actual values are close to the theoretical values, it does appear that the rockets were fired at random.

Chapter 6

The Normal Distribution

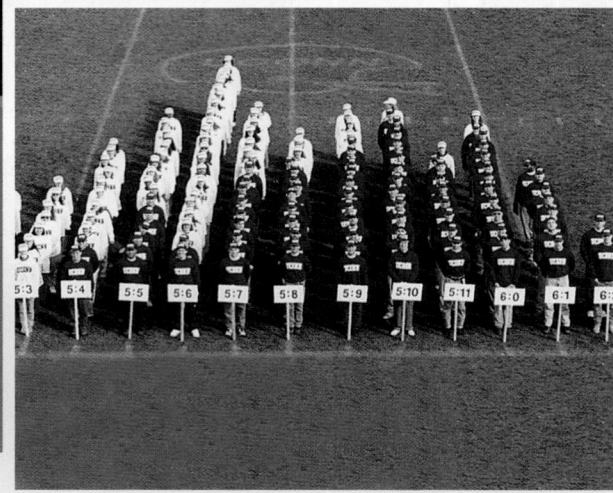

Statistics Today

What Is Normal?

Medical researchers have determined so-called normal intervals for a person's blood pressure, cholesterol level, body temperature, and the like. For example, the normal range of systolic blood pressure is 110 to 140 millimetres of mercury (mmHg). The normal interval for a person's total cholesterol is 5.2 to 6.2 millimoles per litre (mmol/L). The normal core body temperature for healthy adults ranges from 36.1°C to 37.8°C. By measuring these variables, a physician can determine if a patient's vital statistics are within the normal interval or if some type of treatment is needed to correct a condition and avoid future illnesses. The question then is, How does one determine the so-called normal intervals? See Statistics Today—Revisited, page 296.

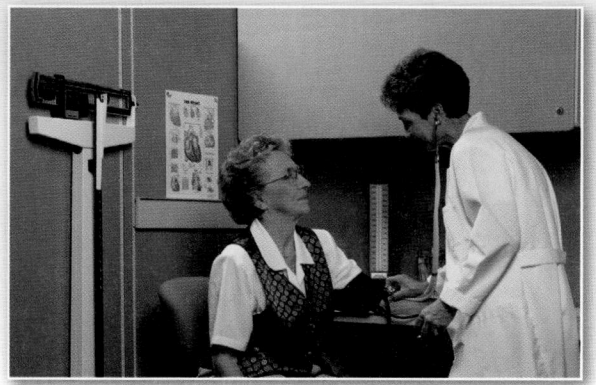

In this chapter, you will learn how researchers determine normal intervals for specific medical tests by using a normal distribution. You will see how the same methods are used to determine the lifetimes of batteries, the strength of ropes, and many other traits.

Introduction >

Random variables can be either discrete or continuous. Discrete variables and their distributions were explained in Chapter 5. Recall that a discrete variable cannot assume all values between any two given values of the variables. On the other hand, a continuous variable can assume all values between any two given values of the variables. Examples of continuous variables are the heights of adult men, body temperatures of rats, and cholesterol levels of adults. Many continuous variables, such as the examples just mentioned, have distributions that are bell-shaped, and these are called *approximately normally distributed variables.* For example, if a researcher selects a random sample of 100 adult women, measures their heights, and constructs a histogram, the researcher gets a graph similar to the one shown in Figure 6–1(a). Now, if the researcher increases the sample size and decreases the width of the classes, the histograms will look like the ones shown in Figures 6–1(b) and (c). Finally, if it were possible to measure exactly the heights of all adult females in Canada and plot them, the histogram would very closely approximate a continuous curve referred to as the *normal distribution curve,* shown in Figure 6–1(d). This distribution is a *bell curve,* also known as a *Gaussian distribution,* named for the German mathematician Carl Friedrich Gauss (1777–1855), who derived its equation.

No variable fits a normal distribution perfectly, since a normal distribution is a theoretical distribution. However, a normal distribution can be used to describe many variables, because the deviations from a normal distribution are very small. This concept will be explained further in Section 6–1.

When the data values are evenly distributed about the mean, a distribution is said to be a **symmetric distribution.** (A normal distribution is symmetric.) Figure 6–2(a) shows a symmetric distribution. When the majority of the data values fall to the left or right of the mean, the distribution is said to be *skewed.* When the majority of the data

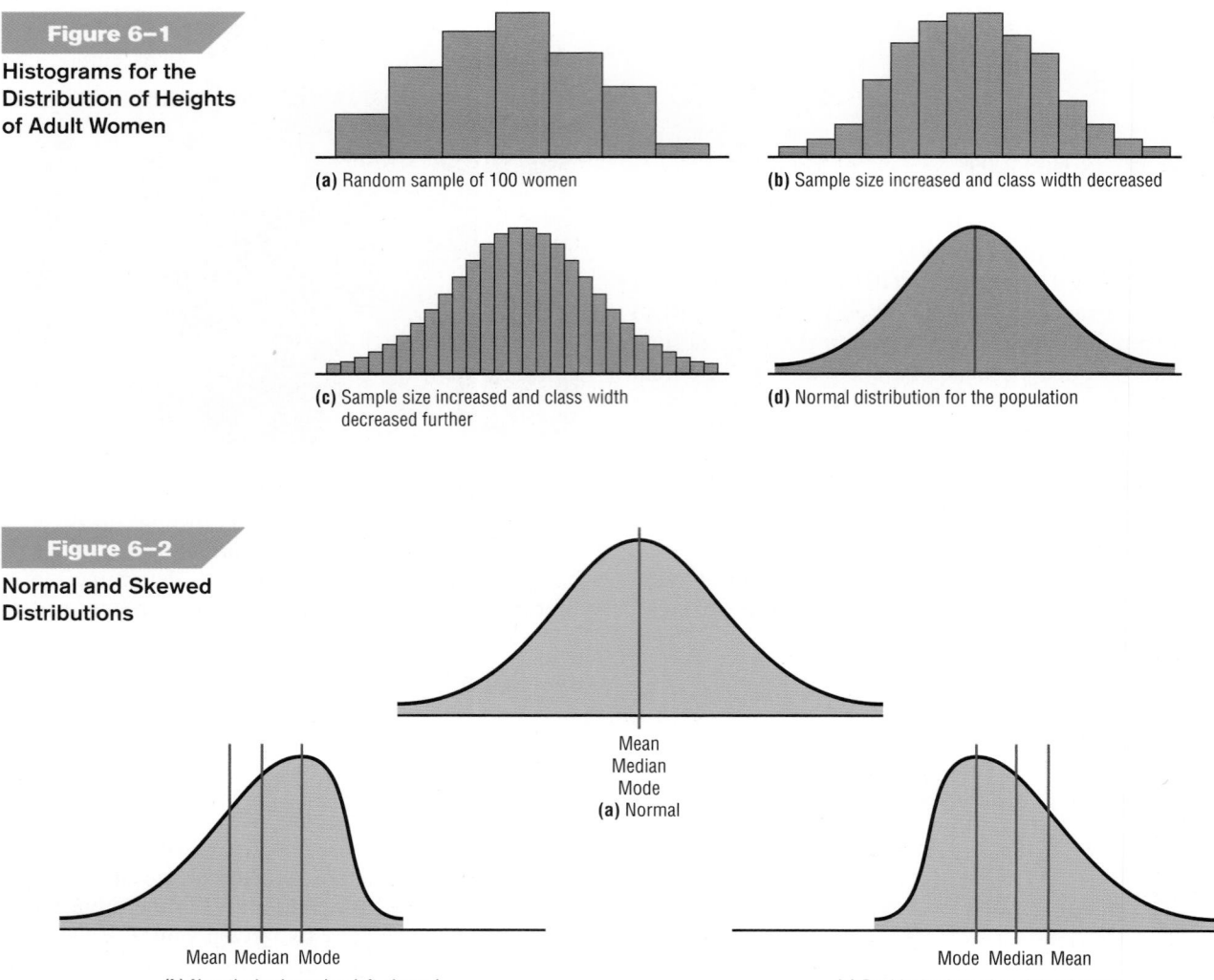

Figure 6–1

Histograms for the Distribution of Heights of Adult Women

(a) Random sample of 100 women

(b) Sample size increased and class width decreased

(c) Sample size increased and class width decreased further

(d) Normal distribution for the population

Figure 6–2

Normal and Skewed Distributions

Mean
Median
Mode
(a) Normal

Mean Median Mode
(b) Negatively skewed or left-skewed

Mode Median Mean
(c) Positively skewed or right-skewed

values fall to the right of the mean, the distribution is said to be a **negatively or left-skewed distribution.** Typically the mean is to the left of the median, and the mean and the median are to the left of the mode. See Figure 6–2(b). When the majority of the data values fall to the left of the mean, a distribution is said to be a **positively or right-skewed distribution.** Generally the mean falls to the right of the median, and both the mean and the median fall to the right of the mode. See Figure 6–2(c).

The "tail" of the curve indicates the direction of skewness (right is positive, left negative). These distributions can be compared with the ones shown in Figure 3–1 on page 94. Both types follow the same principles.

This chapter will present the properties of a normal distribution and discuss its applications. Then a very important fact about a normal distribution called the *central limit theorem* will be explained. Finally, the chapter will explain how a normal distribution curve can be used as an approximation to other distributions, such as the binomial distribution. Since a binomial distribution is a discrete distribution, a correction for continuity may be employed when a normal distribution is used for its approximation.

6–1 | Normal Distributions ›

LO1

Identify distribution shapes and normal distribution properties, and find areas under the standard normal distribution, given various z scores.

Historical Note

The discovery of the equation for a normal distribution can be traced to three mathematicians. In 1733, the French mathematician Abraham DeMoivre derived an equation for a normal distribution based on the random variation of the number of heads appearing when a large number of coins were tossed. Not realizing any connection with the naturally occurring variables, he showed this formula to only a few friends. About 100 years later, two mathematicians, Pierre Laplace in France and Carl Gauss in Germany, derived the equation of the normal curve independently and without any knowledge of DeMoivre's work. In 1924, Karl Pearson found that DeMoivre had discovered the formula before Laplace or Gauss.

The *normal distribution curve* can be used to study many variables that are approximately normal. The equation to generate a normal, bell-shaped curve is derived using mathematical methods beyond the scope of an introductory statistics text. In applied statistics, tables or technology will be used to solve specific problems instead of equations.

The area under the normal curve is most important in determining statistical probabilities for continuous random variables located on the x axis. The height of the normal curve is not relevant for calculating probabilities using tables or technology. Subsequently the y axis is often omitted in the illustration of the normal curve.

The shape and position of a normal distribution curve depend on two parameters, the *mean* and *standard deviation*. This results in unique distributions for each normally distributed random variable. Figure 6–3(a) shows two normal distributions with the same mean but different standard deviations. The larger the standard deviation, the more dispersed, or spread out, the distribution is. Figure 6–3(b) shows two normal distributions with the same standard deviation but different means. These curves have the same shapes but are located at different positions on the x axis. Figure 6–3(c) shows two normal distributions with different means and different standard deviations affecting both position and shape.

> A **normal distribution** is a continuous, symmetric, bell-shaped distribution of a variable.

Properties of a Normal Distribution

The properties of a normal distribution, including those mentioned in the definition, are explained next.

Summary of the Properties of the Normal Distribution

1. A normal distribution is bell-shaped with the two tails continuing indefinitely in both directions, never touching the x axis.
2. The normal curve is a continuous unimodal distribution that is symmetric about the centre—mean, median, and mode.
3. The total area under the normal distribution curve is equal to 1 or 100%.

Figure 6–3

Shapes of Normal Distributions

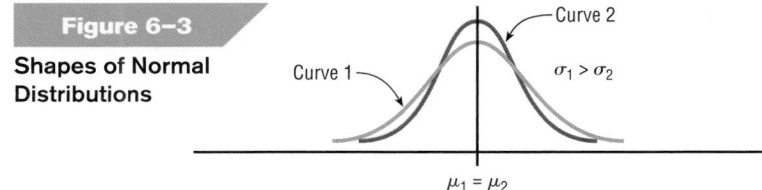

(a) Same means but different standard deviations

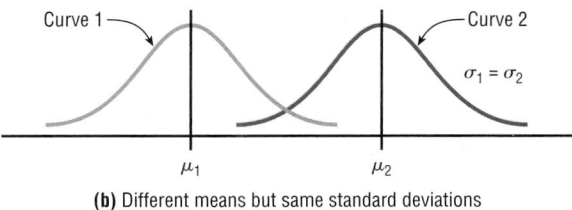

(b) Different means but same standard deviations

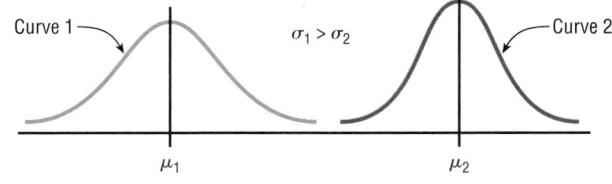

(c) Different means and different standard deviations

Empirical Rule and Areas under the Normal Curve

Section 3–2 discussed the *empirical rule* for bell-shaped data distributions. Using empirical-cal rule methods and normal distribution properties, areas under the normal curve within 1, 2, and 3 standard deviations (σ) of the population mean (μ), can be determined. Refer to Figure 6–4. *Note:* Areas above and below ± 3 standard deviations from the mean are 0.13%, respectively.

Figure 6–4

Areas under a Normal Distribution Curve

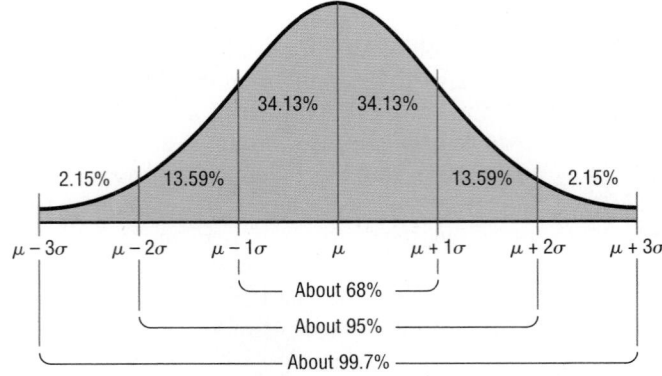

The following example will illustrate the relationship between the population mean and standard deviation and a normally distributed continuous random variable.

Example 6–1

Cellphone Battery Life

Assume that cellphone battery life is normally distributed with a mean of 4.5 hours and a standard deviation of 1.25 hours. Determine the life of the cellphone batteries within 0, ± 1, ± 2, and ± 3 standard deviations of the mean. Sketch, and then interpret your answer.

Solution

Given $\mu = 4.50$ hours and $\sigma = 1.25$ hours. Refer to Figure 6–4.

$$\mu - 3\sigma = 4.50 - 3(1.25) = 0.75$$
$$\mu - 2\sigma = 4.50 - 2(1.25) = 2.00$$
$$\mu - 1\sigma = 4.50 - 1(1.25) = 3.25$$
$$\mu - 0\sigma = 4.50 - 0(1.25) = 4.50$$
$$\mu + 1\sigma = 4.50 + 1(1.25) = 5.75$$
$$\mu + 2\sigma = 4.50 + 2(1.25) = 7.00$$
$$\mu + 3\sigma = 4.50 + 3(1.25) = 8.25$$

The *X* values that correspond to $-3, -2, -1, 0, +1, +2, +3$ standard deviations from the mean are illustrated in Figure 6–5.

Figure 6–5

Normal Distribution Curve ($\mu = 4.50, \sigma = 1.25$)

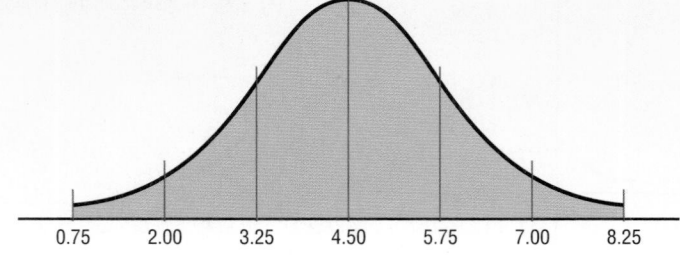

Referring to Figure 6–4, about 68% of the cellphone batteries will last between 3.25 and 5.75 hours, about 95% will last between 2.00 and 7.00 hours, and about 99.7% will last between 0.75 and 8.25 hours. These percentages also represent the probabilities that the cellphones will last in the range indicated.

The Standard Normal Distribution

Since each normally distributed variable has its own mean and standard deviation, as stated earlier, the shape and location of these curves will vary. In practical applications, then, one would require a table of areas under the curve for each variable. To simplify this situation, statisticians use the *standard normal distribution*.

> The **standard normal distribution** is a normal distribution with a mean of 0 and a standard deviation of 1.

The standard normal distribution as shown in Figure 6–6 should be compared with the areas under the normal distribution curve in Figure 6–4. The values under the curve indicate the proportion of area in each section. For example, the area between the mean and 1 standard deviation above the mean is about 0.3413, or 34.13%. In other words, if continuous data are normally distributed, there is a probability of 0.3413 that a data value will fall between the mean and 1 standard deviation above the mean.

Figure 6–6

Standard Normal Distribution

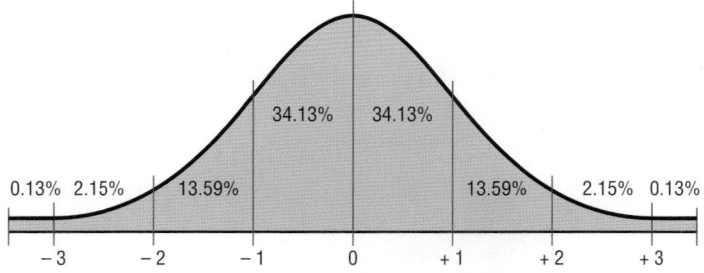

Formula for Standard Score

The *standard score* indicates the number of standard deviations that a data value is located above (positive z score) or below (negative z score) the mean. To convert a continuous random variable X to a standard score z, use the following formula.

$$z = \frac{X - \mu}{\sigma}$$

z = standard score
X = continuous random variable or X value
μ = population mean
σ = population standard deviation

Example 6–2

Test Scores

A student scored 85 on a statistics test with a test mean of 67 and a standard deviation of 9. Assuming that the test is normally distributed, convert the test score to a standard score. Interpret.

Solution

Given $X = 85$, $\mu = 67$, $\sigma = 9$, substitute into the standard score formula.

$$z = \frac{X - \mu}{\sigma} = \frac{85 - 67}{9} = 2.0$$

The student score of 85 is 2.0 standard deviations above the mean of 67. Also, approximately 47.72% (34.13% + 13.59%) of all scores fall between the mean of 67 and the score of 85. Another interpretation would be the probability that a student scores between 67 and 85 on the statistics test is 0.4772.

A few practical applications of the standard normal distribution method include:

- Locating the cutoff point for admission into a graduate program of study
- Determining the percentage of women who weigh between 50 and 60 kilograms
- Finding the probability that a cellphone battery will last longer than 4.5 hours

The next section will focus on procedures to find percentages and probabilities for continuous random variables using standard score tables and areas under the normal distribution curve. Additional applications of the normal distribution using X values will be shown in Section 6–2.

Finding Areas under the Standard Normal Distribution Curve

For the solution of problems using the standard normal distribution, the following procedure will provide a useful guideline.

Step 1   Sketch and label the normal curve shading the desired area.

Step 2   Look up the cumulative area to the left of each z score in the sketch using Table E–1, Negative z Scores, and Table E–2, Positive z Scores, in Appendix C.

Step 3   If necessary, perform the appropriate operation to obtain the desired area.

Rounding Areas

Tables E–1 and E–2 display the z scores rounded to one decimal place and the probabilities rounded to four decimal places. If converting area to a percentage, round to two decimal places.

Interesting Fact

Bell-shaped distributions occurred quite often in early coin-tossing and die-rolling experiments.

| Example 6–3 | **Area to the Left of z** |

Find the area under the standard normal distribution curve to the left of $z = 1.25$.

Solution

Sketch the curve and represent the area as shown in Figure 6–7.

Figure 6–7

Area under the Standard Normal Distribution Curve for Example 6–3

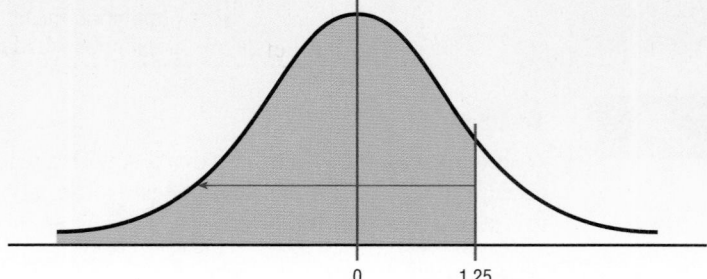

Refer to Table E–2, Positive z Scores, in Appendix C, which indicates the cumulative area to the **left** of the z score. In the column labelled z to $z = 1.2$, look to the right of the row labelled z to $z = 0.05$. Read to the right of $z = 1.2$ and below $z = 0.05$ and locate where they intersect: 0.8944, which represents the cumulative area to the **left** of $z = 1.25$. Refer to Figure 6–8. Therefore, the desired area is 0.8944, or 89.44%.

Figure 6–8

Using Table E–2 in Appendix C for Example 6–3

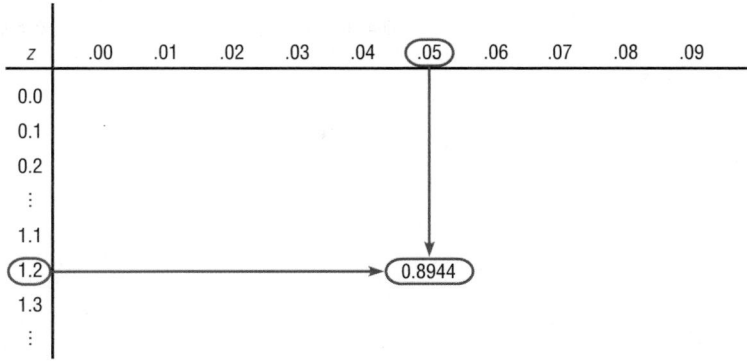

Example 6–4

Area to the Right of z

Find the area under the standard normal distribution curve to the right of $z = -2.33$.

Solution

Sketch the curve and represent the area as shown in Figure 6–9.

Figure 6–9

Area under the Standard Normal Distribution Curve for Example 6–4

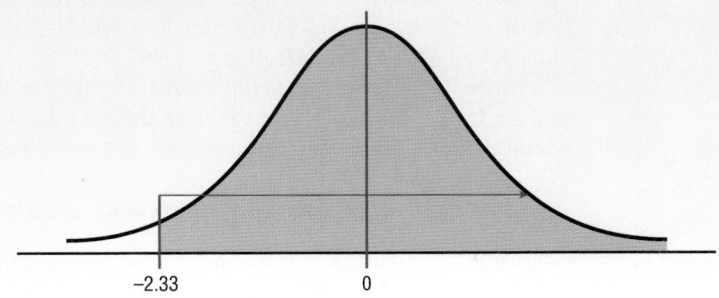

Refer to Table E–1, Negative z Scores, in Appendix C, which indicates the cumulative area to the **left** of the z score. In the column labelled z to $z = -2.3$, look to the right of the row labelled z to $z = 0.03$. Read to the right of $z = -2.3$ and below $z = 0.03$ and locate where they intersect: 0.0099, which represents the cumulative area to the **left** of $z = -2.33$. Refer to Figure 6–10.

Figure 6–10

Using Table E–1 in Appendix C for Example 6–4

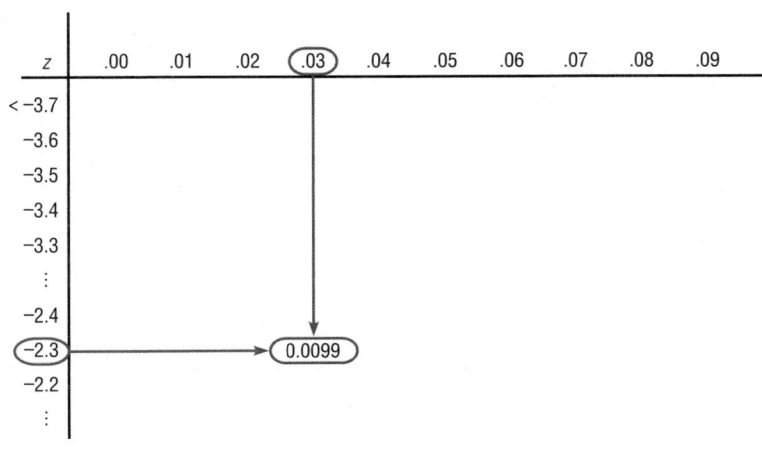

Since the area desired is to the **right** of $z = -2.33$ and the total area under the normal curve is 1.0, subtract 0.0099 from 1.0000 to obtain 0.9901. Therefore, the area to the right of $z = -2.33$ is 0.9901, or 99.01%.

Example 6–5

Area between z Scores

Find the area under the normal curve between $z = -0.67$ and $z = 1.96$.

Solution

Sketch the curve and shade the desired area as shown in Figure 6–11.

Figure 6–11

Area under the Standard Normal Distribution Curve for Example 6–5

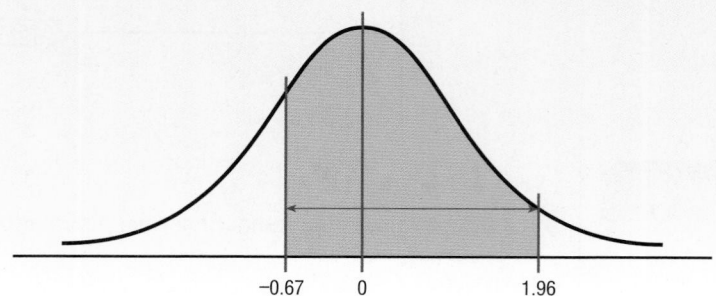

-0.67   0   1.96

Refer to Table E–1, Negative z Scores, in Appendix C. The cumulative area to the **left** of $z = -0.67$ is 0.2514. Refer to Table E–2, Positive z Scores, in Appendix C. The cumulative area to the **left** of $z = 1.96$ is 0.9750.

Since the area desired is **between** $z = -0.67$ and $z = 1.96$, subtract the cumulative area to the left of $z = -0.67$ (0.2514) from the cumulative area to the left of $z = 1.96$ (0.9750) to obtain 0.7236. Therefore, the area between $z = -0.67$ and $z = 1.96$ is 0.7236, or 72.36%.

A Normal Distribution Curve as a Probability Distribution Curve

A normal distribution curve can be used as a probability distribution curve for normally distributed variables. Recall that a normal distribution is a *continuous distribution,* as opposed to a discrete probability distribution, as explained in Chapter 5. The fact that it is continuous means that there are no gaps in the curve. In other words, for every z score on the x axis, there is a corresponding height, or frequency, value.

The area under the standard normal distribution curve can also be thought of as a probability. That is, if it were possible to select any z score at random, the probability of choosing one, say, between 0 and 2.00 would be the same as the area under the curve between 0 and 2.00. In this case, the area is 0.4772. Therefore, the probability of randomly selecting any z score between 0 and 2.00 is 0.4772. The problems involving probability are solved in the same manner as the previous examples involving areas in this section. Referring to Example 6–5, the area under the curve between $z = -0.67$ and $z = 1.96$ is 0.7236 can be written as the probability of randomly selecting a score between $z = -0.67$ and $z = 1.96$ is 0.7236.

Probability Notation

Problems involving continuous probability distributions are written using the following format.

$P(z > a)$ refers to the probability that a z score is greater than a.

$P(z < a)$ refers to the probability that a z score is less than a.

$P(a < z < b)$ refers to the probability the z score is between a and b.

Note: In continuous distributions, the probability of any exact z score is 0 since the area would be represented by a vertical line above the value. In theory, vertical lines have no area. Therefore, $P(a \leq z \leq b) = P(a < z < b)$.

| Example 6–6 | **Area between z Scores** |

Find the probability of randomly selecting a value with a z score that is between $z = 0.44$ and $z = 1.22$.

Solution

Sketch the curve and shade the desired area as shown in Figure 6–12.

Figure 6–12

Area under the Standard Normal Distribution Curve for Example 6–6

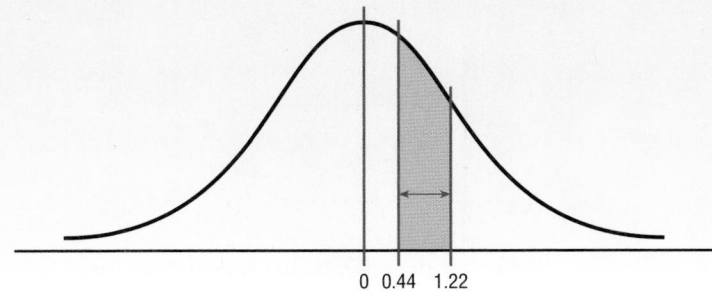

Refer to Table E–2, Positive z Scores, in Appendix C. Since the area desired is **between** $z = 0.44$ and $z = 1.22$, subtract the cumulative area to the **left** of $z = 0.44$ (0.6700) from the cumulative area to the **left** of $z = 1.22$ (0.8888) to obtain 0.2138.

Using probability notation, $P(0.44 < z < 1.22) = 0.2138$, or 21.38% of all values fall between 0.44 and 1.22 standard deviations above the mean.

Finding z Scores When Given Areas

Some statistical applications involve finding z scores when the area under the standard normal distribution curve is given. The procedure involves working from inside Table E–1, Negative z Scores (cumulative areas to the left from 0.001 to 0.5000) or Table E–2, Positive z Scores (cumulative areas to the left from 0.5000 to 0.9999) in Appendix C. Locate the desired area or the area **closest to** the desired area and then read the corresponding z score on the outside margins that intersect with this area. Refer to Example 6–7.

| Example 6–7 | **z Score for a Given Area** |

Find the z score that corresponds to a cumulative area to the left of 0.7500.

Solution

Sketch the curve and shade the desired area as shown in Figure 6–13.

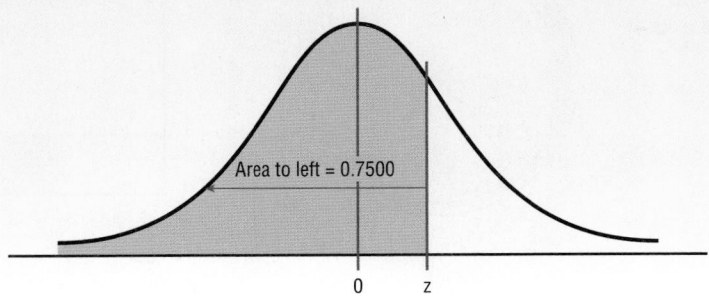

Area to left = 0.7500

Refer to Table E–2, Positive z Scores, in Appendix C as the cumulative areas to the left range from 0.5000 to 0.9999 and the desired area (0.7500) is in this range. Locate the area inside the table **closest to** 0.7500 (0.7486). Read out to the z scores in the margin above and to the left of 0.7486. The z score that intersects with 0.7486 is $z = 0.67$. Refer to Figure 6–13.

Figure 6–13

Using Table E–2 in Appendix C for Example 6–7

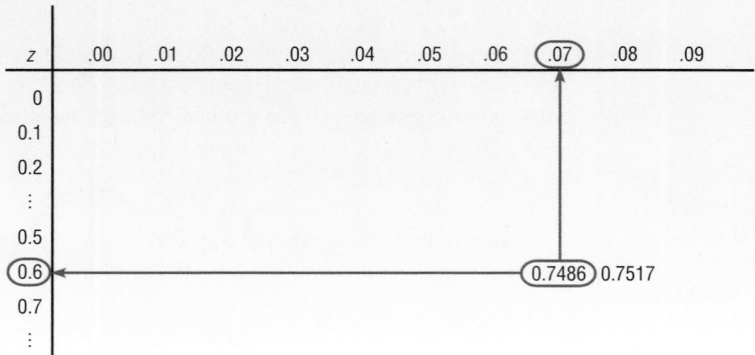

Note: If the desired area is **exactly** halfway between two areas in the table, find the average of the z scores that correspond to the areas below and above the desired area. For example, the area 0.9500 is **exactly** halfway between 0.9495 and 0.9505, which correspond to z scores of $z = 1.64$ and $z = 1.65$, respectively. Therefore, the average of these two z scores is $z = 1.645$. Also 0.9950 is equidistant from 0.9949 ($z = 2.57$) and 0.9951 ($z = 2.58$), therefore the average of $z = 2.575$ will be used. In a similar manner use z scores for 0.0500 ($z = -1.645$) and 0.0050 ($z = -2.575$). Refer to Tables E–1 and E–2 in Appendix C.

Area and Probability Relationship

The rationale for using an area under a continuous curve to determine a probability can be understood by considering the example of a watch that is powered by a battery. When the battery goes dead, what is the probability that the minute hand will stop somewhere between the numbers 2 and 5 on the face of the watch? In this case, the values of the variable constitute a continuous variable since the hour hand can stop anywhere on the dial's face between 0 and 12 (one revolution of the minute hand). Hence, the sample space can be considered to be 12 units long, and the distance between the numbers 2 and 5 is $5 - 2$, or 3 units. Hence, the probability that the minute hand stops on a number between 2 and 5 is $\frac{3}{12} = \frac{1}{4}$. See Figure 6–14(a).

Figure 6–14

The Relationship between Area and Probability

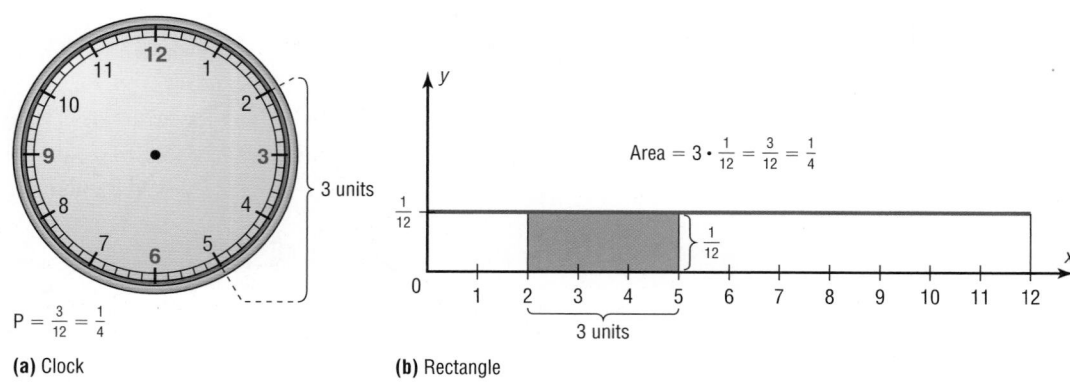

The problem could also be solved by using a graph of a continuous variable. Let us assume that since the watch can stop anytime at random, the values where the minute hand would land are spread evenly over the range of 0 through 12. The graph would then consist of a *continuous uniform distribution* with a range of 12 units. Now if we require the area under the curve to be 1 (like the area under the standard normal distribution), the height of the rectangle formed by the curve and the x axis would need to be $\frac{1}{12}$. The reason is that the area of a rectangle is equal to the base times the height. If the base is 12 units long, then the height would have to be $\frac{1}{12}$ since $12 \cdot \frac{1}{12} = 1$.

The area of the rectangle with a base from 2 through 5 would be $3 \cdot \frac{1}{12}$, or $\frac{1}{4}$. See Figure 6–14(b). Notice that the area of the small rectangle is the same as the probability found previously. Hence the area of this rectangle corresponds to the probability of this event. The same reasoning can be applied to the standard normal distribution curve shown in Example 6–6.

Finding the area under the standard normal distribution curve is the first step in solving a wide variety of practical applications in which the variables are normally distributed. Some of these applications will be presented in Section 6–2.

6–1 Applying the Concepts

Assessing Normality

Many times in statistics it is necessary to see if a distribution of data values is approximately normally distributed. There are special techniques that can be used. One technique is to draw a histogram for the data and see if it is approximately bell-shaped. (*Note:* It does not have to be exactly symmetric to be bell-shaped.)

The numbers of branches of the 50 top libraries are shown.

67	84	80	77	97	59	62	37	33	42
36	54	18	12	19	33	49	24	25	22
24	29	9	21	21	22	24	31	17	21
13	19	19	22	22	30	41	22	18	20
26	33	14	14	16	22	26	10	16	24

Source: The World Almanac and Book of Facts.

1. Construct a frequency distribution for the data.

2. Construct a histogram for the data.

3. Describe the shape of the histogram.

4. Based on your answer to question 3, do you feel that the distribution is approximately normal?

In addition to the histogram, distributions that are approximately normal have about 68% of the values fall within 1 standard deviation of the mean, about 95% of the data values fall within 2 standard deviations of the mean, and almost 100% of the data values fall within 3 standard deviations of the mean. (Refer back to Figure 6–4.)

5. Find the mean and standard deviation for the data.

6. What percentage of the data values fall within 1 standard deviation of the mean?

7. What percentage of the data values fall within 2 standard deviations of the mean?

8. What percentage of data values fall within 3 standard deviations of the mean?

9. How do your answers to questions 6, 7, and 8 compare to 68, 95, and 100%, respectively?

10. Does your answer help support the conclusion you reached in question 4? Explain.

(More techniques for assessing normality are explained in Section 6–2.)
See page 300 for the answers.

Exercises 6–1

1. What are the properties of a normal distribution?

2. Why is the standard normal distribution important in statistical analysis?

3. What is the total area under the standard normal distribution curve?

4. What percentage of the area falls below the mean? Above the mean?

5. About what percentage of the area under the normal distribution curve falls within 1 standard deviation above and below the mean? 2 standard deviations? 3 standard deviations?

For Exercises 6 through 25, find the area under the standard normal distribution curve.

6. Between $z = 0$ and $z = 1.66$

7. Between $z = 0$ and $z = 0.75$

8. Between $z = 0$ and $z = -0.35$

9. Between $z = 0$ and $z = -2.07$

10. To the right of $z = 1.10$

11. To the right of $z = 0.23$

12. To the left of $z = -0.48$

13. To the left of $z = -1.43$

14. Between $z = 1.23$ and $z = 1.90$

15. Between $z = 0.79$ and $z = 1.28$

16. Between $z = -0.96$ and $z = -0.36$

17. Between $z = -1.56$ and $z = -1.83$

18. Between $z = 0.24$ and $z = -1.12$

19. Between $z = 2.47$ and $z = -1.03$

20. To the left of $z = 1.31$

21. To the left of $z = 2.11$

22. To the right of $z = -1.92$

23. To the right of $z = -0.15$

24. To the left of $z = -2.15$ and to the right of $z = 1.62$

25. To the right of $z = 1.92$ and to the left of $z = -0.44$

In Exercises 26 through 39, find probabilities for each, using the standard normal distribution.

26. $P(0 < z < 1.69)$

27. $P(0 < z < 0.67)$

28. $P(-1.23 < z < 0)$

29. $P(-1.57 < z < 0)$

30. $P(z > 1.16)$

31. $P(z > 2.83)$

32. $P(z < -1.77)$

33. $P(z < -1.21)$

34. $P(-0.05 < z < 1.10)$

35. $P(-2.46 < z < 1.74)$

36. $P(1.12 < z < 1.43)$

37. $P(1.46 < z < 2.97)$

38. $P(z > -1.39)$

39. $P(z < 1.42)$

For Exercises 40 through 45, find the z score that corresponds to the given area.

40.

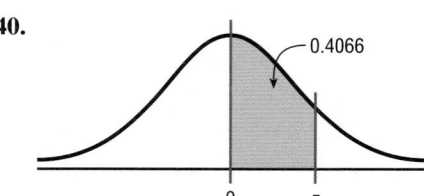

41.

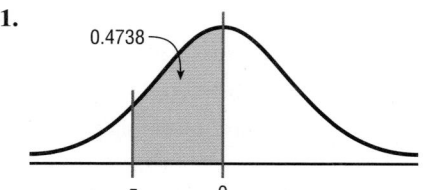

42.

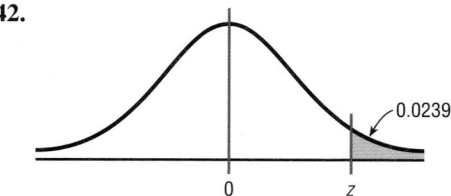

43.

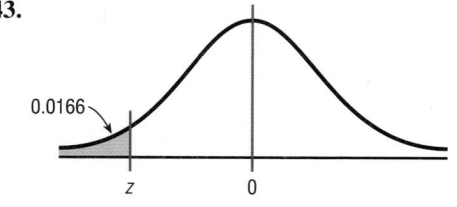

44.

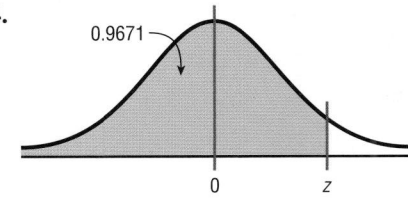

45.

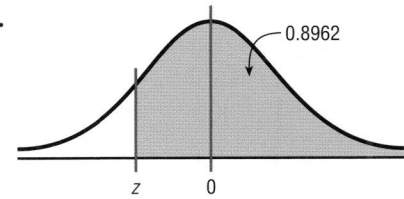

46. Find the z score to the right of the mean so that

    a. 53.98% of the area under the distribution curve lies to the left of it.

    b. 71.90% of the area under the distribution curve lies to the left of it.

    c. 96.78% of the area under the distribution curve lies to the left of it.

47. Find the z score to the left of the mean so that

    a. 98.87% of the area under the distribution curve lies to the right of it.

    b. 82.12% of the area under the distribution curve lies to the right of it.

    c. 60.64% of the area under the distribution curve lies to the right of it.

48. Find two z scores so that 44% of the middle area is bounded by them.

49. Find two z scores, one positive and one negative, so that the areas in the two tails total the following values.

    a. 5%

    b. 10%

    c. 1%

Extending the Concepts »

50. In the standard normal distribution, find the values of z for the 75th, 80th, and 92nd percentiles.

51. Find $P(-1 < z < 1)$, $P(-2 < z < 2)$, and $P(-3 < z < 3)$. How do these values compare with the empirical rule?

52. Find z_0 such that $P(z > z_0) = 0.1234$.

53. Find z_0 such that $P(-1.2 < z < z_0) = 0.8671$.

54. Find z_0 such that $P(z_0 < z < 2.5) = 0.7672$.

55. Find z_0 such that the area between z_0 and $z = -0.5$ is 0.2345 (two answers).

56. Find z_0 such that $P(-z_0 < z < z_0) = 0.86$.

57. The mathematical equation for a normal distribution is

$$y = \frac{e^{-(X-\mu)^2/(2\sigma^2)}}{\sigma\sqrt{2\pi}}$$

Where $\pi \approx 3.14$, $e \approx 2.718$
μ = population mean
σ = population standard deviation

Given $\mu = 0$ and $\sigma = 1$, solve for $X = \{-2, -1.5, -1, -0.5, 0, 0.5, 1, 1.5, 2.0\}$.

58. Use the results in Exercise 57 to graph the normal distribution.

6–2   Applications of the Normal Distribution ›

LO2

Find specific data values for given percentages, using the standard normal distribution.

The standard normal distribution curve can be used to solve a wide variety of practical problems. The only requirement is that the variable be normally or approximately normally distributed. There are several mathematical tests to determine whether a variable is normally distributed. See the Critical Thinking Challenges on page 298. For all the problems presented in this chapter, one can assume that the variable is normally or approximately normally distributed.

    To solve problems using the standard normal distribution, the continuous random variable X must be converted to a standard score z, a quantity without units derived by subtracting the population mean μ from the X value and then dividing the difference by the population standard deviation σ. This is the same formula previously presented in Sections 3–3 and 6–2.

$$z = \frac{X - \mu}{\sigma}$$

After X values have been converted, procedures learned in Section 6–1 using Tables E–1 and E–2 in Appendix C can be used to solve problems involving proportion, percentage, and probability.

For example, suppose that the scores for a standardized test are normally distributed, have a mean of 100, and have a standard deviation of 15. When the scores are transformed to z scores, the two distributions coincide, as shown in Figure 6–15. (Recall that the z distribution has a mean of 0 and a standard deviation of 1.)

Figure 6–15

Test Scores and Their Corresponding z Values

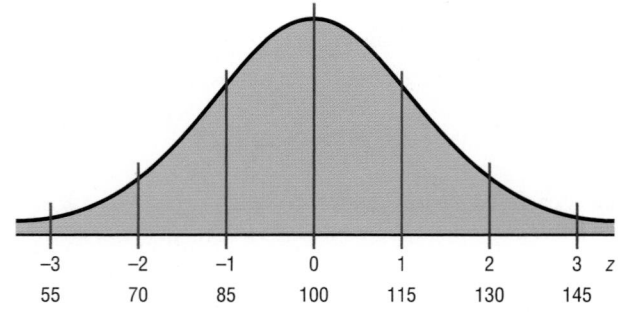

To solve the application problems in this section, transform the values of the variable to z scores and then find the areas under the standard normal distribution, as explained in Section 6–1.

Example 6–8

Internet Usage

The amount of time that Canadians spend on the Internet per week is a variable that is normally distributed with a mean of 13.8 hours and a standard deviation of 1.2 hours. Find the percentage of Canadians who spend less than 15.3 hours online per week.

Source: Canadian Radio-television and Telecommunications Commission, *4.0 Broadcasting,* "4.5 New Media," August 5, 2009.

Solution

Step 1   Sketch the curve and represent the area as shown in Figure 6–16.

Figure 6–16

Area under a Normal Curve for Example 6–8

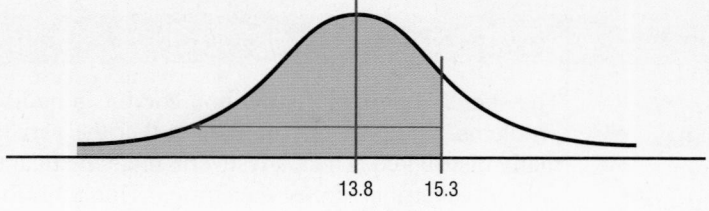

Step 2   Find the z score for $X = 15.3$.

$$z = \frac{X - \mu}{\sigma} = \frac{15.3 - 13.8}{1.2} = 1.25$$

Hence, 15.3 is 1.25 standard deviations above the mean of 13.8, as shown for the z distribution in Figure 6–17.

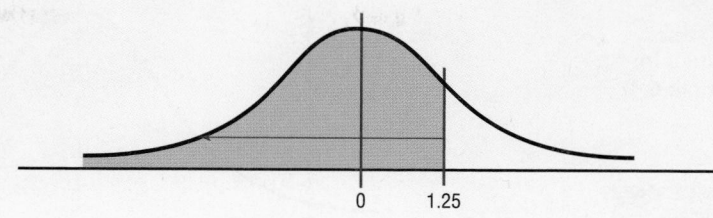

0   1.25

Step 3   Find the area by using Table E–2, Positive z Scores. The cumulative area to the left of $z = 1.25$ is 0.8944.

Therefore, 89.44% of Canadians Internet users spend less than 15.3 hours per week online.

Example 6–9

Recycling e-Waste

British Columbians recycled an average of 2.52 kilograms of electronics products (e-waste) per capita in a recent year. Assume the variable is normally distributed with a standard deviation of 0.48 kilogram. Find the probability that a randomly selected British Columbian recycles

   a. Between 1.8 and 3.6 kilograms of e-waste per year

   b. More than 3.0 kilograms of e-waste per year

Source: Government of British Columbia, *BCStats,* "Electronic-Waste Recycling in British Columbia," September 2009.

Solution *a*

Step 1   Sketch the figure and represent the area. See Figure 6–18.

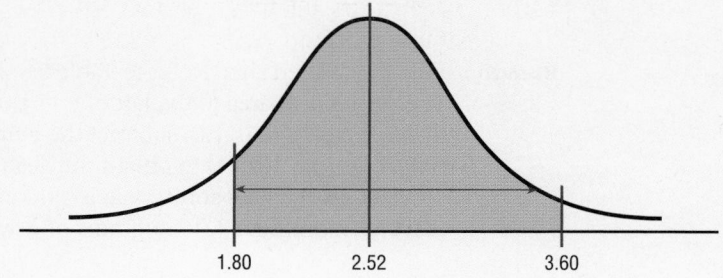

1.80   2.52   3.60

Step 2   Convert $X = 1.8$ and $X = 3.6$ to z scores.

$$z_1 = \frac{X - \mu}{\sigma} = \frac{1.80 - 2.52}{0.48} = -1.50$$

$$z_2 = \frac{X - \mu}{\sigma} = \frac{3.60 - 2.52}{0.48} = 2.25$$

Step 3   Find the desired area. Refer to Table E–1, Negative z Scores, in Appendix C. The cumulative area to the left of $z = -1.50$ is 0.0668. Refer to Table E–2, Positive z Scores, in Appendix C. The cumulative area to the left of $z = 2.25$ is 0.9878. Subtract the cumulative area to the left of $z = -1.50$ (0.0668) from the cumulative area to the left of $z = 2.25$ (0.9878) to obtain the desired area 0.9210. Refer to Figure 6–19.

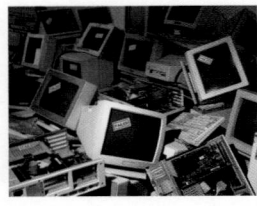

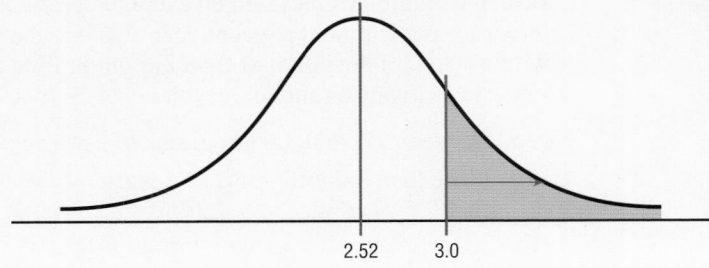

| 1.80 | 2.52 | 3.60 |
| -1.50 | 0 | 2.25 |

Hence, the probability that a randomly selected British Columbian recycles between 1.8 and 3.6 kilograms of e-waste per year is 0.9210, or 92.10%.

Solution b

Step 1 Sketch the figure and represent the area. See Figure 6–20.

| 2.52 | 3.0 |

Step 2 Convert $X = 3.0$ to a z score.

$$z = \frac{X - \mu}{\sigma} = \frac{3.0 - 2.52}{0.48} = 1.0$$

Step 3 Find the desired area. Refer to Table E–2, Positive z Scores, in Appendix C. The cumulative area to the left of $z = 1.0$ is 0.8413. Since the total area under the normal curve is 1.0, subtract the cumulative area to the left of $z = 1.0$ (0.8413) from 1.0000 to obtain the desired area to the right of 0.1587.

Hence, the probability that a randomly selected British Columbian recycles more than 3.0 kilograms of e-waste per year is 0.1587, or 15.87%.

A normal distribution can also be used to answer questions of "How many?" This application is shown in Example 6–10.

Example 6–10

EMS Response Time

The Canadian Association of Emergency Physicians collates data for emergency medical services (EMS) response times for 911 calls. The average time to respond to an emergency call was 13 minutes. Assume that the variable is normally distributed, with a standard deviation of 3.2 minutes. If 50 emergency 911 calls are randomly selected, for approximately how many calls would you expect the response time to be less than 10 minutes?

Source: Canadian Association of Emergency Physicians.

Solution

Step 1   Draw a figure and represent the area as shown in Figure 6–21.

Figure 6–21

Area under a
Normal Curve for
Example 6–10

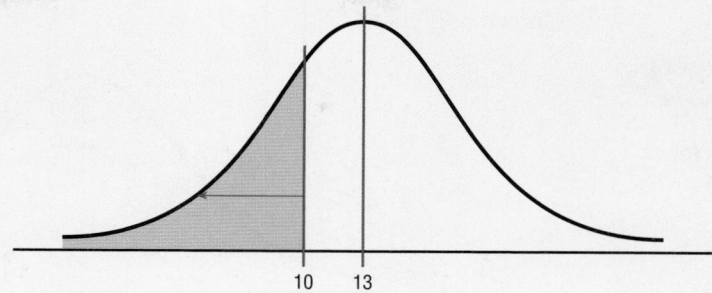

10   13

Step 2   Find the z score for $X = 10$.

$$z = \frac{X - \mu}{\sigma} = \frac{10 - 13}{3.2} = -0.94$$

Step 3   Find the desired area. Refer to Table E–1, Negative z Scores, in Appendix C. The cumulative area to the left of $z = -0.94$ is 0.1736.

Step 4   To find out how many emergency calls will be responded to in less than 10 minutes, multiply the sample size 50 by 0.1736 to obtain 8.68. Hence, 8.68 or approximately 9 of the emergency calls will have a response time of less than 10 minutes.

Note: For problems using percentages, be sure to change the percentage to a decimal before multiplying. Also, round the answer to the nearest whole number, since it is not possible to have 8.68 calls.

Finding Data Values Given Specific Probabilities

A normal distribution can also be used to find the specific data values for given percentages. This X value represents the desired cutoff point separating the specified area from the remainder of the curve. Simply determine the z score that corresponds to the area to the **left** of the X value using Table E–1 or Table E–2 as previously illustrated. Substitute the z score and the given mean (μ) and standard deviation (σ) into the standard score formula and solve for X.

To simplify the calculation, the standard score formula $z = \dfrac{X - \mu}{\sigma}$ has been rearranged and can be used to solve for X.

$$X = z \cdot \sigma + \mu$$

This application is shown in Example 6–11.

Example 6–11

Police Academy Qualifications

To qualify for a police academy, candidates must score in the top 10% on a general abilities test. The test has a mean of 200 and a standard deviation of 20. Find the lowest possible score to qualify. Assume the test scores are normally distributed.

Solution

Since the test scores are normally distributed, the test value X that cuts off the upper 10% of the area under a normal distribution curve is desired. This area is shown in Figure 6–22.

Figure 6–22

Area under a Normal Curve for Example 6–11

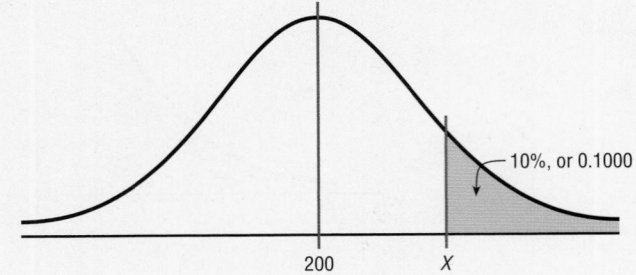

10%, or 0.1000

200   X

Work backward to solve this problem.

Step 1   Subtract 0.1000 from the total area under the normal curve, 1.000 to obtain 0.9000.

Step 2   Find the z score from Table E–2, Positive z Scores, in Appendix C that corresponds to the cumulative area to the left **closest to** the desired area 0.9000. The **closest** value to 0.9000 is 0.8997, which corresponds to a z score of 1.28. Refer to Figure 6–23.

Figure 6–23

Finding the z Score from Table E–2, Positive z Scores, in Appendix C

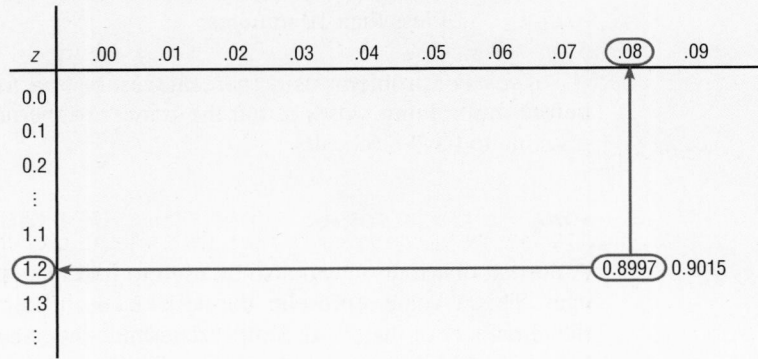

Step 3   Substitute in the rearranged standard score formula.

$$X = z \cdot \sigma + \mu$$
$$X = (1.28)(20) + 200$$
$$X = 225.6$$
$$X = 226 \text{ (rounded)}$$

A score of 226 should be used as a cutoff. Anybody scoring 226 or higher qualifies.

Interesting Fact

The average CEO reaches the Canadian average annual earnings by 9:46 A.M. on January 2.

Example 6–12

Blood Pressure Readings

For a medical study, a researcher wishes to select people in the middle 60% of the population, based on blood pressure. If the mean systolic blood pressure is 120 millimetres of mercury (mmHg) and the standard deviation is 8 mmHg, find the upper and lower readings that would qualify people to participate in the study.

Solution

Assume that blood pressure readings are normally distributed; then cutoff points are as shown in Figure 6–24.

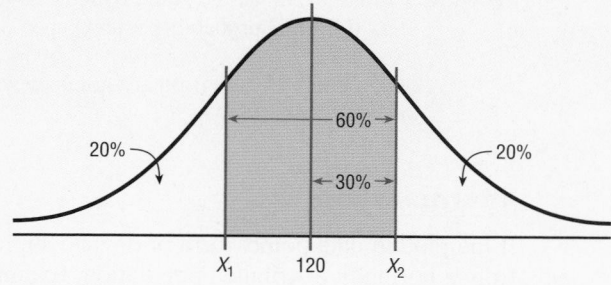

The two X values enclosing the middle 60% of the population have cumulative areas of 20% and 80% to the left, respectively. The z score that corresponds to X_1 with a cumulative area to the left closest to 0.2000 (0.2005) is $z = -0.84$. The z score that corresponds to X_2 with a cumulative area to the left closest to 0.8000 (0.7995) is $z = 0.84$.

Substitute into the standard score formula rearranged for X.

$$X_1 = z \cdot \sigma + \mu = (-0.84)(8) + 120 = 113.28$$
$$X_2 = z \cdot \sigma + \mu = (0.84)(8) + 120 = 126.72$$

Therefore, the middle 60% of the population will have blood pressure readings, mmHg, of between 113.28 and 126.72, or $113.28 < X < 126.72$.

As shown in this section, a normal distribution is a useful tool in answering many questions about variables that are normally or approximately normally distributed.

Normality Assumption

The key assumption made when determining probabilities for continuous random variables is that the data are drawn randomly from a population that approximates a normal distribution. Methods will be learned in later chapters that will allow normal distribution tables to be used for populations that are not normal. Other methods will assume normality without providing proof. Statistical methods have been developed to test if a population is normal. The simplest test of normality, if data are available, is to plot the data frequencies and construct a histogram. If the histogram is bell-shaped, then the data are considered normally distributed. If the data are uniform, skewed, or not bell-shaped, then the data are not normally distributed. Applying the Concepts 6–1 discussed the histogram method for assessing normality.

Another method to test for normality is to construct a normal probability plot. This method plots data points on a graph. The x axis represents the observed data values and the y axis represents the standard score (z) scale or percentile rank (P_k) of each data value. If the plotted data points form a straight line, the data are normally distributed. The following procedure illustrates the steps for creating a normal probability plot.

Procedure to Construct a Normal Probability Plot

Step 1: Sort and rank the data in ascending order (smallest to largest).

Step 2: Calculate the percentile rank (P_k) for each data value, using the percentile formula. (Refer to Section 3–3.)

(continued)

Procedure to Construct a Normal Probability Plot *(continued)*

Step 3: Convert each percentile rank to a z-score using Tables E–1 and E–2.

Step 4: Plot the data on the graph with the X-values on the horizontal axis.
    a. If normal probability graph paper is available, plot the percentiles on the vertical axis.
    b. Otherwise, use ordinary graph paper and plot the z-scores on the vertical axis.

Interpretation

If the plotted data points form or deviate slightly from a straight line, the data are likely from a normally distributed population. Example 6–13 illustrates the steps for creating a normal probability plot using ordinary graph paper.

Example 6–13

Laptop Battery Life

The data represent battery life, in minutes, for laptop computers while watching live-broadcast streaming video. Check for normality using a normal probability plot. (See Figure 6–25.)

| 320 | 395 | 380 | 295 | 305 | 330 | 260 | 285 | 360 | 410 |

Solution

X	(1) Rank	(2) P_k	(3) z
260	1	5%	−1.645
285	2	15%	−1.04
295	3	25%	−0.67
305	4	35%	−0.39
320	5	45%	−0.13
330	6	55%	0.13
360	7	65%	0.39
380	8	75%	0.67
395	9	85%	1.04
410	10	95%	1.645

Figure 6–25

Normal Probability Plot for Laptop Battery Life

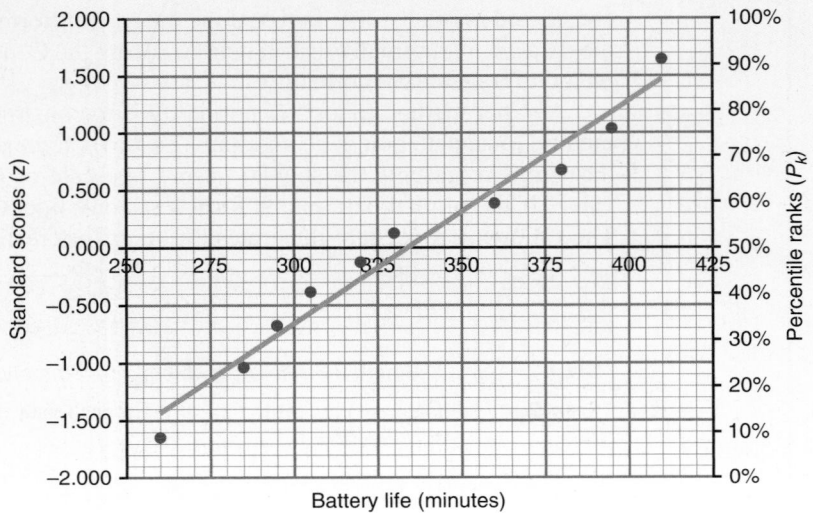

Battery life (minutes)

Interpretation

The data deviate slightly from a straight line, which indicates that the battery life data are approximately normally distributed.

Another test for normality is to check data for a distribution's symmetry or skewness. *Pearson's Index (PI) of Skewness* uses the rule that if the index value is between -1 and $+1$, then the distribution is symmetric. A PI of skewness value of < -1 signifies a negatively or left-skewed distribution and $> +1$ a positively or right-skewed distribution. To compute the index value, use the formula

$$\text{PI of skewness} = \frac{(\overline{X} - \text{median})}{s}$$

Yet another method to test for normality is the check for *outliers,* as explained in Section 3–3. Several other methods are used to test for normality, such as the Kolmogorov-Smirnov test and the Lilliefors test. An explanation of these tests can be found in advanced textbooks.

Graphing calculators (TI-83 Plus and TI-84 Plus) and software applications (Excel, Minitab, and SPSS) include procedures to quickly test for normality using the normal quantile plot. For step-by-step guidance on the use of TI-83 Plus/TI-84 Plus calculators, see Appendix E at the back of this textbook. For summary procedures for Minitab, SPSS, and Excel, see the full version of Appendix E on *Connect.*

6–2 Applying the Concepts

Smart People

Assume you are thinking about starting a Mensa chapter in your hometown, which has a population of about 10,000 people. You need to know how many people would qualify for Mensa, which requires an IQ of at least 130. You realize that IQ is normally distributed with a mean of 100 and a standard deviation of 15. Complete the following.

1. Find the approximate number of people in your hometown that are eligible for Mensa.
2. Is it reasonable to continue your quest for a Mensa chapter there?
3. How would you proceed to find out how many of the eligible people would actually join the new chapter? Be specific about your methods of gathering data.
4. What would be the minimum IQ score needed if you wanted to start an Ultra-Mensa club that included only the top 1% of IQ scores?

See page 300 for the answers.

Exercises 6–2

1. **Admission Charge for Movies** The average admission charge in Canada for new-release movies is $11.42. If the distribution of admission charges is normal with a standard deviation of $1.32, what is the probability that less than $10.00 is charged for admission to a randomly selected new-release movie?
Source: MovieTickets.com: www.movietickets.com/default.asp.

2. **Youth Work Week** Recent statistics indicate that Canadian employed youth work an average of 28.8 hours per week. Assume a standard deviation of 3.5 hours and a normally distributed population. What is the probability that a randomly selected Canadian employed youth has the following workweek?

   a. Between 25 and 30 hours
   b. Less than 25 hours
   c. More than 30 hours
   Source: Human Resources and Skills Development Canada, *Indicators of Well-Being in Canada,* "Work: Weekly Hours Worked."

3. **Prison Inmate Population** The average number of male inmates in Canada's provincial and federal prison system, over a 12-year period, was 100,809 with a standard deviation of 15,488. Assume that prison inmate numbers are normally distributed. Find the probability that in a randomly selected year the inmate population is

   a. Greater than 110,000.
   b. Between 80,000 and 90,000.
   Source: Correctional Service, Canada.

4. **SAT Scores** The SAT Reasoning Test, formerly the Scholastic Aptitude Test, is used by colleges and universities in the United States to aid in the selection of incoming national and international students. If the average score is 1019 and the scores are normally distributed with $\sigma = 90$, what is the 90th percentile score? What is the probability that a randomly selected score exceeds 1200?

   Source: N.Y. Times Almanac.

5. **Chocolate Bar Calories** The average number of calories in a 50-gram chocolate bar is 225. Suppose that the distribution of calories is approximately normal with $\sigma = 10$. Find the probability that a randomly selected chocolate bar will have

   a. Between 200 and 220 calories.

   b. Less than 200 calories.

   Source: The Doctor's Pocket Calorie, Fat, and Carbohydrate Counter.

6. **Age of CEOs** The average age of CEOs is 56 years. Assume the variable is normally distributed. If the standard deviation is 4 years, find the probability that the age of a randomly selected CEO will be in the following range.

   a. Between 53 and 59 years old

   b. Between 58 and 63 years old

   c. Between 50 and 55 years old

   Source: Michael D. Shook and Robert L. Shook, The Book of Odds.

7. **Employee Hourly Wage** The average hourly wage in 2010 for employees in the natural and applied sciences and related occupations was $31.65. Assume a normally distributed population with a standard deviation of $3.90. If one employee is randomly selected from this occupation, find the probability that the employee earns

   a. At least $30 per hour.

   b. At most $25 per hour.

   c. Between $35 and $40 per hour.

   Source: Statistics Canada, Summary Tables, "Average Hourly Wages of Employees by Selected Characteristics and Profession, Unadjusted Data, by Province (monthly)."

8. **Labourer Work Hours** Construction industry labourers work an average of 38.4 hours per week. Assume the variable is from a normally distributed population with a standard deviation of 4.5 hours. If a construction industry labourer is selected at random, find the probability that the labourer works

   a. More than 40 hours per week.

   b. Less than 36 hours per week.

   c. Between 36 and 40 hours per week.

   Source: Statistics Canada, Summary Tables, "Weekly Hours of Hourly Paid Employees, Average, by Industry (all industries)," March 31, 2010.

9. **Appliance Energy Consumption** The average annual energy consumption of residential dishwashers is 352.5 kilowatt hours per year (kWh/year). If the data are normally distributed with a standard deviation of

41.2 kWh/year, find the probability that a randomly selected dishwasher will consume

   a. More than 400 kWh/year.

   b. Between 350 and 375 kWh/year.

   c. What percentage of dishwashers would qualify for the Energy Star efficiency rating of less than 324 kWh/year?

   Sources: Natural Resources Canada, Office of Energy Efficiency, Energy Consumption of Major House Appliances, "Trends for 1990–2007," and Personal: Residential, "Major Appliance Requirements," December 2009.

10. **Work Commute Time** Canadians spend an average of 63 minutes each day commuting to work. If we assume that commuting times are normally distributed with a standard deviation of 15.4 minutes, what is the probability that a randomly selected commuter spends more than 60 minutes commuting? Less than 45 minutes?

    Source: CBC News, "Commuters Spending More Time in Transit: Statistics Canada," July 12, 2006.

11. **Ph.D. Time to Completion** The *Survey of Earned Doctorates* published by Statistics Canada revealed that doctoral candidates required, on average, 70 months to earn their Ph.D. degrees. If time to completion is normally distributed with a standard deviation of 17 months, find the probability that a doctoral candidate will earn a Ph.D. degree in

    a. Less than 5 years.

    b. Between 5 and 6 years.

    c. More than 6 years.

    Source: University Affairs, "Maybe Our Doctoral Students Are Starting Too Late," Jon Driver, October 10, 2005.

12. **Lake Water Temperature** British Columbia's Lake Osoyoos is Canada's warmest lake, with mean summer water temperatures of 24°C. Assume the summer temperatures are normally distributed with a standard deviation of 1.9°C. For a randomly selected summer day, find the probability that the water temperature will be as follows.

    a. Above 26°C

    b. Below 27.5°C

    c. Between 21°C and 23°C

    d. If the lake temperature was above 27.5°C, would you consider the water to be warmer than usual?

    Source: www.olwgs.org.

13. **Restaurant Seating Time** The average waiting time to be seated for dinner at a popular restaurant is 23.5 minutes, with a standard deviation of 3.6 minutes. Assume the variable is normally distributed. When a patron arrives at the restaurant for dinner, find the probability that the patron will have to wait the following time.

    a. Between 15 and 22 minutes

    b. Less than 18 minutes or more than 25 minutes

    c. Is it likely that a person will be seated in less than 15 minutes?

14. Price of Gasoline The average pump price for regular gasoline across Canada on a given day was $1.03 per litre. If gas prices are normally distributed with a standard deviation of $0.19, calculate the 15th and 85th percentile of Canadian gas prices.

Source: gasticker.com, "Canada's Gasoline Price Tracker," March 7, 2010.

15. Hospital Wait Times A report on hospital wait times from general practitioner referrals to surgical and other therapeutic treatments in Canada was 17.3 weeks. If wait times are normally distributed with a standard deviation of 1.9 weeks, find the cutoff for the middle 60% of hospital wait times.

Source: Fraser Institute, Waiting Your Turn: Hospital Waiting Lists in Canada, 2008.

16. Student Tuition Fees On average, undergraduate students in Ontario paid the highest tuition fees in Canada at $5951. If the data are normally distributed with a standard deviation of $654, find the cutoff for the top and bottom 5% of tuition fees.

Source: Statistics Canada, The Daily, "University Tuition Fees, 2009/2010," October 20, 2009.

17. Used Boat Prices A marine sales dealer finds that the average price of a previously owned boat is $6492. He decides to sell boats that will appeal to the middle 66% of the market in terms of price. Find the maximum and minimum prices of the boats the dealer will sell. The standard deviation is $1025, and the variable is normally distributed. Would a boat priced at $5550 be sold in this store?

18. Charitable Donations The Fraser Institute reports that British Columbia ranks first in Canada for charitable donations, with the average taxpayer claiming a charitable donation of $1194. Suppose that the distribution of contributions is normal with a standard deviation of $149. Find the limits for the middle 50% of contributions.

Source: The Fraser Institute.

19. New-Home Sizes A contractor decided to build homes that will include the middle 80% of the market. The average single-family detached home in Canada is 149 square metres (m^2). Find the maximum and minimum sizes of the homes the contractor should build. Assume that the standard deviation is 7.2 m^2 and that the variable is normally distributed.

Source: Natural Resources Canada, Office of Energy Efficiency, Survey of Household Energy Use, 2007.

20. Home Energy Efficiency The average annual energy consumption is 138 gigajoules (GJ) for a single-family home in Canada. Assuming normally distributed data with a standard deviation of 6.9 GJ, find the middle 50% energy consumption for single-family homes.

Source: Natural Resources Canada, Office of Energy Efficiency, Survey of Household Energy Use, 2007.

21. Wedding Costs Canadian couples spend an average of $19,038 to cover the cost of their weddings. Determine the cutoff for the top 10% of wedding costs if the stan-

dard deviation is $2094 and the data is normally distributed.

Source: Weddingbells, "Wedding Trends in Canada," 2008.

22. Reading Improvement Program To help students improve their reading, a school district decides to implement a reading program. It is to be administered to the bottom 5% of the students in the district, based on the scores on a reading achievement exam. If the average score for the students in the district is 122.6, find the cutoff score that will make a student eligible for the program. The standard deviation is 18. Assume the variable is normally distributed.

23. Used Car Prices An automobile dealer finds that the average price of a previously owned vehicle is $8256. He decides to sell cars that will appeal to the middle 60% of the market in terms of price. Find the maximum and minimum prices of the cars the dealer will sell. The standard deviation is $1150, and the variable is normally distributed.

24. Age of Railway Cars The Canadian locomotive fleet railway cars' average age is 17.1 years. Assuming that the distribution of railway cars is normal and that 20% of the fleet is older than 20 years, find the standard deviation.

Source: www.railway.ca.

25. Length of Hospital Stays The average length of stay for acute inpatients in Canada is 6.7 days. If we assume that the lengths of hospital stays are normally distributed with a variance of 2.1, then 10% of acute inpatient hospital stays are longer than how many days? Thirty percent of inpatient stays are less than how many days?

Source: Canadian Institute for Health Information, Analysis in Brief, "Inpatient Hospitalizations and Average Length of Stay: Trends in Canada, 2003–2004 and 2004–2005," November 30, 2005.

26. High School Competency Test A mandatory competency test for second-year high school students has a normal distribution with a mean of 400 and a standard deviation of 100.

a. The top 3% of students receive $500. What is the minimum score you would need to receive this award?

b. The bottom 1.5% of students must go to summer school. What is the minimum score you would need to stay out of this group?

27. Product Marketing An advertising company plans to market a product to low-income families. A study states that for a particular area, the average income per family is $24,596 and the standard deviation is $6256. If the company plans to target the bottom 18% of the families based on income, find the cutoff income. Assume the variable is normally distributed.

28. Food Expenditure On average, a Canadian household spends $7435 annually on food. Assume the variable is normal, with a standard deviation of $817.

Find the maximum and minimum dollar amounts that the middle 50% of Canadian households spend annually on food.

Source: Statistics Canada, Summary Tables, "Average Household Expenditures by Province and Territory, 2008."

29. Wristwatch Lifetimes The mean lifetime of a wristwatch is 25 months, with a standard deviation of 5 months. If the distribution is normal, for how many months should a guarantee be made if the manufacturer does not want to exchange more than 10% of the watches? Assume the variable is normally distributed.

30. Security Officer Stress Tolerance To qualify for security officers' training, recruits are tested for stress tolerance. The scores are normally distributed, with a mean of 62 and a standard deviation of 8. If only the top 15% of recruits are selected, find the cutoff score.

31. In the distributions shown, state the mean and standard deviation for each. *Hint:* See Figures 6–4 and 6–6. Also the vertical lines are 1 standard deviation apart.

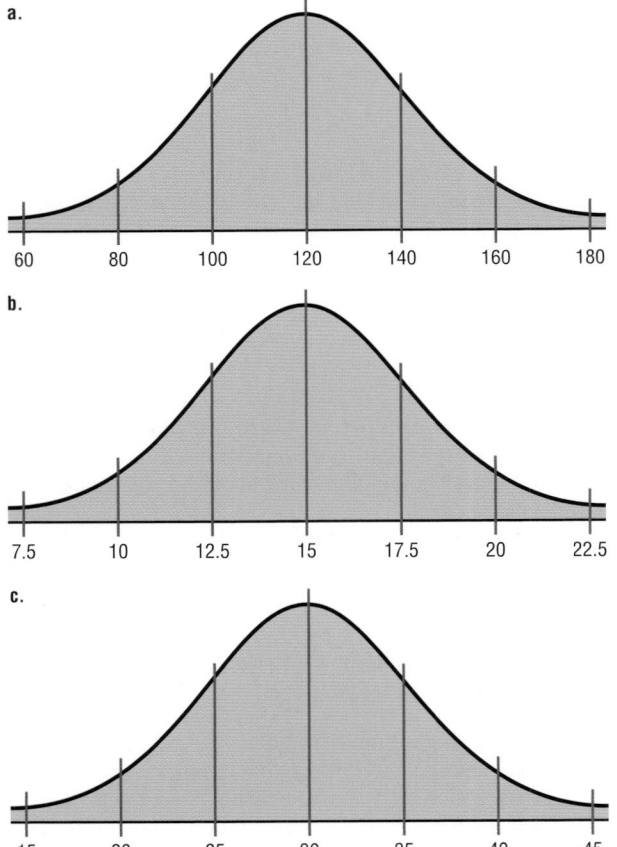

a.

| 60 | 80 | 100 | 120 | 140 | 160 | 180 |

b.

| 7.5 | 10 | 12.5 | 15 | 17.5 | 20 | 22.5 |

c.

| 15 | 20 | 25 | 30 | 35 | 40 | 45 |

32. SAT Scores Suppose that the mathematics SAT scores for high school seniors for a specific year have a mean of 456 and a standard deviation of 100 and are approximately normally distributed. If a subgroup of these high school seniors, those who are in the National Honour Society, is selected, would you expect the distribution of scores to have the same mean and standard deviation? Explain your answer.

33. Given a data set, how could you decide if the distribution of the data was approximately normal?

34. If a distribution of raw scores was plotted and then the scores were transformed to z scores, would the shape of the distribution change? Explain your answer.

35. In a normal distribution, find σ when $\mu = 110$ and 2.87% of the area lies to the right of 112.

36. In a normal distribution, find μ when σ is 6 and 3.75% of the area lies to the left of 85.

37. In a certain normal distribution, 1.25% of the area lies to the left of 42, and 1.25% of the area lies to the right of 48. Find μ and σ.

38. Exam Scores An instructor gives a 100-point examination in which the grades are normally distributed. The mean is 60 and the standard deviation is 10. If there are 5% As and 5% Fs, 15% Bs and 15% Ds, and 60% Cs, find the scores that divide the distribution into those categories.

39. Fire Deaths The data shown represent fire deaths in Canada during a 26-year period. Check for normality.

811	844	733	833	694	675	539	598	550	553
539	535	519	481	406	401	417	377	400	374
416	337	388	327	338	304

Source: Council of Canadian Fire Marshals and Fire Commissioners, Canadian Fire Statistics, "Annual Reports of Fire Losses in Canada."

40. Currency Exchange Rate The data shown represent a random selection over a 10-year period of the daily exchange rate of one Canadian dollar expressed in United States currency. Check for normality.

| 0.69 | 0.67 | 0.66 | 0.63 | 0.64 | 0.73 | 0.76 | 0.82 | 0.80 | 0.85 |
| 0.87 | 0.89 | 0.87 | 0.94 | 1.00 | 1.01 | 0.84 | 0.79 | 0.90 | 0.95 |

Source: Bank of Canada, Rates and Statistics, "Exchange Rates."

41. Box Office Revenues The data shown represent the domestic box-office receipts (in millions of dollars) for a randomly selected sample of the top-grossing films in 2009. Check for normality.

402	155	138	37	296	63	80	94	714	177
46	33	32	22	150	164	293	146	41	43
38	80	32	43	37	108	52	277	36	23

Source: Box Office Mojo, Yearly Box Office, "2009 Domestic Grosses."

42. Number of Goals Scored The data shown represent the number of goals scored by Wayne Gretzky during each season of his National Hockey League career. Check for normality.

| 51 | 55 | 92 | 71 | 87 | 73 | 52 | 62 | 40 | 54 |
| 40 | 41 | 31 | 16 | 38 | 11 | 15 | 8 | 25 | 23 |

Source: hockeyDB.com, Internet Hockey Database, "Wayne Gretzky."

6–3	The Central Limit Theorem >

LO3

Use the central limit theorem to solve problems involving sample means for large samples.

In addition to knowing how individual data values vary about the mean for a population, statisticians are interested in knowing how the means of samples of the same size taken from the same population vary about the population mean.

Sampling Distribution of Means

Suppose a researcher selects a sample of 30 adult males and finds the mean of the measure of the triglyceride levels for the sample subjects to be 187 milligrams/decilitre. Then suppose a second sample is selected, and the mean of that sample is found to be 192 milligrams/decilitre. Continue the process for 100 samples. What happens then is that the mean becomes a random variable, and the sample means 187, 192, 184, . . . , 196 constitute a *sampling distribution of means.*

> A **sampling distribution of means** is a distribution using the means computed from all possible random samples of a specific size taken from a population.

If the samples are randomly selected with replacement, the sample means, for the most part, will be somewhat different from the population mean μ. These differences are caused by sampling error.

> **Sampling error** is the difference between the sample measure and the corresponding population measure due to the fact that the sample is not a perfect representation of the population.

When all possible samples of a specific size are selected with replacement from a population, the sampling distribution of means for a variable has two important properties, which are explained next.

Properties of the Sampling Distribution of Means

1. The mean of the sample means will be the same as the population mean.
2. The standard deviation of the sample means will be smaller than the standard deviation of the population, and it will be equal to the population standard deviation divided by the square root of the sample size.

The following example illustrates these two properties. Suppose a professor gave an 8-point quiz to a small class of four students. The results of the quiz were 2, 6, 4, and 8. For the sake of discussion, assume that the four students constitute the population. The mean of the population is

$$\mu = \frac{2 + 6 + 4 + 8}{4} = 5$$

The standard deviation of the population is

$$\sigma = \sqrt{\frac{(2 - 5)^2 + (6 - 5)^2 + (4 - 5)^2 + (8 - 5)^2}{4}} = 2.236$$

The graph of the original distribution is shown in Figure 6–26. This is called a *uniform distribution.*

Figure 6–26

**Distribution of Quiz
Scores**

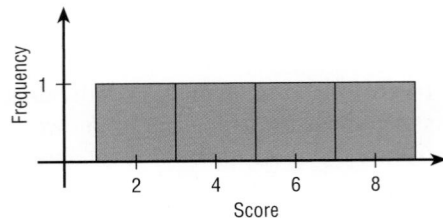

Now, if all samples of size 2 are taken with replacement and the mean of each sample is found, the distribution is as shown.

Sample	Mean	Sample	Mean
2, 2	2	6, 2	4
2, 4	3	6, 4	5
2, 6	4	6, 6	6
2, 8	5	6, 8	7
4, 2	3	8, 2	5
4, 4	4	8, 4	6
4, 6	5	8, 6	7
4, 8	6	8, 8	8

A frequency distribution of sample means is as follows.

$\overline{X}$	f
2	1
3	2
4	3
5	4
6	3
7	2
8	1

Historical Note

Two mathematicians who contributed to the development of the central limit theorem were Abraham DeMoivre (1667–1754) and Pierre Simon Laplace (1749–1827). DeMoivre was once jailed for his religious beliefs. After his release, DeMoivre made a living by consulting on the mathematics of gambling and insurance. He wrote two books, *Annuities Upon Lives* and *The Doctrine of Chance.*

Laplace held a government position under Napoleon and later under Louis XVIII. He once computed the probability of the sun rising to be 18,226,214/ 18,226,215.

For the data from the example just discussed, Figure 6–27 shows the graph of the sample means. The histogram appears to be approximately normal.

The mean of the sample means, denoted by $\mu_{\overline{X}}$, is

$$\mu_{\overline{X}} = \frac{2 + 3 + \cdots + 8}{16} = \frac{80}{16} = 5$$

which is the same as the population mean. Hence,

$$\mu_{\overline{X}} = \mu$$

The standard deviation of sample means, denoted by $\sigma_{\overline{X}}$, is

$$\sigma_{\overline{X}} = \sqrt{\frac{(2 - 5)^2 + (3 - 5)^2 + \cdots + (8 - 5)^2}{16}} = 1.581$$

which is the same as the population standard deviation, divided by $\sqrt{2}$:

$$\sigma_{\overline{X}} = \frac{2.236}{\sqrt{2}} = 1.581$$

(*Note:* Rounding rules were not used here in order to show that the answers coincide.)

In summary, if all possible samples of size n are taken with replacement from the same population, the mean of the sample means, denoted by $\mu_{\overline{X}}$, equals the population mean μ;

Figure 6–27

Figure 6–27

Sampling Distribution of Means

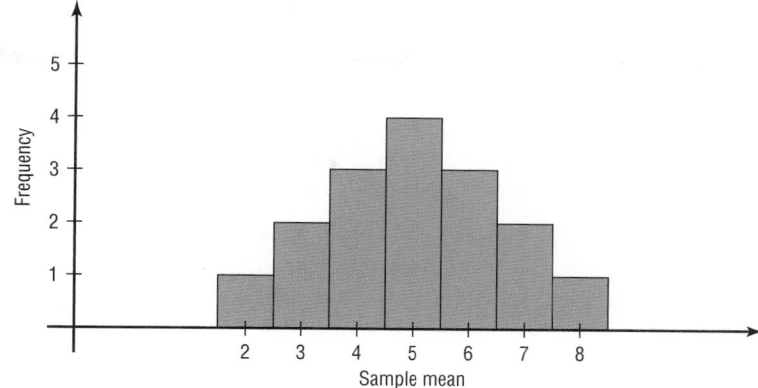

and the standard deviation of the sample means, denoted by $\sigma_{\overline{X}}$, equals $\sigma/\sqrt{n}$. The standard deviation of the sample means is called the **standard error of the mean.** Hence,

$$\sigma_{\overline{X}} = \frac{\sigma}{\sqrt{n}}$$

A third property of the sampling distribution of means pertains to the shape of the distribution and is explained by the **central limit theorem.**

The Central Limit Theorem

As the sample size n increases without limit, the shape of the sampling distribution of means taken with replacement from a population with mean μ and standard deviation σ will approach a normal distribution. As previously shown, this distribution will have a mean μ and a standard deviation $\sigma/\sqrt{n}$.

If the sample size is sufficiently large, the central limit theorem can be used to answer questions about sample means in the same manner that a normal distribution can be used to answer questions about individual values. The only difference is that a new formula must be used for the z scores. It is

$$z = \frac{\overline{X} - \mu}{\sigma/\sqrt{n}}$$

Notice that $\overline{X}$ is the sample mean, and the denominator must be adjusted since means are being used instead of individual data values. The denominator is the standard deviation of the sample means.

If a large number of samples of a given size are selected from a normally distributed population, or if a large number of samples of a given size that is greater than or equal to 30 are selected from a population that is not normally distributed, and the sample means are computed, then the sampling distribution of means will look like the one shown in Figure 6–28. Their percentages indicate the areas of the regions.

Interesting Fact

McMaster University researchers discovered that Albert Einstein's brain was 15% wider than normal in the area responsible for mathematical thought.

Figure 6–28

Sampling Distribution of Means for Large Number of Samples

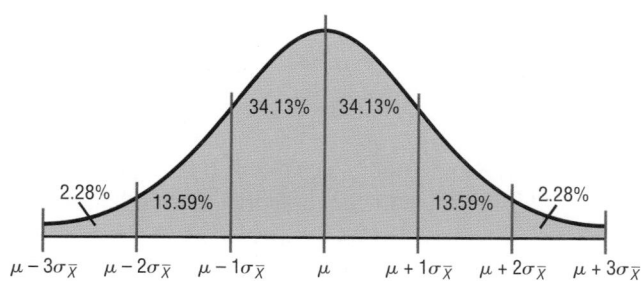

It's important to remember two things when you use the central limit theorem:

1. When the original variable is normally distributed, the distribution of the sample means will be normally distributed for any sample size n.

2. When the distribution of the original variable might not be normal, a sample size of 30 or more is needed to use a normal distribution to approximate the distribution of the sample means. The larger the sample, the better the approximation will be.

Examples 6–14 through 6–16 show how the standard normal distribution can be used to answer questions about sample means.

Example 6–14

Hours That Children Watch Television

A. C. Neilsen reported that children between the ages of 2 and 5 watch an average of 25 hours of television per week. Assume the variable is normally distributed and the standard deviation is 3 hours. If 20 children between the ages of 2 and 5 are randomly selected, find the probability that the mean of the number of hours they watch television will be greater than 26.3 hours.

Source: Michael D. Shook and Robert L. Shook, *The Book of Odds.*

Solution

Since the variable is normally distributed, the sampling distribution of means will be normal, with a mean of 25. The standard deviation of the sample means is

$$\sigma_{\overline{X}} = \frac{\sigma}{\sqrt{n}} = \frac{3}{\sqrt{20}} = 0.671$$

The distribution of the means is shown in Figure 6–29, with the appropriate area shaded.

Figure 6–29

Distribution of the Means for Example 6–14

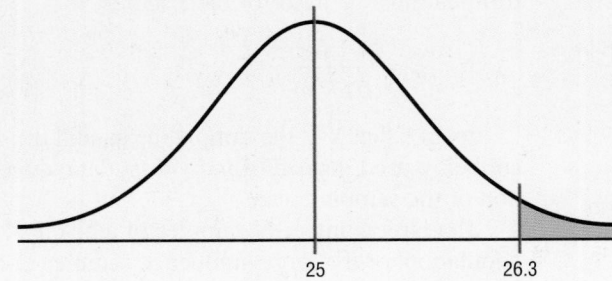

The z score is

$$z = \frac{\overline{X} - \mu}{\sigma/\sqrt{n}} = \frac{26.3 - 25}{3/\sqrt{20}} = \frac{1.3}{0.671} = 1.94$$

The cumulative area to the left for $z = 1.94$ is 0.9738. Since the desired area is to the right of $z = 1.94$, subtract 0.9738 from the total area under the curve, 1.000. Hence, $1.000 - 0.9738 = 0.0262$, or 2.62%.

One can conclude that the probability of obtaining a sample mean larger than 26.3 hours is 2.62% [i.e., $P(\overline{X} > 26.3) = 2.62\%$].

Example 6–15

Age of Light-Duty Vehicles

The average age of light-duty vehicles in Canada is 8.5 years, or 102 months. Assume a standard deviation of 16 months. If a random sample of 36 vehicles is selected, find the probability that the mean of their age is between 96 and 106 months

Source: DesRosiers Automotive Consultants Inc.

Solution

Since the sample is 30 or larger, the normality assumption is not necessary. The desired area is shown in Figure 6–30.

Figure 6–30

Area under a
Normal Curve for
Example 6–15

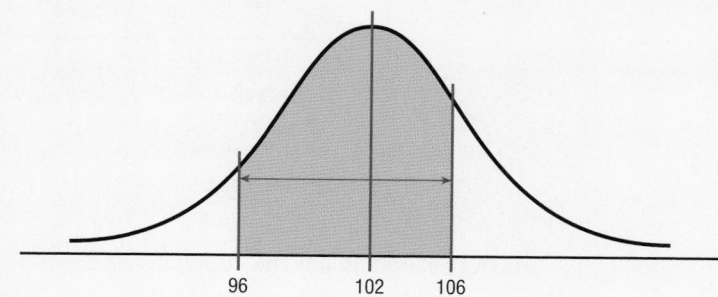

Convert $\overline{X}_1 = 96$ and $\overline{X}_2 = 106$ to z scores.

$$z_1 = \frac{\overline{X}_1 - \mu}{\frac{\sigma}{\sqrt{n}}} = \frac{96 - 102}{\frac{16}{\sqrt{36}}} = -2.25$$

$$z_2 = \frac{\overline{X}_2 - \mu}{\frac{\sigma}{\sqrt{n}}} = \frac{106 - 102}{\frac{16}{\sqrt{36}}} = 1.5$$

The cumulative area to the left of $z_1 = -2.25$ is 0.0122. The cumulative area to the left of $z_2 = 1.5$ is 0.9332. Hence, the desired area is $0.9332 - 0.0122 = 0.9210$, or 92.1%.

Therefore, the probability of obtaining a sample mean between 96 and 106 months is 92.1%; that is, $P(96 < \overline{X} < 106) = 92.1\%$.

Example 6–16

Meat Consumption

The average annual Canadian consumption of red meat is 62.9 kilograms per person. Assume a standard deviation of 7 kilograms and an approximately normal distribution.

    a. Find the probability that a person selected at random consumes less than 65 kilograms per year.

    b. If a sample of 40 individuals is selected, find the probability that the mean of the sample will be less than 65 kilograms per year.

Sources: Adapted from Statistics Canada, *Food Consumption in Canada* (Part 1), Catalogue 32–229, and *Food Consumption in Canada* (Part 2), Catalogue 32–230.

Solution

a. Since the question asks about an individual person, the formula $z = (X - \mu)/\sigma$ is used. The distribution is shown in Figure 6–31.

Figure 6–31

Area under a Normal
Curve for Part *a* of
Example 6–16

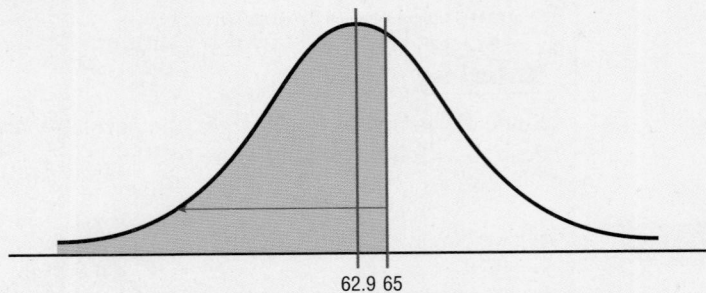

62.9 65
Distribution of individual data values for the population

Convert the X value to a z score.

$$z = \frac{X - \mu}{\sigma} = \frac{65 - 62.9}{7} = 0.3$$

The desired area is the cumulative area to the left of $z = 0.3$, which is 0.6179.
Hence, the probability of selecting a Canadian who consumes less than 65 kilograms of red meat per year is 0.6179, or 61.79%; that is, $P(X < 65) = 0.6179$.

b. Since the question concerns the mean of a sample with size 40, the formula $z = (\overline{X} - \mu)/(\sigma \sqrt{n})$ is used. The distribution is shown in Figure 6–32.

Figure 6–32

Area under a Normal
Curve for Part *b* of
Example 6–16

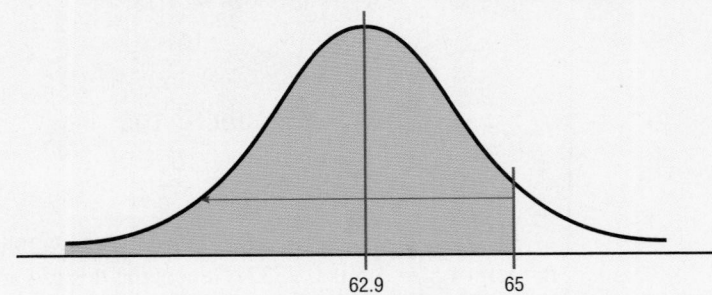

62.9   65
Distribution of means for all samples of size 40 from the population

Convert the $\overline{X}$ value to a z score.

$$z = \frac{\overline{X} - \mu}{\dfrac{\sigma}{\sqrt{n}}} = \frac{65 - 62.9}{\dfrac{7}{\sqrt{40}}} = 1.90$$

The desired area is the cumulative area to the left of $z = 1.90$, which is 0.9713.
Hence, the probability that the mean of a sample of 40 Canadians who consume less than 65 kilograms of red meat per year is 0.9713, or 97.13%; that is, $P(\overline{X} < 65) = 0.9713$.

Comparing the two probabilities, one can see that the probability of selecting an individual who consumes less than 65 kilograms of red meat per year is 61.79%, but the probability of selecting 40 people with a mean consumption of red meat that is less than 65 kilograms per year is 97.13%. This rather large difference is due to the fact that the sampling distribution of means is much less variable than the distribution of individual data values. (*Note:* An individual person is the equivalent of saying $n = 1$.)

Finite Population Correction Factor (Optional)

The formula for the standard error of the mean $\sigma/\sqrt{n}$ is accurate when the samples are drawn with replacement or are drawn without replacement from a very large or infinite population. Since sampling with replacement is for the most part unrealistic, a *correction factor* is necessary for computing the standard error of the mean for samples drawn without replacement from a finite population. Compute the correction factor by using the expression

$$\sqrt{\frac{N-n}{N-1}}$$

Interesting Fact

The bubonic plague killed more than 25 million people in Europe between 1347 and 1351.

where N is the population size and n is the sample size.

This correction factor is necessary if relatively large samples are taken from a small population, because the sample mean will then more accurately estimate the population mean and there will be less error in the estimation. Therefore, the standard error of the mean must be multiplied by the correction factor to adjust for large samples taken from a small population. That is,

$$\sigma_{\bar{X}} = \frac{\sigma}{\sqrt{n}} \cdot \sqrt{\frac{N-n}{N-1}}$$

Finally, the formula for the z score becomes

$$z = \frac{\bar{X} - \mu}{\dfrac{\sigma}{\sqrt{n}} \cdot \sqrt{\dfrac{N-n}{N-1}}}$$

The rule of thumb is to use the finite population correction factor if the sample size is greater than 5% of the population size, that is if $n > 0.05N$. When the population is large and the sample is small, the correction factor is generally not used, since it will be very close to 1.00.

The formulas and their uses are summarized in Table 6–1.

Table 6–1	Summary of Formulas and Their Uses
Formula	**Use**
1. $z = \dfrac{\bar{X} - \mu}{\sigma}$	Used to gain information about an individual data value when the variable is normally distributed.
2. $z = \dfrac{\bar{X} - \mu}{\sigma/\sqrt{n}}$	Used to gain information when applying the central limit theorem about a sample mean when the variable is normally distributed or when the sample size is 30 or more.

6–3   Applying the Concepts

Central Limit Theorem

Twenty students from a statistics class each collected a random sample of times on how long it took students to get to class from their homes. All the sample sizes were 30. The resulting means are listed.

Student	Mean	Std. Dev.	Student	Mean	Std. Dev.
1	22	3.7	11	27	1.4
2	31	4.6	12	24	2.2
3	18	2.4	13	14	3.1
4	27	1.9	14	29	2.4
5	20	3.0	15	37	2.8
6	17	2.8	16	23	2.7
7	26	1.9	17	26	1.8
8	34	4.2	18	21	2.0
9	23	2.6	19	30	2.2
10	29	2.1	20	29	2.8

1. The students noticed that everyone had different answers. If you randomly sample over and over from any population, with the same sample size, will the results ever be the same?

2. The students wondered whose results were right. How can they find out what the population mean and standard deviation are?

3. Input the means into the computer and check to see if the distribution is normal.

4. Check the mean and standard deviation of the means.

5. Is the distribution of the means a sampling distribution?

6. Check the sampling error for students 3, 7, and 14.

7. Compare the standard deviation of the sample of the 20 means with the standard deviation from each student's sample.

See page 301 for the answers.

Exercises 6–3

1. If samples of a specific size are selected from a population and the means are computed, what is this distribution of means called?

2. Why do most of the sample means differ somewhat from the population mean? What is this difference called?

3. What is the mean of the sample means?

4. What is the standard deviation of the sample means called? What is the formula for this standard deviation?

5. What does the central limit theorem say about the shape of the sampling distribution of means?

6. What formula is used to gain information about an individual data value when the variable is normally distributed?

7. What formula is used to gain information about a sample mean when the variable is normally distributed or when the sample size is 30 or more?

For Exercises 8 through 25, assume that the sample is taken from a large population and the correction factor can be ignored.

8. **Disposal of Nonhazardous Material** The waste management industry reports that Canadian individuals dispose of an average of 760 kilograms of nonhazardous material in a given year. Assume a standard deviation of 90 kilograms. Find the probability that the mean of a sample of 55 Canadians will be between 750 and 775 kilograms.
   Source: Statistics Canada, *Waste Management Industry Survey.*

9. **Cost of Dog Ownership** The average yearly cost per household of owning a dog is $186.80. Suppose that we randomly select 50 households that own a dog. What is the probability that the sample mean for these 50 households is less than $175.00? Assume $\sigma = \$32$.
   Source: *N.Y. Times Almanac.*

10. **Social Networking User Ages** In 2010, the average age of users of the social networking Web site *Facebook* was 37 years. Assume a normally distributed population with a standard deviation of 5 years.

a. What is the probability that a randomly selected *Facebook* user is younger than 35 years old?

b. In a random sample of 30 *Facebook* users, what is the probability that the sample mean is younger than 35 years?

Source: OhMyGov! "6 Social Media Stats You Can't Live Without," Briana Kerensky, February 24, 2010.

11. **Weight of 15-Year-Old Males** The mean weight of 15-year-old males is 64.4 kilograms, and the standard deviation is 5.6 kilograms. If a random sample of thirty-six 15-year-old males is selected, find the probability that the mean of the sample will be greater than 65.5 kilograms. Assume the variable is normally distributed. Based on your answer, would you consider the group overweight?

12. **Experienced Teachers' Salaries** For the 2009/2010 school year, the average salary for experienced Alberta teachers with 4 years of university education and 10 years of experience was $84,800. Assume a normal distribution with $\sigma = \$8050$.

a. What is the probability that a randomly selected experienced Alberta teacher earned less than $85,000 in the 2009/2010 school year?

b. In a random sample of 100 experienced Alberta teachers, what is the probability that the 2009/2010 mean salary of the sample is less than $85,000?

Source: The Alberta Teachers' Association.

13. **Food Expenditure** Canadian households spend an average of $124 per week on food in either stores or restaurants. Assume a standard deviation of $11 per week. If a sample of 40 households is randomly selected, find the probability that the mean of the sample is less than $120.
Source: Statistics Canada.

14. **SAT Score** The national average SAT score is 1019. Suppose that nothing is known about the shape of the distribution and that the standard deviation is 100. If a random sample of 200 scores was selected and the sample mean was calculated to be 1050, would you be surprised? Explain.
Source: N.Y. Times Almanac.

15. **Sodium in Frozen Food** The average number of milligrams (mg) of sodium in a certain brand of low-salt microwave frozen dinners is 660 mg, and the standard deviation is 35 mg. Assume the variable is normally distributed.

a. If a single dinner is selected, find the probability that the sodium content will be more than 670 mg.

b. If a sample of 10 dinners is selected, find the probability that the mean of the sample will be larger than 670 mg.

c. Why is the probability for part a greater than that for part b?

16. **Engineers' Ages** The average age of chemical engineers is 37 years with a standard deviation of 4 years. If an engineering firm employs 25 chemical engineers, find the probability that the average age of the group is greater than 38.2 years old. If this is the case, would it be safe to assume that the engineers in this group are generally much older than average?

17. **Water Intake** Health Canada reports that the average adult drinks 1.5 litres of water daily, including water used in drinks such as coffee, tea, and juice. Assume a normally distributed variable with a standard deviation of 0.3 litres per day. If 15 Canadian adults are selected at random, find the probability that the sample mean of daily water consumption will be between 1.3 and 1.6 litres.
Source: Health Canada.

18. **Students in Elementary Schools** The average public elementary school has 458 students. Assume the standard deviation is 97. If a random sample of 36 public elementary schools is selected, find the probability that the number of students enrolled is between 450 and 465.

19. **Vision Care Expenses** *The Globe and Mail* reported that the average annual Canadian out-of-pocket expense on vision care was $1701 per household. If the standard deviation is $205, find the probability that the sample mean of 50 household vision care expenditures randomly selected will be between $1650 and $1750.
Source: www.theglobeandmail.com.

20. **Student Tuition Fees** In 2010, Canadian university undergraduate students paid an average of $4917 per year for tuition fees. Assume that tuition fees are normally distributed with a standard deviation of $541.

a. If an undergraduate student is selected at random, find the probability that the student pays less than $4750 tuition fees.

b. If a random sample of 25 students is selected, find the probability that the sample mean tuition fee is less than $4750.

c. Why is the probability for part b higher than the probability for part a?

Source: Statistics Canada, *The Daily*, "University Tuition Fees, 2009/2010," October 20, 2009.

21. **Time to Complete an Exam** The average time it takes a group of adults to complete a certain achievement test is 46.2 minutes. The standard deviation is 8 minutes. Assume the variable is normally distributed.

a. Find the probability that a randomly selected adult will complete the test in less than 43 minutes.

b. Find the probability that, if 50 randomly selected adults take the test, the mean time it takes the group to complete the test will be less than 43 minutes.

c. Does it seem reasonable that an adult would finish the test in less than 43 minutes? Explain.

d. Does it seem reasonable that the mean of the 50 adults could be less than 43 minutes?

22. **Systolic Blood Pressure** Assume that the mean systolic blood pressure of normal adults is 120 millimetres of

mercury (mm Hg) and the standard deviation is 5.6. Assume the variable is normally distributed.

a. If an individual is selected, find the probability that the individual's pressure will be between 120 and 121.8 mm Hg.

b. If a sample of 30 adults is randomly selected, find the probability that the sample mean will be between 120 and 121.8 mm Hg.

c. Why is the answer to part *a* so much smaller than the answer to part *b*?

23. Cholesterol Content The average cholesterol content of a certain brand of eggs is 5.56 millimoles per litre (mmol/L), and the standard deviation is 0.39 mmol/L. Assume the variable is normally distributed.

a. If a single egg is selected, find the probability that the cholesterol content will be greater than 5.70 mmol/L.

b. If a sample of two dozen eggs is selected, find the probability that the mean of the sample will be larger than 5.70 mmol/L.

Source: Living Fit.

24. Age of Proofreaders At a large publishing company, the mean age of proofreaders is 36.2 years, and the standard deviation is 3.7 years. Assume the variable is normally distributed.

a. If a proofreader from the company is randomly selected, find the probability that his or her age will be between 36 and 37.5 years.

b. If a random sample of 15 proofreaders is selected, find the probability that the mean age of the proofreaders in the sample will be between 36 and 37.5 years.

25. Egg Consumption Statistics Canada reports the per capita (average) annual consumption of eggs in Canada was 15.5 dozen, or 186 eggs. Assume the standard deviation of egg consumption is 18 eggs. If 35 Canadian consumers are selected, find the probability that the mean number of eggs consumed is between 180 and 190.

Source: Statistics Canada.

Extending the Concepts »

For Exercises 26 and 27, check to see whether the correction factor should be used. If so, be sure to include it in the calculations.

26. Life Expectancies In a study of the life expectancy of 500 people in a certain geographic region, the mean age at death was 72.0 years, and the standard deviation was 5.3 years. If a sample of 50 people from this region is selected, find the probability that the mean life expectancy will be less than 70 years.

27. Home Values A study of 800 homeowners in Ontario showed that the average value of their homes was $329,000, and the standard deviation was $20,000. If 50 homes are for sale, find the probability that the mean of the values of these homes is greater than $334,500.

Source: Canadian Real Estate Association, MLS Statistics.

28. Breaking Strength of Steel Cable The average breaking strength of a certain brand of steel cable is 907 kilograms, with a standard deviation of 45 kilograms. A sample of 20 cables is selected and tested. Find the sample mean that will cut off the upper 95% of all samples of size 20 taken from the population. Assume the variable is normally distributed.

29. The standard deviation of a variable is 15. If a sample of 100 individuals is selected, compute the standard error of the mean. What sample size is necessary to double the standard error of the mean?

30. In Exercise 29, what sample size is needed to cut the standard error of the mean in half?

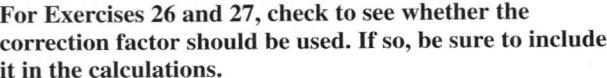

6–4   The Normal Approximation to the Binomial Distribution (Optional) ›

Use the normal approximation to compute probabilities for a binomial variable.

A normal distribution may be used to solve complex problems that involve the binomial distribution when *n* is large and technological tools are not readily available. Recall from Chapter 5 that a binomial distribution has the following characteristics:

1. There must be a fixed number of trials.

2. The outcome of each trial must be independent.

3. Each experiment can have only two outcomes or outcomes that can be reduced to two outcomes.

4. The probability of a success must remain the same for each trial.

Also, recall that a binomial distribution is determined by n (the number of trials) and p (the probability of a success). When p is approximately 0.5, and as n increases, the shape of the binomial distribution becomes similar to that of a normal distribution. The larger n is and the closer p is to 0.5, the more similar the shape of the binomial distribution is to that of a normal distribution.

But when p is close to 0 or 1 and n is relatively small, a normal approximation is inaccurate. As a rule of thumb, statisticians generally agree that a normal approximation should be used only when $n \cdot p$ and $n \cdot q$ are both greater than or equal to 5. (*Note:* $q = 1 - p$.) For example, if p is 0.3 and n is 10, then $np = (10)(0.3) = 3$, and a normal distribution should not be used as an approximation. On the other hand, if $p = 0.5$ and $n = 10$, then $np = (10)(0.5) = 5$ and $nq = (10)(0.5) = 5$, and a normal distribution can be used as an approximation. See Figure 6–33.

In addition to the previous condition of $np \geq 5$ and $nq \geq 5$, a correction for continuity may be used in the normal approximation.

A **correction for continuity** is a correction employed when a continuous distribution is used to approximate a discrete distribution.

Figure 6–33

Comparison of the Binomial Distribution and a Normal Distribution

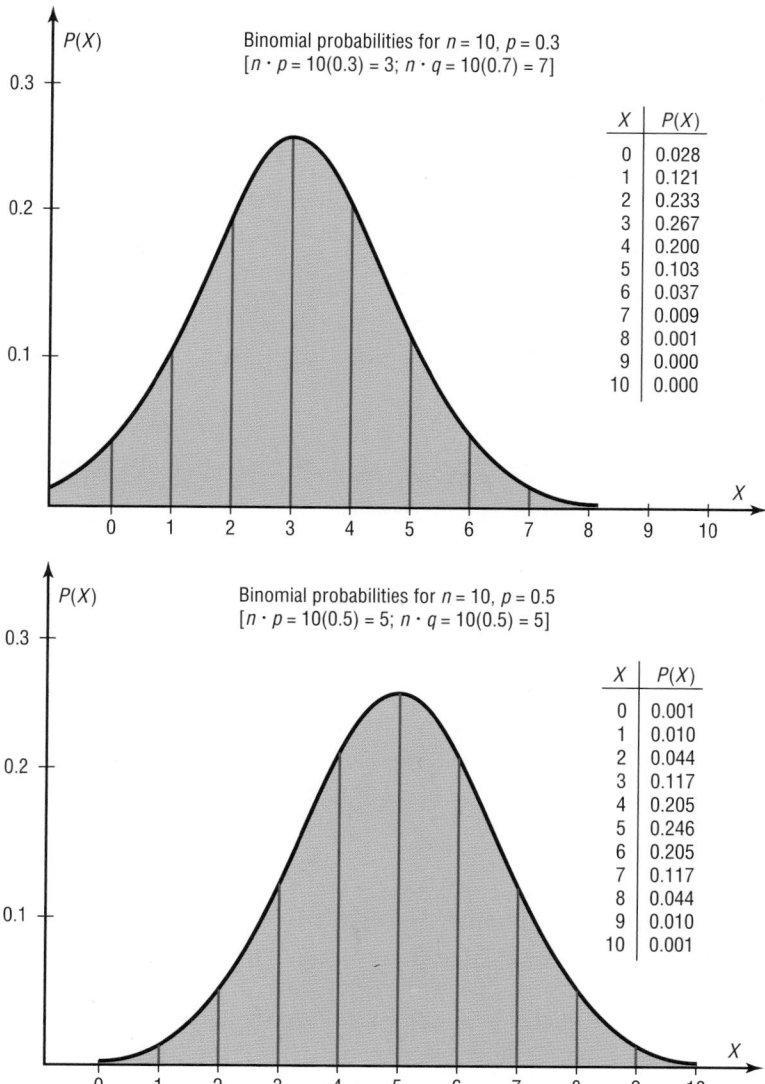

The continuity correction means that for any specific value of X, say 8, the boundaries of X in the binomial distribution (in this case, 7.5 to 8.5) must be used. (See Section 1–2.) Hence, when one employs a normal distribution to approximate the binomial, the boundaries of any specific value X must be used as they are shown in the binomial distribution. For example, for $P(X = 8)$, the correction is $P(7.5 < X < 8.5)$ For $P(X \leq 7)$, the correction is $P(X < 7.5)$. For $P(X \geq 3)$, the correction is $P(X > 2.5)$.

Students sometimes have difficulty deciding whether to add 0.5 or subtract 0.5 from the data value for the correction factor. Table 6–2 summarizes the different situations.

Table 6–2	Summary of the Normal Approximation to the Binomial Distribution
Binomial	**Normal**
When finding	Use
1. $P(X = a)$	$P(a - 0.5 < X < a + 0.5)$
2. $P(X \geq a)$	$P(X > a - 0.5)$
3. $P(X > a)$	$P(X > a + 0.5)$
4. $P(X \leq a)$	$P(X < a + 0.5)$
5. $P(X < a)$	$P(X < a - 0.5)$

For all cases, $\mu = n \cdot p$, $\sigma = \sqrt{n \cdot p \cdot q}$, $n \cdot p \geq 5$, and $n \cdot q \geq 5$.

The formulas for the mean and standard deviation for the binomial distribution are necessary for calculations. They are

$$\mu = n \cdot p \qquad \text{and} \qquad \sigma = \sqrt{n \cdot p \cdot q}$$

The steps for using the normal distribution to approximate the binomial distribution are shown in this Procedure Table.

Procedure Table

Procedure for the Normal Approximation to the Binomial Distribution

Step 1   Check to see whether the normal approximation can be used.

Step 2   Find the mean μ and the standard deviation σ.

Step 3   Write the problem in probability notation, using X.

Step 4   Rewrite the problem by using the continuity correction factor, and show the corresponding area under the normal distribution.

Step 5   Find the corresponding z scores.

Step 6   Find the solution.

Example 6–17

Cellphone Use while Driving

A marketing study reported that 26% of Canadian drivers surveyed talk on cellphones while driving. If 300 drivers are selected at random, find the probability that exactly 90 have talked on their cellphones while driving.

Source: Leger Marketing.

Solution

Step 1 Here, $p = 0.26$, $q = 0.74$, and $n = 300$.

$$np = (300)(0.26) = 78 \qquad nq = (300)(0.74) = 222$$

Since $np \geq 5$ and $nq \geq 5$, the normal distribution can be used.

Step 2 Find the mean and standard deviation.

$$\mu = np = (300)(0.26) = 78$$
$$\sigma = \sqrt{npq} = \sqrt{(300)(0.26)(0.74)} = \sqrt{57.72} = 7.6$$

Step 3 Write the problem in probability notation $P(X = 90)$.

Step 4 Rewrite the problem by using the continuity correction factor. See approximation number 1 in Table 6–2; $P(90 - 0.5 < X < 90 + 0.5) = P(89.5 < X < 90.5)$. Show the corresponding area under the normal distribution curve. See Figure 6–34.

Figure 6–34

Area under a Normal Curve and X Values for Example 6–17

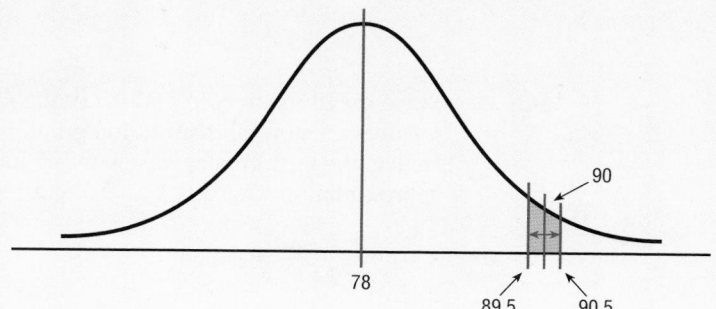

Step 5 Find the corresponding z scores. Since 90 represents any value between $X_1 = 89.5$ and $X_2 = 90.5$, find both z scores.

$$z_1 = \frac{89.5 - 78}{7.6} = 1.51 \qquad z_2 = \frac{90.5 - 78}{7.6} = 1.64$$

Step 6 Find the desired area. The cumulative area to the left of $z = 1.51$ is 0.9345 and the cumulative area to the left of $z = 1.64$ is 0.9495. Hence, the desired area is $0.9495 - 0.9345 = 0.4495 - 0.4245 = 0.015$, or 1.5%.

Therefore, the probability that exactly 90 out of 300 Canadian drivers are talking on their cellphones is 1.5%.

Example 6–18

Widowed Bowlers

Of the members of a bowling league, 10% are widowed. If 200 bowling league members are selected at random, find the probability that 10 or more will be widowed.

Solution

Here, $p = 0.10$, $q = 0.90$, and $n = 200$.

Step 1 Since $np = (200)(0.10) = 20$ and $nq = (200)(0.90) = 180$, the normal approximation can be used.

Step 2 $\mu = np = (200)(0.10) = 20$

$\sigma = \sqrt{npq} = \sqrt{(200)(0.10)(0.90)} = \sqrt{18} = 4.24$

Step 3 $P(X \geq 10)$.

Step 4   See approximation number 2 in Table 6–2: $P(X > 10 - 0.5) = P(X > 9.5)$. The desired area is shown in Figure 6–35.

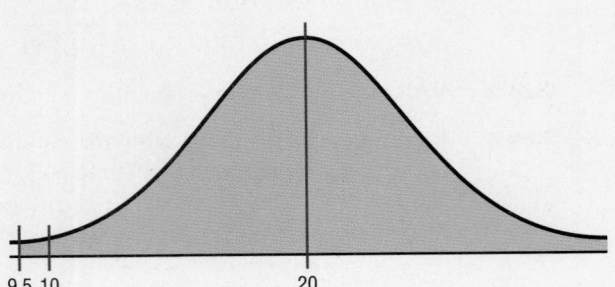

Figure 6–35

Area under a Normal Curve and X Value for Example 6–18

9.5 10   20

Step 5   Since the problem is to find the probability of 10 or more widowed members, a normal distribution graph is as shown in Figure 6–35. Hence, the area greater then $X = 9.5$ must be used to get the correct approximation. Convert $X = 9.5$ to a z score.

$$z = \frac{9.5 - 20}{4.24} = -2.48$$

Step 6   Find the desired area. The cumulative area to the left of $z = -2.48$ is 0.0066. Hence, the desired area is $1.000 - 0.0066 = 0.9934$, or 99.34%.

It can be concluded, then, that the probability of 10 or more widowed people in a random sample of 200 bowling league members is 99.34%.

Example 6–19

Baseball Batting Average

If a baseball player's batting average is 0.320 (32% hit safely to batting attempts made), find the probability that the player will get at most 26 hits in 100 times at bat.

Solution

Here, $p = 0.32$, $q = 0.68$, and $n = 100$.

Step 1   Since $np = (100)(0.320) = 32$ and $nq = (100)(0.680) = 68$, the normal distribution can be used to approximate the binomial distribution.

Step 2 $\mu = np = (100)(0.320) = 32$

$\sigma = \sqrt{npq} = \sqrt{(100)(0.32)(0.68)} = \sqrt{21.76} \approx 4.66$

Step 3 $P(X \leq 26)$.

Step 4   See approximation number 4 in Table 6–2: $P(X < 26 + 0.5) = P(X < 26.5)$. The desired area is shown in Figure 6–36.

Figure 6–36

Area under a
Normal Curve for
Example 6–19

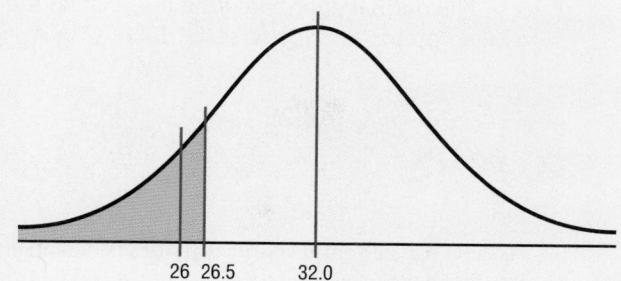

26 26.5   32.0

Step 5   The z score is

$$z = \frac{26.5 - 32}{4.66} = -1.18$$

Step 6   The cumulative area to the left of $z = -1.18$ is 0.1190. Therefore, the desired area is 0.1190, or 11.90%.

Hence the probability that the player will get at most 26 hits is 11.90%.

The closeness of the normal approximation is illustrated in Example 6–20.

Example 6–20

Comparing Binomial Distribution Table and Normal Approximation Methods
When $n = 10$ and $p = 0.5$, use the binomial distribution table (Table B in Appendix C) to find the probability that $X = 6$. Then use the normal approximation to find the probability that $X = 6$.

Solution

From Table B, for $n = 10$, $p = 0.5$, and $X = 6$, the probability is 0.205.
   For a normal approximation,

$$\mu = np = (10)(0.5) = 5$$
$$\sigma = \sqrt{npq} = \sqrt{(10)(0.5)(0.5)} \approx 1.58$$

Now, $X = 6$ is represented by the boundaries 5.5 and 6.5. So the z scores are

$$z_1 = \frac{6.5 - 5}{1.58} = 0.95 \qquad z_2 = \frac{5.5 - 5}{1.58} = 0.32$$

The cumulative areas to the left of $z = 0.95$ is 0.8289 and $z = 0.32$ is 0.6255, respectively.
   The solution is $0.8289 - 0.6255 = 0.2034$, which is very close to the binomial table value of 0.205. The desired area is shown in Figure 6–37.

Figure 6–37

Area under a
Normal Curve for
Example 6–20

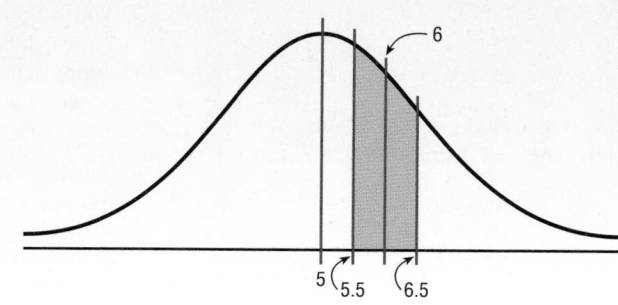

5   6.5
  5.5   6.5

The normal approximation also can be used to approximate other distributions, such as the Poisson distribution (see Table C in Appendix C).

6–4   Applying the Concepts

How Safe Are You?

Assume one of your favourite activities is mountain climbing. When you go mountain climbing, you have several safety devices to keep you from falling. You notice that attached to one of your safety hooks is a reliability rating of 97%. You estimate that throughout the next year you will be using this device about 100 times. Answer the following questions.

1. Does a reliability rating of 97% mean that there is a 97% chance that the device will not fail any of the 100 times?
2. What is the probability of at least one failure?
3. What is the complement of this event?
4. Can this be considered a binomial experiment?
5. Can you use the binomial probability formula? Why or why not?
6. Find the probability of at least two failures.
7. Can you use a normal distribution to accurately approximate the binomial distribution? Explain why or why not.
8. Is correction for continuity needed?
9. How much safer would it be to use a second safety hook independently of the first?

See page 301 for the answers.

Exercises 6–4

1. Explain why a normal distribution can be used as an approximation to a binomial distribution. What conditions must be met to use the normal distribution to approximate the binomial distribution? Why is a correction for continuity necessary?

2. **(ans)** Use the normal approximation to the binomial to find the probabilities for the specific value(s) of X.

   a. $n = 30, p = 0.5, X = 18$
   b. $n = 50, p = 0.8, X = 44$
   c. $n = 100, p = 0.1, X = 12$
   d. $n = 10, p = 0.5, X \geq 7$
   e. $n = 20, p = 0.7, X \leq 12$
   f. $n = 50, p = 0.6, X \leq 40$

3. Check each binomial distribution to see whether it can be approximated by a normal distribution (i.e., are $np \geq 5$ and $nq \geq 5$?).

   a. $n = 20, p = 0.5$
   b. $n = 10, p = 0.6$
   c. $n = 40, p = 0.9$

   d. $n = 50, p = 0.2$
   e. $n = 30, p = 0.8$
   f. $n = 20, p = 0.85$

4. **High School Graduation** The BC Ministry of Education reports that the six-year Grade 12 graduation rate for all students is 79.2%. If a random sample of former British Columbia high school students is selected, find the probability that at least 400 completed Grade 12 within six years.
   Source: BC Ministry of Education.

5. **Youth Smoking Habit** Two out of 5 adult smokers acquired the habit by age 14. If 400 smokers are randomly selected, find the probability that 170 or more acquired the habit by age 14.
   Source: Harper's Index.

6. **Theatre No-Shows** A theatre owner has found that 5% of patrons do not show up for the performance for which they purchased tickets. If the theatre has 100 seats, find the probability that 6 or more patrons will not show up for a sold-out performance.

7. **High School Graduates** The percentage of Canadians 15 years and older with at least a high school graduate certificate is 66.8%. In a random sample of 300 Canadians 15 years old and older, what is the probability that more than 200 have at least a high school graduate certificate?
Source: Statistics Canada.

8. **Home Internet** A Media Awareness Network study, *Young Canadians in a Wired World,* researched online behaviours of children and youth from Grades 4 to 11. One finding was that 94% of the respondents connect to the Internet from home. If a random sample of 90 young Canadians was taken, find the probability that all 90 respondents have a home Internet connection.

9. **Post-Secondary Credentials** Statistics Canada's study on education attainment reports that 61% of Canadian adults aged 25 to 34 years have post-secondary documentation, i.e., university degree, college diploma, or trade credential. If 250 Canadian adults, aged 25 to 34 years, are randomly selected, find the probability that fewer than 150 have post-secondary documentation.
Source: Statistics Canada.

10. **Women in the Work Force** Women make up 24% of the science and engineering work force. In a random sample of 400 science and engineering employees, what is the probability that more than 120 are women?
Source: Science and Engineering Indicators: www.nsf.gov.

11. **Elementary School Teachers** Women comprise 83.3% of all elementary school teachers. In a random sample of 300 elementary school teachers, what is the probability that more than 50 are men?
Source: N.Y. Times Almanac.

12. **Self-Employed Workers** Canada's labour force consists of 11.9% workers who are self-employed. If 150 workers from across Canada are selected at random, what is the probability that more than 20 workers are self-employed?
Source: Statistics Canada.

13. **Parking Lot Construction** The mayor of a small town estimates that 35% of the residents in his town favour the construction of a municipal parking lot. If there are 350 people at a town meeting, find the probability that at least 100 favour construction of the parking lot. Based on your answer, is it likely that 100 or more people would favour the parking lot?

14. **Home Region of Immigrants** In 2008, 45.6% of immigrants to Canada claiming permanent residency were from the Asia and South Pacific region. If 250 permanent resident immigrants are selected at random, find the probability that fewer than 100 are from the Asia and South Pacific region.
Source: Citizenship and Immigration Canada, Facts and Figures, "Immigration Overview: Permanent and Temporary Residents, 2008."

Extending the Concepts »

15. Recall that for use of a normal distribution as an approximation to the binomial distribution, the conditions $np \geq 5$ and $nq \geq 5$ must be met. For each given probability, compute the minimum sample size needed for use of the normal approximation.

    a. $p = 0.1$ *d.* $p = 0.8$

    b. $p = 0.3$ *e.* $p = 0.9$

    c. $p = 0.5$

Summary >

A normal distribution can be used to describe a variety of variables, such as heights, weights, and temperatures. A normal distribution is bell-shaped, unimodal, symmetric, and continuous; its mean, median, and mode are equal. Since each variable has its own distribution with mean μ and standard deviation σ, mathematicians use the standard normal distribution, which has a mean of 0 and a standard deviation of 1. Other approximately normally distributed variables can be transformed to the standard normal distribution with the formula $z = (X - \mu)/\sigma$.

A normal distribution can also be used to describe a sampling distribution of means. These samples must be of the same size and randomly selected with replacement from the population. The means of the samples will differ somewhat from the population mean, since samples are generally not perfect representations of the population from which they came. The mean of the sample means will be equal to the population mean, and the standard deviation of the sample means will be equal to the population standard deviation, divided by the square root of the sample size. The central limit theorem states that as the size of the samples increases, the sampling distribution of means will be approximately normal.

A normal distribution can be used to approximate other distributions, such as a binomial distribution. For a normal distribution to be used as an approximation, the conditions $np \geq 5$ and $nq \geq 5$ must be met. Also, a correction for continuity may be used for more accurate results.

For step-by-step guidance on the use of Texas Instruments TI-83 Plus/TI-84 Plus programmable calculators, see Appendix E at the back of this textbook. For summary procedures for Minitab, SPSS, and Excel, see the full version of Appendix E on *Connect*.

Important Terms >>

central limit theorem 279

correction for continuity 287

negatively or left-skewed distribution 254

normal distribution 255

positively or right-skewed distribution 254

sampling distribution of means 277

sampling error 277

standard error of the mean 279

standard normal distribution 257

symmetric distribution 253

Important Formulas >>

Formula for the z score (or standard score):

$$z = \frac{X - \mu}{\sigma}$$

Formula for finding a specific data value:

$$X = z \cdot \sigma + \mu$$

Formula for the mean of the sample means:

$$\mu_{\bar{X}} = \mu$$

Formula for the standard error of the mean:

$$\sigma_{\bar{X}} = \frac{\sigma}{\sqrt{n}}$$

Formula for the z score for the central limit theorem:

$$z = \frac{\bar{X} - \mu}{\sigma/\sqrt{n}}$$

Formulas for the mean and standard deviation for the binomial distribution:

$$\mu = n \cdot p \qquad \sigma = \sqrt{n \cdot p \cdot q}$$

Mc Graw Hill **connect**™ Practise and learn online with *Connect* with data sets and algorithmic questions related to concepts covered in this chapter. Questions and tables with online data sets are marked with ⬈.

Review Exercises »

1. Find the area under the standard normal distribution curve for each.

    a. Between $z = 0$ and $z = 1.95$
    b. Between $z = 0$ and $z = 0.37$
    c. Between $z = 1.32$ and $z = 1.82$
    d. Between $z = -1.05$ and $z = 2.05$
    e. Between $z = -0.03$ and $z = 0.53$
    f. Between $z = +1.10$ and $z = -1.80$
    g. To the right of $z = 1.99$
    h. To the right of $z = -1.36$
    i. To the left of $z = -2.09$
    j. To the left of $z = 1.68$

2. Using the standard normal distribution, find each probability.

    a. $P(0 < z < 2.07)$
    b. $P(-1.83 < z < 0)$
    c. $P(-1.59 < z < +2.01)$
    d. $P(1.33 < z < 1.88)$
    e. $P(-2.56 < z < 0.37)$
    f. $P(z > 1.66)$
    g. $P(z < -2.03)$
    h. $P(z > -1.19)$
    i. $P(z < 1.93)$
    j. $P(z > -1.77)$

3. **Salaries for Non-High School Graduates** The average annual salary of employed Canadians, aged 15 to 24, with less than a high school graduate certificate is $19,476. Assume the variable is normally distributed with a standard deviation of $2050. Find these probabilities for a randomly selected 15- to 24-year-old worker with less than high school completion.

    a. The worker earns more than $19,476.
    b. The worker earns less than $18,000.
    c. If you were offered a job at $18,000, how would you compare your salary with the salaries of the population of 15- to 24-year-olds without a high school graduate certificate?

    Source: Statistics Canada.

4. **Doctor Fee-for-Service Billing** Canadian medical doctors' average fee-for-service billing to their provincial health-care systems is $202,000 per annum. If the billings of medical doctors are normally distributed with a standard deviation of $13,700, find the probability that

    a. An individual medical doctor fee-for-service billing is more than $210,000.
    b. A random sample of 9 medical doctors' fee-for-service billing is more than $210,000.

    Source: Canadian Institute for Health Information.

5. **Speeding Vehicles** A vehicular fatality inquest in Ontario monitored a section of highway in which the posted speed limit was 80 kilometres per hour (km/h). The report indicated that during the monitored time

period the average speed of vehicles in this section of highway was 98 km/h. Assume speeds are normally distributed with a standard deviation of 9.7 km/h. What percentage of vehicles that were monitored exceeded the posted speed limit? If police decided to ticket only motorists exceeding 85 km/h, what percentage of motorists would be ticketed?

Source: Ontario Legislature—Hansard Debates.

6. **Monthly Cellphone Subscriptions** On average, cellphone users in Canada spend $57.95 in monthly subscription fees. Assume that the subscription fees are normally distributed, with a standard deviation of $8.47. Find the probability that a randomly selected cellphone subscriber spends

    a. More than $60 per month.
    b. Between $50 and $60 per month.
    c. Less than $50 per month.

    Source: Canadian Radio-television and Telecommunications Commission, *5.0 Telecommunications*, "5.5 Wireless," August 5, 2009.

7. **Average Precipitation** During a 6-month period the average monthly precipitation in Vancouver was 116.4 millimetres (mm). If the average precipitation is normally distributed with a standard deviation of 32.8 mm, find these probabilities:

    a. A randomly selected year will have precipitation greater than 100 mm for the same 6-month period.
    b. Five randomly selected years will have an average precipitation greater than 100 mm for the same 6-month period.

    Source: Environment Canada.

8. **Suitcase Weights** The average weight of an airline passenger's suitcase is 20 kg. The standard deviation is 0.9 kg. If 15% of the suitcases are overweight, find the maximum weight allowed by the airline. Assume the variable is normally distributed.

9. **Fish Consumption** Annual average Canadian consumption of fish products per capita is 9.48 kilograms. Assume that fish consumption is normally distributed with a standard deviation of 1.23 kilograms. Find the following probabilities.

    a. A randomly selected Canadian consumes more than 10 kilograms of fish products.
    b. In a random sample of 50 Canadians, the sample mean for fish consumption is more than 10 kilograms.

    Source: Statistics Canada, *Summary Tables*, "Food Available, by Major Food Groups."

10. **Paid Maternity Leave** A 2010 report stated that 80% of mothers employed in the work force reported receiving paid maternity and/or parental leave benefits after giving birth. In a random sample of 120 employed new mothers, find the probability that between 90 and 95 (inclusive) received paid maternity and/or parental leave benefits.

    Source: Statistics Canada, *Perspectives*, "Employer Top-Ups," Katherine Marshall, February 2010.

11. Plasma TV Lifespan Plasma HDTV manufacturers claim an average lifespan of 60,000 hours before the panel reaches half-brightness. Assume the variable is normally distributed, with a standard deviation of 7500 hours. If a random sample of 30 plasma HDTVs is selected, find the probability that the sample mean lifespan to half-brightness will be less than 58,000 hours.
Source: CBS, *CNET Reviews,* "Quick Guide: Four Styles of HDTV," David Katzmaier, February 20, 2009.

12. Slot Machines The probability of winning on a slot machine is 5%. If a person plays the machine 500 times, find the probability of winning 30 times. Use the normal approximation to the binomial distribution.

13. Trade-Related Employment Census information indicates that 14.1% of the Canadian labour force is employed in a trade-related occupation. If 400 working Canadians are selected at random, find the probability that at least 50 are employed in a trade-related occupation.
Source: Statistics Canada.

14. Personal Finance Course Enrollment In a large university, 30% of first-year students elect to enroll in a personal finance course offered by the university. Find the probability that of 800 randomly selected first-year students, at least 260 have elected to enroll in the course.

15. Gold Medal Hockey Viewers The 2010 Olympic men's hockey final gold medal game was watched, in whole or in part, by 80% of the Canadian population. If 200 Canadians are randomly selected, find the probability that at least 150 watched the Olympic gold medal hockey game.
Source: TSN.ca. *NHL,* "Oh Canada! 80% of Canadians Watch Gold Medal Game," March 1, 2010.

16. Heights of Active Volcanoes The heights (in metres above sea level) of a random sample of the world's active volcanoes are shown here. Check for normality.

4095	1565	3456	3726	2277
2890	3774	2339	1592	1716
1087	2168	1783	1731	3836
1703	2462	2911	2458	819
1600	1936	1400	799	2849
1833	731	1725	654	926

Source: N.Y. Times Almanac.

17. School Enrollment A random sample of enrollments based on full-time equivalency (FTE) in Toronto School District schools is listed here. Check for normality.

1409	223	452	159	247
594	289	273	172	390
1324	411	229	187	486
447	874	558	368	478

Source: National Post.

Statistics Today

What Is Normal?—Revisited

Many of the variables measured in medical tests—blood pressure, cholesterol level, body temperature, etc.—are approximately normally distributed for the majority of the population in Canada. Thus, researchers can find the mean and standard devia-tion of these variables. Then, using these two mea-sures along with the z scores, they can find normal intervals for healthy individuals. For example, 95% of the systolic blood pressures of healthy individu-als fall within 2 standard deviations of the mean. If an individual's blood pressure is outside the deter-mined normal range (either above or below), the physician will look for a possible cause and pre-scribe treatment if necessary.

Chapter Quiz »

Determine whether each statement is true or false. If the statement is false, explain why.

1. The total area under a normal distribution is infinite.

2. The standard normal distribution is a continuous distribution.

3. All variables that are approximately normally distrib-uted can be transformed to standard normal variables.

4. The z score corresponding to a number below the mean is always negative.

5. The area under the standard normal distribution to the left of $z = 0$ is negative.

6. The central limit theorem applies to means of samples selected from different populations.

Select the best answer.

7. The mean of the standard normal distribution is

a. 0   *c.* 100
b. 1   *d.* Variable

8. Approximately what percentage of normally distributed data values will fall within 1 standard deviation above or below the mean?

   a. 68%
   b. 95%
   c. 99.7%
   d. Variable

9. Which is not a property of the standard normal distribution?

   a. It's symmetric about the mean.
   b. It's uniform.
   c. It's bell-shaped.
   d. It's unimodal.

10. When a distribution is positively skewed, the usual relationship of the mean, median, and mode from left to right will be

    a. Mean, median, mode
    b. Mode, median, mean
    c. Median, mode, mean
    d. Mean, mode, median

11. The standard deviation of all possible sample means equals

    a. The population standard deviation.
    b. The population standard deviation divided by the population mean.
    c. The population standard deviation divided by the square root of the sample size.
    d. The square root of the population standard deviation.

Complete the following statements with the best answer.

12. When one is using the standard normal distribution, $P(z < 0) =$ _____.

13. The difference between a sample mean and a population mean is due to _____.

14. The mean of the sample means equals _____.

15. The standard deviation of all possible sample means is called _____.

16. The normal distribution can be used to approximate the binomial distribution when $n \cdot p$ and $n \cdot q$ are both greater than or equal to _____.

17. The correction factor for the central limit theorem should be used when the sample size is greater than _____ the size of the population.

18. Find the area under the standard normal distribution for each.

    a. Between 0 and 1.50
    b. Between 0 and −1.25
    c. Between 1.56 and 1.96
    d. Between −1.20 and −2.25
    e. Between −0.06 and 0.73

    f. Between 1.10 and −1.80
    g. To the right of $z = 1.75$
    h. To the right of $z = -1.28$
    i. To the left of $z = -2.12$
    j. To the left of $z = 1.36$

19. Using the standard normal distribution, find each probability.

    a. $P(0 < z < 2.16)$
    b. $P(-1.87 < z < 0)$
    c. $P(-1.63 < z < 2.17)$
    d. $P(1.72 < z < 1.98)$
    e. $P(-2.17 < z < 0.71)$
    f. $P(z > 1.77)$
    g. $P(z < -2.37)$
    h. $P(z > -1.73)$
    i. $P(z < 2.03)$
    j. $P(z > -1.02)$

20. **Annual Rainfall** The average annual rainfall in St. John's, Newfoundland and Labrador, is 69.9 mm. Assume the variable is normally distributed, with a standard deviation of 24.7 mm. Find the probability that next year St. John's will receive the following amount of rainfall.

    a. At most 65 mm of rain
    b. At least 80 mm of rain
    c. Between 60 mm and 75 mm of rain
    d. How many millimetres of rain would you consider to constitute an extremely wet year?

    Source: Environment Canada.

21. **Heights of Women** The average height of adult women in Canada is 163 cm. Assume a standard deviation of 6.3 cm and a normally distributed variable. Find the probability that a randomly selected, Canadian adult female's height will be

    a. Greater than 170 cm.
    b. Less than 160 cm.
    c. Between 160 cm and 170 cm.
    d. Find the 5th and 95th percentiles of heights.

    Source: Canadian Fitness and Lifestyle Research Institute.

22. **Coffee Consumption** Statistics Canada reports that the average Canadian consumes 90.5 litres of coffee per year. Suppose coffee consumption is normally distributed with a standard deviation of 11 litres per year. If a Canadian is randomly selected, find the probability that the amount of coffee consumed per year is

    a. Between 80 and 90 litres.
    b. Less than 80 litres.
    c. At least 70 litres.
    d. At most 100 litres.

    Source: Statistics Canada.

23. **Years to Complete Graduate Program** The average number of years a person takes to complete a graduate degree program is 3. The standard deviation is 4 months. Assume the variable is normally distributed. If an

individual enrolls in the program, find the probability that it will take

a. More than 4 years to complete the program.
b. Less than 2.5 years to complete the program.
c. Between 3.25 and 3.75 years to complete the program.
d. Between 2.5 and 3.5 years to complete the program.

24. **Bus Passengers** On the daily run of an express bus, the average number of passengers is 48. The standard deviation is 3. Assume the variable is normally distributed. Find the probability that the bus will have

a. Between 36 and 40 passengers.
b. Fewer than 42 passengers.
c. More than 48 passengers.
d. Between 43 and 47 passengers.

25. **Thickness of Library Books** The average thickness of books on a library shelf is 8.3 centimetres. The standard deviation is 0.6 centimetre. If 20% of the books are oversized, find the minimum thickness of the oversized books on the library shelf. Assume the variable is normally distributed.

26. **Membership in an Organization** Membership in an elite organization requires a test score in the upper 30% range. If $\mu = 115$ and $\sigma = 12$, find the lowest acceptable score that would enable a candidate to apply for membership. Assume the variable is normally distributed.

27. **Microwave Oven Repair Costs** The average repair cost of a microwave oven is $55, with a standard deviation of $8. The costs are normally distributed. If 12 ovens are repaired, find the probability that the mean of the repair bills will be greater than $60.

28. **Electric Bills** The average electric bill in a residential area is $72 for the month of April. The standard deviation is $6. If the amounts of the electric bills are normally distributed, find the probability that the mean of the bill for 15 residents will be less than $75.

29. **Insomnia Survey** A study on insomnia, a sleep disorder, indicates that 14% of Canadians 15 years of age and older are affected. If 50 Canadians, aged

15 years and older, are randomly selected, find the probability that 7 or more suffer from insomnia.
Source: Statistics Canada.

30. **Factory Union Membership** If 10% of the people in a certain factory are members of a union, find the probability that, in a sample of 2000, fewer than 180 people are union members.

31. **Households Online** The proportion of Canadian households online remains steady at 73%. In a random sample of 420 households, what is the probability that fewer than 300 are connected online?
Source: TNS Canadian Facts.

32. **Sales and Service Workers** A Statistics Canada report indicates that 24.5% of the Canadian work force is employed in sales and services occupations. If 75 Canadian workers are randomly selected, find the probability that at most 20 are employed in these occupations.
Source: Statistics Canada.

33. **Calories in Fast-Food Sandwiches** The number of calories contained in a selection of fast-food sandwiches is shown here. Check for normality.

390	405	580	300	320
540	225	720	470	560
535	660	530	290	440
390	675	530	1010	450
320	460	290	340	610
430	530			

Source: The Doctor's Pocket Calorie, Fat, and Carbohydrate Counter.

34. **GMAT Scores** Thousands of Canadians applying to U.S. graduate schools have written the Graduate Management Admissions Test (GMAT). The average GMAT scores for the top 30-ranked graduate schools of business are listed here. Check for normality.

718	703	703	703	700	690	695	705	690	688
676	681	689	686	691	669	674	652	680	670
651	651	637	662	641	645	645	642	660	636

Source: U.S. News & World Report Best Graduate Schools.

Critical Thinking Challenges »

Sometimes a researcher must decide whether a variable is normally distributed. There are several ways to do this. One simple but very subjective method uses special graph paper, which is called *normal probability paper*. For the distribution of systolic blood pressure readings measured in millimetres of mercury (mmHg) given in Chapter 3 of the textbook, the following method can be used.

1. Make a table, as shown.

Boundaries	Frequency	Cumulative frequency	Cumulative percent frequency
89.5–104.5	24		
104.5–119.5	62		
119.5–134.5	72		
134.5–149.5	26		
149.5–164.5	12		
164.5–179.5	4		
	200		

2. Find the cumulative frequencies for each class, and place the results in the third column.

3. Find the cumulative percentages for each class by dividing each cumulative frequency by 200 (the total frequencies) and multiplying by 100%. (For the first class, it would be 24/200 × 100% = 12%.) Place these values in the last column.

4. Using the normal probability paper shown in Table 6–3, label the *x* axis with the class boundaries as shown and plot the percentages.

5. If the points fall approximately in a straight line, it can be concluded that the distribution is normal. Do you feel that this distribution is approximately normal? Explain your answer.

6. To find an approximation of the mean or median, draw a horizontal line from the 50% point on the *y* axis over to the curve and then a vertical line down to the *x* axis. Compare this approximation of the mean with the computed mean.

7. To find an approximation of the standard deviation, locate the values on the *x* axis that correspond to the 16 and 84% values on the *y* axis. Subtract these two values and divide the result by 2. Compare this approximate standard deviation to the computed standard deviation.

8. Explain why the method used in step 7 works.

Table 6–3	Normal Probability Paper

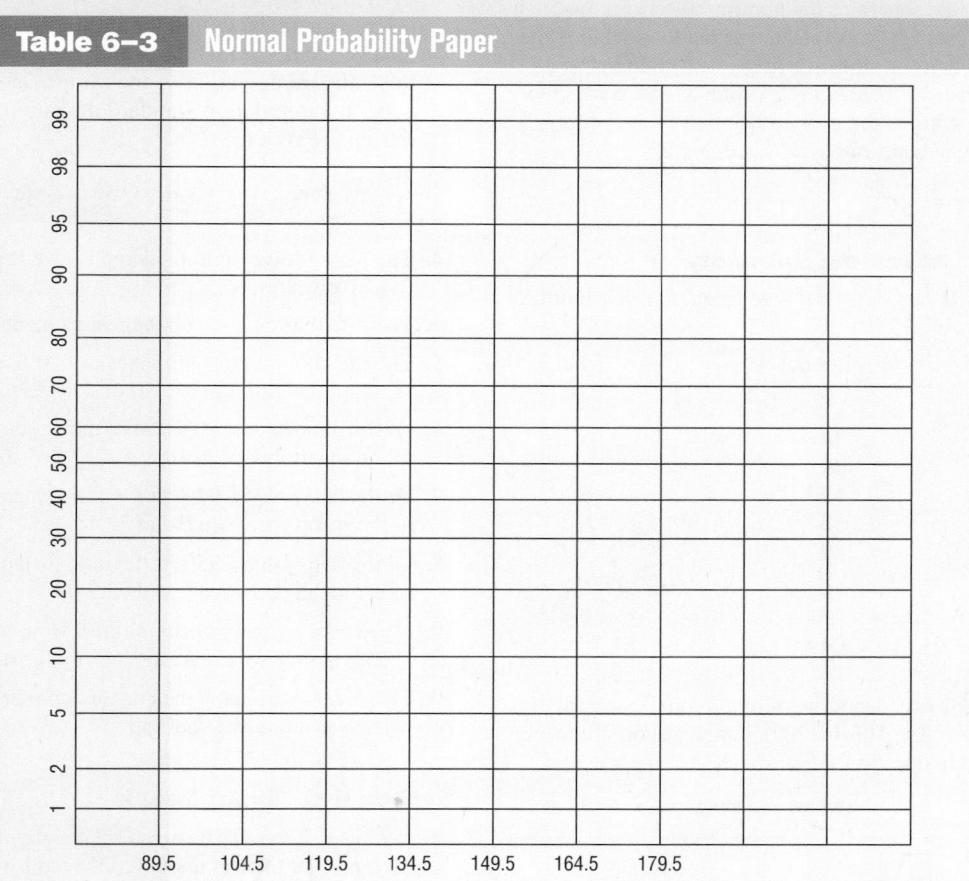

Data Projects »

Where appropriate, use Minitab, SPSS, TI-83 Plus, TI-84 Plus, Excel, or a computer program of your choice to complete the following exercises.

1. **Business and Finance** Use the data collected for Data Project 1 in Chapter 2 regarding earnings per share to complete this problem. Use the mean and standard deviation computed in Data Project 1 of Chapter 3 as

estimates for the population parameters. What value separates the top 5% of stocks from the others?

2. **Sports and Leisure** Find the mean and standard deviation for the batting average for a player in the most recently completed Major League Baseball season. What batting average would separate the top 5% of all hitters from the rest? What is the probability that a randomly

selected player bats over 0.300? What is the probability that a team of 25 players has a mean that is above 0.275?

3. **Technology** Use the data collected for Data Project 3 in Chapter 2 regarding song lengths. If the sample estimates for mean and standard deviation are used as replacements for the population parameters for this data set, what song length separates the bottom 5% and top 5% from the other values?

4. **Health and Wellness** Use the data regarding heart rates collected for Data Project 6 in Chapter 2 for this problem. Use the sample mean and standard deviation as estimates of the population parameters. For the before-exercise data, what heart rate separates the top 10% from the other values? For the after-exercise data, what heart rate separates the bottom 10% from the other values? If a student was selected at random, what is the probability that the student's mean heart rate before exercise was less than 72? If 25 students were selected at random, what is the probability that their before-exercise mean heart rate was less than 72?

5. **Politics and Economics** Research the gender and age of Canada's members of Parliament (MPs). Calculate the mean and standard deviation of MP ages. Compare the age statistics to Canada's senators. Determine the 10th and 90th percentile of MP and senator ages. What is the probability that a randomly selected MP is younger than 40 years old? What is the probability that a randomly selected senator is over 60 years old?

6. **Your Class** Confirm that the two formulas hold true for the central limit theorem for the population containing the elements {1, 5, 10}. First, compute the population mean and standard deviation for the data set. Next, create a list of all 9 of the possible two-element samples that can be created with replacement: {1, 1}, {1, 5}, etc. For each of the 9, compute the sample mean. Now find the mean of the sample means. Does it equal the population mean? Compute the standard deviation of the sample means. Does it equal the population standard deviation, divided by the square root of n?

Answers to Applying the Concepts »

Section 6–1 Assessing Normality

1. Answers will vary. One possible frequency distribution is the following:

Branches	Frequency
0–9	1
10–19	14
20–29	17
30–39	7
40–49	3
50–59	2
60–69	2
70–79	1
80–89	2
90–99	1

2. Answers will vary according to the frequency distribution in question 1. This histogram matches the frequency distribution in question 1.

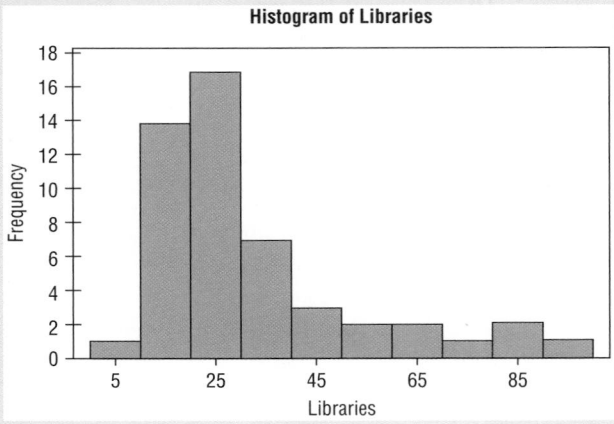

3. The histogram is unimodal and skewed to the right (positively skewed).

4. The distribution does not appear to be normal.

5. The mean number of branches is $\bar{x} = 31.4$, and the standard deviation is $s = 20.6$.

6. Of the data values, 80% fall within 1 standard deviation of the mean (between 10.8 and 52).

7. Of the data values, 92% fall within 2 standard deviations of the mean (between 0 and 72.6).

8. Of the data values, 98% fall within 3 standard deviations of the mean (between 0 and 93.2).

9. My values in questions 6–8 differ from the 68, 95, and 100% that we would see in a normal distribution.

10. These values support the conclusion that the distribution of the variable is not normal.

Section 6–2 Smart People

1. $z = \frac{130 - 100}{15} = 2$. The area to the right of 2 in the standard normal table is about 0.0228, so I would expect about 10,000(0.0228) = 228 people in my hometown to qualify for Mensa.

2. It does seem reasonable to continue my quest to start a Mensa chapter in my hometown.

3. Answers will vary. One possible answer would be to randomly call telephone numbers (both home and cellphone) in town, ask to speak to an adult, and ask whether the person would be interested in joining Mensa.

4. To have an Ultra-Mensa club, I would need to find the people in town who have IQs that are at least 2.326

standard deviations above average. This means that I would need to recruit those with IQs that are at least 135:

$$2.326 = \frac{x - 100}{15} \Rightarrow x = 100 + 2.326(15) = 134.89$$

Section 6–3 Central Limit Theorem

1. It is very unlikely that we would ever get the same results for any of our random samples. While it is a remote possibility, it is highly unlikely.

2. A good estimate for the population mean would be to find the average of the students' sample means. Similarly, a good estimate for the population standard deviation would be to find the average of the students' sample standard deviations.

3. The distribution appears to be somewhat left (negatively) skewed.

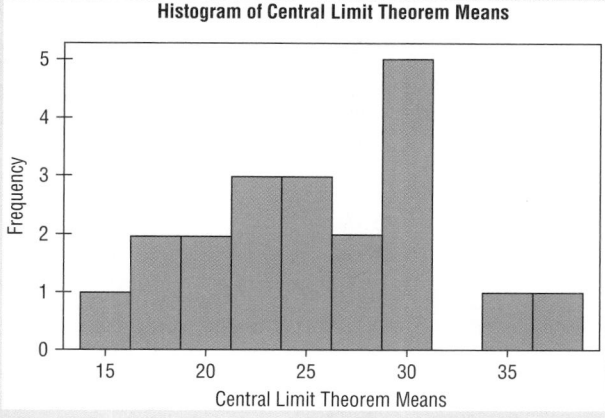

Histogram of Central Limit Theorem Means

4. The mean of the students' means is 25.4, and the standard deviation is 5.8.

5. The distribution of the means is not a sampling distribution, since it represents just 20 of all possible samples of size 30 from the population.

6. The sampling error for student 3 is $18 - 25.4 = -7.4$; the sampling error for student 7 is $26 - 25.4 = +0.6$; the sampling error for student 14 is $29 - 25.4 = +3.6$.

7. The standard deviation for the sample of the 20 means is greater than the standard deviations for each of the individual students.

Section 6–4 How Safe Are You?

1. A reliability rating of 97% means that, on average, the device will not fail 97% of the time. We do not know how many times it will fail for any particular set of 100 climbs.

2. The probability of at least 1 failure in 100 climbs is $1 - (0.97)^{100} = 1 - 0.0476 = 0.9524$ (about 95%).

3. The complement of the event in question 2 is the event of "no failures in 100 climbs."

4. This can be considered a binomial experiment. We have two outcomes: success and failure. The probability of the equipment working (success) remains constant at 97%. We have 100 independent climbs. And we are counting the number of times the equipment works in these 100 climbs.

5. We could use the binomial probability formula, but it would be very messy computationally.

6. The probability of at least two failures *cannot* be estimated with the normal distribution (see below). So the probability is $1 - [(0.97)^{100} + 100(0.97)^{99}(0.03)] = 1 - 0.1946 = 0.8054$ (about 80.5%).

7. We *should not* use the normal approximation to the binomial since nq is not ≥ 5.

8. If we had used the normal approximation, we would have needed a correction for continuity, since we would have been approximating a discrete distribution with a continuous distribution.

9. Since a second safety hook will be successful or fail independently of the first safety hook, the probability of failure drops from 3% to $(0.03)(0.03) = 0.0009$, or 0.09%.

Chapter 7

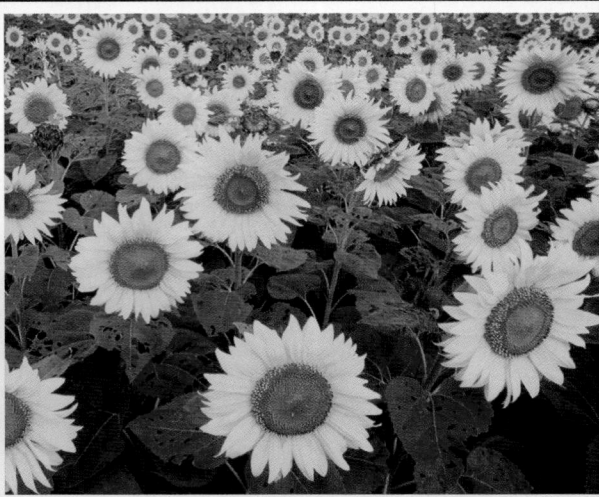

Confidence Intervals and Sample Size

Statistics Today

Do You Waste Water?

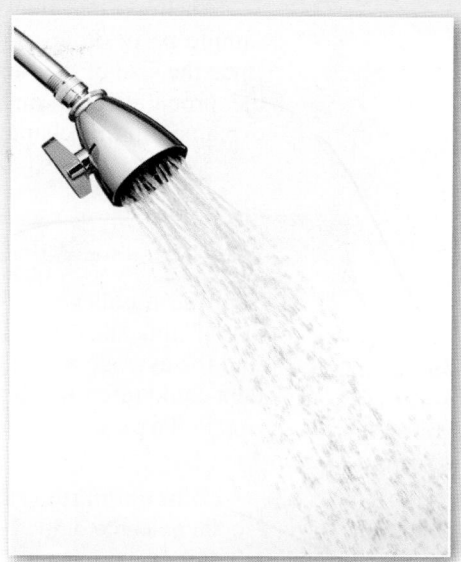

An Ipsos Reid market research survey found that 89% of Canadians are concerned about water usage after being told that the average Canadian consumes 329 litres of water per person each day. In fact, 49% of survey respondents felt that water was Canada's most precious natural resource. The *2010 Canadian Water Attitudes Study* included a sample of 2022 adult Canadians across Canada. The results are considered accurate to within ±2.2%, 19 times out of 20.

Several questions arise:

1. How do these estimates compare with the true population percentages?

2. What is meant by accurate to within ±2.2%, 19 times out of 20?

3. Is the sample of 2022 large enough to represent the water attitudes for the population of all Canadian adults?

After reading this chapter, you will be able to answer these questions, since this chapter explains how statisticians can use statistics to make estimates of parameters.

See Statistics Today—Revisited, page 336, for the answers.

Source: Ipsos Reid, *2010 Canadian Water Attitudes Study,* February 2010.

Introduction >

One aspect of inferential statistics is **estimation,** which is the process of estimating the value of a parameter from information obtained from a sample. For example, Statistics Canada and other public as well as private agencies collect economic, societal, and cultural data of the people and resources of the country. Examples of data disseminated through these sources include the following.

> *The average after-tax income for male single-parent families is $54,200, compared to $41,300 for female single-parent families. (Statistics Canada)[1]*
> *1 in 5 Canadians list talking on cellphones as their biggest grievance with other drivers on the road, yet 1 in 4 are guilty of it themselves. (Leger Marketing)*
> *Television viewing by Canadians averages 21 hours per week. (Statistics Canada)[2]*
> *44% of Canadian drivers change their own vehicle spark plugs. (DesRosiers Automotive Consultants)*
> *Cannabis dependence is significantly higher among youth (27%) than adults (5%). (Canadian Community Epidemiology Network on Drug Use)*

Since the populations from which these values were obtained are large, these values are only *estimates* of the true parameters and are derived from data collected from samples.

---

[1] Adapted from Statistics Canada, *Summary Tables,* "Average Income after Tax by Economic Family Type, 2004–2008."
[2] Adapted from Statistics Canada, *The Daily,* "Television Viewing," March 31, 2006.

The statistical procedures for estimating the population mean, proportion, variance, and standard deviation will be explained in this chapter.

An important question in estimation is that of sample size. How large should the sample be in order to make an accurate estimate? This question is not easy to answer since the size of the sample depends on several factors, such as the accuracy desired and the probability of making a correct estimate. The question of sample size will be explained in this chapter also.

7–1	Confidence Intervals for the Mean When σ Is Known >

Find the confidence interval for the mean when σ is known and determine the minimum sample size.

Suppose a college president wishes to estimate the average age of students attending classes this semester. The president could select a random sample of 100 students and find the average age of these students, say, 22.3 years. From the sample mean, the president could infer that the average age of all the students is 22.3 years. This type of estimate is called a *point estimate.*

> A **point estimate** is a specific numerical value that approximates a parameter. The best point estimate of the population mean μ is the sample mean $\overline{X}$.

One might ask why other measures of central tendency, such as the median and mode, are not used to estimate the population mean. The reason is that the means of samples vary less than other statistics (such as medians and modes) when many samples are selected from the same population. Therefore, the sample mean is the best estimate of the population mean.

Sample measures (i.e., statistics) are used to estimate population measures (i.e., parameters). These statistics are called **estimators.** As previously stated, the sample mean is a better estimator of the population mean than the sample median or sample mode.

A good estimator should satisfy the three properties described now.

Three Properties of a Good Estimator

1. The estimator should be an **unbiased estimator.** That is, the expected value or the mean of the estimates obtained from samples of a given size is equal to the parameter being estimated.
2. The estimator should be consistent. For a **consistent estimator,** as sample size increases, the value of the estimator approaches the value of the parameter estimated.
3. The estimator should be a **relatively efficient estimator.** That is, of all the statistics that can be used to estimate a parameter, the relatively efficient estimator has the smallest variance.

Confidence Intervals

As stated in Chapter 6, the sample mean will be, for the most part, somewhat different from the population mean due to sampling error. Therefore, one might ask a second question: How good is a point estimate? The answer is that there is no way of knowing how close a particular point estimate is to the population mean.

This answer places some doubt on the accuracy of point estimates. For this reason, statisticians prefer another type of estimate, called an *interval estimate.*

> An **interval estimate** of a parameter is a range of values used to approximate a population parameter. The interval may or may not contain the value of the parameter being estimated.

In an interval estimate, the parameter is specified as being between two values. For example, an interval estimate for the average age of all students might be $26.9 < \mu < 27.7$, or 27.3 ± 0.4 years.

Either the interval contains the parameter or it does not. A degree of confidence (usually a percentage) can be assigned before an interval estimate is made. For instance, one may wish to be 95% confident that the interval contains the true population mean. Another question then arises: Why 95%? Why not 99 or 99.5%?

If one wants to be more confident, such as 99 or 99.5% confident, then the interval must be larger. For example, a 99% confidence interval for the mean age of college students might be $26.7 < \mu < 27.9$, or 27.3 ± 0.6. Hence, a tradeoff occurs. To be more confident that the interval contains the true population mean, one must make the interval wider.

Historical Note

Point and interval estimates were known as long ago as the late 1700s. However, it wasn't until 1937 that a mathematician, Jerzy Neyman, formulated practical applications for them.

> The **confidence level** of an interval estimate of a parameter is the probability that the interval estimate will contain the parameter, assuming that a large number of samples are selected and that the estimation process on the same parameter is repeated.
>
> A **confidence interval** is a specific interval estimate of a parameter determined by using data obtained from a sample and by using the specific confidence level of the estimate.

Intervals constructed in this way are called *confidence intervals*. Three common confidence intervals are used: the 90, the 95, and the 99% confidence intervals.

The algebraic derivation of the formula for determining a confidence interval for a mean will be shown later. A brief intuitive explanation will be given first.

The central limit theorem states that when the sample size is large, approximately 95% of the sample means will fall within ± 1.96 standard errors of the population mean, that is,

$$\mu \pm 1.96\left(\frac{\sigma}{\sqrt{n}}\right)$$

Now, if a specific sample mean is selected, say, $\overline{X}$, there is a 95% probability that it falls within the range of $\mu \pm 1.96(\sigma/\sqrt{n})$. Likewise, there is a 95% probability that the interval specified by

$$\overline{X} \pm 1.96\left(\frac{\sigma}{\sqrt{n}}\right)$$

will contain μ, as will be shown later. Stated another way,

$$\overline{X} - 1.96\left(\frac{\sigma}{\sqrt{n}}\right) < \mu < \overline{X} + 1.96\left(\frac{\sigma}{\sqrt{n}}\right)$$

Interesting Fact

Golfers walk, on average, 8 kilometres and burn 1750 calories per round.

Hence, one can be 95% confident that the population mean is contained within that interval when the values of the variable are normally distributed in the population.

For example, in order to target new account advertising, a researcher would like an estimate of the average age and household income of all online stock traders at a confidence level of 95%. Using techniques presented in this chapter, the researcher selects a random sample of new accounts and discovers that, on average, online stock traders are between 39.5 and 46.5 years old with household incomes between \$89,750 and \$110,250. With a 95% degree of confidence in the estimates of the true population mean, the researcher will target these demographics for new accounts.

The value used for the 95% confidence interval, 1.96, is obtained from Table E–2 in Appendix C. For a 99% confidence interval, the value 2.575 is used instead of 1.96 in the formula. This value is also obtained from Table E–2 and is based on the standard normal distribution. Since other confidence intervals are used in statistics, the symbol $z_{\alpha/2}$ (read "zed sub alpha over two") is used in the general formula for confidence intervals. The Greek letter α (alpha) represents the total area in both tails of the standard normal distribution curve, and $\alpha/2$ represents the area in each one of the tails. More will be said following Examples 7–1 and 7–2 about finding other values for $z_{\alpha/2}$.

The relationship between α and the confidence level is that the stated confidence level is the percentage equivalent to the decimal value of $1 - \alpha$, and vice versa. When the 95% confidence interval is to be found, $\alpha = 0.05$, since $1 - 0.05 = 0.95$, or 95%. When $\alpha = 0.01$, then $1 - \alpha = 1 - 0.01 = 0.99$, and the 99% confidence interval is being calculated.

Formula for the Confidence Interval of the Mean for a Specific α When σ Is Known

$$\overline{X} - z_{\alpha/2}\left(\frac{\sigma}{\sqrt{n}}\right) < \mu < \overline{X} + z_{\alpha/2}\left(\frac{\sigma}{\sqrt{n}}\right)$$

For a 90% confidence interval, $z_{\alpha/2} = 1.645$; for a 95% confidence interval, $z_{\alpha/2} = 1.96$; and for a 99% confidence interval, $z_{\alpha/2} = 2.575$.

The term $z_{\alpha/2}(\sigma/\sqrt{n})$ is called the *margin of error,* also referred to as the *maximum error of estimate.* For a specific value, say, $\alpha = 0.05$, 95% of the sample means will fall within this error value on either side of the population mean, as previously explained. See Figure 7–1.

Figure 7–1

95% Confidence Interval

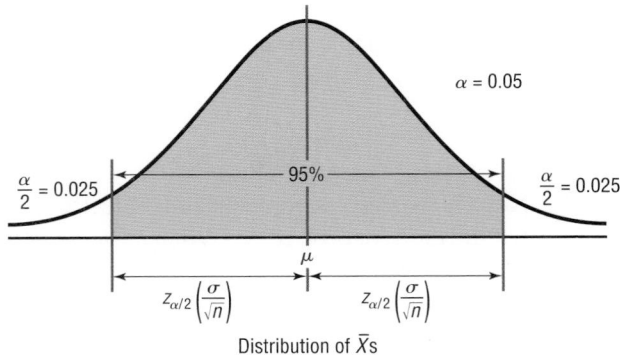

Distribution of $\overline{X}$s

The **margin of error** is the maximum likely difference between the point estimate of a parameter and the actual value of the parameter.

A more detailed explanation of the margin of error follows Examples 7–1 and 7–2, which illustrate the computation of confidence intervals.

Assumptions for Finding a Confidence Interval for a Mean When α Is Known

1. The sample is a random sample.
2. Either $n \geq 30$ or the population is normally distributed if $n < 30$.

Rounding Rule for a Confidence Interval for a Mean   When you are computing a confidence interval for a population mean by using *raw data,* round off to one more decimal place than the number of decimal places in the original data. When you are computing a confidence interval for a population mean by using a sample mean and a standard deviation, round off to the same number of decimal places as given for the mean.

Example 7–1

Life Expectancy

A recent report stated that Canadian life expectancy, on average, is 80.7 years—better than in the United States (78.1 years) but not as good as Japan (82.7 years). Assume that Canadian life expectancies are approximately normal, with a standard deviation of 9.3 years. A random sample of 35 death certificates drawn from a national Canadian vital statistics database indicated a mean age at death of 79.5 years. Find the best point estimate and the 95% confidence interval estimate of the population mean. Do these results support the report of average Canadian life expectancy?

Source: Conference Board of Canada, *Health*, "Life Expectancy," 2006.

Solution

The best point estimate of the population mean is the sample mean of 79.5 years. For the 95% confidence interval, use $z = 1.96$. See Figure 7–2.

$$79.5 - 1.96\left(\frac{9.3}{\sqrt{35}}\right) < \mu < 79.5 + 1.96\left(\frac{9.3}{\sqrt{35}}\right)$$

$$79.5 - 3.08 < \mu < 79.5 + 3.08$$

$$76.42 < \mu < 82.58$$

or

$$79.5 \pm 3.1 \text{ (rounded)}$$

Figure 7–2

Confidence Interval for Life Expectancies

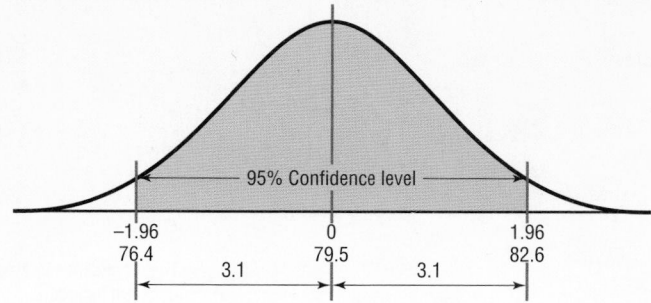

Therefore, we are 95% confident that the average Canadian life expectancy based on a random sample of 50 people is between 76.4 and 82.6 years. The reported figure of 80.7 years is supported, as it falls within this range.

Example 7–2

Health Care Spending

The cost of Canada's health care system continues to escalate, increasing the tax burden for all citizens. A study of 70 Canadians showed a sample mean health care expenditure of $5170. Assume the variable is normally distributed, with a population standard deviation of $687. Find the best point estimate and 99% confidence interval estimate of the population mean.

Source: Canadian Institute for Health Care Information, *National Health Expenditure Trends*, "Spending on Health Care to Reach $5170 per Canadian in 2008," November 13, 2008.

Solution

The best point estimate of the population mean is $5170. For the 99% confidence interval, use $z = 2.575$.

$$\$5170 - 2.575\left(\frac{\$687}{\sqrt{70}}\right) < \mu < \$5170 + 2.575\left(\frac{\$687}{\sqrt{70}}\right)$$

$$\$5170 - \$211.44 < \mu < \$5170 + \$211.44$$

$$\$4958.56 < \mu < \$5381.44$$

or $$\$4958.6 < \mu < \$5381.4 \, (\text{rounded})$$

Hence, we are 99% confident that the mean expenditure by Canadians on health care is between $4958.60 and $5381.40.

Another way of looking at a confidence interval is shown in Figure 7–3. According to the central limit theorem, approximately 95% of the sample means fall within 1.96 standard deviations of the population mean if the sample size is 30 or more or if σ is known when n is less than 30 and the population is normally distributed. If it was possible to build a confidence interval about each sample mean, as was done in Examples 7–1 and 7–2 for μ, 95% of these intervals would contain the population mean, as shown in Figure 7–4. Hence, one can be 95% confident that an interval built around a specific sample mean would contain the population mean. If one wants to be 99% confident, the confidence intervals must be enlarged so that 99 out of every 100 intervals contain the population mean.

Figure 7–3

95% Confidence Interval for Sample Means

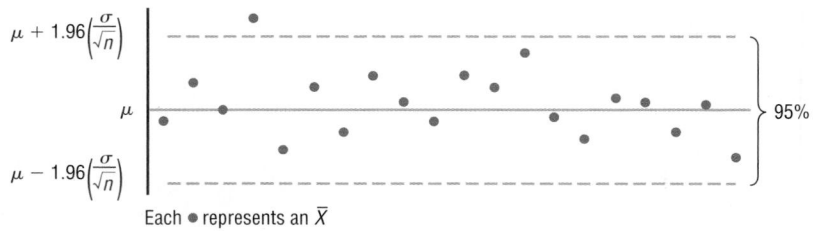

Figure 7–4

95% Confidence Intervals for Each Sample Mean

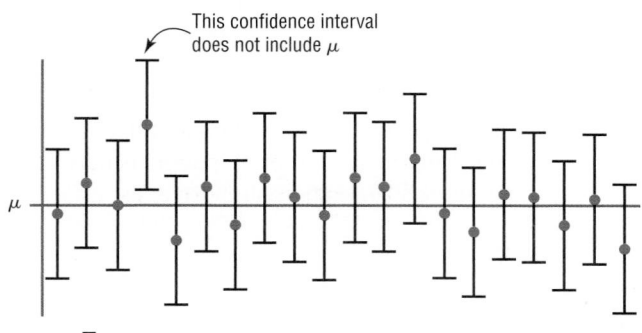

Since other confidence intervals (besides 90, 95, and 99%) are sometimes used in statistics, an explanation of how to find the values for $z_{\alpha/2}$ is necessary. As stated previously, the Greek letter α represents the total of the areas in both tails of the normal distribution. The value for α is found by subtracting the decimal equivalent for the desired confidence level from 1. For example, if one wanted to find the 98% confidence interval, one would change 98% to 0.98 and find $\alpha = 1 - 0.98$, or 0.02. Then $\alpha/2$ is obtained by dividing α by 2. So $\alpha/2$ is 0.02/2, or 0.01. Finally, $z_{0.01}$ is the z value that will give an area of 0.01 in both the left and right tails of the standard normal distribution curve. See Figure 7–5.

Figure 7–5

Finding $\alpha/2$ for a 98% Confidence Interval

$\alpha = 0.02$

$\frac{\alpha}{2} = 0.01$ $\frac{\alpha}{2} = 0.01$

0.98

$-z_{\alpha/2}$ 0 $z_{\alpha/2}$

Once $\alpha/2$ is determined, the corresponding $z_{\alpha/2}$ score can be found by using the procedure shown in Section 6–2, "Finding z Scores When Given Areas." In summary, to obtain the $z_{\alpha/2}$ score for a 98% confidence level, subtract 0.9800 from 1.000 to obtain $\alpha = 0.02$, therefore $\alpha/2 = 0.02/2 = 0.01$. In Table E–2, Positive z Scores, the area 0.0100 to the right is the cumulative area 0.9900 (1.0000 − 0.0100) to the left, where $z = 2.33$. Refer to Figure 7–6.

Figure 7–6

Finding $z_{a/2}$ for a 98% Confidence Interval

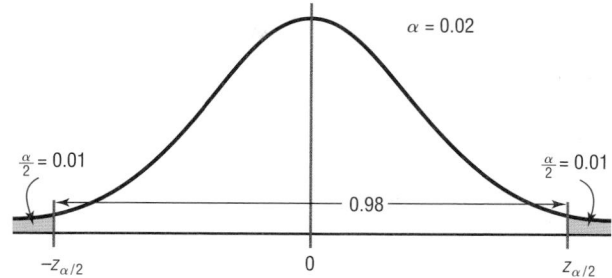

Table E.2						
The Standard Normal Distribution						
z	.00	.01	.02	.03	...	.09
0.0						
0.1						
⋮						
2.3				0.9901		

For confidence intervals, only the positive z score is used in the formula.

When the original variable is normally distributed and σ is known, the standard normal distribution can be used to find confidence intervals regardless of the size of the sample. When $n \geq 30$, the distribution of means will be approximately normal even if the original distribution of the variable departs from normality. When σ is unknown, s can be used as an estimate of σ but a different distribution is used for the critical values, as explained below.

Revised Method for σ Unknown

The previous edition of this text used the sample standard deviation, s, in place of the population standard deviation, σ, when σ was unknown and $n \geq 30$. In most research studies, the population standard deviation is not known. Modern methods use the Student's t distribution (introduced in the next section) in situations in which σ is unknown to estimate the population parameter μ, regardless of the sample size. This method of determining critical values is explained in Section 7–2.

Example 7–3

House Prices

The following data represent a random sample of 30 house prices (in thousands of dollars) in Calgary based on MLS sales for the current year. Find the 90% confidence interval estimate of the mean price of all Calgary houses. Assume $\sigma = 176.95$ based on population data from the previous year.

318.3	507.5	351.9	292.2	487.7	587.2
373.9	261.5	261.5	350.6	381.0	782.3
508.0	262.8	289.3	360.9	447.7	795.8
437.3	276.2	300.0	441.4	545.0	337.0
450.8	317.5	332.5	634.6	945.3	393.6

Source: Calgary Real Estate Board.

Solution

Step 1 Find the sample mean for the data. Use the formula shown in Chapter 3 or use your calculator. The mean $\overline{X} = 434.38$.

Step 2 Find $\alpha/2$. Since the 90% confidence interval is to be used, $\alpha = 1 - 0.90 = 0.10$, and $\dfrac{\alpha}{2} = \dfrac{0.10}{2} = 0.05$.

Step 3 Find $z_{\alpha/2}$. Subtract 0.05 (area in right tail) from 1.0000 to get 0.9500 (cumulative area to the left). The corresponding z score obtained from Table E–2 for 0.9500 is $z = 1.645$, as this value is exactly halfway between $z = 1.64$ (0.9495) and $z = 1.65$ (0.9505).

Step 4 Substitute in the formula

$$\overline{X} - z_{\alpha/2}\left(\frac{\sigma}{\sqrt{n}}\right) < \mu < \overline{X} + z_{\alpha/2}\left(\frac{\sigma}{\sqrt{n}}\right)$$

$$434.38 - 1.645\left(\frac{176.95}{\sqrt{30}}\right) < \mu < 434.38 + 1.645\left(\frac{176.95}{\sqrt{30}}\right)$$

$$434.38 - 53.144 < \mu < 434.38 + 53.144$$

$$381.236 < \mu < 487.524$$

Therefore, one can be 90% confident that the population mean of Calgary house prices for the current year is between $381,236 and $487,524, based on a sample of 30 house sales.

Comment to Computer and Statistical Calculator Users

This chapter and subsequent chapters include examples using raw data. If you are using computer or calculator programs to find the solutions, the answers you get may vary somewhat from the ones given in the textbook. This is so because computers and calculators do not round the answers in the intermediate steps and can use 12 or more decimal places for computation. Also, they use more exact values than those given in the tables at the back of this book. These discrepancies are part and parcel of statistics.

Sample Size

Sample size determination is closely related to statistical estimation. Quite often, one asks, How large a sample is necessary to make an accurate estimate? The answer is not simple, since it depends on three things: the margin of error, the population standard deviation, and the degree of confidence. For example, how close to the true mean does one want to be (2 units, 5 units, etc.), and how confident does one wish to be (90, 95, 99%, etc.)? For the purpose of this chapter, it will be assumed that the population standard deviation of the variable is known or has been estimated from a previous study.

The formula for sample size is derived from the margin of error formula

$$E = z_{\alpha/2}\left(\frac{\sigma}{\sqrt{n}}\right)$$

and this formula is solved for n as follows:

$$E\sqrt{n} = z_{\alpha/2}(\sigma)$$

$$\sqrt{n} = \frac{z_{\alpha/2} \cdot \sigma}{E}$$

Hence, $n = \left(\frac{z_{\alpha/2} \cdot \sigma}{E}\right)^2$

Formula for the Minimum Sample Size Needed for an Interval Estimate of the Population Mean

$$n = \left(\frac{z_{\alpha/2} \cdot \sigma}{E}\right)^2$$

where E is the margin of error. If necessary, round the answer *up* to obtain a whole number. That is, if there is any fraction or decimal portion in the answer, use the next whole number for sample size n.

Example 7–4

Depth of Lake

A scientist wants to estimate the average depth of a freshwater lake in the Muskoka region of central Ontario. He wants to be 98% confident that the estimate is accurate within 0.5 metres. From a previous study, the standard deviation of the depths measured was 1.25 metres.

Solution

Since $1 - \alpha = 0.02$ (or $1 - 0.98$), $z_{\alpha/2} = 2.33$ and $E = 0.5$. Substituting in the formula,

$$n = \left(\frac{z_{\alpha/2} \cdot \sigma}{E}\right)^2 = \left(\frac{(2.33) \cdot (1.25)}{0.5}\right)^2 = 33.93$$

Round the value 33.93 up to 34. Therefore, to be 98% confident that the estimate is within 0.5 metres of the true mean depth, the scientist needs to sample at least 34 measurements. *In most cases in statistics, a number is rounded off. However, when determining sample size, always round up to the next whole number.*

Notice that when one is finding the sample size, the size of the population is irrelevant when the population is large or infinite or when sampling is done with replacement. In other cases, an adjustment is made in the formula for computing sample size. This adjustment is beyond the scope of this book.

The formula for determining sample size requires the use of the population standard deviation. What happens when σ is unknown? In this case, an attempt is made to estimate σ. One such way is to use the standard deviation s obtained from a sample taken previously as an estimate for σ. The standard deviation can also be estimated by dividing the standard deviation by 4, as explained in Section 3–2, using the range rule of thumb.

Interesting Fact

Canadian households with post-secondary students spend more on tuition fees than on food in a year.

Sometimes, interval estimates rather than point estimates are reported. For instance, one may read a statement: "On the basis of a sample of 200 families, the survey estimates that a Canadian family of two spends an average of $84 per week for groceries. One can be 95% confident that this estimate is accurate within $3 of the true mean." This statement means that the 95% confidence interval of the true mean is

$$\$84 - \$3 < \mu < \$84 + \$3$$
$$\$81 < \mu < \$87$$

The algebraic derivation of the formula for a confidence interval is shown next. As explained in Chapter 6, the sampling distribution of the mean is approximately normal when large samples ($n \geq 30$) are taken from a population. Also,

$$z = \frac{\overline{X} - \mu}{\sigma/\sqrt{n}}$$

Furthermore, there is a probability of $1 - \alpha$ that a z will have a value between $-z_{\alpha/2}$ and $+z_{\alpha/2}$. Hence,

$$-z_{\alpha/2} < \frac{\overline{X} - \mu}{\sigma/\sqrt{n}} < z_{\alpha/2}$$

Using algebra, one finds

$$-z_{\alpha/2} \cdot \frac{\sigma}{\sqrt{n}} < \overline{X} - \mu < z_{\alpha/2} \cdot \frac{\sigma}{\sqrt{n}}$$

Subtracting $\overline{X}$ from both sides and from the middle, one gets

$$-\overline{X} - z_{\alpha/2} \cdot \frac{\sigma}{\sqrt{n}} < -\mu < -\overline{X} + z_{\alpha/2} \cdot \frac{\sigma}{\sqrt{n}}$$

Multiplying by -1, one gets

$$\overline{X} + z_{\alpha/2} \cdot \frac{\sigma}{\sqrt{n}} > \mu > \overline{X} - z_{\alpha/2} \cdot \frac{\sigma}{\sqrt{n}}$$

Reversing the inequality, one gets the formula for the confidence interval:

$$\overline{X} - z_{\alpha/2} \cdot \frac{\sigma}{\sqrt{n}} < \mu < \overline{X} + z_{\alpha/2} \cdot \frac{\sigma}{\sqrt{n}}$$

7–1 Applying the Concepts

Making Decisions with Confidence Intervals

Assume you work for Kimberly Clark Corporation, the makers of Kleenex. The job you are presently working on requires you to decide how many Kleenexes are to be put into the new automobile glove compartment boxes. Complete the following.

1. How will you decide on a reasonable number of Kleenexes to put into the boxes?
2. When do people usually need Kleenexes?
3. What type of data collection technique would you use?
4. Assume you found out that from your sample of 85 people, on average about 57 Kleenexes are used throughout the duration of a cold, with a standard deviation of 15. Use a confidence interval to help you decide how many Kleenexes will go into the boxes.
5. Explain how you decided on how many Kleenexes will go into the boxes.

See page 339 for the answers.

Exercises 7–1

1. What is the difference between a point estimate and an interval estimate of a parameter? Which is better? Why?

2. What information is necessary to calculate a confidence interval?

3. What is the margin of error?

4. What is meant by the 95% confidence interval of the mean?

5. What are three properties of a good estimator?

6. What statistic best estimates μ?

7. What is necessary to determine the sample size?

8. When one is determining the sample size for a confidence interval, is the size of the population relevant?

9. Find each.

   a. $z_{\alpha/2}$ for the 99% confidence interval
   b. $z_{\alpha/2}$ for the 98% confidence interval
   c. $z_{\alpha/2}$ for the 95% confidence interval
   d. $z_{\alpha/2}$ for the 90% confidence interval
   e. $z_{\alpha/2}$ for the 94% confidence interval

10. **Freshmen's GPA** First-semester GPAs for a random selection of freshmen at a large university are shown below. Estimate the true mean GPA of the freshman class with 99% confidence. Assume $\sigma = 0.62$, based on prior year results.

1.9	3.2	2.0	2.9	2.7	3.3
2.8	3.0	3.8	2.7	2.0	1.9
2.5	2.7	2.8	3.2	3.0	3.8
3.1	2.7	3.5	3.8	3.9	2.7
2.0	2.8	1.9	4.0	2.2	2.8
2.1	2.4	3.0	3.4	2.9	2.1

11. **Reading Scores** A sample of the reading scores of 35 Grade 5 students has a mean of 82. The standard deviation of the sample is 15.

    a. Find the best point estimate of the mean.
    b. Find the 95% confidence interval of the mean reading scores of all Grade 5 students.
    c. Find the 99% confidence interval of the mean reading scores of all Grade 5 students.
    d. Which interval is larger? Explain why.

12. **House Sales** Find the 90% confidence interval of the population mean for the number of detached house sales in Toronto districts over a one-year period. A random sample of 40 districts is shown. A prior study indicated $\sigma = 550$.

941	573	2864	739
920	759	889	928
1461	799	667	1991
988	718	1280	1137
1278	921	272	624
546	1106	1019	913
1285	535	1463	1377
910	1208	435	2124
1145	538	855	888
650	1105	455	2306

Source: Toronto Real Estate Board.

13. **Time to Grade Term Papers** A study of 40 English composition professors showed that they spent, on average, 12.6 minutes correcting a student's term paper.

    a. Find the best point estimate of the mean.
    b. Find the 90% confidence interval of the mean time for all composition papers when $\sigma = 2.5$ minutes.
    c. If a professor stated that he spent, on average, 30 minutes correcting a term paper, what would be your reaction?

14. **Average Golf Scores** A study of 35 golfers showed that their average score on a particular course was 92. The standard deviation of the population is 5.

    a. Find the best point estimate of the mean.
    b. Find the 95% confidence interval of the mean score for all golfers.
    c. Find the 95% confidence interval of the mean score if a sample of 60 golfers is used instead of a sample of 35.
    d. Which interval is smaller? Explain why.

15. **Actuarial Exams** A survey of 35 individuals who passed the seven exams and obtained the rank of Fellow in the actuarial field finds the average salary to be $150,000. If the standard deviation for the population is $15,000, construct a 95% confidence interval for all Fellows.

    Source: Society of Actuaries/Casualty Actuarial Society, *Be an Actuary.*

16. **Residential Taxation** A *Maclean's* survey of 31 cities across Canada yielded an average residential tax burden (per dwelling) of $1445. Assume a normally distributed variable with $\sigma = \$321$. Estimate the average Canadian residential tax burden with 95% confidence.

    Source: Macleans.ca, "Quizzes—Cities: NMPR Taxation."

17. **Distractions at Work** A recent study showed that the modern working person experiences an average of 2.1 hours per day of distractions (phone calls, e-mails, impromptu visits, etc.). A random sample of 50 workers for a large corporation found that these workers were distracted an average of 1.8 hours per day, and the population standard deviation was 20 minutes. Estimate

the true mean population distraction time with 90% confidence, and compare your answer to the results of the study.

Source: Time Almanac.

18. **Children's TV Viewing Habits** A survey of 40 Canadian children found that, on average, they spend 14.1 hours per week viewing television programs. Assume $\sigma = 1.9$ hours. Determine the true population mean of children's TV viewing hours per week at a 98% confidence level.

Source: Canadian Paediatric Society.

19. **Rave Noise Levels** Police monitoring rave parties suggest that the average noise level is 135 decibels (dB). A sample of 30 raves across Canada measured the average noise level at 131 dB. Assume a population standard deviation, $\sigma = 13$ dB. Estimate the true population mean noise level at raves with 90% confidence. Comment on the police-reported noise level.

Source: Calgary Police Service, Safe Raving Advice, June 2, 2010.

20. **Length of Growing Season** The growing seasons for a random sample of 35 Canadian cities were recorded, yielding a sample mean of 128.3 days, If the population standard deviation is 31.8 days, estimate the true population mean of the growing season in Canada with 95% confidence.

Source: The Old Farmer's Almanac, "Frost Chart for Canada."

21. **Homework Study Hours** A university dean of students wishes to estimate the average number of hours students spend doing homework per week. The standard deviation from a previous study is 6.2 hours. How large a sample must be selected if he wants to be 99% confident of finding whether the true mean differs from the sample mean by 1.5 hours?

22. **Body Mass Index** One measure of the health of Canadians is the *body mass index* (BMI) calculated as a

person's weight (kg)/height (m)^2. The reported average BMI for 20- to 39-year-old Canadians is 26.2 kg/m^2. Assume that a random sample of BMI readings were taken from 75 people, aged 20 to 39, at fitness clubs across the country. Given $\sigma = 3.9$ kg/m^2, and a sample mean of 19.7 kg/m^2, determine the 99% confidence interval estimate for the population mean of fitness club members in the defined age group. Compare these results to the reported BMI average reading.

Source: Statistics Canada, Body Composition of Canadian Adults, 2007 to 2009, Catalogue No. 82-625-X.

23. **Sick Days Study** An insurance company is trying to estimate the average number of sick days that full-time food service workers use per year. A pilot study found the standard deviation to be 2.5 days. How large a sample must be selected if the company wants to be 95% confident of getting an interval that contains the true mean with a maximum error of 1 day?

24. **Cost of Pizzas** A pizza shop owner wishes to find the 95% confidence interval of the true mean cost of a large plain pizza. How large should the sample be if she wants to be accurate to within $0.15? A previous study showed that the standard deviation of the price was $0.26.

25. **National Accounting Examination** If the variance of a national accounting examination is 900, how large a sample is needed to estimate the true mean score within 5 points with 99% confidence?

26. **Vehicle Travel Distances** The 95% confidence interval estimate of the distance travelled in Canada in a recent year is $299.2 < \mu < 331.4$ billion vehicle-kilometres. Construct a 98% confidence interval based on the same data.

Source: Natural Resources Canada, Office of Energy Efficiency, Canadian Vehicle Survey, 2009: Summary Report.

7–2 Confidence Intervals for the Mean When σ Is Unknown >

Find the confidence interval for the mean when σ is unknown.

When σ is known and the variable is normally distributed, the standard normal distribution is used to find confidence intervals for the mean. However, in most situations, the population standard deviation, σ, is not known. Regardless of the sample size, the standard deviation from the sample, *s,* is used in place of the population standard deviation, for confidence interval estimates of μ. When *s* is used, especially when the sample size is small, critical values greater than the values for $z_{\alpha/2}$ are used in confidence intervals in order to keep the interval at a given confidence level, such as 95%. These values are taken from the *Student's t distribution,* most often called the *t* **distribution.**

To use this method, the samples must be simple random samples, and the population from which the samples were taken must be normally or approximately normally distributed, or the sample size must be 30 or more.

Some important characteristics of the *t* distribution are described now.

Characteristics of the t Distribution

The t distribution shares some characteristics of the normal distribution and differs from it in others. The t distribution is similar to the standard normal distribution in these ways.

1. It is bell-shaped.
2. It is symmetric about the mean.
3. The mean, median, and mode are equal to 0 and are located at the centre of the distribution.
4. The curve never touches the x axis.

The t distribution differs from the standard normal distribution in the following ways.

1. The variance is greater than 1.
2. The t distribution is actually a group of curves with different dispersions and heights based on the concept of *degrees of freedom,* which is related to sample size.
3. As the sample size increases, the t distribution approaches the standard normal distribution. See Figure 7–7.

Figure 7–7

The t Family of Curves

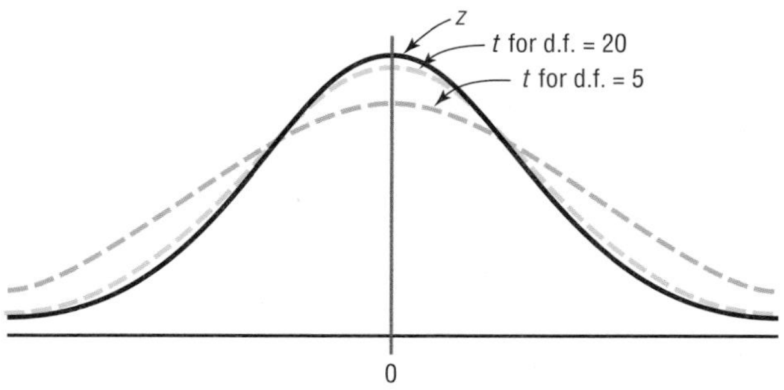

Historical Note

The t distribution was formulated in 1908 by an Irish brewing company employee named W. S. Gosset. Gosset was involved in researching new methods of manufacturing ale. Because brewing company employees were not allowed to publish results, Gosset published his finding using the pseudonym *Student;* hence, the t distribution is sometimes called *Student's t distribution.*

Many statistical distributions use the concept of degrees of freedom, and the formulas for finding the degrees of freedom vary for different statistical tests. The **degrees of freedom** are the number of values that are free to vary after a sample statistic has been computed, and they tell the researcher which specific curve to use when a distribution consists of a family of curves.

For example, if the mean of 5 values is 10, then 4 of the 5 values are free to vary. But once 4 values are selected, the fifth value must be a specific number to get a sum of 50, since $50 \div 5 = 10$. Hence, the degrees of freedom are $5 - 1 = 4$, and this value tells the researcher which t curve to use.

The symbol d.f. will be used for degrees of freedom. The degrees of freedom for a confidence interval for the mean are found by subtracting 1 from the sample size. That is, d.f. $= n - 1$. *Note:* For some statistical tests used later in this book, the degrees of freedom are not equal to $n - 1$.

The formula for finding a confidence interval about the mean by using the t distribution is given now.

Formula for a Specific Confidence Interval for the Mean When σ Is Unknown and $n < 30$

$$\overline{X} - t_{\alpha/2}\left(\frac{s}{\sqrt{n}}\right) < \mu < \overline{X} + t_{\alpha/2}\left(\frac{s}{\sqrt{n}}\right)$$

The degrees of freedom are $n - 1$.

The values for $t_{\alpha/2}$ are found in Table F in Appendix C. The top row of Table F, labelled *Confidence Intervals,* is used to get these values. The other two rows, labelled *One tail* and *Two tails,* will be explained in Chapter 8 and should not be used here.

Example 7–5 shows how to find the value in Table F for $t_{\alpha/2}$.

Example 7–5

Find the $t_{\alpha/2}$ value for a 95% confidence interval when the sample size is 22.

Solution

The d.f. = 22 − 1, or 21. Find 21 in the left column and 95% in the row labelled Confidence Intervals. The intersection where the two meet gives the value for $t_{\alpha/2}$, which is 2.080. See Figure 7–8.

Figure 7–8

Finding $t_{\alpha/2}$ for Example 7–5

	Table F The t Distribution						
Degrees of Freedom	Confidence Intervals	50%	80%	90%	95%	98%	99%
d.f.	One tail, α	0.25	0.10	0.05	0.02	0.01	0.005
	Two tails, α	0.50	0.20	0.10	0.05	0.02	0.01
1		1.000	3.078	6.314	12.706	31.821	63.657
2		0.816	1.886	2.920	4.303	6.965	9.925
⋮							
20		0.687	1.325	1.725	2.086	2.528	2.845
21		0.686	1.323	1.721	2.080	2.518	2.831
22		0.686	1.321	1.717	2.074	2.508	2.819
⋮							
$(z)\infty$		0.674	1.282	1.645	1.960	2.326	2.576

Note: At the bottom of Table F where d.f. = ∞, the $z_{\alpha/2}$ values can be found for specific confidence intervals. The reason is that as the degrees of freedom increase, the t distribution approaches the standard normal distribution. Also, if the desired degrees of freedom value is not on the t distribution table, use the closest d.f. value. For example, if d.f. = 32 for a 95% confidence level, use d.f. = 30 (closest value) and $t_{\alpha/2} =$ 2.042. If the degrees of freedom value is exactly halfway between two d.f. values, use the average of the two d.f. values. For example, if d.f. = 45 for a 95% confidence level, use d.f. = 40 and d.f. = 50. Hence $t_{\alpha/2} = (2.021 + 2.009)/2 = 2.015$.

Examples 7–6 and 7–7 show how to find the confidence interval when one is using the t distribution.

Assumptions for Finding a Confidence Interval for a Mean When σ Is Unknown

1. The sample is a random sample.
2. Either $n \geq 30$ or the population is normally distributed if $n < 30$.

Example 7–6

Impaired Driving

An RCMP Checkstop program reported that 32 drivers charged with impaired driving had a mean blood alcohol concentration (BAC) of 165 mg per 100 mL of blood. The legal BAC limit is 80 mg/100 mL. If the sample standard deviation was 17.5 mg/100 mL, estimate a 98% confidence interval estimate of BAC for the population mean of impaired drivers. Assume the variable is approximately normally distributed.

Solution

Since σ is unknown, use s and the t distribution (Table F) for the 98% confidence interval.

Since a degrees of freedom value of 31 is not in Table F, use the value closest to d.f. = 31, which is d.f. = 30. Therefore, $t_{\alpha/2} = 2.457$.

The 98% confidence interval of the population mean is found by substituting in the formula

$$\overline{X} - t_{\alpha/2}\left(\frac{s}{\sqrt{n}}\right) < \mu < \overline{X} + t_{\alpha/2}\left(\frac{s}{\sqrt{n}}\right)$$

Hence, $165 - (2.457)\left(\dfrac{17.5}{\sqrt{32}}\right) < \mu < 165 + (2.457)\left(\dfrac{17.5}{\sqrt{32}}\right)$

$$165 - 7.6 < \mu < 165 + 7.6$$
$$157.4 < \mu < 172.6$$

Therefore, one can be 98% confident that the population mean BAC reading for impaired drivers is between 157.4 and 172.6 mg/100 mL of blood.

Source: CBC News, "Drinking Drivers More Drunk, RCMP Report," January 5, 2009.

Example 7–7

Home Fires Started by Smoking

The data represent a sample of the number of home fires in Canada started by smoking for selected years. Find the 99% confidence interval for the mean number of home fires started by smoking each year. Assume the data is from a normally distributed population.

3929	3260	1019	2535	3175
2968	3448	3790	2532	4185

Source: Council of Canadian Fire Marshals and Fire Commissioners.

Solution

Step 1   Find the mean and standard deviation for the data. Use the formula in Chapter 3 or your calculator. The mean $\overline{X} = 3084.1$. The standard deviation $s = 911.7$.

Step 2   Find $t_{\alpha/2}$ in Table F. Use the 99% confidence interval with d.f. = 9. It is 3.250.

Step 3   Substitute in the formula and solve.

$$\overline{X} - t_{\alpha/2}\left(\frac{s}{\sqrt{n}}\right) < \mu < \overline{X} + t_{\alpha/2}\left(\frac{s}{\sqrt{n}}\right)$$

$$3084.1 - 3.250\left(\frac{911.7}{\sqrt{10}}\right) < \mu < 3084.1 + 3.250\left(\frac{911.7}{\sqrt{10}}\right)$$

$$3084.1 - 3.250\left(\frac{911.7}{\sqrt{10}}\right) < \mu < 3084.1 + 3.250\left(\frac{911.7}{\sqrt{10}}\right)$$

$$3084.1 - 937.0 < \mu < 3084.1 + 937.0$$

$$2147.1 < \mu < 4021.1$$

Step 4   One can be 99% confident that the population mean number of home fires started by smoking each year is between 2147.1 and 4021.1, based on a sample of home fires occurring over a 10-year period.

Students sometimes have difficulty deciding whether to use *z* scores or *t* values when finding confidence intervals for the mean. As stated previously, when σ is known, $z_{\alpha/2}$, or *z* scores, can be used *no matter what the sample size is,* as long as the variable is normally distributed. When σ is unknown, *s* is used in the formula and $t_{\alpha/2}$ values are used, as long as the variable is approximately normally distributed. These rules are summarized in Figure 7–9.

Figure 7–9

When to Use the z or t Distribution

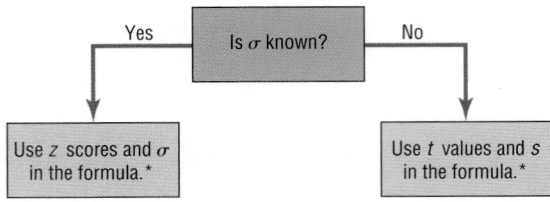

Yes   Is σ known?   No

Use *z* scores and σ in the formula.*

Use *t* values and *s* in the formula.*

*If *n* < 30, the variable must be normally distributed. If not, refer to Chapter 13, Nonparametric Statistics.

7–2 Applying the Concepts

Sports Drink Decision

Assume you get a new job as a coach for a sports team, and one of your first decisions is to choose the sports drink that the team will use during practices and games. You obtain a *Sports Report* magazine so that you can use your statistical background to help you make the best decision. The following table lists the most popular sports drinks and some important information about each of them. Answer the questions that follow the table.

Drink	Calories	Sodium	Potassium	Cost
Gatorade	60	110	25	$1.29
Powerade	68	77	32	1.19
All Sport	75	55	55	0.89
10-K	63	55	35	0.79
Exceed	69	50	44	1.59
1st Ade	58	58	25	1.09
Hydra Fuel	85	23	50	1.89

1. Would this be considered a small sample?
2. Compute the mean cost per container, and create a 90% confidence interval about that mean. Do all the costs per container fall inside the confidence interval? If not, which ones do not?
3. Are there any you would consider outliers?
4. How many degrees of freedom are there?
5. If cost is a major factor influencing your decision, would you consider cost per container or cost per serving?
6. List which drink you would recommend and why.

See page 339 for the answers.

Exercises 7–2

1. What are the properties of the t distribution?

2. What is meant by *degrees of freedom*?

3. When should the t distribution be used to find a confidence interval for the mean?

4. Find the values for each.

   a. $t_{\alpha/2}$ and $n = 18$ for the 99% confidence interval for the mean

   b. $t_{\alpha/2}$ and $n = 23$ for the 95% confidence interval for the mean

   c. $t_{\alpha/2}$ and $n = 15$ for the 98% confidence interval for the mean

   d. $t_{\alpha/2}$ and $n = 10$ for the 90% confidence interval for the mean

   e. $t_{\alpha/2}$ and $n = 20$ for the 95% confidence interval for the mean

For Exercises 5 through 20, assume that all variables are approximately normally distributed.

5. **Blood Hemoglobin** The average hemoglobin reading for a sample of 20 teachers was 16 grams per 100 millilitres, with a sample standard deviation of 2 grams. Find the 99% confidence interval of the true mean.

6. **Professors' Salaries** The following data represent annual salaries of a random selection of academics with the rank of professor (or full professor) in Ontario universities. Estimate the mean salary of all Ontario university professors at a 95% confidence level.

$119,843	$149,749	$152,311
$115,914	$132,184	$153,454
$159,845	$150,261	$178,068

   Source: Ontario Ministry of Finance, *Universities,* "Disclosure for 2008 under the *Public Sector Salary Disclosure Act, 1996.*"

7. **Tuition Fees** A sample of undergraduate university tuition fees across Canada is listed below. Estimate, with 98% confidence, the true population tuition fees for all undergraduate students.

$1968	$4673	$4988
$2550	$4920	$5101
$3108	$4872	$5630
$4638	$5004	$4989
$4719	$5008	$2911

   Source: Macleans.ca, "On Campus: The Bottom Line," November 5, 2009.

8. **Oil Production** A random sample of oil-producing countries lists oil production measured in barrels of oil per day (bbl/day). Estimate the true population mean oil consumption for all oil-producing countries in the world at a 90% confidence level. Data shown are thousands of bbl/day.

33	2,422	3186	11	368
20	115	36	2466	305
2531	133	797	287	71
586	10,780	4174	30	12
18	51	1584	359	38

   Source: Central Intelligence Agency, *The World Factbook,* "Country Comparison: Oil Production," (2009 est.).

9. **College Wrestler Weights** A sample of 6 university wrestlers had an average weight of 125 kg with a standard deviation of 5.5 kg. Find the 90% confidence interval of the true mean weight of all university wrestlers. If a coach claimed that the average weight of the wrestlers on his team was 141 kg, would the claim be believable?

10. **Charitable Donations** Different regions of Canada were sampled to determine per capita charitable donations. Results are listed below. At a 98% level of confidence, estimate the mean charitable donations for all Canadians.

$253	$333	$322	$299	$150
$415	$387	$367	$426	$397

    Source: Human Resources and Skills Development Canada, *Indicators of Well-Being in Canada,* "Social Participation—Charitable Donations, 2004."

11. **Distance Travelled to Work** A recent study of 28 employees of XYZ company showed that the mean of the distance they travelled to work was 23 km. The standard deviation of the sample mean was 3 km. Find the 95% confidence interval of the true mean. If a manager wanted to be sure that most of his employees would not be late, how much time would he suggest they allow for the commute if the average speed was 48 km per hour?

12. **Sunny Days** A random selection of Canadian cities yielded the following annual number of sunny days. Estimate the average number of sunny days for all Canadian cities at a 99% confidence level.

272	299	320	324	275
300	277	294	287	323
292	293	307	274	312
286	292	306	300	277

    Source: Environment Canada.

13. **Student Gas Consumption** A study of 25 students showed that they spent an average of $18.53 for gasoline per week. The standard deviation of the sample was $3.00. Find the 95% confidence interval of the true mean.

14. **Male Stress Test** For a group of 10 men subjected to a stress situation, the mean number of heartbeats per minute was 126, and the standard deviation was 4. Find the 95% confidence interval of the true mean.

15. **Female Stress Test** For the stress test described in Exercise 14, six women had an average heart rate of 115 beats per minute. The standard deviation of the sample was 6 beats. Find the 95% confidence interval of the true mean for the women.

16. **Foggy Days** A random selection of Canadian cities yielded the following number of annual foggy days. Estimate the average number of foggy days for all Canadian cities at a 95% confidence level.

30	119	19	2	10
76	27	26	10	49
15	35	20	118	32

Source: Environment Canada.

17. **Carbohydrates in Soft Drinks** The number of grams of carbohydrates in a 340-mL serving of a regular soft drink is listed here for a random sample of sodas. Estimate the mean number of carbohydrates in all brands of soda with 95% confidence.

48	37	52	40	43	46	41	38
41	45	45	33	35	52	45	41
30	34	46	40				

Source: The Doctor's Pocket Calorie, Fat, and Carbohydrate Counter.

18. **Football Player Heart Rates** For a group of 22 college football players, the mean heart rate after a morning workout session was 86 beats per minute, and the standard deviation was 5. Find the 90% confidence interval of the true mean for all college football players after a workout session. If a coach did not want to work his team beyond its capacity, what would be the maximum value he should use for the mean number of heartbeats per minute?

19. **Grooming Time for Men and Women** It has been reported that 20- to 24-year-old men spend an average of 37 minutes per day grooming, and 20- to 24-year-old women spend an average of 49 minutes per day grooming. Ask your classmates for their individual grooming times per day, and use the data to estimate the true mean grooming time for your school with 95% confidence.

Source: Time magazine.

20. **Smog in Cities** The number of unhealthy days based on the AQI (Air Quality Index) for a random sample of metropolitan areas is shown. Construct a 98% confidence interval based on the data.

61	12	6	40	27	38	93	5	13	40

Source: N.Y. Times Almanac.

Extending the Concepts »

21. A *one-sided confidence* interval can be found for a mean by using

$$\mu > \overline{X} - t_\alpha \frac{s}{\sqrt{n}} \quad \text{or} \quad \mu < \overline{X} + t_\alpha \frac{s}{\sqrt{n}}$$

where t_α is the value found under the row labelled One tail. Find two one-sided 95% confidence intervals of the population mean for the data shown, and interpret the

answers. The data represent the daily revenues in dollars from 20 parking meters in a small municipality.

2.60	1.05	2.45	2.90
1.30	3.10	2.35	2.00
2.40	2.35	2.40	1.95
2.80	2.50	2.10	1.75
1.00	2.75	1.80	1.95

7-3 Confidence Intervals for Proportions ›

LO3

Find the confidence interval for a proportion and determine the minimum sample size.

Transport Canada's National Occupant Restraint Program surveyed seat belt use among Canadians. Occupants of pickup trucks were least likely to "buckle up" with a rate of 85%. The parameter 85% is called a **proportion.** It means that 17 out of 20 occupants of pickup trucks in Canada wear their seat belts. A proportion represents a part of a whole. It can be expressed as a fraction, decimal, or percentage. In this case, 85% = 0.85 = 85/100 or 17/20. Proportions can also represent probabilities. In this case, if an occupant of a pickup truck is selected at random, the probability that the occupant is wearing a seat belt is 0.85.

Proportions can be obtained from samples or populations. The following symbols will be used.

Symbols Used in Proportion Notation

p = population proportion

$\hat{p}$ (read "p hat") = sample proportion

For a sample proportion,

$$\hat{p} = \frac{X}{n} \qquad \text{and} \qquad \hat{q} = \frac{n - X}{n} \qquad \text{or} \qquad 1 - \hat{p}$$

where X = number of sample units that possess the characteristics of interest
n = sample size

For example, in a study, 200 people were asked if they were satisfied with their job or profession; 162 said that they were. In this case, $n = 200$, $X = 162$, and $\hat{p} = X/n = 162/200 = 0.81$. It can be said that for this sample, 0.81, or 81%, of those surveyed were satisfied with their job or profession. The sample proportion is $\hat{p} = 0.81$.

The proportion of people who did not respond favourably when asked if they were satisfied with their job or profession constituted $\hat{q}$, where $\hat{q} = (n - X)/n$. For this survey, $\hat{q} = (200 - 162)/200 = 38/200$, or 0.19, or 19%.

When $\hat{p}$ and $\hat{q}$ are given in decimals or fractions, $\hat{p} + \hat{q} = 1$. When $\hat{p}$ and $\hat{q}$ are given in percentages, $\hat{p} + \hat{q} = 100\%$. It follows, then, that $\hat{q} = 1 - \hat{p}$, or $\hat{p} = 1 - \hat{q}$, when $\hat{p}$ and $\hat{q}$ are in decimal or fraction form. For the sample survey on job satisfaction, $\hat{q}$ can also be found by using $\hat{q} = 1 - \hat{p}$, or $1 - 0.81 = 0.19$.

Similar reasoning applies to population proportions; that is, $p = 1 - q$, $q = 1 - p$, and $p + q = 1$, when p and q are expressed in decimal or fraction form. When p and q are expressed as percentages, $p + q = 100\%$, $p = 100\% - q$, and $q = 100\% - p$.

Example 7–8

Impaired Driving

In Manitoba, the RCMP pulled over 18,918 vehicles in their province-wide Checkstop program over a 4-week holiday period. There were 105 people charged with impaired driving. Find $\hat{p}$ and $\hat{q}$, where $\hat{p}$ is the proportion of impaired drivers.

Source: Winnipeg Sun, "Checkstops Yield 105 Impaired Drivers," January 5, 2010.

Solution

Since $X = 105$ and $n = 18,914$,

$$\hat{p} = \frac{X}{n} = \frac{105}{18,918} \approx 0.006 = 0.6\%$$

$$\hat{q} = \frac{n - X}{n} = \frac{18,918 - 105}{18,918} = \frac{18,813}{18,918} \approx 0.994 = 99.4\%$$

One can also find $\hat{q}$ by using the formula $\hat{q} = 1 - \hat{p}$. In this case $\hat{q} = 1 - 0.006 = 0.994$.

As with means, the statistician, given the sample proportion, tries to estimate the population proportion. Point and interval estimates for a population proportion can be made by using the sample proportion. For a point estimate of p (the population proportion), $\hat{p}$ (the sample proportion) is used. On the basis of the three properties of a good estimator, $\hat{p}$ is unbiased, consistent, and relatively efficient. But as with means, one is not able to decide how good the point estimate of p is. Therefore, statisticians also use an interval estimate for a proportion, and they can assign a probability that the interval will contain the population proportion.

For example, in early 2010 as Canada recovered from the 2009 recession, pollsters published the following results. If an election was held, support for the Conservatives would be 33.3%; Liberals, 27.7%; NDP, 15.9%; Green, 10.4%; Bloc Québécois, 9.8%; and Other, 2.8%. The margin of error was $\pm 1.8\%$ at a 95% confidence level. That is, the Conservatives would conceivably garner between 31.5% and 35.1% of the popular vote, the Liberals between 25.9% and 29.5%, and so on. (Source: *Ekos Politics*, "Liberals Falling Back," March 25, 2010.)

The confidence interval for a particular p is based on the sampling distribution of $\hat{p}$. When the sample size n is no more than 5% of the population size, the sampling distribution of $\hat{p}$ is approximately normally distributed with a mean of p and a standard deviation of $\sqrt{\frac{pq}{n}}$, where $q = 1 - p$.

Confidence Intervals

To construct a confidence interval about a proportion, one must use the margin of error, which is

$$E = z_{\alpha/2}\sqrt{\frac{\hat{p}\hat{q}}{n}}$$

Confidence intervals about proportions must meet the criteria that $np \geq 5$ and $nq \geq 5$.

Formula for a Specific Confidence Interval for a Proportion

$$\hat{p} - z_{\alpha/2}\sqrt{\frac{\hat{p}\hat{q}}{n}} < p < \hat{p} + z_{\alpha/2}\sqrt{\frac{\hat{p}\hat{q}}{n}}$$

when np and nq are each greater than or equal to 5.

Assumptions for Finding a Confidence Interval for a Population Proportion

1. The sample is a random sample.
2. The conditions for a binomial experiment are satisfied. (See Chapter 5.)

Rounding Rule for a Confidence Interval for a Proportion Round off to three decimal places.

Example 7–9

Male Nursing Applicants

A sample of 500 nursing applications included 60 from men. Find the 90% confidence interval of the true proportion of men who applied to the nursing program.

Solution

Since $\alpha = 1 - 0.90 = 0.10$ and $z_{\alpha/2} = 1.645$, substituting in the formula

$$\hat{p} - z_{\alpha/2}\sqrt{\frac{\hat{p}\hat{q}}{n}} < p < \hat{p} + z_{\alpha/2}\sqrt{\frac{\hat{p}\hat{q}}{n}}$$

when $\hat{p} = 60/500 = 0.12$ and $\hat{q} = 1 - \hat{p} = 1 - 0.12 = 0.88$, one gets

$$0.12 - 1.645\sqrt{\frac{(0.12)(0.88)}{500}} < p < 0.12 + 1.645\sqrt{\frac{(0.12)(0.88)}{500}}$$

$$0.12 - 0.024 < p < 0.12 + 0.024$$

$$0.096 < p < 0.144$$

or

$$9.6\% < p < 14.4\%$$

Hence, one can be 90% confident that the percentage of nursing applicants who are men is between 9.6 and 14.4%.

When a specific percentage is given, the percentage becomes $\hat{p}$ when it is changed to a decimal. For example, if the problem states that 12% of the applicants were men, then $\hat{p} = 0.12$.

Example 7–10

Online Voting Support

A survey of 1200 Canadians indicated that 64% would support online voting in the next federal election if Elections Canada offered a safe and secure Internet platform. Construct a 95% confidence interval of the true proportion of Canadian online-voting support.

Source: CBC News, "Canadians Support Online Voting: Poll," December 17, 2009.

Solution

From the survey, $\hat{p} = 0.64$ (i.e., 64%), $\hat{q} = 1 - \hat{p} = 1 - 0.64 = 0.36$, and $n = 1200$. Since $z_{\alpha/2} = 1.96$, substituting in the formula

$$\hat{p} - z_{\alpha/2}\sqrt{\frac{\hat{p}\hat{q}}{n}} < p < \hat{p} + z_{\alpha/2}\sqrt{\frac{\hat{p}\hat{q}}{n}}$$

yields

$$0.64 - 1.96\sqrt{\frac{(0.64)(0.36)}{1200}} < p < 0.64 - 1.96\sqrt{\frac{(0.64)(0.36)}{1200}}$$

$$0.64 - 0.027 < p < 0.64 + 0.027$$

$$0.613 < p < 0.667$$

Hence, one can say with 95% confidence that the true proportion of Canadians who support online voting is between 61.3% and 66.7%.

Sample Size for Proportions

To find the sample size needed to determine a confidence interval about a proportion, use the following formula.

Formula for Minimum Sample Size Needed for Interval Estimate of a Population Proportion

$$n = \hat{p}\hat{q}\left(\frac{z_{\alpha/2}}{E}\right)^2$$

If necessary, round up to obtain a whole number.

This formula can be found by solving the margin of error value for n:

$$E = z_{\alpha/2}\sqrt{\frac{\hat{p}\hat{q}}{n}}$$

There are two situations to consider. First, if some approximation of $\hat{p}$ is known (e.g., from a previous study), that value can be used in the formula.

Second, if no approximation of $\hat{p}$ is known, one should use $\hat{p} = 0.5$. This value will give a sample size sufficiently large to guarantee an accurate prediction, given the confidence interval and the error of estimate. The reason is that when $\hat{p}$ and $\hat{q}$ are each 0.5, the product $\hat{p}\hat{q}$ is at maximum, as shown here.

$\hat{p}$	$\hat{q}$	$\hat{p}\hat{q}$
0.1	0.9	0.09
0.2	0.8	0.16
0.3	0.7	0.21
0.4	0.6	0.24
0.5	**0.5**	**0.25**
0.6	0.4	0.24
0.7	0.3	0.21
0.8	0.2	0.16
0.9	0.1	0.09

Example 7–11

Home Broadband Internet

A researcher wants to estimate with 98% confidence the proportion of Canadians who have a high-speed broadband Internet connection at home. A previous study showed that 52% of Canadian homes had broadband Internet. The researcher wants to be accurate within 3% of the true proportion. Find the minimum sample size necessary.

Solution

Since $z_{\alpha/2} = 2.33$, $E = 0.03$, $\hat{p} = 0.52$, and $\hat{q} = 0.48$, then

$$n = \hat{p}\hat{q}\left(\frac{z_{\alpha/2}}{E}\right)^2 = (0.48)(0.52)\left(\frac{2.33}{0.03}\right)^2 = 1505.6$$

which, when rounded up, indicates that 1506 homes need to be sampled.

Example 7–12

Mobile Internet Access

The same researcher wants to estimate the proportion of Canadians who access the Internet on their mobile phones. She wants to be 90% confident and be accurate within 5% of the true proportion. Find the minimum sample size necessary.

Solution

Since there is no prior knowledge of $\hat{p}$, statisticians assign the values $\hat{p} = 0.5$ and $\hat{q} = 0.5$. The sample size obtained by using these values will be large enough to ensure the specified level of confidence. Hence,

$$n = \hat{p}\hat{q}\left(\frac{z_{\alpha/2}}{E}\right)^2 = (0.5)(0.5)\left(\frac{1.645}{0.05}\right)^2 = 270.60$$

which, when rounded up, indicates that 271 Canadians need to be sampled.

In determining the sample size, the size of the population is irrelevant. Only the degree of confidence and the maximum error are necessary to make the determination.

Speaking of Statistics

Does Success Bring Happiness?

W. C. Fields said, "Start every day off with a smile and get it over with."

Do you think people are happy because they are successful, or are they successful because they are just happy people? A recent survey conducted by *Money* magazine showed that 34% of the people surveyed said that they were happy because they were successful; however, 63% said that they were successful because they were happy individuals. The people surveyed had an average household income of $75,000 or more. The margin of error was ±2.5%. Based on the information in this article, what would be the confidence interval for each percentage?

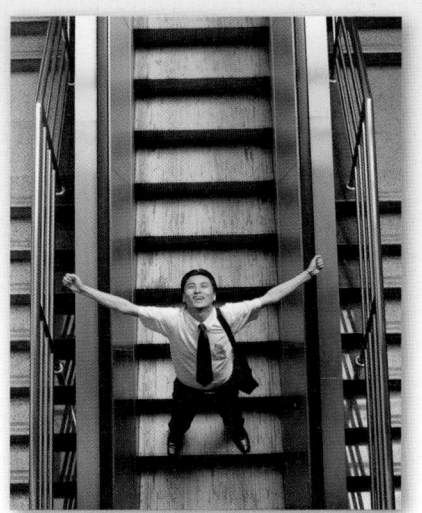

7–3 Applying the Concepts

Contracting Influenza

To answer the questions, use the following table describing the percentage of Americans who reported contracting influenza, by gender and race/ethnicity.

	Influenza	
Characteristic	**Percentage**	**(95% CI)**
Gender		
Men	48.8	(47.1–50.5%)
Women	51.5	(50.2–52.8%)
Race/ethnicity		
Caucasian	52.2	(51.1–53.3%)
African American	33.1	(29.5–36.7%)
Hispanic	47.6	(40.9–54.3%)
Other	39.7	(30.8–48.5%)
Total	50.4	(49.3–51.5%)

Forty-nine states and the District of Columbia participated in the study. Weighted means were used. The sample size was 19,774. There were 12,774 women and 7000 men.

1. Explain what (95% CI) means.
2. How large is the error for men reporting influenza?
3. What is the sample size?
4. How does sample size affect the size of the confidence interval?
5. Would the confidence intervals be larger or smaller for a 90% CI, using the same data?
6. Where does the 51.5% under influenza for women fit into its associated 95% CI?

See page 339 for the answers.

Exercises 7–3

1. In each case, find $\hat{p}$ and $\hat{q}$.
   a. $n = 80$ and $X = 40$
   b. $n = 200$ and $X = 90$
   c. $n = 130$ and $X = 60$
   d. $n = 60$ and $X = 35$
   e. $n = 95$ and $X = 43$

2. (ans) Find $\hat{p}$ and $\hat{q}$ for each percentage. (Use each percentage for $\hat{p}$.)
   a. 15%   d. 51%
   b. 37%   e. 79%
   c. 71%

3. **Social Networking** In a survey of 2356 Canadian Internet users aged 12 years and older, 919 were reported to visit a social networking Web site at least monthly. Find the 95% confidence interval for the true proportion of Canadian Internet users who visit social networking Web sites at least monthly.
   Source: Canadian Internet Project, *Canada Online!* "The Internet, Media and Emerging Technologies: Uses, Attitudes, Trends and International Comparisons," 2007.

4. **Diabetics** A study of diabetes in Canada reported that of 4345 people surveyed, 2.7% reported to be diagnosed with diabetes. Find the 90% confidence interval of the population proportion of Canadians with diabetes.
   Source: Campbell Survey on Well-Being in Canada.

5. **Drinking Tap Water** A survey of 2165 adult Canadians revealed that 33% will not drink tap water from their municipal or regional water supply. Find the 90% confidence interval of the true proportion of adult Canadians who will not drink water directly from the tap.
   Source: Royal Bank of Canada and Unilever: *2009 Canadian Water Attitudes Survey.*

6. **Automated Shopping** In a global survey of 4600 primary household shoppers, 55% of Canadians believe that by 2015, networked refrigerators and online devices will be available to prepare shopping lists and order goods that require replenishing. Estimate with 99% confidence the true proportion of Canadian shoppers who hold this belief.
   Source: TNS Canadian Facts, *New Future in Store,* "Consumers Predict Fridges Will Prepare Shopping Lists and Arrange Deliveries by 2015: Global Survey," July 7, 2008.

7. **Speeding and Climate Change** Transport Canada surveyed 2002 adult Canadians on their attitudes toward speeding. One finding was that 55% of respondents felt that speeding had no impact on climate change. At a 98% confidence level, estimate the true proportion of adult Canadians who hold the belief that speeding does not affect climate change.
   Source: Transport Canada, *Driver Attitude to Speeding and Speed Management: A Quantitative and Qualitative Study—Final Report,* May 2005.

8. **Space Travel** A *CBS News/New York Times* poll found that 329 out of 763 adults said they would travel to outer space in their lifetime, given the chance. Estimate with 92% confidence the true proportion of adults who would like to travel to outer space.
   Source: www.pollingreport.com.

9. **Youth Smokers** A study by Health Canada found that 10% of Canadians aged 15 to 17 years old are current smokers. A rural school board decided to survey regional high schools to compare its results with the national smoking rate. Two hundred 15- to 17-year-old youth were surveyed, and 13% said they smoked on occasion. Find the 98% confidence interval of the true proportion of 15- to 17-year-old youth who smoke, and compare the results with Health Canada's national smoking rates.
   Source: Health Canada, *Health Concerns,* "Canadian Tobacco Use Monitoring Survey, 2008."

10. **White-Water Canoe Experience** A survey of 50 first-time white-water canoers showed that 23 did not want to repeat the experience. Find the 90% confidence interval of the true proportion of canoers who did not wish to canoe the rapids a second time. If a rafting company wants to distribute brochures for repeat trips, what is the minimum number it should print?

11. **Blu-ray Players** A survey of 125 households found that 9% own a Blu-ray player primarily to play Blu-ray movies on high-definition television. At a 90% confidence level, estimate the true proportion of households that own a Blu-ray player.

Source: CDRinfo, Blu-Ray Penetration on Rise, Report Says, April 3, 2008.

12. **Food Bank Usage** A random sample of 600 Canadians showed that 2.4% have visited a food bank to supplement their daily food requirements. Estimate with 96% confidence the true proportion of Canadians who have visited a food bank.

Source: Food Banks Canada, HungerCount 2009.

13. **Financial Well-Being** In a Gallup Poll of 1005 individuals, 452 thought they were worse off financially than a year ago. Find the 95% confidence interval for the true proportion of individuals who feel they are worse off financially.

Source: Gallup Poll.

14. **Avian Flu Health Threat** In a survey of 1023 Canadian adults, 614 respondents are not concerned about the health threat of avian flu. Find the 95% confidence interval for the true proportion of Canadians who do not feel threatened by the avian flu.

Source: CTV.ca.

15. **Vitamins for Women** A medical researcher wishes to determine the percentage of females who take vitamins. He wants to be 99% confident that the estimate is within 2 percentage points of the true proportion. A recent study of 180 females showed that 25% took vitamins.

   a. How large should the sample size be?

   b. If no estimate of the sample proportion is available, how large should the sample be?

16. **Widows** A recent study indicated that 29% of the 100 women over age 55 in the study were widows.

   a. How large a sample must one take to be 90% confident that the estimate is within 0.05 of the true proportion of women over age 55 who are widows?

   b. If no estimate of the sample proportion is available, how large should the sample be?

17. **Greenhouse Gas Reductions** A researcher wishes to estimate the proportion of Canadians who are in favour of the Kyoto Protocol's call for the reduction of emissions of greenhouse gases. She wants to be 99% confident that her estimate is within 5% of the true proportion.

   a. How large a sample should be taken if in a prior survey of Canadians, 70% were in favour of the Kyoto Protocol?

   b. If no estimate of the sample proportion is available, how large should the sample be?

18. **Obesity** Health Canada classifies obesity using the body mass index (BMI) scale of weight (kg)/height (m)^2 as 30 kg/m^2 or more. A study on chronic diseases in Canada stated with 95% confidence that between 16.68% and 17.95% of Canadians aged 25 to 64 were obese. What was the sample size?

Source: Public Health Agency of Canada, Chronic Diseases in Canada, "Socio-Demographic and Geographic Analysis of Overweight and Obesity in Canadian Adults Using the Canadian Community Health Survey (2005)," December 2009.

19. **Women Playing Hockey** A national sports governing organization wants to determine the percentage of active females, aged 15 years and older, who participate in ice hockey. The national organization would like to be accurate within 2.5 percentage points with 90% confidence of the true proportion of female ice hockey participants. How large a sample would be required if

   a. No prior research results are available?

   b. A prior study indicated that 12.2% of active females participate in ice hockey?

Source: Statistics Canada, Culture, Tourism and the Centre for Education Statistics, Sport Participation in Canada, 2005, Fidelis Ifedi.

20. **Welfare Recipients** The Canadian Council on Social Development would like to update its statistics on the percentage of Canadians receiving welfare. A previous study found that 4.2% of Canadians were on welfare. How large a sample is required to estimate the true proportion of Canadian welfare recipients within 1.5% at a 95% confidence level?

Source: Canadian Council on Social Development, Estimated Number of People on Welfare by Province and Territory, 1993–1994.

Extending the Concepts »

21. **Gun Control** If a sample of 600 people is selected and the researcher decides to have a maximum error of estimate of 4% on the specific proportion who favour gun control, find the level of confidence. A recent study showed that 50% were in favour of some form of gun control.

22. **Fight for the Arctic** QMI Agency and Sun Media reported that 49.6% of 1510 Canadians polled believe that Canada should exercise military power to assert sovereignty in the resource-rich Arctic. If the margin of error was 3.0 percentage points, what was the confidence level used for the estimate?

Source: Leger Marketing.

Speaking of Statistics

Here is a survey about college students' credit card usage. Suggest several ways that the study could have been more meaningful if confidence intervals had been used.

OTHER PEOPLE'S MONEY

Undergrads love their plastic. That means—you guessed it—students are learning to become debtors. According to the Public Interest Research Groups, only half of all students pay off card balances in full each month, 36% sometimes do and 14% never do. Meanwhile, 48% have paid a late fee. Here's how undergrads stack up, according to Nellie Mae, a provider of college loans:

Undergrads with a credit card **78%**

Average number of cards owned . . **3**

Average student card debt **$1236**

Students with 4 or more cards. . . . **32%**

Balances of $3000 to $7000 . . . . . **13%**

Balances over $7000. . . . . **9%**

Reprinted with permission from the January 2002 *Reader's Digest*.
Copyright © 2002 by The Reader's Digest Assn. Inc.

7–4	Confidence Intervals for Variances and Standard Deviations ›

Find a confidence interval for a variance and a standard deviation.

Historical Note

The χ^2 distribution with 2 degrees of freedom was formulated by a mathematician named Hershel in 1869 while he was studying the accuracy of shooting arrows at a target. Many other mathematicians have since contributed to its development.

In Sections 7–1 through 7–3, confidence intervals were calculated for means and proportions. This section will explain how to find confidence intervals for variances and standard deviations. In statistics, the variance and standard deviation of a variable are as important as the mean. For example, when products that fit together (such as pipes) are manufactured, it is important to keep the variations of the diameters of the products as small as possible; otherwise, they will not fit together properly and will have to be scrapped. In the manufacture of medicines, the variance and standard deviation of the medication in the pills play an important role in making sure patients receive the proper dosage. For these reasons, confidence intervals for variances and standard deviations are necessary.

To calculate these confidence intervals, a new statistical distribution is needed. It is called the **chi-square distribution.**

The chi-square variable is similar to the t variable in that its distribution is a family of curves based on the number of degrees of freedom. The symbol for chi-square is χ^2 (Greek letter chi, pronounced "ki"). Several of the distributions are shown in Figure 7–10, along with the corresponding degrees of freedom. The chi-square distribution is obtained from the values of $(n - 1)s^2/\sigma^2$ when random samples are selected from a normally distributed population whose variance is σ^2.

A chi-square variable cannot be negative, and the distributions are positively skewed. As degrees of freedom increase, the chi-square distribution approaches but never attains symmetry. The area under each chi-square distribution is equal to 1.00, or 100%.

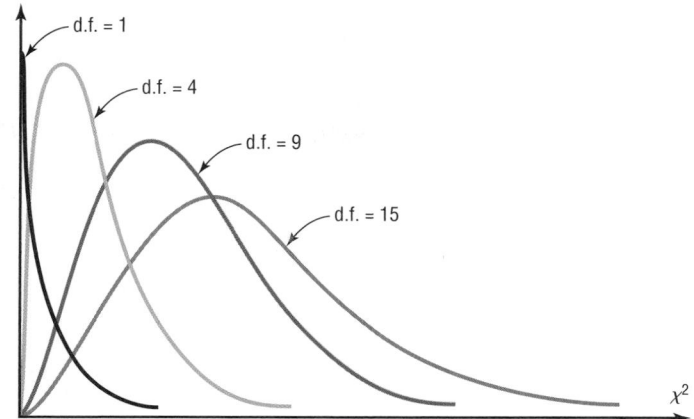

Figure 7–10

The Chi-Square Family of Curves

Table G in Appendix C gives the values for the chi-square distribution. These values are used in the denominators of the formulas for confidence intervals. Two different values are used in the formula. One value is found on the left side of the table, and the other is on the right. See Figure 7–11. For example, to find the table values corresponding to the 95% confidence interval, one must first change 95% to a decimal and subtract it from 1 $(1 - 0.95 = 0.05)$. Then divide the answer by 2 $(\alpha/2 = 0.05/2 = 0.025)$. This is the column on the

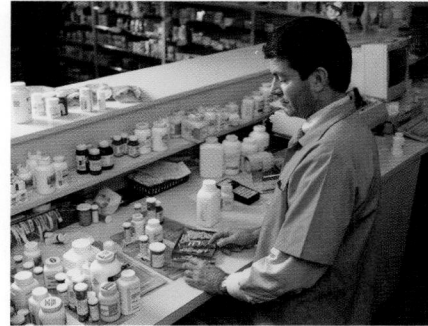

right side of the table, used to get the values for χ^2_{right}. To get the value for χ^2_{left}, subtract the value of $\alpha/2$ from 1 $(1 - 0.05/2 = 0.975)$. Finally, find the appropriate row corresponding to the degrees of freedom $n - 1$. A similar procedure is used to find the values for a 90 or 99% confidence interval.

Figure 7–11

Chi-Square Distribution for d.f. = $n - 1$

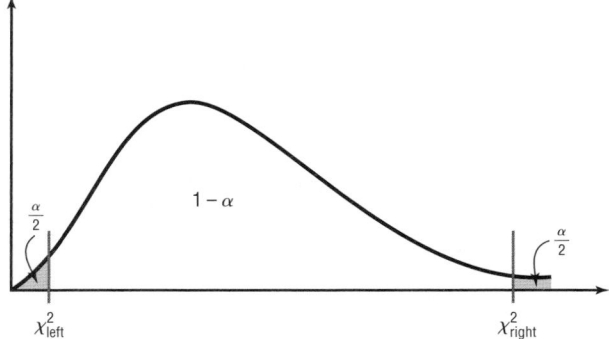

Example 7–13

Find the values for χ^2_{right} and χ^2_{left} for a 90% confidence interval when $n = 25$.

Solution

To find χ^2_{right}, subtract $1 - 0.90 = 0.10$ and divide by 2 to get 0.05.

To find χ^2_{left}, subtract $1 - 0.05$ to get 0.95. Hence, use the 0.95 and 0.05 columns and the row corresponding to 24 d.f. See Figure 7–12.

Figure 7–12

χ^2 **Table for Example 7–13**

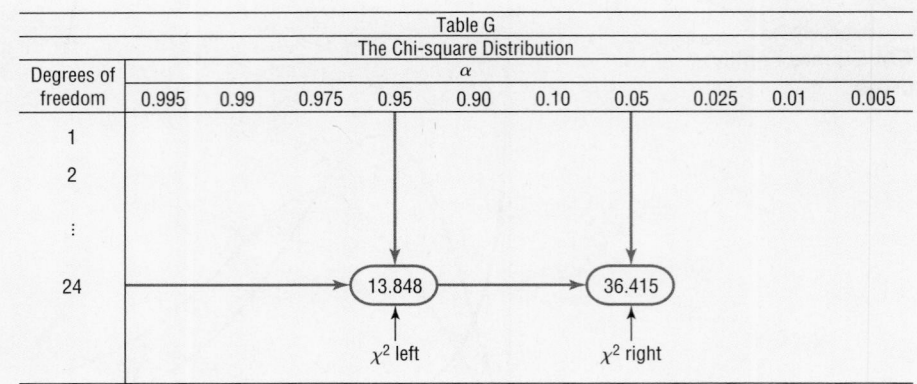

Table G The Chi-square Distribution										
Degrees of freedom	α									
	0.995	0.99	0.975	0.95	0.90	0.10	0.05	0.025	0.01	0.005
1										
2										
⋮										
24				13.848			36.415			

χ^2 left χ^2 right

The answers are

$$\chi^2_{\text{right}} = 36.415$$

$$\chi^2_{\text{left}} = 13.848$$

See Figure 7–13.

Figure 7–13

χ^2 **Distribution for Example 7–13**

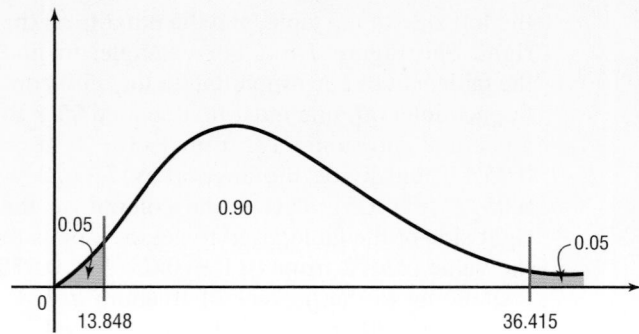

Useful estimates for σ^2 and σ are s^2 and s, respectively.

To find confidence intervals for variances and standard deviations, one must assume that the variable is normally distributed.

The formulas for the confidence intervals are shown here.

Formula for the Confidence Interval for a Variance

$$\frac{(n-1)s^2}{\chi^2_{\text{right}}} < \sigma^2 < \frac{(n-1)s^2}{\chi^2_{\text{left}}}$$

d.f. $= n - 1$

Formula for the Confidence Interval for a Standard Deviation

$$\sqrt{\frac{(n-1)s^2}{\chi^2_{\text{right}}}} < \sigma < \sqrt{\frac{(n-1)s^2}{\chi^2_{\text{left}}}}$$

d.f. $= n - 1$

Recall that s^2 is the symbol for the sample variance and s is the symbol for the sample standard deviation. If the problem gives the sample standard deviation s, be sure to *square it* when you are using the formula. But if the problem gives the sample variance s^2, *do not square it* when using the formula, since the variance is already in square units.

Assumptions for Finding a Confidence Interval for a Variance or Standard Deviation

1. The sample is a random sample.
2. The population must be normally distributed.

Rounding Rule for a Confidence Interval for a Variance or Standard Deviation

When you are computing a confidence interval for a population variance or standard deviation by using raw data, round off to one more decimal place than the number of decimal places in the original data.

When you are computing a confidence interval for a population variance or standard deviation by using a sample variance or standard deviation, round off to the same number of decimal places as given for the sample variance or standard deviation.

Example 7–14 shows how to find a confidence interval for a variance and standard deviation.

Example 7–14

Nicotine Content

Find the 95% confidence interval for the variance and standard deviation of the nicotine content of cigarettes manufactured if a sample of 20 cigarettes has a standard deviation of 1.6 milligrams.

Solution

Since $\alpha = 0.05$, the two critical values, respectively, for the 0.025 and 0.975 levels for 19 degrees of freedom are 32.852 and 8.907. The 95% confidence interval for the variance is found by substituting in the formula.

$$\frac{(n-1)s^2}{\chi^2_{\text{right}}} < \sigma^2 < \frac{(n-1)s^2}{\chi^2_{\text{left}}}$$

$$\frac{(20-1)(1.6)^2}{32.852} < \sigma^2 < \frac{(20-1)(1.6)^2}{8.907}$$

$$1.5 < \sigma^2 < 5.5$$

Hence, one can be 95% confident that the true variance for the nicotine content is between 1.5 and 5.5.

For the standard deviation, the confidence interval is

$$\sqrt{1.5} < \sigma < \sqrt{5.5}$$

$$1.2 < \sigma < 2.3$$

Hence, one can be 95% confident that the true standard deviation for the nicotine content of all cigarettes manufactured is between 1.2 and 2.3 milligrams, based on a sample of 20 cigarettes.

Example 7–15

Cost of Ski Lift Tickets

Find the 90% confidence interval for the variance and standard deviation for the price in dollars of an adult single-day ski lift ticket. The data represent a selected sample of American ski resorts. Assume the variable is normally distributed.

59	54	53	52	51
39	49	46	49	48

Source: USA TODAY.

Solution

Step 1   Find the variance for the data. Use the formulas in Chapter 3 or your calculator. The variance $s^2 = 28.2$.

Step 2   Find χ^2_{right} and χ^2_{left} from Table G in Appendix C. Since $\alpha = 0.10$, the two critical values are 3.325 and 16.919, using d.f. = 9 and 0.95 and 0.05.

Step 3   Substitute in the formula and solve.

$$\frac{(n-1)s^2}{\chi^2_{\text{right}}} < \sigma^2 < \frac{(n-1)s^2}{\chi^2_{\text{left}}}$$

$$\frac{(10-1)(28.2)}{16.919} < \sigma^2 < \frac{(10-1)(28.2)}{3.325}$$

$$15.0 < \sigma^2 < 76.3$$

For the standard deviation

$$\sqrt{15} < \sigma < \sqrt{76.3}$$

$$3.87 < \sigma < 8.73$$

Hence one can be 90% confident that the standard deviation for the price of all single-day ski lift tickets of the population is between $3.87 and $8.73, based on a sample of 10 American ski resorts. (Two decimal places are used since the data are in dollars and cents.)

Note: If you are using the standard deviation instead (as in Example 7–14) of the variance, be sure to square the standard deviation when substituting in the formula.

7–4   Applying the Concepts

Confidence Interval for Standard Deviation

Shown are the ages (in years) of Canadian prime ministers at the time of their deaths.

76	49	77	75	91
70	94	82	86	83
72	93	76	75	80

Source: Parliament of Canada, Prime Ministers of Canada, "Biographical Information," January 15, 2007.

1. Do the data represent a population or a sample?

2. Select a random sample of 7 ages and find the variance and standard deviation.

3. Find the 95% confidence interval of the standard deviation.

4. Find the standard deviation of all the data values.

5. Does the confidence interval calculated in question 3 contain the mean?

6. If it does not, give a reason why.

7. What assumption(s) must be considered for constructing the confidence interval in step 3?

See page 340 for the answers.

Exercises 7–4

1. What distribution must be used when computing confidence intervals for variances and standard deviations?

2. What assumption must be made when computing confidence intervals for variances and standard deviations?

3. Using Table G, find the values for χ^2_{left} and χ^2_{right}.

   a. $\alpha = 0.05$, $n = 12$
   b. $\alpha = 0.10$, $n = 20$
   c. $\alpha = 0.05$, $n = 27$
   d. $\alpha = 0.01$, $n = 6$
   e. $\alpha = 0.10$, $n = 41$

4. **Lifetimes of Smartphone Batteries** Find the 90% confidence interval for the variance and standard deviation for the lifetime of Smartphone batteries if a sample of 16 Smartphone batteries has a standard deviation of 2.1 months. Assume the variable is normally distributed. Do you feel that the lifetimes of the batteries are relatively consistent?

5. **Online Orders** Find the 95% confidence interval for the variance and standard deviation for the time it takes a customer to place an online order at an electronics Web site if a sample of 23 online orders has a standard deviation of 3.8 minutes. Assume the variable is normally distributed. Do you think that the times are relatively consistent?

6. **Carbohydrates in Yogurt** The number of carbohydrates (in grams) per 227-gram serving of yogurt for each of a random selection of brands is listed below. Assume a normally distributed variable. Estimate the true population variance and standard deviation for the number of carbohydrates per 227-gram serving of yogurt with 95% confidence.

   17 42 41 20 39 41 35 15 43
   25 38 33 42 23 17 25 34

7. **Applesauce Sugar Content** The sugar content (in grams) for a random sample of 113-ml containers of applesauce is shown. Find the 99% confidence interval for the population variance and standard deviation. Assume the variable is normally distributed.

18.6	19.5	20.2	20.4	19.3
21.0	20.3	19.6	20.7	18.9
22.1	19.7	20.8	18.9	20.7
21.6	19.5	20.1	20.3	19.9

8. **College Student Ages** Find the 90% confidence interval for the variance and standard deviation of the ages of seniors at Oak Park College if a sample of 24 students has a standard deviation of 2.3 years. Assume the variable is normally distributed.

9. **Calories in Cheese** The number of calories in a 28-mL serving of various kinds of regular cheese is shown. Estimate the population variance and standard deviation with 90% confidence.

110	45	100	95	110
110	100	110	95	120
130	100	80	105	105
90	110	70	125	108

Source: *The Doctor's Pocket Calorie, Fat, and Carbohydrate Counter.*

10. **Stock Prices** A random sample of stock prices per share (in dollars) is shown. Find the 90% confidence interval for the variance and standard deviation for the prices. Assume the variable is normally distributed.

26.69	13.88	28.37	12.00
75.37	7.50	47.50	43.00
3.81	53.81	13.62	45.12
6.94	28.25	28.00	60.50
40.25	10.87	46.12	14.75

Source: *Pittsburgh Tribune Review.*

11. **Time for Oil Change** A service station advertises that customers will have to wait no more than 30 minutes for an oil change. A sample of 28 oil changes has a standard deviation of 5.2 minutes. Assume a normally distributed variable. Find the 95% confidence interval of the population standard deviation of the time spent waiting for an oil change.

12. **Bottle-Filling Machine** Find the 95% confidence interval for the variance and standard deviation of the litres of water that a bottle-filling machine dispenses in 500-mL bottles. Assume the variable is normally distributed. The data are given.

   503 495 499 494 500 504 503 496 501 498

Extending the Concepts

13. **Lifetimes of Calculator Batteries** A confidence interval for a standard deviation for large samples taken from a normally distributed population can be approximated by

$$s - z_{\alpha/2}\frac{s}{\sqrt{2n}} < \sigma < s + z_{\alpha/2}\frac{s}{\sqrt{2n}}$$

Find the 95% confidence interval for the population standard deviation of calculator batteries. A sample of 200 calculator batteries has a standard deviation of 18 months.

Summary >

An important aspect of inferential statistics is estimation. Estimations of parameters of populations are accomplished by selecting a random sample from that population and choosing and computing a statistic that is the best estimator of the parameter. A good estimator must be unbiased, consistent, and relatively efficient. The best estimators of μ and p are $\overline{X}$ and $\hat{p}$, respectively. The best estimators of σ^2 and σ are s^2 and s, respectively.

There are two types of estimates of a parameter: point estimates and interval estimates. A point estimate is a specific value. For example, if a researcher wishes to estimate the average length of a certain adult fish, a sample of the fish is selected and measured. The mean of this sample is computed; for example, 3.2 centimetres. From this sample mean, the researcher estimates the population mean to be 3.2 centimetres.

The problem with point estimates is that the accuracy of the estimate cannot be determined. For this reason, statisticians prefer to use the interval estimate. By computing an interval about the sample value, statisticians can be 95 or 99% (or some other percentage) confident that their estimate contains the true parameter. The confidence level is determined by the researcher. The higher the confidence level, the wider the interval of the estimate must be. For example, a 95% confidence interval of the true mean length of a certain species of fish might be

$$3.17 < \mu < 3.23$$

whereas the 99% confidence interval might be

$$3.15 < \mu < 3.25$$

When the confidence interval of the mean is computed, the z scores or t values are used, depending on whether the population standard deviation is known. If σ is known, the z scores can be used. If σ is not known, the t values are used. When the sample size is less than 30, the population should be normally distributed.

Closely related to computing confidence intervals is the determination of the sample size to make an estimate of the mean. This information is needed to determine the minimum sample size necessary.

1. The degree of confidence must be stated.

2. The population standard deviation must be known or be able to be estimated.

3. The margin of error must be stated.

Confidence intervals and sample sizes can also be computed for proportions, using the normal distribution; and confidence intervals for variances and standard deviations can be computed, using the chi-square distribution. A confidence interval is given as the point estimate ± the margin of error.

For step-by-step guidance on the use of Texas Instruments TI-83 Plus/TI-84 Plus programmable calculators, see Appendix E at the back of this book. For summary procedures for Minitab, SPSS, and Excel, please see the full version of Appendix E available on *Connect*.

Important Terms

chi-square distribution 328	degrees of freedom 315	margin of error 306	relatively efficient estimator 304
confidence interval 305	estimation 303		
confidence level 305	estimator 304	point estimate 304	t distribution 314
consistent estimator 304	interval estimate 304	proportion 320	unbiased estimator 304

Important Formulas »

Formula for the confidence interval of the mean when σ is known:

$$\overline{X} - z_{\alpha/2}\left(\frac{\sigma}{\sqrt{n}}\right) < \mu < \overline{X} + z_{\alpha/2}\left(\frac{\sigma}{\sqrt{n}}\right)$$

Formula for the sample size for means:

$$n = \left(\frac{z_{\alpha/2} \cdot \sigma}{E}\right)^2$$

where E is the margin of error.

Formula for the confidence interval of the mean when σ is unknown:

$$\overline{X} - t_{\alpha/2}\left(\frac{s}{\sqrt{n}}\right) < \mu < \overline{X} + t_{\alpha/2}\left(\frac{s}{\sqrt{n}}\right)$$

Formula for the confidence interval for a proportion:

$$\hat{p} - z_{\alpha/2}\sqrt{\frac{\hat{p}\hat{q}}{n}} < p < \hat{p} + z_{\alpha/2}\sqrt{\frac{\hat{p}\hat{q}}{n}}$$

where $\hat{p} = X/n$ and $\hat{q} = 1 - \hat{p}$.

Formula for the sample size for proportions:

$$n = \hat{p}\hat{q}\left(\frac{z_{\alpha/2}}{E}\right)^2$$

Formula for the confidence interval for a variance:

$$\frac{(n-1)s^2}{\chi^2_{\text{right}}} < \sigma^2 < \frac{(n-1)s^2}{\chi^2_{\text{left}}}$$

Formula for confidence interval for a standard deviation:

$$\sqrt{\frac{(n-1)s^2}{\chi^2_{\text{right}}}} < \sigma < \sqrt{\frac{(n-1)s^2}{\chi^2_{\text{left}}}}$$

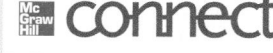 **connect**™ Practise and learn online with *Connect* with data sets and algorithmic questions related to concepts covered in this chapter. Questions and tables with online data sets are marked with .

Review Exercises »

1. **Marathon Runners' Speeds** A study of 36 marathon runners showed that they could run at an average rate of 12.6 kilometres per hour (km/h). The sample standard deviation is 0.9 km/h. Find a point estimate of the population mean. Find the 90% confidence interval for the mean of all runners.

2. **Product Recycling** A survey of 1275 Canadians indicated that 1224 prefer buying products that can be recycled. Find a 95% confidence interval for the true population proportion.

   Source: Sharp Canada.

3. **Hospital Length of Stay** A survey of 1100 hospital admissions reports that the average length of stay for seniors aged 65 and over who are hospitalized for falls is 13 days. Find a point estimate of the population mean. Find the 95% confidence interval of the true mean. Assume the population standard deviation from a prior study was 1.3 days.

   Source: Canadian Institute for Health Information.

4. **Condo Rents** A sample of 14 districts in Toronto found the following monthly rental payments for a 1-bedroom condominium (in dollars). Assume rental payments are normally distributed.

   | 1511 | 1605 | 2025 | 1275 | 1100 | 1203 | 1462 |
   | 1563 | 1488 | 1100 | 1447 | 1254 | 1259 | 1323 |

   Find a point estimate of the population mean. Find the 95% confidence interval for the population mean.

   Source: Toronto Real Estate Board.

5. **Mail Carriers' Dog Bites** For a certain urban area, in a sample of 5 months, an average of 28 mail carriers were bitten by dogs each month. The standard deviation of the sample was 3. Find the 90% confidence interval of the true mean number of mail carriers who are bitten by dogs each month. Assume the variable is normally distributed.

6. **Teachers' Salaries** A researcher is interested in estimating the average salary of teachers in a large urban school district. She wants to be 95% confident that her estimate is correct. If the standard deviation is $1050, how large a sample is needed to be accurate within $200?

7. **Postage Costs** A researcher wishes to estimate, within $25, the true average amount that a college spends on postage each year. If she wishes to be 90% confident, how large a sample is necessary? The standard deviation is known to be $80.

8. **Canadian Content TV Programming** The Friends of Canadian Broadcasting commissioned a poll of 1100 adult Canadians. On the question of Canadian content, 61% of respondents felt that there should be a specified minimum amount of Canadian programming on television. Find the 95% confidence interval of the true proportion of all adults who favour a defined minimum Canadian television content.

   Source: Friends of Canadian Broadcasting.

9. **Snow Removal Survey** In a recent study of 75 people, 41 said they were dissatisfied with their community's snow removal service. Find the 95% confidence interval of the true proportion of individuals who are dissatisfied with their community's snow removal service. Based on the results, should the supervisor consider making improvements in the snow removal service?

10. **Lengths of Children's Animated Films** The lengths (in minutes) of a random selection of popular children's

animated films are listed below. Estimate the true mean length of all children's animated films with 95% confidence.

93 83 76 92 77 81 78 100 78 76 75

11. Household Gambling A 2006 report on gambling indicated that 74% of Canadian households participated in at least one gambling activity (e.g., lotteries, casinos, bingo). How large a sample is needed to estimate the true proportion of households that participate in at least one gambling activity, with 90% confidence and at most a 2.5% margin of error?

Source: Statistics Canada, *Perspectives,* July 2009, Catalogue No. 75-001-X.

12. Child-Care Programs A study found that 73% of pre-kindergarten children aged 3 to 5 whose mothers had a bachelor's degree or higher were enrolled in centre-based early childhood care and education programs. How large a sample is needed to estimate the true proportion within 3 percentage points with 95% confidence? How large a sample is needed if you had no prior knowledge of the proportion?

13. Baseball Diameters The standard deviation of the diameter of 18 baseballs was 0.29 cm. Assume a normally distributed variable. Find the 95% confidence interval of the true standard deviation of the diameters

of the baseballs. Do you think the manufacturing process should be checked for inconsistency?

14. Truck Fuel Efficiency A random sample of 15 new pickup trucks was selected, and the vehicles were tested to determine their fuel efficiency in litres per 100 kilometres (L/100 km). The variance of the measurements was 3.5. Find the 95% confidence interval of the true variance. Assume fuel efficiency is normally distributed.

Source: Natural Resources Canada, Office of Energy Efficiency, *Personal: Transportation,* "Fuel Consumption Ratings."

15. Snowmobile Batteries Lifetimes A random sample of 15 snowmobiles was selected, and the lifetime (in months) of the batteries was measured. The variance of the sample was 8.6. Find the 90% confidence interval of the true variance. Assume the variable is normally distributed.

16. Health Risk of PCBs Health Canada does not consider the small quantities of PCBs (polychlorinated biphenyls) in fish and seafood to be a health risk. A sample of 28 salmon was measured for PCB contamination. The standard deviation of PCB levels was 10.6 parts per billion (ppb). Assume PCB levels are normally distributed. Find the 95% confidence interval of the standard deviation of the PCB contaminants.

Source: Health Canada, *Fish & Seafood Survey, 2002.*

 Statistics Today

Do You Waste Water?–Revisited

The estimates given in the survey are point estimates. However, since the margin of error (i.e., accurate to within ± 2.2%) is stated, an interval estimate can easily be obtained. For example, if 89% of Canadians are concerned about water usage, then the confidence interval of the true percentage of all Canadians, the population proportion, is between 86.8% and 91.2%. Using the same procedure, between 46.8% and 51.2% (that is, 49% ± 2.2%) of Canadians feel that water is Canada's

most important natural resource. In both cases, we are 95% confident—accurate 19 times out of 20—that our confidence interval contains the true population proportion of Canadians' attitude toward water.

Using the formula given in Section 7–3, a minimum sample size of 1985 would be needed to obtain a 95% confidence interval for *p,* as shown. *Use $\hat{p}$ and $\hat{q}$ as 0.5, since no value is known for $\hat{p}$.*

$$n = \hat{p} \cdot \hat{q} \cdot \left(\frac{z_{\alpha/2}}{E}\right)^2$$
$$= (0.5)(0.5)\left(\frac{1.96}{0.022}\right)^2$$
$$= 1985 \text{ (rounded up)}$$

Data Analysis »

The databanks for these questions can be found in Appendix D near the back of the textbook and also on ▦ **connect**.

1. From the databank choose a variable, find the mean, and construct the 95 and 99% confidence intervals of the population mean. Use a sample of at least 30 subjects. Find the mean of the population, and determine whether it falls within the confidence interval.

2. Repeat Exercise 1, using a different variable and a sample of 15.

3. Repeat Exercise 1, using a proportion. For example, construct a confidence interval for the proportion of individuals who did not complete high school.

4. From Data Set III in Appendix D, select a sample of 30 values and construct the 95 and 99% confidence intervals of the mean length in kilometres of major North American rivers. Find the mean of all the values, and determine if the confidence intervals contain the mean.

5. From Data Set VI in Appendix D, select a sample of 20 values and find the 90% confidence interval of the mean of the number of square kilometres. Find the mean of all the values, and determine if the confidence interval contains the mean.

6. Select a random sample of 20 of the record high temperatures found in Data Set I in Appendix D in both

Canada and the United States (North America). Find the proportion of temperatures below 44°C. Construct a 95% confidence interval for this proportion. Then find the true proportion of temperatures below 44°C, using all the data. Is the true proportion contained in the confidence interval? Explain record low temperatures below −44°C in North America. Repeat the procedure for the record low temperatures for North America.

Chapter Quiz »

Determine whether each statement is true or false. If the statement is false, explain why.

1. Interval estimates are preferred over point estimates since a confidence level can be specified.

2. For a specific confidence interval, the larger the sample size, the smaller the margin of error will be.

3. An estimator is consistent if, as the sample size decreases, the value of the estimator approaches the value of the parameter estimated.

4. To determine the sample size needed to estimate a parameter, one must know the margin of error.

Select the best answer.

5. When a 99% confidence interval is calculated instead of a 95% confidence interval with n being the same, the margin of error will be

   a. Smaller.
   b. Larger.
   c. The same.
   d. It cannot be determined.

6. The best point estimate of the population mean is

   a. The sample mean.
   b. The sample median.
   c. The sample mode.
   d. The sample midrange.

7. In a normally distributed population with unknown standard deviation and a sample size less than 30, what table value should be used in computing a confidence interval for a mean?

   a. z
   b. t
   c. χ^2
   d. None of the above

Complete the following statements with the best answer.

8. A good estimator should be _____, _____, and _____.

9. The maximum difference between the point estimate of a parameter and the actual value of the parameter is called _____.

10. The statement "The average height of an adult male is 178 centimetres" is an example of a(n) _____ estimate.

11. The three confidence intervals used most often are the _____%, _____%, and _____%.

12. **Shopping Survey** A random sample of 49 shoppers showed that they spent an average of $23.45 per visit at the Saturday Mornings Bookstore. The standard deviation of the sample was $2.80. Find a point estimate of the population mean. Find the 90% confidence interval of the true mean.

13. **Dentist's Fees** A random selection of 20 dental patients found that the mean amount of money they spent each year on visits to the dentist was $364.40. The standard deviation of the sample was $49.98. Find a point estimate of the population mean. Find the 95% confidence interval of the population mean. Assume the variable is normally distributed.
   Source: Canadian Dental Association, *Dental Statistics*.

14. **Weight of Minivans** The average weight of 40 randomly selected minivans is 1882 kilograms. Assume the variable is normally distributed and the population standard deviation is 218 kilograms. Find the best point estimate of the population mean. Find the 99% confidence interval of the true mean weight of the minivans.

15. **Insurance Representatives' Ages** In a study of 10 insurance sales representatives from a certain large city, the average age of the group was 48.6 years and the standard deviation was 4.1 years. Assume the variable is normally distributed. Find the 95% confidence interval of the population mean age of all insurance sales representatives in that city.

16. **Hospital Emergency Room Patients** In a hospital, a sample of 8 weeks was selected, and it was found that an average of 438 patients were treated in the emergency room each week. The standard deviation was 16. Find the 99% confidence interval of the true mean. Assume the variable is normally distributed.

17. **Burglaries** For a certain urban area, it was found that in a sample of 4 months, an average of 31 burglaries occurred each month. The standard deviation was 4. Assume the variable is normally distributed. Find the 90% confidence interval of the true mean number of burglaries each month.

18. **Hours Spent Studying** A university dean wants to estimate the average number of hours that freshmen study

each week. The standard deviation from a previous study is 2.6 hours. How large a sample must be selected if he wants to be 99% confident of finding whether the true mean differs from the sample mean by 0.5 hour?

19. **Money Spent on Road Repairs** A researcher wishes to estimate within $300 the true average amount of money a county spends on road repairs each year. If she wants to be 90% confident, how large a sample is necessary? The standard deviation is known to be $900.

20. **Bus Ridership** A study of 75 workers found that 53 people rode the bus to work each day. Find the 95% confidence interval of the proportion of all workers who rode the bus to work.

21. **Children's Serious Accidents** In a study of 150 accidents that required treatment in an emergency room, 36% involved children under 6 years of age. Find the 90% confidence interval of the true proportion of accidents that involve children under the age of 6.

22. **HDTV Ownership** A survey of 90 families showed that 41 owned at least one high-definition television (HDTV). Find the 95% confidence interval of the true proportion of families who own at least one HDTV.

23. **Skipping Lunch** A nutritionist wants to determine, within 3%, the true proportion of adults who do not eat any lunch. If he wishes to be 95% confident that his estimate contains the population proportion, how large a sample will be necessary? A previous study found that 15% of the 125 people surveyed said they did not eat lunch.

24. **Novel Pages** A sample of 25 novels has a standard deviation of 9 pages. Find the 95% confidence interval of the population standard deviation. Assume a normally distributed variable.

25. **Import Car Safety Inspection** Before licensing, a car imported from the United States to Canada requires a safety inspection. Find the 90% confidence interval for the variance and standard deviation for the time it takes for a safety inspection if a sample of 27 imported vehicles has a standard deviation of 6.8 minutes. Assume the variable is normally distributed.

26. **Automobile Pollution** A sample of 20 automobiles has a pollution by-product release standard deviation of 15 mL when 1 litre of gasoline is used. Find the 90% confidence interval of the population standard deviation. Assume a normally distributed variable.

Critical Thinking Challenges »

A confidence interval for a median can be found by using these formulas

$$U = \frac{n + 1}{2} + \frac{z_{\alpha/2}\sqrt{n}}{2} \quad \text{(round up)}$$

$$L = n - U + 1$$

to define positions in the set of ordered data values.

Suppose a data set has 30 values, and one wants to find the 95% confidence interval for the median. Substituting in the formulas, one gets

$$U = \frac{30 + 1}{2} + \frac{1.96\sqrt{30}}{2} = 21 \quad \text{(rounded up)}$$

$$L = 30 - 21 + 1 = 10$$

when $n = 30$ and $z_{\alpha/2} = 1.96$.

Arrange the data in order from smallest to largest, and then select the 10th and 21st values of the data array; hence, $X_{10} <$ median $< X_{21}$.

Find the 90% confidence interval for the median for the given data.

84	49	3	133	85	4340	461	60	28	97
14	252	18	16	24	346	254	29	254	6
31	104	72	29	391	19	125	10	6	17
72	31	23	225	72	5	61	366	77	8
26	8	55	138	158	846	123	47	21	82

Data Projects »

Where appropriate use Minitab, SPSS, TI-83 Plus, TI-84 Plus, Excel or a computer program of your choice to complete these exercises.

1. **Business and Finance** Use 30 Dow Jones industrial stocks as the sample. Note the amount each stock has gained or lost in the last quarter. Compute the mean and standard deviation for the data set. Compute the 95%

confidence interval for the mean and the 95% confidence interval for the standard deviation. Compute the percentage of stocks that had a gain in the last quarter. Find a 95% confidence interval for the percentage of stocks with a gain.

2. **Sports and Leisure** Use the top home run hitter from each major league baseball team as the data set. Find the

mean and the standard deviation for the number of home runs hit by the top hitter on each team. Find a 95% confidence interval for the mean number of home runs hit.

3. **Technology** Use the data collected in Data Project 3 of Chapter 2 regarding song lengths. Select a specific genre and compute the percentage of songs in the sample that are of that genre. Create a 95% confidence interval for the true percentage. Use the entire music library and find the population percentage of the library with that genre. Does the population percentage fall within the confidence interval?

4. **Health and Wellness** Use your class as the sample. Have each student take her or his temperature on a healthy day. Compute the mean and standard deviation for the sample. Create a 95% confidence interval for the mean temperature. Does the confidence interval

obtained support the long-held belief that the average body temperature is 37.0°C?

5. **Politics and Economics** Select five recent political polls and note the margin of error, sample size, and percentage favouring each federal political party. For each poll, determine the level of confidence that must have been used to obtain the margin of error given. Does a trend emerge?

6. **Your Class** Have each student compute his or her body mass index (BMI) [weight (kg)/height (m)^2]. For example, an adult who weighs 70 kg and whose height is 1.75 m will have a BMI of 22.9 kg/m^2. Find the mean and standard deviation for the data set. Compute a 95% confidence interval for the mean BMI of a student. A BMI score over 30 is considered obese. Does the confidence interval indicate that the mean for BMI could be in the obese range?

Answers to Applying the Concepts »

Section 7–1 Making Decisions with Confidence Intervals

1. Answers will vary. One possible answer is to find out the average number of Kleenexes that a group of randomly selected individuals uses in a 2-week period.

2. People usually need Kleenexes when they have a cold or when their allergies are acting up.

3. If we want to concentrate on the number of Kleenexes used when people have colds, we select a random sample of people with colds and have them keep a record of how many Kleenexes they use during their colds.

4. Answers may vary. I will use a 95% confidence interval:

$$\overline{X} \pm 1.96\frac{s}{\sqrt{n}} = 57 \pm 1.96\frac{15}{\sqrt{85}} = 57 \pm 3.2$$

I am 95% confident that the interval 53.8–60.2 contains the true mean number of Kleenexes used by people when they have colds. It seems reasonable to put 60 Kleenexes in the new automobile glove compartment boxes.

5. Answers will vary. Since I am 95% confident that the interval contains the true average, any number of Kleenexes between 54 and 60 would be reasonable. Sixty seemed to be the most reasonable answer, since it is close to 2 standard deviations above the sample mean.

Section 7–2 Sports Drink Decision

1. Answers will vary. One possible answer is that this is a small sample since we are looking at only seven popular sports drinks.

2. The mean cost per container is $1.25, with standard deviation of $0.39. The 90% confidence interval is

$$\overline{X} \pm t_{\alpha/2}\frac{s}{\sqrt{n}} = 1.25 \pm 1.943\frac{0.39}{\sqrt{7}} = 1.25 \pm 0.29$$

or $0.96 < \mu < 1.54$.

The 10-K, All Sport, Exceed, and Hydra Fuel all fall outside of the confidence interval.

3. None of the values appear to be outliers.

4. There are $7 - 1 = 6$ degrees of freedom.

5. Cost per serving would impact my decision on purchasing a sports drink, since this would allow me to compare the costs on an equal scale.

6. Answers will vary.

Section 7–3 Contracting Influenza

1. (95% CI) means that these are the 95% confidence intervals constructed from the data.

2. The margin of error for men reporting influenza is $\frac{50.5 - 47.1}{2} = 1.7\%$

3. The total sample size was 19,774.

4. The larger the sample size, the smaller the margin of error (all other things being held constant).

5. A 90% confidence interval would be narrower (smaller) than a 95% confidence interval, since we need to include fewer values in the interval.

6. The 51.5% is the middle of the confidence interval, since it is the point estimate for the confidence interval.

Section 7–4 Confidence Interval for Standard Deviation

1. The data represent a population, since we have the ages at death for all deceased Canadian prime ministers (at the time of the writing of this book).

2. Answers will vary. One possible sample is 76, 75, 91, 82, 80, 49, 77, which results in a standard deviation of 12.96 years and a variance of 167.9.

3. Answers will vary. The 95% confidence interval for the standard deviation is $\sqrt{\frac{(n-1)s^2}{\chi^2_{\text{right}}}}$ to $\sqrt{\frac{(n-1)s^2}{\chi^2_{\text{left}}}}$. In this case, we have $\sqrt{\frac{(7-1)\cdot(12.96)^2}{14.449}} = \sqrt{69.747} = 8.4$ to $\sqrt{\frac{(7-1)\cdot(12.96)^2}{1.237}} = \sqrt{814.688} = 28.5$ or 8.4 to 28.5 years.

4. The standard deviation for all the data values is 11.1 years.

5. Answers will vary. Yes, the confidence interval does contain the population standard deviation.

6. Answers will vary.

7. We need to assume that the distribution of ages at death is normal.

|Chapter 8

Hypothesis Testing

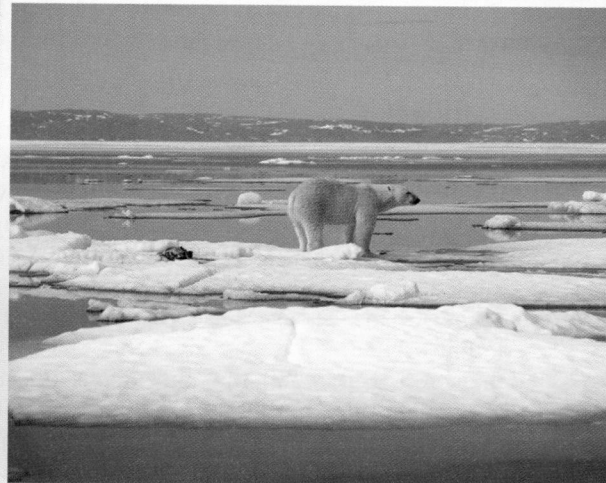

connect™ Practise and learn online with *Connect* with data sets and algorithmic questions related to concepts covered in this chapter. Throughout this chapter, questions and tables with online data sets are marked with ↗.

Statistics Today

How Much Better Is Better?

Suppose a provincial minister of Education reviews test results of the Program for International Student Assessment (PISA), a project of the Organisation for Economic Co-operation and Development (OECD). The OECD average from all countries taking the PISA test was 500. Furthermore, assume a sample of students writing the PISA test in the minister's province scored, on average, 530. Can the provincial minister conclude that the students in his province scored higher than the average? At first glance, you might be inclined to say yes, since 530 is higher than 500. But recall that the means of samples vary about the population mean when samples are selected from a specific population. So the question arises, Is there a real difference in the means, or is the difference simply due to chance (i.e., sampling error)? In this chapter, you will learn how to answer that question by using statistics that explain hypothesis testing. See Statistics Today—Revisited, page 401, for the answer. In this chapter, you will learn how to answer many questions of this type by using statistics that are explained in the theory of hypothesis testing.

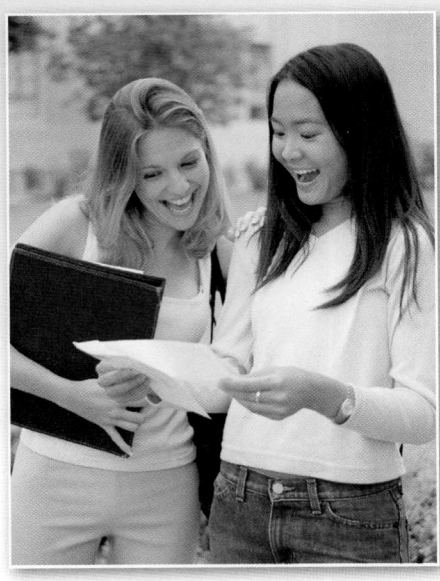

Source: Human Resources and Skills Development Canada/ Council of Ministers of Education, Canada, *Measuring Up: Canadian Results of the OECD PISA Study.*

Introduction >

Researchers are interested in answering many types of questions. For example, a scientist might want to know whether the earth is warming up. A physician might want to know whether a new medication will lower a person's blood pressure. An educator might wish to see whether a new teaching technique is better than a traditional one. A retail merchant might want to know whether the public prefers a certain colour in a new line of fashion. Automobile manufacturers are interested in determining whether seat belts will reduce the severity of injuries caused by accidents. These types of questions can be addressed through statistical **hypothesis testing,** which is a decision-making process for evaluating claims about a population. In hypothesis testing, the researcher must define the population under study, state the particular hypotheses that will be investigated, assign an acceptable error level, select a sample from the population, collect the data, perform the calculations required for the statistical test, and reach a conclusion.

Hypotheses concerning parameters such as means and proportions can be investigated. Two specific statistical tests are used for hypotheses concerning means: the *z test* and the *t test*. This chapter will explain in detail the hypothesis-testing procedure along with the *z* test and the *t* test. In addition, a hypothesis-testing procedure for testing a single variance or standard deviation using the chi-square distribution is explained in Section 8–5.

The three methods used to test hypotheses are

1. The traditional method
2. The *P*-value method
3. The confidence interval method

The *traditional method* will be explained first. It has been used since the hypothesis-testing method was formulated. A newer method, called the *P-value method,* has become popular with the advent of modern computers and high-powered statistical calculators. It will be explained at the end of Section 8–2. The third method, the *confidence interval method,* is explained in Section 8–6 and illustrates the relationship between hypothesis testing and confidence intervals.

8–1 Steps in Hypothesis Testing—Traditional Method >

Understand hypothesis-testing concepts, terminology, and procedures.

Every hypothesis-testing situation begins with the statement of a hypothesis.

A **statistical hypothesis** is a conjecture about a population parameter. This conjecture may or may not be true.

There are two types of statistical hypotheses for each situation: the null hypothesis and the alternative hypothesis.

The **null hypothesis,** symbolized by H_0, is a statistical hypothesis that states that a parameter is equal to a specific value, or that there is no difference between two parameters.

The **alternative hypothesis,** symbolized by H_1, is a statistical hypothesis that states a parameter is either less than, not equal to, or greater than a specific value, or states that there is a difference between two parameters.

(*Note:* Although the definitions of null and alternative hypotheses given here use the word *parameter,* these definitions can be extended to include other terms such as *distributions* and *randomness.* This is explained in later chapters.)

As an illustration of how hypotheses should be stated, three different statistical studies will be used as examples.

Situation A A medical researcher is interested in finding out whether a new medication will have any undesirable side effects. The researcher is particularly concerned with the pulse rate of the patients who take the medication. Will the pulse rate increase, decrease, or remain unchanged after a patient takes the medication?

Since the researcher knows that the mean pulse rate for the population under study is 82 beats per minute, the hypotheses for this situation are

$$H_0: \mu = 82 \quad \text{and} \quad H_1: \mu \neq 82$$

The null hypothesis specifies that the mean will remain unchanged, and the alternative hypothesis states that it will be different. This test is called a *two-tailed test* (a term that will be formally defined later in this section), since the possible side effects of the medicine could be to raise or lower the pulse rate.

Situation B A chemist invents an additive to increase the life of an automobile battery. If the mean lifetime of the automobile battery without the additive is 36 months, then her hypotheses are

$$H_0: \mu = 36 \quad \text{and} \quad H_1: \mu > 36$$

In this situation, the chemist is interested only in increasing the lifetime of the batteries, so her alternative hypothesis is that the mean is greater than 36 months. The null hypothesis is that the mean is less than or equal to 36 months. This test is called *right-tailed,* since the interest is in an increase only.

Situation C A contractor wishes to lower heating bills by using a special type of insulation in houses. If the average of the monthly heating bills is $78, her hypotheses about heating costs with the use of insulation are

$$H_0\colon \mu = \$78 \quad \text{and} \quad H_1\colon \mu < \$78$$

This test is a *left-tailed test,* since the contractor is interested only in lowering heating costs.

To state hypotheses correctly, researchers must translate the *conjecture* or *claim* from words into mathematical symbols. The basic symbols used are as follows:

Equal to	$=$	Not equal to	$\neq$
Less than	$<$	Greater than	$>$

The null and alternative hypotheses are stated together, and the null hypothesis contains the equals sign, as shown (where k represents a specified number).

Two-tailed test	Right-tailed test	Left-tailed test
$H_0\colon \mu = k$	$H_0\colon \mu = k$	$H_0\colon \mu = k$
$H_1\colon \mu \neq k$	$H_1\colon \mu > k$	$H_1\colon \mu < k$

The formal definitions of the different types of tests are given later in this section.

This text will follow the convention of displaying the null hypothesis, H_0, with an equals sign. This method is consistent with most professional journals. When the null hypothesis is tested, the assumption is that the mean, proportion, or standard deviation is equal to a given specific value. Also, when a researcher conducts a study, he or she is generally looking for evidence to support a claim. Therefore, the claim is most often stated as the alternative hypothesis; that is the claim H_1 may be $<$ or $\neq$ or $>$. Because of this, the alternative hypothesis is sometimes referred to as the **research hypothesis.**

A claim, though, can be stated as either the null hypothesis or the alternative hypothesis; however, the statistical evidence can support the claim only if it is the alternative hypothesis. It is uncommon to see new research studies use $\leq$ or $=$ or $\geq$, even when H_0 is the claim. Statistical evidence can be used to reject the claim if the claim is the null hypothesis. These facts are important when you are stating the conclusion of a statistical study.

| Example 8–1 | State the null and alternative hypotheses for each conjecture. |

a. A researcher thinks that if expectant mothers use vitamin pills, the birth weight of the babies will increase. The average birth weight of the population is 3.9 kilograms.

b. An engineer hypothesizes that the mean number of defects can be decreased in a manufacturing process of compact discs by using robots instead of humans for certain tasks. The mean number of defective discs per 1000 is 18.

c. A psychologist feels that playing soft music during a test will change the results of the test. The psychologist is not sure whether the grades will be higher or lower. In the past, the mean of the scores was 73.

Solution

a. $H_0\colon \mu = 3.9$ and $H_1\colon \mu > 3.9$

b. $H_0\colon \mu = 18$ and $H_1\colon \mu < 18$

c. $H_0\colon \mu = 73$ and $H_1\colon \mu \neq 73$

After stating the hypothesis, the researcher designs the study. The researcher selects the correct *statistical test,* chooses an appropriate *level of significance,* and formulates a plan for conducting the study. In situation A, for instance, the researcher will select a sample of patients who will be given the drug. After allowing a suitable time for the drug to be absorbed, the researcher will measure each person's pulse rate.

Recall that when samples of a specific size are selected from a population, the means of these samples will vary about the population mean, and the distribution of the sample means will be approximately normal when the sample size is 30 or more. (See Section 6–4.) So even if the null hypothesis is true, the mean of the pulse rates of the sample of patients will not, in most cases, be exactly equal to the population mean of 82 beats per minute. There are two possibilities. Either the null hypothesis is true and the difference between the sample mean and the population mean is due to chance, *or* the null hypothesis is false and the sample came from a population whose mean is not 82 beats per minute but is some other value that is not known. These situations are shown in Figure 8–1.

The farther away the sample mean is from the population mean, the more evidence there would be for rejecting the null hypothesis. The probability that the sample came from a population whose mean is 82 decreases as the distance between the means increases.

If the mean pulse rate of the sample was, say, 83, the researcher would probably conclude that this difference was due to chance and would not reject the null hypothesis. But if the sample mean was, say, 90, then in all likelihood the researcher would conclude that the medication increased the pulse rate of the users and would reject the null hypothesis. The question is: Where does the researcher draw the line? This decision is not made on feelings or intuition; it is made statistically. That is, the difference must be significant and in all likelihood not due to chance. Statistical tests and significance levels are essential to credible decision making.

A **statistical test** uses the data obtained from a sample to make a decision about whether the null hypothesis should be rejected.

The numerical value calculated from the sample data in a statistical test is called the **test statistic.**

Figure 8–1

Situations in Hypothesis Testing

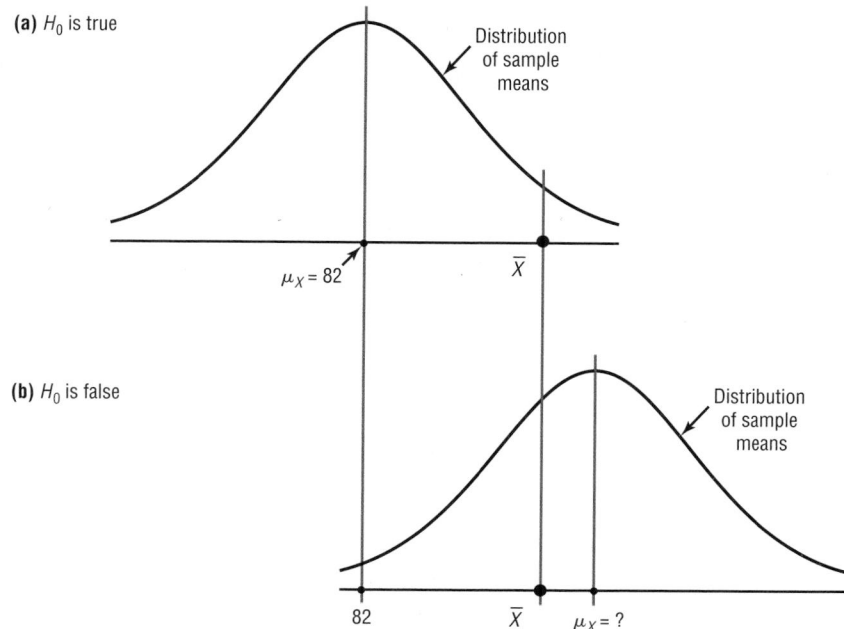

(a) H_0 is true

Distribution of sample means

$\mu_{\overline{X}} = 82$ $\overline{X}$

(b) H_0 is false

Distribution of sample means

82    $\overline{X}$ $\mu_{\overline{X}} = ?$

In this type of statistical test, the mean is computed for the data obtained from the sample and is compared with the population mean. Then a decision is made to reject or not reject the null hypothesis on the basis of the value obtained from the statistical test. If the difference is significant, the null hypothesis is rejected. If it is not, then the null hypothesis is not rejected.

In the hypothesis-testing situation, there are four possible outcomes. In reality, the null hypothesis may or may not be true, and a decision is made to reject or not reject it on the basis of the data obtained from a sample. The four possible outcomes are shown in Figure 8–2. Notice that there are two possibilities for a correct decision and two possibilities for an incorrect decision.

Figure 8–2

Possible Outcomes of a Hypothesis Test

	H_0 true	H_0 false
Reject H_0	**Error** Type I	Correct decision
Do not reject H_0	Correct decision	**Error** Type II

If a null hypothesis is true and it is rejected, then a *type I error* is made. In situation A, for instance, the medication might not significantly change the pulse rate of all the users in the population, but it might change the rate, by chance, of the subjects in the sample. In this case, the researcher will reject the null hypothesis when it is really true, thus committing a type I error.

On the other hand, the medication might not change the pulse rate of the subjects in the sample, but when it is given to the general population, it might cause a significant increase or decrease in the pulse rate of users. The researcher, on the basis of the data obtained from the sample, will not reject the null hypothesis, thus committing a *type II error.*

In situation B, the additive might not significantly increase the lifetimes of automobile batteries in the population, but it might increase the lifetimes of the batteries in the sample. In this case, the null hypothesis would be rejected when it was really true. This would be a type I error. On the other hand, the additive might not work on the batteries selected for the sample, but if it was to be used in the general population of batteries, it might significantly increase their lifetimes. The researcher, on the basis of information obtained from the sample, would not reject the null hypothesis, thus committing a type II error.

A **type I error** occurs if one rejects the null hypothesis when it is true.

A **type II error** occurs if one does not reject the null hypothesis when it is false.

The hypothesis-testing situation can be compared to a jury trial. In a jury trial, there are four possible outcomes. The defendant is either guilty or innocent, and he or she will be convicted or acquitted. See Figure 8–3.

Now the hypotheses are

H_0: The defendant is innocent

H_1: The defendant is not innocent (i.e., guilty)

Figure 8–3

Hypothesis Testing and a Jury Trial

H_0: The defendant is innocent.
H_1: The defendant is not innocent.

The results of a trial can be shown as follows:

	H_0 true (innocent)	H_0 false (not innocent)
Reject H_0 (convict)	1. Type I error	2. Correct decision
Do not reject H_0 (acquit)	3. Correct decision	4. Type II error

Next, the evidence is presented in court by the prosecutor, and based on this evidence, the jury decides the verdict, innocent or guilty.

If the defendant is convicted but he or she did not commit the crime, then a type I error has been committed. See block 1 of Figure 8–3. On the other hand, if the defendant is convicted and he or she has committed the crime, then a correct decision has been made. See block 2.

If the defendant is acquitted and he or she did not commit the crime, a correct decision has been made by the jury. See block 3. However, if the defendant is acquitted and he or she did commit the crime, then a type II error has been made. See block 4.

The decision of the jury does not prove that the defendant did or did not commit the crime. The decision is based on the evidence presented. If the evidence is strong enough, the defendant will be convicted in most cases. If the evidence is weak, the defendant will be acquitted in most cases. Nothing is proved absolutely. Likewise, the decision to reject or not reject the null hypothesis does not prove anything. *The only way to prove anything statistically is to use the entire population,* which, in most cases, is not possible. The decision, then, is made on the basis of probabilities. That is, when there is a large difference between the mean obtained from the sample and the hypothesized mean, the null hypothesis is probably not true. The question is: How large a difference is necessary to reject the null hypothesis? Here is where the level of significance is used.

Unusual Stat

The average Canadian adult watches over 25,000 TV commercials annually.

The **level of significance** is the maximum probability of committing a type I error. This probability is symbolized by α (Greek letter **alpha**). That is, P (type I error) $= \alpha$.

The probability of a type II error is symbolized by β, the Greek letter **beta.** That is, P (type II error) $= \beta$. In most hypothesis-testing situations, β cannot easily be computed; however, α and β are related in that decreasing one increases the other. The probability of rejecting a false null hypothesis, that is making a correct decision, is referred to as the **power of a test.** Refer to Section 8–6 for further discussion of the relationship between type I and type II errors and the power of a test.

Statisticians generally agree on using three arbitrary significance levels: the 0.10, 0.05, and 0.01 levels. That is, if the null hypothesis is rejected, the probability of a type I error will be 10, 5, or 1%, depending on which level of significance is used. Here is another way of putting it: When $\alpha = 0.10$, there is a 10% chance of rejecting a true null hypothesis; when $\alpha = 0.05$, there is a 5% chance of rejecting a true null hypothesis; and when $\alpha = 0.01$, there is a 1% chance of rejecting a true null hypothesis.

In a hypothesis-testing situation, the researcher decides what level of significance to use. It does not have to be the 0.10, 0.05, or 0.01 level. It can be any level, depending on the seriousness of the type I error. After a significance level is chosen, a *critical value* is selected from a table for the appropriate test. If a z test is used, for example, the z tables (Tables E–1 and E–2 in Appendix C) are consulted to find the critical value. The critical value determines the critical and noncritical regions. The symbol C.V. or CV may be used for critical value.

> The **critical value** separates the critical region from the noncritical region.
>
> The **critical** or **rejection region** is the range of values of the test statistic that indicates that there is a significant difference and that the null hypothesis should be rejected.
>
> The **noncritical or nonrejection region** is the range of values of the test statistic that indicates that the difference was probably due to chance and that the null hypothesis should not be rejected.

The critical value can be on the right side of the mean or on the left side of the mean for a *one-tailed test*. Its location depends on the inequality sign of the alternative hypothesis. For example, in situation B, where the chemist is interested in increasing the average lifetime of automobile batteries, the alternative hypothesis is H_1: $\mu > 36$. Since the inequality sign is $>$, the null hypothesis will be rejected only when the sample mean is significantly greater than 36. Hence, the critical value must be on the right side of the mean. Therefore, this test is called a *right-tailed test*.

> A **one-tailed test** indicates that the null hypothesis should be rejected when the test statistic is in the critical region on one side of the mean. A one-tailed test is either a **right-tailed test** or **left-tailed test,** depending on the direction of the inequality of the alternative hypothesis.

To obtain the critical value, the researcher must choose an alpha level. In situation B, suppose the researcher chose $\alpha = 0.01$. Then the researcher must find a z score such that 1% of the area falls to the right of the z score and 99% falls to the left of the z score, as shown in Figure 8–4(a).

Next, the researcher must find the value in Table E–2 closest to 0.9900 (0.9901), which corresponds to a z score of 2.33. Therefore the critical z value is 2.33 as shown in Figure 8–4(b).

The critical and noncritical regions and the critical value are shown in Figure 8–5.

Figure 8–4

Finding the Critical Value for $\alpha = 0.01$ (Right-Tailed Test)

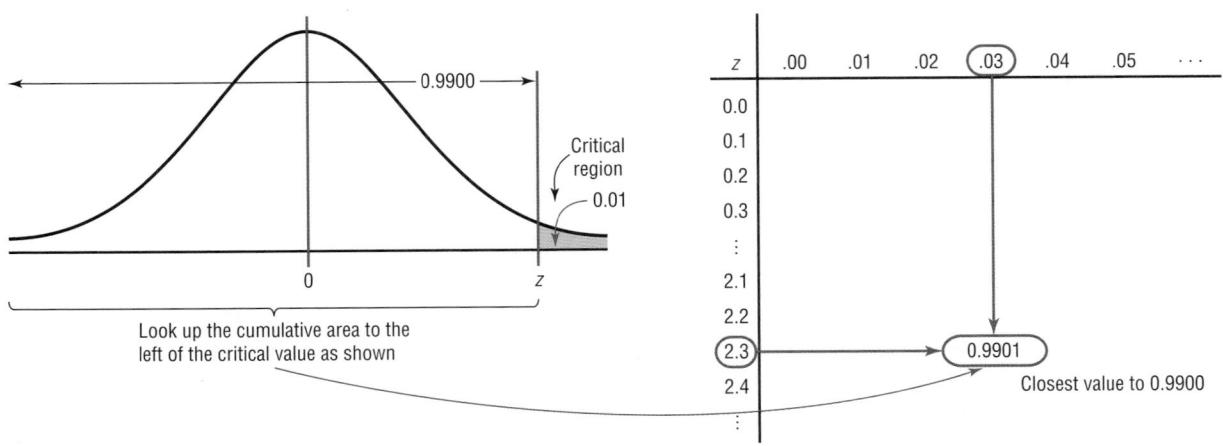

(a) The critical region

(b) The critical value from Table E–2

Figure 8–5

Critical and Noncritical Regions for $\alpha = 0.01$ (Right-Tailed Test)

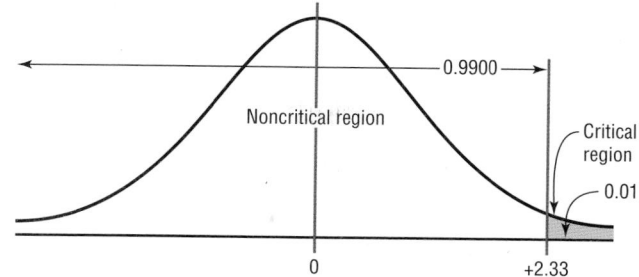

Now, move on to situation C, where the contractor is interested in lowering the heating bills. The alternative hypothesis is H_1: $\mu < \$78$. Hence, the critical value falls to the left of the mean. This test is thus a left-tailed test. At $\alpha = 0.01$, the critical value is -2.33, as shown in Figure 8–6. Refer to Table E–1 in Appendix C.

Figure 8–6

Critical and Noncritical Regions for $\alpha = 0.01$ (Left-Tailed Test)

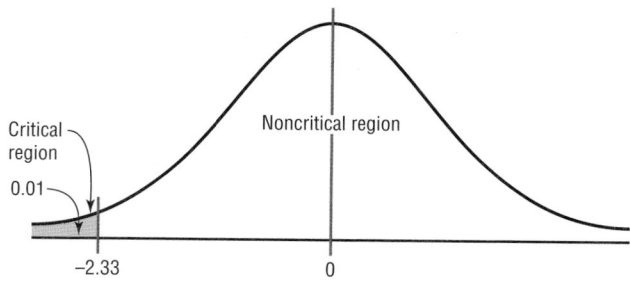

When a researcher conducts a two-tailed test, as in situation A, the null hypothesis can be rejected when there is a significant difference in either direction, above or below the mean.

In a **two-tailed test,** the null hypothesis should be rejected when the test statistic is in either of the two critical regions.

For a two-tailed test, then, the critical region must be split into two equal parts. If $\alpha = 0.01$, then one-half of the area, or $\alpha/2 = 0.005$, must be to the right of the mean and one-half must be to the left of the mean, as shown in Figure 8–7.

In this case, the area to be found in Table E–1 is 0.0050 (area in left tail is 0.005) with a critical z value of -2.575. The cumulative area to the left in Table E–2 is 0.9950 (area in right tail is 0.005) with a critical z value of $+2.575$, as shown in Figure 8–8.

Figure 8–7

Finding the Critical Values for $\alpha = 0.01$ (Two-Tailed Test)

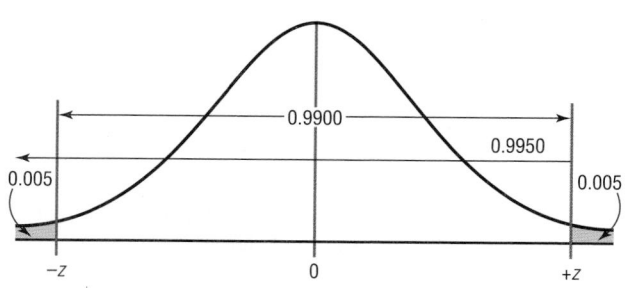

Figure 8–8

Critical and Noncritical Regions for $\alpha = 0.01$ (Two-Tailed Test)

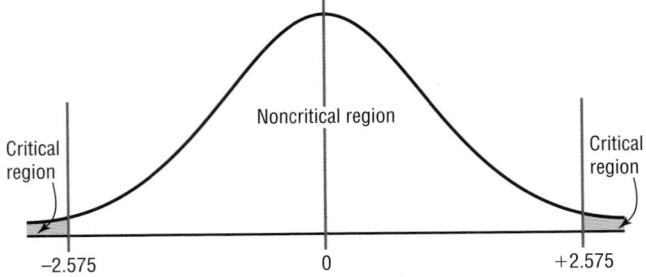

A similar procedure is used for other values of α.

Figure 8–9 with rejection regions shaded shows the critical value for the three situations discussed in this section for values of $\alpha = 0.10$, $\alpha = 0.05$, and $\alpha = 0.01$. The procedure for finding critical values is outlined in the Procedure Table (where k is a specified number).

Figure 8–9

Summary of Hypothesis Testing and Critical Values

α	Critical Value
0.10	−1.28
0.05	−1.645
0.01	−2.33

$H_0: \mu = k$
$H_1: \mu < k$

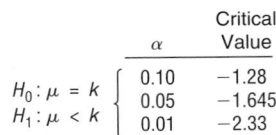

(a) Left-tailed

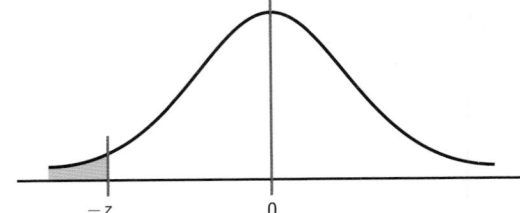

α	Critical Value
0.10	1.28
0.05	1.645
0.01	2.33

$H_0: \mu = k$
$H_1: \mu > k$

(b) Right-tailed

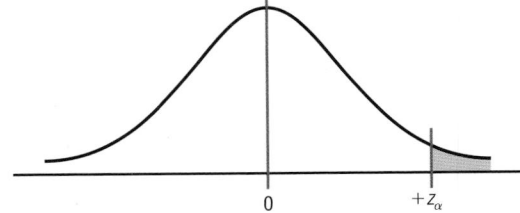

α	$\alpha/2$	Critical Value
0.10	0.05	±1.645
0.05	0.025	±1.96
0.01	0.005	±2.575

$H_0: \mu = k$
$H_1: \mu \neq k$

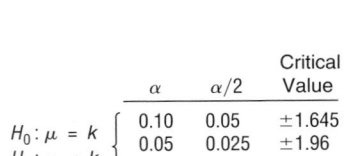

(c) Two-tailed

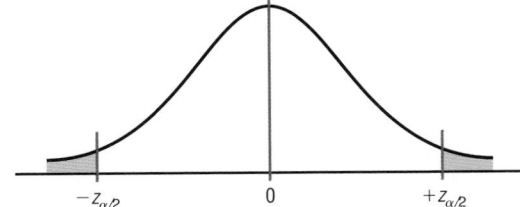

Procedure Table

Finding the Critical Values for Specific α Values, Using Tables E–1 and E–2

Step 1   Draw the figure and indicate the appropriate area.

    a.   If the test is left-tailed, the critical region, with an area equal to *a*, will be on the left side of the mean.

    b.   If the test is right-tailed, the critical region, with an area equal to *a*, will be on the right side of the mean.

> c. If the test is two-tailed, α must be divided by 2; one-half of the area will be to the right of the mean, and one-half will be to the left of the mean.
>
> **Step 2** a. For a left-tailed test, look up the area (equivalent to α) in Table E–1, Negative z Scores.
>
> b. For a right-tailed test, look up the area (equivalent to $1 - \alpha$) in Table E–2, Positive z Scores.
>
> c. For a two-tailed test, look up the area (equivalent to $\alpha/2$) in Table E–1, Negative z Scores, and look up the area (equivalent to $1 - \alpha/2$) in Table E–2, Positive z Scores.
>
> **Step 3** Find the z score that corresponds to the area. This will be the critical value.

Example 8–2

Using Tables E–1 and E–2 in Appendix C, find the critical value(s) for each situation and draw the appropriate figure, showing the critical region.

a. A left-tailed test with $\alpha = 0.10$.

b. A two-tailed test with $\alpha = 0.02$.

c. A right-tailed test with $\alpha = 0.005$.

Solution *a*

Step 1 Draw the figure and indicate the appropriate area. Since this is a left-tailed test, the area of 0.10 is located in the left tail, as shown in Figure 8–10.

Step 2 Look up the area closest to 0.1000 in Table E–1; in this case, 0.1003.

Step 3 Find the z score that corresponds to this area. The z score for 0.1003 is -1.28. Hence, the critical value is -1.28 on the left-tail. See Figure 8–10.

Figure 8–10

Critical Value and Critical Region for Part *a* of Example 8–2

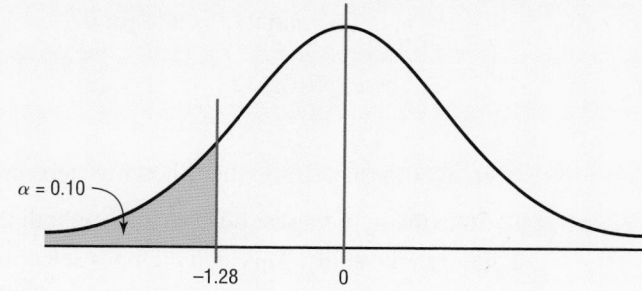

$\alpha = 0.10$

$-1.28 \qquad 0$

Solution *b*

Step 1 Draw the figure and indicate the appropriate area. In this case, there are two areas equivalent to $\alpha/2$, or $0.02/2 = 0.01$.

Step 2 For the left tail, look up the area closest to 0.0100 in Table E–1; in this case, 0.0099. For the right tail, look up the area closest to 0.9900 ($1 - 0.01$) in Table E–2; in this case, 0.9901.

Step 3 Find the z scores that correspond to each area. The z score for 0.0099 is -2.33 and the z score for 0.9901 is $+2.33$. Hence, the two critical values are -2.33 on the left-tail and $+2.33$ on the right-tail. See Figure 8–11.

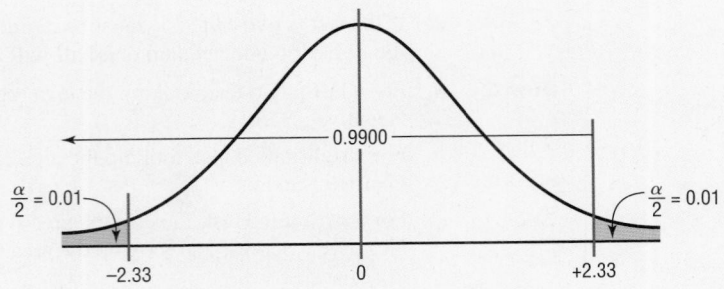

Solution c

Step 1 Draw the figure and indicate the appropriate area. Since this is a right-tailed test, the area 0.005 is located in the right tail, as shown in Figure 8–12.

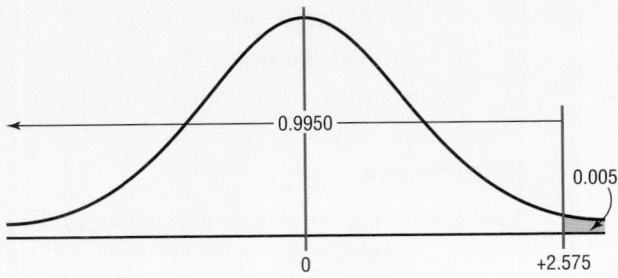

Step 2 Look up the area closest to 0.9950 $(1 - 0.005)$ in Table E–2; in this case, equal distance to 0.9949 and 0.9951.

Step 3 Find the z score that corresponds to each area. The z score for 0.9949 is $+2.57$ and the z score for 0.9951 is $+2.58$. The average of the two z scores is $+2.575$. Hence, the critical value is $+2.575$ on the right-tail. See Figure 8–12.

In hypothesis testing, the following steps are recommended.

1. State the hypotheses. Be sure to state both the null and the alternative hypotheses.
2. Design the study. This step includes selecting the correct statistical test, choosing a level of significance, and formulating a plan to carry out the study. The plan should include information such as the definition of the population, the way the sample will be selected, and the methods that will be used to collect the data.
3. Conduct the study and collect the data.
4. Evaluate the data. The data should be tabulated in this step, and the statistical test should be conducted. Finally, decide whether to reject or not reject the null hypothesis.
5. Summarize the results.

For the purposes of this chapter, a simplified version of the hypothesis-testing procedure will be used, since designing the study and collecting the data will be omitted. The steps are summarized in the following Procedure Table.

Procedure Table

Solving Hypothesis-Testing Problems (Traditional Method)

Step 1   State the hypotheses and identify the claim.

Step 2   Find the critical value(s) from the appropriate table in Appendix C.

Step 3   Compute the test statistic.

Step 4   Make the decision to reject or not reject the null hypothesis.

Step 5   Summarize the results.

8–1   Applying the Concepts

Eggs and Your Health

The Incredible Edible Egg company recently found that eating eggs does not increase a person's blood serum cholesterol. Five hundred subjects participated in a study that lasted for two years. The participants were randomly assigned to either a no-egg group or a moderate-egg group. The blood serum cholesterol levels were checked at the beginning and at the end of the study. Overall, the groups' levels were not significantly different. The company reminds us that eating eggs is healthy if done in moderation. Many of the previous studies relating eggs and high blood serum cholesterol jumped to improper conclusions.

Using this information, answer these questions.

1. What prompted the study?
2. What is the population under study?
3. Was a sample collected?
4. What was the hypothesis?
5. Were data collected?
6. Were any statistical tests run?
7. What was the conclusion?

See page 404 for the answers.

Exercises 8–1

1. Define *null* and *alternative hypotheses,* and give an example of each.

2. What is meant by a type I error? A type II error? How are they related?

3. What is meant by a statistical test?

4. Explain the difference between a one-tailed and a two-tailed test.

5. What is meant by the critical region? The noncritical region?

6. What symbols are used to represent the null hypothesis and the alternative hypothesis?

7. What symbols are used to represent the probabilities of type I and type II errors?

8. Explain what is meant by a significant difference.

9. When should a one-tailed test be used? A two-tailed test?

10. List the steps in hypothesis testing.

11. In hypothesis testing, why can't the hypothesis be proved true?

12. (ans) Using the z tables (Tables E–1 and E–2), find the critical value (or values) for each.

a. $\alpha = 0.05$, two-tailed test
b. $\alpha = 0.01$, left-tailed test
c. $\alpha = 0.005$, right-tailed test
d. $\alpha = 0.01$, right-tailed test
e. $\alpha = 0.05$, left-tailed test
f. $\alpha = 0.02$, left-tailed test
g. $\alpha = 0.05$, right-tailed test
h. $\alpha = 0.01$, two-tailed test
i. $\alpha = 0.04$, left-tailed test
j. $\alpha = 0.02$, right-tailed test

13. For each conjecture, state the null and alternative hypotheses:

a. The average age of college students is 24.6 years.
b. The average income of accountants is $51,497.
c. The average age of attorneys is greater than 25.4 years.
d. The average score of 50 high school basketball games is less than 88.
e. The average pulse rate of male marathon runners is less than 70 beats per minute.
f. The average cost in Canada to raise a child from birth to one year old is $10,000.
g. The average weight loss for a sample of people who exercise 30 minutes per day for 6 weeks is 3.7 kilograms.

8–2 | z Test for a Mean >

Test means when σ is known, using the z test.

In this chapter, two statistical tests for means will be explained: the z test, used to test for the mean when the population standard deviation is known, and the t test, used to test for the mean when the population standard deviation is not known. This section explains the z test, and Section 8–3 explains the t test.

Many hypotheses are tested using a statistical test based on the following general formula:

$$\text{Test statistic} = \frac{(\text{Observed value}) - (\text{Expected value})}{\text{Standard error}}$$

The observed value is the statistic (such as the mean) that is computed from the sample data. The expected value is the parameter (such as the mean) that one would expect to obtain if the null hypothesis was true—in other words, the hypothesized value. The denominator is the standard error of the statistic being tested (in this case, the standard error of the mean).

The z test definition and formula are shown below.

> The **z test** is a statistical test for the mean of a population. It is used when the population standard deviation, σ, is known and the population is approximately normally distributed or $n \geq 30$.

Formula for the z Test for a Mean

The formula for the test statistic, z, is

$$z = \frac{\overline{X} - \mu}{\sigma/\sqrt{n}}$$

where

$\overline{X}$ = sample mean
μ = hypothesized population mean
σ = population standard deviation
n = sample size

For the z test, the observed value is the value of the sample mean. The expected value is the value of the population mean, assuming that the null hypothesis is true. The denominator $\sigma/\sqrt{n}$ is the standard error of the mean.

The formula for the z test is the same formula shown in Chapter 6 for the situation where one is using a distribution of sample means. When σ is known, the z test is robust for samples that satisfy normality conditions, even for small samples where $n < 30$. In nonnormal conditions, the standard normal distribution can be approximated with larger samples, such as $n \geq 30$, by applying the central limit theorem. If σ is unknown, use the sample standard deviation, s, and the t distribution for critical value(s), regardless of the sample size. This is explained in Section 8-3.

Assumptions for the z Test for a Mean When s Is Known

1. The sample is a random sample.
2. Either $n \geq 30$ or the population is normally distributed if $n < 30$.

As stated in Section 8-1, there are five steps for solving *hypothesis-testing* problems:

Step 1   State the hypotheses and identify the claim.

Step 2   Find the critical value(s).

Step 3   Compute the test statistic.

Step 4   Make the decision to reject or not reject the null hypothesis.

Step 5   Summarize the results.

Example 8-3 illustrates these five steps.

Speaking of Statistics

This study found that people who used pedometers reported having increased energy, mood improvement, and weight loss. State possible null and alternative hypotheses for the study. What would be a likely population? What is the sample size? Comment on the sample size.

RD HEALTH

Step to It

IT FITS in your hand, costs less than $30, and will make you feel great. Give up? A pedometer. Brenda Rooney, an epidemiologist at Gundersen Lutheran Medical Center in LaCrosse, Wis., gave 500 people pedometers and asked them to take 10,000 steps—about 8 kilometres or five miles—a day. (Office workers typically average about 4000 steps a day.) By the end of eight weeks, 56 percent reported having more energy, 47 percent improved their mood and 50 percent lost weight. The subjects reported that seeing their total step-count motivated them to take more.

— JENNIFER BRAUNSCHWEIGER

Source: Reprinted with permission from the April 2002 *Reader's Digest.* Copyright © 2002 by The Reader's Digest Assn. Inc.

Example 8–3

Professors' Salaries

A researcher reports that the average salary of full professors in Canadian universities is \$100,735. A sample of 30 full professors has a mean of \$103,746. At $\alpha = 0.05$, test the claim that full professors earn more than \$100,735 a year. From a prior study, the standard deviation of the population is known to be \$12,499.

Source: Excerpt adapted from Statistics Canada, *Salaries and Salary Scales of Full-Time Teaching Staff at Canadian Universities 2004/2005: Final Report.* Catalogue 81-595, No. 48, page 11. Released December 5, 2006.

Solution

Step 1 State the hypothesis and identify the claim.

$$H_0: \mu = \$100,735 \quad \text{and} \quad H_1: \mu > \$100,735 \text{ (claim)}$$

Step 2 Find the critical value. Since $\alpha = 0.05$ and the test is a right-tailed test, the critical value is $z = +1.645$

Step 3 Compute the test statistic.

$$z = \frac{\overline{X} - \mu}{\sigma/\sqrt{n}} = \frac{\$103,746 - \$100,735}{\$12,499/\sqrt{30}} \approx 1.319$$

Step 4 Make the decision. Since the test statistic, $+1.319$, is less than the critical value, $+1.645$, and is not in the critical region, the decision is to not reject the null hypothesis. This test is summarized in Figure 8–13.

Figure 8–13

Summary of the z Test of Example 8–3

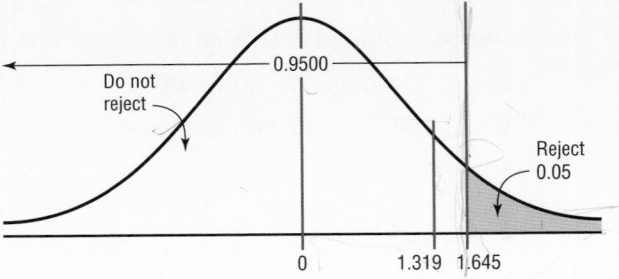

Step 5 Summarize the results. There is not enough evidence to support the claim that full professors earn more on average than \$100,735 a year.

Comment: Even though in Example 8–3 the sample mean, \$103,746, is higher than the hypothesized population mean of \$100,735, it is not *significantly* higher. Hence, the difference may be due to chance. When the null hypothesis is not rejected, there is still a chance of a type II error, i.e., of not rejecting the null hypothesis when it is false.

The probability of a type II error is not easily ascertained. Further explanation about the type II error is given in Section 8–6. For now, it is only necessary to realize that the probability of type II error exists when the decision is not to reject the null hypothesis.

Also note that when the null hypothesis is not rejected, it cannot be accepted as true. There is merely not enough evidence to say that it is false. This guideline may sound a little confusing, but the situation is analogous to a jury trial. The verdict is either guilty or not guilty and is based on the evidence presented. If a person is judged not guilty, it does not mean that the person is proved innocent; it only means that there was not enough evidence to reach the guilty verdict.

Example 8–4

Cost of Men's Athletic Shoes 🏃

A researcher claims that the average cost of men's athletic shoes is less than $80. He selects a random sample of 36 pairs of shoes from a catalogue and finds the following costs (in dollars). (The costs have been rounded to the nearest dollar.) Is there enough evidence to support the researcher's claim at $\alpha = 0.10$? Assume $\sigma = 19.2$.

60	70	75	55	80	55
50	40	80	70	50	95
120	90	75	85	80	60
110	65	80	85	85	45
75	60	90	90	60	95
110	85	45	90	70	70

Solution

Step 1 State the hypotheses and identify the claim

$$H_0: \mu = \$80 \qquad \text{and} \qquad H_1: \mu < \$80 \text{ (claim)}$$

Step 2 Find the critical value. Since $\alpha = 0.10$ and the test is a left-tailed test, the critical value is -1.28.

Step 3 Compute the test statistic. Since the exercise gives raw data, it is necessary to find the mean of the data. Using the formulas in Chapter 3 or your calculator gives $\overline{X} = 75.0$ and $\sigma = 19.2$. Substitute in the formula

$$z = \frac{\overline{X} - \mu}{\sigma/\sqrt{n}} = \frac{75 - 80}{19.2/\sqrt{36}} \approx -1.56$$

Step 4 Make the decision. Since the test statistic, -1.56, falls in the critical region, the decision is to reject the null hypothesis. See Figure 8–14.

Figure 8–14

Critical Value and Test Statistic for Example 8–4

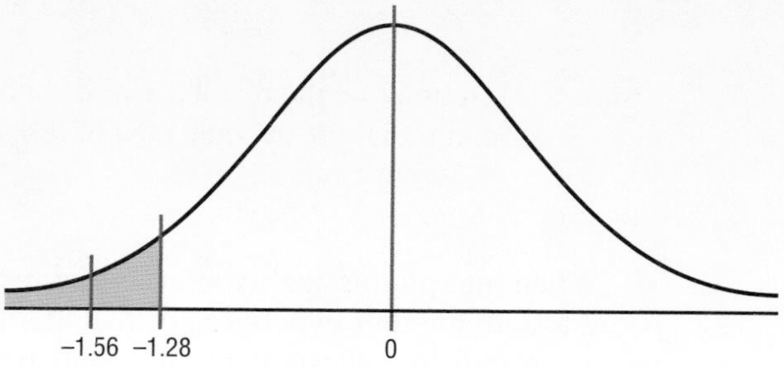

-1.56 -1.28 0

Step 5 Summarize the results. There is enough evidence to support the claim that the average cost of men's athletic shoes is less than $80.

Comment: In Example 8–4, the difference is said to be significant. However, when the null hypothesis is rejected, there is always a chance of a type I error. In this case, the probability of a type I error is at most 0.10, or 10%.

Example 8–5

Cost of Rehabilitation

The Medical Rehabilitation Education Foundation reports that the average cost of rehabilitation for stroke victims is $24,672. To see if the average cost of rehabilitation is different at a particular hospital, a researcher selects a random sample of 35 stroke victims at the hospital and finds that the average cost of their rehabilitation is

$25,226. The standard deviation of the population is $3251. At $\alpha = 0.01$, can it be concluded that the average cost of stroke rehabilitation at a particular hospital is different from $24,672?

Source: Snapshot, *USA TODAY.*

Solution

Step 1 State the hypotheses and identify the claim.

$$H_0: \mu = \$24{,}672 \quad \text{and} \quad H_1: \mu \neq \$24{,}672 \text{ (claim)}$$

Step 2 Find the critical values. Since $\alpha = 0.01$ and the test is a two-tailed test, the critical values are $+2.575$ and -2.575.

Step 3 Compute the test statistic.

$$z = \frac{\overline{X} - \mu}{\sigma/\sqrt{n}} = \frac{25{,}226 - 24{,}672}{3251/\sqrt{35}} \approx 1.01$$

Step 4 Make the decision. Do not reject the null hypothesis, since the test statistic falls in the noncritical region, as shown in Figure 8–15.

Figure 8–15

Critical Values and
Test Statistic for
Example 8–5

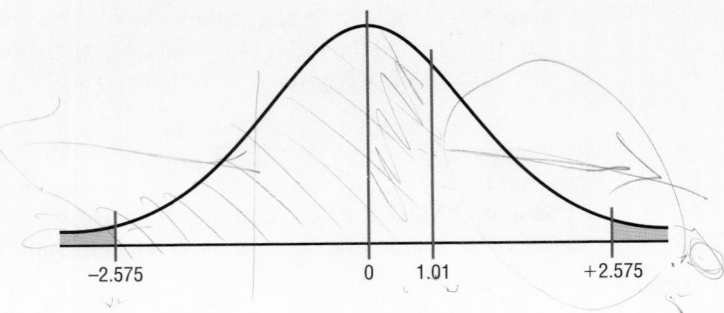

Step 5 Summarize the results. There is not enough evidence to support the claim that the average cost of rehabilitation at the particular hospital is different from $24,672.

When interpreting the hypothesis test results, it is important to know what claim is being tested, the null hypothesis or the alternative hypothesis. In either case, we would reject the null hypothesis if the test statistic falls in the critical region; otherwise we would fail to reject the null hypothesis. The four possible outcomes and summary statements are shown.

Outcomes of a Hypothesis-Testing Situation

1. Claim is H_0 and H_0 is rejected, then there is sufficient evidence to reject the claim.
2. Claim is H_0 and H_0 is not rejected, then there is not sufficient evidence to reject the claim.
3. Claim is H_1 and H_0 is rejected, then there is sufficient evidence to support the claim.
4. Claim is H_1 and H_0 is not rejected, then there is not sufficient evidence to support the claim.

For example, suppose a researcher claims that the mean daily maximum temperature of Ottawa in July is 27°C. In this case, the claim would be the null hypothesis, $H_0: \mu = 27$, since the researcher is asserting that the parameter is a specific value. If the null hypothesis is rejected, the conclusion would be that there is enough evidence to reject the claim that the mean maximum temperature of Ottawa in July is 27°C.

On the other hand, suppose the researcher claims that the mean maximum temperature of Ottawa in July is not 27°C. The claim would be the alternative hypothesis $H_1: \mu \neq 27$. Furthermore, suppose that the null hypothesis is not rejected. The conclusion, then, would be that there is not enough evidence to support the claim that the mean maximum temperature of Ottawa in July is not 27°C.

Again, remember that nothing is being proven true or false. The statistician is only stating that there is or is not enough evidence to say that a claim is *probably* true or false. As noted previously, the only way to prove something would be to use the entire population under study, and usually this cannot be done, especially when the population is very large.

P-Value Method for Hypothesis Testing

Statisticians usually test hypotheses at the common α levels of 0.05 or 0.01 and sometimes at 0.10. Recall that the choice of the level depends on the seriousness of the type I error. Besides listing an α value, many computer statistical packages give a P-value for hypothesis tests.

> The **P-value** (or probability value) is the likelihood of obtaining a sample statistic (such as the mean) or a more extreme sample statistic in the direction of the alternative hypothesis when the null hypothesis is true.

In other words, the P-value is the actual area under the standard normal distribution curve (or other curve, depending on what statistical test is being used) representing the probability of a particular sample statistic or a more extreme sample statistic occurring if the null hypothesis is true.

For example, suppose that an alternative hypothesis is $H_1: \mu > 50$ and the mean of a sample is $\overline{X} = 52$. If the statistical software displayed a P-value of 0.0356 for a statistical test, then the probability of getting a sample mean of 52 or greater is 0.0356 if the true population mean is 50 (for the given sample size and standard deviation). The relationship between the P-value and the α value can be explained in this manner. For a P-value $- 0.0356$, the null hypothesis would be rejected at $\alpha = 0.05$ but not rejected at $\alpha = 0.01$. See Figure 8–16.

Figure 18–16

Decision Rule for α and P-Values

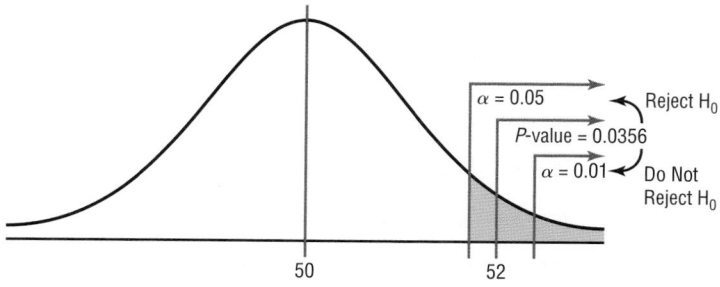

When the hypothesis test is two-tailed, the area in one tail must be doubled. For a two-tailed test, if α is 0.05 and the area in one tail is 0.0356, the P-value will be 2(0.0356) = 0.0712. That is, the null hypothesis should not be rejected at $\alpha = 0.05$, since 0.0712 is greater than 0.05. In summary, the null hypothesis is rejected only if the P-value is less than or equal to the significance level (α); otherwise, if the P-value is greater than the significance level (α), do not reject the null hypothesis.

The P-value for the z test can be found by using Table E–1 or Table E–2 in Appendix C. First find the cumulative area to the left under the standard normal curve that corresponds to the calculated test statistic or z score.

- For a left-tailed test, H_1: $\mu < k$, the P-value is the cumulative area to the left associated with the z score.
- For a right-tailed test, H_1: $\mu > k$, the P-value is 1 minus the cumulative area to the left (or cumulative area to the right) associated with the z score.
- For a two-tailed test, H_1: $\mu \neq k$, the P-value is twice the cumulative area to the left if the z score is negative or twice the cumulative area to the right if the z score is positive.

This procedure is shown in step 3 of Examples 8–6 and 8–7.

The P-value method for testing hypotheses differs from the traditional method somewhat. The steps for the P-value method are summarized next.

Procedure Table

Solving Hypothesis-Testing Problems (P-Value Method)

Step 1   State the hypotheses and identify the claim.

Step 2   Compute the test statistic.

Step 3   Find the P-value.

Step 4   Make the decision.

Step 5   Summarize the results.

Examples 8–6 and 8–7 show how to use the P-value method to test hypotheses.

Example 8–6

Age of Education Infrastructure

A published report states that the average age of Canada's education infrastructure (elementary and secondary schools, colleges and universities) is 20.1 years. A provincial Education minister suggests that her province's education infrastructure is older than the national average. A random sample of 36 educational institutions is selected, with a mean age of 21.2 years. Assume a population standard deviation of 2.9 years. At $\alpha = 0.05$, is there enough evidence to support the minister's claim? Use the P-value method.

Source: Statistics Canada, Trends in the Age of Education Infrastructure in Canada, Valérie Gaudreault, Donald Overton, and John Trstenjak, December 16, 2009.

Solution

Step 1   State the hypotheses and identify the claim.

$$H_0: \mu = 20.1 \quad \text{and} \quad H_1: \mu > 20.1 \text{ (claim)}$$

Step 2   Compute the test statistic.

$$z = \frac{21.2 - 20.1}{2.9/\sqrt{36}} \approx 2.28$$

Step 3 Find the *P*-value. Since the test statistic (*z* score) in step 2 is positive, look up the corresponding area in Table E–2 in Appendix C. For *z* = 2.28, the cumulative area to the left is 0.9887. Since the alternative hypothesis indicates a right-tailed test, subtract this area from 1 to obtain the cumulative area to the right.

$$1.0000 - 0.9887 = 0.0113$$

Hence, the *P*-value is 0.0113.

Step 4 Make the decision. Since the *P*-value is less than 0.05, the decision is to reject the null hypothesis. See Figure 8–17.

Figure 8–17

P-Value and α Value for Example 8–6

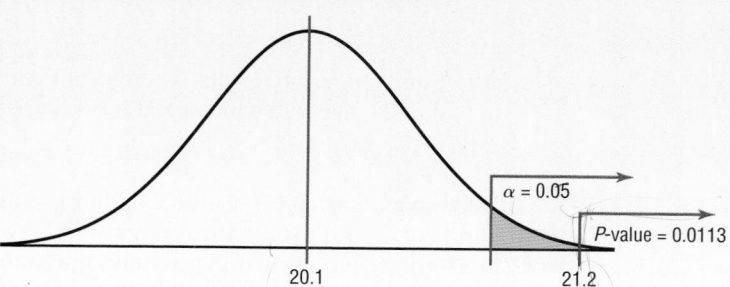

Step 5 Summarize the results. There is enough evidence to support the minister's claim that the average age of the province's educational institutions is greater than 20.1 years.

Note: Had the researcher chosen α = 0.01, the null hypothesis would not have been rejected, since the *P*-value (0.0113) is greater than 0.01.

Example 8–7

Wind Speed

A researcher claims that the average wind speed in a certain city is 8 kilometres per hour. A sample of 32 days has an average wind speed of 8.2 kilometres per hour. The population standard deviation of the sample is 0.6 kilometre per hour. At α = 0.05, is there enough evidence to reject the claim? Use the *P*-value method.

Solution

Step 1 State the hypotheses and identify the claim.

$$H_0: \mu = 8 \text{ (claim)} \qquad \text{and} \qquad H_1: \mu \neq 8$$

Step 2 Compute the test statistic.

$$z = \frac{8.2 - 8}{0.6/\sqrt{32}} \approx 1.89$$

Step 3 Find the *P*-value. Since the test statistic (*z* score) in step 2 is positive, look up the corresponding area in Table E–2 in Appendix C. For *z* = 1.89, the area to the left is 0.9706. Subtract the value from 1.0000 to obtain the area to the right.

$$1.0000 - 0.9706 = 0.0294$$

Since this is a two-tailed test and the *z* score is positive, calculate twice the area to the right to obtain the *P*-value.

$$2(0.0294) = 0.0588$$

Step 4 Make the decision. The decision is to not reject the null hypothesis, since the *P*-value is greater than 0.05. See Figure 8–18.

Figure 8–18

P-Values and α Values
for Example 8–7

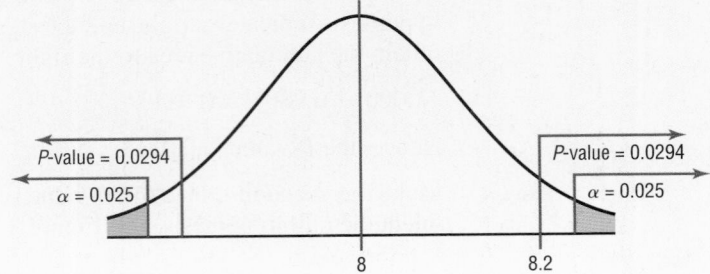

Step 5 Summarize the results. There is not enough evidence to reject the claim that the average wind speed is 8 kilometres per hour.

In Examples 8–6 and 8–7, the *P*-value and the α value were shown on a normal distribution curve to illustrate the relationship between the two values; however, it is not necessary to draw the normal distribution curve to make the decision whether to reject the null hypothesis. One can use the following rule.

Decision Rule When Using a *P*-Value

If *P*-value $\leq \alpha$, reject the null hypothesis.
If *P*-value $> \alpha$, fail to reject the null hypothesis.

In Example 8–6, *P*-value = 0.0113 and α = 0.05. Since *P*-value $\leq \alpha$, the null hypothesis was rejected. In Example 8–7, *P*-value = 0.0588 and α = 0.05. Since *P*-value $> \alpha$, the null hypothesis was not rejected.

The *P*-values given on calculators and computers are slightly different from those found with Tables E–1 and E–2. This is due to the fact that *z* scores and the values in Tables E–1 and E–2 have been rounded. *Also, most calculators and computers give the exact P-value for two-tailed tests, so it should not be doubled (as it should when the area found in Tables E–1 and E–2 is used).*

A clear distinction between the α value and the *P*-value should be made. The α value is chosen by the researcher before the statistical test is conducted. The *P*-value is computed after the sample mean has been found.

There are two schools of thought on *P*-values. Some researchers do not choose an α value but report the *P*-value and allow the reader to decide whether the null hypothesis should be rejected.

In this case, the following guidelines can be used, but be advised that these guidelines are not written in stone, and some statisticians may have other opinions.

Guidelines for *P*-Values

If *P*-value ≤ 0.01, reject the null hypothesis. The difference is highly significant.
If *P*-value > 0.01 but *P*-value ≤ 0.05, reject the null hypothesis. The difference is significant.
If *P*-value > 0.05 but *P*-value ≤ 0.10, consider the consequences of type I error before rejecting the null hypothesis.
If *P*-value > 0.10, do not reject the null hypothesis. The difference is not significant.

Others decide on the α value in advance and use the *P*-value to make the decision, as shown in Examples 8–6 and 8–7. A note of caution is needed here: If a researcher selects $\alpha = 0.01$ and the *P*-value is 0.03, the researcher may decide to change the α value from 0.01 to 0.05 so that the null hypothesis will be rejected. This, of course, should not be done. If the α level is selected in advance, it should be used in making the decision.

One additional note on hypothesis testing is that the researcher should distinguish between *statistical significance* and *practical significance*. When the null hypothesis is rejected at a specific significance level, it can be concluded that the difference is probably not due to chance and thus is statistically significant. However, the results may not have any practical significance. For example, suppose that a new fuel additive decreases the litres per 100 kilometres that a car consumes by 0.15 litres for a sample of 1000 automobiles. The results may be statistically significant at the 0.05 level, but it would hardly be worthwhile to market the product for such a small increase. Hence, there is no practical significance to the results. It is up to the researcher to use common sense when interpreting the results of a statistical test.

8–2   Applying the Concepts

Car Thefts

You recently obtained a job with a company that manufactures an automobile anti-theft device. To conduct an advertising campaign for your product, you need to make a claim about the number of automobile thefts per year. Since the population of cities in Canada varies, you decide to use rates per 10,000 people. (The rates are based on the number of people living in the cities.) Your boss said that last year the theft rate was 50 vehicles. Assume the population standard deviation is known to be 42.5. You want to see if it has changed. The following are rates per 10,000 people for 36 randomly selected locations in Canada.

37	75	41	18	20	160
78	29	51	57	42	34
115	158	35	34	12	16
49	82	50	83	29	35
30	71	58	51	100	23
58	54	200	44	23	49

Source: Adapted from Statistics Canada, *Juristat,* "Crime Statistics in Canada, 2005," Catalogue 85-002, Vol. 26, No. 4.

Using this information, answer these questions and follow the instructions.

1. What are the hypotheses that you would use?
2. Is the sample considered large or small?
3. What assumption must be met before the hypothesis test can be conducted?
4. Which probability distribution would you use?
5. Would you select a one- or two-tailed test? Why?
6. What critical value(s) would you use?
7. Conduct a hypothesis test.
8. What is your decision?
9. What is your conclusion?
10. Write a brief statement summarizing your conclusion.
11. If you lived in a city with a population of about 50,000, how many automobile thefts per year would you expect to occur?

See page 404 for the answers.

Exercises 8–2

For Exercises 1 through 13, perform each of the following steps.

    a. State the hypotheses and identify the claim.

    b. Find the critical value(s).

    c. Compute the test statistic.

    d. Make the decision.

    e. Summarize the results.

Use diagrams to show the critical region (or regions), and use the traditional method of hypothesis testing unless otherwise specified.

1. **Walking with a Pedometer** An increase in walking has been shown to contribute to a healthier lifestyle. A sedentary Canadian takes an average of 5000 steps per day (and 59% of Canadians are overweight). A group of health-conscious employees at a regional clinic volunteered to wear pedometers for a month to record their steps. It was found that a random sample of 40 walkers took an average of 5430 steps per day. Assume a population standard deviation from a previous study is 600 steps per day. At $\alpha = 0.05$, can it be concluded that they walked more than the sedentary average of 5000 steps per day?
   Source: MSN Health and Fitness.

2. **Graduating Student Debt** It has been reported that the average student graduating with a bachelor's degree left school with a debt of \$19,500. The student council at a large university feels that the school's recent graduates have a debt much less than this, so it conducts a study of 50 randomly selected graduates and finds that the average debt is \$17,900. Assume a population standard deviation of \$6,575. With $\alpha = 0.05$, is the student council correct?
   Source: CBC News, "Buy Now, Pay Later: Canadians and Debt," Tom McFeat, September 12, 2006.

3. **Revenues of Top Companies** A researcher states that the average revenue of the top 1000 Canadian companies is less than \$15 billion. A sample of 50 companies is randomly selected, and the revenues (rounded to the nearest billion dollars) are shown. At $\alpha = 0.05$, is there enough evidence to support the researcher's claim? From a prior study $\sigma = 9.2$.

29	2	32	5	28
24	32	2	26	23
19	27	5	19	4
4	3	10	5	9
8	17	9	18	7
6	10	7	15	5
2	5	21	10	4
22	27	18	1	7
18	2	14	8	18
14	3	1	6	11

Source: The Globe and Mail Report on Business.

4. **University Gender Salary Comparison** Male full-time university teaching staff members receive an average salary of \$104,091, according to a report on Canadian university teaching staff salary scales. A women's advocate group feels that female full-time university teaching staff members earn significantly less than the male average salary. Random selections of 75 university female teaching staff members find that their mean salary was \$91,868. Assume $\sigma = \$11,555$. At $\alpha = 0.01$, is there evidence to support the claim of the women's advocate group?
   Source: Statistics Canada, *Section B: Financing Education Systems,* "Table D.3.4: Number and Salary of Full-Time University Teaching Staff, by Academic Rank and Sex, Canada and Provinces, 1996/1997 and 2006/2007," March 9, 2009.

5. **Age of Commercial Airline Fleet** A recent industry report claimed that the age of Air Canada's commercial airline fleet averaged 9.8 years. An aviation news editor suggests that the fleet's age was less than the age claimed by the report due to new aircraft purchases. A random sample of 36 aircraft from Air Canada's fleet is selected, and the average age of the aircraft is 8.1 years. From a previous report, $\sigma = 1.8$ years. At $\alpha = 0.01$, can it be concluded that the average fleet age is less than the industry report?

6. **Potato Production** The average production of potatoes on Prince Edward Island is 29.1 tonnes per hectare. A new plant food has been developed and is tested on 60 individual plots of land. The mean yield with the new plant food is 30.6 tonnes of potatoes per hectare. A previous study indicated $\sigma = 5.7$ tonnes per hectare. At $\alpha = 0.05$, can one conclude that the average potato production has increased?

7. **Height of One-Year-Olds** Popular growth charts indicate that the average height of one-year-old toddlers (both genders) is 73.7 cm. Thirty toddlers are measured on their first birthday, randomly selected from multiple day-care centres in northern communities. Given the toddler height sample data, in cm, at $\alpha = 0.05$, can it be concluded that the average one-year-old toddler height in northern communities differs from the average growth-chart height of 73.7 cm? Assume $\sigma = 6.51$ cm.

64	89	76	66	75
76	76	71	74	76
74	69	84	69	74
81	64	67	65	81
72	81	80	75	86
81	71	71	81	75

Source: www.keepkidshealthy.com.

8. **University Student Parental Income** At a certain university, the mean income of parents of the freshman class is reported to be \$91,600. The president of another university feels that the parents' mean income for her school's freshman class is greater than \$91,600. She surveys 100 randomly

selected families and finds the mean income to be $96,321. Given $\sigma = \$9555$ and $\alpha = 0.05$, is she correct?

Source: The Chronicle of Higher Education.

9. **Undergraduate School Expenses** Average undergraduate cost for tuition, fees, room, and board for all institutions last year was $19,410. A random sample of costs this year for 40 institutions of higher learning indicated that the sample mean was $22,098. From a prior study, $\sigma = \$6050$. At the 0.01 level of significance, is there sufficient evidence to conclude that the cost of attendance has increased?

Source: The New York Times Almanac.

10. **Real Estate Prices** A real estate agent claims that the average price of a single-family home in British Columbia's capital of Victoria is $475,000. A random sample of 36 homes sold in Victoria is selected, and the prices in dollars are shown. Is there enough evidence to reject the agent's claim at $\alpha = 0.05$? Assume $\sigma = \$133,183$.

488,800	399,000	509,000	449,900	599,000	327,500
539,900	479,900	598,000	799,000	469,000	349,500
579,900	485,000	625,000	309,000	439,900	349,900
599,000	499,900	754,900	374,900	379,900	519,000
634,900	529,000	769,500	479,000	379,900	439,900
635,000	533,500	775,000	369,900	364,900	379,000

Source: The Canadian Real Estate Association.

11. **TV Viewing Hours** On average, Canadians watch 21.4 hours of television per week. A sociologist claims that TV viewers in Quebec differ from the Canadian national average. A random sample of 35 Quebec households during a one-week period had a mean of 23.3 hours. A previous report showed the population standard deviation to be 3.2 hours per week. Is there sufficient evidence at the 0.01 level of significance that the average weekly television viewing hours for Quebecers differs from the national average of all Canadians?

Source: Statistics Canada.

12. **Construction Worker Wages** The Canadian average weekly wage for construction workers was $1030 in 2009. An economist believes that due to a downturn in the economy, construction workers' wages have decreased. A random sample of 50 construction workers had a mean weekly wage of $998. Assume $\sigma = \$129$. Is there sufficient evidence at the $\alpha = 0.05$ level to conclude that the mean weekly wage has decreased?

Source: Living in Canada, "Canadian Salary Survey," 2009.

13. **Expenditures on Health** A Canadian Nursing Association (CNA) position paper states that, on average, Canadians spent $850 per person on health insurance and out-of-pocket costs for health services in a one-year period. A provincial health authority disputes this claim. A random sample of 64 people determines an average health expenditure of $818. Assume $\sigma = \$117$. At

$\alpha = 0.01$, can the CNA statement be disproved. Repeat the test using $\alpha = 0.05$ and compare the results.

Source: Canadian Nursing Association, Financing Canada's Health System, June 2001.

14. What is meant by a *P*-value?

15. State whether the null hypothesis should be rejected on the basis of the given *P*-value.

  a. *P*-value = 0.258, $\alpha = 0.05$, one-tailed test
  b. *P*-value = 0.0684, $\alpha = 0.10$, two-tailed test
  c. *P*-value = 0.0153, $\alpha = 0.01$, one-tailed test
  d. *P*-value = 0.0232, $\alpha = 0.05$, two-tailed test
  e. *P*-value = 0.002, $\alpha = 0.01$, one-tailed test

16. **Consumption of Bottled Water** A researcher claims that the average yearly consumption of bottled water in Canada is equal to 27 litres per capita. In a sample of 50 randomly selected Canadians, the mean yearly consumption of bottled water was 29.3 litres. The standard deviation of the sample was 1.8 litres. Find the *P*-value for the test. On the basis of the *P*-value, is the researcher's claim valid?

Source: Statistics Canada.

17. **Vehicle Winter Stopping Distances** In winter driving conditions, it takes all vehicles longer to stop on snow-covered roads. Travelling at 90 kilometres per hour (km/h), the stopping distance for the average passenger vehicle on loose snow is 213 metres. A tire manufacturer claims that its winter tires decrease vehicle stopping distance on snow-covered roads. A sample of 20 vehicles equipped with the manufacturer's tires was tested in winter on a test track. The average stopping distance at a speed of 90 km/h on loose snow was 211.6 metres. Assume a population standard deviation of 2.4 metres. Test the claim that the average stopping distance decreased with the new winter tires. Find the *P*-value. On the basis of the *P*-value, should the null hypothesis be rejected at $\alpha = 0.01$? Assume that the variable is normally distributed.

Source: Government of Ontario.

18. **Copy Machine Use** A store manager hypothesizes that the average number of pages a person copies on the store's copy machine is less than 40. A sample of 50 customers' orders is selected. At $\alpha = 0.01$, is there enough evidence to support the claim? Use the *P*-value hypothesis-testing method. Assume $\sigma = 30.9$.

2	2	2	5	32
5	29	8	2	49
21	1	24	72	70
21	85	61	8	42
3	15	27	113	36
37	5	3	58	82
9	2	1	6	9
80	9	51	2	122
21	49	36	43	61
3	17	17	4	1

19. **Burning Calories Playing Tennis** A health researcher read that a 91-kilogram male can burn an average of 546 calories per hour playing tennis. Thirty-six males were randomly selected and tested. The mean of the number of calories burned per hour was 544.8. Test the claim that the average number of calories burned is actually less than 546, and find the P-value. On the basis of the P-value, should the null hypothesis be rejected at $\alpha = 0.01$? The standard deviation of the sample is 3. Can it be concluded that the average number of calories burned is less than originally thought?

20. **Breaking Strength of Cable** A special cable has a breaking strength of 363 kilograms. The standard deviation of the population is 5.5 kilograms. A researcher selects a sample of 20 cables and finds that the average breaking strength is 360 kilograms. Can one reject the claim that the breaking strength is 363 kilograms? Find the P-value. Should the null hypothesis be rejected at $\alpha = 0.01$? Assume that the variable is normally distributed.

21. **National Farm Sizes** Several years ago the Agriculture Division of Statistics Canada reported that the average size of farms in Canada was 246 hectares (ha). A random sample of 50 farms was selected, and the mean farm size was 296 ha. From the previous report, the population standard deviation was 59 ha. Use the P-value method to test the claim at $\alpha = 0.05$ that the average farm size is larger today. Should the Agriculture Division update its information?

    Source: Statistics Canada.

22. **Provincial Farm Sizes** Ten years ago the average farm size in Ontario was 81 ha. The standard deviation of the population was 7 ha. A recent study consisting of 22 Ontario farms showed that the average farm size was 83.9 ha. Use the P-value method to test the claim, at $\alpha = 0.10$, that the average farm size has not changed in the past 10 years. Use $\sigma = 7$ ha and assume that the variable is normally distributed.

    Source: Statistics Canada.

23. **Vehicle Transmission Service** A car manufacturer recommends that new-vehicle transmissions be serviced at 48,000 km to maintain proper function. To see whether its customers are adhering to this recommendation, a car dealership selects a random sample of 40 customers and finds that the average distance driven by the serviced automobiles was 48,730 km. A prior study indicated a population standard deviation of 2694 km. Using the P-value method, test the claim that the owners are having their transmissions serviced at 48,000 km. Use $\alpha = 0.10$.

24. **Speeding Tickets** A motorist claims that the local police issue an average of 60 speeding tickets per day. These data show the number of speeding tickets issued each day for a period of one month. Assume σ is 13.42. Is there enough evidence to reject the motorist's claim at $\alpha = 0.05$? Use the P-value method.

72	45	36	68	69	71	57	60
83	26	60	72	58	87	48	59
60	56	64	68	42	57	57	
58	63	49	73	75	42	63	

25. **Sick Days** A manager states that in his factory, the average number of days per year missed by employees due to illness is less than the national average of 10. The following data show the number of days missed by 40 employees last year. Is there sufficient evidence to believe the manager's statement at $\alpha = 0.05$? Assume $\sigma = 3.63$. Use the P-value method.

0	6	12	3	3	5	4	1
3	9	6	0	7	6	3	4
7	4	7	1	0	8	12	3
2	5	10	5	15	3	2	5
3	11	8	2	2	4	1	9

Extending the Concepts »

26. Suppose a statistician chose to test a hypothesis at $\alpha = 0.01$. The critical value for a right-tailed test is $+2.33$. If the test statistic was 1.97, what would the decision be? What would happen if, after seeing the test statistic, she decided to choose $\alpha = 0.05$? What would the decision be? Explain the contradiction, if there is one.

27. **Hourly Wage** The president of a company states that the average hourly wage of her employees is $8.65. A sample of 50 employees has the distribution shown. At $\alpha = 0.05$, is the president's statement believable? Assume $\sigma = 0.105$.

Class	Frequency
8.35–8.43	2
8.44–8.52	6
8.53–8.61	12
8.62–8.70	18
8.71–8.79	10
8.80–8.88	2

| 8–3 | *t* Test for a Mean **>** |

Test means when σ is unknown, using the *t* test.

When the population standard deviation, σ, is unknown, the *z* test is not generally used for testing hypotheses involving means. A different test, called the *t test,* is used. The distribution of the variable should be approximately normal.

As stated in Chapter 7, the *t* distribution is similar to the standard normal distribution in the following ways.

1. It is bell-shaped.
2. It is symmetric about the mean.
3. The mean, median, and mode are equal to 0 and are located at the centre of the distribution.
4. The curve never touches the *x* axis.

The *t* distribution differs from the standard normal distribution in the following ways.

1. The variance is greater than 1.
2. The *t* distribution is a family of curves based on the *degrees of freedom,* which is a number related to sample size. (Recall that the symbol for degrees of freedom is d.f. See Section 7–2 for an explanation of degrees of freedom.)
3. As the sample size increases, the *t* distribution approaches the normal distribution.

The *t* test definition and formula are shown below.

> The **t test** is a statistical test for the mean of a population and is used when σ is unknown and the population is normally or approximately normally distributed.

Formula for the *t* Test for a Mean

The formula for the *t* test is

$$t = \frac{\overline{X} - \mu}{s/\sqrt{n}}$$

The degrees of freedom are d.f. $= n - 1$ and where

$\overline{X}$ = sample mean
μ = hypothesized population mean
s = sample standard deviation
n = sample size

The formula for the *t* test is similar to the formula for the *z* test. But since the population standard deviation σ is unknown, the sample standard deviation *s* is used instead.

The critical values for the *t* test are given in Table F in Appendix C. For a one-tailed test, find the α level by looking at the top row of the table and finding the appropriate column. Find the degrees of freedom by looking down the left-hand column.

Notice that the degrees of freedom are given for values from 1 through 30 and then at select intervals above 30 up to 1000. In the intervals above 30, select the degrees of freedom closest to the calculated d.f. value. For example, if d.f. = 37, use the d.f. = 35 table value. If d.f. is exactly between two degrees of freedom values on Table F, use the average of the two table d.f. values above and below. For example, if d.f. = 45, look up the d.f. = 40 *t* value and the d.f. = 50 *t* value for the desired α, and average the two *t* values.

As the degrees of freedom get larger, the critical values approach the *z* scores. At (z) ∞, the *t* values and *z* scores are very similar, and either may be used.

| Example 8–8 | Find the critical t value for $\alpha = 0.05$ with d.f. = 16 for a right-tailed t test. |

Solution

Find the 0.05 column in the top row and 16 in the left-hand column. Where the row and column meet, the appropriate critical value is found; it is $+1.746$. See Figure 8–19.

Figure 8–19

Finding the Critical Value for the t Test in Table F (Example 8–8)

Table F							
		The t Distribution					
Degrees of Freedom	Confidence Intervals	50%	80%	90%	95%	98%	99%
d.f.	One tail, α	0.25	0.10	0.05	0.025	0.01	0.005
	Two tails, α	0.50	0.20	0.10	0.05	0.02	0.01
1		1.000	3.078	6.314	12.706	31.821	63.657
2		0.816	1.886	2.920	4.303	6.965	9.925
⋮							
15		0.691	1.341	1.753	2.131	2.602	2.947
16		0.690	1.337	1.746	2.120	2.583	2.921
17		0.689	1.333	1.740	2.110	2.567	2.898
⋮							
$(z)\infty$		0.674	1.282	1.645	1.960	2.326	2.576

| Example 8–9 | Find the critical t value for $\alpha = 0.01$ with d.f. = 22 for a left-tailed test. |

Solution

Find the 0.01 column in the row labelled "One tail," and find 22 in the left column. The critical value is -2.508 since the test is a one-tailed left test.

| Example 8–10 | Find the critical values for $\alpha = 0.10$ with d.f. = 18 for a two-tailed t test. |

Solution

Find the 0.10 column in the row labelled "Two tails," and find 18 in the column labelled "d.f." The critical values are $+1.734$ and -1.734.

| Example 8–11 | Find the critical value for $\alpha = 0.05$ with d.f. = 37 for a right-tailed t test. |

Solution

Find the 0.05 column in the "One tail" row. Since d.f. = 37 is not in Table F, use the d.f. value closest to 37, which is d.f. = 35. The critical value is $+1.690$.

Assumptions for the t Test for a Mean When σ Is Unknown

  1. The sample is a random sample.
  2. Either $n \geq 30$ or the population is normally distributed if $n < 30$.

When you test hypotheses by using the t test (traditional method), follow the same procedure as for the z test, except use Table F in Appendix C.

Step 1   State the hypotheses and identify the claim.

Step 2   Find the critical value(s) from Table F.

Step 3   Compute the test statistic.

Step 4   Make the decision to reject or not reject the null hypothesis.

Step 5   Summarize the results.

Remember that the t test should be used when the population is approximately normally distributed and the population standard deviation is unknown.

Examples 8–12 through 8–14 illustrate the application of the *t* test.

Example 8–12

Practical Nursing Salaries

A health-care recruitment agency claims that the average starting salary for Canada's practical nursing graduates is $39,500. Suppose a random sample of 10 nursing graduates yields an average salary of $38,554 and a standard deviation of $750. At $\alpha = 0.05$, is there enough evidence to reject the recruitment agency's claim? Assume the variable is approximately normally distributed.

Solution

Step 1 H_0: $\mu = \$39,500$ (claim) and H_1: $\mu \neq \$39,500$

Step 2   The critical values are $+2.262$ and -2.262 for $\alpha = 0.05$ (two tails) and d.f. = 9.

Step 3   The test statistic is

$$t = \frac{\overline{X} - \mu}{s/\sqrt{n}} = \frac{\$38,554 - \$39,500}{\$750/\sqrt{10}} \approx -3.989$$

Step 4   Reject the null hypothesis, since $-3.989 < -2.262$ as shown in Figure 8–20.

Figure 8–20

Summary of the *t* Test in Example 8–12

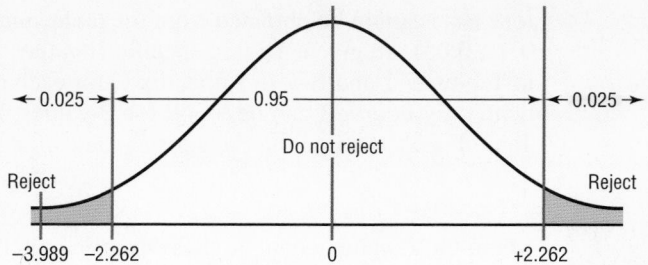

Step 5   There is enough evidence to reject the claim that the starting salary of practical nurses is $39,500.

Example 8–13

Substitute Teachers' Salaries

A union representative claims that the average salary for substitute teachers is less than $185 per day in southern Ontario school districts. A sample of 8 school districts is randomly selected, and the daily salaries (in dollars) are shown. Is there enough evidence to support the union representative's claim at $\alpha = 0.10$? Assume that the population data is normally distributed.

185   179   185   173   198   171   185   172

Solution

Step 1 H_0: $\mu = \$185$ and H_1: $\mu < \$185$ (claim)

Step 2   At $\alpha = 0.10$ and d.f. $= 7$, the critical value is -1.415.

Step 3   To compute the test statistic, the mean and standard deviation must be found. Using either the formulas in Chapter 3 or your calculator, $\overline{X} = \$181$ and $s = \$9.15$.

$$t = \frac{\overline{X} - \mu}{s/\sqrt{n}} = \frac{\$181 - \$185}{\$9.15/\sqrt{8}} \approx -1.237$$

Step 4   Do not reject the null hypothesis, since -1.237 falls in the noncritical region. See Figure 8–21.

Figure 8–21

Critical Value and
Test Statistic for
Example 8–13

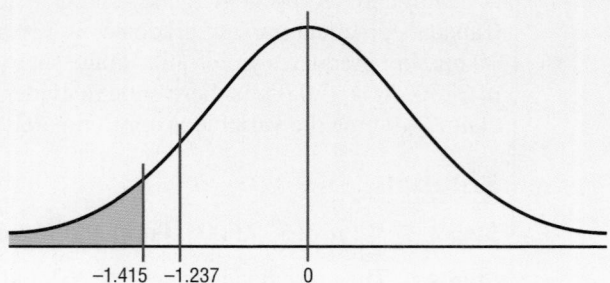

-1.415 -1.237 0

Step 5   There is not enough evidence to support the union's claim that the average salary of substitute teachers in southern Ontario school districts is less than $185 per day.

    The P-values for the t test can be found by using Table F; however, specific P-values for t tests cannot be obtained from the table since only selected values of α (for example, 0.01, 0.05) are given. To find specific P-values for t tests, one would need tables similar to Tables E–1 and E–2 in Appendix C for each degree of freedom. Since this is not practical, only *intervals* can be found for P-values. Examples 8–14 to 8–16 show how to use Table F to determine intervals for P-values for the t test.

Example 8–14

Find the P-value when the t test statistic is 2.056, the sample size is 11, and the test is right-tailed.

Solution

To get the P-value, look across the row with 10 degrees of freedom (d.f. $= n - 1$) in Table F and find the two values that 2.056 falls between. They are 1.812 and 2.228. Since this is a right-tailed test, look up to the row labelled "One tail, α" and find the two α values corresponding to 1.812 and 2.228. They are 0.05 and 0.025, respectively. See Figure 8–22. Hence, the P-value would be contained in the interval $0.025 < P\text{-value} < 0.05$. This means that the P-value is between 0.025 and 0.05. If α was 0.05, one would reject the null hypothesis since the P-value is less than 0.05. But if α was 0.01, one would not reject the null hypothesis since the P-value is greater than 0.01. (Actually, it is greater than 0.025.)

Figure 8–22

Finding the P-Value for Example 8–14

	Confidence intervals	50%	80%	90%	95%	98%	99%
	One tail, α	0.25	0.10	(0.05)	(0.025)	0.01	0.005
d.f.	Two tails, α	0.50	0.20	0.10	0.05	0.02	0.01
1		1.000	3.078	6.314	12.706	31.821	63.657
2		0.816	1.886	2.920	4.303	6.965	9.925
3		0.765	1.638	2.353	3.182	4.541	5.841
4		0.741	1.533	2.132	2.776	3.747	4.604
5		0.727	1.476	2.015	2.571	3.365	4.032
6		0.718	1.440	1.943	2.447	3.143	3.707
7		0.711	1.415	1.895	2.365	2.998	3.499
8		0.706	1.397	1.860	2.306	2.896	3.355
9		0.703	1.383	1.833	2.262	2.821	3.250
(10)		0.700	1.372	(1.812) *	(2.228)	2.764	3.169
11		0.697	1.363	1.796	2.201	2.718	3.106
12		0.695	1.356	1.782	2.179	2.681	3.055
13		0.694	1.350	1.771	2.160	2.650	3.012
14		0.692	1.345	1.761	2.145	2.624	2.977
15		0.691	1.341	1.753	2.131	2.602	2.947
⋮		⋮	⋮	⋮	⋮	⋮	⋮
$(z)\ \infty$		0.674	1.282	1.645	1.960	2.326	2.576

*2.056 falls between 1.812 and 2.228.

Example 8–15

Find the P-value when the t test value is 2.983, the sample size is 6, and the test is two-tailed.

Solution

To get the P-value, look across the row with d.f. = 5 and find the two values that 2.983 falls between. They are 2.571 and 3.365. Then look up to the row labelled "Two tails, α" to find the corresponding α values.

In this case, they are 0.05 and 0.02. Hence the P-value is contained in the interval $0.02 < P\text{-value} < 0.05$. This means that the P-value is between 0.02 and 0.05. In this case, if $\alpha = 0.05$, the null hypothesis can be rejected since $P\text{-value} < 0.05$; but if $\alpha = 0.01$, the null hypothesis cannot be rejected since $P\text{-value} > 0.01$ (actually $P\text{-value} > 0.02$).

Note: **Since many students will be using calculators or computer programs that give the specific P-value for the t test and other tests presented later in this textbook, these specific values, in addition to the intervals, will be given for the answers to the examples and exercises.**

The P-value obtained from a calculator for Example 8–14 is 0.033. The P-value obtained from a calculator for Example 8–15 is 0.031.

To test hypotheses using the P-value method, follow the same steps as explained in Section 8–2. These steps are repeated here.

Step 1   State the hypotheses and identify the claim.

Step 2   Compute the test statistic.

Interesting Fact

Canada has 4000 centenarians, 3400 of whom are women.

Step 3 Find the *P*-value.

Step 4 Make the decision.

Step 5 Summarize the results.

This method is shown in Example 8–16.

| Example 8–16 | **Joggers' Oxygen Uptake** |

Joggers' Oxygen Uptake

A physician claims that joggers' maximal volume oxygen uptake is greater than the average of all adults. A sample of 15 joggers has a mean of 40.6 millilitres per kilogram (mL/kg) and a standard deviation of 6 mL/kg. If the average of all adults is 36.7 mL/kg, is there enough evidence to support the physician's claim at $\alpha = 0.05$? Use the *P*-value method.

Solution

Step 1 State the hypotheses and identify the claim.

$$H_0: \mu = 36.7 \qquad \text{and} \qquad H_1: \mu > 36.7 \text{ (claim)}$$

Step 2 Compute the test statistic. The test statistic is

$$t = \frac{\overline{X} - \mu}{s/\sqrt{n}} = \frac{40.6 - 36.7}{6/\sqrt{15}} \approx 2.517$$

Step 3 Find the *P*-value. Looking across the row with d.f. = 14 in Table F, one sees that 2.517 falls between 2.145 and 2.624, corresponding to $\alpha = 0.025$ and $\alpha = 0.01$ since this is a right-tailed test. Hence, *P*-value > 0.01 and *P*-value < 0.025 or 0.01 < *P*-value < 0.025. That is, the *P*-value is somewhere between 0.01 and 0.025. (The *P*-value obtained from a calculator is 0.012.)

Step 4 Reject the null hypothesis since *P*-value < 0.05 (that is, *P*-value < α).

Step 5 There is enough evidence to support the claim that the joggers' maximal volume oxygen uptake is greater than 36.7 mL/kg.

Students sometimes have difficulty deciding whether to use the *z* test or *t* test. The rules are the same as those pertaining to confidence intervals.

1. If σ is known, use the **z test.** The variable must be normally distributed if $n < 30$.
2. If σ is unknown but $n \geq 30$, use the **t test.**
3. If σ is unknown and $n < 30$, use the **t test.** (The population must be approximately normally distributed.)

These rules are summarized in Figure 8–23.

| **Figure 8–23** |

When to Use *z* or *t* Test

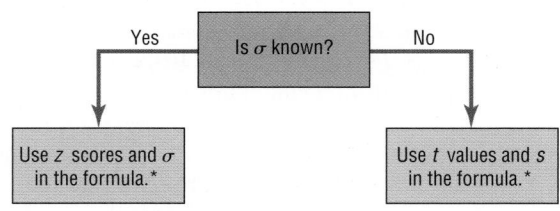

*If $n < 30$, the variable must be normally distributed. If not, refer to Chapter 13, Nonparametric Statistics.

Speaking of Statistics

Can Sunshine Relieve Pain?

A study conducted at the University of Pittsburgh showed that hospital patients in rooms with lots of sunlight required less pain medication the day after surgery and during their total stay in the hospital than patients who were in darker rooms.

Patients in the sunny rooms averaged 3.2 milligrams of pain reliever per hour for their total stay as opposed to 4.1 milligrams per hour for those in darker rooms. This study compared two groups of patients. Although no statistical tests were mentioned in the article, what statistical test do you think the researchers used to compare the groups?

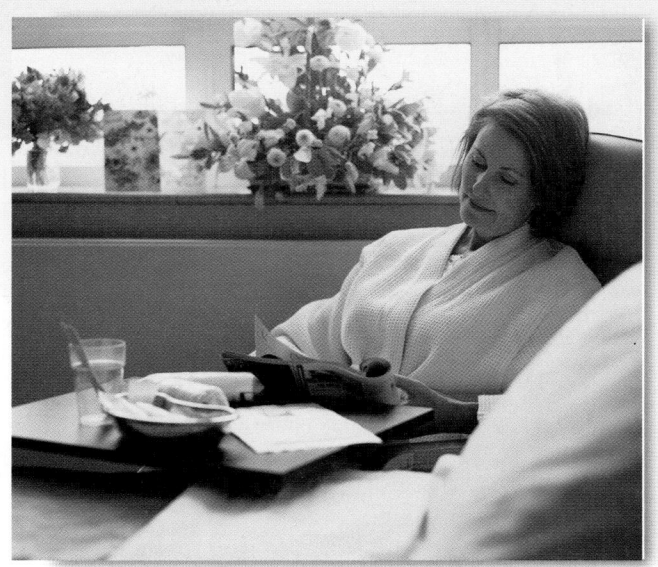

8–3 Applying the Concepts

How Much Nicotine Is in Those Cigarettes?

A tobacco company claims that its best-selling cigarettes contain at most 40 mg of nicotine. This claim is tested at the 1% significance level by using the results of 15 randomly selected cigarettes. The mean was 42.6 mg and the standard deviation was 3.7 mg. Evidence suggests that nicotine is normally distributed. Information from a computer output of the hypothesis test is listed.

Sample mean = 42.6   *P*-value = 0.008
Sample standard deviation = 3.7   Significance level = 0.01
Sample size = 15   Test statistic *t* = 2.72155
Degrees of freedom = 14   Critical value *t* = 2.62610

1. What are the degrees of freedom?
2. Is this a large or small sample test?
3. Is this a comparison of one or two samples?
4. Is this a right-tailed, left-tailed, or two-tailed test?
5. From observing the *P*-value, what would you conclude?
6. By comparing the test statistic to the critical value, what would you conclude?
7. Is there a conflict in this output? Explain.
8. What has been proved in this study?

See page 404 for the answers.

Exercises 8–3

1. In what ways is the *t* distribution similar to the standard normal distribution? In what ways is the *t* distribution different from the standard normal distribution?

2. What are the degrees of freedom for the *t* test?

3. Find the critical value (or values) for the *t* test for each.

   a. $n = 10$, $\alpha = 0.05$, right-tailed
   b. $n = 18$, $\alpha = 0.10$, two-tailed
   c. $n = 6$, $\alpha = 0.01$, left-tailed
   d. $n = 9$, $\alpha = 0.025$, right-tailed
   e. $n = 15$, $\alpha = 0.05$, two-tailed
   f. $n = 23$, $\alpha = 0.005$, left-tailed
   g. $n = 36$, $\alpha = 0.01$, right-tailed
   h. $n = 45$, $\alpha = 0.05$, two-tailed

4. Using Table F, find the *P*-value interval for each test value.

   a. $t = 2.321$, $n = 15$, right-tailed
   b. $t = 1.945$, $n = 28$, two-tailed
   c. $t = -1.267$, $n = 8$, left-tailed
   d. $t = 1.562$, $n = 17$, two-tailed
   e. $t = 3.025$, $n = 24$, right-tailed
   f. $t = -1.145$, $n = 5$, left-tailed
   g. $t = 2.179$, $n = 13$, two-tailed
   h. $t = 0.665$, $n = 10$, right-tailed

For Exercises 5 through 18, perform each of the following steps.

   a. State the hypotheses and identify the claim.
   b. Find the critical value(s).
   c. Find the test statistic.
   d. Make the decision.
   e. Summarize the results.

Use the traditional method of hypothesis testing unless otherwise specified.

Assume that the population is approximately normally distributed.

5. **Maritimes' Summer Rainfall** The average amount of rainfall reported during the summer months for the Maritime provinces is 281.5 mm. An environmental researcher believes the current average summer rainfall is different from the historical average. He selects a random sample of 10 cities in the Maritimes and determines that the mean summer rainfall was 265.2 mm. The sample standard deviation was 17.4 mm. At $\alpha = 0.05$, can it be concluded that the mean summer rainfall for the current year is different from the historical average of 281.5 mm?
   Source: Environment Canada.

6. **Provincial Park Area** A provincial minister claims that the average area of British Columbia's provincial parks is 137.6 km². An environmental group believes that the actual area is less than the reported figure. The group selects a random sample of provincial parks, and the areas, in km², are shown. At $\alpha = 0.01$, is there enough evidence to support the provincial minister's claim?

   280 32 109 68 155 205 542 6 78 49
   Source: British Columbia Ministry of the Environment.

7. **Mayors' Salaries** The average salary of mayors of Canada's cities is reported to be equal to $120,000. To test this claim, 5 Canadian cities are selected and it is found that the average salary is $132,389. Assume the population standard deviation is $12,121. Using $\alpha = 0.05$, test the claim that the reported salary is incorrect.
   Source: Calgary Herald.

8. **Work Commute Times** A survey finds that urban Canadians average 62.1 minutes commuting to and from work. A Chamber of Commerce executive claims that the average commute time in her city is less than the Canadian average commute time and she wants to publicize this. She randomly selects 25 commuters and finds the average commute time is 53.9 minutes with a standard deviation of 12.9 minutes. At $\alpha = 0.10$, test the executive's claim.
   Source: Statistics Canada.

9. **Heights of Tall Buildings** An architect designing a new office tower estimates that the average height of Canada's tallest buildings of 30 or more storeys is at least 200 metres. A random sample of 10 buildings is selected and the heights in metres are shown. At $\alpha = 0.025$, is there enough evidence to reject the claim?

   155 195 224 183 167 177 190 263 155 215
   Source: www.architecture.about.com.

10. **Condo Rental Rates** A report on Toronto's real estate market indicated that a two-bedroom condominium unit's rental rate averaged $1765 per month. A company subsidizing new employee housing selected a random sample of 15 similar rental units and found the average rent was $1924 with a standard deviation of $374. At $\alpha = 0.05$, test the claim that there is no difference in the average rents.
    Source: MLS Rental Market Report.

11. **Undergraduate Tuition Cost** The average undergraduate cost for tuition, fees, and room and board for two-year institutions last year was $13,252. The following year, a random sample of 20 two-year institutions had a mean of $15,560 and a standard deviation of $3500. Is there sufficient evidence at the $\alpha = 0.01$ level to conclude that the mean cost has increased?
    Source: The New York Times Almanac.

12. **Men's Exercise and Reading Time** On average, men spend 29 minutes per day on weekends and holidays

exercising and playing sports. They spend an average of 23 minutes per day reading. A random sample of 25 men resulted in a mean of 35 minutes exercising, with a standard deviation of 6.9 minutes, and an average of 20.5 minutes reading, with $s = 7.2$ minutes. At $\alpha = 0.05$ for both, is there sufficient evidence that these two results differ from the national means?

Source: Time magazine.

13. **Cost of Making Movies** During a recent year the average cost of making a movie was $54.8 million. This year, a random sample of 15 recent action movies had an average production cost of $62.3 million with a variance of $90.25 million. At the 0.05 level of significance, can it be concluded that it costs more than average to produce an action movie?

Source: The New York Times Almanac.

14. **Cookie Calories** An average serving of 30-gram cookies contains 150 calories. A random sample of 15 different brands of 30-gram cookies resulted in the following calorie amounts. At the $\alpha = 0.01$ level, is there sufficient evidence that the average calorie content of 30-gram cookies is greater than 150 calories?

140	165	190	200	225	165	195	185
200	140	190	180	185	160	150	

Source: Health Canada.

15. **Broadway Show Running Times** The average running time for current Broadway shows is 2 hours and 12 minutes. A producer in another city claims that the length of time of productions in his city is the same. He samples 8 shows and finds the time to be 2 hours and 5 minutes with a standard deviation of 11 minutes. Using $\alpha = 0.05$, is the producer correct?

Source: The New York Times, Arts and Leisure.

16. **Water Usage** The *National Post* reported that Canadians use an average of 329 litres of water per person per day. A researcher believes that Canadians are becoming more environmentally sensitive and that the current water consumption is less than the report claims. A random selection of 80 people found a mean water consumption of 318 litres of per day with $s = 36.5$ litres. At $\alpha = 0.01$, is there enough evidence to support the researcher's claim? Use the *P*-value method.

Source: National Post, "New Study Calls Average Water Use by Canadians 'Alarming,'" Thomas Jolicoeur, March 18, 2009.

17. **Visits to Doctor** A report by the Gallup Poll stated that on average a woman visits her physician 5.8 times a year. A researcher randomly selects 20 women and obtains these data.

3	2	1	3	7	2	9	4	6	6
8	0	5	6	4	2	1	3	4	1

At $\alpha = 0.05$ can it be concluded that the average is still 5.8 visits per year? Use the *P*-value method.

18. **Job Tenure** Statistics Canada published a study on *Changes in Job Tenure and Job Stability in Canada.* The study reported that on average workers aged 25 to 34 years worked for 4.3 years before changing jobs. To see if this average is correct, a researcher selected a sample of 8 workers aged 25 to 34 years who completed a job term. The worker job tenures (in years) are listed.

2.1	5.9	7.2	4.3	5.3	11.1	1.5	2.7

At $\alpha = 0.05$ can it be concluded that the mean job tenure for workers aged 25 to 34 years is 4.3 years? Use the *P*-value method. Give one reason why the respondents might not have given the exact number of years that they have worked.

Source: Statistics Canada.

19. **Teaching Assistant Stipends** A random sample of stipends of teaching assistants in economics is listed. Is there sufficient evidence at the $\alpha = 0.05$ level to conclude that the average stipend differs from $15,000? The stipends listed (in dollars) are for the academic year.

14,000	18,000	12,000	14,356	13,185
13,419	14,000	11,981	17,604	12,283
16,338	15,000			

Source: The Chronicle of Higher Education.

20. **Farm Family Size** The average farm family size in Canada was reported as 3.2. A random sample of farm families in a particular rural community resulted in the following family sizes.

5	4	5	4	4	3	6	4	3	3	5	2
6	3	3	2	7	4	5	2	2	2	3	5

At $\alpha = 0.05$, does the average farm family size differ from the national average?

Source: Statistics Canada, Summary Tables, "Census Families on Farms, by Family Size, by Province (2001 and 2006 Census of Agriculture and Census of Population)."

8–4 *z* Test for a Proportion

LO4

Test proportions, using the *z* test.

Many hypothesis-testing situations involve proportions. Recall from Chapter 7 that a *proportion* is the same as a percentage of the population.

These data were adapted from the book *What Canadians Think* by Darrell Bricker and John Wright (Doubleday Canada, 2005):

- 33% of Canadians feel that Newfoundlanders have the best sense of humour.
- 69% of pet owners allow their pets in bed at night.

- 57% of Albertans will barbecue all year round.
- 94% of Canadians would put their trust in a firefighter.

A hypothesis test involving a population proportion can be considered as a binomial experiment when there are only two outcomes and the probability of a success does not change from trial to trial. Recall from Section 5–3 that the mean is $\mu = np$ and the standard deviation is $\sigma = \sqrt{npq}$ for the binomial distribution.

Since a normal distribution can be used to approximate the binomial distribution when $np \geq 5$ and $nq \geq 5$, the standard normal distribution can be used to test hypotheses for proportions.

Formula for the *z* Test for Proportions

$$z = \frac{\hat{p} - p}{\sqrt{pq/n}}$$

where

$\hat{p} = \dfrac{X}{n}$ (sample proportion)

p = hypothesized population proportion

$q = 1 - p$

n = sample size

The formula is derived from the normal approximation to the binomial and follows the general formula

$$\text{Test statistic} = \frac{(\text{Observed value}) - (\text{Expected value})}{\text{Standard error}}$$

We obtain $\hat{p}$ from the sample (i.e., observed value), p is the expected value (i.e., hypothesized population proportion), and $\sqrt{pq/n}$ is the standard error.

The formula $z = \dfrac{\hat{p} - p}{\sqrt{pq/n}}$ can be derived from the formula $z = \dfrac{X - \mu}{\sigma}$ by substituting $\mu = np$ and $\sigma = \sqrt{npq}$ and then dividing both numerator and denominator by n. Some algebra is used. See Exercise 23 in this section.

Assumptions for Testing a Proportion

1. The sample is a random sample.
2. The conditions for a binomial experiment are satisfied. (See Chapter 5.)
3. Both $np \geq 5$ and $nq \geq 5$.

The steps for hypothesis testing are the same as those shown in Section 8–2. Tables E–1 and E–2 are used to find critical values and *P*-values.

Examples 8–17 to 8–19 show the traditional method of hypothesis testing. Example 8–20 illustrates the *P*-value method.

Sometimes it is necessary to find $\hat{p}$, as shown in Examples 8–17, 8–19, and 8–20, and sometimes $\hat{p}$ is given in the exercise. See Example 8–18.

Example 8–17

High School Diploma Deficiency

A Quebec adult educator estimates that 15% of adults, aged 25 to 34 years, have yet to obtain their high school diplomas. The educator surveys a random sample of 200 Quebec adults, aged 25 to 34 years, and discovers that 38 have not obtained their high school diplomas. At $\alpha = 0.05$, is there significant evidence to reject the educator's claim?

Source: Excerpt from 30 Years of Education: Canada's Language Groups, adapted from Statistics Canada, Canadian Social Trends, Catalogue 11-008, Winter 2003.

Solution

Step 1 State the hypothesis and identify the claim.

$$H_0: p = 0.15 \text{ (claim)} \quad \text{and} \quad H_1: p \neq 0.15$$

Step 2 Find the critical value. Since $\alpha = 0.05$ and the test is a two-tailed test, the critical values are $z = \pm 1.96$.

Step 3 Compute the test statistic. First, it is necessary to find $\hat{p}$.

$$\hat{p} = \frac{X}{n} = \frac{38}{200} = 0.19 \quad \text{and} \quad p = 0.15 \quad \text{and} \quad q = 1 - 0.15 = 0.85$$

Substitute the formula and solve.

$$z = \frac{\hat{p} - p}{\sqrt{pq/n}} = \frac{0.19 - 0.15}{\sqrt{(0.15)(0.85)/200}} \approx 1.584$$

Step 4 Make the decision. Do not reject the null hypothesis, since the test statistic falls outside the critical region, as shown in Figure 8–24.

Figure 8–24

Critical Values and Test Statistic for Example 8–17

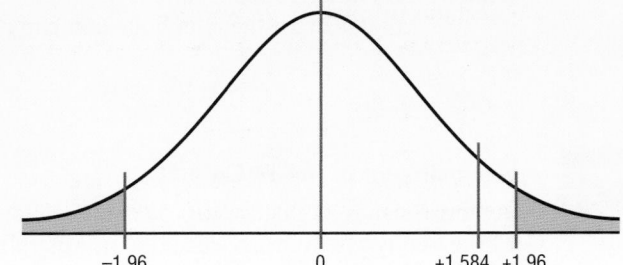

−1.96   0   +1.584 +1.96

Step 5 Summarize the results. There is not enough evidence to reject the claim that the 15% of Quebec adults, aged 25 to 34 years, have yet to obtain their high school diplomas.

Example 8–18

Call-Waiting Service Survey

A telephone company representative estimates that 40% of its customers have call-waiting service. To test this hypothesis, she selected a sample of 100 customers and found that 37% had call-waiting. At $\alpha = 0.01$, is there enough evidence to reject the claim?

Solution

Step 1 State the hypotheses and identify the claim.

$$H_0: p = 0.40 \text{ (claim)} \quad \text{and} \quad H_1: p \neq 0.40$$

Step 2 Find the critical value(s). Since $\alpha = 0.01$ and this test is two-tailed, the critical values are ± 2.575.

Step 3 Compute the test statistic. It is not necessary to find $\hat{p}$ since it is given in the exercise; $\hat{p} = 0.37$. Substitute in the formula and solve.

$$p = 0.40 \quad \text{and} \quad q = 1 - 0.40 = 0.60$$

$$z = \frac{\hat{p} - p}{\sqrt{pq/n}} = \frac{0.37 - 0.40}{\sqrt{(0.40)(0.60)/100}} = -0.612$$

Step 4 Make the decision. Do not reject the null hypothesis, since the test statistic falls in the noncritical region, as shown in Figure 8–25.

Figure 8–25

Critical Values and
Test Statistic for
Example 8–18

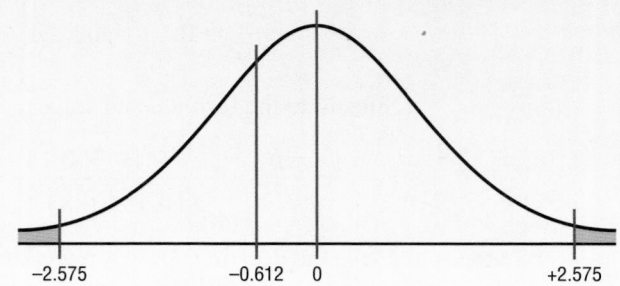

$$-2.575 \qquad -0.612 \quad 0 \qquad\qquad +2.575$$

Step 5 Summarize the results. There is not enough evidence to reject the claim that 40% of the telephone company's customers have call-waiting.

Example 8–19

Abolishment of the 1¢ Coin

A statistician read that at least 59% of Canada's population opposes the abolishment of the penny (1¢ coin) as was done in Australia and New Zealand. To see if this claim is valid, the statistician selected a random sample of 80 Canadians and found that 41 were opposed to abolishing the penny. At $\alpha = 0.01$, test the claim that at least 59% oppose the penny's abolishment.

Source: Harris Poll.

Solution

Step 1 State the hypothesis and identify the claim. (*Note:* At least infers $\geq$ and the null hypothesis assumes a state of equality; therefore the alternative is $<$.)

$$H_0: p = 0.59 \text{ (claim)} \quad \text{and} \quad H_1: p < 0.59$$

Step 2 Find the critical value. Since $\alpha = 0.01$ and the test is left-tailed test, the critical value is -2.33.

Step 3 Compute the test statistic.

$$\hat{p} = \frac{X}{n} = \frac{41}{80} = 0.5125$$

$$p = 0.59 \qquad \text{and} \qquad q = 1 - 0.59 = 0.41$$

$$z = \frac{\hat{p} - p}{\sqrt{pq/n}} = \frac{0.5125 - 0.59}{\sqrt{(0.59)(0.41)/80}} \approx -1.409$$

Step 4 Do not reject the null hypothesis, since the test statistic does not fall in the critical region, as shown in Figure 8–26.

Figure 8–26

Critical Value and
Test Statistic for
Example 8–19

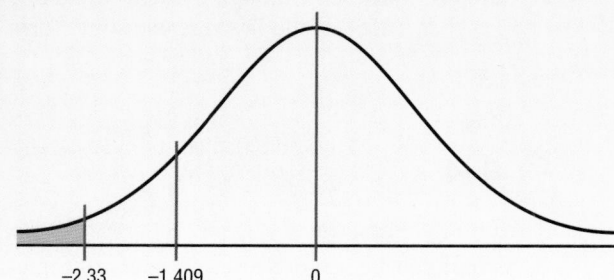

-2.33 -1.409 0

Step 5 There is not enough evidence to reject the claim that at least 59% of the population opposes the abolishment of the penny coin.

Example 8–20

Advertising by Lawyers

A lawyer claims that more than 25% of all lawyers advertise. A sample of 200 lawyers in a certain city showed that 63 had used some form of advertising. At $\alpha = 0.05$, is there enough evidence to support the lawyer's claim? Use the P-value method.

Interesting Fact

Lightning is the second most common killer among storm-related hazards. On average, 73 people are killed each year by lightning. Of people who are struck by lightning, 90% do survive; however, they usually have lasting medical problems or disabilities.

Solution

Step 1 State the hypotheses and identify the claim.

$$H_0: p = 0.25 \qquad \text{and} \qquad H_1: p > 0.25 \text{ (claim)}$$

Step 2 Compute the test statistic.

$$\hat{p} = \frac{X}{n} = \frac{63}{200} = 0.315$$

$$p = 0.25 \qquad \text{and} \qquad q = 1 - 0.25 = 0.75$$

$$z = \frac{\hat{p} - p}{\sqrt{pq/n}} = \frac{0.315 - 0.25}{\sqrt{(0.25)(0.75)/200}} \approx 2.12$$

Step 3 Find the P-value. The area under the curve for $z = 2.12$ is 0.9830. Subtracting the area from 1.000, one gets $1.000 - 0.983 = 0.0170$. The P-value is 0.0170.

Step 4 Reject the null hypothesis, since $0.0170 < 0.05$ (that is, P-value < 0.05). See Figure 8–27.

Figure 8-27

P-Value and α Value for Example 8–20

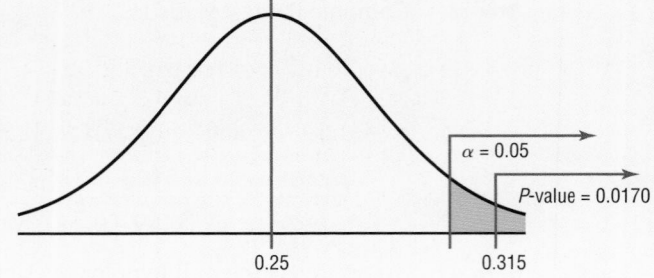

Step 5 There is enough evidence to support the attorney's claim that more than 25% of the lawyers use some form of advertising.

8-4 Applying the Concepts

Quitting Smoking

Assume you are part of a research team that compares products designed to help people quit smoking. The Condor Consumer Products Company would like more specific details about the study to be made available to the scientific community. Review the following and then answer the questions about how you would have conducted the study.

New StopSmoke

No method has been proved more effective. StopSmoke provides significant advantages to all other methods. StopSmoke is simpler to use, and it requires no weaning. StopSmoke is also significantly less expensive than the leading brands. StopSmoke's superiority has been proved in two independent studies.

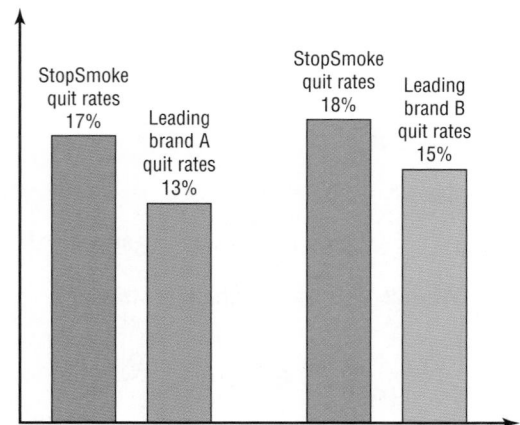

1. What were the statistical hypotheses?
2. What were the null hypotheses?
3. What were the alternative hypotheses?
4. Were any statistical tests run?
5. Were one- or two-tailed tests run?
6. What were the levels of significance?
7. If a type I error was committed, explain what it would have been.

8. If a type II error was committed, explain what it would have been.

9. What did the studies prove?

10. Two statements are made about significance. One states that StopSmoke provides significant advantages, and the other states that StopSmoke is significantly less expensive than other leading brands. Are they referring to statistical significance? What other type of significance is there?

See page 404 for the answers.

Exercises 8–4

1. Give three examples of proportions.

2. Why is a proportion considered a binomial variable?

3. When one is testing hypotheses by using proportions, what are the necessary requirements?

4. What formulas for the mean and standard deviation of a binomial distribution are used to derive the formula for the z test for proportions?

For Exercises 5 through 15, perform each of the following steps.

  a. State the hypotheses and identify the claim.
  b. Find the critical value(s).
  c. Compute the test statistic.
  d. Make the decision.
  e. Summarize the results.

Use the traditional method of hypothesis testing unless otherwise specified.

5. **Home Ownership** National census data indicate that 68.4% of heads of households report that they own their homes. A municipal real estate company wants to see if home ownership rates are the same in its city. In a random sample of 150 heads of households, 92 responded that they owned their homes. At the 0.02 level of significance, is the city household ownership rate the same as the national proportion?
Source: CBC News, "More Homeowners, Fewer Renters, StatsCan Says," June 4, 2008.

6. **RRSP Contributions** A news article stated that 38% of Canadian adults contributed to their registered retirement savings plans (RRSPs). A bank executive believes that this figure was low for his bank customers, so he surveyed 95 customers and found that 43 had contributed to their RRSPs. At $\alpha = 0.05$, do these results support the bank manager's claim that his customers contributed at a higher rate than reported in the news article?
Source: Financial Post, "Only 38% of 'Cash Strapped' Canadians Contributed to Their RRSPs This Season," Jonathan Chevreau, March 3, 2010.

7. **Computer Hobbies** It has been reported that 40% of the adult population participate in computer hobbies during their leisure time. A random sample of 180 adults found that 65 engaged in computer hobbies. At $\alpha = 0.01$, is there sufficient evidence to conclude that the proportion differs from 40%?
Source: The New York Times Almanac.

8. **Female Physicians** The Canadian Institute for Health Information (CIHI) reports that in a recent year, 33.3% of Canadian physicians were female. A regional health authority feels that its region employs a higher percentage of female physicians. In a random sample of 110 health region physicians, 45 were women. Is there sufficient evidence at the 0.05 level of significance to conclude that the proportion of women physicians in the region is higher than the 33.3% reported nationally?
Source: CIHI, Health Human Resources: Physicians.

9. **Households with Cellphones** Industry Canada reports indicated that 71% of Canadian households have cellphones for personal use. A mobile communication service wants to test this claim in a new city earmarked for expansion. A survey of 250 households shows that 189 have cellphones. At $\alpha = 0.05$, does the new city have the same proportion as the Industry Canada report?
Source: Industry Canada, Canada's Office of Consumer Affairs, Cellphone Services—Recent Consumer Trends, 2006.

10. **Performing Arts Attendance** The Canada Council reported that 35% of adults attended a Canadian performing arts performance in the past year. To test this claim, a researcher surveyed 90 people and found that 40 people had attended a performance in the past year. At $\alpha = 0.05$, test the claim that this figure is correct.
Source: Canada Council.

11. **Fatalities Involving Motorcyclists** A published report claims that 7.3% of vehicle fatalities involve motorcyclists. An insurance investigator studies 50 randomly selected accidents and finds that 4 fatalities implicated motorcyclists. Using $\alpha = 0.05$, can the report be disproved?
Source: Transport Canada.

12. **Exercise to Reduce Stress** A report on the Web site *Women's Health Matters* claims that 26% of Canadian women exercise regularly as a way to reduce stress. In

order to test the claim, a random sample of 100 women was taken and 21 indicated that exercise was used to relieve stress. Use $\alpha = 0.10$ and the P-value method. Could the results be generalized to all Canadian women?

13. Food Bank Usage The Canadian Association of Food Banks (CAFB) claims that 13.3% of food bank users have jobs. To test the claim a random sample of 60 patrons at food banks were surveyed and 10 had jobs. Use $\alpha = 0.01$ and the P-value method. On the basis of the results, would you agree with CAFB's claim?
Source: CAFB, *HungerCount 2004.*

14. Natural Gas Heating Statistics Canada reports that 50.1% of homes in Canada were heated by natural gas. A random sample of 200 homes found that 111 were heated by natural gas. Does the evidence support the claim, or has the percentage changed? Use $\alpha = 0.05$ and the P-value method.
Source: Statistics Canada.

15. Youth Smoking Researchers suspect that 18% of all high school students smoke at least one pack of cigarettes a day. At Wilson High School, with an enrollment of 300 students, a study found that 50 students smoked at least one pack of cigarettes a day. At $\alpha = 0.05$, test the claim that 18% of all high school students smoke at least one pack of cigarettes a day. Use the P-value method.

16. Public Transit Ridership A census report on public transportation stated that Ottawa–Gatineau public transit ridership was at 19.4% of the employed labour force. A civic official claims that transit ridership has increased since the census was taken. A survey of 150 workers confirmed that 38 used public transit. At $\alpha = 0.05$, test the civic official's claim.
Source: Statistics Canada, *Canada Year Book,* "Transportation," Chart 30.4, 2008.

17. Library Book Borrowing For Canadians using library services, a national survey by Canadian Heritage claims that 44% borrow books. A library director feels that this is not true so he randomly selects 100 library service users and finds that 59 borrowed library books. Can he show that the Canadian Heritage survey is incorrect? Use $\alpha = 0.05$.
Source: Canadian Heritage, *Reading and Buying Books for Pleasure.*

18. Ph.D. Teaching Assistantships In a survey of earned doctorates in Canadian universities, 64% of respondents indicated that paid teaching assistantships aided in financing their studies. A university dean feels that this figure is high for her province. A random sample of 50 Ph.D. students finds that 27 have assistantships. At $\alpha = 0.05$, is the dean correct?
Source: Statistics Canada.

19. Firearm-Related Fatalities A gun control advocacy study published research indicating that firearm-related fatalities account for 10% of all injury deaths in the province. Believing this figure to be high, a researcher selects a random sample of 37 injury deaths and discovers that 3 deaths were firearm-related. Is the researcher's claim correct, at $\alpha = 0.05$?
Source: Alberta Centre for Injury Control & Research, *Firearm Deaths and Injuries.*

20. Online Learning The 2008 *Canada Year Book* states that 26% of Canadians use the Internet at home for education, training, or school work. A Ministry of Education researcher feels that her province has a higher online learning participation rate. A random sample of 75 Internet users reveals that 27 search the Web for educational purposes. At $\alpha = 0.01$, is there enough evidence to support the researcher's claim. Would the results change at $\alpha = 0.05$?
Source: Statistics Canada, Catalogue No. 81-004-XIE.

Extending the Concepts >>

When np or nq is not 5 or more, the binomial table (Table B in Appendix C) must be used to find critical values in hypothesis tests involving proportions.

21. Coin-Tossing Experiment A coin is tossed 9 times and 3 heads appear. Can one conclude that the coin is not balanced? Use $\alpha = 0.10$. [*Hint:* Use the binomial table and find $2P(X \leq 3)$ with $p = 0.5$ and $n = 9$.]

22. First-Class Airline Passengers In the past, 20% of all airline passengers flew first class. In a sample of 15 passengers, 5 flew first class. At $\alpha = 0.10$, can one conclude that the proportions have changed?

23. Show that $z = \dfrac{\hat{p} - p}{\sqrt{pq/n}}$ can be derived from $z = \dfrac{X - \mu}{\sigma}$ by substituting $\mu = np$ and $\sigma = \sqrt{npq}$ and dividing both numerator and denominator by n.

8–5 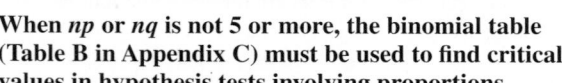 χ^2 Test for a Variance or Standard Deviation >

Test variances or standard deviations, using the chi-square test.

In Chapter 7, the chi-square distribution was used to construct a confidence interval for a single variance or standard deviation. This distribution is also used to test a claim about a single variance or standard deviation.

To find the area under the chi-square distribution, use Table G in Appendix C. There are three cases to consider:

1. Finding the chi-square critical value for a specific α when the hypothesis test is right-tailed.
2. Finding the chi-square critical value for a specific α when the hypothesis test is left-tailed.
3. Finding the chi-square critical values for a specific α when the hypothesis test is two-tailed.

Example 8–21

Find the critical chi-square value for 15 degrees of freedom when $\alpha = 0.05$ and the test is right-tailed.

Solution

The distribution is shown in Figure 8–28.

Figure 8–28

Chi-Square Distribution for Example 8–21

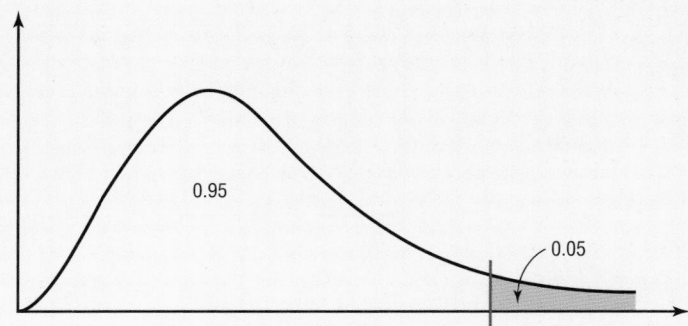

Find the α value at the top of Table G, and find the corresponding degrees of freedom in the left column. The critical value is located where the two columns meet—in this case, 24.996. See Figure 8–29.

Figure 8–29

Locating the Critical Value in Table G for Example 8–21

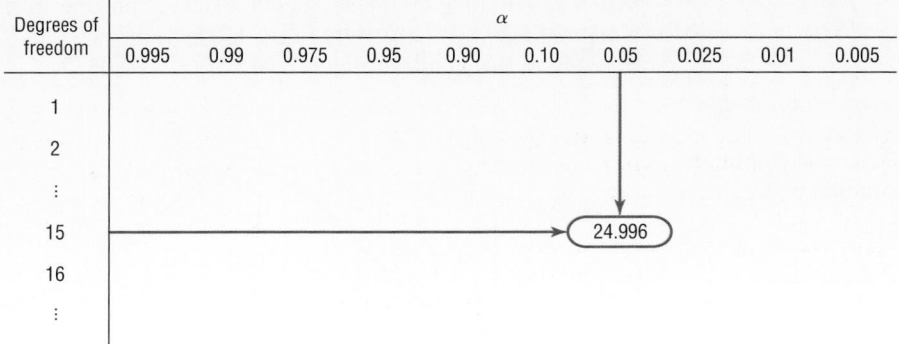

Example 8–22

Find the critical chi-square value for 10 degrees of freedom when $\alpha = 0.05$ and the test is left-tailed.

Solution

This distribution is shown in Figure 8–30.

Figure 8–30

Chi-Square Distribution for Example 8–22

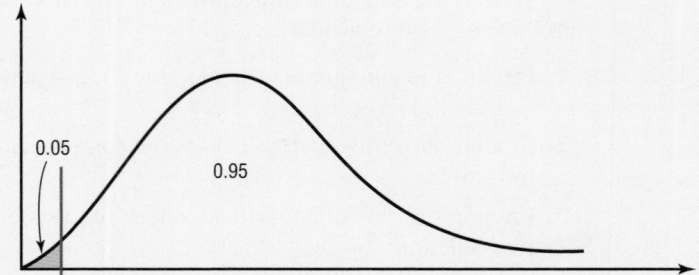

When the test is left-tailed, the α value must be subtracted from 1, that is, $1 - 0.05 = 0.95$. The left side of the table is used, because the chi-square table gives the area to the right of the critical value, and the chi-square statistic cannot be negative. The table is set up so that it gives the values for the area to the right of the critical value. In this case, 95% of the area will be to the right of the value.

For 0.95 and 10 degrees of freedom, the critical value is 3.940. See Figure 8–31.

Figure 8–31

Locating the Critical Value in Table G for Example 8–22

Degrees of freedom					α					
	0.995	0.99	0.975	0.95	0.90	0.10	0.05	0.025	0.01	0.005
1										
2										
⋮										
10				3.940						
⋮										

Example 8–23

Find the critical chi-square values for 22 degrees of freedom when $\alpha = 0.05$ and a two-tailed test is conducted.

Solution

When a two-tailed test is conducted, the area must be split, as shown in Figure 8–32. Note that the area to the right of the larger value is 0.025 (0.05/2), and the area to the right of the smaller value is 0.975 (1.00 − 0.05/2).

Figure 8–32

Chi-Square Distribution for Example 8–23

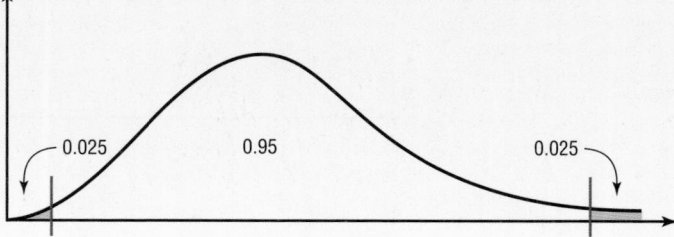

Remember that chi-square values cannot be negative. Hence, one must use α values in the table of 0.025 and 0.975. With 22 degrees of freedom, the critical values are 36.781 and 10.982, respectively.

After the degrees of freedom reach 30, Table G gives values only for multiples of 10 (40, 50, 60, etc.). When the exact degrees of freedom one is seeking are not specified in the table, the closest smaller value should be used. For example, if the given degrees of freedom are 36, use the table value for 30 degrees of freedom. This guideline keeps the type I error equal to or below the α value.

When one is testing a claim about a single variance using the **chi-square test**, there are three possible test situations: right-tailed test, left-tailed test, and two-tailed test.

If a researcher believes the variance of a population to be greater than some specific value, say, 225, then the researcher states the hypotheses as

$$H_0: \sigma^2 = 225 \qquad \text{and} \qquad H_1: \sigma^2 > 225$$

and conducts a right-tailed test.

If the researcher believes the variance of a population to be less than 225, then the researcher states the hypotheses as

$$H_0: \sigma^2 = 225 \qquad \text{and} \qquad H_1: \sigma^2 < 225$$

and conducts a left-tailed test.

Finally, if a researcher does not wish to specify a direction, he or she states the hypotheses as

$$H_0: \sigma^2 = 225 \qquad \text{and} \qquad H_1: \sigma^2 \neq 225$$

and conducts a two-tailed test.

Formula for the Chi-Square Test for a Single Variance

$$\chi^2 = \frac{(n-1)s^2}{\sigma^2}$$

with degrees of freedom equal to $n - 1$ and where

n = sample size
s^2 = sample variance
σ^2 = hypothesized population variance

One might ask, Why is it important to test variances? There are several reasons. First, in any situation where consistency is required, such as in manufacturing, one would like to have the smallest variation possible in the products. For example, when bolts are manufactured, the variation in diameters due to the process must be kept to a minimum, or the nuts will not fit them properly. In education, consistency is required on a test. That is, if the same students take the same test several times, they should get approximately the same grades, and the variance of each of the student's grades should be small. On the other hand, if the test is to be used to judge learning, the overall standard deviation of all the grades should be large so that one can differentiate those who have learned the subject from those who have not learned it.

Three assumptions are made for the chi-square test, as outlined here.

Interesting Fact

2% of Canada's farms account for 35% of gross farm receipts.

Assumptions for the Chi-Square Test for a Single Variance

1. The sample must be randomly selected from the population.
2. The population must be normally distributed for the variable under study.
3. The observations must be independent of one another.

The traditional method for hypothesis testing follows the same five steps listed earlier. They are repeated here.

Step 1   State the hypotheses and identify the claim.

Step 2   Find the critical value(s).

Step 3 Compute the test statistic.

Step 4 Make the decision.

Step 5 Summarize the results.

Examples 8–24 through 8–26 illustrate the traditional hypothesis-testing procedure for variances.

Example 8–24

Variation of Test Scores

An instructor wishes to see whether the variation in scores of the 23 students in her class is less than the variance of the population. The variance of the class is 198. Is there enough evidence to support the claim that the variation of the students is less than the population variance ($\sigma^2 = 225$) at $\alpha = 0.05$? Assume that the scores are normally distributed.

Solution

Step 1 State the hypotheses and identify the claim.

$$H_0: \sigma^2 = 225 \qquad \text{and} \qquad H_1: \sigma^2 < 225 \,(\text{claim})$$

Step 2 Find the critical value. Since this test is left-tailed and $\alpha = 0.05$, use the value $1 - 0.05 = 0.95$. The degrees of freedom are $n - 1 = 23 - 1 = 22$. Hence, the critical value is 12.338. Note that the critical region is on the left, as shown in Figure 8–33.

Figure 8–33

Critical Value for Example 8–24

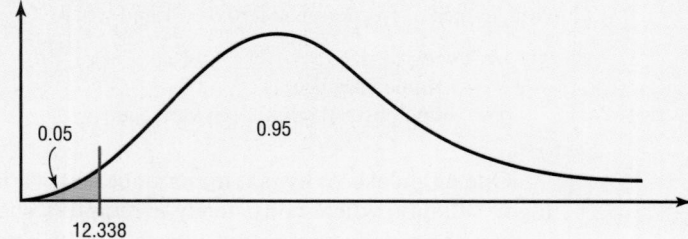

Step 3 Compute the test statistic.

$$\chi^2 = \frac{(n - 1)s^2}{\sigma^2} = \frac{(23 - 1)(198)}{225} = 19.36$$

Step 4 Make the decision. Since the test statistic, 19.36, falls in the noncritical region, as shown in Figure 8–34, the decision is to not reject the null hypothesis.

Figure 8–34

Critical Value and Test Statistic for Example 8–24

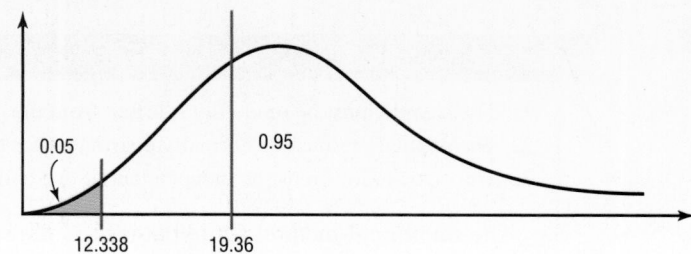

Step 5 Summarize the results. There is not enough evidence to support the claim that the variation in test scores of the instructor's students is less than the variation in scores of the population.

Example 8–25

Outpatient Surgery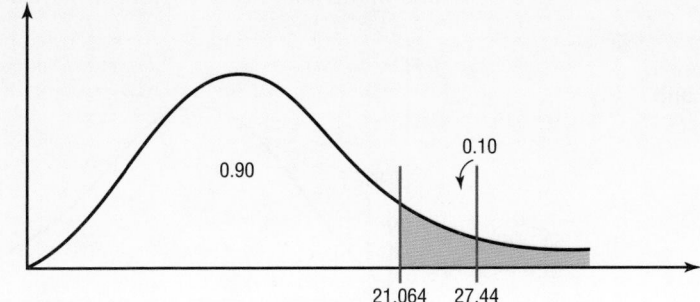

A hospital administrator believes that the standard deviation of the number of people using outpatient surgery per day is greater than 8. A random sample of 15 days is selected. The data are shown. At $\alpha = 0.10$, is there enough evidence to support the administrator's claim? Assume the variable is normally distributed.

25	30	5	15	18
42	16	9	10	12
12	38	8	14	27

Solution

Step 1   State the hypotheses and identify the claim.

$$H_0: \sigma^2 = 64 \qquad \text{and} \qquad H_1: \sigma^2 > 64 \text{ (claim)}$$

Since the standard deviation is given, it should be squared to get the variance.

Step 2   Find the critical statistic. Since this test is right-tailed with d.f. of $15 - 1 = 14$ and $\alpha = 0.10$, the critical value is 21.064.

Step 3   Compute the test value. Since raw data are given, the standard deviation of the sample must be found by using the formula in Chapter 3 or your calculator. It is $s = 11.2$.

$$\chi^2 = \frac{(n-1)s^2}{\sigma^2} = \frac{(15-1)(11.2)^2}{64} = 27.44$$

Step 4   Make the decision. The decision is to reject the null hypothesis since the test statistic, 27.44, is greater than the critical value, 21.064, and falls in the critical region. See Figure 8–35.

Figure 8–35

Critical Value and Test Statistic for Example 8–25

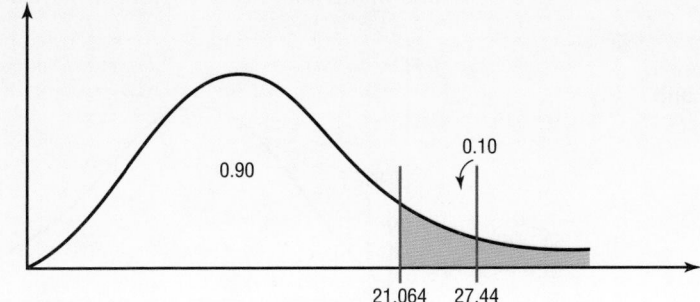

Step 5   Summarize the results. There is enough evidence to support the claim that the standard deviation is greater than 8.

Example 8–26

Nicotine Content of Cigarettes

A cigarette manufacturer wants to test the claim that the variance of the nicotine content of its cigarettes is 0.644. Nicotine content is measured in milligrams, and assume that it is normally distributed. A sample of 20 cigarettes has a standard deviation of 1.00 milligram. At $\alpha = 0.05$, is there enough evidence to reject the manufacturer's claim?

Solution

Step 1   State the hypotheses and identify the claim.

$$H_0: \sigma^2 = 0.644 \text{ (claim)} \quad \text{and} \quad H_1: \sigma^2 \neq 0.644$$

Step 2   Find the critical values. Since this test is a two-tailed test at $\alpha = 0.05$, the critical values for 0.025 and 0.975 must be found. The degrees of freedom are 19; hence, the critical values are 32.852 and 8.907, respectively. The critical or rejection regions are shown in Figure 8–36.

Figure 8–36

Critical Values for Example 8–26

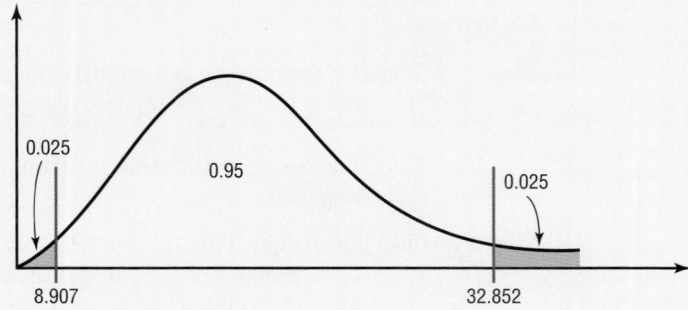

Step 3   Compute the test statistic.

$$\chi^2 = \frac{(n-1)s^2}{\sigma^2} = \frac{(20-1)(1.0)^2}{0.644} \approx 29.503$$

Since the standard deviation s is given in the problem, it must be squared for the formula.

Step 4   Make the decision. Do not reject the null hypothesis, since the test statistic falls between the critical values ($8.907 < 29.503 < 32.852$) and in the noncritical region, as shown in Figure 8–37.

Figure 8–37

Critical Values and Test Statistic for Example 8–26

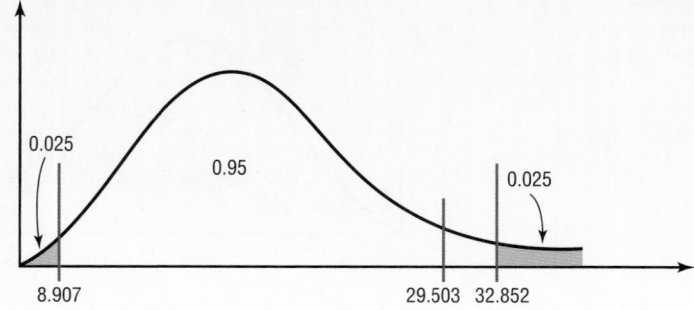

Step 5   Summarize the results. There is not enough evidence to reject the manufacturer's claim that the variance of the nicotine content of the cigarettes is equal to 0.644.

Approximate *P*-values for the chi-square test can be found by using Table G in Appendix C. The procedure is somewhat more complicated than the previous procedures for finding *P*-values for the *z* and *t* tests since the chi-square distribution is not exactly symmetric and χ^2 values cannot be negative. As we did for the *t* test, we will determine an *interval* for the *P*-value based on the table. Examples 8–27 through 8–29 show the procedure.

Example 8–27

Find the P-value when $\chi^2 = 19.274$, $n = 8$, and the test is right-tailed.

Solution

To get the P-value, look across the row with d.f. $= 7$ in Table G and find the two values that 19.274 falls between. They are 18.475 and 20.278. Look up to the top row and find the α values corresponding to 18.475 and 20.278. They are 0.01 and 0.005, respectively. See Figure 8–38. Hence the P-value is contained in the interval $0.005 < P\text{-value} < 0.01$. (The P-value obtained from a calculator is 0.007.)

Figure 8–38

P-Value Interval for Example 8–27

Degrees of freedom	α									
	0.995	0.99	0.975	0.95	0.90	0.10	0.05	0.025	0.01	0.005
1	—	—	0.001	0.004	0.016	2.706	3.841	5.024	6.635	7.879
2	0.010	0.020	0.051	0.103	0.211	4.605	5.991	7.378	9.210	10.597
3	0.072	0.115	0.216	0.352	0.584	6.251	7.815	9.348	11.345	12.838
4	0.207	0.297	0.484	0.711	1.064	7.779	9.488	11.143	13.277	14.860
5	0.412	0.554	0.831	1.145	1.610	9.236	11.071	12.833	15.086	16.750
6	0.676	0.872	1.237	1.635	2.204	10.645	12.592	14.449	16.812	18.548
7	0.989	1.239	1.690	2.167	2.833	12.017	11.067	16.013	18.475	20.278
8	1.344	1.646	2.180	2.733	3.490	13.362	15.507	17.535	20.090	21.955
9	1.735	2.088	2.700	3.325	4.168	14.684	16.919	19.023	21.666	23.589
10	2.156	2.558	3.247	3.940	4.865	15.987	18.307	20.483	23.209	25.188
$\vdots$	$\vdots$	$\vdots$	$\vdots$	$\vdots$	$\vdots$	$\vdots$	$\vdots$	$\vdots$	$\vdots$	$\vdots$
100	67.328	70.065	74.222	77.929	82.358	118.498	124.342	129.561	135.807	140.169

*19.274 falls between 18.475 and 20.278.

Example 8–28

Find the P-value when $\chi^2 = 3.823$, $n = 13$, and the test is left-tailed.

Solution

To get the P-value, look across the row with d.f. $= 12$ and find the two values that 3.823 falls between. They are 3.571 and 4.404. Look up to the top row and find the values corresponding to 3.571 and 4.404. They are 0.99 and 0.975, respectively. When the χ^2 test value falls on the left side, each of the values must be subtracted from 1 to get the interval that P-value falls between.

$$1 - 0.99 = 0.01 \qquad \text{and} \qquad 1 - 0.975 = 0.025$$

Hence the P-value falls in the interval

$$0.01 < P\text{-value} < 0.025$$

(The P-value obtained from a calculator is 0.014.)

When the χ^2 test is two-tailed, both interval values must be doubled. If a two-tailed test was being used in Example 8–28, then the interval would be $2(0.01) < P\text{-value} < 2(0.025)$, or $0.02 < P\text{-value} < 0.05$.

The P-value method for hypothesis testing for a variance or standard deviation follows the same steps shown in the preceding sections.

Step 1   State the hypotheses and identify the claim.

Step 2   Compute the test statistic.

Step 3   Find the P-value.

Step 4   Make the decision.

Step 5   Summarize the results.

Example 8–29 shows the P-value method for variances or standard deviations.

Example 8–29

Car Inspection Times

A researcher knows from past studies that the standard deviation of the time it takes to inspect a car is 16.8 minutes. A sample of 24 cars is selected and inspected. The standard deviation was 12.5 minutes. At $\alpha = 0.05$, can it be concluded that the standard deviation has changed? Use the P-value method.

Solution

Step 1   State the hypotheses and identify the claim.

$$H_0: \sigma = 16.8 \qquad \text{and} \qquad H_1: \sigma \neq 16.8 \ (\text{claim})$$

Step 2   Compute the test statistic.

$$\chi^2 = \frac{(n-1)s^2}{\sigma^2} = \frac{(24-1)(12.5)^2}{(16.8)^2} \approx 12.733$$

Step 3   Find the P-value. Using Table G with d.f. = 23, the value 12.733 falls between 11.689 and 13.091, corresponding to 0.975 and 0.95, respectively. Since these values are found on the left side of the distribution, each value must be subtracted from 1. Hence $1 - 0.975 = 0.025$ and $1 - 0.95 = 0.05$. Since this is a two-tailed test, the area must be doubled to obtain the P-value interval. Hence $0.05 < P\text{-value} < 0.10$, or somewhere between 0.05 and 0.10. (The P-value obtained from a calculator is 0.085.)

Step 4   Make the decision. Since $\alpha = 0.05$ and the P-value is between 0.05 and 0.10, the decision is to not reject the null hypothesis since $P\text{-value} > \alpha$.

Step 5   Summarize the results. There is not enough evidence to support the claim that the standard deviation has changed.

8–5   Applying the Concepts

Testing Fuel Consumption Claims

Assume that you are working for the Office of Consumer Affairs and have recently been getting complaints about the highway fuel consumption of the new Dodge Caravan. Chrysler Corporation agrees to allow you to select at random 40 of its new Dodge Caravans to test the highway gas consumption. Chrysler claims that the Caravans consume 9.6 L/100 km. Your results show a mean fuel consumption of 10.1 L/100 km and a standard deviation 1.5. You support Chrysler's claim.

Source: Natural Resources Canada, Office of Energy Efficiency, *Fuel Consumption Guide, 2007*. Reproduced with the permission of the Minister of Public Works and Government Services Canada, courtesy of the Department of Natural Resources Canada, 2007.

1. Show why you support Chrysler's claim by listing the P-value from your output. After more complaints, you decide to test the variability of the L/100 km on the highway. From further questioning of Chrysler's quality control engineers, you find they are claiming a standard deviation of 0.5 L/100 km.

2. Test the claim about the standard deviation.

3. Write a short summary of your results and any necessary action that Chrysler must take to remedy customer complaints.

4. State your position about the necessity to perform tests of variability along with tests of the means.

See page 405 for the answers.

Exercises 8–5

1. Using Table G, find the critical value(s) for each, show the critical and noncritical regions, and state the appropriate null and alternative hypotheses. Use $\sigma^2 = 225$.

   a. $\alpha = 0.05$, $n = 18$, right-tailed
   b. $\alpha = 0.10$, $n = 23$, left-tailed
   c. $\alpha = 0.05$, $n = 15$, two-tailed
   d. $\alpha = 0.10$, $n = 8$, two-tailed
   e. $\alpha = 0.01$, $n = 17$, right-tailed
   f. $\alpha = 0.025$, $n = 20$, left-tailed
   g. $\alpha = 0.01$, $n = 13$, two-tailed
   h. $\alpha = 0.025$, $n = 29$, left-tailed

2. Using Table G, find the P-value interval for each χ^2 test value.

   a. $\chi^2 = 29.321$, $n = 16$, right-tailed
   b. $\chi^2 = 10.215$, $n = 25$, left-tailed
   c. $\chi^2 = 24.672$, $n = 11$, two-tailed
   d. $\chi^2 = 23.722$, $n = 9$, right-tailed
   e. $\chi^2 = 13.974$, $n = 28$, two-tailed
   f. $\chi^2 = 10.571$, $n = 19$, left-tailed
   g. $\chi^2 = 12.144$, $n = 6$, two-tailed
   h. $\chi^2 = 8.201$, $n = 23$, two-tailed

For Exercises 3 through 9, assume that the variables are normally or approximately normally distributed. Use the traditional method of hypothesis testing unless otherwise specified.

3. **Calories in Pancake Syrup** A nutritionist claims that the standard deviation of the number of calories in 15 millilitres of the major brands of pancake syrup is 60. A sample of major brands of syrup is selected, and the number of calories is shown. At $\alpha = 0.10$, can the claim be rejected?

53	210	100	200	100	220
210	100	240	200	100	210
100	210	100	210	100	60

   Source: Based on information from *The Complete Book of Food Counts* by Corrine T. Netzer, Dell Publishers, New York.

4. **Forest Fires** A researcher claims that the standard deviation of the number of yearly forest fires in Canada is greater than 400. For a 15-year period, the standard deviation of the number of forest fires in Canada is 403. Test the claim at $\alpha = 0.01$. What factor would influence the variation of the number of forest fires that occurred in Canada?

   Source: National Forestry Database Program.

5. **Motor Vehicle Theft Rate** Test the claim that the standard deviation of the motor vehicle theft rate per year in Canada is less than 500 if a sample of 21 years had a standard deviation of 448.9. Theft rates are expressed per 100,000 population. Use $\alpha = 0.05$.

   Source: Statistics Canada, *Juristat.*

6. **CFL Player Weights** A random sample of weights (in kilograms) of Canadian Football League (CFL) players is listed. At $\alpha = 0.05$, is there sufficient evidence that the variance of all football players in the CFL is less than 500?

90.7	78	104.8	126.6
101.2	79.4	136.1	95.3
78.9	93.0	133.8	122.5
96.2	92.5	136.1	133.8

   Source: Canadian Football League.

7. **Transferring Phone Calls** The manager of a large company claims that the standard deviation of the time (in minutes) that it takes a telephone call to be transferred to the correct office in her company is 1.2 minutes or less. A sample of 15 calls is selected, and the calls are timed. The standard deviation of the sample is 1.8 minutes. At $\alpha = 0.01$, test the claim that the standard deviation is less than or equal to 1.2 minutes. Use the P-value method.

8. **Soda Bottle Contents** A machine fills 355-millilitre (mL) bottles with soda. For the machine to function properly, the standard deviation must be less than or equal to 0.9 mL. A sample of 8 bottles is selected, and the number of millilitres of soda in each bottle is given. At $\alpha = 0.05$, can we reject the claim that the machine is functioning properly? Use the P-value method.

355.8	357.8	355.5	354.3
325.3	356.4	354.0	354.6

9. **Calories in Doughnuts** A random sample of 20 different kinds of doughnuts had the following calorie counts. At $\alpha = 0.01$, is there sufficient evidence to conclude that the standard deviation is greater than 20 calories?

290	320	260	220	300	310	310	270	250	230
270	260	310	200	250	250	270	210	260	300

   Source: The Doctor's Pocket Calorie, Fat, and Carbohydrate Counter.

10. **Record High Temperatures** The highest temperatures (°C) on record for randomly selected days in July in Toronto are listed.

36.7   39.4   37.2   40.6   35.4   35.0   35.6

At $\alpha = 0.05$, is there sufficient evidence to conclude that the standard deviation for high temperatures is less than 2.5°C?

Source: Environment Canada.

11. **Fire Deaths** A researcher claims that the standard deviation of the number of deaths annually from fires in Canada is less than 150. If a sample of 11 randomly selected years had a standard deviation of 147.5, is the claim believable? Use $\alpha = 0.05$.

Source: Council of Canadian Fire Marshals and Fire Commissioners.

12. **Speeding Tickets** A survey by the City of Chilliwack in British Columbia indicated that almost one-half of motorists would agree to speeding tickets of vehicles over 5 kilometres per hour (km/h) over the posted 30 km/h. Assume that 5 km/h is claimed to be the standard deviation of driver speeds. A speed watch is established in a 30 km/h zone. The standard deviation of 50 vehicles through the zone is 7 km/h. Test the 5 km/h claim at $\alpha = 0.05$.

Source: City of Chilliwack Web site.

13. **Home Run Totals** A random sample of home run totals for Major League Baseball's National League Home Run Champions from 1938 to 2001 is shown. At the 0.05 level of significance, is there sufficient evidence to conclude that the variance is greater than 25?

34	47	43	23	36	50	42
44	43	40	39	41	47	45

Source: The New York Times Almanac.

14. **French Fry Fat Content** Are some fast-food restaurants healthier than others? The number of grams of fat in a regular serving of French fries for a random sample of restaurants is shown. Is there sufficient evidence to conclude that the standard deviation exceeds 4 grams of fat? Use $\alpha = 0.05$.

15	13	15	22	13	21	10	20
10	17	11	17	15	18	24	18

Source: The Doctor's Pocket Calorie, Fat, and Carbohydrate Counter.

15. **Volcano Heights** A sample of heights (in metres) of active volcanoes in the United States, outside of Alaska, is listed below. Is there sufficient evidence that the standard deviation in heights of volcanoes outside Alaska is less than the standard deviation in heights of Alaskan volcanoes, which is 727.2 metres? Use $\alpha = 0.05$.

3284.8   2486.9   3426.0   3187.0
4316.9   2549.0

Source: Time Almanac.

16. **Manufactured Machine Parts** A manufacturing process produces machine parts, the measurements of which must have a standard deviation of no more than 0.52 mm. A random sample of 20 parts in a given lot revealed a standard deviation in measurement of 0.568 mm. Is there sufficient evidence at $\alpha = 0.05$ to conclude that the standard deviation of the parts is outside the required guidelines?

8–6 Additional Topics Regarding Hypothesis Testing ❯

LO6

Test hypotheses, using confidence intervals, and explain type II errors and the power of a test.

In hypothesis testing, several other concepts might be of interest to students in elementary statistics. These topics include the relationship between hypothesis testing and confidence intervals, and some additional information about the type II error.

Confidence Intervals and Hypothesis Testing

There is a relationship between confidence intervals and two-tailed hypothesis testing. When the null hypothesis is rejected in a hypothesis-testing situation, the confidence interval for the mean using the same level of significance *will not* contain the hypothesized mean. Likewise, when the null hypothesis is not rejected, the confidence interval computed using the same level of significance *will* contain the hypothesized mean. Examples 8–30 and 8–31 show this concept for two-tailed tests.

Example 8–30

Sugar Production

Sugar is packed in 2-kg bags. An inspector suspects the bags may not contain 2 kg. A sample of 50 bags produces a mean of 1.85 kg. Assume a population standard deviation of 0.3 kg. Is there enough evidence to conclude that the bags do not contain 2 kg as stated at $\alpha = 0.05$? Also, find the 95% confidence interval of the true mean.

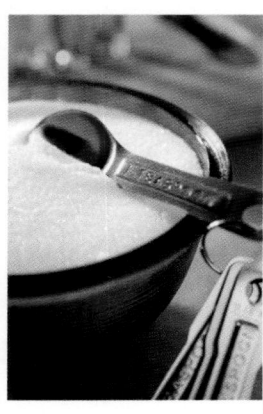

Solution

Now H_0: $\mu = 2$ and H_1: $\mu \neq 2$ (claim). The critical values are $+1.96$ and -1.96. The test statistic is

$$z = \frac{\overline{X} - \mu}{\sigma/\sqrt{n}} = \frac{1.85 - 2}{0.3/\sqrt{50}} \approx -3.54$$

Since $-3.54 < -1.96$, the null hypothesis is rejected. There is enough evidence to support the claim that the bags do not weigh 2 kilograms.

The 95% confidence for the mean is given by

$$\overline{X} - z_{\alpha/2}\frac{\sigma}{\sqrt{n}} < \mu < \overline{X} + z_{\alpha/2}\frac{\sigma}{\sqrt{n}}$$

$$1.85 - 1.96\frac{0.3}{\sqrt{50}} < \mu < 1.85 + 1.96\frac{0.3}{\sqrt{50}}$$

$$1.77 < \mu < 1.93$$

Notice that the 95% confidence interval of μ does *not* contain the hypothesized value $\mu = 2$. As expected, the hypothesis test and the confidence interval are in agreement.

Example 8–31

Hog Weights

A researcher claims that adult hogs fed a special diet will have an average weight of 91 kilograms. A sample of 10 hogs has an average weight of 90.2 kilograms and a standard deviation of 1.5 kilograms. At $\alpha = 0.05$, can the claim be rejected? Also, find the 95% confidence interval of the true mean. Assume the population is approximately normally distributed.

Solution

Now H_0: $\mu = 91$ kilograms (claim) and H_1: $\mu \neq 91$ kilograms. The t test must be used since σ is unknown. The critical values for two-tails at $\alpha = 0.05$ with 9 degrees of freedom are -2.262 and $+2.262$. The test statistic is

$$t = \frac{\overline{X} - \mu}{s/\sqrt{n}} = \frac{90.2 - 91}{1.5/\sqrt{10}} \approx -1.687$$

Thus, the null hypothesis is not rejected. There is not enough evidence to reject the claim that the weight of the adult hogs is 91 kilograms.

The 95% confidence for the mean is given by

$$\overline{X} - t_{\alpha/2}\frac{s}{\sqrt{n}} < \mu < \overline{X} + t_{\alpha/2}\frac{s}{\sqrt{n}}$$

$$90.2 - (2.262)\left(\frac{1.5}{\sqrt{10}}\right) < \mu < 90.2 + (2.262)\left(\frac{1.5}{\sqrt{10}}\right)$$

$$89.1 < \mu < 91.3$$

The 95% confidence interval does contain the hypothesized mean $\mu = 91$. Again there is agreement between the hypothesis test and the confidence interval.

In summary, then, when the null hypothesis is rejected, the confidence interval computed at the same significance level will not contain the value of the mean that is stated in the null hypothesis. On the other hand, when the null hypothesis is not rejected, the confidence interval computed at the same significance level will contain the value of the mean stated in the null hypothesis. These results are true for other hypothesis-testing situations and are not limited to means tests.

The relationship between confidence intervals and hypothesis testing presented here is valid for two-tailed tests. The relationship between one-tailed hypothesis tests and one-sided or one-tailed confidence intervals is also valid; however, this technique is beyond the scope of this textbook.

Hypothesis-Testing Errors and the Power of a Test

Recall that in hypothesis-testing scenarios, there are four possible outcomes. Two of the outcomes are correct decisions (i.e., reject a false hypothesis and do not reject a true hypothesis) and two of the outcomes represent errors (i.e., reject a true hypothesis and do not reject a false hypothesis).

A **type I error,** α, is when H_0 is true and is rejected.

A **type II error,** β, is when H_0 is false and is not rejected.

The **power of a test,** $1 - \beta$, is the probability of rejecting a false hypothesis.

The researcher determines a type I error by assigning an acceptable level of significance, such as $\alpha = 0.01$ or 0.05. The type II error relies on additional information besides α, including the sample size, standard deviation, and both the hypothesized and true population parameter. Unfortunately, the true population parameter is unknown and therefore must be estimated. Subsequently, a type II error is typically calculated for many possible true population parameters. The procedure shown below is performed after a formal hypothesis test, using any method, and illustrates how to calculate the power of a test, including the type II error calculation. *Note:* The procedure is similar for a left-tail or two-tail hypothesis test as well as a z test for proportions (*not shown*). Refer to Figure 8–39.

Figure 8–39

Relationship between α, β, and the Power of a Test for a Right-Tail Hypothesis Test

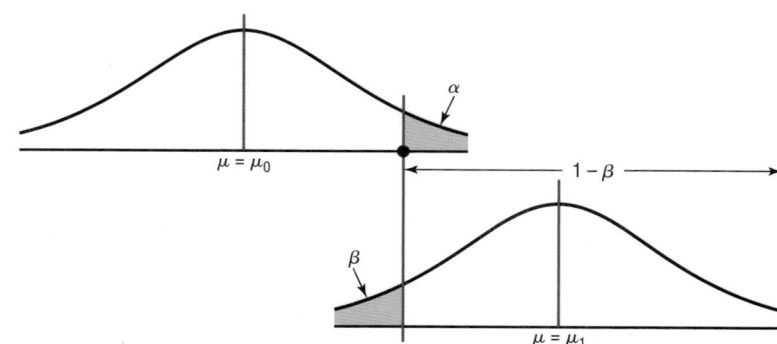

Procedure to Calculate a Type II Error and Power of a Test

Step 1 For a specific value of α, find the corresponding critical value(s) of $\overline{X}$ using
$$z = \frac{\overline{X} - \mu_0}{\sigma/\sqrt{n}} \text{ or } t = \frac{\overline{X} - \mu_0}{s/\sqrt{n}} \text{ where } \mu \text{ is the hypothesized value, } \mu_0, \text{ given in } H_0.$$

Step 2 Using the critical value(s) of $\overline{X}$ from step 1 and the assumed true hypothesized value, μ_1, find the appropriate area to obtain β, using the formula $z = \dfrac{\overline{X} - \mu_1}{\sigma/\sqrt{n}} \text{ or } t = \dfrac{\overline{X} - \mu_1}{s/\sqrt{n}}$

Step 3 Subtract the value of β from 1 to obtain the power of a test.

Example 8–32

CFL Bulbs

Test a manufacturer's claim that its compact fluorescent light (CFL) bulbs last longer than the average rating of 6000 hours. Assume the variable is normally distributed. A random selection of 36 CFL bulbs yields a sample mean of 6250 hours, with a standard deviation of 900 hours. Using an estimated population parameter of $\mu = 6500$ hours, calculate the type II error and power of the test.

Solution

First let's perform a hypothesis test for $\mu_0 = 6000$ hours.

H_0: $\mu_0 = 6000$ hours and H_1: $\mu_0 > 6000$ hours (claim). The critical value for a right-tail test at $\alpha = 0.05$ with d.f. $= 36 - 1 = 35$ is 1.690. The test statistic is 1.67 as shown.

$$t = \frac{\overline{X} - \mu}{s/\sqrt{n}} = \frac{6250 - 6000}{900/\sqrt{36}} \approx 1.67$$

Since $t = 1.67$ is not in the critical regions, the null hypothesis is not rejected. There is not enough evidence to support the manufacturer's claim that the average light bulb life expectancy is greater than 6000 hours.

Now, let's solve for the type II error, β, and the power of the test, $1 - \beta$, using $\mu_1 = 6500$ hours. Refer to Figure 8–40.

Figure 8–40

Type II Error and Power of a Test for Example 8–32

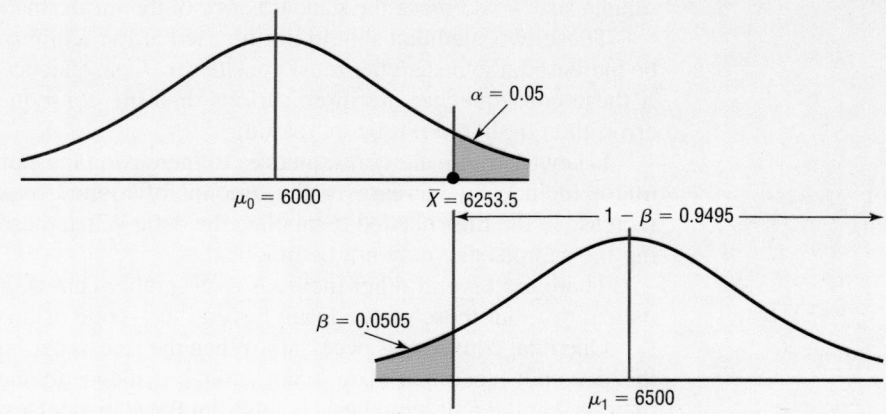

Step 1 Convert the critical value for $t = 1.690$ into an average CFL bulb life expectancy. Solve for $\overline{X}$.

$$t = \frac{\overline{X} - \mu_0}{s/\sqrt{n}}$$

$$1.690 = \frac{\overline{X} - 6000}{900/\sqrt{36}}$$

$$\overline{X} = 6000 + 1.690 \cdot \frac{900}{\sqrt{36}}$$

$$\overline{X} = 6000 + 253.5$$

$$\overline{X} = 6253.5 \text{ hours}$$

Step 2 Find the type II error (β) by calculating the area in the left tail for the assumed true population mean, $\mu_1 = 6500$ hours.

$$t = \frac{\overline{X} - \mu_1}{s/\sqrt{n}} = \frac{6253.5 - 6500}{900/\sqrt{36}} \approx -1.64$$

$$\beta = P(z < -1.64) = 0.0505$$

Step 3 Obtain the power of the hypothesis test by subtracting β from 1.

$$1 - \beta = 1 - 0.0505 = 0.9495$$

Interpretation

If the true population mean of CFL bulbs is 6500 hours, the probability of a type II error, failing to reject a manufacturer's false claim, is 0.0505. The probability of correctly rejecting a manufacturer's false claim is the power of the test, which is 0.9495. The hypothesis test procedure can be repeated with other assumed true population means, such as 6400 hours, 6300 hours, and so on, to obtain different type II errors and power of a test probabilities.

A statistical test should try to maximize the power of a test probability. The power of a test can be increased by increasing the value of α. For example, instead of using $\alpha = 0.01$, use $\alpha = 0.05$. Recall that as α increases, β decreases. So if β is decreased, then $1 - \beta$ will increase, thus increasing the power of the test.

Another way to increase the power of a test is to select a larger sample size. A larger sample size would make the standard error of the mean smaller and consequently reduce β.

These two methods should not be used at the whim of the researcher. Before α can be increased, the researcher must consider the consequences of committing a type I error. If these consequences are more serious than the consequences of committing a type II error, then α should not be increased.

Likewise, there are consequences to increasing the sample size. These consequences might include an increase in the amount of money required to do the study and an increase in the time needed to tabulate the data. When these consequences result, increasing the sample size may not be practical.

There are several other methods a researcher can use to increase the power of a statistical test, but these methods are beyond the scope of this book.

One final comment is necessary. When the researcher fails to reject the null hypothesis, this does not mean that there is not enough evidence to support alternative hypotheses. It may be that the null hypothesis is false but the statistical test has too low a power to detect the real difference; hence, one can conclude only that in this study, there is not enough evidence to reject the null hypothesis.

The relationship among α, β, and the power of a test can be analyzed in greater detail than the explanation given here. However, it is hoped that this explanation will show the student that there is no magic formula or statistical test that can guarantee foolproof results when a decision is made about the validity of H_0. Whether the decision is to reject H_0 or not to reject H_0, there is in either case a chance of being wrong. The goal, then, is to try to keep the probabilities of type I and type II errors as small as possible.

8–6 Applying the Concepts

Confidence Intervals and Hypothesis Testing

Hypothesis testing and testing claims with confidence intervals are two different approaches that lead to the same conclusion. In the following activities, you will compare and contrast those two approaches.

Assume that you are working for the Office of Consumer Affairs and have recently been getting complaints about the highway fuel consumption of the new Dodge Caravan. Chrysler Corporation agrees to allow you to randomly select 40 of its new Dodge Caravans to test the highway gas consumption. Chrysler claims that the Caravans consume 9.6 L/100 km. Your results show a mean fuel consumption 10.1 L/100 km, with a standard deviation of 2.0 L/100 km. Uncertain whether to generate a confidence interval estimate or run a hypothesis test, you decide to do both at the same time.

1. Draw a normal curve labelling the critical values, critical regions, test statistic, and population mean. List the significance level and the null and alternative hypotheses.

2. Draw a confidence interval directly below the normal distribution, labelling the sample mean, error, and boundary values.

3. Explain which parts from each approach are the same and which parts are different.

4. Draw a picture of a normal curve and confidence interval where the sample and hypothesized means are equal.

5. Draw a picture of a normal curve and confidence interval where the lower boundary of the confidence interval is equal to the hypothesized mean.

See page 405 for the answers.

Exercises 8–6

1. **Ski Shop Sales** A ski shop manager claims that the average of the sales for her shop is $1800 a day during the winter months. Ten winter days are selected at random, and the mean of the sales is $1830. The standard deviation of the population is $200. Can one reject the claim at $\alpha = 0.05$? Find the 95% confidence interval of the mean. Does the confidence interval interpretation agree with the hypothesis test results? Explain. Assume that the variable is normally distributed.

2. **Charter Bus Trips** Charter bus records show that in past years, the buses carried an average of 42 people per trip to Niagara Falls. The standard deviation of the population in the past was found to be 8. This year, the average of 10 trips showed a mean of 48 people booked. Can one reject the claim, at $\alpha = 0.10$, that the average is still the same? Find the 90% confidence interval of the mean. Does the confidence interval interpretation agree with the hypothesis-testing results? Explain. Assume that the variable is normally distributed.

3. **Condo Monthly Maintenance Fees** The sales manager of a rental agency claims that the monthly maintenance fee for a condominium in the Lakewood region is $86. Past surveys showed that the standard deviation of the population is $6. A sample of 15 owners shows that they pay an average of $84. Test the manager's claim at $\alpha = 0.01$. Find the 99% confidence interval of the mean. Does the confidence interval interpretation agree with the results of the hypothesis test? Explain. Assume that the variable is normally distributed.

4. **Canoe Trip Times** The average time it takes a person in a one-person canoe to complete a certain river course is 47 minutes. Because of rapid currents in the spring, a group of 10 people traverse the course in 42 minutes. The standard deviation, known from previous trips, is 7 minutes. Test the claim that this group's time was different because of the strong currents. Use $\alpha = 0.10$. Find the 90% confidence level of the true mean. Does the confidence interval interpretation agree with the results of the hypothesis test? Explain. Assume that the variable is normally distributed.

5. **College Study Times** From past studies the average time college freshmen spend studying is 22 hours per week. The standard deviation is 4 hours. This year, 60 students were surveyed, and the average time that they spent studying was 20.8 hours. Test the claim that the time students spend studying has changed. Use $\alpha = 0.01$. It is believed that the standard deviation is unchanged. Find the 99% confidence interval of the mean. Do the results agree? Explain.

6. **Newspaper Reading Times** A survey taken several years ago found that the average time a person spent reading the local daily newspaper was 10.8 minutes. The standard deviation of the population was 3 minutes. To see whether the average time had changed since the newspaper's format was revised, the newspaper editor surveyed 36 individuals. The average time that the 36 people spent reading the paper was 12.2 minutes. At $\alpha = 0.02$, is there a change in the average time an individual spends reading the newspaper? Find the 98% confidence interval of the mean. Do the results agree? Explain.

7. What is meant by the power of a test?

8. How is the power of a test related to the type II error?

9. How can the power of a test be increased?

Summary >

This chapter introduces the basic concepts of hypothesis testing. A statistical hypothesis is a conjecture about a population. There are two types of statistical hypotheses: the null and the alternative hypotheses. The null hypothesis states that there is no difference, and the alternative hypothesis specifies a difference. To test the null hypothesis, researchers use a statistical test. Many test statistics are computed by using

$$\text{Test statistic} = \frac{(\text{Observed value}) - (\text{Expected value})}{\text{Standard error}}$$

Two common statistical tests for hypotheses about a mean are the z test and the t test. The z test is used either when the population standard deviation is known and the variable is normally distributed, or when σ is known and the sample size is greater than or equal to 30. When the population standard deviation is not known and the variable is normally distributed, the sample standard deviation is used, but a t test should be conducted instead. The z test is also used to test proportions when $np \geq 5$ and $nq \geq 5$.

There is a relationship between confidence intervals and hypothesis testing. When the null hypothesis is rejected, the confidence interval for the mean using the same level of significance will not contain the hypothesized mean. When the null hypothesis is not rejected, the confidence interval, using the same level of significance, will contain the hypothesized mean.

Researchers compute a test statistic from the sample data in order to decide whether the null hypothesis should be rejected. Statistical tests can be one-tailed or two-tailed, depending on the hypotheses.

The null hypothesis is rejected when the difference between the population parameter and the sample statistic is said to be significant. The difference is significant when the test statistic falls in the critical region of the distribution. The critical region is determined by α, the level of significance of the test. The significance level is the probability of rejecting the null hypothesis when it is true or committing a type I error. The most common values of α are 0.10, 0.05 and 0.01. A type II error, β, is committed when the null hypothesis is not rejected when it is false. The power of a test, $1 - \beta$, is the correct decision of rejecting a null hypothesis when it is false. The power of a statistical test measures the sensitivity of the test to detect a real difference in parameters if one actually exists. $1 - \beta$ is called the power of a test.

Finally, one can test a single variance by using a chi-square test.

All hypothesis-testing situations using the traditional method should include the following steps:

1. State the null and alternative hypotheses and identify the claim.
2. State an alpha level and find the critical value(s).
3. Compute the test statistic.
4. Make the decision to reject or not reject the null hypothesis.
5. Summarize the results.

All hypothesis-testing situations using the P-value method should include the following steps:

1. State the hypotheses and identify the claim.
2. Compute the test statistic.
3. Find the P-value.
4. Make the decision.
5. Summarize the results.

For step-by-step guidance on the use of Texas Instruments TI-83 Plus/TI-84 Plus programmable calculators, see Appendix E at the back of this book. For summary procedures for Minitab, SPSS, and Excel, please see the full version of Appendix E on *Connect*.

Important Terms »

α (alpha) 347

alternative hypothesis 343

β (beta) 347

chi-square test 385

critical or rejection
region 348

critical value 348

hypothesis testing 342

left-tailed test 348

level of significance 347

noncritical or nonrejection
region 348

null hypothesis 343

one-tailed test 348

power of a test 347, 394

P-value 359

research hypothesis 344

right-tailed test 348

statistical hypothesis 343

statistical test 345

t test 367

test statistic 345

two-tailed test 349

type I error 346, 394

type II error 346, 394

z test 354

Important Formulas »

Formula for the z test for means:

$$z = \frac{\overline{X} - \mu}{\sigma/\sqrt{n}}$$

If $n < 30$, variable must be normally distributed.

Formula for the t test for means:

$$t = \frac{\overline{X} - \mu}{s/\sqrt{n}}$$

If $n < 30$, variable must be normally distributed.

Formula for the z test for proportions:

$$z = \frac{X - \mu}{\sigma} \quad \text{or} \quad z = \frac{\hat{p} - p}{\sqrt{pq/n}}$$

Formula for the chi-square test for variance or standard deviation:

$$\chi^2 = \frac{(n-1)s^2}{\sigma^2}$$

McGraw Hill **Connect**™ Practise and learn online with *Connect* with data sets and algorithmic questions related to concepts covered in this chapter. Questions and tables with online data sets are marked with 🏹.

Review Exercises »

For Exercises 1 through 19, perform each of the following steps.

   a. State the hypotheses and identify the claim.
   b. Find the critical value(s).
   c. Compute the test statistic.
   d. Make the decision.
   e. Summarize the results.

Use the traditional method of hypothesis testing unless otherwise specified.

1. **High Temperatures in Eastern Canada** A meteorolo-
 gist claims that the average of the highest temperatures in eastern Canada is 37°C. A random sample of 50 cities is selected, and the highest temperatures are recorded. The data are shown. At $\alpha = 0.05$, can the claim be rejected? Assume $\sigma = 2.31$°C.

38.3	35.6	37.0	40.3	35.0
37.6	39.0	36.1	38.5	32.2
36.0	38.3	38.5	35.1	34.5
37.8	39.0	37.0	36.0	35.5
35.0	36.7	35.4	30.6	36.5
38.0	38.0	36.8	37.0	35.5
33.9	37.0	36.1	36.5	31.1
37.4	37.0	40.6	39.1	33.3
32.2	34.0	38.4	32.8	38.9
36.7	34.0	35.6	32.8	32.8

Source: Environment Canada Climate Data.

2. **Stock Market Shares Traded** A stockbroker thought that the average number of shares of stocks traded daily in the stock market was about 500 million. To test the claim, a researcher selected a random sample of 40 days and found the mean number of shares traded each day was 506 million shares. Assume the population standard deviation was 10.3. At $\alpha = 0.05$, is there enough evidence to reject the broker's claim? Based on the results, do you agree or disagree with the broker?

3. **Salaries of Actuarial Graduates** Nationwide, graduates entering the actuarial field earn \$40,000. A college placement officer feels that this number is too low. She surveys 36 graduates entering the actuarial field and finds the average salary to be \$41,000. From a prior study $\sigma = \$3000$. Can her claim be supported at $\alpha = 0.05$?
Source: BeAnActuary.org.

4. **Salaries of Actuarial Fellows** Nationwide, the average salary of actuaries who achieve the rank of Fellow is \$150,000. An insurance executive wants to see how this compares with Fellows within his company. He checks the salaries of eight Fellows and finds the average salary to be \$155,500 with a standard deviation of \$15,000. Can he conclude that Fellows in his company make more than the national average, using $\alpha = 0.05$?
Source: BeAnActuary.org.

5. **July High Temperatures** The normal July maximum temperature for Metropolitan Toronto is 26.8°C. News

reports indicated that July 2006 was hotter than normal. A random sample of 10 days in July 2006 shows an average daily maximum temperature of 28.6°C with a standard deviation of 3.5°C. At $\alpha = 0.10$, can it be concluded that July 2006 was hotter than normal? Assume the variable is normally distributed.

Source: Environment Canada Climate Data.

6. **Age of Tennis Fans** The Tennis Industry Association stated that the average age of a tennis fan is 32 years. To test the claim, a researcher selected a random sample of 18 tennis fans and found that the mean of their ages was 31.3 years and the standard deviation was 2.8 years. At $\alpha = 0.05$ does it appear that the average age is lower than that stated by the Tennis Industry Association? Use the *P*-value method, and assume the variable is approximately normally distributed.

7. **College Graduate Debt** A random sample of the average debt (in dollars) at graduation from a selection of public colleges and universities is listed below. Is there sufficient evidence at $\alpha = 0.01$ to conclude that the population mean debt at graduation is less than $18,000?

16,012	15,784	16,597	18,105	12,665	14,734
17,225	16,953	15,309	15,297	14,437	14,835
13,607	13,374	19,410	18,385	22,312	16,656
20,142	17,821	12,701	22,400	15,730	17,673
18,978	13,661	12,580	14,392	16,000	15,176

Source: The Kiplinger Washington Editors: www.Kiplinger.com.

8. **Women Executives** A 2009 report stated that 40.6% of executive positions in Canada were held by women. The president of a nationwide retail chain claims that more women have executive positions in their company. A survey of 75 executives finds that 36 are women. At $\alpha = 0.05$, is the president correct?

Source: Statistics Canada, *Statistics Canada's Integrated Business and Human Resources Plan, 2009/2010,* "B. Employment Equity."

9. **Union Membership** Nationwide, 25.6% of the civilian labour forces are members of organized unions. A random sample of 300 local workers showed that 85 belonged to a union. At $\alpha = 0.05$, is there sufficient evidence to conclude that the proportion of union membership differs from 25.6%?

Source: Human Resources and Skills Development Canada, *Labour Relations,* "Union Membership in Canada—2008."

10. **Aboriginals in Prison** In 2007/2008, Aboriginal adults accounted for 22% of admissions to sentenced custody, while representing 3% of the Canadian population. A warden feels that in his prison, the percentage is even higher. He surveys 400 inmates' records and finds that 103 of the inmates are Aboriginal. At $\alpha = 0.05$, is he correct?

Source: Statistics Canada, *Juristat,* "The Incarceration of Aboriginal People in Adult Correctional Services," Samuel Perreault, July 2009, Vol. 29, No. 3.

11. **Religious Service Attendance** Results of a recent Ipsos poll suggest that 67% of Canadians attend a religious service at least once a year (34% monthly and 17% weekly). A theological researcher claims that the annual figures are low for his constituency. He randomly samples 90 people and discovers that 66 attended a religious service in the past year. At $\alpha = 0.05$, should the claim be rejected? Use the *P*-value method.

Source: Canadian Christianity, *The State of the Canadian Church—Part I: A Nation of Believers?*

12. **Weights of Football Players** A football coach claims that the average weight of all the opposing teams' members is 102 kg. To test the claim, a sample of 50 players is taken from all the opposing teams. The mean is found to be 104 kg, and the standard deviation is 7 kg. At $\alpha = 0.01$, test the coach's claim. Find the *P*-value and make the decision.

13. **Time until Indigestion Relief** An advertisement claims that Fasto Stomach Calm will provide relief from indigestion in less than 10 minutes. For a test of the claim, 35 individuals were given the product; the average time until relief was 9.25 minutes. From past studies, the standard deviation is known to be 2 minutes. Can one conclude that the claim is justified? Find the *P*-value and let $\alpha = 0.05$.

14. **Video Times** A film editor feels that the standard deviation for the number of minutes in a video is 3.4 minutes. A sample of 24 videos has a standard deviation of 4.2 minutes. At $\alpha = 0.05$, is the sample standard deviation different from what the editor hypothesized?

15. **Fuel Consumption** The standard deviation of the fuel consumption of a certain automobile is hypothesized to be greater than or equal to 1.6 litres per 100 kilometres (L/100 km). A sample of 20 automobiles produced a standard deviation of 0.9 L/100 km. Is the standard deviation really less than previously thought? Use $\alpha = 0.05$ and the *P*-value method.

16. **Condo Rental Rates** A real estate agent claims that the standard deviation of the rental rates of condominiums in Metropolitan Toronto is $500. A random sample of rental rates in dollars is shown. At $\alpha = 0.02$, can the claim be refuted? Assume the variable is normally distributed.

2258	1658	2151	1100	1677	1988
3007	1244	2653	2230	1757	1550
2692	1544	2140	1519	1969	1450

Source: MLS Rental Report, Toronto Real Estate Board.

17. **Games Played by NBA Scoring Leaders** A random sample of the number of games played by individual NBA scoring leaders is shown below. Is there sufficient evidence to conclude that the variance in games played differs from 40? Use $\alpha = 0.05$.

72	79	80	74	82
79	82	78	60	75

Source: Time Almanac.

18. **Drying Time of Paint** A manufacturer claims that the standard deviation of the drying time of a certain type of paint is 18 minutes. A sample of five test panels produced a standard deviation of 21 minutes. Test the claim at $\alpha = 0.05$.

19. **Tire Inflation** To see whether people are keeping their car tires inflated to the correct level at 241.3 kilopascals (kPa), a tire company manager selects a sample of 36 tires and checks the pressure. The mean of the sample is 230.9 kPa, and the standard deviation is 20.7 kPa. Are the tires properly inflated? Use $\alpha = 0.10$. Find the 90% confidence interval of the mean. Do the results agree? Explain.

20. **Plant Leaf Length** A biologist knows that the average length of a leaf of a certain full-grown plant is 10.2 centimetres. The standard deviation of the population is 1.5 cm. A sample of 20 leaves of that type of plant given a new type of plant food had an average length of 10.7 cm. Is there reason to believe that the new food is responsible for a change in the growth of the leaves? Use $\alpha = 0.01$. Find the 99% confidence interval of the mean. Do the results concur? Explain. Assume that the variable is approximately normally distributed.

Statistics Today

How Much Better Is Better?—Revisited

Now that you have learned the techniques of hypothesis testing presented in this chapter, you realize that the difference between the sample mean and the population mean must be *significant* before one can conclude that the students really scored above average. The minister of Education should follow the steps in the hypothesis-testing procedure and be able to reject the null hypothesis before announcing that his students scored higher than average.

Data Analysis »

The databank for these questions can be found in Appendix D at the back of the text and on ▤ **connect**.

1. From the databank, select a random sample of at least 30 individuals, and test one or more of the following hypotheses by using the z test. Use $\alpha = 0.05$.

    a. For serum cholesterol, H_0: $\mu = 220$ milligram percentage (mg%). Assume $\sigma = 21.86$.

    b. For systolic pressure, H_0: $\mu = 120$ millimetres of mercury (mm Hg). Assume $\sigma = 12.68$.

    c. For IQ, H_0: $\mu = 100$. Assume $\sigma = 9.63$.

    d. For sodium level, H_0: $\mu = 140$ milliequivalents per litre (mEq/L). Assume $\sigma = 6.02$.

2. Select a random sample of 15 individuals and test one or more of the hypotheses in Exercise 1 by using the t test. Use $\alpha = 0.05$.

3. Select a random sample of at least 30 individuals and, using the z test for proportions, test one or more of the following hypotheses. Use $\alpha = 0.05$.

    a. For educational level, H_0: $p = 0.50$ for level 2.

    b. For smoking status, H_0: $p = 0.20$ for level 1.

    c. For exercise level, H_0: $p = 0.10$ for level 1.

    d. For gender, H_0: $p = 0.50$ for males.

4. Select a sample of 20 individuals and test the hypothesis H_0: $\sigma^2 = 225$ for IQ level. Use $\alpha = 0.05$.

5. Using the data from Data Set XIII, select a sample of 10 hospitals and test H_0: $\mu = 250$ and H_1: $\mu < 250$ for the number of beds. Use $\alpha = 0.05$.

6. Using the data obtained in Exercise 5, test the hypothesis H_0: $\sigma = 150$ and H_1: $\sigma < 150$. Use $\alpha = 0.05$.

Chapter Quiz »

Determine whether each statement is true or false. If the statement is false, explain why.

1. No error is committed when the null hypothesis is rejected when it is false.

2. When one is conducting the t test, the population must be approximately normally distributed.

3. The test statistic separates the critical region from the noncritical region.

4. The values of a chi-square test cannot be negative.

5. The chi-square test for variances is always one-tailed.

Select the best answer.

6. When the value of α is increased, the probability of committing a type I error is

    a. Decreased

    b. Increased

    c. The same

    d. None of the above

7. If one wishes to test the claim that the mean of the population is 100, the appropriate alternative hypothesis is

   a. $\overline{X} \neq 100$
   b. $\mu > 100$
   c. $\mu < 100$
   d. $\mu \neq 100$

8. The degrees of freedom for the chi-square test for variances or standard deviations are

   a. 1
   b. n
   c. $n - 1$
   d. None of the above

9. The correct hypothesis test to use when $n = 40$, σ is unknown, and H_0: $\mu = 100$ is

   a. t test for a mean
   b. z test for a mean
   c. z test for a proportion
   d. χ^2 test for a variance

Complete the following statements with the best answer.

10. Rejecting the null hypothesis when it is true is called a(n) _____ error.

11. The probability of a type II error is referred to as _____.

12. A conjecture about a population parameter is called a(n) _____.

13. To test the claim that the mean is greater than 87, one would use a(n) _____-tailed test.

14. The degrees of freedom for the t test are _____.

For the following exercises where applicable:

   a. State the hypotheses and identify the claim.
   b. Find the critical value(s).
   c. Compute the test statistic.
   d. Make the decision.
   e. Summarize the results.

Use the traditional method of hypothesis testing unless otherwise specified.

15. **First Child for Professional Women** A sociologist wishes to see if it is true that for a certain group of professional women, the average age at which they have their first child is 28.6 years. From a prior study, $\sigma = 4.18$ years. A random sample of 36 women is selected, and their ages at the birth of their first children are recorded. At $\alpha = 0.05$, does the evidence refute the sociologist's assertion?

32	28	26	33	35	34
29	24	22	25	26	28
28	34	33	32	30	29
30	27	33	34	28	25
24	33	25	37	35	33
34	36	38	27	29	26

16. **Home Closing Costs** A real estate agent believes that the average closing cost of purchasing a new home is $6500. She selects 40 new home sales at random and finds that the average closing costs are $6600. The standard deviation of the population is $120. Test her belief at $\alpha = 0.05$.

17. **Teen Text Messaging** According to a recent Nielsen survey, teenagers send an average of 80 text messages per day. The local board of health decides to test this claim and surveys the community schools. Of the 49 teenagers surveyed, the average number of text messages sent per day was 83. From a previous study, $\sigma = 9.82$. At $\alpha = 0.02$, is there evidence to reject the Nielsen report?
   Source: HealthNews.com, *Child Health*, "Average Teen Output—Eighty Text Messages per Day," Neomi Heroux, May 27, 2009.

18. **Hotel Rooms** A travel agent claims that the average of the number of rooms in hotels in a large city is 500. At $\alpha = 0.01$ is the claim realistic? The data for a sample of hotels are shown. Assume the variable is approximately normally distributed.

713	300	292	311	598	401	618

   Give a reason why the claim might be deceptive.

19. **Heights of Models** In a Montreal modelling agency, a researcher wishes to see if the average height of female models is really less than 170 cm, as the chief claims. A sample of 20 models has an average of 167.1 cm. The standard deviation of the sample is 4.3 cm. At $\alpha = 0.05$, is the average height of the models really less than 170 cm? Use the P-value method. Assume the population data is normally distributed.

20. **Experience of Taxi Drivers** A taxi company claims that its drivers have an average of at least 12.4 years' experience. In a study of 15 taxi drivers, the average experience was 11.2 years. The standard deviation was 2. At $\alpha = 0.10$, is the number of years' experience of the taxi drivers really less than the taxi company claimed?

21. **Age of Robbery Victims** A recent study in a small city stated that the average age of robbery victims was 63.5 years. A sample of 20 recent victims had a mean of 63.7 years and a standard deviation of 1.9 years. At $\alpha = 0.05$, is the average age higher than originally believed? Use the P-value method. Assume the variable is approximately normally distributed.

22. **First-Time Marriages** A magazine article stated that the average age of women who are getting married for the first time is 26 years. A researcher decided to test this hypothesis at $\alpha = 0.02$. She selected a sample of 25 women who were recently married for the first time and found the average was 25.1 years. The standard deviation was 3 years. Should the null hypothesis be rejected on the basis of the sample? Assume the variable is approximately normally distributed.

23. **Survey on Vitamin Usage** A survey in *Men's Health* magazine reported that 39% of cardiologists said that they took vitamin E supplements. To see if this is still

true, a researcher randomly selected 100 cardiologists and found that 36 said that they took vitamin E supplements. At $\alpha = 0.05$ test the claim that 39% of the cardiologists took vitamin E supplements. A recent study said that taking too much vitamin E might be harmful. How might this study make the results of the previous study invalid?

24. **Breakfast Survey** A dietitian read a magazine's survey results claiming that at least 55% of adults do not eat breakfast 3 or more days a week. To verify this, she selected a random sample of 80 adults and asked them how many days a week they skipped breakfast. A total of 50% responded that they skipped breakfast 3 or more days a week. At $\alpha = 0.10$, test the survey's claim.

25. **Caffeinated Beverage Survey** A Harris Poll found that 35% of people said that they drink a caffeinated beverage to combat midday drowsiness. A recent survey found that 19 out of 48 people stated that they drank a caffeinated beverage to combat midday drowsiness. At $\alpha = 0.02$ is the claim of the percentage found in the Harris Poll believable?

26. **Cellphone Ban** A social research firm claimed that 27% of Canadians, aged 18 to 24 years, support a cellphone ban while driving. To test this claim, the student's union at a university sampled 80 students, aged 18 to 24 years, and found that 29 supported a cellphone ban. At $\alpha = 0.01$, is there enough evidence to reject the claim?
Source: TNS Canadian Facts, Ban on Using Hand-Held Cellphones While Driving, November 3, 2009.

27. Find the P-value for the z test in Exercise 15.

28. Find the P-value for the z test in Exercise 16.

29. **Pages in Romance Novels** A copy editor thinks the standard deviation for the number of pages in a romance novel is greater than 6. A sample of 25 novels has a standard deviation of 9 pages. At $\alpha = 0.05$, is it higher, as the editor hypothesized?

30. **Seed Germination Time** It has been hypothesized that the standard deviation of the germination time of radish seeds is 8 days. The standard deviation of a sample of 60 radish plants' germination times was 6 days. At $\alpha = 0.01$, test the claim.

31. **Pollution By-Products** The standard deviation of the pollution by-products released in the burning of 1 litre of gas is 18 mL. A sample of 20 automobiles tested produced a standard deviation of 15 mL. Is the standard deviation really less than previously thought? Use $\alpha = 0.05$.

32. **Strength of Wrapping Cord** A manufacturer claims that the standard deviation of the strength of wrapping cord is 4.1 kg. A sample of 10 wrapping cords produced a standard deviation of 5.0 kg. At $\alpha = 0.05$, test the claim. Use the P-value method.

33. Find the 90% confidence interval of the mean in Exercise 15. Is μ contained in the interval?

34. Find the 95% confidence interval for the mean in Exercise 16. Is μ contained in the interval?

Critical Thinking Challenges

1. The *operating characteristic (OC) curve* plots the probability of a type II error, β, on the vertical axis versus different assumed values of the true population mean, μ_1, on the horizontal axis. Software applications (Excel, Minitab, SPSS, etc.) simplify the task of creating these charts but they can also be created manually. Refer to Example 8–32, CFL Bulbs, and calculate β for μ_1 of 6000 hours to 7000 hours in 200-hour increments. Plot β versus μ_1 using a line chart. Interpret the OC chart.

2. For question 1, repeat the hypothesis test using the original hypothesis, μ_0, with $\alpha = 0.01$. Construct a table comparing each assumed value of the true population mean, μ_1, from 6000 hours to 7000 hours in 200-hour increments for type II error, β, and the power of the test, $1 - \beta$. Interpret the table.

Data Projects

Where appropriate, use Minitab, SPSS, TI-83 Plus, TI-84 Plus, Excel, or a computer program of your choice to complete the following exercises.

Use a significance level of 0.05 for all tests below.

1. **Business and Finance** Use the Dow Jones industrial stocks in Data Project 1 in Chapter 7 as your data set. Find the gain or loss for each stock over the last quarter. Test the claim that the mean is that the stocks broke even (no gain or loss indicates a mean of 0).

2. **Sports and Leisure** Use the most recent NFL season for your data. For each team, find the quarterback rating for the number one quarterback. Test the claim that the mean quarterback rating for a number one quarterback is more than 80.

3. **Technology** Use your last month's itemized cellphone bill for your data. Determine the percentage of your text messages that were outgoing. Test the claim that a majority of your text messages were outgoing. Determine the mean, median, and standard deviation for the

length of a call. Test the claim that the mean length of a call is longer than the median length value.

4. **Health and Wellness** Use the data collected in Data Project 4 in Chapter 7 for this exercise. Test the claim that the mean body temperature is less than 37.0°C.

5. **Politics and Economics** Use the most recent results of the federal elections for the top two parties. Determine what percentage of voters in your province voted for the eventual ruling party and what percentage voted for the eventual opposition party. Test the claim that a majority of your province favoured the party who won the election.

6. **Your Class** Use the data collected in Data Project 6 in Chapter 7 for this exercise. Test the claim that the mean BMI for a student is more than 25 kg/m^2.

Answers to Applying the Concepts ≫

Section 8–1 Eggs and Your Health

1. The study was prompted by claims that linked foods high in cholesterol to high blood serum cholesterol.

2. The population under study is people in general.

3. A sample of 500 subjects was collected.

4. The hypothesis was that eating eggs did not increase blood serum cholesterol.

5. Blood serum cholesterol levels were collected.

6. Most likely but we are not told which test.

7. The conclusion was that eating a moderate amount of eggs will not significantly increase blood serum cholesterol level.

Section 8–2 Car Thefts

1. H_0: $\mu = 50$ and H_1: $\mu \neq 50$

2. This sample can be considered large for our purposes.

3. The variable is derived from a normally distributed population or the central limit theorem applies.

4. We will use the z distribution.

5. Since we are interested in whether the automobile theft rate has changed, we use a two-tailed test.

6. Answers may vary. At the $\alpha = 0.05$ significance level, the critical values are $z = \pm 1.96$.

7. The sample mean is $\overline{X} = 58.3$, and the population standard deviation is 42.5. Our test statistic is

$$z = \frac{58.3 - 50}{42.5/\sqrt{36}} \approx 1.17$$

8. Since 1.17 is between ± 1.96, we do not reject the null hypothesis.

9. There is not enough evidence to conclude that the automobile theft rate has changed.

10. Answers will vary. Based on our sample data, it appears that the automobile theft rate has not changed from 50 vehicles per 10,000 people. Although the sample data suggest an increase, the evidence is insufficient to indicate a change has occurred.

11. Based on our sample, we would expect 58.3 automobile thefts per 10,000 people, so we would expect (58.3)(5) = 291.5, or about 292 automobile thefts in the city.

Section 8–3 How Much Nicotine Is in Those Cigarettes?

1. We have $15 - 1 = 14$ degrees of freedom.

2. This is a small-sample test.

3. We are testing only one sample.

4. This is a right-tailed test, since the hypotheses of the tobacco company are H_0: $\mu = 40$ and H_1: $\mu > 40$.

5. The P-value is 0.008, which is less than the significance level of 0.01. We reject the tobacco company's claim.

6. Since the test statistic (2.72) is greater than the critical value (2.62), we reject the tobacco company's claim.

7. There is no conflict in this output, since the results based on the P-value and on the critical value agree.

8. Answers will vary. It appears that the company's claim is false and that there is more than 40 mg of nicotine in its cigarettes.

Section 8–4 Quitting Smoking

1. The statistical hypotheses were that StopSmoke helps more people quit smoking than the other leading brands.

2. The null hypotheses were that StopSmoke has the same effectiveness as or is not as effective as the other leading brands.

3. The alternative hypotheses were that StopSmoke helps more people quit smoking than the other leading brands. (The alternative hypotheses are the statistical hypotheses.)

4. No statistical tests were run that we know of.

5. Had tests been run, they would have been one-tailed tests.

6. Some possible significance levels are 0.01, 0.05, and 0.10.

7. A type I error would be concluding that StopSmoke is better when it really is not.

8. A type II error would be concluding that StopSmoke is not better when it really is.

9. These studies proved nothing. Had statistical tests been used, we could have tested the effectiveness of StopSmoke.

10. Answers will vary. One possible answer is that more than likely the statements are talking about practical significance and not statistical significance, since we have no indication that any statistical tests were conducted.

Section 8–5 Testing Fuel Consumption Claims

1. The hypotheses are H_0: $\mu = 9.6$ and H_1: $\mu > 9.6$. The value of the test statistic is $t = 2.108$, and the associated P-value is 0.021. At $\alpha = 0.05$, we would fail to reject Chrysler's claim but at $\alpha = 0.01$, we would reject Chrysler's claim of getting 9.6 L/100 km and conclude that the vehicles actually use more than 9.6 L/100 km.

2. The hypotheses are H_0: $\sigma = 0.5$ and H_1: $\sigma > 0.5$. The value of our test statistic is

$$\chi^2 = \frac{(n-1)s^2}{\sigma^2} = \frac{(40-1)(1.5)^2}{(0.5)^2} = 351.0$$

and the associated P-value is approximately zero. We would reject Chrysler's claim that the standard deviation is 0.5 L/100 km.

3. Answers will vary. It is recommended that Chrysler increase its claim about the vehicle fuel consumption in L/100 km of the Dodge Caravans. Chrysler should also try to increase variability in L/100 km and provide confidence intervals for the highway fuel consumption.

4. Answers will vary. There are cases when a mean may be fine, but if there is a lot of variability about the mean, there will be complaints (due to the lack of consistency).

Section 8–6 Confidence Intervals and Hypothesis Testing

1. Answers will vary.

2. Answers will vary.

3. Answers will vary.

4. Answers will vary.

5. Answers will vary.

6. Answers will vary.

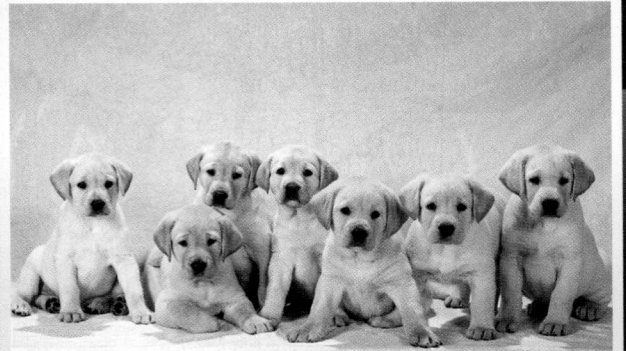

Chapter 9

Testing the Difference between Two Means, Two Proportions, and Two Variances

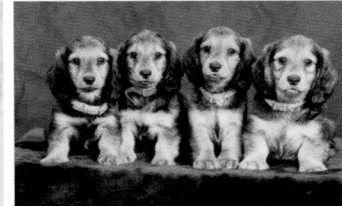

Objectives >

After completing this chapter, you should be able to

LO1 Test the difference between sample means, using the *z* test.

LO2 Test the difference between two means for independent samples, using the *t* test.

LO3 Test the difference between two means for dependent samples.

LO4 Test the difference between two proportions.

LO5 Test the difference between two variances or standard deviations.

Outline >

Mc Graw Hill **connect**™ Practise and learn online with *Connect* with data sets and algorithmic questions related to concepts covered in this chapter. Throughout this chapter, questions and tables with online data sets are marked with 🏹.

Statistics Today

A Woman's Path to Pay Equity

Women in Canada earn less than their male counterparts employed in many comparable labour

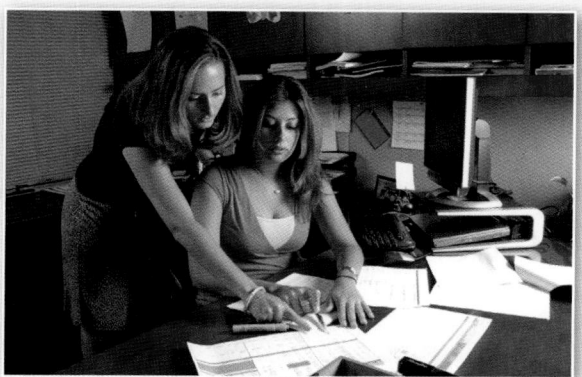

activities. Statistics Canada has reported that the gender earnings gap was even larger with self-employed than with the wage work force. In order to study gender differences in wage and self-employed earnings, census data from the two groups was collected. Unlike techniques used in Chapter 8, this study used procedures explained in this chapter and found some interesting results. Refer to Statistics Today—Revisited, page 448, to see the techniques used and the results of the study.

Sources: Neil Wolff, School of Business, Ryerson University, "Earning Equity: A Comparative Study of Changing Gender Earnings Differentials between Earners and Self-Employed," paper submitted to the Conference on Gender & Diversity in Organization, Halifax, Nova Scotia, 2002; "Excerpts from A Profile of the Self-Employed, 1997," adapted from Statistics Canada, *Canadian Economic Observer,* November 1997, Vol. 10, No. 11. Released October 24, 1997.

Introduction >

The basic concepts of hypothesis testing were explained in Chapter 8. With the z, t, and χ^2 tests, a sample mean, variance, or proportion can be compared to a specific population mean, variance, or proportion to determine whether the null hypothesis should be rejected.

There are, however, many instances when researchers wish to compare two sample means, using experimental and control groups. For example, the average lifetimes of two different brands of bus tires might be compared to see whether there is any difference in tread wear. Two different brands of fertilizer might be tested to see whether one is better than the other for growing plants. Or two brands of cough syrup might be tested to see whether one brand is more effective than the other.

In the comparison of two means, the same basic steps for hypothesis testing shown in Chapter 8 are used, and the z and t tests are also used. When comparing two means by using the t test, the researcher must decide if the two samples are *independent* or *dependent.* The concepts of independent and dependent samples will be explained in Sections 9–2 and 9–3.

The z test can be used to compare two proportions, as shown in Section 9–4. Finally, two variances can be compared by using an F test, as shown in Section 9–5.

9–1	Testing the Difference between Two Means: Using the *z* Test >

Test the difference between sample means, using the *z* test.

Suppose a researcher wishes to determine whether there is a difference in the average age of nursing students who enroll in a nursing program at a college and those who enroll in a nursing program at a university. In this case, the researcher is not interested in the average age of all beginning nursing students; instead, he is interested in *comparing* the means of the two groups. His research question is: Does the mean age of nursing students who enroll at a college differ from the mean age of nursing students who enroll at a university? Here, the hypotheses are

$$H_0: \mu_1 = \mu_2$$
$$H_1: \mu_1 \neq \mu_2$$

where

μ_1 = mean age of all beginning nursing students at the college
μ_2 = mean age of all beginning nursing students at the university

Another way of stating the hypotheses for this situation is

$$H_0: \mu_1 - \mu_2 = 0$$
$$H_1: \mu_1 - \mu_2 \neq 0$$

If there is no difference in population means, subtracting them will give a difference of zero. If they are different, subtracting will give a number other than zero. Both methods of stating hypotheses are correct and will be illustrated in this chapter.

Assumptions for the z Test to Determine the Difference between Two Means

1. Both samples are random samples.
2. The samples must be independent of each other. That is, there can be no relationship between the subjects in each sample.
3. The standard deviations of both populations must be known, and if the sample sizes are less than 30, the populations must be normally or approximately normally distributed.

The theory behind testing the difference between two means is based on selecting pairs of samples and comparing the means of the pairs. The population means are not typically known.

All possible pairs of samples are taken from populations. The means for each pair of samples are computed and then subtracted, and the differences are plotted. If both populations have the same mean, then most of the differences will be zero or close to zero. Occasionally, there will be a few large differences due to chance alone, some positive and others negative. If the differences are plotted, the curve will be shaped like a normal distribution and have a mean of zero, as shown in Figure 9–1.

The variance of the difference $\overline{X}_1 - \overline{X}_2$ is equal to the sum of the individual variances of $\overline{X}_1$ and $\overline{X}_2$. That is,

$$\sigma^2_{\overline{X}_1 - \overline{X}_2} = \sigma^2_{\overline{X}_1} + \sigma^2_{\overline{X}_2}$$

Figure 9–1

Differences of Means of Pairs of Samples

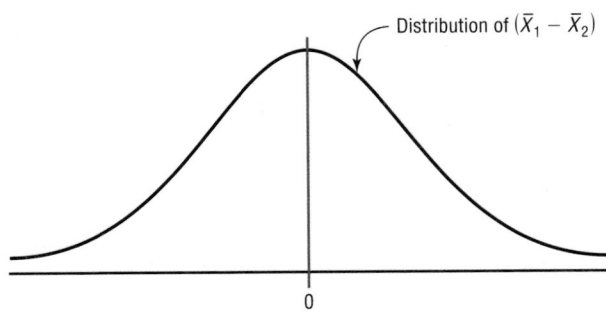

Distribution of $(\overline{X}_1 - \overline{X}_2)$

0

where $\qquad \sigma_{\overline{X}_1}^2 = \dfrac{\sigma_1^2}{n_1} \qquad$ and $\qquad \sigma_{\overline{X}_2}^2 = \dfrac{\sigma_2^2}{n_2}$

So the standard deviation of $\overline{X}_1 - \overline{X}_2$ is

$$\sqrt{\frac{\sigma_1^2}{n_1} + \frac{\sigma_2^2}{n_2}}$$

Formula for the *z* Test for Comparing Two Means from Independent Populations

$$z = \frac{(\overline{X}_1 - \overline{X}_2) - (\mu_1 - \mu_2)}{\sqrt{\dfrac{\sigma_1^2}{n_1} + \dfrac{\sigma_2^2}{n_2}}}$$

This formula is based on the general format of

$$\text{Test statistic} = \frac{(\text{Observed value}) - (\text{Expected value})}{\text{Standard error}}$$

where $\overline{X}_1 - \overline{X}_2$ is the observed difference, and the expected difference $\mu_1 - \mu_2$ is zero when the null hypothesis is $\mu_1 = \mu_2$, since that is equivalent to $\mu_1 - \mu_2 = 0$. Finally, the standard deviation of the difference, referred to as the standard error of the difference is

$$\sqrt{\frac{\sigma_1^2}{n_1} + \frac{\sigma_2^2}{n_2}}$$

In the comparison of two sample means, the difference may be due to chance, in which case the null hypothesis will not be rejected, and the researcher can assume that the means of the populations are basically the same. The difference in this case is not significant. See Figure 9–2(a). On the other hand, if the difference is significant, the null hypothesis is rejected and the researcher can conclude that the population means are different. See Figure 9–2(b).

These tests can also be one-tailed, using the following hypotheses:

Right-tailed			**Left-tailed**		
$H_0: \mu_1 = \mu_2$	or	$H_0: \mu_1 - \mu_2 = 0$	$H_0: \mu_1 = \mu_2$	or	$H_0: \mu_1 - \mu_2 = 0$
$H_1: \mu_1 > \mu_2$		$H_1: \mu_1 - \mu_2 > 0$	$H_1: \mu_1 < \mu_2$		$H_1: \mu_1 - \mu_2 < 0$

Figure 9–2

Hypothesis-Testing Situations in the Comparison of Means

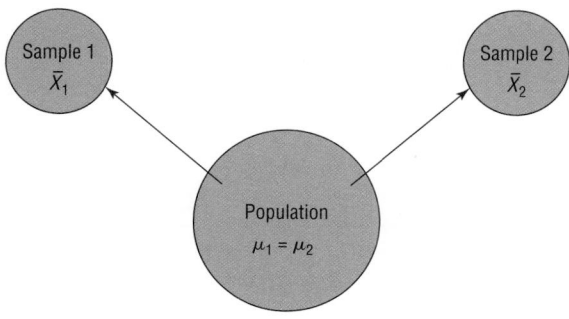

(a) Difference is not significant

Do not reject H_0: $\mu_1 = \mu_2$ since $\overline{X}_1 - \overline{X}_2$ is not significant.

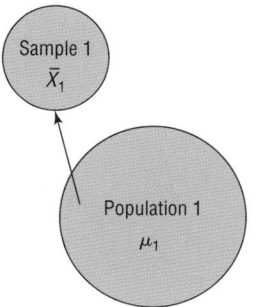
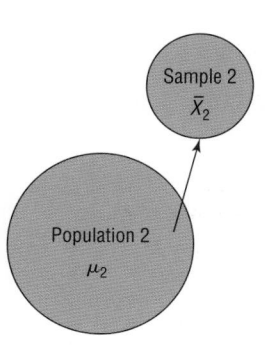

(b) Difference is significant

Reject H_0: $\mu_1 = \mu_2$ since $\overline{X}_1 - \overline{X}_2$ is significant.

The same critical values used in Section 8–2 are used here. They can be obtained from Tables E–1 and E–2 in Appendix C.

If σ_1^2 and σ_2^2 are not known, the researcher can use the variances from each sample s_1^2 and s_2^2, but a t test must be used. This will be explained in Section 9–2.

The basic format for hypothesis testing using the traditional method is reviewed here.

Step 1 State the hypotheses and identify the claim.

Step 2 Find the critical value(s).

Step 3 Compute the test statistic.

Step 4 Make the decision.

Step 5 Summarize the results.

Example 9–1

Hotel Room Cost

A survey found that the average hotel room rate in Toronto was $175.53 and the average room rate in Vancouver was $171.31. Assume that the data were obtained from two samples of 50 hotels each and the standard deviations of the populations are $9.52 and $10.89, respectively. At $\alpha = 0.05$, can it be concluded that there was a significant difference in the rates?

Source: Canadian Lodging Outlook, June 2006.

Solution

Step 1 State the hypotheses and identify the claim.

$$H_0: \mu_1 = \mu_2 \quad \text{and} \quad H_1: \mu_1 \neq \mu_2 \text{(claim)}$$

Step 2 Find the critical values. Since $\alpha = 0.05$, the critical values are $+1.96$ and -1.96.

Step 3 Compute the test statistic.

$$z = \frac{(\overline{X}_1 - \overline{X}_2) - (\mu_1 - \mu_2)}{\sqrt{\dfrac{\sigma_1^2}{n_1} + \dfrac{\sigma_2^2}{n_2}}} = \frac{(175.53 - 171.31) - 0}{\sqrt{\dfrac{9.52^2}{50} + \dfrac{10.89^2}{50}}} \approx 2.06$$

Step 4 Make the decision. Reject the null hypothesis at $\alpha = 0.05$, since $2.06 > 1.96$. See Figure 9–3.

Figure 9–3

Critical Values and Test Statistic for Example 9–1

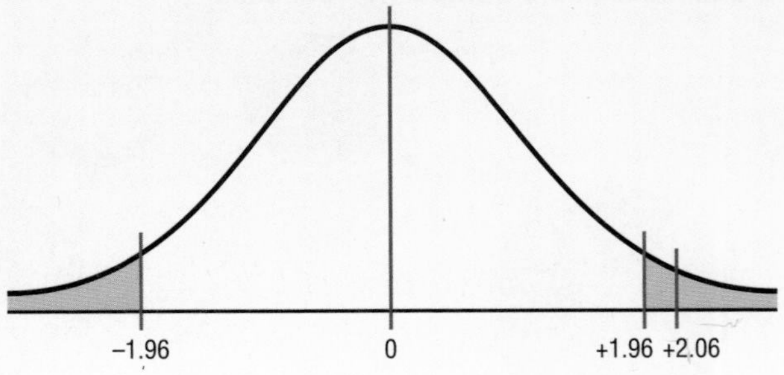

Step 5 Summarize the results. There is enough evidence to support the claim that the means are not equal. Hence, there is a significant difference in the rates.

P-Value Method

The P-values for this test can be determined by using the same procedure shown in Section 8–2. For example, if the test statistics for a two-tailed test is +2.06, then the P-value obtained from Table E–2 is 0.0394. This value is obtained by looking up the area for $z = 2.06$, which is 0.9803. Then 0.9803 is subtracted from 1.0000 to get 0.0197. Finally, this value is doubled to get 0.0394, since the test is two-tailed. If $\alpha = 0.05$, the decision would be to reject the null hypothesis, since the P-value $< \alpha$.

The P-value method for hypothesis testing for this chapter also follows the same format as stated in Chapter 8. The steps are reviewed here.

Step 1   State the hypotheses and identify the claim.

Step 2   Compute the test statistic.

Step 3   Find the P-value.

Step 4   Make the decision.

Step 5   Summarize the results.

Example 9–2 illustrates these steps.

Example 9–2

College Sports Offerings

A researcher hypothesizes that the average number of sports that colleges offer for males is greater than the average number of sports that colleges offer for females. A sample of the number of sports offered by colleges is shown. At $\alpha = 0.10$, is there enough evidence to support the claim? Assume σ_1 and $\sigma_2 = 3.3$.

Males					Females				
6	11	11	8	15	6	8	11	13	8
6	14	8	12	18	7	5	13	14	6
6	9	5	6	9	6	5	5	7	6
6	9	18	7	6	10	7	6	5	5
15	6	11	5	5	16	10	7	8	5
9	9	5	5	8	7	5	5	6	5
8	9	6	11	6	9	18	13	7	10
9	5	11	5	8	7	8	5	7.	6
7	7	5	10	7	11	4	6	8	7
10	7	10	8	11	14	12	5	8	5

Source: USA TODAY.

Solution

Step 1   State the hypotheses and identify the claim.

$$H_0: \mu_1 = \mu_2 \qquad \text{and} \qquad H_1: \mu_1 > \mu_2 \text{ (claim)}$$

Step 2   Compute the test statistic. Using a calculator or the formulas in Chapter 3, find the mean and standard deviation for each data set.

For the males $\overline{X}_1 = 8.6$ and $\sigma_1 = 3.3$

For the females $\overline{X}_1 = 7.9$ and $\sigma_2 = 3.3$

Substitute in the formula.

$$z = \frac{(\overline{X}_1 - \overline{X}_2) - (\mu_1 - \mu_2)}{\sqrt{\dfrac{\sigma_1^2}{n_1} + \dfrac{\sigma_2^2}{n_2}}} = \frac{(8.6 - 7.9) - 0}{\sqrt{\dfrac{3.3^2}{50} + \dfrac{3.3^2}{50}}} \approx 1.06^*$$

Step 3 Find the *P*-value. For $z = +1.06$, the cumulative area to the left from Table E–2 is 0.8554. For a right-tailed test, the required area is $1.0000 - 0.8554 = 0.1446$ or a *P*-value of 0.1446.

Step 4 Make the decision. Since the *P*-value is larger than α (that is, $0.1446 > 0.10$), the decision is to not reject the null hypothesis. See Figure 9–4.

Figure 9–4

P-Value and α Value for Example 9–2

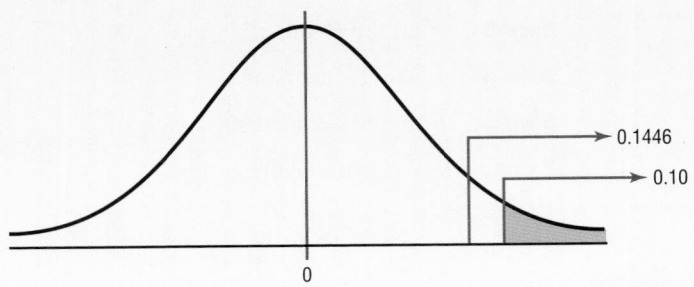

Note: Calculator results may differ due to rounding.

Step 5 Summarize the results. There is not enough evidence to support the claim that colleges offer more sports for males than they do for females.

Sometimes, the researcher is interested in testing a specific difference in means other than zero. For example, he or she might hypothesize that the nursing students at a college are, on the average, 3.2 years older than those at a university. In this case, the hypotheses are

$$H_0: \mu_1 - \mu_2 = 3.2 \qquad \text{and} \qquad H_1: \mu_1 - \mu_2 > 3.2$$

The formula for the *z* test is still

$$z = \frac{(\overline{X}_1 - \overline{X}_2) - (\mu_1 - \mu_2)}{\sqrt{\dfrac{\sigma_1^2}{n_1} + \dfrac{\sigma_2^2}{n_2}}}$$

where $\mu_1 - \mu_2$ is the hypothesized difference or expected value. In this case, $\mu_1 - \mu_2 = 3.2$.

Confidence intervals for the difference between two means can also be found. When one is hypothesizing a difference of zero, if the confidence interval contains zero, the null hypothesis is not rejected. If the confidence interval does not contain zero, the null hypothesis is rejected.

Confidence intervals for the difference between two means can be found by using the following formula.

Formula for the *z* Confidence Interval for Difference between Two Means

$$(\overline{X}_1 - \overline{X}_2) - z_{\alpha/2}\sqrt{\frac{\sigma_1^2}{n_1} + \frac{\sigma_2^2}{n_2}} < \mu_1 - \mu_2 < (\overline{X}_1 - \overline{X}_2) + z_{\alpha/2}\sqrt{\frac{\sigma_1^2}{n_1} + \frac{\sigma_2^2}{n_2}}$$

Example 9–3

Hotel Room Cost

Find the 95% confidence interval for the difference between the means for the data in Example 9–1.

Solution

$$(\overline{X}_1 - \overline{X}_2) - z_{\alpha/2}\sqrt{\frac{\sigma_1^2}{n_1} + \frac{\sigma_2^2}{n_2}} < \mu_1 - \mu_2 < (\overline{X}_1 - \overline{X}_2) + z_{\alpha/2}\sqrt{\frac{\sigma_1^2}{n_1} + \frac{\sigma_2^2}{n_2}}$$

$$(175.53 - 171.31) - 1.96\sqrt{\frac{9.52^2}{50} + \frac{10.89^2}{50}} < \mu_1 - \mu_2$$

$$< (175.53 - 171.31) + 1.96\sqrt{\frac{9.52^2}{50} + \frac{10.89^2}{50}}$$

$$4.22 - 4.01 < \mu_1 - \mu_2 < 4.22 + 4.01$$

$$0.21 < \mu_1 - \mu_2 < 8.23$$

Since the confidence interval does not contain zero, the decision is to reject the null hypothesis, which agrees with the previous result.

9–1   Applying the Concepts

Home Runs

For a sports radio talk show, you are asked to research the question whether more home runs are hit by Major League Baseball players in the National League or by players in the American League. You decide to use the home run leaders from each league for the last 40 years as your data. The numbers are shown. Assume $\sigma_1 = 8.8$ and $\sigma_2 = 7.8$.

National League

47	49	73	50	65	70	49	47	40	43
46	35	38	40	47	39	49	37	37	36
40	37	31	48	48	45	52	38	38	36
44	40	48	45	45	36	39	44	52	47

American League

47	57	52	47	48	56	56	52	50	40
46	43	44	51	36	42	49	49	40	43
39	39	22	41	45	46	39	32	36	32
32	32	37	33	44	49	44	44	49	32

Using the data given, answer the following questions.

1. Define a population.
2. What kind of sample was used?
3. Do you feel that it is representative?
4. What are your hypotheses?
5. What significance level will you use?
6. What statistical test will you use?
7. What are the test results?
8. What is your decision?
9. What can you conclude?
10. Do you feel that using the data given really answers the original question asked?
11. What other data might be used to answer the question?

See page 452 for the answers.

Exercises 9–1

1. Explain the difference between testing a single mean and testing the difference between two means.

2. When a researcher selects all possible pairs of samples from a population in order to find the difference between the means of each pair, what will be the shape of the distribution of the differences when the original distributions are normally distributed? What will be the mean of the distribution? What will be the standard deviation of the distribution?

3. What two assumptions must be met when one is using the z test to test differences between two means? When can the sample standard deviations s_1 and s_2 be used in place of the population standard deviations σ_1 and σ_2?

4. Show two different ways to state that the means of two populations are equal.

For Exercises 5 through 17, use the following traditional method of hypothesis testing unless otherwise specified.

   a. State the hypotheses and identify the claim.
   b. Find the critical value(s).
   c. Compute the test statistic.
   d. Make the decision.
   e. Summarize the results.

5. **Comparison of River Lengths** A researcher wishes to see if the average length of the major rivers in North America is the same as the average length of the major rivers in Europe. The data (in kilometres) of a sample of rivers are shown. At $\alpha = 0.01$, is there enough evidence to reject the claim? Assume $\sigma_1 = 724$ and $\sigma_2 = 763$.

North America			Europe		
1173	901	698	774	1165	1320
529	531	579	856	575	813
724	3726	1392	2858	1806	798
531	660	1667	1970	1020	370
529	1287	719	2285	525	1007
966	2108	1049	1411	933	338
2000	974	579	719	912	406
845	1490	1162	1326	1500	966
1368	499	692	1020	1809	2535
856	604	3185	909	652	3685
1143	877	417	1086	731	
483	756	684			

Source: The World Almanac and Book of Facts.

6. **Coping Skills with the Disabled** A study was conducted to see if there was a difference between spouses and significant others in coping skills when living with

or caring for a person with multiple sclerosis. These skills were measured by questionnaire responses. The results of the two groups are given on one factor, ambivalence. At $\alpha = 0.10$, is there a difference in the means of the two groups?

Spouses	Significant others
$\overline{X}_1 = 2.0$	$\overline{X}_2 = 1.7$
$\sigma_1 = 0.6$	$\sigma_2 = 0.7$
$n_1 = 120$	$n_2 = 34$

Source: Elsie E. Gulick, "Coping Among Spouses or Significant Others of Persons with Multiple Sclerosis," Nursing Research.

7. **Pulse Rates of Smokers/Nonsmokers** A medical researcher wishes to see whether the pulse rates of smokers are higher than the pulse rates of nonsmokers. Samples of 100 smokers and 100 nonsmokers are selected. The results are shown here. Can the researcher conclude, at $\alpha = 0.05$, that smokers have higher pulse rates than nonsmokers?

Smokers	Nonsmokers
$\overline{X}_1 = 90$	$\overline{X}_2 = 88$
$\sigma_1 = 5$	$\sigma_2 = 6$
$n_1 = 100$	$n_2 = 100$

8. **Heights of Nine-Year Olds** At age 9 the average weight (21.3 kg) and the average height (124.5 cm) for both boys and girls are exactly the same. A random sample of 9-year-olds yielded these results. Estimate the mean difference in height between boys and girls with 95% confidence. Does your interval support the given claim?

	Boys	Girls
Sample size	60	50
Mean height, cm	123.5	126.2
Population variance	98	120

Source: www.healthepic.com.

9. **Length of Hospital Stays** The average length of "short" hospital stays for men is slightly longer than that for women: 5.2 days versus 4.5 days. A random sample of recent hospital stays for both men and women revealed the following. At $\alpha = 0.01$, is there sufficient evidence to conclude that the average hospital stay for men is longer than the average hospital stay for women?

	Men	Women
Sample size	32	30
Sample mean	5.5 days	4.2 days
Population standard deviation	1.2 days	1.5 days

Source: National Center for Health Statistics.

10. **Home Prices** A real estate agent compares the selling prices of Alberta homes in Calgary and Edmonton to see if there is a difference in the price. The results of the study are shown. Is there enough evidence to reject the claim that the average cost of a home in both locations is the same? Use $\alpha = 0.01$.

Calgary	Edmonton
$\overline{X}_1 = \$358,103*$	$\overline{X}_2 = \$303,304*$
$\sigma_1 = \$21,471$	$\sigma_2 = \$14,636$
$n_1 = 35$	$n_2 = 40$

*Based on data from the Multiple Listing Service.

11. **Women Science Majors** In a study of women science majors, the following data were obtained on two groups, those who left their profession within a few months after graduation (leavers) and those who remained in their profession after they graduated (stayers). Test the claim that those who stayed had a higher science grade point average than those who left. Use $\alpha = 0.05$.

Leavers	Stayers
$\overline{X}_1 = 3.16$	$\overline{X}_2 = 3.28$
$\sigma_1 = 0.52$	$\sigma_2 = 0.46$
$n_1 = 103$	$n_2 = 225$

Source: Paula Rayman and Belle Brett, "Women Science Majors: What Makes a Difference in Persistence after Graduation?" *The Journal of Higher Education.*

12. **University Entrance Grades** A published survey of Canada's universities nationwide indicated an average entering grade of 82.9 based on 2683 responses. Assume that a survey of 500 Saint Mary's University students shows a mean grade of 80.6. If the population standard deviation in each case is 3.1, can we conclude that Saint Mary's University has a lower average entry grade than the national average? Use $\alpha = 0.05$.

Source: *Maclean's* university survey.

13. **Money Spent on College Sports** A school administrator hypothesizes that colleges spend more for male sports than they do for female sports. A sample of two different colleges is selected, and the annual expenses (in dollars) per student at each school are shown. At $\alpha = 0.01$, is there enough evidence to support the claim? Assume $\sigma_1 = 3830$ and $\sigma_2 = 2745$.

Males				
7,040	6,576	1,664	12,919	8,605
22,220	3,377	10,128	7,723	2,063
8,033	9,463	7,656	11,456	12,244
6,670	12,371	9,626	5,472	16,175
8,383	623	6,797	10,160	8,725
14,029	13,763	8,811	11,480	9,544
15,048	5,544	10,652	11,267	10,126
8,796	13,351	7,120	9,505	9,571
7,551	5,811	9,119	9,732	5,286
5,254	7,550	11,015	12,403	12,703

Females				
10,333	6,407	10,082	5,933	3,991
7,435	8,324	6,989	16,249	5,922
7,654	8,411	11,324	10,248	6,030
9,331	6,869	6,502	11,041	11,597
5,468	7,874	9,277	10,127	13,371
7,055	6,909	8,903	6,925	7,058
12,745	12,016	9,883	14,698	9,907
8,917	9,110	5,232	6,959	5,832
7,054	7,235	11,248	8,478	6,502
7,300	993	6,815	9,959	10,353

Source: *USA TODAY.*

14. **Taxi Weekly Kilometres** Is there a difference in average kilometres for each of two taxi companies during a randomly selected week? The data are shown. Use $\alpha = 0.05$. Assume that the populations are normally distributed. Use the *P*-value method.

Black Top Taxi Company	Yellow Cab Company
$\overline{X}_1 = 1347$	$\overline{X}_2 = 1212$
$\sigma_1 = 48$	$\sigma_2 = 64$
$n_1 = 35$	$n_2 = 40$

15. **Self-Esteem Scores** In the study cited in Exercise 11, the researchers collected the data shown here on a self-esteem questionnaire. At $\alpha = 0.05$, can it be concluded that there is a difference in the self-esteem scores of the two groups? Use the *P*-value method.

Leavers	Stayers
$\overline{X}_1 = 3.05$	$\overline{X}_2 = 2.96$
$\sigma_1 = 0.75$	$\sigma_2 = 0.75$
$n_1 = 103$	$n_2 = 225$

Source: Paula Rayman and Belle Brett, "Women Science Majors: What Makes a Difference in Persistence after Graduation?" *The Journal of Higher Education.*

16. **Age of College Students** The dean of students wants to see whether there is a significant difference in ages of resident students and commuting students. She selects a sample of 50 students from each group. The ages are shown here. At $\alpha = 0.05$, decide if there is enough evidence to reject the claim of no difference in the ages of the two groups. Use the *P*-value method. Assume $\sigma_1 = 3.68$ and $\sigma_2 = 4.7$.

Resident students							
22	25	27	23	26	28	26	24
25	20	26	24	27	26	18	19
18	30	26	18	18	19	32	23
19	19	18	29	19	22	18	22
26	19	19	21	23	18	20	18
22	21	19	21	21	22	18	20
19	23						

Commuter students

18	20	19	18	22	25	24	35
23	18	23	22	28	25	20	24
26	30	22	22	22	21	18	20
19	26	35	19	19	18	19	32
29	23	21	19	36	27	27	20
20	21	18	19	23	20	19	19
20	25						

17. Problem-Solving Ability Two groups of students are given a problem-solving test, and the results are compared. Find the 90% confidence interval of the true difference in means.

Mathematics majors	Computer science majors
$\overline{X}_1 = 83.6$	$\overline{X}_2 = 79.2$
$\sigma_1 = 4.3$	$\sigma_2 = 3.8$
$n_1 = 36$	$n_2 = 36$

18. Credit Card Debt The average credit card debt for a recent year was \$9205. Five years earlier the average credit card debt was \$6618. Assume sample sizes of 35 were used and the population standard deviations of both samples were \$1928. Is there enough evidence to believe that the average credit card debt has increased? Use $\alpha = 0.05$. Give a possible reason as to why or why not the debt was increased.

Source: CardWeb.com.

19. Cigarette Nicotine Content Two brands of cigarettes are selected, and their nicotine content is compared. The data are shown here. Find the 99% confidence interval of the true difference in the means.

Brand A	Brand B
$\overline{X}_1 = 28.6$ milligrams	$\overline{X}_2 = 32.9$ milligrams
$\sigma_1 = 5.1$ milligrams	$\sigma_2 = 4.4$ milligrams
$n_1 = 30$	$n_2 = 40$

20. Battery Voltage Two brands of batteries are tested, and their voltage is compared. The data follow. Find the 95% confidence interval of the true difference in the means. Assume that both variables are normally distributed.

Brand X	Brand Y
$\overline{X}_1 = 9.2$ volts	$\overline{X}_2 = 8.8$ volts
$\sigma_1 = 0.3$ volt	$\sigma_2 = 0.1$ volt
$n_1 = 27$	$n_2 = 30$

Extending the Concepts

21. Exam Scores at Private and Public Schools A researcher claims that students in a private school have exam scores that are at most 8 points higher than those of students in public schools. Random samples of 60 students from each type of school are selected and given an exam. The results are shown. At $\alpha = 0.05$, test the claim.

Private school	Public school
$\overline{X}_1 = 110$	$\overline{X}_2 = 104$
$\sigma_1 = 15$	$\sigma_2 = 15$
$n_1 = 60$	$n_2 = 60$

9–2 | ## Testing the Difference between Two Means of Independent Samples: Using the *t* Test >

Test the difference between two means for independent samples, using the *t* test.

In Section 9–1, the *z* test was used to test the difference between two means when the population standard deviations were known and the variables were normally or approximately normally distributed, or when both sample sizes were greater than or equal to 30. In many situations, however, these conditions cannot be met—that is, the population standard deviations are not known. In these cases, a *t* test is used to test the difference between means when the two samples are independent and when the samples are taken from two normally or approximately normally distributed populations. Samples are **independent samples** when they are not related. Also, it will be assumed that the variances are not equal.

> **Formula for the *t* Test—For Testing the Difference between Two Means—Independent Samples**
>
> Variances are assumed to be unequal:
>
> $$t = \frac{(\overline{X}_1 - \overline{X}_2) - (\mu_1 - \mu_2)}{\sqrt{\dfrac{s_1^2}{n_1} + \dfrac{s_2^2}{n_2}}}$$
>
> where the degrees of freedom are equal to the smaller of $n_1 - 1$ or $n_2 - 1$.

The formula

$$t = \frac{(\overline{X}_1 - \overline{X}_2) - (\mu_1 - \mu_2)}{\sqrt{\dfrac{s_1^2}{n_1} + \dfrac{s_2^2}{n_2}}}$$

follows the format of

$$\text{Test statistic} = \frac{(\text{Observed value}) - (\text{Expected value})}{\text{Standard error}}$$

where $\overline{X}_1 - \overline{X}_2$ is the observed difference between sample means and where the expected value $\mu_1 - \mu_2$ is equal to zero when no difference between population means is hypothesized. The denominator $\sqrt{s_1^2/n_1 + s_2^2/n_2}$ is the standard error of the difference between two means. Since mathematical derivation of the standard error is somewhat complicated, it will be omitted here.

Assumptions for the t Test for Two Independent Means When σ_1 and σ_2 Are Unknown

1. The samples are random samples.
2. The sample data are independent of each other.
3. When the sample sizes are less than 30, the population must be normally or approximately normally distributed.

Example 9–4

Farm Sizes

The average size of a farm in Ontario is 85 hectares (ha). The average size of a farm in Quebec is 93 ha. Assume the data were obtained from two samples with standard deviations of 17 ha and 6 ha, respectively, and sample sizes of 8 and 10, respectively. Can it be concluded at $\alpha = 0.05$ that the average size of the farms in the two provinces is different? Assume the populations are normally distributed.

Source: Adapted from Statistics Canada, *Farming Facts, 2002*, Catalogue 21-522-XPE.

Solution

Step 1 State the hypotheses and identify the claim for the means.

$$H_0: \mu_1 = \mu_2 \qquad \text{and} \qquad H_1: \mu_1 \neq \mu_2 \text{ (claim)}$$

Step 2 Find the critical values. Since the test is two-tailed, since $\alpha = 0.05$, and since the variances are unequal, the degrees of freedom are the smaller of $n_1 - 1$ or $n_2 - 1$. In this case the degrees of freedom are $8 - 1 = 7$. Hence, from Table F, the critical values are $+2.365$ and -2.365.

Step 3 Compute the test statistic. Since the variances are unequal, use the first formula.

$$t = \frac{(\overline{X}_1 - \overline{X}_2) - (\mu_1 - \mu_2)}{\sqrt{\dfrac{s_1^2}{n_1} + \dfrac{s_2^2}{n_2}}} = \frac{(85 - 93) - 0}{\sqrt{\dfrac{17^2}{8} + \dfrac{6^2}{10}}} \approx -1.269$$

Step 4 Make the decision. Do not reject the null hypothesis, since $-1.269 > -2.365$. See Figure 9–5.

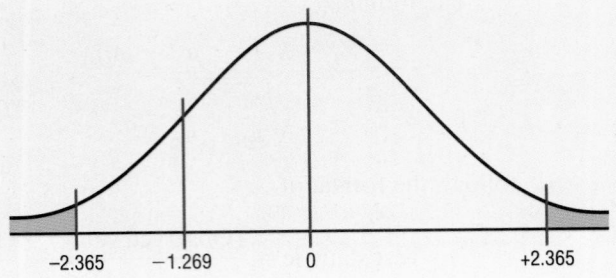

$-2.365 \quad -1.269 \quad 0 \quad +2.365$

Step 5 Summarize the results. There is not enough evidence to support the claim that the average size of the farms is different.

Unusual Stat

On average, women's interpersonal space measures 6 centimetres closer than men's.

When raw data are given in the exercises, use your calculator or the formulas in Chapter 3 to find the means and variances for the data sets. Then follow the procedures shown in this section to test the hypotheses.

Confidence intervals can also be found for the difference between two means with the following formula.

Formula for the Confidence Intervals for the Difference of Two Means: Independent Samples

Variances are assumed to be unequal.

$$(\overline{X}_1 - \overline{X}_2) - t_{\alpha/2}\sqrt{\frac{s_1^2}{n_1} + \frac{s_2^2}{n_2}} < \mu_1 - \mu_2 < (\overline{X}_1 - \overline{X}_2) + t_{\alpha/2}\sqrt{\frac{s_1^2}{n_1} + \frac{s_2^2}{n_2}}$$

d.f. = smaller value of $n_1 - 1$ or $n_2 - 1$

Example 9–5

Find the 95% confidence interval for the data in Example 9–4.

Solution

Substitute in the formula.

$$(\overline{X}_1 - \overline{X}_2) - t_{\alpha/2}\sqrt{\frac{s_1^2}{n_1} + \frac{s_2^2}{n_2}} < \mu_1 - \mu_2 < (\overline{X}_1 - \overline{X}_2) + t_{\alpha/2}\sqrt{\frac{s_1^2}{n_1} + \frac{s_2^2}{n_2}}$$

$$(85 - 93) - 2.365\sqrt{\frac{17^2}{8} + \frac{6^2}{10}} < \mu_1 - \mu_2 < (85 - 93) + 2.365\sqrt{\frac{17^2}{8} + \frac{6^2}{10}}$$

$$-22.91 < \mu_1 - \mu_2 < 6.91$$

Since 0 is contained in the interval, the decision is to not reject the null hypothesis $H_0: \mu_1 = \mu_2$.

In many statistical software packages, a different method is used to compute the degrees of freedom for this t test. They are determined by the formula

$$\text{d.f.} = \frac{(s_1^2/n_1 + s_2^2/n_2)^2}{(s_1^2/n_1)^2/(n_1 - 1) + (s_2^2/n_2)^2/(n_2 - 1)}$$

This formula will not be used in this textbook.

There are actually two different options for the use of t tests. *One option is used when the variances of the populations are not equal, and the other option is used when the variances are equal.* To determine whether two sample variances are equal, the researcher can use an *F* test, as shown in Section 9–5.

When the variances are assumed to be equal, this formula is used and

$$t = \frac{(\overline{X}_1 - \overline{X}_2) - (\mu_1 - \mu_2)}{\sqrt{\dfrac{(n_1 - 1)s_1^2 + (n_2 - 1)s_2^2}{n_1 + n_2 - 2}} \sqrt{\dfrac{1}{n_1} + \dfrac{1}{n_2}}}$$

follows the format of

$$\text{Test statistic} = \frac{(\text{Observed value}) - (\text{Expected value})}{\text{Standard error}}$$

For the numerator, the terms are the same as in the previous formula. However, a note of explanation is needed for the denominator of the second test statistic. Since both populations are assumed to have the same variance, the standard error is computed with what is called a *pooled estimate of the variance.* A **pooled estimate of the variance** is a weighted average of the variance, using the two sample variances and the *degrees of freedom* of each variance as the weights. Again, since the algebraic derivation of the standard error is somewhat complicated, it is omitted.

Note, however, that not all statisticians are in agreement about using the *F* test before using the *t* test. Some believe that conducting the *F* and *t* tests at the same level of significance will change the overall level of significance of the *t* test. Their reasons are beyond the scope of this textbook. Because of this, we will assume that $\sigma_1 \neq \sigma_2$ in this textbook.

9–2   Applying the Concepts

Too Long on the Telephone

A company collects data on the lengths of telephone calls made by employees in two different divisions. The mean and standard deviation for the sales division are 10.26 and 8.56, respectively. The mean and standard deviation for the shipping and receiving division are 6.93 and 4.93, respectively. A hypothesis test was run, and the computer output follows.

Degrees of freedom = 56
Confidence interval limits = −0.18979, 6.84979
Test statistic $t = 1.89566$
Critical value $t = -2.0037, 2.0037$
P-value = 0.06317
Significance level = 0.05

1. Are the samples independent or dependent?
2. What assumption is made about the population variances?
3. Which number from the output is compared to the significance level to check if the null hypothesis should be rejected?
4. Which number from the output gives the probability of a type I error that is calculated from the sample data?
5. What decision rule is used for the confidence interval limits?
6. Was a right-, left-, or two-tailed test done? Why?
7. What are your conclusions?
8. What would your conclusions be if the level of significance was initially set at 0.10?

See page 453 for the answers.

For these exercises, use the following traditional method of hypothesis testing unless otherwise specified.

    a. State the hypotheses and identify the claim.

    b. Find the critical value(s).

    c. Compute the test statistic.

    d. Make the decision.

    e. Summarize the results.

For all exercises, assume normally or approximately normally distributed variables and unequal variances.

1. **Assessed Home Values** A real estate agent wishes to determine whether tax assessors and real estate appraisers agree on the values of homes. A random sample of the two groups appraised 10 homes. The data are shown here. Is there a significant difference in the values of the homes for each group? Let $\alpha = 0.05$. Find the 95% confidence interval for the difference of the means.

Real estate appraisers	Tax assessors
$\overline{X}_1 = \$83{,}256$	$\overline{X}_2 = \$88{,}354$
$s_1 = \$3256$	$s_2 = \$2341$
$n_1 = 10$	$n_2 = 10$

2. **Hours Spent Watching Television** According to Nielsen media research, children (ages 2–11) spend an average of 21 hours and 30 minutes watching television per week, while teens (ages 12–17) spend an average of 20 hours and 40 minutes. Based on the sample statistics obtained below, is there sufficient evidence to conclude a difference in average television watching times between the two groups? Use $\alpha = 0.01$.

	Children	Teens
Sample mean	22.45	18.50
Sample variance	16.4	18.2
Sample size	15	15

Source: Time Almanac.

3. **NFL Salaries** An agent claims that there is no difference between the pay of safeties and linebackers in the National Football League. A survey of 15 safeties found an average salary of $501,580, and a survey of 15 linebackers found an average salary of $513,360. If the standard deviation in each case was $20,000, is the agent correct? Use $\alpha = 0.05$.

Source: NFL Players Assn./USA TODAY.

4. **Cyber School Enrollment** The data show the number of students attending cyber charter schools in Allegheny County and the number of students attending cyber schools in counties surrounding Allegheny County. At $\alpha = 0.01$ is there enough evidence to support the claim that the average number of students in school districts in Allegheny County who attend cyber schools is greater than those who attend cyber schools in school districts outside Allegheny County?

Give a factor that should be considered in interpreting this answer.

Allegheny County	Outside Allegheny County
25 75 38 41 27 32	57 25 38 14 10 29

Source: Pittsburgh Tribune-Review.

5. **Hockey's Highest Scorers** The number of points held by a sample of the NHL's highest scorers for both the Eastern Conference and the Western Conference is shown below. At $\alpha = 0.05$, can it be concluded that there is a difference in means based on these data?

Eastern Conference				Western Conference			
83	60	75	58	77	59	72	58
78	59	70	58	37	57	66	55
62	61	59	61				

Source: Fox Sports.

6. **Missing Persons** A researcher wishes to test the claim that, on average, more juveniles than adults are classified as missing persons. Records for the last 5 years are shown. At $\alpha = 0.10$, is there enough evidence to support the claim?

Juveniles	65,513	65,934	64,213	61,954	59,167
Adults	31,364	34,478	36,937	35,946	38,209

Source: USA TODAY.

7. **Tax Return Help** The local branch of the Canada Revenue Agency spent an average of 21 minutes helping each of 10 people prepare their tax returns. The standard deviation was 5.6 minutes. A volunteer tax preparer spent an average of 27 minutes helping 14 people prepare their taxes. The standard deviation was 4.3 minutes. At $\alpha = 0.02$, is there a difference in the average time spent by the two services? Find the 98% confidence interval for the two means.

8. **College Students' Volunteer Work** Females and males alike from the general adult population volunteer an average of 4.2 hours per week. A random sample of 20 female college students and 18 male college students indicated these results concerning the amount of time spent in volunteer service per week. At the 0.01 level of significance, is there sufficient evidence to conclude that a difference exists between the mean number of volunteer hours per week for male and female college students?

	Male	Female
Sample mean	2.5	3.8
Sample variance	2.2	3.5
Sample size	18	20

Source: The New York Times Almanac.

9. **Moisture Content of Fruits and Vegetables** Following is a list of the moisture content (by percentage) for random samples of different fruits and vegetables. At the 0.05 level of significance, can it be concluded that fruits differ from vegetables in average moisture content?

Fruits		Vegetables	
Apricot	86	Artichoke	85
Banana	75	Bamboo shoot	91
Avocado	72	Beets	88
Blackberry	88	Broccoli	89
Clementine	87	Cucumber	95
Fig	79	Iceberg lettuce	96
Pink grapefruit	92	Mushroom	92
Mango	84	Radish	95
		Tomato	94

Source: Nutrition Data: www.nutritiondata.com.

10. **Maternity Patients' Hospital Stays** Health Care Knowledge Systems reported that an insured woman spends on average 2.3 days in the hospital for a routine childbirth, while an uninsured woman spends on average 1.9 days. Assume that two samples of 16 women each were used in both samples. The standard deviation of the first sample is equal to 0.6 day, and the standard deviation of the second sample is 0.3 day. At $\alpha = 0.01$, test the claim that the means are equal. Find the 99% confidence interval for the differences of the means. Use the *P*-value method.
Source: Michael D. Shook and Robert L. Shook, *The Book of Odds.*

11. **Mice Maze Run Times** The times (in minutes) it took 6 white mice to learn to run a simple maze and the times it took 6 brown mice to learn to run the same maze are given here. At $\alpha = 0.05$, does the colour of the mice make a difference in their learning rate? Find the 95% confidence interval for the difference of the means.

White mice	18	24	20	13	15	12
Brown mice	25	16	19	14	16	10

12. **Medical School Enrollments** A random sample of enrollments from medical schools that specialize in research and from those that are noted for primary care is listed. Find the 90% confidence interval for the difference in the means.

Research				Primary care			
474	577	605	663	783	605	427	728
783	467	670	414	546	474	371	107
813	443	565	696	442	587	293	277
692	694	277	419	662	555	527	320
884							

Source: U.S. News & World Report Best Graduate Schools.

13. **Student Tuition Fees** Tuition fees for a random sample of Canadian and international undergraduate students (in dollars) are listed. Find the 95% confidence interval for the difference in the means.

Canadian		International	
4,092	4,184	16,620	11,079
6,557	4,133	20,981	12,450
4,689	1,668	8,765	11,970
2,700		5,700	8,780

Source: Association of Universities and Colleges of Canada.

9–3 Testing the Difference between Two Means: Dependent Samples >

LO3

Test the difference between two means for dependent samples.

In Section 9–2, the *t* test was used to compare two sample means when the samples were independent. In this section, a different version of the *t* test is explained. This version is used when the samples are dependent. Samples are considered to be **dependent samples** when the subjects are paired or matched in some way.

For example, suppose a medical researcher wants to see whether a drug will affect the reaction time of its users. To test this hypothesis, the researcher must pretest the subjects in the sample first. That is, they are given a test to ascertain their normal reaction times. Then after taking the drug, the subjects are tested again, using a posttest. Finally, the means of the two tests are compared to see whether there is a difference. Since the same subjects are used in both cases, the samples are *related;* subjects scoring high on the pretest will generally score high on the posttest, even after consuming the drug. Likewise, those scoring lower on the pretest will tend to score lower on the posttest. To take this effect into account, the researcher employs a *t* test, using the differences between the pretest values and the posttest values. Thus, only the gain or loss in values is compared.

Here are some other examples of dependent samples. A researcher may want to design an SAT Reasoning Test preparation course to help students raise their test scores the second time they take the SAT Reasoning Test. Hence, the differences between the two exams are compared. A medical specialist may want to see whether a new counselling program will help subjects lose weight. Therefore, the preweights of the subjects will be compared with the postweights.

Besides samples in which the same subjects are used in a pre–post situation, there other cases where the samples are considered dependent. For example, students might be matched or paired according to some variable that is pertinent to the study; then one student is assigned to one group, and the other student is assigned to a second group. For instance, in a study involving learning, students can be selected and paired according to their IQs. That is, two students with the same IQ will be paired. Then one will be assigned to one sample group (which might receive instruction by computers), and the other student will be assigned to another sample group (which might receive instruction by the lecture discussion method). These assignments will be done randomly. Since a student's IQ is important to learning, it is a variable that should be controlled. By matching subjects on IQ, the researcher can eliminate the variable's influence, for the most part. Matching, then, helps to reduce type II error by eliminating extraneous variables.

Two notes of caution should be mentioned. First, when subjects are matched according to one variable, the matching process does not eliminate the influence of other variables. Matching students according to IQ does not account for their mathematical ability or their familiarity with computers. Since not all variables influencing a study can be controlled, it is up to the researcher to determine which variables should be used in matching. Second, when the same subjects are used for a pre–post study, sometimes the knowledge that they are participating in a study can influence the results. For example, if people are placed in a special program, they may be more highly motivated to succeed simply because they have been selected to participate; the program itself may have little effect on their success.

When the samples are dependent, a special t test for dependent means is used. This test employs the difference in values of the matched pairs. The hypotheses are as follows:

Two-tailed	Left-tailed	Right-tailed
$H_0: \mu_D = 0$	$H_0: \mu_D = 0$	$H_0: \mu_D = 0$
$H_1: \mu_D \neq 0$	$H_1: \mu_D < 0$	$H_1: \mu_D > 0$

where μ_D is the symbol for the expected mean of the difference of the matched pairs. The general procedure for finding the test statistic involves several steps.

First, find the differences of the values of the pairs of data.

$$D = X_1 - X_2$$

Second, find the mean $\overline{D}$ of the differences, using the formula

$$\overline{D} = \frac{\Sigma D}{n}$$

where n is the number of data pairs. Third, find the standard deviation s_D of the differences, using the formula

$$s_D = \sqrt{\frac{n\Sigma D^2 - (\Sigma D)^2}{n(n-1)}}$$

Fourth, find the estimated standard error $s_{\overline{D}}$ of the differences, which is

$$s_{\overline{D}} = \frac{s_D}{\sqrt{n}}$$

Finally, find the test statistic, using the formula

$$t = \frac{\overline{D} - \mu_D}{s_D/\sqrt{n}} \qquad \text{with d.f.} = n - 1$$

The formula in the final step follows the basic format of

$$\text{Test statistic} = \frac{(\text{Observed value}) - (\text{Expected value})}{\text{Standard error}}$$

Unusual Stat

Canadians consume, on average, 45 kilograms of sugar per year.

where the observed value is the mean of the differences. The expected value μ_D is zero if the hypothesis is $\mu_D = 0$. The standard error of the difference is the standard deviation of the difference, divided by the square root of the sample size. Both populations must be normally or approximately normally distributed. Example 9–6 illustrates the hypothesis testing procedure in detail.

> **Assumptions for the t Test for Two Means When the Samples Are Dependent**
>
> 1. The sample or samples are random.
> 2. The sample data are dependent.
> 3. When the sample size or sample sizes are less than 30, the population or populations must be normally or approximately normally distributed.

Example 9–6

Vitamin for Increased Strength

A physical education director claims that by taking a special vitamin, a weightlifter can increase his strength. Eight athletes are selected and given a test of strength, using the standard bench press. After 2 weeks of regular training, supplemented with the vitamin, they are tested again. Test the effectiveness of the vitamin regimen at $\alpha = 0.05$. Each value in these data represents the maximum number of kilograms the athlete can bench-press. Assume that the variable is approximately normally distributed.

Athlete	1	2	3	4	5	6	7	8
Before (X_1)	95	104	83	92	119	115	99	98
After (X_2)	99	107	81	93	122	113	101	98

Solution

Step 1 State the hypotheses and identify the claim. For the vitamin to be effective, the *before* weights must be significantly less than the *after* weights; hence, the mean of the differences must be less than zero.

$H_0: \mu_D = 0$ and $H_1: \mu_D < 0$ (claim)

Step 2 Find the critical value. The degrees of freedom are $n - 1$. In this case, d.f. $= 8 - 1 = 7$. The critical value for a left-tailed test with $\alpha = 0.05$ is -1.895.

Step 3 Compute the test statistic.
a. Make a table.

Before (X_1)	After (X_2)	Column A $D = X_1 - X_2$	Column B $D^2 = (X_1 - X_2)^2$
95	99		
104	107		
83	81		
92	93		
119	122		
115	113		
99	101		
98	98		

b. Find the differences and place the results in column A.

$$95 - 99 = -4$$
$$104 - 107 = -3$$
$$83 - 81 = 2$$
$$92 - 93 = -1$$
$$119 - 122 = -3$$
$$115 - 113 = 2$$
$$99 - 101 = -2$$
$$98 - 98 = 0$$
$$\Sigma D = -9$$

c. Find the mean of the differences.

$$\overline{D} = \frac{\Sigma D}{n} = \frac{-9}{8} = -1.125$$

d. Square the differences and place the results in column B.

$$(-4)^2 = 16$$
$$(-3)^2 = 9$$
$$(2)^2 = 4$$
$$(-1)^2 = 1$$
$$(-3)^2 = 9$$
$$(2)^2 = 4$$
$$(-2)^2 = 4$$
$$(0)^2 = 0$$
$$\overline{\Sigma D^2 = 47}$$

The completed table is shown.

		Column A	Column B
Before (X_1)	After (X_2)	$D = X_1 - X_2$	$D^2 = (X_1 - X_2)^2$
95	99	-4	16
104	107	-3	9
83	81	2	4
92	93	-1	1
119	122	-3	9
115	113	2	4
99	101	-2	4
98	98	0	0
		$\Sigma D = -9$	$\Sigma D^2 = 47$

e. Find the standard deviation of the differences.

$$s_D = \sqrt{\frac{n\Sigma D^2 - (\Sigma D)^2}{n(n-1)}} = \sqrt{\frac{8 \cdot (47) - (-9)^2}{8(8-1)}} \approx 2.295$$

f. Find the test statistic.

$$t = \frac{\overline{D} - \mu_0}{s_D/\sqrt{n}} = \frac{-1.125 - 0}{2.295/\sqrt{8}} \approx -1.386$$

Step 4   Make the decision. The decision is to not reject the null hypothesis at $\alpha = 0.05$, since $-1.386 > -1.895$, as shown in Figure 9–6.

Figure 9–6

Critical Value and
Test Statistic for
Example 9–6

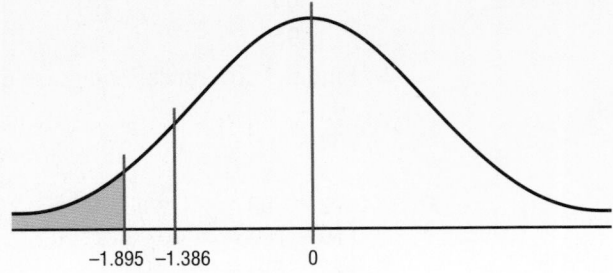

-1.895 -1.386   0

Step 5   Summarize the results. There is not enough evidence to support the claim that the vitamin supplement increases the strength of weightlifters.

The formulas for this t test are summarized next.

Formulas for the t Test for Dependent Samples

$$t = \frac{\overline{D} - \mu_D}{s_D/\sqrt{n}}$$

with d.f. $= n - 1$ and where

$$\overline{D} = \frac{\Sigma D}{n} \quad \text{and} \quad s_D = \sqrt{\frac{n \Sigma D^2 - (\Sigma D)^2}{n(n - 1)}}$$

Example 9–7

Mineral Supplement and Cholesterol Level

A dietitian wants to see if a person's cholesterol level will change if the diet is supplemented by a certain mineral. Six subjects were pretested, and then they took the mineral supplement for a 6-week period. The results are shown in the table. (Cholesterol level is measured in millimoles per litre, mmol/L) Can it be concluded that the cholesterol level has been changed at $\alpha = 0.10$? Assume the variable is approximately normally distributed.

Subject	1	2	3	4	5	6
Before (X_1)	5.44	6.09	5.39	4.92	4.46	6.32
After (X_2)	4.92	4.40	5.44	4.87	4.48	5.91

Solution

Step 1 State the hypotheses and identify the claim. If the diet is effective, the *before* cholesterol levels should be different from the *after* levels.

H_0: $\mu_D = 0$ and H_1: $\mu_D \neq 0$ (claim)

Step 2 Find the critical value. The degrees of freedom are 5. At $\alpha = 0.10$, the critical values are ± 2.015.

Step 3 Compute the test statistic.
a. Make a table.

Before (X_1)	After (X_2)	Column A $D = X_1 - X_2$	Column B $D^2 = (X_1 - X_2)^2$
5.44	4.92		
6.09	4.40		
5.39	5.44		
4.92	4.87		
4.46	4.48		
6.32	5.91		

b. Find the differences and place the results in column A.

$$
\begin{aligned}
5.44 - 4.92 &= 0.52 \\
6.09 - 4.40 &= 1.69 \\
5.39 - 5.44 &= -0.05 \\
4.92 - 4.87 &= 0.05 \\
4.46 - 4.48 &= -0.02 \\
6.32 - 5.91 &= \underline{0.41} \\
\Sigma D &= 2.60
\end{aligned}
$$

c. Find the mean of the differences.

$$\overline{D} = \frac{\Sigma D}{n} = \frac{2.60}{6} \approx 0.43$$

d. Square the differences and place the results in column B.

$$(0.52)^2 = 0.270$$
$$(1.69)^2 = 2.856$$
$$(-0.05)^2 = 0.003$$
$$(0.05)^2 = 0.002$$
$$(-0.02)^2 = 0.000$$
$$\underline{(0.41)^2 = 0.168}$$
$$\Sigma D^2 = 6.760$$

Then complete the table as shown.

Before (X_1)	After (X_2)	Column A $D = X_1 - X_2$	Column B $D^2 = (X_1 - X_2)^2$
5.44	4.92	0.52	0.270
6.09	4.40	1.69	2.856
5.39	5.44	−0.05	0.003
4.92	4.87	0.05	0.002
4.46	4.48	−0.02	0.000
6.32	5.91	0.41	0.168
		$\Sigma D = 2.60$	$\Sigma D^2 = 3.300$

e. Find the standard deviation of the differences.

$$s_D = \sqrt{\frac{n\Sigma D^2 - (\Sigma D)^2}{n(n-1)}} = \sqrt{\frac{6 \cdot (3.300) - (2.60)^2}{6(6-1)}} \approx 0.659$$

f. Find the test statistic.

$$t = \frac{\overline{D} - \mu_D}{s_D/\sqrt{n}} = \frac{0.43 - 0}{0.659/\sqrt{6}} \approx 1.598$$

Step 4 Make the decision. The decision is to not reject the null hypothesis, since the test statistic 1.598 is in the noncritical region, as shown in Figure 9−7.

Figure 9−7

Critical Values and Test Statistic for Example 9−7

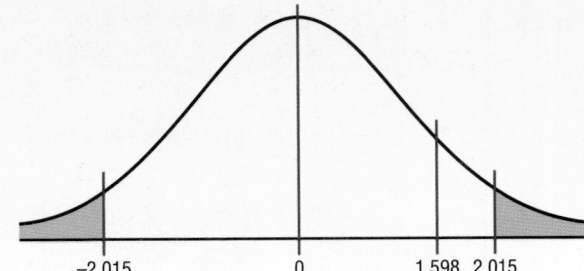

−2.015   0   1.598 2.015

Step 5 Summarize the results. There is not enough evidence to support the claim that the mineral changes a person's cholesterol level.

The steps for this t test are summarized in the Procedure Table.

Procedure Table

Testing the Difference between Means for Dependent Samples

Step 1 State the hypotheses and identify the claim.

Step 2 Find the critical value(s).

Step 3 Compute the test statistic.

    a. Make a table, as shown.

X_1	X_2	Column A $D = X_1 - X_2$	Column B $D^2 = (X_1 - X_2)^2$
⋮	⋮		
		$\Sigma D = \underline{\quad}$	$\Sigma D^2 = \underline{\quad}$

    b. Find the differences and place the results in column A.

$$D = X_1 - X_2$$

    c. Find the mean of the differences.

$$\overline{D} = \frac{\Sigma D}{n}$$

    d. Square the differences and place the results in column B. Complete the table.

$$D^2 = (X_1 - X_2)^2$$

    e. Find the standard deviation of the differences.

$$s_D = \sqrt{\frac{n\Sigma D^2 - (\Sigma D)^2}{n(n-1)}}$$

    f. Find the test statistic.

$$t = \frac{\overline{D} - \mu_D}{s_D/\sqrt{n}} \quad \text{with d.f.} = n - 1$$

Step 4 Make the decision.

Step 5 Summarize the results.

Unusual Stat

2% of Canadian women younger than 45 years of age are grandparents.

The P-values for the t test are found in Table F in Appendix C. For a two-tailed test with d.f. $= 5$ and $t = 1.610$, the P-value is found between 1.476 and 2.015; hence, $0.10 < P\text{-value} < 0.20$. Thus, the null hypothesis cannot be rejected at $\alpha = 0.10$.

If a specific difference is hypothesized, this formula should be used

$$t = \frac{\overline{D} - \mu_D}{s_D/\sqrt{n}}$$

where μ_D is the hypothesized difference.

For example, if a dietitian claims that people on a specific diet will lose an average of 1.5 kilograms in a week, the hypotheses are

$$H_0: \mu_D = 1.5 \quad \text{and} \quad H_1: \mu_D \neq 1.5$$

The value 1.5 will be substituted in the test statistic formula for μ_D.

Confidence intervals can be found for the mean differences with this formula.

Formula for the Confidence Interval for the Mean Difference

$$\overline{D} - t_{\alpha/2}\frac{s_D}{\sqrt{n}} < \mu_D < \overline{D} + t_{\alpha/2}\frac{s_D}{\sqrt{n}}$$

d.f. $= n - 1$

Example 9–8

Find the 90% confidence interval for the data in Example 9–7.

Solution

Substitute in the formula.

$$\overline{D} - t_{\alpha/2}\frac{s_D}{\sqrt{n}} < \mu_D < \overline{D} + t_{\alpha/2}\frac{s_D}{\sqrt{n}}$$

$$16.7 - 2.015 \cdot \frac{25.4}{\sqrt{6}} < \mu_D < 16.7 + 2.015 \cdot \frac{25.4}{\sqrt{6}}$$

$$16.7 - 20.89 < \mu_D < 16.7 + 20.89$$

$$-4.19 < \mu_D < 37.59$$

Since 0 is contained in the interval, the decision is to not reject the null hypothesis H_0: $\mu_D = 0$.

Speaking of Statistics

Can Video Games Save Lives?

Can playing video games help doctors perform surgery? The answer is yes. A study showed that surgeons who played video games for at least 3 hours each week made about 37% fewer mistakes and finished operations 27% faster than those who did not play video games.

The type of surgery that they performed is called *laparoscopic* surgery, where the surgeon inserts a tiny video camera into the body and uses a joystick to manoeuvre the surgical instruments while watching the results on a television monitor. This study compared two groups and used proportions. What statistical test do you think was used to compare the percentages? (See Section 9–4.)

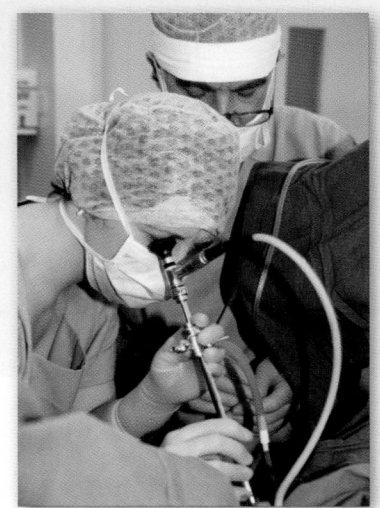

9–3 Applying the Concepts

Air Quality

As a researcher for the Ontario Ministry of the Environment, you have been asked to determine if Ontario's air quality index (AQI) has changed in the past 2 years. You select a random sample of 10 cities and find the air quality index on the same day in two consecutive years. The data are shown. (*Note:* The lower the AQI, the better the air quality.)

Year 1	25	39	29	33	42	17	35	10	21	30
Year 2	42	28	48	46	44	32	48	30	25	46

Source: Ontario Ministry of the Environment.

Based on the data, answer the following questions.

1. What is the purpose of the study?
2. Are the samples independent or dependent?
3. What are the hypotheses that you would use?
4. What is (are) the critical value(s) that you would use?
5. What statistical test would you use?
6. How many degrees of freedom are there?
7. What is your conclusion?
8. Could an independent means test have been used?
9. Do you think this was a good way to answer the original question?

See page 453 for the answers.

Exercises 9–3

1. Classify each as independent or dependent samples.

   a. Heights of identical twins
   b. Test scores of the same students in English and psychology
   c. The effectiveness of two different brands of pain reliever
   d. Effects of a drug on reaction time, measured by a *before* and an *after* test
   e. The effectiveness of two different diets on two different groups of individuals

For Exercises 2 through 10, use the following traditional method of hypothesis testing unless otherwise specified.

   a. State the hypotheses and identify the claim.
   b. Find the critical value(s).
   c. Compute the test statistic.
   d. Make the decision.
   e. Summarize the results.

Assume that all variables are normally or approximately normally distributed.

2. **Retention Test Scores** A sample of non-English majors at a selected college was used in a study to see if the students retained more from reading a nineteenth-century novel or by watching it in DVD form. Each student was assigned one novel to read and a different one to watch, and then they were given a 20-point written quiz on each novel. The test results are shown below. At $\alpha = 0.05$, can it be concluded that the book scores are higher than the DVD scores?

Book	90	80	90	75	80	90	84
DVD	85	72	80	80	70	75	80

3. **Improving Study Habits** As an aid for improving students' study habits, nine students were randomly selected to attend a seminar on the importance of education in life. The table shows the number of hours each student studied per week before and after the seminar. At $\alpha = 0.10$, did attending the seminar increase the number of hours the students studied per week?

Before	9	12	6	15	3	18	10	13	7
After	9	17	9	20	2	21	15	22	6

4. **Obstacle Course Times** An obstacle course was set up on a campus, and 10 volunteers were given a chance to complete it while they were being timed. They then sampled a new energy drink and were given the opportunity to run the course again. The *before* and *after* times in seconds are shown below. Is there sufficient evidence at $\alpha = 0.05$ to conclude that the students did better the second time? Discuss possible reasons for your results.

Student	1	2	3	4	5	6	7	8
Before	67	72	80	70	78	82	69	75
After	68	70	76	65	75	78	65	68

5. Sleep Report Students in a statistics class were asked to report the number of hours they slept on weeknights and on weekends. At $\alpha = 0.05$, is there sufficient evidence that there is a difference in the mean number of hours slept?

Student	1	2	3	4	5	6	7	8
Hours, Sun.–Thurs.	8	5.5	7.5	8	7	6	6	8
Hours, Fri.–Sat.	4	7	10.5	12	11	9	6	9

6. PGA Golf Scores At a PGA tournament (the Honda Classic at Palm Beach Gardens, Florida) the following scores were posted for eight randomly selected golfers for two consecutive days. At $\alpha = 0.05$, is there evidence of a difference in mean scores for the two days?

Golfer	1	2	3	4	5	6	7	8
Thursday	67	65	68	68	68	70	69	70
Friday	68	70	69	71	72	69	70	70

7. Reducing Grammatical Errors A composition teacher wishes to see whether a new grammar program will reduce the number of grammatical errors her students make when writing a two-page essay. The data are shown here. At $\alpha = 0.025$, can it be concluded that the number of errors has been reduced?

Student	1	2	3	4	5	6
Errors before	12	9	0	5	4	3
Errors after	9	6	1	3	2	3

8. Amounts of Shrimp Caught According to the National Marine Fisheries Service, the amounts of shrimp landed during the month of January (in thousands of kilograms) are shown below for several Gulf Coast states for three selected years. At the 0.05 level of significance, is there sufficient evidence to conclude a difference in the mean production between 2007 and 2006? Between 2006 and 2005?

	Florida	Alabama	Mississippi	Louisiana	Texas
2007	156	94	77	776	391
2006	572	435	240	893	637
2005	428	245	150	1043	278

Source: NOAA Fisheries, Office of Science and Technology.

9. Pulse Rate of Identical Twins A researcher wanted to compare the pulse rates of identical twins to see whether there was any difference. Eight sets of twins were selected. The rates are given in the table as number of beats per minute. At $\alpha = 0.01$, is there a significant difference in the average pulse rates of twins? Find the 99% confidence interval for the difference of the two. Use the P-value method.

Twin A	87	92	78	83	88	90	84	93
Twin B	83	95	79	83	86	93	80	86

10. House Sales A real estate reporter hypothesizes that house sales in Canada have changed during a 4-year period. A selection of city house sales (in thousands of units) is shown below. At $\alpha = 0.05$, can it be concluded that house sales have changed? Use the P-value method.

City	Vancouver	Calgary	Edmonton	Toronto	Ottawa	Montreal	Halifax
2005	42	32	19	86	13	50	7
2009	36	25	19	89	15	43	6

Source: Scotiabank Group, *Global Real Estate Trends.*

Extending the Concepts »

11. Instead of finding the mean of the differences between X_1 and X_2 by subtracting $X_1 - X_2$, one can find it by finding the means of X_1 and X_2 and then subtracting the means. Show that these two procedures will yield the same results.

9–4 | Testing the Difference between Proportions »

LO4

Test the difference between two proportions.

The z test with some modifications can be used to test the equality of two proportions. For example, a researcher might ask, Is the proportion of men who exercise regularly less than the proportion of women who exercise regularly? Is there a difference in the percentage of students who own a personal computer and the percentage of nonstudents who own one? Is there a difference in the proportion of college graduates who pay cash for purchases and the proportion of non-college graduates who pay cash?

Recall from Chapter 7 that the symbol $\hat{p}$ ("p hat") is the sample proportion used to estimate the population proportion, denoted by p. For example, if in a sample of 30 college students, 9 are on probation, then the sample proportion is $\hat{p} = \frac{9}{30}$, or 0.3. The population proportion p is the number of all students who are on probation, divided by the number of students who attend the college. The formula for $\hat{p}$ is

$$\hat{p} = \frac{X}{n}$$

where

X = number of units that possess the characteristic of interest
n = sample size

When one is testing the difference between two population proportions p_1 and p_2, the hypotheses can be stated thus, if no difference between the proportions is hypothesized.

$$H_0: p_1 = p_2 \qquad \text{or} \qquad H_0: p_1 - p_2 = 0$$
$$H_1: p_1 \neq p_2 \qquad\qquad H_1: p_1 - p_2 \neq 0$$

Similar statements in the alternative hypothesis using $<$ or $>$ can be formed for one-tailed tests.

For two proportions, $\hat{p}_1 = X_1/n_1$ is used to estimate p_1 and $\hat{p}_2 = X_2/n_2$ is used to estimate p_2. The standard error of the difference is

$$\sigma_{(\hat{p}_1 - \hat{p}_2)} = \sqrt{\sigma_{p_1}^2 + \sigma_{p_2}^2} = \sqrt{\frac{p_1 q_1}{n_1} + \frac{p_2 q_2}{n_2}}$$

where $\sigma_{p_1}^2$ and $\sigma_{p_2}^2$ are the variances of the proportions, $q_1 = 1 - p_1$, $q_2 = 1 - p_2$, and n_1 and n_2 are the respective sample sizes.

Since p_1 and p_2 are unknown, a weighted estimate of p can be computed by using the formula

$$\bar{p} = \frac{n_1 \hat{p}_1 + n_2 \hat{p}_2}{n_1 + n_2}$$

and $\bar{q} = 1 - \bar{p}$. This weighted estimate is based on the hypothesis that $p_1 = p_2$. Hence, $\bar{p}$ is a better estimate than either $\hat{p}_1$ or $\hat{p}_2$, since it is a combined average using both $\hat{p}_1$ and $\hat{p}_2$.

Since $\hat{p}_1 = X_1/n_1$ and $\hat{p}_2 = X_2/n_2$, $\bar{p}$ can be simplified to

$$\bar{p} = \frac{X_1 + X_2}{n_1 + n_2}$$

Finally, the standard error of the difference in terms of the weighted estimate is

$$\sigma_{(\hat{p}_1 - \hat{p}_2)} = \sqrt{\bar{p}\,\bar{q}\left(\frac{1}{n_1} + \frac{1}{n_2}\right)}$$

The formula for the test statistic is shown next.

Formula for the z Test for Comparing Two Proportions

$$z = \frac{(\hat{p}_1 - \hat{p}_2) - (p_1 - p_2)}{\sqrt{\bar{p}\,\bar{q}\left(\dfrac{1}{n_1} + \dfrac{1}{n_2}\right)}}$$

where

$$\bar{p} = \frac{X_1 + X_2}{n_1 + n_2} \qquad \hat{p}_1 = \frac{X_1}{n_1}$$

$$\bar{q} = 1 - \bar{p} \qquad \hat{p}_2 = \frac{X_2}{n_2}$$

This formula follows the format

$$\text{Test statistic} = \frac{(\text{Observed value}) - (\text{Expected value})}{\text{Standard error}}$$

Assumptions for the z Test for Two Proportions

1. The samples must be random samples.
2. The sample data are independent of each other.
3. For both samples $np \geq 5$ and $nq \geq 5$.

Example 9–9

Vaccination Rates in Nursing Homes

Researchers found that 12 out of 34 small nursing homes had a resident vaccination rate of less than 80%, while 17 out of 24 large nursing homes had a vaccination rate of less than 80%. At $\alpha = 0.05$, test the claim that there is no difference in the proportions of the small and large nursing homes with a resident vaccination rate of less than 80%.

Source: Nancy Arden, Arnold S. Monto, and Suzanne E. Ohmit, "Vaccine Use and the Risk of Outbreaks in a Sample of Nursing Homes During an Influenza Epidemic," *American Journal of Public Health.*

Solution

Let $\hat{p}_1$ be the proportion of the small nursing homes with a vaccination rate of less than 80% and $\hat{p}_2$ be the proportion of the large nursing homes with a vaccination rate of less than 80%. Then

$$\hat{p}_1 = \frac{X_1}{n_1} = \frac{12}{34} = 0.35 \qquad \text{and} \qquad \hat{p}_2 = \frac{X_2}{n_2} = \frac{17}{24} = 0.71$$

$$\bar{p} = \frac{X_1 + X_2}{n_1 + n_2} = \frac{12 + 17}{34 + 24} = \frac{29}{58} = 0.5$$

$$\bar{q} = 1 - \bar{p} = 1 - 0.5 = 0.5$$

Now, follow the steps in hypothesis testing.

Step 1 State the hypotheses and identify the claim.

$$H_0: p_1 = p_2 \text{ (claim)} \qquad \text{and} \qquad H_1: p_1 \neq p_2$$

Step 2 Find the critical values. Since $\alpha = 0.05$, the critical values are $+1.96$ and -1.96.

Step 3 Compute the test statistic.

$$z = \frac{(\hat{p}_1 - \hat{p}_2) - (p_1 - p_2)}{\sqrt{\bar{p}\,\bar{q}\left(\dfrac{1}{n_1} + \dfrac{1}{n_2}\right)}}$$

$$= \frac{(0.35 - 0.71) - 0}{\sqrt{(0.5)(0.5)\left(\dfrac{1}{34} + \dfrac{1}{24}\right)}} = \frac{-0.36}{0.1333} = -2.7$$

Step 4 Make the decision. Reject the null hypothesis, since $-2.7 < -1.96$. See Figure 9–8.

Figure 9–8

Critical Values and Test Statistic for Example 9–9

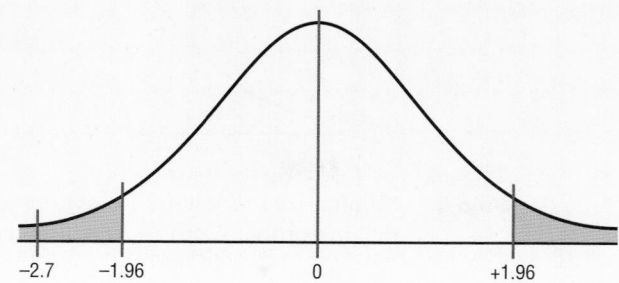

Step 5 Summarize the results. There is enough evidence to reject the claim that there is no difference in the proportions of small and large nursing homes with a resident vaccination rate of less than 80%.

Example 9–10

Text-Messaging While Driving

A survey of 1000 drivers this year showed that 29% text-message while driving. Last year, a survey of 1000 drivers showed that 17% text-messaged while driving. At $\alpha = 0.01$, can it be concluded that there has been an increase in the number of drivers who text-message while driving?

Source: FindLaw.com.

Solution

Since the statistics are given in percentages, $\hat{p}_1 = 29\%$, or 0.29, and $\hat{p}_2 = 17\%$, or 0.17. To compute $\bar{p}$, you must find X_1 and X_2.

$$X_1 = \hat{p}_1 n_1 = 0.29(1000) = 290$$

$$X_2 = \hat{p}_2 n_2 = 0.17(1000) = 170$$

$$\bar{p} = \frac{X_1 + X_2}{n_1 + n_2} = \frac{290 + 170}{1000 + 1000} = \frac{460}{2000} = 0.23$$

$$\bar{q} = 1 - \bar{p} = 1 - 0.23 = 0.77$$

Step 1 State the hypotheses and identify the claim.

$$H_0: p_1 = p_2 \qquad \text{and} \qquad H_1: p_1 > p_2 \text{ (claim)}$$

Step 2 Find the critical values. Since $\alpha = 0.01$, the critical value is 2.33.

Step 3 Compute the test statistic.

$$z = \frac{(\hat{p}_1 - \hat{p}_2) - (p_1 - p_2)}{\sqrt{\bar{p}\,\bar{q}\left(\dfrac{1}{n_1} + \dfrac{1}{n_2}\right)}} = \frac{(0.29 - 0.17) - 0}{\sqrt{(0.23)(0.77)\left(\dfrac{1}{1000} + \dfrac{1}{1000}\right)}} = 6.38$$

Step 4 Make the decision. Reject the null hypothesis, since $6.38 > 2.33$. See Figure 9–9.

Figure 9–9

Critical Values and
Test Statistic for
Example 9–10

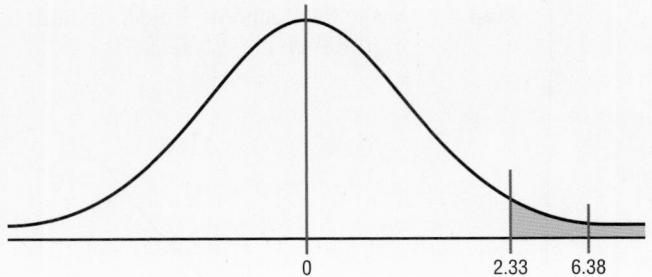

Step 5 Summarize the results. There is enough evidence to support the claim that the proportion of drivers who text-message is larger than it was last year.

The P-value for the difference of proportions can be found from Tables E–1 and E–2, as shown in Section 8–3. For Example 9–10, the null hypothesis is rejected, as the P-value for $z = 6.38$ is less than 0.0001 $(1 - 0.9999)$, which is less than α, 0.01.

The formula for the confidence interval for the difference between two proportions is shown next.

Formula for the Confidence Interval for the Difference between Two Proportions

$$(\hat{p}_1 - \hat{p}_2) - z_{\alpha/2}\sqrt{\frac{\hat{p}_1\hat{q}_1}{n_1} + \frac{\hat{p}_2\hat{q}_2}{n_2}} < p_1 - p_2 < (\hat{p}_1 - \hat{p}_2) + z_{\alpha/2}\sqrt{\frac{\hat{p}_1\hat{q}_1}{n_1} + \frac{\hat{p}_2\hat{q}_2}{n_2}}$$

Example 9–11

Vaccination Rates in Nursing Homes

Find the 95% confidence interval for the difference of proportions for the data in Example 9–9.

Solution

$$\hat{p}_1 = \frac{12}{34} = 0.35 \qquad \hat{q}_1 = 0.65$$

$$\hat{p}_2 = \frac{17}{24} = 0.71 \qquad \hat{q}_2 = 0.29$$

Substitute in the formula.

$$(\hat{p}_1 - \hat{p}_2) - z_{\alpha/2}\sqrt{\frac{\hat{p}_1\hat{q}_1}{n_1} + \frac{\hat{p}_2\hat{q}_2}{n_2}} < p_1 - p_2$$

$$< (\hat{p}_1 - \hat{p}_2) + z_{\alpha/2}\sqrt{\frac{\hat{p}_1\hat{q}_1}{n_1} + \frac{\hat{p}_2\hat{q}_2}{n_2}}$$

$$(0.35 - 0.71) - 1.96\sqrt{\frac{(0.35)(0.65)}{34} + \frac{(0.71)(0.29)}{24}}$$

$$< p_1 - p_2 < (0.35 - 0.71) + 1.96\sqrt{\frac{(0.35)(0.65)}{34} + \frac{(0.71)(0.29)}{24}}$$

$$-0.36 - 0.242 < p_1 - p_2 < -0.36 + 0.242$$

$$-0.602 < p_1 - p_2 < -0.118$$

Since 0 is not contained in the interval, the decision is to reject the null hypothesis $H_0: p_1 = p_2$.

9–4 Applying the Concepts

Smoking and Education

You are researching the hypothesis that there is no difference in the percentage of public school students who smoke and the percentage of private school students who smoke. You find these results from a recent survey.

School	Percentage who smoke
Public	32.3
Private	14.5

Based on these figures, answer the following questions.

1. What hypotheses would you use if you wanted to compare percentages of the public school students who smoke with the private school students who smoke?
2. What critical value(s) would you use?
3. What statistical test would you use to compare the two percentages?
4. What information would you need to complete the statistical test?
5. Suppose you found that 1000 individuals in each group were surveyed. Could you perform the statistical test?
6. If so, complete the test and summarize the results.

See page 453 for the answers.

Exercises 9–4

1a. Find the proportions $\hat{p}$ and $\hat{q}$ for each.

   a. $n = 48, X = 34$
   b. $n = 75, X = 28$
   c. $n = 100, X = 50$
   d. $n = 24, X = 6$
   e. $n = 144, X = 12$

1b. Find each X, given $\hat{p}$.

   a. $\hat{p} = 0.16, n = 100$
   b. $\hat{p} = 0.08, n = 50$
   c. $\hat{p} = 6\%, n = 800$
   d. $\hat{p} = 52\%, n = 200$
   e. $\hat{p} = 20\%, n = 150$

2. Find $\bar{p}$ and $\bar{q}$ for each.

   a. $X_1 = 60, n_1 = 100, X_2 = 40, n_2 = 100$
   b. $X_1 = 22, n_1 = 50, X_2 = 18, n_2 = 30$
   c. $X_1 = 18, n_1 = 60, X_2 = 20, n_2 = 80$
   d. $X_1 = 5, n_1 = 32, X_2 = 12, n_2 = 48$
   e. $X_1 = 12, n_1 = 75, X_2 = 15, n_2 = 50$

For Exercises 3 through 14, use the following traditional method of hypothesis testing unless otherwise specified.

   a. State the hypotheses and identify the claim.
   b. Find the critical value(s).
   c. Compute the test statistic.
   d. Make the decision.
   e. Summarize the results.

3. Lung Disease in Industrial/Rural Communities A sample of 150 people from a certain industrial community showed that 80 people suffered from a lung disease. A sample of 100 people from a rural community showed that 30 suffered from the same lung disease. At $\alpha = 0.05$, is there a difference between the proportions of people who suffer from the disease in the two communities?

4. Undergraduate Financial Aid A study is conducted to determine if the percentage of women who receive financial aid in undergraduate school is different from the percentage of men who receive financial aid in undergraduate school. A random sample of undergraduates revealed these results. At $\alpha = 0.01$, is there significant evidence to reject the null hypothesis?

	Women	Men
Sample size	250	300
Number receiving aid	200	180

Source: U.S. Department of Education, National Center for Education Statistics.

5. **Female Cashiers and Servers** Labour statistics indicate that 77% of cashiers and servers are women. A random sample of cashiers and servers in a large metropolitan area found that 112 of 150 cashiers and 150 of 200 servers were women. At the 0.05 level of significance, is there sufficient evidence to conclude that a difference exists between the proportion of servers and the proportion of cashiers who are women?

Source: The New York Times Almanac.

6. **Dog Bites in Two Cities** An Edmonton report indicated that in a sample of 284 dog bites, 31 were from the Rottweiler breed. In a Winnipeg survey, a sample of 166 dog bites revealed that 11 were from the Rottweiler breed. Is there a significant difference in the proportions from the two cities? Use $\alpha = 0.05$. Find the 95% confidence interval for the difference of the two proportions.

Source: Dog Legislation Council of Canada.

7. **Lecture versus Computer-Assisted Instruction** A survey found that 83% of the men questioned preferred computer-assisted instruction to lecture and 75% of the women preferred computer-assisted instruction to lecture. There were 100 individuals in each sample. At $\alpha = 0.05$, test the claim that there is no difference in the proportion of men and the proportion of women who favour computer-assisted instruction over lecture. Find the 95% confidence interval for the difference of the two proportions.

8. **Leisure Time** In a sample of 50 men, 44 said that they had less leisure time today than they had 10 years ago. In a sample of 50 women, 48 women said that they had less leisure time than they had 10 years ago. At $\alpha = 0.10$ is there a difference in the proportion? Find the 90% confidence interval for the difference of the two proportions. Does the confidence interval contain 0? Give a reason why this information would be of interest to a researcher.

Source: Based on statistics from *Market Directory.*

9. **Desire to Be Rich** In a sample of 80 North Americans, 55% wished that they were rich. In a sample of 90 Europeans, 45% wished that they were rich. At $\alpha = 0.01$, is there a difference in the proportions? Find

the 99% confidence interval for the difference of the two proportions.

10. **Seat Belt Use** In a sample of 200 men, 130 said they used seat belts. In a sample of 300 women, 63 said they used seat belts. Test the claim that men are more safety conscious than women, at $\alpha = 0.01$. Use the P-value method.

11. **Dog Ownership** A survey found that in a sample of 75 families, 26 owned dogs. A survey done 15 years ago found that in a sample of 60 families, 26 owned dogs. At $\alpha = 0.05$, has the proportion of dog owners changed over the 15-year period? Find the 95% confidence interval of the true difference in the proportions. Does the confidence interval contain 0? Why would this fact be important to a researcher?

Source: Based on statistics from the American Veterinary Medical Association.

12. **Bullying** Bullying is a problem at any age but especially for students aged 12 to 18. A study showed that 7.2% of all students in this age bracket reported being bullied at school during the past six months, with Grade 6 having the highest incidence at 13.9% and Grade 12 the lowest at 2.2%. To see if there is a difference between public and private schools, 200 students were randomly selected from each. At the 0.05 level of significance, can a difference be concluded?

	Private	Public
Sample size	200	200
No. bullied	13	16

Source: National Center for Education Statistics, U.S. Department of Education.

13. **Survey on Inevitability of War** A sample of 200 teenagers shows that 50 believe that war is inevitable, and a sample of 300 people over age 60 shows that 93 believe war is inevitable. Is the proportion of teenagers who believe war is inevitable different from the proportion of people over age 60 who do? Use $\alpha = 0.01$. Find the 99% confidence interval for the difference of the two proportions.

14. **Hypertension** It has been found that 26% of men 20 years and older suffer from hypertension (high blood pressure) and 31.5% of women are hypertensive. A random sample of 150 of each gender was selected from recent hospital records, and the following results were obtained. Can you conclude that a higher percentage of women have high blood pressure? Use $\alpha = 0.05$.

Men	43 patients had high blood pressure
Women	52 patients had high blood pressure

Source: National Center for Health Statistics.

15. **Elected Senate** Find the 99% confidence interval for the difference in the population proportions for the data of a study in which 43% of 150 respondents in Atlantic Canada are in favour of replacing the existing Senate with an elected Senate and 57% of 125 Alberta respondents favour an elected Senate.

Source: CanWest News Service, Ottawa Citizen.

16. **Percentage of Female Workers** The City of Hamilton councillors feel that a higher percentage of women work there than in the neighbouring Regional Municipality of Niagara. To test this, they randomly selected 1000 women in each area and found that in Hamilton, 579 women work, and in Niagara, 557 women work. Using $\alpha = 0.05$, do you think that City of Hamilton councillors are correct?

Source: Statistics Canada, 2001 Census.

17. **Credit Card Use** In a sample of 100 store customers, 43 used a MasterCard. In another sample of 100, 58 used a Visa card. At $\alpha = 0.05$, is there a difference in the proportion of people who use each type of credit card?

18. **Death Penalty Support** Find the 95% confidence interval for the true difference in proportions for the data of a study in which 40% of the 200 males surveyed opposed the death penalty and 56% of the 100 females surveyed opposed the death penalty.

19. **College Education** The percentages of adults 25 years of age and older who have completed 4 or more years of college are 23.6% for females and 27.8% for males. A random sample of women and men who were 25 years old or older was surveyed with these results. Estimate the true difference in proportions with 95% confidence, and compare your interval with the *Almanac* statistics.

	Women	Men
Sample size	350	400
No. who completed 4 or more years	100	115

Source: The New York Times Almanac.

Extending the Concepts »

20. If there is a significant difference between p_1 and p_2 and between p_2 and p_3, can one conclude that there is a significant difference between p_1 and p_3?

9–5 Testing the Difference between Two Variances ›

LO5

Test the difference between two variances or standard deviations.

In addition to comparing two means, statisticians are interested in comparing two variances or standard deviations. For example, is the variation in the temperatures for a certain month for two cities different?

In another situation, a researcher may be interested in comparing the variance of the cholesterol of men with the variance of the cholesterol of women. For the comparison of two variances or standard deviations, an *F* **test** is used. The *F* test should not be confused with the chi-square test, which compares a single sample variance to a specific population variance, as shown in Chapter 8.

If two independent samples are selected from two normally distributed populations in which the variances are equal ($\sigma_1^2 = \sigma_2^2$) and if the variances s_1^2 and s_2^2 are compared as $\dfrac{s_1^2}{s_2^2}$, the sampling distribution of the variances is called the *F* **distribution.**

Characteristics of the *F* Distribution

1. The values of *F* cannot be negative, because variances are always positive or zero.
2. The distribution is positively skewed.
3. The mean value of *F* is approximately equal to 1.
4. The *F* distribution is a family of curves based on the degrees of freedom of the variance of the numerator and the degrees of freedom of the variance of the denominator.

Figure 9–10 shows the shapes of several curves for the F distribution.

Figure 9–10

The F Family of Curves

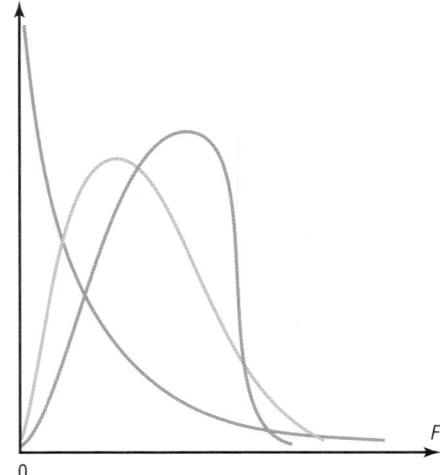

Formula for the F Test

$$F = \frac{s_1^2}{s_2^2}$$

where the larger of the two variances is placed in the numerator regardless of the subscripts. (See note on page 443.)

The F test has two terms for the degrees of freedom: that of the numerator, $n_1 - 1$, and that of the denominator, $n_2 - 1$, where n_1 is the sample size from which the larger variance was obtained.

When one is finding the F test statistic, *the larger of the variances is placed in the numerator of the F formula;* this is not necessarily the variance of the larger of the two sample sizes.

Table H in Appendix C gives the F critical values for $\alpha = 0.005$, 0.01, 0.025, 0.05, and 0.10 (each α value involves a separate table in Table H). These are one-tailed values; if a two-tailed test is being conducted, then the $\alpha/2$ value must be used. For example, if a two-tailed test with $\alpha = 0.05$ is being conducted, then the $0.05/2 = 0.025$ table of Table H should be used.

Example 9–12

Find the critical value for a right-tailed F test when $\alpha = 0.05$, the degrees of freedom for the numerator (abbreviated d.f.N.) are 15, and the degrees of freedom for the denominator (d.f.D.) are 21.

Solution

Since this test is right-tailed with $\alpha = 0.05$, use the 0.05 table. The d.f.N. is listed across the top, and the d.f.D. is listed in the left column. The critical value is found where the row and column intersect in the table. In this case, it is 2.18. See Figure 9–11.

Figure 9–11

Finding the Critical Value in Table H for Example 9–12

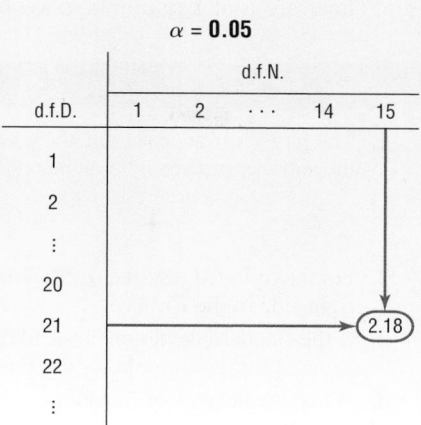

$\alpha = \mathbf{0.05}$

As noted previously, when the F test is used, the larger variance is always placed in the numerator of the formula. When one is conducting a two-tailed test, α is split; and even though there are two values, only the right tail is used. The reason is that the F test statistic is always greater than or equal to 1.

Example 9–13

Find the critical value for a two-tailed F test with $\alpha = 0.05$ when the sample size from which the variance for the numerator was obtained was 21 and the sample size from which the variance for the denominator was obtained was 12.

Solution

Since this is a two-tailed test with $\alpha = 0.05$, the $0.05/2 = 0.025$ table must be used. Here, d.f.N. $= 21 - 1 = 20$, and d.f.D. $= 12 - 1 = 11$; hence, the critical value is 3.23. See Figure 9–12.

Figure 9–12

Finding the Critical Value in Table H for Example 9–13

$\alpha = \mathbf{0.025}$

	d.f.N.			
d.f.D.	1	2	$\cdots$	20
1				
2				
$\vdots$				
10				
11				3.23
12				
$\vdots$				

When the degree of freedom values cannot be found in the table, the closest value on the smaller side should be used. For example, if d.f.N. $= 14$, this value is between the given table values of 12 and 15; therefore, 12 should be used, to be on the safe side.

When one is testing the equality of two variances, these hypotheses are used:

Right-tailed	**Left-tailed**	**Two-tailed**
H_0: $\sigma_1^2 = \sigma_2^2$	H_0: $\sigma_1^2 = \sigma_2^2$	H_0: $\sigma_1^2 = \sigma_2^2$
H_1: $\sigma_1^2 > \sigma_2^2$	H_1: $\sigma_1^2 < \sigma_2^2$	H_1: $\sigma_1^2 \neq \sigma_2^2$

There are four key points to keep in mind when one is using the F test.

Notes for the Use of the F Test

1. The larger variance should always be placed in the numerator of the formula regardless of the subscripts. (See note on page 443.)

$$F = \frac{s_1^2}{s_2^2}$$

2. For a two-tailed test, the α value must be divided by 2 and the critical value placed on the right side of the F curve.
3. If the standard deviations instead of the variances are given in the problem, they must be squared for the formula for the F test.
4. When the degrees of freedom cannot be found in Table H, the closest value on the smaller side should be used.

Assumptions for Testing the Difference between Two Variances

1. The samples must be random samples.
2. The populations from which the samples were obtained must be normally distributed. (*Note:* The test should not be used when the distributions depart from normality.)
3. The samples must be independent of each other.

Remember also that in tests of hypotheses using the traditional method, these five steps should be taken:

Step 1 State the hypotheses and identify the claim.

Step 2 Find the critical value.

Step 3 Compute the test statistic.

Step 4 Make the decision.

Step 5 Summarize the results.

Example 9–14

Heart Rates of Smokers

A medical researcher wishes to see whether the variance of the heart rates (in beats per minute) of smokers is different from the variance of heart rates of people who do not smoke. Two samples are selected, and the data are as shown. Using $\alpha = 0.05$, is there enough evidence to support the claim?

Smokers	Nonsmokers
$n_1 = 26$	$n_2 = 18$
$s_1^2 = 36$	$s_2^2 = 10$

Solution

Step 1 State the hypotheses and identify the claim.

$$H_0: \sigma_1^2 = \sigma_2^2 \qquad \text{and} \qquad H_1: \sigma_1^2 \neq \sigma_2^2 \text{ (claim)}$$

Step 2 Find the critical value. Use the 0.025 table in Table H since $\alpha = 0.05$ and this is a two-tailed test. Here, d.f.N. $= 26 - 1 = 25$, and d.f.D. $= 18 - 1 = 17$. The critical value is 2.56 (d.f.N. $= 24$ was used). See Figure 9–13.

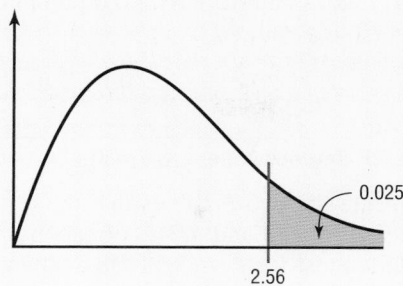

Figure 9–13

Critical Value for
Example 9–14

0.025

2.56

Step 3   Compute the test statistic.

$$F = \frac{s_1^2}{s_2^2} = \frac{36}{10} = 3.6$$

Step 4   Make the decision. Reject the null hypothesis, since $3.6 > 2.56$.

Step 5   Summarize the results. There is enough evidence to support the claim that the variance of the heart rates of smokers and nonsmokers is different.

Example 9–15

Waiting Time to See a Doctor

The standard deviation of the average waiting time to see a doctor for nonlife-threatening problems in the emergency room at an urban hospital is 32 minutes. At a second hospital, the standard deviation is 28 minutes. If a sample of 16 patients was used in the first case and 18 in the second case, is there enough evidence to conclude that the standard deviation of the waiting times in the first hospital is greater than the standard deviation of the waiting times in the second hospital? Use $\alpha = 0.01$.

Solution

Step 1   State the hypotheses and identify the claim.

$$H_0: \sigma_1^2 = \sigma_2^2 \qquad \text{and} \qquad H_1: \sigma_1^2 > \sigma_2^2 \text{ (claim)}$$

Step 2   Find the critical value. Here, d.f.N. $= 16 - 1 = 15$, and d.f.D. $= 18 - 1 = 17$. From the 0.01 table, the critical value is 3.31.

Step 3   Compute the test statistic.

$$F = \frac{s_1^2}{s_2^2} = \frac{32^2}{28^2} \approx 1.31$$

Step 4   Do not reject the null hypothesis since $1.31 < 3.31$.

Step 5   Summarize the results. There is not enough evidence to support the claim that the standard deviation of the waiting times of the first hospital is greater than the standard deviation of the waiting times of the second hospital.

Finding *P*-values for the *F* test statistic is somewhat more complicated since it requires looking through all the *F* tables (Table H in Appendix C) using the specific d.f.N. and d.f.D. values. For example, suppose that a certain test has $F = 3.58$, d.f.N. $= 5$, and d.f.D. $= 10$. To find the *P*-value interval for $F = 3.58$, one must first find the corresponding *F* values for d.f.N. $= 5$ and d.f.D. $= 10$ for α equal to 0.005 on page 676, 0.01 on page 677, 0.025 on page 678, 0.05 on page 679, and 0.10 on page 680 in Table H. Then make a table as shown.

α	0.10	0.05	0.025	0.01	0.005
F	2.52	3.33	4.24	5.64	6.87
Reference page	680	679	678	677	676

Now locate the two F values that the test statistic 3.58 falls between. In this case, 3.58 falls between 3.33 and 4.24, corresponding to 0.05 and 0.025. Hence, the P-value for a right-tailed test for $F = 3.58$ falls between 0.025 and 0.05 (that is, $0.025 < P\text{-value} < 0.05$). For a right-tailed test, then, one would reject the null hypothesis at $\alpha = 0.05$ but not at $\alpha = 0.01$. The P-value obtained from a calculator is 0.0408. Remember that for a two-tailed test the values found in Table H for α must be doubled. In this case, $0.05 < P\text{-value} < 0.10$ for $F = 3.58$.

Once you understand the concept, you can dispense with making a table as shown and find the P-value directly from Table H.

Example 9–16

Airport Passengers

The CEO of an airport hypothesizes that the variance in the number of passengers for American airports is greater than the variance in the number of passengers for Canadian airports. At $\alpha = 0.10$, is there enough evidence to support the hypothesis? The data in millions of passengers per year are shown for selected airports. Use the P-value method. Assume the variable is normally distributed.

American airports		Canadian airports	
76.0	66.7	23.8	13.4
56.2	52.8	7.5	7.3
35.6	35.5		

Sources: Transport Canada; and Statistics Canada, Air Carrier Statements St. 2, 4 & 6 dated February 2002 and updated September 30, 2003. Reproduced with the permission of the Minister of Public Works and Government Services Canada, 2007.

Solution

Step 1 State the hypotheses and identify the claim.

$$H_0: \sigma_1^2 = \sigma_2^2 \qquad \text{and} \qquad H_0: \sigma_1^2 > \sigma_2^2 \text{ (claim)}$$

Step 2 Compute the test statistic. Using the formula in Chapter 3 or a calculator, find the variance for each group.

$$s_1^2 \approx 266.43 \qquad \text{and} \qquad s_2^2 \approx 59.85$$

Substitute in the formula and solve.

$$F = \frac{s_1^2}{s_2^2} = \frac{266.43}{59.85} \approx 4.45$$

Step 3 Find the P-value in Table H, using d.f.N. = 5 and d.f.D. = 3.

α	0.10	0.05	0.025	0.01	0.005
F	5.31	9.01	14.88	28.24	45.39

Since 4.45 is less than 5.31, the P-value is greater than 0.10. (The P-value obtained from a calculator is 0.124.)

Step 4 Make the decision. The decision is to not reject the null hypothesis since $P\text{-value} > 0.10$.

Step 5   Summarize the results. There is not enough evidence to support the claim that the variance in the number of passengers for American airports is greater than the variance in the number of passengers for Canadian airports.

If the exact degrees of freedom are not specified in Table H, the closest smaller value should be used. For example, if $\alpha = 0.05$ (right-tailed test), d.f.N. = 18, and d.f.D. = 20, use the column d.f.N. = 15 and the row d.f.D. = 20 to get $F = 2.20$.

Note: It is not absolutely necessary to place the larger variance in the numerator when one is performing the F test. Critical values for left-tailed hypotheses tests can be found by interchanging the degrees of freedom and taking the reciprocal of the value found in Table H.

Also, one should use caution when performing the F test since the data can run contrary to the hypotheses on rare occasions. For example, if the hypotheses are H_0: $\sigma_1^2 = \sigma_2^2$ and H_1: $\sigma_1^2 > \sigma_2^2$, but if $s_1^2 < s_2^2$, then the F test should not be performed and one would not reject the null hypothesis.

9–5   Applying the Concepts

Variability and Automatic Transmissions

Assume the following data values are from the June 1996 issue of *Automotive Magazine*. An article compared various parameters of North American- and Japanese-made sports cars. This report centres on the price of an optional automatic transmission. Which sector has the greater variability in the price of automatic transmissions? Input the data and answer the following questions.

Japanese cars		North American cars	
Nissan 300ZX	$1940	Dodge Stealth	$2363
Mazda RX7	1810	Saturn	1230
Mazda MX6	1871	Mercury Cougar	1332
Nissan NX	1822	Ford Probe	932
Mazda Miata	1920	Eagle Talon	1790
Honda Prelude	1730	Chevy Lumina	1833

1. What is the null hypothesis?
2. What test statistic is used to test for any significant differences in the variances?
3. Is there a significant difference in the variability in the prices between the two car sectors?
4. What effect does a small sample size have on the standard deviations?
5. What degrees of freedom are used for the statistical test?
6. Could two sets of data have significantly different variances without having significantly different means?

See page 453 for the answers.

Exercises 9–5

1. When one is computing the F test statistic, what condition is placed on the variance that is in the numerator?

2. Why is the critical region always on the right side in the use of the F test?

3. What are the two different degrees of freedom associated with the F distribution?

4. What are the characteristics of the F distribution?

5. Using Table H, find the critical value for each.

    a. Sample 1: $s_1^2 = 128$, $n_1 = 23$
        Sample 2: $s_2^2 = 162$, $n_2 = 16$
        Two-tailed, $\alpha = 0.01$

    b. Sample 1: $s_1^2 = 37$, $n_1 = 14$
        Sample 2: $s_2^2 = 89$, $n_2 = 25$
        Right-tailed, $\alpha = 0.01$

    c. Sample 1: $s_1^2 = 232$, $n_1 = 30$
        Sample 2: $s_2^2 = 387$, $n_2 = 46$
        Two-tailed, $\alpha = 0.05$

    d. Sample 1: $s_1^2 = 164$, $n_1 = 21$
        Sample 2: $s_2^2 = 53$, $n_2 = 17$
        Two-tailed, $\alpha = 0.10$

    e. Sample 1: $s_1^2 = 92.8$, $n_1 = 11$
        Sample 2: $s_2^2 = 43.6$, $n_2 = 11$
        Right-tailed, $\alpha = 0.05$

6. (ans) Using Table H, find the *P*-value interval for each *F* test statistic.

    a. $F = 2.97$, d.f.N. $= 9$, d.f.D. $= 14$, right-tailed
    b. $F = 3.32$, d.f.N. $= 6$, d.f.D. $= 12$, two-tailed
    c. $F = 2.28$, d.f.N. $= 12$, d.f.D. $= 20$, right-tailed
    d. $F = 3.51$, d.f.N. $= 12$, d.f.D. $= 21$, right-tailed
    e. $F = 4.07$, d.f.N. $= 6$, d.f.D. $= 10$, two-tailed
    f. $F = 1.65$, d.f.N. $= 19$, d.f.D. $= 28$, right-tailed
    g. $F = 1.77$, d.f.N. $= 28$, d.f.D. $= 28$, right-tailed
    h. $F = 7.29$, d.f.N. $= 5$, d.f.D. $= 8$, two-tailed

For Exercises 7 through 20, use the following traditional method of hypothesis testing unless otherwise specified.

    a. State the hypotheses and identify the claim.
    b. Find the critical value.
    c. Compute the test statistic.
    d. Make the decision.
    e. Summarize the results.

Assume that all variables are normally distributed.

7. Fiction Bestsellers The standard deviation for the number of weeks 15 *New York Times* hardcover fiction books spent on its bestseller list is 6.17 weeks. The standard deviation for the 15 *New York Times* hardcover nonfiction list is 13.12 weeks. At $\alpha = 0.10$, can we conclude that there is a difference in the variances?
Source: The New York Times.

8. Cat and Dog Ages A researcher claims that the standard deviation of the ages of cats is smaller than the standard deviation of the ages of dogs that are owned by families in a large city. A randomly selected sample of 29 cats has a standard deviation of 2.7 years, and a random sample of 16 dogs has a standard deviation of 3.5 years. Is the researcher correct? Use $\alpha = 0.05$. If there is a difference, suggest a reason for the difference.

9. Tax-Exempt Properties A tax collector wishes to see if the variances of the values of the tax-exempt properties are different for two large cities. The values of the tax-exempt properties for two samples are shown. The data are given in millions of dollars. At $\alpha = 0.05$, is there enough evidence to support the tax collector's claim that the variances are different?

City A				City B			
113	22	14	8	82	11	5	15
25	23	23	30	295	50	12	9
44	11	19	7	12	68	81	2
31	19	5	2	20	16	4	5

10. Hospital Noise Levels In a hospital study it was found that the standard deviation of the sound levels from 20 areas designated as "casualty doors" was 4.1 decibels acoustic (dBA) and the standard deviation of 24 areas designated as operating theatres was 7.5 dBA. At $\alpha = 0.05$, can you substantiate the claim that there is a difference in the standard deviations?
Source: M. Bayo, A. Garcia, and A. Garcia, "Noise Levels in an Urban Hospital and Workers' Subjective Responses," Archives of Environmental Health 50, No. 3, p. 249, May–June 1995.

11. Calories in Ice Cream The numbers of calories contained in 113-gram servings of randomly selected flavours of ice cream from two national brands are listed here. At the 0.05 level of significance, is there sufficient evidence to conclude that the variance in the number of calories differs between the two brands?

Brand A		Brand B	
330	300	280	310
310	350	300	370
270	380	250	300
310	300	290	310

Source: The Doctor's Pocket Calorie, Fat and Carbohydrate Counter.

12. International Border Vehicle Crossings A researcher wants to see if the variance in the number of passenger vehicles crossing the Canada–U.S. border southbound each year is different from the variance in the number of vehicles crossing the border northbound. Recent annual data (in thousands) are shown. At $\alpha = 0.05$, can it be concluded that the variances are different?

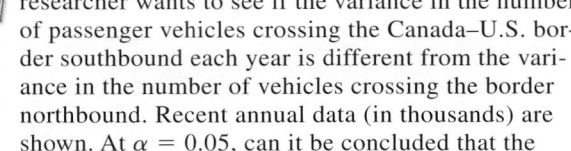

Southbound	Northbound
39,146	38,584
39,531	38,858
38,950	38,950
36,597	36,693
37,220	36,460
36,915	36,172
34,308	34,012
32,539	32,020
30,220	29,953

Source: North American Transportation Statistics.

13. Slot Machine and Roulette Players The standard deviation of the ages of a sample of people who were playing the slot machines is 6.8 years. The standard deviation of the ages of a sample of people who were playing roulette is 3.2 years. If each sample contained 25 people, can it be concluded that the standard deviations of the ages are different? Use $\alpha = 0.05$. If there is a difference, suggest a reason for the difference.

14. Carbohydrates in Candy The number of grams of carbohydrates contained in 30-gram servings of randomly selected chocolate and nonchocolate candy is listed here. Is there sufficient evidence to conclude that the variance in carbohydrate content varies between chocolate and nonchocolate candy? Use $\alpha = 0.10$.

Chocolate	29	25	17	36	41	25	32	29
	38	34	24	27	29			
Nonchocolate	41	41	37	29	30	38	39	10
	29	55	29					

Source: The Doctor's Pocket Calorie, Fat and Carbohydrate Counter.

15. Medical School Tuition Costs The yearly tuition costs in dollars for random samples of medical schools that specialize in research and in primary care are listed. At $\alpha = 0.05$, can it be concluded that a difference between the variances of the two groups exists?

Research			Primary care		
30,897	34,280	31,943	26,068	21,044	30,897
34,294	31,275	29,590	34,208	20,877	29,691
20,618	20,500	29,310	33,783	33,065	35,000
21,274			27,297		

Source: U.S. News & World Report Best Graduate Schools.

16. Number of Farms A researcher wants to find out if the variance of the number of small farms (<73 hectares) in Saskatchewan is less than the variance of the number of small farms in Alberta. A random sample of farm geographical divisions is selected, and the data are shown. At $\alpha = 0.01$, can it be concluded that the variance of the number of small farms in Saskatchewan is less than the variance of the number of small farms in Alberta?

Saskatchewan			Alberta		
3006	3388	2849	1971	1804	1031
1956	4424	2004	3540	6436	4347
3169	4605	5400	3911	3323	1228

Source: Statistics Canada—Census 2001—Farm Data.

17. Heights of Tall Buildings Test the claim that the variance of heights of the tallest buildings in Montreal is equal to the variance in heights of the tallest buildings in Calgary at $\alpha = 0.10$. The data are given in metres.

Montreal			Calgary		
205	188	158	250	197	167
195	180	181	215	191	164
190	173	198	191	177	162

Source: www.answers.com.

18. Teachers' Salaries A researcher claims that the variation in the salaries of elementary school teachers is greater than the variation in the salaries of secondary school teachers. A sample of the salaries of 30 elementary school teachers has a variance of $8324, and a sample of the salaries of 30 secondary school teachers has a variance of $2862. At $\alpha = 0.05$, can the researcher conclude that the variation in the elementary school teachers' salaries is greater than the variation in the secondary teachers' salaries? Use the P-value method.

19. Weights of Running Shoes The weights, in grams, of a sample of running shoes for men and women are shown. Calculate the variances for each sample, and test the claim that the variances are equal at $\alpha = 0.05$. Use the P-value method.

Men			Women		
370.1	323.5	391.9	329.7	317.3	273.7
382.6	345.2	457.2	298.6	295.5	295.5
286.2	335.9	401.2	314.1	348.4	289.3
348.4	363.9	413.7	292.4	320.4	295.5
429.2	398.1	451.0	304.8	320.4	342.1

20. Daily Stock Prices Two portfolios were randomly assembled from the New York Stock Exchange and the daily stock prices are shown below. At the 0.05 level of significance, can it be concluded that a difference in variance in price exists between the two portfolios?

Portfolio A	36.44	44.21	12.21	59.60	55.44
Portfolio B	32.69	47.25	49.35	36.17	63.04
Portfolio A	39.42	51.29	48.68	41.59	19.49
Portfolio B	17.74	4.23	34.98	37.02	31.48

Source: Washington Observer-Reporter.

Summary ❯

Many times, researchers are interested in comparing two parameters such as two means, two proportions, or two variances. These measures are obtained from two samples and then compared using a z test, t test, or an F test.

- If two sample means are compared, when the samples are independent and the population standard deviations are known, a z test is used. If the sample sizes are less than 30, the populations should be normally distributed.
- If the two means are compared when the samples are independent and the sample standard deviations are used, then a t test is used. Both variances are assumed to be unequal.
- When the two samples are dependent or related, such as using the same subjects and comparing the means of before and after tests, then the t test for dependent samples is used.
- Two proportions can be compared by using a z test for proportions. In this case, $n_1 p_1$ and $n_1 q_1$ must be 5 or more and, $n_2 p_2$ and $n_2 q_2$ must be 5 or more.
- Two variances can be compared by using an F test. The critical values for the F test are obtained from the F distribution.
- Confidence intervals for differences between two parameters can also be found.

For step-by-step guidance on the use of Texas Instruments TI-83 Plus/TI-84 Plus programmable calculators, see Appendix E at the back of this book. For summary procedures for Minitab, SPSS, and Excel, please see the full version of Appendix E on *Connect*.

Important Terms ❯❯

dependent samples 421	F distribution 437	independent samples 416	pooled estimate of the variance 419
	F test 437		

Important Formulas ❯❯

Formula for the z test for comparing two means from independent populations; σ_1 and σ_2 are known:

$$z = \frac{(\overline{X}_1 - \overline{X}_2) - (\mu_1 - \mu_2)}{\sqrt{\dfrac{\sigma_1^2}{n_1} + \dfrac{\sigma_2^2}{n_2}}}$$

Formula for the confidence interval for difference of two means when σ_1 and σ_2 are known:

$$(\overline{X}_1 - \overline{X}_2) - z_{\alpha/2}\sqrt{\frac{\sigma_1^2}{n_1} + \frac{\sigma_2^2}{n_2}} < \mu_1 - \mu_2$$
$$< (\overline{X}_1 - \overline{X}_2) + z_{\alpha/2}\sqrt{\frac{\sigma_1^2}{n_1} + \frac{\sigma_2^2}{n_2}}$$

Formula for the t test for comparing two means (independent samples, variances not equal); σ_1 and σ_2 are unknown:

$$t = \frac{(\overline{X}_1 - \overline{X}_2) - (\mu_1 - \mu_2)}{\sqrt{\dfrac{s_1^2}{n_1} + \dfrac{s_2^2}{n_2}}}$$

and d.f. = the smaller of $n_1 - 1$ or $n_2 - 1$.

Formula for the confidence interval for the difference of two means (independent samples, variances unequal); σ_1 and σ_2 are unknown:

$$(\overline{X}_1 - \overline{X}_2) - t_{\alpha/2}\sqrt{\frac{s_1^2}{n_1} + \frac{s_2^2}{n_2}} < \mu_1 - \mu_2$$
$$< (\overline{X}_1 - \overline{X}_2) + t_{\alpha/2}\sqrt{\frac{s_1^2}{n_1} + \frac{s_2^2}{n_2}}$$

and d.f. = the smaller of $n_1 - 1$ or $n_2 - 1$.

Formula for the t test for comparing two means from dependent samples:

$$t = \frac{\overline{D} - \mu_D}{s_D/\sqrt{n}}$$

where $\overline{D}$ is the mean of the differences

$$\overline{D} = \frac{\Sigma D}{n}$$

and s_D is the standard deviation of the differences

$$s_D = \sqrt{\frac{n\Sigma D^2 - (\Sigma D)^2}{n(n-1)}}$$

Formula for confidence interval for the mean of the difference for dependent samples:

$$\overline{D} - t_{\alpha/2}\frac{s_D}{\sqrt{n}} < \mu_D < \overline{D} + t_{\alpha/2}\frac{s_D}{\sqrt{n}}$$

and d.f. $= n - 1$.

Formula for the z test for comparing two proportions:

$$z = \frac{(\hat{p}_1 - \hat{p}_2) - (p_1 - p_2)}{\sqrt{\overline{p}\,\overline{q}\left(\dfrac{1}{n_1} + \dfrac{1}{n_2}\right)}}$$

where

$$\overline{p} = \frac{X_1 + X_2}{n_1 + n_2} \qquad \hat{p}_1 = \frac{X_1}{n_1}$$

$$\overline{q} = 1 - \overline{p} \qquad \hat{p}_2 = \frac{X_2}{n_2}$$

Formula for confidence interval for the difference of two proportions:

$$(\hat{p}_1 - \hat{p}_2) - z_{\alpha/2}\sqrt{\frac{\hat{p}_1\hat{q}_1}{n_1} + \frac{\hat{p}_2\hat{q}_2}{n_2}} < p_1 - p_2$$

$$< (\hat{p}_1 - \hat{p}_2) + z_{\alpha/2}\sqrt{\frac{\hat{p}_1\hat{q}_1}{n_1} + \frac{\hat{p}_2\hat{q}_2}{n_2}}$$

Formula for the F test for comparing two variances:

$$F = \frac{s_1^2}{s_2^2} \qquad \begin{array}{l} \text{d.f.N.} = n_1 - 1 \\ \text{d.f.D.} = n_2 - 1 \end{array}$$

McGraw Hill Connect™ Practise and learn online with *Connect* with data sets and algorithmic questions related to concepts covered in this chapter. Questions and tables with online data sets are marked with ➤.

Review Exercises »

For each exercise, use the following traditional method of hypothesis testing unless otherwise specified.

   a. State the hypotheses and identify the claim.
   b. Find the critical value(s).
   c. Compute the test statistic.
   d. Make the decision.
   e. Summarize the results.

Assume that all variables are normally or approximately normally distributed.

1. **Driving for Pleasure** Two groups of drivers are surveyed to see how many kilometres per week they drive for pleasure trips. The data are shown. At $\alpha = 0.01$, can it be concluded that single drivers do more driving for pleasure trips on average than married drivers? Assume that $\sigma_1 = 27.0$ and $\sigma_2 = 25.8$.

Single drivers					Married drivers				
171	177	185	195	212	156	167	222	164	185
192	156	190	196	217	214	193	192	219	154
177	188	187	222	229	224	174	188	233	183
185	183	166	158	159	225	219	182	182	241
174	188	245	237	188	163	183	187	182	217
248	138	185	187	167	185	175	237	171	142
172	214	222	229	225	182	192	159	174	169

2. **Average Earnings of College Graduates** The average yearly earnings of male college graduates (with at least a bachelor's degree) are $58,500 for men aged 25 to 34. The average yearly earnings of female college graduates with the same qualifications are $49,339. Based on the following results, can it be concluded that there is a difference in mean earnings between male and female college graduates? Use the 0.01 level of significance.

	Male	Female
Sample mean	$59,235	$52,487
Population standard deviation	8,945	10,125
Sample size	40	35

Source: *The New York Times Almanac.*

3. **Communication Times** According to a time-use survey, married persons spend an average of 8 minutes per day on phone calls, mail, and e-mail, while single persons spend an average of 14 minutes per day on these same tasks. Based on the following information, is there sufficient evidence to conclude that single persons spend, on average, a greater amount of time each day communicating? Use the 0.05 level of significance.

	Single	Married
Sample size	26	20
Sample mean	16.7 min.	12.5 min.
Sample variance	8.41	10.24

Source: *Time* magazine.

4. **Average Temperatures** The average temperatures (°C) for a 25-day period for Victoria, British Columbia, and St. John's, Newfoundland, are shown. Based on the samples, at $\alpha = 0.10$, can it be concluded that it is warmer in Victoria?

Victoria					St. John's				
22.4	25.3	24.8	24.4	25.9	20.5	24.7	20.5	23.5	20.5
21.9	17.3	23.2	25.6	24.8	18.0	23.2	21.4	20.1	17.8
21.8	21.4	20.2	24.7	25.9	15.3	18.9	22.4	19.6	14.6
22.3	20.7	20.3	17.3	23.8	15.5	15.5	22.2	20.9	12.8
25.7	18.8	18.1	19.6	20.4	16.7	23.7	22.6	23.8	19.3
25.6	22.6	24.9	20.7	20.0	22.9	17.9	18.9	22.7	16.6

Source: Environment Canada.

5. **Teachers' Salaries** A sample of 15 teachers from Nova Scotia has an average salary of $44,168 with a standard

deviation of $4077. A sample of 30 teachers from New Brunswick has an average salary of $40,482 with a standard deviation of $1964. Is there a significant difference in teachers' salaries between the two provinces? Use $\alpha = 0.02$. Find the 98% confidence interval for the difference of the two means.

Source: Education Canada Network: Canadian Teacher Salaries.

6. **Soft Drinks in School** The data show the amounts (in thousands of dollars) of the contracts for soft drinks in local school districts. At $\alpha = 0.10$, can it be concluded that there is a difference in the averages? Use the *P*-value method. Give a reason why the result would be of concern to a cafeteria manager.

Pepsi						Coca-Cola		
46	120	80	500	100	59	420	285	57

Source: Local school districts.

7. **Vocabulary Skills** In order to improve the vocabulary of 10 students, a teacher provides a weekly 1-hour tutoring session for them. A pretest is given before the sessions, and a posttest is given afterward. The results are shown in the table. At $\alpha = 0.01$, can the teacher conclude that the tutoring sessions helped to improve the students' vocabularies?

Before	1	2	3	4	5	6	7	8	9	10
Pretest	83	76	92	64	82	68	70	71	72	63
Posttest	88	82	100	72	81	75	79	68	81	70

8. **Automobile Part Production** In an effort to increase production of an automobile part, the factory manager decides to play music in the manufacturing area. Eight workers are selected, and the number of items each produced for a specific day is recorded. After one week of music, the same workers are monitored again. The data are given in the table. At $\alpha = 0.05$, can the manager conclude that the music has increased production?

Worker	1	2	3	4	5	6	7	8
Before	6	8	10	9	5	12	9	7
After	10	12	9	12	8	13	8	10

9. **Foggy Days** St. Petersburg, Russia, has 207 foggy days out of 365 days while Stockholm, Sweden, has 166 foggy days out of 365. At $\alpha = 0.02$, can it be concluded that the proportions of foggy days for the two cities are different? Find the 98% confidence interval for the difference of the two proportions.

Source: Jack Williams, USA TODAY.

10. **Adopted Pets** According to a recent National Pet Owners Survey, only 16% of pet dogs were adopted from an animal shelter and 15% of pet cats were adopted. To test this difference in proportions of adopted pets, a survey was taken in a local region. Is there sufficient evidence to conclude that there is a difference in proportions? Use $\alpha = 0.05$.

	Dogs	Cats
Number	180	200
Adopted	36	30

Source: The Humane Society of the United States.

11. **Noise Levels in Hospitals** In a hospital study, the standard deviation of the noise levels of 11 intensive care units was 4.1 dBA (decibels acoustic), and the standard deviation of the noise levels of 24 nonmedical care areas, such as kitchens and machine rooms, was 13.2 dBA. At $\alpha = 0.10$, is there a significant difference between the standard deviations of these two areas?

Source: M. Bayo, A. Garcia, and A. Garcia, "Noise Levels in an Urban Hospital and Workers' Subjective Responses," Archives of Environmental Health 50, No. 3, p. 249, May–June 1995.

12. **Heights of World-Famous Cathedrals** The heights (in metres) for a random sample of world-famous cathedrals are listed below. In addition, the heights for a sample of the tallest buildings in the world are listed. Is there sufficient evidence at $\alpha = 0.05$ to conclude a difference in the variances in height between the two groups?

Cathedrals	21.9	34.7	47.9	17.1	25.3
Tallest buildings	137.8	134.7	126.5	119.2	108.2

Cathedrals	32.9	27.4	46.0	
Tallest buildings	104.9	94.5	92.0	63.7

Source: Infoplease: www.infoplease.com.

Statistics Today

A Woman's Path to Pay Equity–Revisited

Using a *z* test, the researchers compared the difference between gender self-employment and wage compensation gap means. Statistically significant results indicated that the average income gap between self-employed workers was $10,904 compared to an average income gap of $38,626 for wage earners, both in favour of the male gender. Using statistical methods presented in later chapters, the researchers predicted that the gender income gap for both self-employed and wage earners will decrease with age but self-employed females will experience a lesser amount of income gap differential.

Data Analysis »

The databanks for these questions can be found in Appendix D at the back of the textbook and on ▓ connect.

1. From the databank, select a variable and compare the mean of the variable for a random sample of at least 30 men with the mean of the variable for the random sample of at least 30 women. Use a z test.

2. Repeat the experiment in Exercise 1, using a different variable and two samples of size 15. Compare the means by using a t test.

3. Compare the proportion of men who are smokers with the proportion of women who are smokers. Use the data

in the databank. Choose random samples of size 30 or more. Use the z test for proportions.

4. Select two samples of 20 values from the data in Data Set IV. Test the hypothesis that the mean heights of the buildings are equal.

5. Using the same data obtained in Exercise 4, test the hypothesis that the variances are equal.

Chapter Quiz »

Determine whether each statement is true or false. If the statement is false, explain why.

1. When one is testing the difference between two means for small samples, it is not important to distinguish whether the samples are independent of each other.

2. If the same diet is given to two groups of randomly selected individuals, the samples are considered to be dependent.

3. When computing the F test statistic, one always places the larger variance in the numerator of the fraction.

4. Tests for variances are always two-tailed.

Select the best answer.

5. To test the equality of two variances, one would use a(n) _____ test.

   a. z
   b. t
   c. χ^2
   d. F

6. To test the equality of two proportions, one would use a(n) _____ test.

   a. z
   b. t
   c. χ^2
   d. F

7. The mean value of the F is approximately equal to

   a. 0
   b. 0.5
   c. 1
   d. It cannot be determined.

8. What test can be used to test the difference between two sample means when the population variances are known?

   a. z c. χ^2
   b. t d. F

Complete these statements with the best answer.

9. If one hypothesizes that there is no difference between means, this is represented as H_0: _____.

10. When you are testing the difference between two means, the _____ test is used when the population variances are not known.

11. When the t test is used for testing the equality of two means, the populations must be _____.

12. The values of F cannot be _____.

13. The formula for the F test for variances is _____.

odds

For Exercises 14 through 25, use the following traditional method of hypothesis testing unless otherwise specified.

   a. State the hypotheses and identify the claim.
   b. Find the critical value(s).
   c. Compute the test statistic.
   d. Make the decision.
   e. Summarize the results.

Assume that all variables are normally or approximately normally distributed.

14. **Cholesterol Levels** A researcher wishes to see if there is a difference in the cholesterol levels of two groups of men. A random sample of 30 men between the ages of 25 and 40 is selected and tested. The average level is 223. A second sample of 25 men between the ages of 41 and 56 is selected and tested. The average of this group is 229. The population standard deviation for both groups is 6. At $\alpha = 0.01$, is there a difference in the cholesterol levels between the two groups? Find the 99% confidence interval for the difference of the two means.

15. **Apartment Rental Fees** The data shown are the rental fees (in dollars) for two random samples of apartments in a large city. At $\alpha = 0.10$, can it be concluded that the

average rental fee for apartments in the east is greater than the average rental fee in the west?

East					West				
495	390	540	445	420	525	400	310	375	750
410	550	499	500	550	390	795	554	450	370
389	350	450	530	350	385	395	425	500	550
375	690	325	350	799	380	400	450	365	425
475	295	350	485	625	375	360	425	400	475
275	450	440	425	675	400	475	430	410	450
625	390	485	550	650	425	450	620	500	400
685	385	450	550	425	295	350	300	360	400

Source: Pittsburgh Post-Gazette.

16. Prices of Low-Calories Foods The average price of a sample of 12 bottles of diet salad dressing taken from different stores is $1.43. The standard deviation is $0.09. The average price of a sample of 16 low-calorie frozen desserts is $1.03. The standard deviation is $0.10. At $\alpha = 0.01$, is there a significant difference in price? Find the 99% confidence interval of the difference in the means.

17. Aircraft Accidents The data shown represent the number of world aircraft accidents during two periods. At $\alpha = 0.05$, can it be concluded that the average number of accidents per year has decreased from one period to the next?

1999–2004			2005–2009		
211	189	200	185	166	147
185	199	172	156	125	

Source: BAAA–ACRO, Aircraft Crashes Record Office, Geneva, Switzerland.

18. Health-Care Workers' Salaries A sample of 12 health-care workers from British Columbia shows an average annual salary of $39,420 with a standard deviation of $1659, while a sample of 26 health-care workers from Manitoba has an average salary of $30,215 with a standard deviation of $4116. Is there a significant difference between the two provinces in health-care worker salaries at $\alpha = 0.02$? Find the 98% confidence interval of the difference in the means.
Source: Statistics Canada.

19. Urban and Rural Family Incomes The average income of 15 families who reside in a large metropolitan east coast city is $62,456. The standard deviation is $9652. The average income of 11 families who reside in a rural area in the west is $60,213, with a standard deviation of $2009. At $\alpha = 0.05$, can it be concluded that families who live in cities have a higher average income than those who live in rural areas? Use the P-value method.

20. Mathematical Skills In an effort to improve the mathematical skills of 10 students, a teacher provides a weekly 1-hour tutoring session for the students. A pretest is given before the sessions, and a posttest is given after. The results are shown here. At $\alpha = 0.01$,

can it be concluded that the sessions help to improve the students' mathematical skills?

Student	1	2	3	4	5	6	7	8	9	10
Pretest	82	76	91	62	81	67	71	69	80	85
Posttest	88	80	98	80	80	73	74	78	85	93

21. Egg Production To increase egg production, a farmer decided to increase the amount of time the lights in his henhouse were on. Ten hens were selected, and the number of eggs each produced was recorded. After 1 week of lengthened light time, the same hens were monitored again. The data are given here. At $\alpha = 0.05$, can it be concluded that the increased light time increased egg production?

Hen	1	2	3	4	5	6	7	8	9	10
Before	4	3	8	7	6	4	9	7	6	5
After	6	5	9	7	4	5	10	6	9	6

22. Factory Worker Literacy Rates In a sample of 80 workers at a factory in city A, it was found that 5% were unable to read, while in a sample of 50 workers in city B, 8% were unable to read. Can it be concluded that there is a difference in the proportions of non-readers in the two cities? Use $\alpha = 0.10$. Find the 90% confidence interval for the difference of the two proportions.

23. Single Male Head of Household A survey of 200 households showed that 8 had a single male as the head of household. Forty years ago, a survey of 200 households showed that 6 had a single male as the head of household. At $\alpha = 0.05$ can it be concluded that the proportion has changed? Find the 95% confidence interval of the difference of the two proportions. Does the confidence interval contain 0? Why is this important to know?
Source: Based on data from the U.S. Census Bureau.

24. Money Spent on Road Repair A politician wants to compare the variances of the amount of money spent for road repair in two different regions. The data are given here. At $\alpha = 0.05$, is there a significant difference in the variances of the amounts spent in the two regions? Use the P-value method.

County A	County B
$s_1 = \$11{,}596$	$s_2 = \$14{,}837$
$n_1 = 15$	$n_2 = 18$

25. Heights of Basketball Players A researcher wants to compare the variances of the heights (in centimetres) of university basketball players with those of college players. A sample of 30 players from each type of school is selected, and the variances of the heights for each type are 15.68 and 20.32, respectively. At $\alpha = 0.10$, is there a significant difference between the variances of the heights of basketball players in the two types of schools?

Critical Thinking Challenges

1. The study cited in the article below, "Only the Timid Die Young," stated that "Timid rats were 60% more likely to die at any given time than were their outgoing brothers." Based on the results, answer the following questions.

   a. Why were rats used in the study?
   b. What are the variables in the study?
   c. Why were infants included in the article?
   d. What is wrong with extrapolating the results to humans?
   e. Suggest some ways humans might be used in a study of this type.

2. Based on the study presented in the article on the next page entitled "Sleeping Brain, Not at Rest," answer these questions.

   a. What were the variables used in the study?
   b. How were they measured?
   c. Suggest a statistical test that might have been used to arrive at the conclusion.
   d. Based on the results, what would you suggest for students preparing for an exam?

ONLY THE TIMID DIE YOUNG

DO OVERACTIVE STRESS HORMONES DAMAGE HEALTH?

ABOUT 15 OUT OF 100 CHILDREN ARE BORN SHY, BUT ONLY THREE WILL BE SHY AS ADULTS.

FEARFUL TYPES MAY MEET THEIR maker sooner, at least among rats. Researchers have for the first time connected a personality trait—fear of novelty—to an early death.

Sonia Cavigelli and Martha McClintock, psychologists at the University of Chicago, presented unfamiliar bowls, tunnels and bricks to a group of young male rats. Those hesitant to explore the mystery objects were classified as "neophobic."

The researchers found that the neophobic rats produced high levels of stress hormones, called glucocorticoids—typically involved in the fight-or-flight stress response—when faced with strange situations. Those rats continued to have high levels of the hormones at random times throughout their lives, indicating that timidity is a fixed and stable trait. The team then set out to examine the cumulative effects of this personality trait on the rats' health.

Timid rats were 60 percent more likely to die at any given time than were their outgoing brothers. The causes of death were similar for both groups. "One hypothesis as to why the neophobic rats died earlier is that the stress hormones negatively affected their immune system," Cavigelli says. Neophobes died, on average, three months before their rat brothers, a significant gap, considering that most rats lived only two years.

Shyness—the human equivalent of neophobia—can be detected in infants as young as 14 months. Shy people also produce more stress hormones than "average," or thrill-seeking humans. But introverts don't necessarily stay shy for life, as rats apparently do. Jerome Kagan, a professor of psychology at Harvard University, has found that while 15 out of every 100 children will be born with a shy temperament, only three will appear shy as adults. None, however, will be extroverts.

Extrapolating from the doomed fate of neophobic rats to their human counterparts is difficult. "But it means that something as simple as a personality trait could have physiological consequences," Cavigelli says.

—*Carlin Flora*

SLEEPING BRAIN, NOT AT REST

Regions of the brain that have spent the day learning sleep more heavily at night.

In a study published in the journal *Nature*, Giulio Tononi, a psychiatrist at the University of Wisconsin–Madison, had subjects perform a simple point-and-click task with a computer adjusted so that its cursor didn't track in the right direction. Afterward, the subjects' brain waves were recorded while they slept, then examined for "slow wave" activity, a kind of deep sleep.

Compared with people who had completed the same task with normal cursors, Tononi's subjects showed elevated slow wave activity in brain areas associated with spatial orientation, indicating that their brains were adjusting to the day's learning by making cellular-level changes. In the morning, Tononi's subjects performed their tasks better than they had before going to sleep.

—*Richard A. Love*

Reprinted with permission from *Psychology Today*, Copyright © 2004, Sussex Publishers, Inc.

Data Projects ≫

Where appropriate, use Minitab, SPSS, TI-83 Plus, TI-84 Plus, Excel, or a computer program of your choice to complete the following exercises.

Use a significance level of 0.05 for all tests below.

1. **Business and Finance** Use the data collected in Data Project 1 in Chapter 2 to complete this problem. Test the claim that the mean earnings per share for Dow Jones stocks are greater than for Toronto Stock Exchange (TSX) stocks.

2. **Sports and Leisure** Use the data collected in Data Project 2 in Chapter 7 regarding home runs for this problem. Test the claim that the mean number of home runs hit by the American League sluggers is the same as the mean for the National League.

3. **Technology** Use the cellphone data collected for Data Project 3 in Chapter 8 to complete this problem. Test the claim that the mean length for outgoing calls is the same as that for incoming calls. Test the claim that the

standard deviation for outgoing calls is more than that for incoming calls.

4. **Health and Wellness** Use the data regarding BMI that were collected in Data Project 6 in Chapter 7 to complete this problem. Test the claim that the mean BMI for males is the same as that for females. Test the claim that the standard deviation for males is the same as that for females.

5. **Politics and Economics** Use the most recent results of the federal elections for the Liberals and Conservatives to categorize the 13 provinces and territories as Liberal "red" or Conservative "blue," based on the highest percentage of votes for the two parties. Research the average provincial income per capita. Test the claim that the average income for Liberal "red" and Conservative "blue" provinces/territories are equal.

6. **Your Class** Use the data collected in Data Project 6 of Chapter 2 regarding heart rates. Test the claim that the heart rates after exercise are more variable than the heart rates before exercise.

Answers to Applying the Concepts ≫

Section 9–1 Home Runs

1. The population is all home runs hit by Major League Baseball players.

2. A cluster sample was used.

3. Answers will vary. While this sample is not representative of all Major League Baseball players per se, it does allow us to compare the leaders in each league.

4. H_0: $\mu_1 = \mu_2$ and H_1: $\mu_1 \neq \mu_2$

5. Answers will vary. Possible answers include the 0.05 and 0.01 significance levels.

6. We will use the z test for the difference in means.

7. Our test statistic is $z = \dfrac{44.75 - 42.88}{\sqrt{\dfrac{8.88^2}{40} + \dfrac{7.82^2}{40}}} = 1.01$, and our

   P-value is 0.3173.

8. We fail to reject the null hypothesis.

9. There is not enough evidence to conclude that there is a difference in the number of home runs hit by National League versus American League baseball players.

10. Answers will vary. One possible answer is that since we do not have a random sample of data from each league, we cannot answer the original question asked.

11. Answers will vary. One possible answer is that we could get a random sample of data from each league from a recent season.

Section 9–2 Too Long on the Telephone

1. These samples are independent.

2. The population variances are assumed to be unequal.

3. We compare the P-value of 0.06317 to the significance level to check if the null hypothesis should be rejected.

4. The P-value of 0.06317 also gives the probability of a type I error.

5. Since 0 is contained in the interval, the decision is to not reject the null hypothesis.

6. Since two critical values are shown, we know that a two-tailed test was done.

7. Since the P-value of 0.06317 is greater than the significance value of 0.05, we fail to reject the null hypothesis and find that we do not have enough evidence to conclude that there is a difference in the lengths of telephone calls made by employees in the two divisions of the company.

8. If the significance level had been 0.10, we would have rejected the null hypothesis, since the P-value would have been less than the significance level.

Section 9–3 Air Quality

1. The purpose of the study is to determine if the air quality index in Ontario has changed over a 2-year period.

2. These are dependent samples, since we have two readings from each of the 10 cities.

3. The hypotheses we will test are $H_0: \mu_D = 0$ and $H_1: \mu_D \neq 0$.

4. We will use the 0.05 significance level and critical values of $t = \pm 2.262$.

5. We will use the t test for dependent samples.

6. There are $10 - 1 = 9$ degrees of freedom.

7. Our test statistic is $t = \dfrac{-10.8 - 0}{9.682/\sqrt{10}} = -3.527$

   We reject the null hypothesis and find that there is enough evidence to conclude that the air quality in Ontario has changed over the past 2 years.

8. No, we could not use an independent means test since we have two readings from each city.

9. Answers will vary. One possible answer is that there may be other measures of air quality that we could have examined to answer the question.

Section 9–4 Smoking and Education

1. Our hypotheses are $H_0: p_1 = p_2$ and $H_1: p_1 \neq p_2$.

2. At the 0.05 significance level, our critical values are $z = \pm 1.96$.

3. We will use the z test for the difference between proportions.

4. To complete the statistical test, we would need the sample sizes.

5. Knowing the sample sizes were 1000, we can now complete the test.

6. Our test statistic is

   $$z = \frac{0.323 - 0.145}{\sqrt{(0.234)(0.766)\left(\dfrac{1}{1000} + \dfrac{1}{1000}\right)}} = 9.40$$

   and our P-value is very close to zero. We reject the null hypothesis and find that there is enough evidence to conclude that there is a difference in the proportions of public school students and private school students who smoke.

Section 9–5 Variability and Automatic Transmissions

1. The null hypothesis is that the variances are the same: $H_0: \sigma_1^2 = \sigma_2^2$.

2. We will use an F test.

3. The value of the test statistic is $F = \dfrac{s_1^2}{s_2^2} = \dfrac{514.8^2}{77.7^2} = 43.92$,

   and the P-value is 0.0008. There is a significant difference in the variability of the prices between the two car sectors.

4. Small sample sizes are highly impacted by outliers.

5. The degrees of freedom for the numerator and denominator are both 5.

6. Yes, two sets of data can centre on the same mean but have very different standard deviations.

Hypothesis-Testing Summary 1 »

1. Comparison of a sample mean with a specific population mean.

   Example: $H_0: \mu = 100$

   a. Use the z test when σ is known:

   $$z = \frac{\overline{X} - \mu}{\sigma/\sqrt{n}}$$

   b. Use the t test when σ is unknown:

   $$t = \frac{\overline{X} - \mu}{s/\sqrt{n}} \quad \text{with d.f.} = n - 1$$

2. Comparison of a sample variance or standard deviation with a specific population variance or standard deviation.

   Example: $H_0: \sigma^2 = 225$

   Use the chi-square test:

   $$\chi^2 = \frac{(n-1)s^2}{\sigma^2} \quad \text{with d.f.} = n - 1$$

3. Comparison of two sample means.

   Example: $H_0: \mu_1 = \mu_2$

   a. Use the z test when the population variances are known:

   $$z = \frac{(\overline{X}_1 - \overline{X}_2) - (\mu_1 - \mu_2)}{\sqrt{\dfrac{\sigma_1^2}{n_1} + \dfrac{\sigma_2^2}{n_2}}}$$

   b. Use the t test for independent samples when the population variances are unknown and the sample variances are unequal:

   $$t = \frac{(\overline{X}_1 - \overline{X}_2) - (\mu_1 - \mu_2)}{\sqrt{\dfrac{s_1^2}{n_1} + \dfrac{s_2^2}{n_2}}}$$

   with d.f. = the smaller of $n_1 - 1$ or $n_2 - 1$.

   c. Use the t test for means for dependent samples:

   Example: $H_0: \mu_D = 0$

   $$t = \frac{\overline{D} - \mu_D}{s_D/\sqrt{n}} \quad \text{with d.f.} = n - 1$$

   where n = number of pairs.

4. Comparison of a sample proportion with a specific population proportion.

   Example: $H_0: p = 0.32$

   Use the z test:

   $$z = \frac{X - \mu}{\sigma} \quad \text{or} \quad z = \frac{\hat{p} - p}{\sqrt{pq/n}}$$

5. Comparison of two sample proportions.

   Example: $H_0: p_1 = p_2$

   Use the z test:

   $$z = \frac{(\hat{p}_1 - \hat{p}_2) - (p_1 - p_2)}{\sqrt{\overline{p}\,\overline{q}\left(\dfrac{1}{n_1} + \dfrac{1}{n_2}\right)}}$$

   where

   $$\overline{p} = \frac{X_1 + X_2}{n_1 + n_2} \qquad \hat{p}_1 = \frac{X_1}{n_1}$$

   $$\overline{q} = 1 - \overline{p} \qquad \hat{p}_2 = \frac{X_2}{n_2}$$

6. Comparison of two sample variances or standard deviations.

   Example: $H_0: \sigma_1^2 = \sigma_2^2$

   Use the F test:

   $$F = \frac{s_1^2}{s_2^2}$$

   where

   s_1^2 = larger variance   d.f.N. = $n_1 - 1$

   s_2^2 = smaller variance   d.f.D. = $n_2 - 1$

Chapter 10

Correlation and Regression

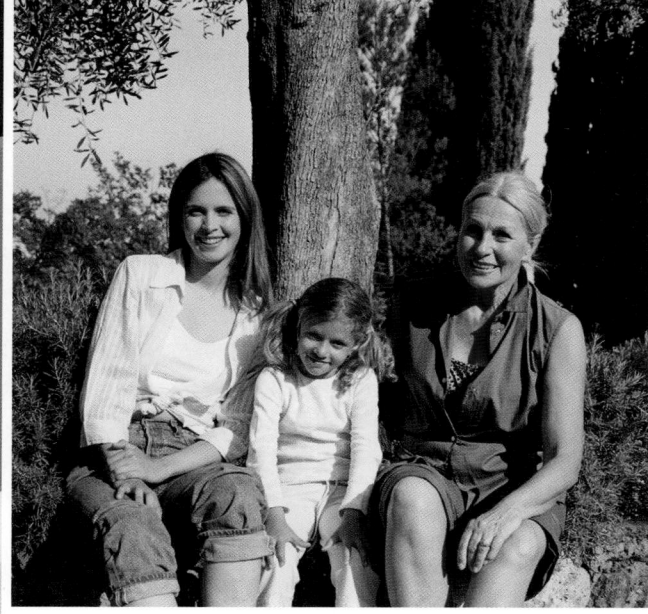

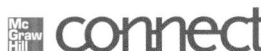 **Connect**™ Practise and learn online with *Connect* with data sets and algorithmic questions related to concepts covered in this chapter. Throughout this chapter, questions and tables with online data sets are marked with 🖱.

Statistics Today

Like Parent, Like Child?

Do parents influence a child's participation in the Employment Insurance (EI) program? A Statistics

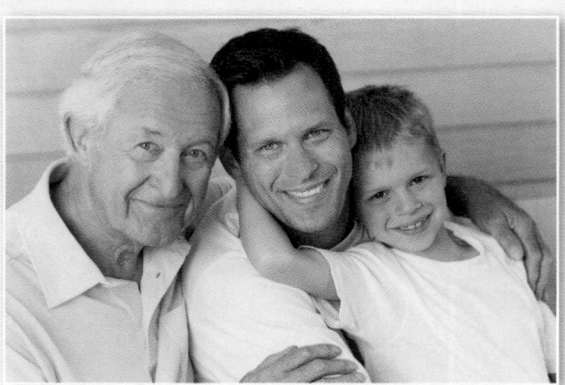

Canada family and labour study examined the relationship between a young adult's use of EI and having a parent who collected EI. The Canada–Sweden joint study also compared other factors, such as past experience with the program and time to a first EI claim, as well as the entire sequence of claims over time. Using methods of correlation and regression, which are explained in this chapter, they were able to determine the effect of parental factors in an offspring's involvement in the EI program. See Statistics Today— Revisited, page 498.

Source: "Excerpts from the Intergenerational Influences on the Receipt of Unemployment Insurance in Canada and Sweden," adapted from Statistics Canada, *Analytical Studies Branch Research Paper Series*.

Introduction >

In Chapters 7 and 8, two areas of inferential statistics—confidence intervals and hypothesis testing—were explained. Another area of inferential statistics involves determining whether a relationship between two or more numerical or quantitative variables exists. For example, a businessperson may want to know whether the volume of sales for a given month is related to the amount of advertising the firm does that month. Educators are interested in determining whether the number of hours a student studies is related to the student's score on a particular exam. Medical researchers are interested in questions such as, Is caffeine related to heart damage? or Is there a relationship between a person's age and his or her blood pressure? A zoologist may want to know whether the birth weight of a certain animal is related to its life span. These are only a few of the many questions that can be answered by using the techniques of correlation and regression analysis. **Correlation** is a statistical method used to determine whether a relationship between variables exists. **Regression** is a statistical method used to describe the nature of the relationship between variables, that is, positive or negative, linear or nonlinear.

The purpose of this chapter is to answer these questions statistically:

1. Are two or more variables related?
2. If so, what is the strength of the relationship?
3. What type of relationship exists?
4. What kind of predictions can be made from the relationship?

To answer the first two questions, statisticians use a numerical measure to determine whether two or more variables are related and to determine the strength of the relationship between or among the variables. This measure is called a *correlation coefficient.* For

Interesting Fact

Using computer models, the Canadian Forest Service predicts that if the climate warms, the average forest area burned in the next 50 years will double.

example, there are many variables that contribute to heart disease, among them lack of exercise, smoking, heredity, age, stress, and diet. Of these variables, some are more important than others; therefore, a physician who wants to help a patient must know which factors are most important.

To answer the third question, one must ascertain what type of relationship exists. There are two types of relationships: *simple* and *multiple*. In a simple relationship, there are two variables—an **independent variable,** also called an *explanatory variable* or a *predictor variable,* and a **dependent variable,** also called a *response variable.* A simple relationship analysis is called *simple regression,* and there is one independent variable that is used to predict the dependent variable. For example, a manager may wish to see whether the number of years the salespeople have been working for the company has anything to do with the amount of sales they make. This type of study involves a simple relationship, since there are only two variables—years of experience and amount of sales.

In a multiple relationship, called *multiple regression,* two or more independent variables are used to predict one dependent variable. For example, an educator may wish to investigate the relationship between a student's success in college and factors such as the number of hours devoted to studying, the student's GPA, and the student's high school background. This type of study involves several variables.

Simple relationships can also be positive or negative. A **positive relationship** exists when both variables increase or decrease at the same time. For instance, a person's height and weight are related and the relationship is positive, since the taller a person is, generally, the more the person weighs. In a **negative relationship,** as one variable increases, the other variable decreases, and vice versa. For example, if one measures the strength of people over 60 years of age, one will find that as age increases, strength generally decreases. The word *generally* is used here because there are exceptions.

Finally, the fourth question asks what type of predictions can be made. Every day, predictions are made in all facets of modern life. Examples include weather forecasting, stock market analyses, sales predictions, crop predictions, gasoline predictions, and sports predictions. Some predictions are more accurate than others, due to the strength of the relationship. That is, the stronger the relationship is between variables, the more accurate the prediction is.

10–1   Scatter Plots and Correlation >

Draw a scatter plot for a set of ordered pairs, calculate the correlation coefficient, and test the hypothesis $H_0: \rho = 0$.

In simple correlation and regression studies, the researcher collects data on two numerical or quantitative variables to see whether a relationship exists between the variables. For example, if a researcher wishes to see whether there is a relationship between number of hours of study and test scores on an exam, she must select a random sample of students, determine the hours each studied, and obtain their grades on the exam. A table can be made for the data, as shown here.

Student	Hours of study x	Grade y (%)
A	6	82
B	2	63
C	1	57
D	5	88
E	2	68
F	3	75

As stated previously, the two variables for this study are called the *independent variable* and the *dependent variable*. The independent variable is the variable in regression that can be controlled or manipulated. In this case, "number of hours of study" is the independent variable and is designated as the x variable. The dependent variable is the variable in regression that cannot be controlled or manipulated. The grade the student received on the exam is the dependent variable, designated as the y variable. The reason for this distinction between the variables is that one assumes that the grade the student earns *depends* on the number of hours the student studied. Also, one assumes that, to some extent, the student can regulate or *control* the number of hours she or he studies for the exam.

The determination of the x and y variables is not always clear-cut and is sometimes an arbitrary decision. For example, if a researcher studies the effects of age on a person's blood pressure, the researcher can generally assume that age affects blood pressure. Hence, the variable *age* can be called the *independent variable,* and the variable *blood pressure* can be called the *dependent variable.* On the other hand, if a researcher is studying the attitudes of husbands on a certain issue and the attitudes of their wives on the same issue, it is difficult to say which variable is the independent variable and which is the dependent variable. In this study, the researcher can arbitrarily designate the variables as independent and dependent.

Scatter Plots

The independent and dependent variables can be plotted on a graph called a *scatter plot.* The independent variable x is plotted on the horizontal axis, and the dependent variable y is plotted on the vertical axis.

> A **scatter plot** is a graph of the ordered pairs (x, y) of numbers consisting of the independent variable x and the dependent variable y.

The scatter plot is a visual way to describe the nature of the relationship between the independent and dependent variables. The scales of the variables can be different, and the coordinates of the axes are determined by the smallest and largest data values of the variables.

The procedure for drawing a scatter plot is shown in Examples 10–1 through 10–3.

| Example 10–1 | **Age and Blood Pressure** |

Construct a scatter plot for the data obtained in a study of age (years) and systolic blood pressure (millimetres of mercury, mmHg) of six randomly selected subjects. The data are shown in the table.

Subject	Age x	Pressure y
A	43	128
B	48	120
C	56	135
D	61	143
E	67	141
F	70	152

Solution

Step 1   Draw and label the x and y axes.

Step 2   Plot each point on the graph, as shown in Figure 10–1.

Figure 10–1

Scatter Plot for
Example 10–1

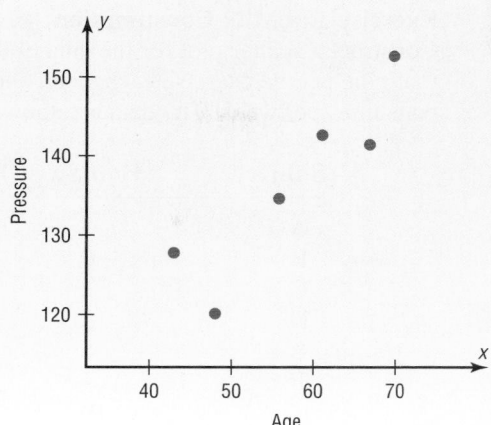

Figure 10–1

Scatter Plot for
Example 10–1

Example 10–2

Absences and Final Grades

Construct a scatter plot for the data obtained in a study on the number of absences and the final grades of seven randomly selected students from a statistics class. The data are shown here.

Student	Number of absences x	Final grade y (%)
A	6	82
B	2	86
C	15	43
D	9	74
E	12	58
F	5	90
G	8	78

Solution

Step 1 Draw and label the x and y axes.

Step 2 Plot each point on the graph, as shown in Figure 10–2.

Figure 10–2

Scatter Plot for
Example 10–2

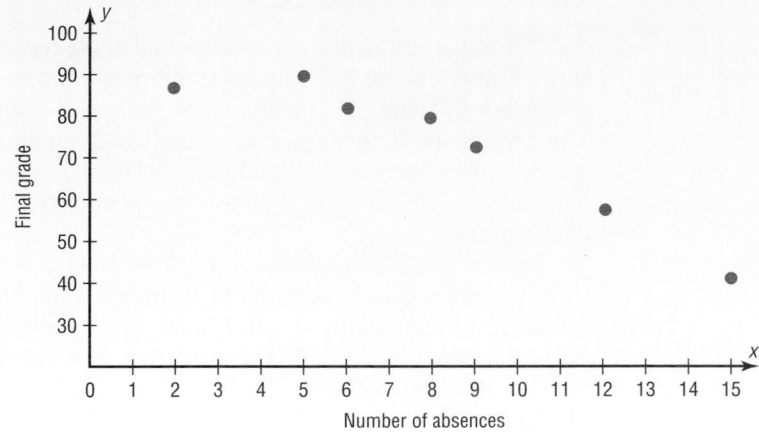

Example 10–3

Exercise and Milk Consumption

Construct a scatter plot for the data obtained in a study on the number of hours that nine people exercise each week and the amount of milk (in litres) each person consumes per week. The data are shown.

Subject	Hours x	Amount y
A	3	1.4
B	0	0.2
C	2	0.9
D	5	1.9
E	8	0.3
F	5	0.9
G	10	1.7
H	2	2.1
I	1	1.4

Solution

Step 1   Draw and label the x and y axes.

Step 2   Plot each point on the graph, as shown in Figure 10–3.

Figure 10–3

Scatter Plot for Example 10–3

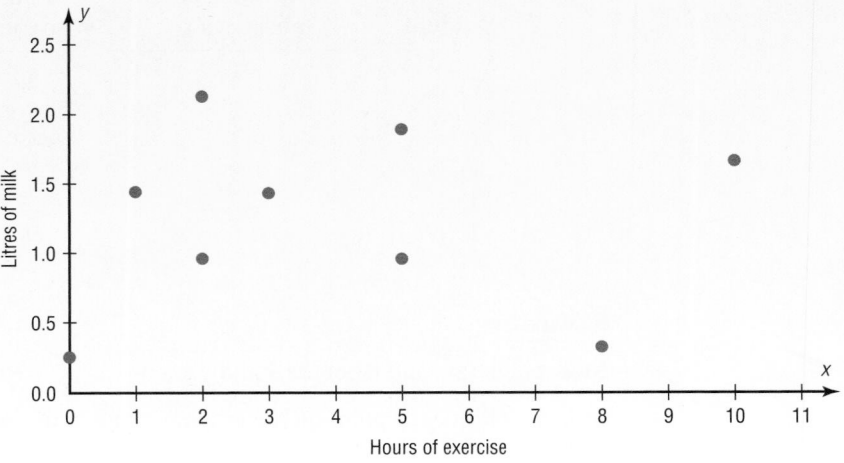

After the plot is drawn, it should be analyzed to determine which type of relationship, if any, exists. For example, the plot shown in Figure 10–1 suggests a positive relationship, since as a person's age increases, blood pressure tends to increase also. The plot of the data shown in Figure 10–2 suggests a negative relationship, since as the number of absences increases, the final grade decreases. Finally, the plot of the data shown in Figure 10–3 shows no specific type of relationship, since no pattern is discernible.

Note that the data shown in Figures 10–1 and 10–2 also suggest a linear relationship, since the points seem to fit a straight line, although not perfectly. Sometimes a scatter plot, such as the one in Figure 10–4, shows a curvilinear or nonlinear relationship between the data. In this situation, the methods shown in this section and in Section 10–2 cannot be used. Methods for nonlinear relationships are beyond the scope of this book.

Figure 10–4

Scatter Plot Suggesting
a Nonlinear Relationship

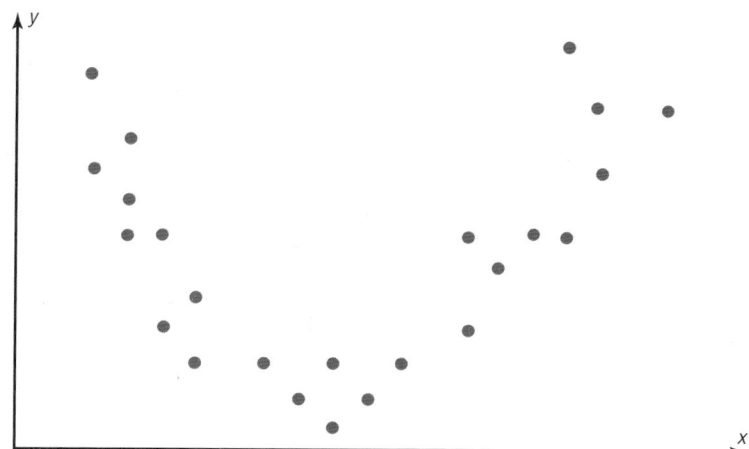

In summary, check the following patterns in a scatter plot to identify possible relationships.

Shape of plot—linear or nonlinear

Direction of data points—direct (positive slope) or indirect (negative slope)

Strength of relationship—strong (minimal or no scatter), weak (scatter with pattern), none (scatter without pattern)

Outliers—extreme data points outside of pattern

Correlation

Correlation Coefficient

As stated in the Introduction, statisticians use a measure called the *correlation coefficient* to determine the strength of the relationship between two variables. There are several types of correlation coefficients. The one explained in this section is called the **Pearson product moment correlation coefficient** (PPMC), named after statistician Karl Pearson, who pioneered the research in this area.

> The **correlation coefficient** computed from the sample data measures the strength and direction of a linear relationship between two variables. The symbol for the sample correlation coefficient is r. The symbol for the population correlation coefficient is ρ (Greek letter *rho*).

The *range of the correlation coefficient* is from -1 to $+1$. If there is a *strong positive linear relationship* between the variables, the value of r will be close to $+1$. If there is a *strong negative linear relationship* between the variables, the value of r will be close to -1. When there is no linear relationship between the variables or only a weak relationship, the value of r will be close to 0. See Figure 10–5.

Figure 10–5

Range of Values for the
Correlation Coefficient

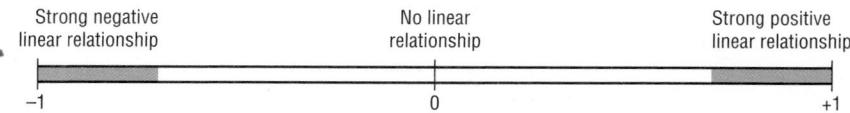

The graphs in Figure 10–6 show the relationship between the correlation coefficients and their corresponding scatter plots. Notice that as the value of the correlation coefficient increases from 0 to +1 (parts *a*, *b*, and *c*), data values become closer to an increasingly stronger relationship. As the value of the correlation coefficient decreases from 0 to −1 (parts *d*, *e*, and *f*), the data values also become closer to a straight line. Again, this suggests a stronger relationship.

Figure 10–6

Relationship between the Correlation Coefficient and the Scatter Plot

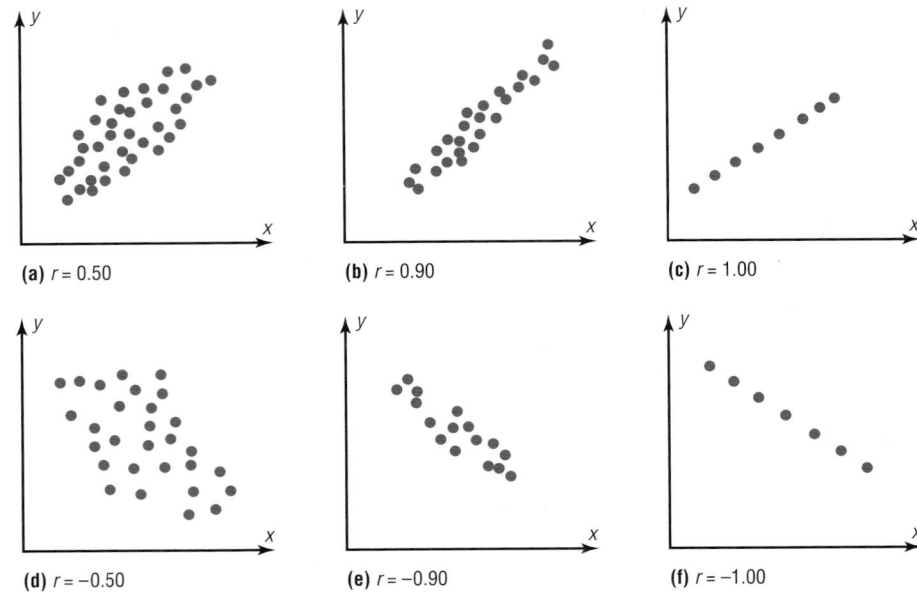

There are several ways to compute the value of the correlation coefficient. One method is to use the formula shown here.

Formula for the Correlation Coefficient *r*

$$r = \frac{n(\Sigma xy) - (\Sigma x)(\Sigma y)}{\sqrt{[n(\Sigma x^2) - (\Sigma x)^2][n(\Sigma y^2) - (\Sigma y)^2]}}$$

where *n* is the number of data pairs.

Assumptions for the Correlation Coefficient

1. The sample is a random sample.
2. Both variables are interval/ratio measurement levels and the data pairs are approximately linear.
3. The variables have a joint normal distribution. (This means that given any specific value of *x*, the *y* values are normally distributed and given any specific value of *y*, the *x* values are normally distributed.)

Rounding Rule for the Correlation Coefficient Round the value of *r* to three decimal places.

The formula looks somewhat complicated, but using a table to compute the values, as shown in Example 10–4, makes it somewhat easier to determine the value of *r*.

Example 10–4

Age and Blood Pressure

Compute the value of the correlation coefficient for the data obtained in the study of age and blood pressure given in Example 10–1.

Solution

Step 1   Make a table, as shown here.

Subject	Age x	Pressure y	xy	x^2	y^2
A	43	128			
B	48	120			
C	56	135			
D	61	143			
E	67	141			
F	70	152			

Step 2   Find the values of xy, x^2, and y^2 and place these values in the corresponding columns of the table.
The completed table is shown.

Subject	Age x	Pressure y	xy	x^2	y^2
A	43	128	5,504	1,849	16,384
B	48	120	5,760	2,304	14,400
C	56	135	7,560	3,136	18,225
D	61	143	8,723	3,721	20,449
E	67	141	9,447	4,489	19,881
F	70	152	10,640	4,900	23,104
	$\Sigma x = 345$	$\Sigma y = 819$	$\Sigma xy = 47,634$	$\Sigma x^2 = 20,399$	$\Sigma y^2 = 112,443$

Step 3   Substitute in the formula and solve for r.

$$r = \frac{n(\Sigma xy) - (\Sigma x)(\Sigma y)}{\sqrt{[n(\Sigma x^2) - (\Sigma x)^2][n(\Sigma y^2) - (\Sigma y)^2]}}$$

$$= \frac{(6)(47,634) - (345)(819)}{\sqrt{[(6)(20,399) - (345)^2][(6)(112,443) - (819)^2]}} \approx 0.897$$

The correlation coefficient suggests a strong positive relationship between age and blood pressure.

Example 10–5

Absences and Final Grades

Compute the value of the correlation coefficient for the data obtained in the study of the number of absences and the final grades of the seven students in the statistics class given in Example 10–2.

Solution

Step 1   Make a table.

Step 2   Find the values of xy, x^2, and y^2 and place these values in the corresponding columns of the table.

Student	Number of absences x	Final grade y (%)	xy	x^2	y^2
A	6	82	492	36	6,724
B	2	86	172	4	7,396
C	15	43	645	225	1,849
D	9	74	666	81	5,476
E	12	58	696	144	3,364
F	5	90	450	25	8,100
G	8	78	624	64	6,084
	$\Sigma x = 57$	$\Sigma y = 511$	$\Sigma xy = 3745$	$\Sigma x^2 = 579$	$\Sigma y^2 = 38,993$

Step 3 Substitute in the formula and solve for r.

$$r = \frac{n(\Sigma xy) - (\Sigma x)(\Sigma y)}{\sqrt{[n(\Sigma x^2) - (\Sigma x)^2][n(\Sigma y^2) - (\Sigma y)^2]}}$$

$$= \frac{(7)(3745) - (57)(511)}{\sqrt{[(7)(579) - (57)^2][(7)(38{,}993) - (511)^2]}} \approx -0.944$$

The value of r suggests a strong negative relationship between a student's final grade and the number of absences a student has. That is, the more absences a student has, the lower is his or her grade.

Example 10–6	**Exercise and Milk Consumption** 🏃

Compute the value of the correlation coefficient for the data given in Example 10–3 for the number of hours a person exercises and the amount of milk a person consumes per week.

Solution

Step 1 Make a table.

Step 2 Find the values of xy, x^2, and y^2 and place these values in the corresponding columns of the table.

Subject	Hours x	Amount y	xy	x^2	y^2
A	3	1.4	4.2	9	1.96
B	0	0.2	0.0	0	0.04
C	2	0.9	1.8	4	0.81
D	5	1.9	9.5	25	3.61
E	8	0.3	2.4	64	0.09
F	5	0.9	4.5	25	0.81
G	10	1.7	17.0	100	2.89
H	2	2.1	4.2	4	4.41
I	1	1.4	1.4	1	1.96
	$\Sigma x = 36$	$\Sigma y = 10.8$	$\Sigma xy = 45$	$\Sigma x^2 = 232$	$\Sigma y^2 = 16.58$

Step 3 Substitute into the formula and solve for r:

$$r = \frac{n(\Sigma xy) - (\Sigma x)(\Sigma y)}{\sqrt{[n(\Sigma x^2) - (\Sigma x)^2][n(\Sigma y^2) - (\Sigma y)^2]}}$$

$$r = \frac{9(45) - (36)(10.8)}{\sqrt{[9(232) - (36)^2][9(16.58) - (10.8)^2]}} \approx 0.101$$

The value of r indicates a very weak positive relationship between the variables.

In Example 10–4, the value of r was high (close to 1.00); in Example 10–6, the value of r was much lower (close to 0). This question then arises: When is the value of r due to chance, and when does it suggest a significant linear relationship between the variables? This question will be answered next.

The Significance of the Correlation Coefficient

As stated before, the range of the correlation coefficient is between -1 and $+1$. When the value of r is near $+1$ or -1, there is a strong linear relationship. When the value of r is near 0, the linear relationship is weak or nonexistent. Since the value of r is computed from data obtained from samples, there are two possibilities when r is not equal to zero: Either the value of r is high enough to conclude that there is a significant linear relationship between the variables, or the value of r is due to chance.

To make this decision, one uses a hypothesis-testing procedure. The traditional method is similar to the one used in previous chapters.

Step 1   State the hypotheses.

Step 2   Find the critical values.

Step 3   Compute the test statistic.

Step 4   Make the decision.

Step 5   Summarize the results.

The population correlation coefficient is computed from taking all possible (x,y) pairs; it is designated by the Greek letter ρ (rho). The sample correlation coefficient can then be used as an estimator of ρ if the following assumptions are valid.

1. The variables x and y are *linearly* related.

2. The variables are *random* variables.

3. The two variables have a *bivariate normal distribution.*

A bivariate normal distribution means that for the pairs of (x, y) data values, the corresponding y values have a bell-shaped distribution for any given x value, and the x values for any given y value have a bell-shaped distribution.

Historical Note

A mathematician named Karl Pearson (1857–1936) became interested in Francis Galton's work and saw that the correlation and regression theory could be applied to other areas besides heredity. Pearson defined the correlation coefficient method that bears his name.

> Formally defined, the **population correlation coefficient** ρ is the correlation computed by using all possible pairs of data values (x, y) taken from a population.

In hypothesis testing, one of these is true:

H_0: $\rho = 0$ This null hypothesis means that there is no correlation between the x and y variables in the population.

H_1: $\rho \neq 0$ This alternative hypothesis means that there is a significant correlation between the variables in the population.

When the null hypothesis is rejected at a specific level, it means that there is a significant difference between the value of r and 0. When the null hypothesis is not rejected, it means that the value of r is not significantly different from 0 (zero) and is probably due to chance.

Several methods can be used to test the significance of the correlation coefficient. Three methods will be shown in this section. The first uses the t test.

Formula for the t Test for the Correlation Coefficient

$$t = r\sqrt{\frac{n-2}{1-r^2}}$$

with degrees of freedom equal to $n - 2$.

Although hypothesis tests can be one-tailed, most hypotheses involving the correlation coefficient are two-tailed. Recall that ρ represents the population correlation coefficient. Also, if there is no linear relationship, the value of the correlation coefficient will be 0. Hence, the hypotheses will be

$$H_0: \rho = 0 \quad \text{and} \quad H_1: \rho \neq 0$$

One does not have to identify the claim here, since the question will always be whether there is a significant linear relationship between the variables.

The two-tailed critical values are used. These values are found in Table F in Appendix C. Also, when one is testing the significance of a correlation coefficient, both variables x and y must come from normally distributed populations.

Example 10–7

Age and Blood Pressure

Test the significance of the correlation coefficient found in Example 10–4. Use $\alpha = 0.05$ and $r = 0.897$.

Solution

Step 1 State the hypotheses.

$$H_0: \rho = 0 \quad \text{and} \quad H_1: \rho \neq 0$$

Step 2 Find the critical values. Since $\alpha = 0.05$ and there are $6 - 2 = 4$ degrees of freedom, the critical values obtained from Table F are ± 2.776, as shown in Figure 10–7.

Figure 10–7

Critical Values for Example 10–7

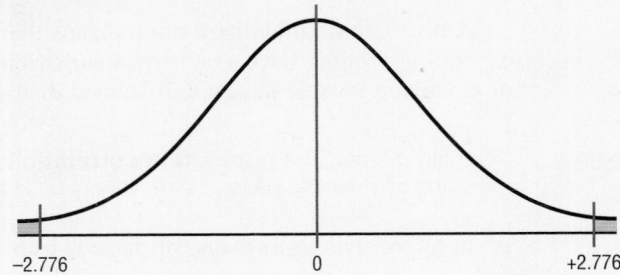

$$-2.776 \qquad 0 \qquad +2.776$$

Step 3 Compute the test statistic.

$$t = r\sqrt{\frac{n-2}{1-r^2}} = (0.897)\sqrt{\frac{6-2}{1-(0.897)^2}} \approx 4.059$$

Step 4 Make the decision. Reject the null hypothesis, since the test statistic falls in the critical region, as shown in Figure 10–8.

Figure 10–8

Critical Values and Test Statistic for Example 10–7

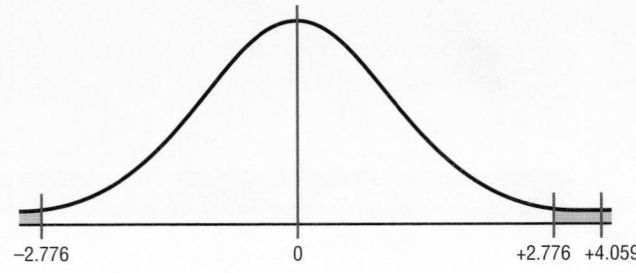

$$-2.776 \qquad 0 \qquad +2.776 \quad +4.059$$

Step 5 Summarize the results. There is a significant relationship between the variables of age and blood pressure.

The second method that can be used to test the significance of r is the P-value method. The method is the same as that shown in Chapters 8 and 9. It uses the following steps.

Step 1   State the hypotheses.

Step 2   Find the test statistic. (In this case, use the t test.)

Step 3   Find the P-value. (In this case, use Table F.)

Step 4   Make the decision.

Step 5   Summarize the results.

Referring to Example 10–7, we see that the t value obtained in step 3 is 4.059 and d.f. = 4. Using Table F with d.f. = 4 and the row "Two tails," the value 4.059 falls between 3.747 and 4.604; hence, $0.01 < P\text{-value} < 0.02$. (The P-value obtained from a calculator is 0.015.) That is, the P-value falls between 0.01 and 0.02. The decision then is to reject the null hypothesis since $P\text{-value} < 0.05$.

The third method of testing the significance of r is to use Table I in Appendix C. This table shows the values of the correlation coefficient that are significant for a specific α level and a specific number of degrees of freedom. For example, for 7 degrees of freedom and $\alpha = 0.05$, the table gives a critical value of 0.666. Any value of r greater than $+0.666$ or less than -0.666 will be significant, and the null hypothesis will be rejected. See Figure 10–9. When Table I is used, one need not compute the t test statistic. Table I is for two-tailed tests only.

Figure 10–9

Finding the Critical Value from Table I

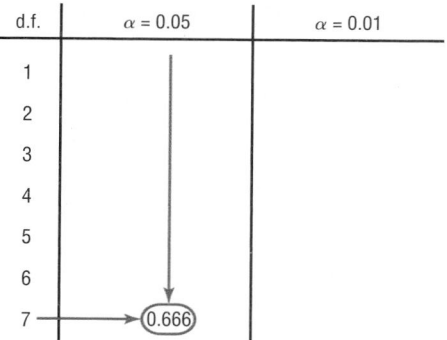

d.f.	$\alpha = 0.05$	$\alpha = 0.01$
1		
2		
3		
4		
5		
6		
7	0.666	

Example 10–8

Exercise and Milk Consumption
Using Table I, test the significance of the correlation coefficient $r = 0.101$, obtained in Example 10–6, at $\alpha = 0.01$.

Solution

$$H_0\!: \rho = 0 \qquad \text{and} \qquad H_1\!: \rho \neq 0$$

Since the sample size is 9, there are 7 degrees of freedom. When $\alpha = 0.01$ and with 7 degrees of freedom, the value obtained from Table I is 0.798. For a significant relationship, a value of r greater than $+0.798$ or less than -0.798 is needed. Since $r = 0.101$, the null hypothesis is not rejected. Hence, there is not enough evidence to say that there is a significant linear relationship between the variables. See Figure 10–10.

Figure 10–10

Critical and Noncritical Regions for Example 10–8

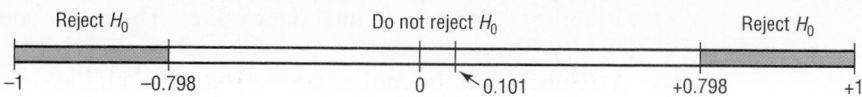

Reject H_0 Do not reject H_0 Reject H_0

-1 -0.798 0 0.101 $+0.798$ $+1$

Correlation and Causation

Researchers must understand the nature of the linear relationship between the independent variable x and the dependent variable y. When a hypothesis test indicates that a significant linear relationship exists between the variables, researchers must consider the possibilities outlined next.

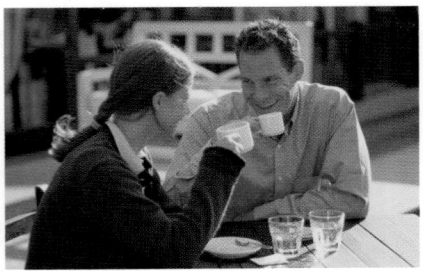

Possible Relationships between Variables

When the null hypothesis has been rejected for a specific α value, any of the following five possibilities can exist.

1. *There is a direct cause-and-effect relationship between the variables.* That is, x causes y. For example, water causes plants to grow, poison causes death, and heat causes ice to melt.

2. *There is a reverse cause-and-effect relationship between the variables.* That is, y causes x. For example, suppose a researcher believes excessive coffee consumption causes nervousness, but the researcher fails to consider that the reverse situation may occur. That is, it may be that an extremely nervous person craves coffee to calm his or her nerves.

3. *The relationship between the variables may be caused by a third variable.* For example, if a statistician correlated the number of deaths due to drowning and the number of cans of soft drink consumed daily during the summer, she or he would probably find a significant relationship. However, the soft drink is not necessarily responsible for the deaths, since both variables may be related to heat and humidity.

4. *There may be a complexity of interrelationships among many variables.* For example, a researcher may find a significant relationship between students' high school grades and university grades. But there probably are many other variables involved, such as IQ, hours of study, influence of parents, motivation, age, and instructors.

5. *The relationship may be coincidental.* For example, a researcher may be able to find a significant relationship between the increase in the number of people who are exercising and the increase in the number of people who are committing crimes. But common sense dictates that any relationship between these two values must be due to coincidence.

When two variables are highly correlated, possibility 3 states that there exists a possibility that the correlation is due to a third variable. If this is the case and the third variable is unknown to the researcher or not accounted for in the study, it is called a **lurking variable.** An attempt should be made by the researcher to identify such variables and to use methods to control their influence.

Also, one should be cautious when the data for one or both of the variables involve averages rather than individual data. It is not wrong to use averages, but the results cannot be generalized to individuals since averaging tends to smooth out the variability among individual data values. The result could be a higher correlation than actually exists.

Thus, when the null hypothesis is rejected, the researcher must consider all possibilities and select the appropriate one as determined by the study. Remember, correlation does not necessarily imply causation.

10–1 Applying the Concepts

Stopping Distances

Manitoba Public Insurance published a brochure entitled *Watch Your Speed.* The purpose of the study was to educate the public on the most common factors associated with vehicle crashes. An area that was focused on in the study was the stopping distance (metres) required to completely stop a vehicle at various speeds (kilometres per hour). Use the following table to answer the questions.

Speed (km/h)	Stopping distance (m)
30	18
50	35
70	57
100	98
110	114

Assume km/h is going to be used to predict stopping distance.

1. Which of the two variables is the independent variable?
2. Which is the dependent variable?
3. What type of variable is the independent variable?
4. What type of variable is the dependent variable?
5. Construct a scatter plot for the data.
6. Is there a linear relationship between the two variables?
7. Redraw the scatter plot and change the distances between the independent-variable numbers. Does the relationship look different?
8. Is the relationship positive or negative?
9. Can stopping distance be accurately predicted from km/h?
10. List some other variables that affect stopping distance.
11. Compute the value of r.
12. Is r significant at $\alpha = 0.05$?

See page 501 for the answers.

Exercises 10–1

1. What is meant by the statement that two variables are related?

2. How is a linear relationship between two variables measured in statistics? Explain.

3. What is the symbol for the sample correlation coefficient? The population correlation coefficient?

4. What is the range of values for the correlation coefficient?

5. What is meant when the relationship between the two variables is positive? Negative?

6. Give examples of two variables that are positively correlated and two that are negatively correlated.

7. Give an example of a correlation study, and identify the independent and dependent variables.

8. What is the diagram of the independent and dependent variables called? Why is drawing this diagram important?

9. What is the name of the correlation coefficient used in this section?

10. What statistical test is used to test the significance of the correlation coefficient?

11. When two variables are correlated, can the researcher be sure that one variable causes the other? Why or why not?

For Exercises 12 through 27, perform the following steps.

a. Draw the scatter plot for the variables.
b. Compute the value of the correlation coefficient.
c. State the hypotheses.
d. Test the significance of the correlation coefficient at $\alpha = 0.05$, using Table I.
e. Give a brief explanation of the type of relationship.

Speaking of Statistics

In correlation and regression studies, it is difficult to control all variables. This study shows some of the consequences when researchers overlook certain aspects in studies. Suggest ways that the extraneous variables might be controlled in future studies.

Source: Reprinted with permission of the Associated Press.

Coffee Not Disease Culprit, Study Says

NEW YORK (AP)—Two new studies suggest that coffee drinking, even up to 5½ cups per day, does not increase the risk of heart disease, and other studies that claim to have found increased risks might have missed the true culprits, a researcher says.

"It might not be the coffee cup in one hand, it might be the cigarette or coffee roll in the other," said Dr. Peter W. F. Wilson, the author of one of the new studies.

He noted in a telephone interview Thursday that many coffee drinkers, particularly heavy coffee drinkers, are smokers. And one of the new studies found that coffee drinkers had excess fat in their diets.

The findings of the new studies conflict sharply with a study reported in November 1985 by Johns Hopkins University scientists in Baltimore.

The Hopkins scientists found that coffee drinkers who consumed five or more cups of coffee per day had three times the heart-disease risk of non-coffee drinkers.

The reason for the discrepancy appears to be that many of the coffee drinkers in the Hopkins study also smoked—and it was the smoking that increased their heart-disease risk, said Wilson.

Wilson, director of laboratories for the Framingham Heart Study in Framingham, Mass., said Thursday at a conference sponsored by the American Heart Association in Charleston, S.C., that he had examined the coffee intake of 3,937 participants in the Framingham study during 1956–66 and an additional 2,277 during the years 1972–1982.

In contrast to the subjects in the Hopkins study, most of these coffee drinkers consumed two or three cups per day, Wilson said. Only 10 percent drank six or more cups per day.

He then looked at blood cholesterol levels and heart and blood vessel disease in the two groups. "We ran these analyses for coronary heart disease, heart attack, sudden death and stroke and in absolutely every analysis, we found no link with coffee," Wilson said.

He found that coffee consumption was linked to a significant decrease in total blood cholesterol in men, and to a moderate increase in total cholesterol in women.

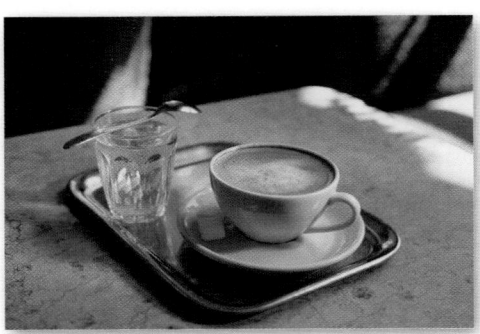

12. **Broadway Productions** A researcher wants to see if there is a relationship between the number of new productions on Broadway in any given year and the attendance for the season. The data shown here were recorded for a selected number of years. Based on these data, can you conclude a relationship between the number of new productions in a season and the attendance?

Number of new productions	54	67	60	54	61	60	50	37
Attendance (millions)	7.4	8.2	7.1	8.8	9.6	11	8.4	7.4

(The information in this exercise will be used for Exercise 12 in Section 10–2.)

Source: World Almanac.

13. Age and Exercise Hours A researcher wishes to determine if a person's age is related to the number of hours he or she exercises per week. The data for the sample are shown here. (The information in this exercise will be used for Exercises 13 and 36 in Section 10–2 and Exercise 13 in Section 10–3.)

Age x	18	26	32	38	52	59
Hours y	10	5	2	3	1.5	1

14. Forest Fires and Hectares Burned An environmentalist wants to determine the relationships between the number (in thousands) of forest fires over the year and the number (in hundreds of thousands) of hectares burned. The data for 8 recent years are shown. Describe the relationship.

Number of fires x	72	69	58	47	84	62	57	45
Number of hectares burned y	25	17	8	11	21	6	12	6

Source: National Emergency Fire Causes.

(The information in this exercise will be used for Exercises 14 and 36 in Section 10–2 and Exercises 14 and 18 in Section 10–3.)

15. Alumni Contributions The director of an alumni association for a small college wants to determine whether there is any type of relationship between the amount of an alumnus's contribution (in dollars) and the years the alumnus has been out of school. The data follow. (The information in this exercise will be used for Exercises 15, 36, and 37 in Section 10–2 and Exercises 15 and 19 in Section 10–3.)

Years x	1	5	3	10	7	6
Contribution y	500	100	300	50	75	80

16. Age and Sick Days A store manager wishes to find out whether there is a relationship between the age of her employees and the number of sick days they take each year. The data for the sample are shown. (The information in this exercise will be used for Exercises 16 and 37 in Section 10–2 and Exercises 16 and 20 in Section 10–3.)

Age x	18	26	39	48	53	58
Days y	16	12	9	5	6	2

17. Robbery and Homicide A criminology student wants to determine if there is a relationship between the robbery and homicide crime rates in Canada. Data is collected from 7 randomly selected cities. Crime rates are calculated per 100,000 population. Is there a relationship between the two types of crimes in Canada's cities?

Robbery crimes x	229	148	141	150	91	88	84
Homicide crimes y	4.9	2.6	3.4	1.7	1.9	1.3	1.1

Source: Statistics Canada.

(The information in this exercise will be used for Exercise 17 of Section 10–2.)

18. Football Pass Attempts A football fan wishes to see how the number of pass attempts (not completions) relates to the number of yards gained for quarterbacks in past National Football League (NFL) season playoff games. The data are shown for five quarterbacks. Describe the relationships.

Pass attempts x	116	90	82	108	92
Yards gained y	1001	823	851	873	839

(The information in this exercise will be used for Exercises 18 and 38 in Section 10–2.)

19. Egg Production Recent agricultural data showed the number of eggs produced and the price received per dozen for a given year. Based on the following data for a random selection of states, can it be concluded that a relationship exists between the number of eggs produced and the price per dozen? (The information in this exercise will be used for Exercise 19 in Section 10–2.)

Number of eggs (millions) x	957	1332	1163	1865	119	273
Price per dozen (dollars) y	0.770	0.697	0.617	0.652	1.080	1.420

Source: World Almanac.

20. Emergency Calls and Temperature An emergency medical service wishes to see whether a relationship exists between the outside temperature (°C) and the number of emergency calls it receives for an 8-hour period. The data are shown. (The information in this exercise will be used for Exercises 20 and 38 in Section 10–2.)

Temperature (°C) x	20	23	28	31	34	37	38
Number of calls y	7	4	8	10	11	9	13

21. Visible Minorities in Cities A random sample of cities in eastern Canada is selected to determine if there is a relationship between the number of Black and number of Asian visible minorities. (The information in this exercise will be used for Exercises 21 and 36 in Section 10–2.)

Black x	350	13,085	1,440	325	3,640
Asian y	1,735	9,665	1,110	425	5,065

Source: Statistics Canada.

22. Apartment Rents The results of a survey of the average monthly rents (in dollars) for one-bedroom apartments and three-bedroom apartments in randomly selected metropolitan areas are shown. Determine if there is a relationship between the rents. (The information in this exercise will be used for Exercise 22 in Section 10–2.)

One-bedroom x	782	486	451	529	618	520	845
Three-bedroom y	1223	902	739	954	1055	875	1455

Source: The New York Times Almanac.

23. Average Temperature and Precipitation The average daily temperature (°C) and the corresponding average monthly precipitation (cm) for the month of July are shown for 7 randomly selected Canadian cities. Determine if there is a relationship between the two variables. (The information in this exercise will be used for Exercise 23 in 10–2.)

Temperature (°C) x	21.8	23.2	26.3	26.1	26.4	24.9	23.1
Precipitation (cm) y	17.6	29.9	58.9	72.0	88.1	118.5	81.6

Source: Environment Canada.

24. Baseball Hall of Fame Pitchers A random sample of Major League Baseball Hall of Fame pitchers' career wins and their total number of strikeouts is shown next. Is there a relationship between the variables? (The information in this exercise will be used for Exercise 24 in Section 10–2.)

Wins x	329	150	236	300	284	207
Strikeouts y	4136	1155	1956	2266	3192	1277

Wins x	247	314	273	324
Strikeouts y	1068	3534	1987	3574

Source: The New York Times Almanac.

25. Calories and Cholesterol The number of calories and the number of milligrams of cholesterol for a random sample of fast-food chicken sandwiches from 7 restau-

rants are shown here. Is there a relationship between the variables? (The information in this exercise will be used in Exercise 25 in Section 10–2.)

Calories x	390	535	720	300	430	500	440
Cholesterol y	43	45	80	50	55	52	60

Source: The Doctor's Pocket Calorie, Fat, and Carbohydrate Counter.

26. Tall Buildings An architect wants to determine if a relationship exists between the number of storeys in a building and the height (in metres) of the building. The data for a random sample of 7 buildings in Vancouver are shown. Explain the relationship. (The information in this exercise will be used in Exercise 26 in Section 10–2.)

Storeys x	48	28	30	37	35	30	32
Height y	150	146	142	141	138	127	122

Source: www.answers.com.

27. Hospital Beds A hospital administrator wants to see if there is a relationship between the number of licensed beds and the number of staffed beds in U.S. hospitals. The data for a specific day are shown. Describe the relationship.

Licensed beds x	144	32	175	185	208	100	169
Staffed beds y	112	32	162	141	103	80	118

Source: Pittsburgh Tribune-Review.

(The information in this exercise will be used for Exercise 28 of this section and Exercise 27 in Section 10–2.)

Extending the Concepts »

28. Hospital Beds One of the formulas for computing r is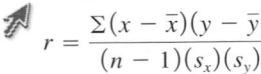

$$r = \frac{\Sigma(x - \bar{x})(y - \bar{y})}{(n-1)(s_x)(s_y)}$$

Using the data in Exercise 27, compute r with this formula. Compare the results.

29. Compute r for the data set shown. Explain the reason for this value of r. Now, interchange the values of x and y and compute r again. Compare this value with the previous one. Explain the results of the comparison.

x	1	2	3	4	5
y	3	5	7	9	11

30. Compute r for the following data and test the hypothesis H_0: $\rho = 0$. Draw the scatter plot and then explain the results.

x	−3	−2	−1	0	1	2	3
y	9	4	1	0	1	4	9

10–2 | Regression ›

Determine the equation of the regression line.

In studying relationships between two variables, collect the data and then construct a scatter plot. The purpose of the scatter plot, as indicated previously, is to determine the nature of the relationship. The possibilities include a positive linear relationship, a negative linear relationship, a nonlinear relationship, or no discernible relationship. After the scatter plot is drawn, the next steps are to compute the value of the correlation coefficient and to test the significance of the relationship. If the value of the correlation coefficient is significant, the next step that is often performed by researchers is to determine the equation of the **regression line,** which is the data's line of best fit. (*Note:* Determining the regression line when r is not significant and then making predictions using the regression line are meaningless.) The purpose of the regression line is to enable the researcher to see the trend and make predictions on the basis of the data.

Line of Best Fit

Figure 10–11 shows a scatter plot for the data of two variables. It shows that several lines can be drawn on the graph near the points. Given a scatter plot, one must be able to draw the *line of best fit*. *Best fit* means that the sum of the squares of the errors in the y direction from each point to the line is at a minimum. The reason one needs a line of best fit is that the values of y will be predicted from the values of x; hence, the closer the points are to the line, the better the fit and the prediction will be. See Figure 10–12. When r is positive, the line slopes upward and to the right. When r is negative, the line slopes downward from left to right.

Determination of the Regression Line Equation

In algebra, the equation of a line is usually given as $y = mx + b$, where m is the slope of the line and b is the y intercept. (Students who need an algebraic review of the properties

Figure 10–11

**Scatter Plot with Three
Lines Fit to the Data**

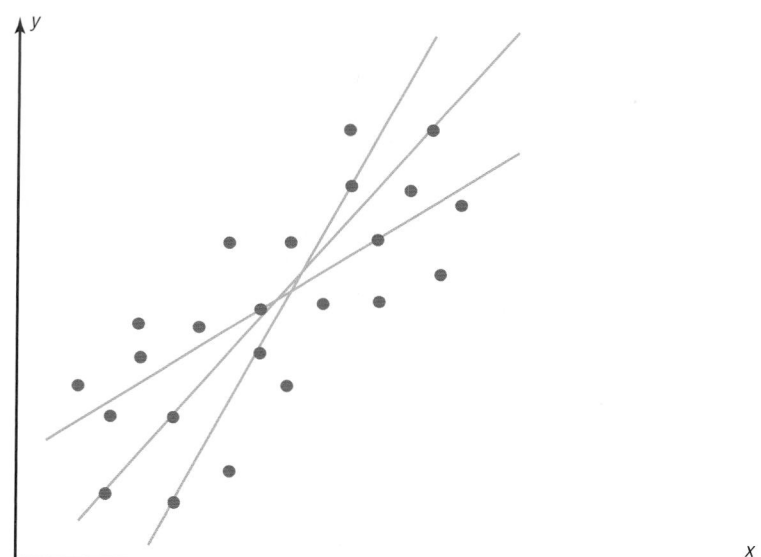

Figure 10–12

**Line of Best Fit for a
Set of Data Points**

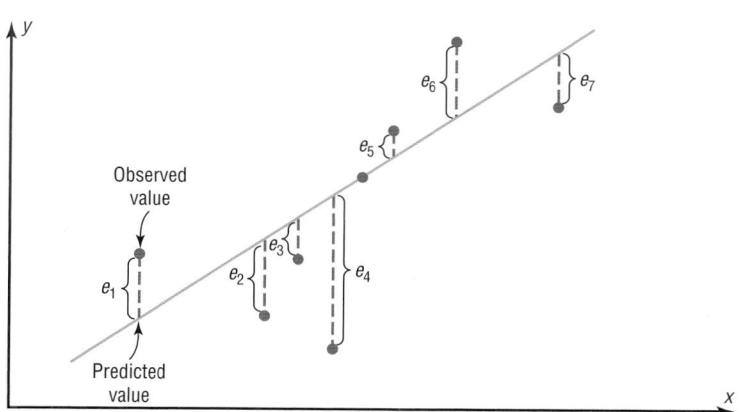

of a line should refer to Appendix A, Section A–3, before studying this section.) In statistics, the equation of the regression line is written as $y' = a + bx$, where a is the y' intercept and b is the slope of the line. See Figure 10–13.

Figure 10–13

A Line as Represented in Algebra and in Statistics

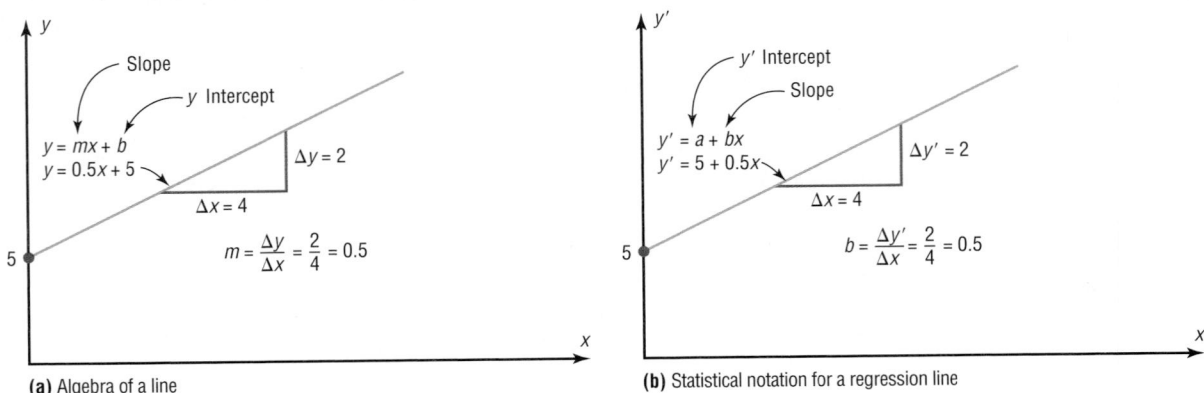

(a) Algebra of a line   **(b)** Statistical notation for a regression line

There are several methods for finding the equation of the regression line. Two formulas are given here. *These formulas use the same values that are used in computing the value of the correlation coefficient.* The mathematical development of these formulas is beyond the scope of this book.

Formulas for the Regression Line $y' = a + bx$

$$a = \frac{(\Sigma y)(\Sigma x^2) - (\Sigma x)(\Sigma xy)}{n(\Sigma x^2) - (\Sigma x)^2}$$

$$b = \frac{n(\Sigma xy) - (\Sigma x)(\Sigma y)}{n(\Sigma x^2) - (\Sigma x)^2}$$

where a is the y' intercept and b is the slope of the line.

Rounding Rule for the Intercept and Slope   Round the values of a and b to three decimal places.

Example 10–9

Age and Blood Pressure

Find the equation of the regression line for the data in Example 10–4, and graph the line on the scatter plot of the data.

Solution

The values needed for the equation are $n = 6$, $\Sigma x = 345$, $\Sigma y = 819$, $\Sigma xy = 47{,}634$, and $\Sigma x^2 = 20{,}399$. Substituting in the formulas, one gets

$$a = \frac{(\Sigma y)(\Sigma x^2) - (\Sigma x)(\Sigma xy)}{n(\Sigma x^2) - (\Sigma x)^2} = \frac{(819)(20{,}399) - (345)(47{,}634)}{(6)(20{,}399) - (345)^2} \approx 81.048$$

$$b = \frac{n(\Sigma xy) - (\Sigma x)(\Sigma y)}{n(\Sigma x^2) - (\Sigma x)^2} = \frac{(6)(47{,}634) - (345)(819)}{(6)(20{,}399) - (345)^2} \approx 0.964$$

Hence, the equation of the regression line $y' = a + bx$ is

$$y' = 81.048 + 0.964x$$

The graph of the line is shown in Figure 10–14.

Figure 10–14

Regression Line for
Example 10–9

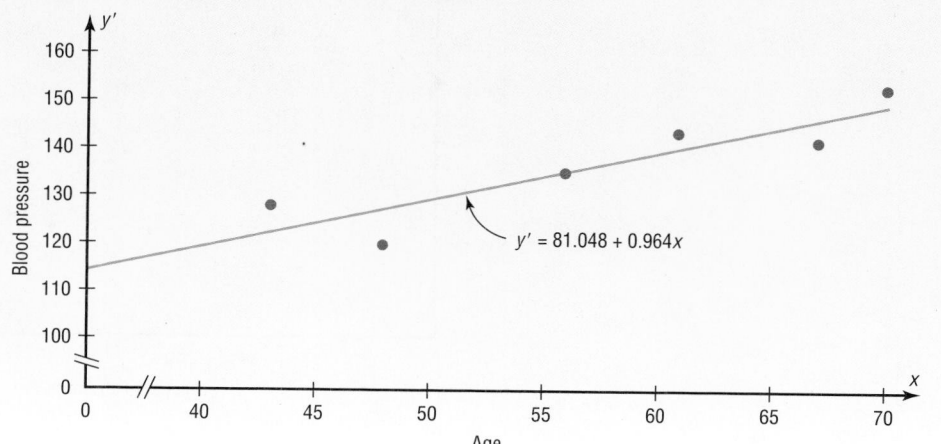

$y' = 81.048 + 0.964x$

Historical Note

In 1805, French mathematician Adrien-Marie Legendre (1752–1833) published the foundation for the modern least-squares approximation. This method was used to refine the measure of the meridian arc, the basis of the metric system.

Note: When one is drawing the scatter plot and the regression line, it is sometimes desirable to *truncate* the graph (see Chapter 2). The motive is to show the line drawn in the range of the independent and dependent variables. For example, the regression line in Figure 10–14 is drawn between the x values of approximately 43 and 82 and the y' values of approximately 120 and 152. The range of the x values in the original data shown in Example 10–4 is $70 - 43 = 27$, and the range of the y' values is $152 - 120 = 32$. Notice that the x axis has been truncated; the distance between 0 and 40 is not shown in the proper scale compared to the distance between 40 and 50, 50 and 60, etc. The y' axis has been similarly truncated.

The important thing to remember is that when the x axis and sometimes the y' axis have been truncated, do not use the y' intercept value a to graph the line. To be on the safe side when graphing the regression line, use a value for x selected from the range of x values.

Example 10–10

Absences and Final Grades

Find the equation of the regression line for the data in Example 10–5, and graph the line on the scatter plot.

Solution

The values needed for the equation are $n = 7$, $\Sigma x = 57$, $\Sigma y = 511$, $\Sigma xy = 3745$, and $\Sigma x^2 = 579$. Substituting in the formulas, one gets

$$a = \frac{(\Sigma y)(\Sigma x^2) - (\Sigma x)(\Sigma xy)}{n(\Sigma x^2) - (\Sigma x)^2} = \frac{(511)(579) - (57)(3745)}{(7)(579) - (57)^2} = 102.493$$

$$b = \frac{n(\Sigma xy) - (\Sigma x)(\Sigma y)}{n(\Sigma x^2) - (\Sigma x)^2} = \frac{(7)(3745) - (57)(511)}{(7)(579) - (57)^2} = -3.622$$

Hence, the equation of the regression line $y' = a + bx$ is

$$y' = 102.493 - 3.622x$$

The graph of the line is shown in Figure 10–15.

Figure 10–15

Regression Line for
Example 10–10

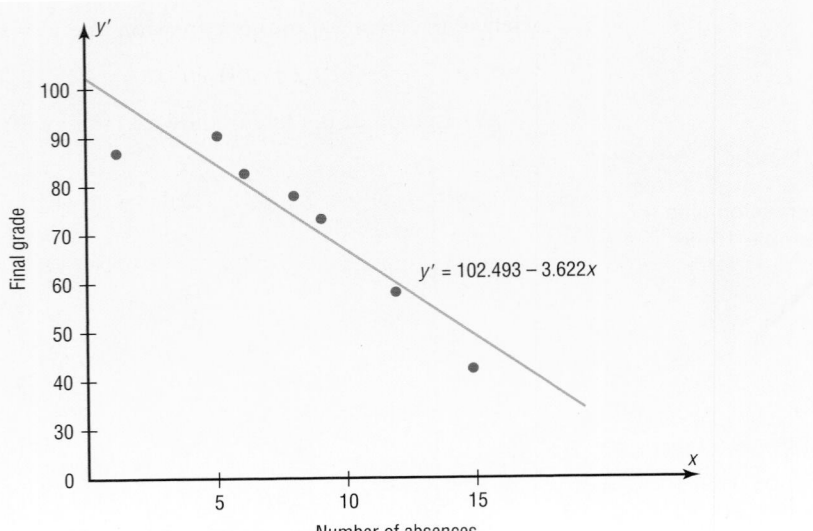

$y' = 102.493 - 3.622x$

The sign of the correlation coefficient and the sign of the slope of the regression line will always be the same. That is, if r is positive, then b will be positive; if r is negative, then b will be negative. The reason is that the numerators of the formulas are the same and determine the signs of r and b, and the denominators are always positive. The regression line will always pass through the point whose x coordinate is the mean of the x values and whose y coordinate is the mean of the y values, that is, $(\bar{x}, \bar{y})$.

The regression line can be used to make predictions for the dependent variable. The method for making predictions is shown in Example 10–11.

Example 10–11

Age and Blood Pressure

Using the equation of the regression line found in Example 10–9, predict the blood pressure for a person who is 50 years old.

Solution

Substituting 50 for x in the regression line $y' = 81.048 + 0.964x$ gives

$$y' = 81.048 + (0.964)(50) = 129.248 \text{ (rounded to 129)}$$

In other words, the predicted systolic blood pressure for a 50-year-old person is 129.

The value obtained in Example 10–11 is a point prediction, and with point predictions, no degree of accuracy or confidence can be determined. More information on prediction is given in Section 10–3.

The magnitude of the change in one variable when the other variable changes exactly 1 unit is called a **marginal change.** The value of slope b of the regression line equation represents the marginal change. For example, the slope of the regression line equation in Example 10–9 is 0.964. This means that for each increase of 1 year, the value of y (systolic blood pressure reading) changes by 0.964 millimetres of mercury, mmHg, on average. In other words, for each year a person ages, her or his blood pressure rises about 1 mmHg.

When r is not significantly different from 0, the best predictor of y is the mean of the data values of y. For valid predictions, the value of the correlation coefficient must be significant. Also, three other assumptions must be met.

Assumptions for Valid Predictions in Regression

1. The sample is a random sample.
2. For any specific value of the independent variable x, the value of the dependent variable y must be normally distributed about the regression line. See Figure 10–16(a).
3. The standard deviation of each of the dependent variables must be the same for each value of the independent variable. See Figure 10–16(b).

Figure 10–16
Assumptions for Predictions

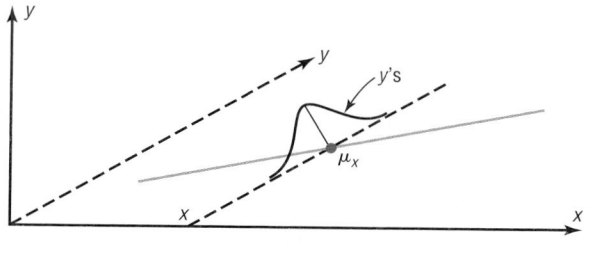

(a) Dependent variable y normally distributed

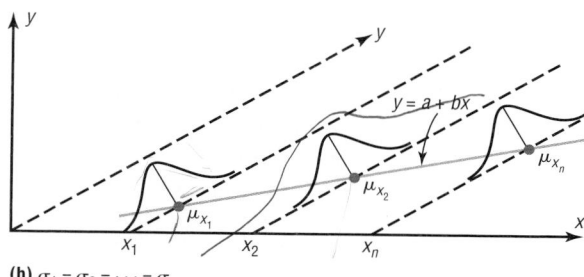

(b) $\sigma_1 = \sigma_2 = \cdots = \sigma_n$

Extrapolation, or making predictions beyond the bounds of the data, must be interpreted cautiously. For example, in 1979, some experts predicted that North America would run out of oil by the year 2003. This prediction was based on the current consumption and on known oil reserves at that time. However, since then, the automobile industry has produced many new fuel-efficient vehicles. Also, there are many as yet undiscovered oil fields. Finally, science may someday discover a way to run a car on something as unlikely but as common as peanut oil. In addition, the price of a litre of gasoline was predicted to reach $2.50 a few years later. Fortunately this has not come to pass. *Remember that when predictions are made, they are based on present conditions or on the premise that present trends will continue.* This assumption may or may not prove true in the future.

The steps for finding the value of the correlation coefficient and the regression line equation are summarized in the following Procedure Table.

Interesting Fact

It is estimated that wearing a motorcycle helmet reduces the risk of a fatal accident by 30%.

Procedure Table

Finding the Correlation Coefficient and the Regression Line Equation

Step 1   Make a table, as shown in step 2.

Step 2   Find the values of xy, x^2, and y^2. Place them in the appropriate columns and sum each column.

x	y	xy	x^2	y^2
.	.	.	.	.
.	.	.	.	.
.	.	.	.	..
$\Sigma x =$ ___	$\Sigma y =$ ___	$\Sigma xy =$ ___	$\Sigma x^2 =$ ___	$\Sigma y^2 =$ ___

(continued)

Procedure Table *(continued)*

Step 3   Substitute in the formula to find the value of r.

$$r = \frac{n(\Sigma xy) - (\Sigma x)(\Sigma y)}{\sqrt{[n(\Sigma x^2) - (\Sigma x)^2][n(\Sigma y^2) - (\Sigma y)^2]}}$$

Step 4   When r is significant, substitute in the formulas to find the values of a and b for the regression line equation $y' = a + bx$.

$$a = \frac{(\Sigma y)(\Sigma x^2) - (\Sigma x)(\Sigma xy)}{n(\Sigma x^2) - (\Sigma x)^2} \qquad b = \frac{n(\Sigma xy) - (\Sigma x)(\Sigma y)}{n(\Sigma x^2) - (\Sigma x)^2}$$

A scatter plot should be checked for outliers. An outlier is a point that seems out of place when compared with the other points (see Chapter 3). Some of these points can affect the equation of the regression line. When this happens, the points are called **influential points** or **influential observations.**

When a point on the scatter plot appears to be an outlier, it should be checked to see if it is an influential point. An influential point tends to "pull" the regression line toward the point itself. To check for an influential point, the regression line should be graphed with the point included in the data set. Then a second regression line should be graphed that excludes the point from the data set. If the position of the second line is changed considerably, the point is said to be an influential point. Points that are outliers in the x direction tend to be influential points.

Researchers should use their judgment as to whether to include influential points in the final analysis of the data. If the researcher has substantive reasons, then an influential point should be excluded so that it does not influence the results of the study. However, if the researcher feels that it is necessary, then he or she may want to obtain additional data values whose x values are near the x value of the influential point and then include them in the study.

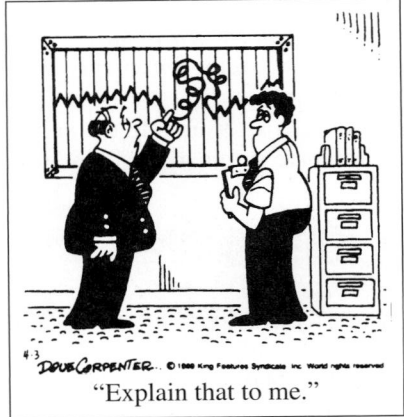

"Explain that to me."

Source: Reprinted with special permission of King Features Syndicate.

10–2   Applying the Concepts

Stopping Distances Revisited

In a study on speed and stopping distance, researchers looked for a method to estimate how fast a person was travelling before an accident by measuring the length of the skid marks. An area that was focused on in the study was the distance required to completely stop a vehicle at various speeds. Use the following table to answer the questions.

Speed (km/h)	Stopping distance (m)
30	18
50	35
70	57
100	98
110	114

Assume km/h is going to be used to predict stopping distance.

1. Determine the linear regression equation.
2. What does the slope tell you about km/h and the stopping distance? How about the y intercept?
3. Estimate the stopping distance when km/h = 60.
4. Estimate the stopping distance when km/h = 120.
5. Comment on predicting beyond the given data values.

See page 501 for the answers.

Exercises 10–2

1. What two things should be done before one performs a regression analysis?

2. What are the assumptions for regression analysis?

3. What is the general form for the regression line used in statistics?

4. What is the symbol for the slope? For the y intercept?

5. What is meant by the *line of best fit?*

6. When all the points fall on the regression line, what is the value of the correlation coefficient?

7. What is the relationship between the sign of the correlation coefficient and the sign of the slope of the regression line?

8. As the value of the correlation coefficient increases from 0 to 1, or decreases from 0 to −1, how do the points of the scatter plot fit the regression line?

9. How is the value of the correlation coefficient related to the accuracy of the predicted value for a specific value of x?

10. If the value of r is not significant, what can be said about the regression line?

11. When the value of r is not significant, what value should be used to predict y?

For Exercises 12 through 27, use the same data as for the corresponding exercises in Section 10–1. For each exercise, find the equation of the regression line and find the y' value for the specified x value. Remember that no regression should be done when r is not significant.

12. **Broadway Productions** New Broadway productions and seasonal attendance are as follows.

Number of new productions	54	67	60	54	61	60	50	37
Attendance (millions)	7.4	8.2	7.1	8.8	9.6	11	8.4	7.4

Find y' when $x = 48$ new productions.

13. **Age and Exercise** Data are shown for a person's age and number of hours of exercise per week.

Age x	18	26	32	38	52	59
Hours y	10	5	2	3	1.5	1

Find y' when $x = 35$ years.

14. **Forest Fires and Hectares Burned** Data are shown for the number (in thousands) of forest fires over the year and the number (in hundreds of thousands) of hectares burned.

Number of fires x	72	69	58	47	84	62	57	45
Number of hectares burned y	25	17	8	11	21	6	12	6

Find y' when $x = 60$.

15. **Alumni Contributions** Data for an alumnus's contribution (in dollars) and the years the alumnus has been out of school are shown.

Years x	1	5	3	10	7	6
Contribution y, $	500	100	300	50	75	80

Find y' when $x = 4$ years.

16. **Age and Sick Days** Data are shown for employee age and the number of sick days per year.

Age x	18	26	39	48	53	58
Days y	16	12	9	5	6	2

Find y' when $x = 47$ years.

17. **Robbery and Homicide** Data for robbery and homicide crime rates (per 100,000 population) in Canada are shown.

Robbery crimes x	229	148	141	150	91	88	84
Homicide crimes y	4.9	2.6	3.4	1.7	1.9	1.3	1.1

Find y', when $x = 100$.

18. **Football Pass Attempts** Data are shown for NFL quarterback pass attempts and the number of yards gained.

Attempts x	116	90	82	108	92
Yards y	1001	823	851	873	837

Find y' when $x = 95$.

19. **Egg Production** Annual data for the number of eggs produced and the price received per dozen are shown.

Number of eggs (millions) x	957	1332	1163	1865	119	273
Price per dozen (dollars) y	0.770	0.697	0.617	0.652	1.080	1.420

Find y' when $x = 1600$ million eggs.

20. **Emergency Calls and Temperature** Data for outside temperature (°C) and the number of emergency calls received during an 8-hour period are shown.

Temperature (°C) x	20	23	28	31	34	37	38
Number of calls y	7	4	8	10	11	9	13

Find y' when $x = 30$°C.

21. **Visible Minorities in Cities** Data are shown for the number of Black and Asian visible minorities in Canadian cities.

Black x	350	13,085	1,440	325	3,640
Asian y	1,735	9,665	1,110	425	5,065

Predict y' when $x = 2,500$.

22. **Apartment Rents** Data for average monthly rents (in dollars) for one- and three-bedroom apartments in metropolitan areas are shown.

One-bedroom x, $	782	486	451	529	618	520	845
Three-bedroom y, $	1223	902	739	954	1055	875	1455

Find y' when $x = \$700$.

23. **Average Temperature and Precipitation** Canadian city data for the average daily temperature (°C) and the average monthly precipitation (cm) for July are shown.

Temperature (°C) x	21.8	23.2	26.3	26.1	26.4	24.9	23.1
Precipitation (cm) y	17.6	29.9	58.9	72.0	88.1	118.5	81.6

Find y' when $x = 25$°C.
Source: Environment Canada.

24. **Hall of Fame Pitchers** Data for Major League Baseball Hall of Fame pitchers' career wins and total number of strikeouts are shown.

Wins x	329	150	236	300	284	207
Strikeouts y	4136	1155	1956	2266	3192	1277
Wins x	247	314	273	324		
Strikeouts y	1068	3534	1987	3574		

Find y' when $x = 260$ wins.

25. **Calories and Cholesterol** Data are shown for fast-food restaurant calories and the milligrams of cholesterol in chicken sandwiches.

Calories x	390	535	720	300	430	500	440
Cholesterol y	43	45	80	50	55	52	60

Find y' when $x = 600$ calories.

26. **Tall Buildings** Data for the number of storeys in a building and the height (in metres) of the building are shown.

Storeys x	48	28	30	37	35	30	32
Height y	150	146	142	141	138	127	122

Find y' when $x = 40$ storeys.

27. **Hospital Beds** Data for the number of licensed and staffed beds in hospitals are shown.

Licensed beds x	144	32	175	185	208	100	169
Staffed beds y	112	32	162	141	103	80	118

Find y' when $x = 44$.

For Exercises 28 through 33, do a complete regression analysis by performing these steps.

a. Draw a scatter plot.

b. Compute the correlation coefficient.

c. State the hypotheses.

d. Test the hypotheses at $\alpha = 0.05$. Use Table I. If the hypothesis test produces a significant result, proceed to steps *e–g*; otherwise, stop.

e. Determine the regression line equation.

f. Plot the regression line on the scatter plot.

g. Summarize the results.

28. SAT Scores Educational researchers wanted to find out if a relationship exists between the average Scholastic Aptitude Test (SAT) verbal score and the average SAT mathematical score. Several regions were randomly selected, and their SAT average scores are recorded below. Is there sufficient evidence to conclude that a relationship exists between the two scores?

Verbal x	526	504	594	585	503	589
Math y	530	522	606	588	517	589

Source: World Almanac.

29. Smoking and Lung Damage These data were obtained from a survey of the number of years people smoked and the percentage of lung damage they sustained. Predict the percentage of lung damage for a person who has smoked for 30 years.

Years x	22	14	31	36	9	41	19
Damage y	20	14	54	63	17	71	23

30. Brand-Name and Generic Prescription Drug Cost A medical researcher wishes to describe the relationship between the prescription cost of a brand-name drug and its generic equivalent. The data (in dollars) are shown.

Brand name x	96	93	59	80	44	47	15	56
Generic y	42	31	17	16	8	12	6	22

31. Business Head Offices The following data compare the number of business head offices in a random sample of Canadian cities between 1999 and 2005. Predict the number of head offices in 2005 for a city with 200 head offices in 1999.

1999 x	596	100	826	114	279	139	355
2005 y	536	101	918	129	316	157	335

Source: Statistics Canada.

32. Television Viewers A television executive selects 10 television shows and compares the average number of viewers the show had last year with the average number of viewers this year. The data (in millions) are shown. Describe the relationship.

Viewers last year x	26.6	17.85	20.3	16.8	20.8
Viewers this year y	28.9	19.2	26.4	13.7	20.2
Viewers last year x	16.7	19.1	18.9	16.0	15.8
Viewers this year y	18.8	25.0	21.0	16.8	15.3

Source: Nielson media research.

33. Absences and Final Grades An educator wants to see how the number of absences for a student in her class affects the student's final grade. The data obtained from a sample are shown.

No. of absences x	10	12	2	0	8	5
Final grade y	70	65	96	94	75	82

For Exercises 34 and 35, do a complete regression analysis and test the significance of r at $\alpha = 0.05$, using the P-value method.

34. Father's and Son's Weights A physician wishes to know whether there is a relationship between a father's weight (in kilograms) and his newborn son's weight (in kilograms). The data are given here.

Father's weight x	79.8	72.6	84.8	95.3	88.9	64.4	93.0	97.5
Son's weight y	3.0	3.7	4.2	3.2	4.0	4.2	3.4	3.9

35. Age and Net Worth Is a person's age related to his or her net worth? A sample of 10 billionaires is selected, and the person's age and net worth are compared. The data are given here.

Age x	56	39	42	60	84	37	68	66	73	55
Net worth (in billions) y	18	14	12	14	11	10	10	7	7	5

Source: The Associated Press.

Extending the Concepts   »

36. For Exercises 13, 15, and 21 in Section 10–1, find the mean of the x and y variables. Then substitute the mean of the x variable into the corresponding regression line equations found in Exercises 13, 15, and 21 in this section and find y'. Compare the value of y' with $\bar{y}$ for each exercise. Generalize the results.

37. The y intercept value a can also be found by using the equation

$$a = \bar{y} - b\bar{x}$$

Verify this result by using the data in Exercises 15 and 16 of Sections 10–1 and 10–2.

38. The value of the correlation coefficient can also be found by using the formula

$$r = \frac{bs_x}{s_y}$$

where s_x is the standard deviation of the x value and s_y is the standard deviation of the y values. Verify this result for Exercises 18 and 20 of Section 10–1.

10–3 | Coefficient of Determination and Standard Error of the Estimate ❯

Compute the coefficient of determination and the standard error of the estimate, and find a prediction interval.

The previous sections stated that if the correlation coefficient is significant, the equation of the regression line can be determined. Also, for various values of the independent variable x, the corresponding values of the dependent variable y can be predicted. Several other measures are associated with the correlation and regression techniques. They include the coefficient of determination, the standard error of the estimate, and the prediction interval. But before these concepts can be explained, the different types of variation associated with the regression model must be defined.

Types of Variation for the Regression Model

Consider the following hypothetical regression model.

x	1	2	3	4	5
y	10	8	12	16	20

The equation of the regression line is $y' = 4.8 + 2.8x$, and $r = 0.919$. The sample y values are 10, 8, 12, 16, and 20. The predicted values, designated by y', for each x can be found by substituting each x value into the regression equation and finding y'. For example, when $x = 1$,

$$y' = 4.8 + 2.8x = 4.8 + (2.8)(1) = 7.6$$

Now, for each x, there is an observed y value and a predicted y' value; for example, when $x = 1$, $y = 10$, and $y' = 7.6$. Recall that the closer the observed values are to the predicted values, the better the fit is and the closer r is to $+1$ or -1.

The *total variation* $\Sigma(y - \bar{y})^2$ is the sum of the squares of the vertical distances that each point is from the mean. The total variation can be divided into two parts: that which is attributed to the relationship of x and y and that which is due to chance. The variation obtained from the relationship (i.e., from the predicted y' values) is $\Sigma(y' - \bar{y})^2$ and is called the *explained variation*. Most of the variations can be explained by the relationship. The closer the value r is to $+1$ or -1, the better the points fit the line and the closer $\Sigma(y' - \bar{y})^2$ is to $\Sigma(y - \bar{y})^2$. In fact, if all points fall on the regression line, $\Sigma(y' - \bar{y})^2$ will equal $\Sigma(y - \bar{y})^2$, since y' would be equal to y in each case.

On the other hand, the variation due to chance, found by $\Sigma(y - y')^2$, is called the *unexplained variation*. This variation cannot be attributed to the relationship. When the unexplained variation is small, the value of r is close to $+1$ or -1. If all points fall on the regression line, the unexplained variation $\Sigma(y - y')^2$ will be 0. Hence, the *total variation* is equal to the sum of the explained variation and the unexplained variation. That is,

$$\Sigma(y - \bar{y})^2 = \Sigma(y' - \bar{y})^2 + \Sigma(y - y')^2$$

These values are shown in Figure 10–17. For a single point, the differences are called *deviations*. For the hypothetical regression model given earlier, for $x = 1$ and $y = 10$, one gets $y' = 7.6$ and $\bar{y} = 13.2$.

The procedure for finding the three types of variation is illustrated next.

Step 1 Find the predicted y' values.

For $x = 1$ $y' = 4.8 + 2.8x = 4.8 + (2.8)(1) = 7.6$

For $x = 2$ $y' = 4.8 + (2.8)(2) = 10.4$

For $x = 3$ $y' = 4.8 + (2.8)(3) = 13.2$

For $x = 4$ $y' = 4.8 + (2.8)(4) = 16.0$

For $x = 5$ $y' = 4.8 + (2.8)(5) = 18.8$

Figure 10–17

**Deviations for the
Regression Equation**

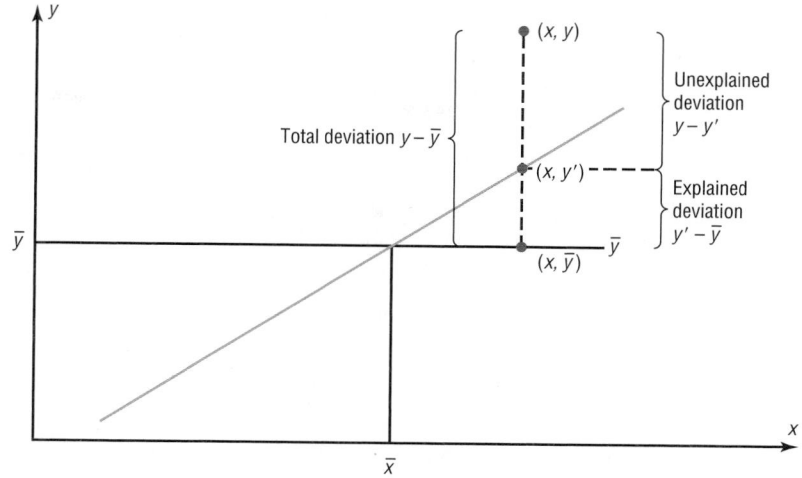

Figure 10–17

**Deviations for the
Regression Equation**

Hence, the values for this example are as follows:

x	y	y'
1	10	7.6
2	8	10.4
3	12	13.2
4	16	16.0
5	20	18.8

Step 2   Find the mean of the y values.

$$\bar{y} = \frac{10 + 8 + 12 + 16 + 20}{5} = 13.2$$

Step 3   Find the total variation $\Sigma(y - \bar{y})^2$.

$$(10 - 13.2)^2 = 10.24$$
$$(8 - 13.2)^2 = 27.04$$
$$(12 - 13.2)^2 = 1.44$$
$$(16 - 13.2)^2 = 7.84$$
$$(20 - 13.2)^2 = \underline{46.24}$$
$$\Sigma(y - \bar{y})^2 = 92.8$$

Step 4   Find the explained variation $\Sigma(y' - \bar{y})^2$.

$$(7.6 - 13.2)^2 = 31.36$$
$$(10.4 - 13.2)^2 = 7.84$$
$$(13.2 - 13.2)^2 = 0.00$$
$$(16 - 13.2)^2 = 7.84$$
$$(18.8 - 13.2)^2 = \underline{31.36}$$
$$\Sigma(y' - \bar{y})^2 = 78.4$$

Step 5   Find the unexplained variation $\Sigma(y - y')^2$.

$$(10 - 7.6)^2 = 5.76$$
$$(8 - 10.4)^2 = 5.76$$
$$(12 - 13.2)^2 = 1.44$$
$$(16 - 16)^2 = 0.00$$
$$\underline{(20 - 18.8)^2 = 1.44}$$
$$\Sigma(y - y')^2 = 14.4$$

Notice that

Total variation = Explained variation + Unexplained variation

$$92.8 = \qquad 78.4 \qquad + \qquad 14.4$$

Note: The values $(y - y')$ are called *residuals*. A **residual** is the difference between the actual value of y and the predicted value y' for a given x value. The mean of the residuals is always zero. As stated previously, the regression line determined by the formulas in Section 10–2 is the line that best fits the points of the scatter plot. The regression line computation minimizes the sum of the squared residuals. For this reason, a regression line is also called a **least-squares line.**

Coefficient of Determination

The *coefficient of determination* is the ratio of the explained variation to the total variation and is denoted by r^2. That is,

$$r^2 = \frac{\text{Explained variation}}{\text{Total variation}}$$

For the example, $r^2 = 78.4/92.8 = 0.845$. The term r^2 is usually expressed as a percentage. So in this case, 84.5% of the total variation is explained by the regression line using the independent variable.

Another way to arrive at the value for r^2 is to square the correlation coefficient. In this case, $r = 0.919$ and $r^2 = 0.845$, which is the same value found by using the variation ratio.

> The **coefficient of determination** is a measure of the percentage of variation of the dependent variable that is explained by the regression line and the independent variable. The symbol for the coefficient of determination is r^2.

Of course, it is usually easier to find the coefficient of determination by squaring r and converting it to a percentage. Therefore, if $r = 0.90$, then $r^2 = 0.81$, which is equivalent to 81%. This result means that 81% of the variation in the dependent variable is accounted for by the variations in the independent variable.

Standard Error of the Estimate

When a y' value is predicted for a specific x value, the prediction is a point prediction. However, a prediction interval about the y' value can be constructed, just as a confidence interval was constructed for an estimate of the population mean. The prediction interval uses a statistic called the *standard error of the estimate.*

> The **standard error of the estimate,** denoted by s_{est}, is the standard deviation of the observed y values about the predicted y' values.

Formula for the Standard Error of the Estimate

$$s_{\text{est}} = \sqrt{\frac{\Sigma(y - y')^2}{n - 2}}$$

The standard error of the estimate is similar to the standard deviation, but the mean is not used. As can be seen from the formula, the standard error of the estimate is the square root of the unexplained variation—that is, the variation due to the difference of the observed values and the expected values—divided by $n - 2$. So the closer the observed values are to the predicted values, the smaller the standard error of the estimate will be.

Example 10–12 shows how to compute the standard error of the estimate.

Example 10–12

Copy Machine Maintenance Costs 🖋

A researcher collects the following data and determines that there is a significant relationship between the age of a copy machine and its monthly maintenance cost. The regression equation is $y' = 55.57 + 8.13x$. Find the standard error of the estimate.

Machine	Age x (years)	Monthly cost y
A	1	$ 62
B	2	78
C	3	70
D	4	90
E	4	93
F	6	103

Solution

Step 1   Make a table, as shown.

x	y	y'	$y - y'$	$(y - y')^2$
1	62			
2	78			
3	70			
4	90			
4	93			
6	103			

Step 2   Using the regression line equation $y' = 55.57 + 8.13x$, compute the predicted values y' for each x and place the results in the column labelled "y'."

$x = 1$ $y' = 55.57 + (8.13)(1) = 63.70$
$x = 2$ $y' = 55.57 + (8.13)(2) = 71.83$
$x = 3$ $y' = 55.57 + (8.13)(3) = 79.96$
$x = 4$ $y' = 55.57 + (8.13)(4) = 88.09$
$x = 6$ $y' = 55.57 + (8.13)(6) = 104.35$

Step 3   For each y, subtract y' and place the answer in the column labelled "$y - y'$."

$62 - 63.70 = -1.70$ $90 - 88.09 = 1.91$
$78 - 71.83 = 6.17$ $93 - 88.09 = 4.91$
$70 - 79.96 = -9.96$ $103 - 104.35 = -1.35$

Step 4   Square the numbers found in step 3 and place the squares in the column labelled "$(y - y')^2$."

Step 5 Find the sum of the numbers in the last column. The completed table is shown.

x	y	y'	$y - y'$	$(y - y')^2$
1	62	63.70	-1.70	2.89
2	78	71.83	6.17	38.0689
3	70	79.96	-9.96	99.2016
4	90	88.09	1.91	3.6481
4	93	88.09	4.91	24.1081
6	103	104.35	-1.35	1.8225
				169.7392

Step 6 Substitute in the formula and find s_{est}.

$$s_{est} = \sqrt{\frac{\Sigma(y - y')^2}{n - 2}} = \sqrt{\frac{169.7392}{6 - 2}} \approx 6.51$$

In this case, the standard deviation of observed values about the predicted values is 6.51.

The following example illustrates another method of computing the standard error of the estimate, using the slope and y intercept.

Alternative Formula for the Standard Error of the Estimate

$$s_{est} = \sqrt{\frac{\Sigma y^2 - a\,\Sigma y - b\,\Sigma xy}{n - 2}}$$

Example 10–13

Copy Machine Maintenance Costs

Find the standard error of the estimate for the data for Example 10–12 by using the preceding formula. The equation of the regression line is $y' = 55.57 + 8.13x$.

Solution

Step 1 Make a table.

Step 2 Find the product of x and y values, and place the results in the third column.

Step 3 Square the y values, and place the results in the fourth column.

Step 4 Find the sums of the second, third, and fourth columns. The completed table is shown here.

x	y	xy	y^2
1	62	62	3,844
2	78	156	6,084
3	70	210	4,900
4	90	360	8,100
4	93	372	8,649
6	103	618	10,609
	$\Sigma y = 496$	$\Sigma xy = 1,778$	$\Sigma y^2 = 42,186$

Step 5 From the regression equation $y' = 55.57 + 8.13x$, $a = 55.57$ and $b = 8.13$.

Step 6   Substitute in the formula and solve for s_{est}.

$$s_{\text{est}} = \sqrt{\frac{\Sigma y^2 - a \Sigma y - b \Sigma xy}{n - 2}}$$

$$= \sqrt{\frac{42{,}186 - (55.57)(496) - (8.13)(1778)}{6 - 2}} \approx 6.48$$

This value is close to the value found in Example 10–12. The difference is due to rounding.

Prediction Interval

The standard error of the estimate can be used for constructing a **prediction interval** (similar to a confidence interval) about a y' value.

When a specific value x is substituted into the regression equation, one gets y', which is a point estimate for y. For example, if the regression line equation for the age of a machine and the monthly maintenance cost is $y' = 55.57 + 8.13x$ (Example 10–12), then the predicted maintenance cost for a 3-year-old machine would be $y' = 55.57 + 8.13(3)$, or \$79.96. Since this is a point estimate, one has no idea how accurate it is. But one can construct a prediction interval about the estimate. By selecting an α value, one can achieve a $(1 - \alpha) \cdot 100\%$ confidence that the interval contains the population mean of the y values that correspond to the given value of x.

The reason is that there are possible sources of prediction errors in finding the regression line equation. One source occurs when finding the standard error of the estimate s_{est}. Two others are errors made in estimating the slope and the y' intercept, since the equation of the regression line will change somewhat if different random samples are used when calculating the equation.

Formula for the Prediction Interval about a Value y'

$$y' - t_{\alpha/2}s_{\text{est}}\sqrt{1 + \frac{1}{n} + \frac{n(x - \overline{X})^2}{n\Sigma x^2 - (\Sigma x)^2}} < y < y' + t_{\alpha/2}s_{\text{est}}\sqrt{1 + \frac{1}{n} + \frac{n(x - \overline{X})^2}{n \Sigma x^2 - (\Sigma x)^2}}$$

with d.f. $= n - 2$

Example 10–14

Copy Machine Maintenance Costs

For the data in Example 10–12, find the 95% prediction interval for the monthly maintenance cost of a machine that is 3 years old.

Solution

Step 1   Find Σx, Σx^2, and $\overline{X}$.

$$\Sigma x = 20 \qquad \Sigma x^2 = 82 \qquad \overline{X} = \frac{20}{6} = 3.3$$

Step 2   Find y' for $x = 3$.

$$y' = 55.57 + 8.13x$$
$$y' = 55.57 + 8.13(3) = 79.96$$

Step 3   Find s_{est}.

$$s_{\text{est}} = 6.48$$

as shown in Example 10–13.

Step 4 Substitute in the formula and solve: $t_{\alpha/2} = 2.776$, d.f. $= 6 - 2 = 4$ for 95%.

$$y' - t_{\alpha/2}S_{est}\sqrt{1 + \frac{1}{n} + \frac{n(x - \overline{X})^2}{n\Sigma x^2 - (\Sigma x)^2}} < y < y'$$

$$+ t_{\alpha/2}S_{est}\sqrt{1 + \frac{1}{n} + \frac{n(x - \overline{X})^2}{n\,\Sigma x^2 - (\Sigma x)^2}}$$

$$79.96 - (2.776)(6.48)\sqrt{1 + \frac{1}{n} + \frac{6(3 - 3.3)^2}{6(82) - (20)^2}} < y < 79.96$$

$$+ (2.776)(6.48)\sqrt{1 + \frac{1}{6} + \frac{6(3 - 3.3)^2}{6(82) - (20)^2}}$$

$$79.96 - (2.776)(6.48)(1.08) < y < 79.96 + (2.776)(6.48)(1.08)$$
$$79.96 - 19.43 < y < 79.96 + 19.43$$
$$60.53 < y < 99.39$$

Hence, one can be 95% confident that the interval $60.53 < y < 99.39$ contains the actual value of y.

10-3 Applying the Concepts

Interpreting Simple Linear Regression

Answer the questions about the following computer-generated information.

Linear correlation coefficient $r = 0.794556$
Coefficient of determination $= 0.631319$
Standard error of the estimate $= 12.9668$
Explained variation $= 5182.41$
Unexplained variation $= 3026.49$
Total variation $= 8208.90$
Equation of regression line $\quad y' = 0.725983x + 16.5523$
Level of significance $= 0.1$
Test statistic $= 0.794556$
Critical value $= 0.378419$

1. Are both variables moving in the same direction?
2. Which number measures the distances from the prediction line to the actual values?
3. Which number is the slope of the regression line?
4. Which number is the y intercept of the regression line?
5. Which number can be found in a table?
6. Which number is the allowable risk of making a type I error?
7. Which number measures the variation explained by the regression?
8. Which number measures the scatter of points about the regression line?
9. What is the null hypothesis?
10. Which number is compared to the critical value to see if the null hypothesis should be rejected?
11. Should the null hypothesis be rejected?

See page 502 for the answers.

Exercises 10–3

1. What is meant by the *explained variation?* How is it computed?

2. What is meant by the *unexplained variation?* How is it computed?

3. What is meant by the *total variation?* How is it computed?

4. Define the coefficient of determination.

5. How is the coefficient of determination found?

For Exercises 6 through 11, find the coefficient of determination and interpret.

6. $r = 0.81$

7. $r = 0.70$

8. $r = 0.45$

9. $r = 0.37$

10. $r = 0.15$

11. $r = 0.05$

12. Define the standard error of the estimate for regression. When can the standard error of the estimate be used to construct a prediction interval about a value y'?

13. **Age and Exercise Hours** Compute the standard error of the estimate for Exercise 13 in Section 10–1. The

regression line equation was found in Exercise 13 in Section 10–2.

14. **Forest Fires and Hectares Burned** Compute the standard error of the estimate for Exercise 14 in Section 10–1. The regression line equation was found in Exercise 14 in Section 10–2.

15. **Alumni Contributions** Compute the standard error of the estimate for Exercise 15 in Section 10–1. The regression line equation was found in Exercise 15 in Section 10–2.

16. **Age and Sick Days** Compute the standard error of the estimate for Exercise 16 in Section 10–1. The regression line equation was found in Exercise 16 in Section 10–2.

17. **Age and Exercise Hours** For the data in Exercise 13 in Sections 10–1, 10–2, and 10–3, find the 90% prediction interval when $x = 20$ years.

18. **Forest Fires and Hectares Burned** For the data in Exercise 14 in Sections 10–1, 10–2, and 10–3, find the 95% prediction interval when $x = 60$.

19. **Alumni Contributions** For the data in Exercise 15 in Sections 10–1, 10–2, and 10–3, find the 90% prediction interval when $x = 4$ years.

20. **Age and Sick Days** For the data in Exercise 16 in Sections 10–1, 10–2, and 10–3, find the 98% prediction interval when $x = 47$ years.

10–4   Multiple Regression (Optional) >

Be familiar with the concept of multiple regression.

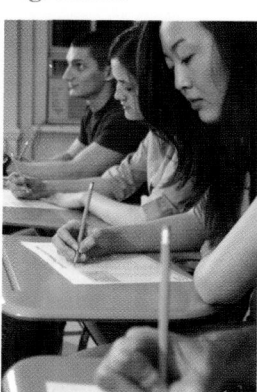

The previous sections explained the concepts of simple linear regression and correlation. In simple linear regression, the regression equation contains one independent variable x and one dependent variable y' and is written as

$$y' = a + bx$$

where a is the y' intercept and b is the slope of the regression line.

In **multiple regression,** there are several independent variables and one dependent variable, and the equation is

$$y' = a + b_1x_1 + b_2x_2 + \cdots + b_kx_k$$

where $x_1, x_2, \ldots, x_k$ are the independent variables.

For example, suppose a dean of Graduate Studies wishes to see whether there is a relationship between a student's grade point average, age, and the GMAT entrance examination. The two independent variables are GPA (denoted by x_1) and age (denoted by x_2). The dean will collect the data for all three variables for a sample of graduate students. Rather than conduct two separate simple regression studies, one using the GPA and GMAT scores and another using ages and GMAT scores, the dean can conduct one study

Speaking of Statistics

In this study, researchers found a correlation between the cleanliness of the homes children are raised in and the years of schooling completed and earning potential for those children. What interfering variables were controlled? How might these have been controlled? Summarize the conclusions of the study.

SUCCESS

HOME SMART HOME

KIDS WHO GROW UP IN A CLEAN HOUSE FARE BETTER AS ADULTS

Good-bye, GPA. So long, SATs. New research suggests that we may be able to predict children's future success from the level of cleanliness in their homes.

A University of Michigan study presented at the annual meeting of the American Economic Association uncovered a surprising correlation: children raised in clean homes were later found to have completed more school and to have higher earning potential than those raised in dirty homes. The clean homes may indicate a family that values organization and similarly helpful skills at school and work, researchers say.

Cleanliness ratings for about 5000 households were assessed between 1968 and 1972, and respondents were interviewed 25 years later to determine educational achievement and professional earnings of the young adults who had grown up there, controlling for variables such as race, socioeconomic status and level of parental education. The data showed that those raised in homes rated "clean" to "very clean" had completed an average of 1.6 more years of school than those raised in "not very clean" or "dirty" homes. Plus, the first group's annual wages averaged about $3100 more than the second's.

But don't buy stock in Mr. Clean and Pine Sol just yet. "We're not advocating that everyone go out and clean their homes right this minute," explains Rachel Dunifon, a University of Michigan doctoral candidate and a researcher on the study. Rather, the main implication of the study, Dunifon says, is that there is significant evidence that non-cognitive factors, such as organization and efficiency, play a role in determining academic and financial success.

— *Jackie Fisherman*

Source: Reprinted with permission from *Psychology Today,* Copyright © (2001) Sussex Publishers, Inc.

using multiple regression analysis with two independent variables—GPA and ages—and one dependent variable—GMAT scores.

A multiple regression correlation R can also be computed to determine if a significant relationship exists between the independent variables and the dependent variable. Multiple regression analysis is used when a statistician thinks there are several independent variables contributing to the variation of the dependent variable. This analysis then can be used to increase the accuracy of predictions for the dependent variable over one independent variable alone.

Two other examples for multiple regression analysis are when a store manager wants to see whether the amount spent on advertising and the amount of floor space used for a display affect the amount of sales of a product, and when a sociologist wants to see whether the amount of time children spend watching television and playing video games is related to their weight. Multiple regression analysis can also be conducted by using more than two independent variables, denoted by $x_1, x_2, x_3, \ldots, x_m$. Since these computations are quite complicated and for the most part would be done on a computer, this chapter will show the computations for two independent variables only.

For example, the dean wishes to see whether a student's grade point average and age are related to the student's score on the GMAT entrance examination. She selects five students and obtains the following data.

Student	GPA x_1	Age x_2	GMAT score y
A	3.2	22	550
B	2.7	27	570
C	2.5	24	525
D	3.4	28	670
E	2.2	23	490

The multiple regression equation obtained from the data is

$$y' = -44.81 + 87.64x_1 + 14.533x_2$$

If a student has a GPA of 3.0 and is 25 years old, her predicted GMAT score can be computed by substituting these values in the equation for x_1 and x_2, respectively, as shown.

$$y' = -44.8 + 87.64(3.0) + 14.533(25)$$
$$= 581.44 \text{ or } 581$$

Hence, if a student has a GPA of 3.0 and is 25 years old, the student's predicted GMAT score is 581.

The Multiple Regression Equation

A multiple regression equation with two independent variables (x_1 and x_2) and one dependent variable would have the form

$$y' = a + b_1x_1 + b_2x_2$$

A multiple regression with three independent variables (x_1, x_2, and x_3) and one dependent variable would have the form

$$y' = a + b_1x_1 + b_2x_2 + b_3x_3$$

General Form of the Multiple Regression Equation

The general form of the multiple regression equation with k independent variables is

$$y' = a + b_1x_1 + b_2x_2 + \cdots + b_kx_k$$

The independent variables are denoted by x. The value for a is more or less an intercept, although a multiple regression equation with two independent variables constitutes a plane rather than a line. *Partial regression coefficients* are denoted by b. Each b represents the amount of change in y' for one unit of change in the corresponding x value when the other x values are held constant. In the example just shown, the regression equation was $y' = -44.81 + 87.64x_1 + 14.533x_2$. In this case, for each unit of change in the student's GPA, there is a change of 87.64 units in the GMAT score with the student's age x_2 being held constant. And for each unit of change in x_2 (the student's age), there is a change of 14.533 units in the GMAT score with the GPA held constant.

Assumptions for Multiple Regression

The assumptions for multiple regression are similar to those for simple regression.

1. For any specific value of the independent variable, the values of the y variable are normally distributed. (This is called the *normality* assumption.)
2. The variances (or standard deviations) for the y variables are the same for each value of the independent variable. (This is called the *equal-variance* assumption.)
3. There is a linear relationship between the dependent variable and the independent variables. (This is called the *linearity* assumption.)
4. The independent variables are not correlated. (This is called the *nonmulticolinearity* assumption.)
5. The values for the y variables are independent. (This is called the *independence* assumption.)

In multiple regression, as in simple regression, the strength of the relationship between the independent variables and the dependent variable is measured by a correlation coefficient. This **multiple correlation coefficient** is symbolized by R. The value of R can range from 0 to $+1$; R can never be negative. The closer to $+1$, the stronger the relationship; the closer to 0, the weaker the relationship. The value of R takes into account all the independent variables and can be computed by using the values of the individual correlation coefficients. The formula for the multiple correlation coefficient when there are two independent variables is shown next.

Formula for the Multiple Correlation Coefficient

The formula for R is

$$R = \sqrt{\frac{r_{yx_1}^2 + r_{yx_2}^2 - 2r_{yx_1} \cdot r_{yx_2} \cdot r_{x_1x_2}}{1 - r_{x_1x_2}^2}}$$

where r_{yx_1} is the value of the correlation coefficient for variables y and x_1; r_{yx_2} is the value of the correlation coefficient for variables y and x_2; and $r_{x_1x_2}$ is the value of the correlation coefficient for variables x_1 and x_2.

In this case, R is 0.989, as shown in Example 10–15. The multiple correlation coefficient is always higher than the individual correlation coefficients. For this specific example, the multiple correlation coefficient is higher than the two individual correlation coefficients computed by using grade point average and GMAT scores ($r_{yx_1} = 0.845$) or age and GMAT scores ($r_{yx_2} = 0.791$). *Note:* $r_{x_1x_2} = 0.371$.

Example 10–15

GMAT Scores

For the data regarding GMAT scores, find the value of R.

Solution

The values of the correlation coefficients are

$$r_{yx_1} = 0.845$$
$$r_{yx_2} = 0.791$$
$$r_{x_1x_2} = 0.371$$

Substituting in the formula, one gets

$$R = \sqrt{\frac{r_{yx_1}^2 + r_{yx_2}^2 - 2r_{yx_1} \cdot r_{yx_2} \cdot r_{x_1x_2}}{1 - r_{x_1x_2}^2}}$$

$$= \sqrt{\frac{(0.845)^2 + (0.791)^2 - 2(0.845)(0.791)(0.371)}{1 - 0.371^2}}$$

$$= \sqrt{\frac{0.8437569}{0.862359}} = \sqrt{0.9784288} = 0.989$$

Hence, the correlation between a student's grade point average and age with the student's GMAT score on the graduate entrance examination is 0.989. In this case, there is a strong relationship among the variables; the value of R is close to 1.00.

As with simple regression, R^2 is the *coefficient of multiple determination,* and it is the amount of variation explained by the regression model. The expression $1 - R^2$ represents the amount of unexplained variation, called the *error* or *residual variation.* Since $R = 0.989$, $R^2 = 0.978$ and $1 - R^2 = 1 - 0.978 = 0.022$.

Testing the Significance of R

An F test is used to test the significance of R. The hypotheses are

$$H_0: \rho = 0 \quad \text{and} \quad H_1: \rho \neq 0$$

where ρ represents the population correlation coefficient for multiple correlation.

Formula for the F Test for Significance of R

The formula for the F test is

$$F = \frac{R^2/k}{(1 - R^2)/(n - k - 1)}$$

where n is the number of data groups $(x_1, x_2, \ldots, y)$ and k is the number of independent variables.

The degrees of freedom are d.f.N. $= n - k$ and d.f.D. $= n - k - 1$.

Example 10–16

GMAT Scores

Test the significance of the R obtained in Example 10–15 at $\alpha = 0.05$.

Solution

$$F = \frac{R^2/k}{(1 - R^2)/(n - k - 1)}$$

$$= \frac{0.978/2}{(1 - 0.978)/(5 - 2 - 1)} = \frac{0.489}{0.011} = 44.45$$

The critical value obtained from Table H with $\alpha = 0.05$, d.f.N. $= 3$, and d.f.D. $= 5 - 2 - 1 = 2$ is 19.16. Hence, the decision is to reject the null hypothesis and conclude that there is a significant relationship among the student's GPA, age, and GMAT score on the graduate entrance examination.

Adjusted R^2

Since the value of R^2 is dependent on n (the number of data pairs) and k (the number of variables), statisticians also calculate what is called an **adjusted R^2,** denoted by R^2_{adj}. This is based on the number of degrees of freedom.

Formula for the Adjusted R^2

The formula for the adjusted R^2 is

$$R^2_{\text{adj}} = 1 - \left[\frac{(1 - R^2)(n - 1)}{n - k - 1} \right]$$

The adjusted R^2 is smaller than R^2 and takes into account the fact that when n and k are approximately equal, the value of R may be artificially high, due to sampling error rather than a true relationship among the variables. This occurs because the chance variations of all the variables are used in conjunction with each other to derive the regression equation. Even if the individual correlation coefficients for each independent variable and the dependent variable were all zero, the multiple correlation coefficient due to sampling error could be higher than zero.

Hence, both R^2 and R^2_{adj} are usually reported in a multiple regression analysis.

Example 10–17

GMAT Scores

Calculate the adjusted R^2 for the data in Example 10–16. The value for R is 0.989.

Solution

$$
\begin{aligned}
R^2_{\text{adj}} &= 1 - \left[\frac{(1 - R^2)(n - 1)}{n - k - 1} \right] \\
&= 1 - \left[\frac{(1 - 0.989^2)(5 - 1)}{5 - 2 - 1} \right] \\
&= 1 - 0.043758 \\
&\approx 0.956
\end{aligned}
$$

In this case, when the number of data pairs and the number of independent variables are accounted for, the adjusted multiple coefficient of determination is 0.956.

10–4 Applying the Concepts

More Math Means More Money

In a study to determine a person's yearly income 10 years after high school, it was found that the two biggest predictors are number of math courses taken and number of hours worked per week during a person's senior year of high school. The multiple regression equation generated from a sample of 20 individuals is

$$y' = 6000 + 4540x_1 + 1290x_2$$

Let x_1 represent the number of mathematics courses taken and x_2 represent hours worked. The correlation between income and mathematics courses is 0.63. The correlation between income and hours worked is 0.84, and the correlation between mathematics courses and hours worked is 0.31. Use this information to answer the following questions.

1. What is the dependent variable?

2. What are the independent variables?

3. What are the multiple regression assumptions?

4. Explain what 4540 and 1290 in the equation tell us.

5. What is the predicted income if a person took 8 math classes and worked 20 hours per week during her senior year in high school?

6. What does a multiple correlation coefficient of 0.77 mean?

7. Compute R^2.

8. Compute the adjusted R^2.

9. Would the equation be considered a good predictor of income?

10. What are your conclusions about the relationship between courses taken, hours worked, and yearly income?

See page 502 for the answers.

Exercises 10–4

1. Explain the similarities and differences between simple linear regression and multiple regression.

2. What is the general form of the multiple regression equation? What does a represent? What does a b represent?

3. Why would a researcher prefer to conduct a multiple regression study rather than separate regression studies using one independent variable and the dependent variable?

4. What are the assumptions for multiple regression?

5. How do the values of the individual correlation coefficients compare to the value of the multiple correlation coefficient?

6. **Age, GPA, and Income** A researcher has determined that a significant relationship exists among an employee's age x_1, grade point average x_2, and income y. The multiple regression equation is $y' = -34{,}127 + 132x_1 + 20{,}805x_2$. Predict the income of a person who is 32 years old and has a GPA of 3.4.

7. **Assembly-Line Work** A manufacturer found that a significant relationship exists among the number of hours an assembly-line employee works per shift x_1, the total number of items produced x_2, and the number of defective items produced y. The multiple regression equation is $y' = 9.6 + 2.2x_1 - 1.08x_2$. Predict the number of defective items produced by an employee who has worked 9 hours and produced 24 items.

8. **Fat, Calories, and Carbohydrates** A nutritionist established a significant relationship among the fat content, the amount of carbohydrates, and the number of calories in a variety of popular 28-gram snacks. She obtained the regression equation $y' = 10.954 + 8.4987x_1 + 4.2982x_2$, where y is the number of calories per snack, x_1 is the number of grams of fat, and x_2 represents the number of carbohydrates in grams. Predict the number of calories in a snack that contains 10 g of fat and 19 g of carbohydrates.

9. **Aspects of Students' Academic Behaviour** A college statistics professor is interested in the relationship among various aspects of a student's academic behaviour and the student's final grade in the class. She found a significant relationship between the number of hours spent studying statistics per week, the number of classes attended per semester, the number of assignments turned in during the semester, and the student's final grade. This relationship is described by the multiple regression equation $y' = -14.9 + 0.93359x_1 + 0.99847x_2 + 5.3844x_3$. Predict the final grade for a student who studies statistics 8 hours per week (x_1), attends 34 classes (x_2), and turns in 11 assignments (x_3).

10. **Age, Cholesterol, and Sodium** A medical researcher found a significant relationship among a person's age x_1, cholesterol level x_2, sodium level of the blood x_3, and systolic blood pressure y. The regression equation is $y' = 97.7 + 0.691x_1 + 219x_2 - 299x_3$. Predict the systolic blood pressure of a person who is 35 years old and has a cholesterol level of 194 milligrams per decilitre (mg/dL) and a sodium blood level of 142 milliequivalents per litre (mEq/L).

11. Explain the meaning of the multiple correlation coefficient R.

12. What is the range of values R can assume?

13. Define R^2 and R^2_{adj}.

14. What are the hypotheses used to test the significance of R?

15. What test is used to test the significance of R?

16. What is the meaning of the adjusted R^2? Why is it computed?

Summary >

Many relationships among variables exist in the real world. One way to determine whether a relationship exists is to use the statistical techniques known as *correlation* and *regression*. The strength and direction of the relationship are measured by the value of the correlation coefficient. It can assume values between and including $+1$ and -1. The closer the value of the correlation coefficient is to $+1$ or -1, the stronger the linear relationship is between the variables. A value of $+1$ or -1 indicates a perfect linear relationship. A positive relationship between two variables means that for small values of the independent variable, the values of the dependent variable will be small, and that for large values of the independent variable, the values of the dependent variable will be large. A negative relationship between two variables means that for small values of the independent variable, the values of the dependent variable will be large, and that for large values of the independent variable, the values of the dependent variable will be small.

Relationships can be linear or curvilinear. To determine the shape, one draws a scatter plot of the variables. If the relationship is linear, the data can be approximated by a straight line, called the *regression line,* or the *line of best fit.* The closer the value of r is to $+1$ or -1, the closer the points will fit the line.

In addition, relationships can be multiple. That is, there can be two or more independent variables and one dependent variable. A coefficient of correlation and a regression equation can be found for multiple relationships, just as they can be found for simple relationships.

The coefficient of determination is a better indicator of the strength of a relationship than the correlation coefficient. It is better because it identifies the percentage of variation of the dependent variable that is directly attributable to the variation of the independent variable. The coefficient of determination is obtained by squaring the correlation coefficient and converting the result to a percentage.

Another statistic used in correlation and regression is the standard error of the estimate, which is an estimate of the standard deviation of the y values about the predicted y' values. The standard error of the estimate can be used to construct a prediction interval about a specific value point estimate y' of the mean of the y values for a given value of x.

Finally, remember that a significant relationship between two variables does not necessarily mean that one variable is a direct cause of the other variable. In some cases this is true, but other possibilities that should be considered include a complex relationship involving other (perhaps unknown) variables, a third variable interacting with both variables, or a relationship due solely to chance.

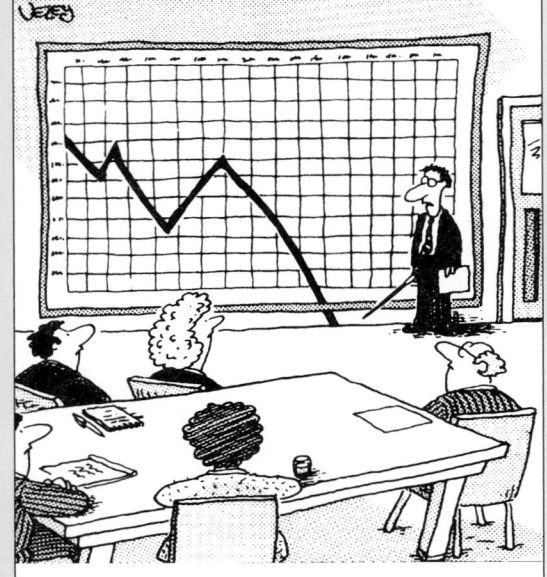

"At this point in my report, I'll ask all of you to follow me to the conference room directly below us!"

Source: Cartoon by Bradford Veley, Marquette, Michigan. Reprinted with permission.

For step-by-step guidance on the use of Texas Instruments TI-83 Plus/TI-84 Plus programmable calculators, see Appendix E at the back of this book. For summary procedures for Minitab, SPSS, and Excel, please see the full version of Appendix E on *Connect.*

Important Terms »

adjusted R^2 494

coefficient of determination 484

correlation 456

correlation coefficient 461

dependent variable 457

extrapolation 477

independent variable 457

influential point or observation 478

least-squares line 484

lurking variable 468

marginal change 476

multiple correlation coefficient 492

multiple regression 489

negative relationship 457

Pearson product moment correlation coefficient 461

Important Formulas »

Formula for the correlation coefficient:

$$r = \frac{n(\Sigma xy) - (\Sigma x)(\Sigma y)}{\sqrt{[n(\Sigma x^2) - (\Sigma x)^2][n(\Sigma y^2) - (\Sigma y)^2]}}$$

Formula for the t test for the correlation coefficient:

$$t = r\sqrt{\frac{n-2}{1-r^2}} \qquad \text{d.f.} = n - 2$$

The regression line equation: $y' = a + bx$, where

$$a = \frac{(\Sigma y)(\Sigma x^2) - (\Sigma x)(\Sigma xy)}{n(\Sigma x^2) - (\Sigma x)^2}$$

$$b = \frac{n(\Sigma xy) - (\Sigma x)(\Sigma y)}{n(\Sigma x^2) - (\Sigma x)^2}$$

Formula for the standard error of the estimate:

$$s_{est} = \sqrt{\frac{\Sigma(y - y')^2}{n-2}}$$

or

$$s_{est} = \sqrt{\frac{\Sigma y^2 - a\,\Sigma y - b\,\Sigma xy}{n-2}}$$

Formula for the prediction interval for a value y':

$$y' - t_{\alpha/2}\, s_{est}\sqrt{1 + \frac{1}{n} + \frac{n(x - \overline{X})^2}{n\Sigma x^2 - (\Sigma x)^2}} < y$$

$$< y' + t_{\alpha/2}\, s_{est}\sqrt{1 + \frac{1}{n} + \frac{n(x - \overline{X})^2}{n\Sigma x^2 - (\Sigma x)^2}}$$

$$\text{d.f.} = n - 2$$

Formula for the multiple correlation coefficient:

$$R = \sqrt{\frac{r_{yx_1}^2 + r_{yx_2}^2 - 2r_{yx_1} \cdot r_{yx_2} \cdot r_{x_1x_2}}{1 - r_{x_1x_2}^2}}$$

Formula for the F test for the multiple correlation coefficient:

$$F = \frac{R^2/k}{(1 - R^2)/(n - k - 1)}$$

with d.f.N $= n - k$ and d.f.D $= n - k - 1$.

Formula for the adjusted R^2:

$$R_{adj}^2 = 1 - \left[\frac{(1 - R^2)(n - 1)}{n - k - 1}\right]$$

Review Exercises »

For Exercises 1 through 7, do a complete regression analysis by performing the following steps.

  a. Draw the scatter plot.
  b. Compute the value of the correlation coefficient.
  c. Test the significance of the correlation coefficient at $\alpha = 0.01$, using Table I.
  d. Determine the regression line equation.
  e. Plot the regression line on the scatter plot.
  f. Predict y' for a specific value of x.

1. **Hockey Shots and Goals Scored** The following data represent the number of shots on goal and the number of goals scored for the top goal scorers in a recent NHL season. If there is a significant relationship between the variables, predict the number of goals scored for a player with 300 shots on goal.

Shots on goal x	363	289	279	272	270
Goals scored y	50	49	48	43	42

Shots on goal x	279	275	279	339	206
Goals scored y	40	39	39	37	35

Source: NHL.com, *Stats*, "Players."

2. **Sports Involvement and Gender** A researcher wishes to determine if there is a relationship between sports involvement and gender in Canada. Statistics Canada collected data on thousands of individuals that included both active and passive participation levels. If a significant relationship exists, predict the number of females participating in sports if 1500 males participate.

Male x	5140	2338	2076	962	537	842	4040
Female y	3169	2261	916	766	399	864	3611

Source: Statistics Canada.

3. **Gasoline and Diesel Pump Price** The data below represent a random selection of regular gasoline and diesel pump prices in Canadian cities. If a significant relationship exists between the variables, predict the diesel pump price if the gasoline price is $1 per litre.

Gasoline (¢ per litre) x	94.2	112.6	98.8	100.7	102.9	103.9
Diesel (¢ per litre) y	88.3	108.4	93.9	103.8	97.9	101.7

Source: Natural Resources Canada, *Energy Sources*, "Retail Fuel Prices by Province [and Territory]."

4. **Driver's Age and Accidents** A study is conducted to determine the relationship between a driver's age and the number of accidents he or she has over a 1-year period. The data are shown here. (This information will be used for Exercise 8.) If there is a significant relationship, predict the number of accidents of a driver who is 28.

Driver's age x	16	24	18	17	23	27	32
No. of accidents y	3	2	5	2	0	1	1

5. **Typing Speed and Word Processing** A researcher desires to know whether the typing speed of a secretary (in words per minute) is related to the time (in hours) that it takes the secretary to learn to use a new word processing program. The data are shown.

Speed x	48	74	52	79	83	56	85	63	88	74	90	92
Time y	7	4	8	3.5	2	6	2.3	5	2.1	4.5	1.9	1.5

If there is a significant relationship, predict the time it will take the average secretary who has a typing speed of 72 words per minute to learn the word processing program. (This information will be used for Exercises 9 and 11.)

6. **Protein and Diastolic Blood Pressure** A study was conducted with vegetarians to see whether the number of grams of protein each ate per day was related to diastolic blood pressure. The data are given here. (This information will be used for Exercises 10 and 12.) If there is a significant relationship, predict the diastolic pressure of a vegetarian who consumes 8 grams of protein per day.

Grams x	4	6.5	5	5.5	8	10	9	8.2	10.5
Pressure y	73	79	83	82	84	92	88	86	95

7. **Vehicle's Age and Repair Costs** An auditor needs to determine if there is a relationship between the age (years) of a vehicle and the annual cost (dollars) of vehicle repair (excluding collision work). A random sample was selected and the vehicle's age and car repair history were obtained. If there is a relationship, what would you expect the annual cost of repair to be for a 7-year-old vehicle?

Vehicle's age x	1	3	4	6	8	9	11	13
Repair cost y	141	510	701	978	1187	1207	1160	1151

Source: DesRosiers Automotive Consultants.

8. **Driver's Age and Accidents** For Exercise 4, find the standard error of the estimate.

9. **Typing Speed and Word Processing** For Exercise 5, find the standard error of the estimate.

10. **Protein and Diastolic Blood Pressure** For Exercise 6, find the standard error of the estimate.

11. **Typing Speed and Word Processing** For Exercise 5, find the 90% prediction interval for time when the speed is 72 words per minute.

12. **Protein and Diastolic Blood Pressure** For Exercise 6, find the 95% prediction interval for pressure when the number of grams is 8.

13. **(Opt.) Job Experience and Workdays Missed** A study found a significant relationship among a person's years of experience on a particular job x_1, the number of workdays missed per month x_2, and the person's age y. The regression equation is $y' = 12.8 + 2.09x_1 + 0.423x_2$. Predict a person's age if he or she has been employed for 4 years and has missed 2 workdays a month.

14. **(Opt.)** Find R when $r_{yx_1} = 0.681$ and $r_{yx_2} = 0.872$ and $r_{x_1x_2} = 0.746$.

15. **(Opt.)** Find R^2_{adj} when $R = 0.873$, $n = 10$, and $k = 3$.

Statistics Today

Like Parent, Like Child?—Revisited

The researchers found that parental use of Employment Insurance (EI) plays a role in shortening the time to the first use of this program by the sample of Canadian men under study. An interesting statistic indicated that 24% of Canadian males who collected EI had parents who were prior recipients. Using the Pearson correlation coefficient, researchers found correlations with statistically significant r values of 0.648, 0.644, and 0.629 in Newfoundland, Prince Edward Island, and Saskatchewan recipients. Researchers also indicated that all of the estimates of parental past and future EI collection are statistically significant, having associated P-values of less than 0.001. It should be noted that the researchers compared Canadian results with a similar Swedish study that found no significant correlation with parental and child Employment Insurance involvement.

Data Analysis »

The databank for these questions can be found in Appendix D at the back of the textbook and on ▨ connect.

1. From the databank, choose two variables that might be related; for example, IQ and educational level; age and cholesterol level; exercise and weight; or weight and systolic blood pressure. Do a complete correlation and regression analysis by performing the following steps. Select a random sample of at least 10 subjects.

   a. Draw a scatter plot.
   b. Compute the correlation coefficient.
   c. Test the hypothesis H_0: $\rho = 0$.
   d. Find the regression line equation.
   e. Summarize the results.

2. Repeat Exercise 1, using samples of values of 10 or more obtained from Data Set V in Appendix D. Let $x =$ the number of suspensions and $y =$ the enrollment size.

3. Repeat Exercise 1, using samples of 10 or more values obtained from Data Set XIII. Let $x =$ the number of beds and $y =$ the number of personnel employed.

Chapter Quiz »

Determine whether each statement is true or false. If the statement is false, explain why.

1. A negative relationship between two variables means that for the most part, as the x variable increases, the y variable increases.

2. A correlation coefficient of -1 implies a perfect linear relationship between the variables.

3. Even if the correlation coefficient is high or low, it may not be significant.

4. When the correlation coefficient is significant, one can assume x causes y.

5. It is not possible to have a significant correlation by chance alone.

6. In multiple regression, there are several dependent variables and one independent variable.

Select the best answer.

7. The strength of the relationship between two variables is determined by the value of

   a. r
   b. a
   c. x
   d. s_{est}

8. To test the significance of r, a(n) _____ test is used.

   a. t
   b. F
   c. χ^2
   d. None of the above

9. The test of significance for r has _____ degrees of freedom.

   a. 1
   b. n
   c. $n - 1$
   d. $n - 2$

10. The equation of the regression line used in statistics is

    a. $x = a + by$
    b. $y = bx + a$
    c. $y' = a + bx$
    d. $x = ay + b$

11. The coefficient of determination is

    a. r
    b. r^2
    c. a
    d. b

Complete the following statements with the best answer.

12. A statistical graph of two variables is called a(n) _____.

13. The x variable is called the _____ variable.

14. The range of r is from _____ to _____.

15. The sign of r and _____ will always be the same.

16. The regression line is called the _____.

17. If all the points fall on a straight line, the value of r will be _____ or _____.

For Exercises 18 through 21, do a complete regression analysis.

   a. Draw the scatter plot.
   b. Compute the value of the correlation coefficient.
   c. Test the significance of the correlation coefficient at $\alpha = 0.05$.
   d. Determine the regression line equation.
   e. Plot the regression line on the scatter plot.
   f. Predict y' for a specific value of x.

18. **Prescription Drug Prices** A medical researcher wants to determine the relationship between the price per dose of prescription drugs in Canada and the price of the same drug in the United States. The data, in Canadian

dollars (C$), are shown. Describe the relationship. Predict the U.S. drug price of $3.75.

Canada price (C$) x	9.17	1.61	1.31	1.70	1.84	0.57	0.96
United States price (C$) y	23.66	2.27	2.93	2.90	1.40	2.12	0.92

Source: CBC News Online.

19. **Driver's Age and Accidents** A study is conducted to determine the relationship between a driver's age and the number of accidents he or she has over a 1-year period. The data are shown here. If there is a significant relationship, predict the number of accidents of a driver who is 64.

Driver's age x	63	65	60	62	66	67	59
No. of accidents y	2	3	1	0	3	1	4

20. **Age and Cavities** A researcher wants to know if the age of a child is related to the number of cavities the child has. The data are shown here. If there is a significant relationship, predict the number of cavities for a child of 11.

Age of child x	6	8	9	10	12	14
No. of cavities y	2	1	3	4	6	5

21. **Fat and Cholesterol Level** A study is conducted with a group of dieters to see if the number of grams of fat each consumes per day is related to cholesterol level. The data are shown here. If there is a significant rela-

tionship, predict the cholesterol level of a dieter who consumes 8.5 grams of fat per day.

Fat grams x	6.8	5.5	8.2	10	8.6	9.1	8.6	10.4
Cholesterol level y	183	201	193	283	222	250	190	218

22. **Age and Cavities** For Exercise 20, find the standard error of the estimate.

23. **Fat and Cholesterol Level** For Exercise 21, find the standard error of the estimate.

24. **Age and Cavities** For Exercise 20, find the 90% prediction interval of the number of cavities for a 7-year-old.

25. **Fat and Cholesterol Level** For Exercise 21, find the 95% prediction interval of the cholesterol level of a person who consumes 10 grams of fat.

26. **(Opt.) Teenage TV and Telephone Habits and Weight** A study was conducted, and a significant relationship was found among the number of hours a teenager watches television per day x_1, the number of hours the teenager talks on the telephone per day x_2, and the teenager's weight y. The regression equation is $y' = 98.7 + 3.82x_1 + 6.51x_2$. Predict a teenager's weight if she averages 3 hours of TV and 1.5 hours on the phone per day.

27. **(Opt.)** Find R when $r_{yx_1} = 0.561$ and $r_{yx_2} = 0.714$ and $r_{x_1x_2} = 0.625$.

28. **(Opt.)** Find R^2_{adj} when $R = 0.774$, $n = 8$, and $k = 2$.

Critical Thinking Challenges »

Product Sales When the points in a scatter plot show a curvilinear trend rather than a linear trend, statisticians have methods of fitting curves rather than straight lines to the data, thus obtaining a better fit and a better prediction model. One type of curve that can be used is the logarithmic regression curve. The data shown are the number of items of a new product sold over a period of 15 months at a certain store. Notice that sales rise during the beginning months and then level off later on.

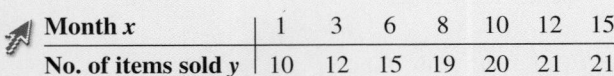

Month x	1	3	6	8	10	12	15
No. of items sold y	10	12	15	19	20	21	21

1. Draw the scatter plot for the data.

2. Find the equation of the regression line.

3. Describe how the line fits the data.

4. Using the log key on your calculator, transform the x values into log x values.

5. Using the log x values instead of the x values, find the equation of a and b for the regression line.

6. Next, plot the curve $y = a + b \log x$ on the graph.

7. Compare the line $y = a + bx$ with the curve $y = a + b \log x$ and decide which one fits the data better.

8. Compute r, using the x and y values; then compute r, using the log x and y values. Which is higher?

9. In your opinion, which (the line or the logarithmic curve) would be a better predictor for the data? Why?

Data Projects »

Where appropriate, use Minitab, SPSS, Excel, TI-83 Plus, TI-84 Plus, or a computer program of your choice to complete the following exercises.

Use a significance level of 0.05 for all tests below.

1. **Business and Finance** Use the Dow Jones industrial stocks in Data Project 1 in Chapter 2 as the sample. For

each, note the current price and the amount of last year's dividends. Are the two variables linearly related? How much variability in amount of dividend is explainable by the price?

2. **Sports and Leisure** For each team in Major League Baseball, note the number of wins the team had last year and the number of home runs by its best home run

hitter. Is the number of wins linearly related to the number of home runs hit? How much variability in total wins is explained by home runs hit? Write a regression equation to determine how many wins you would expect a team to have, knowing their top home run output.

3. **Technology** Use the data collected in Data Project 3 in Chapter 2 for this problem. For the data set, note the length of the song and the year it was released. Is there a linear relationship between the length of a song and the year it was released? Is the sign on the correlation coefficient positive or negative? What does the sign on the coefficient indicate about the relationship?

4. **Health and Wellness** Use a fast-food restaurant to compile your data. For each menu item, note its fat grams and its total calories. Is there a linear relationship between the two variables? How much variance in total calories is explained by fat grams? Write a regression

equation to determine how many total calories you would expect in an item, knowing its fat grams.

5. **Politics and Economics** Research the social assistance rate and unemployment rate of each province and territory for a recent year. Is there a linear relationship between the two rates? Identify another variable that positively correlates with either the social assistance rate or unemployment rate. Identify another variable that negatively correlates with either the social assistance rate or unemployment rate.

6. **Your Class** Use the data collected in Data Project 6 in Chapter 2 regarding heart rates. Is there a linear relationship between the heart rates before and after exercise? How much of the variability in heart rate after exercise is explainable by heart rate before exercise? Write a regression equation to determine what heart rate after exercise you would expect for a person, given the person's heart rate before exercise.

Answers to Applying the Concepts   »

Section 10–1 Stopping Distances

1. The independent variable is kilometres per hour (km/h).

2. The dependent variable is stopping distance (metres).

3. Kilometres per hour is a continuous quantitative variable.

4. Stopping distance is a continuous quantitative variable.

5. A scatter plot of the data is shown.

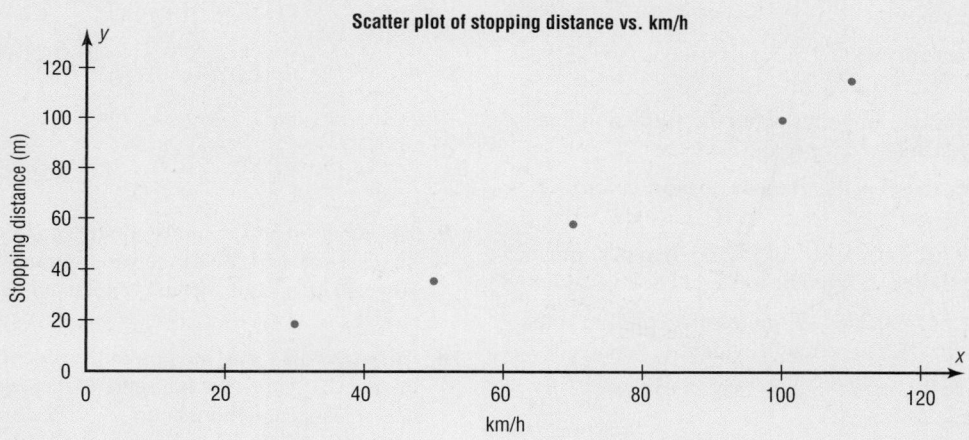

Scatter plot of stopping distance vs. km/h

6. There might be a linear relationship between the two variables, but there is a bit of a curve in the data.

7. Changing the distances between the km/h increments will change the appearance of the relationship.

8. There is a positive relationship between the two variables—higher speeds are associated with longer stopping distances.

9. The strong relationship between the two variables suggests that stopping distance can be accurately predicted from km/h. We might still have some concern about the curve in the data.

10. Answers will vary. Some other variables that might affect stopping distance include road distances, driver response time, and condition of the brakes.

11. The correlation coefficient is $r = 0.995$.

12. The value for $r = 0.995$ is significant at $\alpha = 0.05$. This confirms the strong, positive relationship between the variables.

Section 10–2 Stopping Distances Revisited

1. The linear regression equation is

$$y' = -22.96 + 1.21x.$$

2. The slope says that for each additional kilometre per hour a vehicle is travelling, we expect the stopping distance to increase 1.21 metres, on average. The y intercept is the stopping distance we would expect for a vehicle travelling 0 km/h. Although meaningless in this context, it is an important part of the model.

3. $y' = -22.96 + 1.21(60) = 49.64$. The stopping distance for a vehicle travelling 60 km/h is approximately 50 metres.

4. $y' = -22.96 + 1.21(120) = 122.24$. The stopping distance for a vehicle travelling 120 km/h is approximately 122 metres.

5. Predicting beyond the range of the given data values will become less accurate as the distance from the data set increases. For example, predicting stopping distances for 120 km/h will be more accurate than for 150 km/h.

Section 10–3 Interpreting Simple Linear Regression

1. Both variables are moving in the same direction. In other words, the two variables are positively associated. We know this because the correlation coefficient is positive.

2. The unexplained variation of 3026.49 measures the distances from the prediction line to the actual values.

3. The slope of the regression line is 0.725983.

4. The y intercept is 16.5523.

5. The critical value of 0.378419 can be found in a table.

6. The allowable risk of making a type I error is 0.10, the level of significance.

7. The variation explained by the regression is 0.631319, or about 63.1%.

8. The average scatter of points about the regression line is 12.9668, the standard error of the estimate.

9. The null hypothesis is that there is no correlation, $H_0: \rho = 0$.

10. We compare the test statistic of 0.794556 to the critical value to see if the null hypothesis should be rejected.

11. Since $0.794556 > 0.378419$, we reject the null hypothesis and find that there is enough evidence to conclude that the correlation is not equal to zero.

Section 10–4 More Math Means More Money

1. The dependent variable is yearly income 10 years after high school.

2. The independent variables are number of math courses taken and number of hours worked per week during the senior year of high school.

3. Multiple regression includes normality, equal variance, and linearity assumptions with no correlation for the independent variables and independent values for the y-variables.

4. We expect a person's yearly income 10 years after high school to be $4540 more, on average, for each additional math course taken, all other variables held constant. We expect a person's yearly income 10 years after high school to be $1290 more, on average, for each additional hour worked per week during the senior year of high school, all other variables held constant.

5. $y' = 6000 + 4540(8) + 1290(20) = 68,120$. The predicted yearly income 10 years after high school is $68,120.

6. The multiple correlation coefficient of 0.77 means that there is a fairly strong positive relationship between the independent variables (number of math courses and hours worked during senior year of high school) and the dependent variable (yearly income 10 years after high school).

7. $R^2 = (0.77)^2 = 0.5929$

8. $R^2_{adj} = 1 - \left[\dfrac{(1 - R^2)(n - 1)}{n - k - 1} \right]$

$\qquad = 1 - \left[\dfrac{(1 - 0.5929)(20 - 1)}{20 - 2 - 1} \right]$

$\qquad = 1 - \left[\dfrac{(0.4071)(19)}{17} \right] = 0.5450$

9. The equation appears to be a fairly good predictor of income, since 54.5% of the variation in yearly income 10 years after high school is explained by the regression model.

10. Answers will vary. One possible answer is that yearly income 10 years after high school increases with more math classes and more hours of work during the senior year of high school. The number of math classes has a higher coefficient, so more math does mean more money!

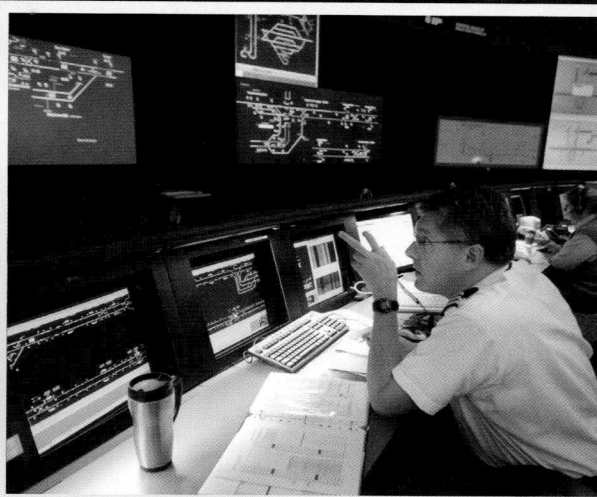

Chapter 11

Other Chi-Square Tests

Statistics Today

Statistics and Heredity

An Austrian monk, Gregor Mendel (1822–1884), studied genetics, and his principles are the foundation for modern genetics. Mendel used his spare time to grow a variety of peas at the monastery. One of his many experiments involved crossbreeding peas that had smooth yellow seeds with peas that had wrinkled green seeds. He noticed that the results occurred with regularity. That is, some of the offspring had smooth yellow seeds, some had smooth green seeds, some had wrinkled yellow seeds, and some had wrinkled green seeds. Furthermore, after several experiments, the percentages of each type seemed to remain approximately the same. Mendel formulated his theory based on the assumption of dominant and recessive traits and tried to predict the results. He then crossbred his peas and examined 556 seeds over the next generation.

Finally, he compared the actual results with the theoretical results to see if his theory was correct. To do this, he used a "simple" chi-square test,

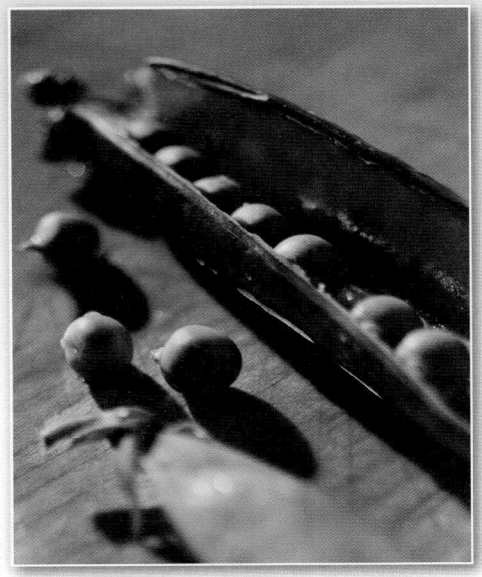

which is explained in this chapter. See Statistics Today—Revisited, page 529.

Source: J. Hodges, Jr., D. Krech, and R. Crutchfield, *Stat Lab, An Empirical Introduction to Statistics* (New York: McGraw-Hill, 1975), pp. 228–229. Used with permission.

Introduction >

The chi-square distribution was used in Chapters 7 and 8 to find a confidence interval for a variance or standard deviation and to test a hypothesis about a single variance or standard deviation.

It can also be used for tests concerning *frequency distributions,* such as "If a sample of buyers is given a choice of automobile colours, will each colour be selected with the same frequency?" The chi-square distribution can be used to test the *independence* of two variables, for example, "Are the opinions of elected members of Parliament on gun control independent of party affiliations?" That is, do the Conservatives feel one way and the Liberals feel differently, or do they have the same opinion?

Finally, the chi-square distribution can be used to test the *homogeneity of proportions.* For example, is the proportion of high school seniors who attend college immediately after graduating the same for western, central, or eastern parts of Canada?"

This chapter explains the chi-square distribution and its applications. In addition to the applications mentioned here, chi-square has many other uses in statistics.

11–1 | Test for Goodness of Fit >

LO1

Test a distribution for goodness of fit, using chi square.

In addition to being used to test a single variance, the chi-square statistic can be used to see whether a frequency distribution fits a specific pattern. For example, to meet customer demands, a manufacturer of running shoes may want to see whether buyers show a preference for a specific style. A traffic engineer may wish to see whether accidents occur more often on some days than on others, so that police patrols can be increased accordingly. An emergency service may want to see whether it receives more calls at certain times of the day than at others, so that it can provide adequate staffing.

When one is testing to see whether a frequency distribution fits a specific pattern, the chi-square **goodness-of-fit test** is used. For example, suppose a market analyst wished to see whether consumers have any preference among five flavours of a new fruit soda. A sample of 100 people provided these data:

Cherry	Strawberry	Orange	Lime	Grape
32	28	16	14	10

If there was no preference, one would expect each flavour to be selected with equal frequency. In this case, each of the five categories would represent 20% of the selections. That is, *approximately* 20 people—100×0.2 or $100/5$—would select each flavour.

Since the frequencies for each flavour were obtained from a sample, these actual frequencies are called the **observed frequencies.** The frequencies obtained by calculation (as if there were no preference) are called the **expected frequencies.** A completed table for the test is shown.

Frequency	Cherry	Strawberry	Orange	Lime	Grape
Observed	32	28	16	14	10
Expected	20	20	20	20	20

The observed frequencies will almost always differ from the expected frequencies due to sampling error; that is, the values differ from sample to sample. But the question is: Are these differences significant (a preference exists), or are they due to chance? The chi-square goodness-of-fit test will enable the researcher to determine the answer.

Before computing the test statistic, one must state the hypotheses. The null hypothesis should be a statement indicating that there is no difference or no change. For this example, the hypotheses are as follows:

H_0: Consumers show no preference for flavours of the fruit soda.

H_1: Consumers show a preference.

In the goodness-of-fit test, the degrees of freedom are equal to the number of categories minus 1. For this example, there are five categories (cherry, strawberry, orange, lime, and grape); hence, the degrees of freedom are $5 - 1 = 4$. This is so because the number of subjects in each of the first four categories is free to vary. But in order for the sum to be 100—the total number of subjects—the number of subjects in the last category is fixed.

Formula for the Chi-Square Goodness-of-Fit Test

$$\chi^2 = \sum \frac{(O - E)^2}{E}$$

with degrees of freedom equal to the number of categories minus 1, and where

O = observed frequency
E = expected frequency

Expected Value

Whether the categories in a χ^2 goodness-of-fit test have equal or unequal proportions, the expected values (or expected frequencies) for each category can be determined as shown.

$E = n \cdot p$ where n = sample size (total number of observations)
p = individual category proportion

Two assumptions are needed for the goodness-of-fit test. These assumptions are given next.

1. The data are obtained from a random sample.
2. The expected frequency for each category must be 5 or more.

This test is a right-tailed test, since when the $O - E$ values are squared, the answer will be positive or zero. This formula is explained in Example 11–1.

Example 11–1

Fruit Soda Flavour Preference

Is there enough evidence to reject the claim that there is no preference in the selection of fruit soda flavours, using the data shown previously? Let $\alpha = 0.05$.

Solution

Step 1   State the hypotheses and identify the claim.

H_0: Consumers show no preference for flavours (claim).

H_1: Consumers show a preference.

Step 2   Find the critical value. The degrees of freedom are $5 - 1 = 4$, and $\alpha = 0.05$. Hence, the critical value from Table G in Appendix C is 9.488.

Step 3   Compute the test statistic by subtracting the expected value from the corresponding observed value, squaring the result and dividing by the expected value, and finding the sum. The expected value for each category is 20, as shown previously.

$$\chi^2 = \sum \frac{(O - E)^2}{E}$$
$$= \frac{(32 - 20)^2}{20} + \frac{(28 - 20)^2}{20} + \frac{(16 - 20)^2}{20} + \frac{(14 - 20)^2}{20}$$
$$+ \frac{(10 - 20)^2}{20} = 18.0$$

Step 4   Make the decision. At $\alpha = 0.05$, the decision is to reject the null hypothesis, since the test statistic ($\chi^2 = 18.0$) is in the critical region, as shown in Figure 11–1. (*P*-value is also shown.)

Figure 11–1

Critical Region and Test Statistic for Example 11–1: χ^2 Distribution (d.f. = 4)

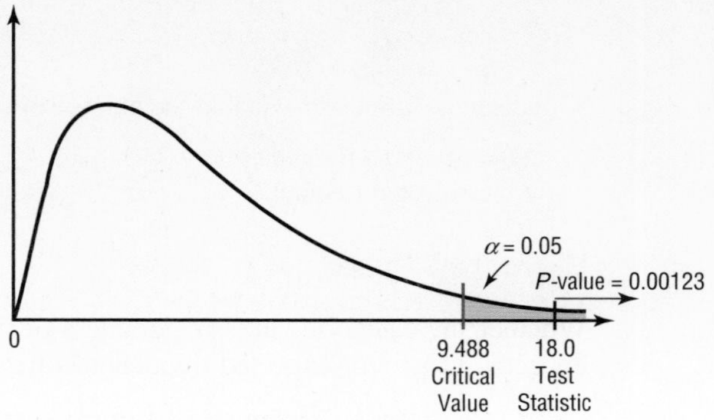

$\alpha = 0.05$

P-value = 0.00123

9.488 Critical Value   18.0 Test Statistic

Step 5   Summarize the results. There is enough evidence to reject the claim that consumers show no preference for the flavours.

P-Value Method

The *P*-value method was explained in Section 8–5, "χ^2 Test for a Variance or Standard Deviation," and is commonly used to make decisions for hypothesis tests. The decision rule for the *P*-value is to reject the null hypothesis if the *P*-value obtained is less than α, the significance level. The approximate *P*-value obtained from Table G for Example 11–1 with d.f. = 4 and the test statistic $\chi^2 = 18.0$ is less than 0.005. The exact *P*-value using technology is 0.00123. Since the *P*-value (0.00123) < significance level ($\alpha = 0.05$), reject H_0. Refer to Figure 11–1. Also, refer to Example 11–3 for a complete solution using the *P*-value method.

To get some idea of why this test is called the goodness-of-fit test, examine graphs of the observed values and expected values. See Figure 11–2. From the graphs, one can see whether the observed values and expected values are close together or far apart.

Figure 11–2

Graphs of the Observed and Expected Values for Soda Flavours

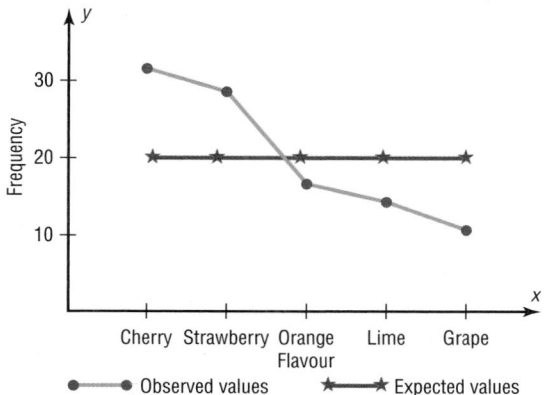

When the observed values and expected values are close together, the chi-square test statistic will be small. Then the decision will be to not reject the null hypothesis—hence, there is "a good fit." See Figure 11–3(a). When the observed values and the expected values are far apart, the chi-square test statistic will be large. Then the null hypothesis will be rejected—hence, there is "not a good fit." See Figure 11–3(b).

Figure 11–3

Results of the Goodness-of-Fit Test

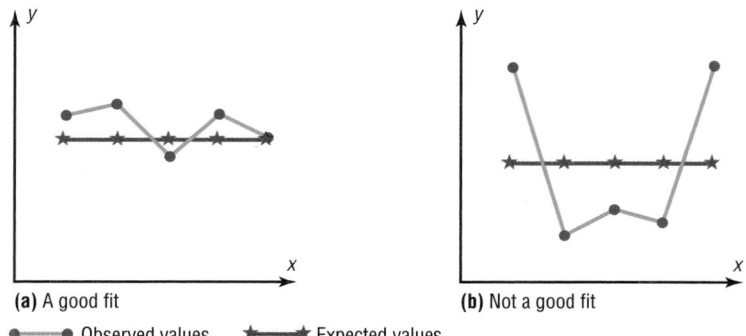

The steps for the chi-square goodness-of-fit test are summarized in this Procedure Table.

Procedure Table

The Chi-Square Goodness-of-Fit Test (Traditional Method)

Step 1 State the hypotheses and identify the claim.

Step 2 Find the critical value. The test is always right-tailed.

(continued)

Procedure Table *(continued)*

Step 3 Compute the test statistic.

Find the sum of the $\dfrac{(O - E)^2}{E}$ values.

Step 4 Make the decision.

Step 5 Summarize the results.

When there is perfect agreement between the observed and the expected values, $\chi^2 = 0$. Also, χ^2 can never be negative. Finally, the test is right-tailed because "H_0: Good fit" and "H_1: Not a good fit" mean that χ^2 will be small in the first case and large in the second case.

Example 11–2

Retiree Reasons for Returning to Work

Canadian retirees returning to paid employment were asked why they did so. Financial considerations were mentioned by 38% of retirees, 22% disliked retirement, 19% alluded to the intrinsic rewards offered by work (challenging tasks, social contacts, sense of purpose), 14% felt they were needed or wanted to help out, and 7% cited other considerations, such as pressure from family members, improved health, or no longer having to provide caregiving. To see if these percentages are consistent with residents of Canada's Atlantic region, a researcher surveyed 300 retirees who had returned to work. The reasons cited were broken down as follows: 128 for financial reasons, 59 disliked retirement, 51 mentioned intrinsic rewards, 37 felt that they were needed, and 25 cited other considerations. At $\alpha = 0.10$, test the claim that the percentages are the same for retirees working in Canada's Atlantic region.

Source: Adapted from Statistics Canada, *Perspectives on Labour and Income,* Catalogue 75-001-XIE, September 2005.

Solution

Step 1 State the hypotheses and identify the claim.

H_0: Canadian retirees' reasons for returning to work are distributed as follows: 38% for financial reasons, 22% disliked retirement, 19% desired intrinsic rewards, 14% felt needed, and 7% cited other considerations (claim).

H_1: The distribution is different than stated in the null hypothesis.

Step 2 Find the critical value. Since $\alpha = 0.10$ and the degrees of freedom are $5 - 1 = 4$, then the critical value is 7.779.

Step 3 Compute the test statistic. Use the formula $E = n \cdot p$ to calculate the expected frequencies for each category.

$E_1 = 300 \times 0.38 = 114 \quad E_2 = 300 \times 0.22 = 66 \quad E_3 = 300 \times 0.19 = 57$
$E_4 = 300 \times 0.14 = 42 \quad E_5 = 300 \times 0.07 = 21$

$$\chi^2 = \sum \frac{(O - E)^2}{E}$$

$$= \frac{(128 - 114)^2}{114} + \frac{(59 - 66)^2}{66} + \frac{(51 - 57)^2}{57} + \frac{(37 - 42)^2}{42} + \frac{(25 - 21)^2}{21}$$

$$\approx 4.450$$

Step 4 Make the decision. At $\alpha = 0.10$, the decision is to not reject the null hypothesis, since the test statistic ($\chi^2 = 4.450$) is not in the critical region, as shown in Figure 11–4. (The P-value is also shown.)

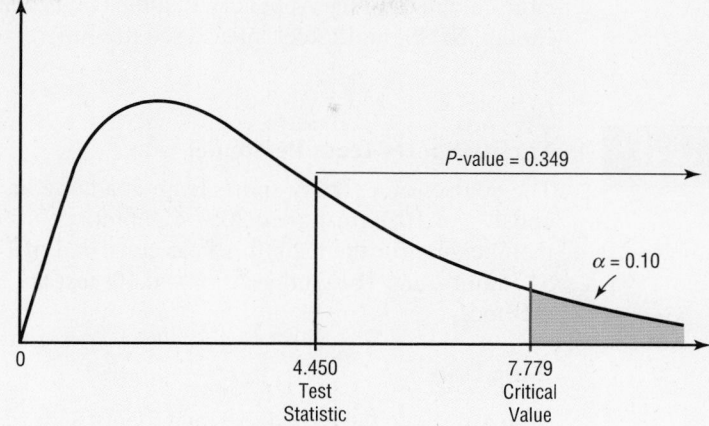

Figure 11–4

Critical Region and Test Statistic for Example 11–2: χ^2 Distribution (d.f. = 4)

P-value = 0.349

$\alpha = 0.10$

0

4.450
Test
Statistic

7.779
Critical
Value

Step 5 Summarize the results. There is not enough evidence to reject the claim. It can be concluded that the proportions are not significantly different from those stated in the null hypothesis.

P-Value Method

The decision rule for the P-value method, as previously explained in Section 8–5, is to reject the null hypothesis if the P-value is less than the significance level, α. The approximate P-value obtained from Table G for Example 11–2 with d.f. = 4 with a test statistic $\chi^2 = 4.450$ is between 0.90 and 0.10. The exact P-value using technology is 0.349. Since the P-value (0.349) > significance level ($\alpha = 0.10$), do not reject H_0. Refer to Figure 11–4. Also, refer to Example 11–3 for a complete solution using the P-value method.

P-Value Method for Chi-Square Tests

The P-value, or probability value, method as explained in Section 8–5, "χ^2 Test for a Variance or Standard Deviation," is commonly used to make decisions for hypothesis tests. The main difference between the traditional method and the P-value method is that the critical value is not required. Instead, the decision rule for the P-value method is to reject the null hypothesis if the P-value is less than the significance level, α, The P-value steps for the χ^2 goodness-of-fit test are shown below.

Procedure Table

The Chi-Square Goodness-of-Fit Test (*P*-Value Method)

Step 1 State the hypotheses and identify the claim.

Step 2 Compute the test statistic.

Step 3 Find the P-value.

Step 4 Make the decision.

Step 5 Summarize the results.

The *P*-value can be approximated using Table G, The Chi-Square Distribution, in Appendix C or more precisely using statistical software (e.g., Minitab, SPSS), a spreadsheet application (e.g., Excel), or a programmable calculator (e.g., TI-83 Plus). For step-by-step guidance on the use of Texas Instruments TI-83 Plus/TI-84 Plus programmable calculators, see Appendix E at the back of this book. For summary procedures for Minitab, SPSS, and Excel, please see the full version of Appendix E on *Connect*.

Example 11–3	**Varsity Sports Team Personnel** 🏹

The adviser of a varsity sports team at a large university believes that the group consists of 10% freshmen, 20% sophomores, 40% juniors, and 30% seniors. The membership for the team this year consisted of 14 freshmen, 19 sophomores, 51 juniors, and 16 seniors. At $\alpha = 0.10$, test the adviser's claim. Use *P*-value method.

Solution

Step 1   State the hypotheses and identify the claim.

H_0: The team consists of 10% freshmen, 20% sophomores, 40% juniors, and 30% seniors (claim).

H_1: The distribution is not the same as stated in the null hypothesis.

Step 2   Compute the test statistic. Use the formula $E = n \cdot p$ to calculate the expected frequencies for each category.

$$E_1 = 100 \times 0.10 = 10 \quad E_2 = 100 \times 0.20 = 20$$
$$E_3 = 100 \times 0.40 = 40 \quad E_4 = 100 \times 0.30 = 30$$

$$\chi^2 = \Sigma \frac{(O - E)^2}{E}$$

$$= \frac{(14 - 10)^2}{10} + \frac{(19 - 20)^2}{20} + \frac{(51 - 40)^2}{40} + \frac{(16 - 30)^2}{30}$$

$$\approx 11.208$$

Step 3   Find the *P*-value.

The approximate *P*-value, obtained from Table G in Appendix C, for the test statistic, $\chi^2 = 11.208$, with d.f. = 3 is between 0.025 and 0.01. See Figure 11–5.

Figure 11–5

Finding the *P*-Value

P-value is between 0.025 and 0.01

Degrees of Freedom	0.995	0.99	0.975	0.95	0.90	0.10	0.05	0.025	0.01	0.005
1	0.000	0.000	0.001	0.004	0.016	2.706	3.841	5.024	6.635	7.879
2	0.010	0.020	0.051	0.103	0.211	4.605	5.991	7.378	9.210	10.597
3	0.072	0.115	0.216	0.352	0.584	6.251	7.815	9.348	11.345	12.838
4	0.207	0.297	0.484	0.711	1.064	7.779	9.486	11.143	13.277	14.860

Test statistic is 11.208

Note: The *P*-value obtained from statistical software, spreadsheet, or calculator is 0.0107.

Step 4   Make the decision. Since the *P*-value (0.0107) is less than the significance level ($\alpha = 0.10$), reject the null hypothesis. Refer to Figure 11–6. (The critical value is also shown.)

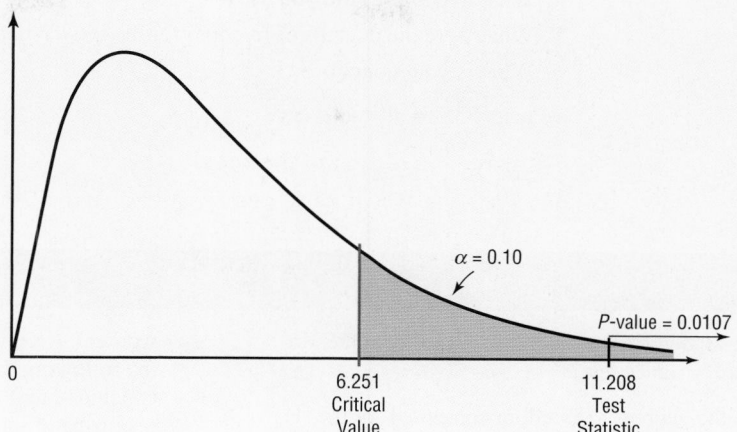

Step 5   Summarize the results. There is enough evidence to reject the adviser's claim.

Traditional Method

The decision rule for the traditional method is to reject the null hypothesis if the test statistic is in the critical region. The critical value at $\alpha = 0.10$ for χ^2 with d.f. $= 3$ is 6.251. Since the test statistic ($\chi^2 = 11.208$) is in the critical region, reject H_0. Refer to Figure 11–6.

For use of the chi-square goodness-of-fit test, statisticians have determined that the expected frequencies should be at least 5, as stated in the assumptions. The reasoning is as follows: The chi-square distribution is continuous, whereas the goodness-of-fit test is discrete. However, the continuous distribution is a good approximation and can be used when the expected value for each class is at least 5. If an expected frequency of a class is less than 5, then that class can be combined with another class so that the expected frequency is 5 or more.

Unusual Stat

Drinking milk may lower your risk of stroke. A 22-year study of men over 55 found that only 4% of men who drank half a litre of milk every day suffered a stroke, compared with 8% of the nonmilk drinkers.

11–1 Applying the Concepts

Never the Same Amounts

M&M/Mars, the makers of Skittles candies, states that the flavour blend is 20% for each flavour. Skittles is a combination of lemon-, lime-, orange-, strawberry-, and grape-flavoured candies. The following data are the results of four randomly selected bags of Skittles and their flavour blends. Use the data to answer the questions.

Bag	Green	Orange	Red	Purple	Yellow
1	7	20	10	7	14
2	20	5	5	13	17
3	4	16	13	21	4
4	12	9	16	3	17
Total	43	50	44	44	52

Flavour (column group header)

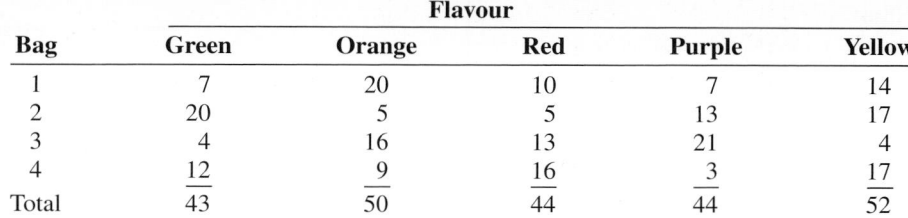

1. Are the variables quantitative or qualitative?

2. What type of test can be used to compare the observed values to the expected values?

3. Perform a chi-square test on the total values.

4. What hypotheses did you use?

5. What were the degrees of freedom for the test? What is the critical value?

6. What is your conclusion?

See page 533 for the answers.

Exercises 11–1

1. How does the goodness-of-fit test differ from the chi-square variance test?

2. How are the degrees of freedom computed for the goodness-of-fit test?

3. How are the expected values computed for the goodness-of-fit test?

4. When the expected frequencies are less than 5 for a specific class, what should be done so that one can use the goodness-of-fit test?

For Exercises 5 through 19, perform these steps.

a. State the hypotheses and identify the claim.

b. Find the critical value.

c. Compute the test statistic.

d. Make the decision.

e. Summarize the results.

Use the traditional method of hypothesis testing unless otherwise specified.

5. **Automobile Age Distribution** A researcher for an automobile manufacturer wants to see if the ages of automobiles are equally distributed among three categories: less than 3 years old, 3 to 7 years old, and 8 years or older. A sample of 30 adult automobile owners is selected, and the results are shown. At $\alpha = 0.05$ can it be considered that the ages of the automobiles are equally distributed among the three categories? What would the results suggest to a tire manufacturer?

Category	Less than three years	3 to 7 years	8 years or older
Number	8	10	12

Source: Based on information from Goodyear.

6. **Combating Midday Drowsiness** A researcher wishes to see if the five ways (drinking caffeinated beverages, taking a nap, going for a walk, eating a sugary snack, other) people use to combat midday drowsiness are equally distributed among office workers. A sample of 60 office workers is selected, and the following data are obtained. At $\alpha = 0.10$ can it be concluded that there is no preference? Why would the results be of interest to an employer?

Method	Beverage	Nap	Walk	Snack	Other
Number	21	16	10	8	5

Source: Based on information from Harris Interactive.

7. **New Vehicle Market Share** An automotive industry report indicates the market share for new vehicles sold in Canada were General Motors, 29.0%; Chrysler, 14.3%; Ford, 14.1%; Toyota, 10.2%; other manufacturers, 32.4%. A recent survey of new car sales in a particular region indicated that of 100 cars sold, 26 were General Motors, 16 were Chrysler, 14 were Ford, 13 were Toyota, and 31 were other manufacturers. At $\alpha = 0.05$, is there sufficient evidence to conclude that the proportions differ from those stated in the report?

Source: DesRosiers Automotive Consultants Inc.

8. **Family Distribution** Recent census data indicates that 38.5% of Canadian families have no children, 27.3% have one child, 24.0% have two children, and 10.3% have three or more children living at home. A random sample of families from a regional school district revealed these results.

Children	0	1	2	3+
Number	51	43	37	9

At $\alpha = 0.05$, is there sufficient evidence to conclude that the proportions of children in the school district's families differ from those reported by the census?

Source: Statistics Canada, *Summary Tables*, "Census Families by Number of Children at Home, by Province and Territory (2006 Census)," September 20, 2007.

9. **Genetically Modified Food** An ABC News poll asked adults whether they felt genetically modified food was safe to eat. Of the respondents, 35% felt it was safe, 52% felt it was not safe, and 13% had no opinion. A random

sample of 120 adults was asked the same question at a local fair; 40 people felt that genetically modified food was safe, 60 felt that it was not safe, and 20 had no opinion. At the 0.01 level of significance, is there sufficient evidence to conclude that the proportions differ from those reported in the survey?

Source: ABCNews.com Poll, www.pollingreport.com.

10. Blood Types Human blood is grouped into four types: A, B, AB, and O. The percentages of Canadians with each blood type are as follows: A, 42%; B, 9%; AB, 3%; and O, 46%. At a recent blood donors' clinic at a local college, the donors were classified as shown below. At the 0.10 level of significance, is there sufficient evidence to conclude that the proportions differ from those stated above?

Blood type	A	B	AB	O
Number	38	12	5	35

Source: Canadian Blood Services, Blood, "Types and Rh System."

11. Credit Union Loans A national publication reported that 21% of loans granted by credit unions were for home mortgages, 39% were for automobile purchases, 20% were for credit card and other unsecured loans, 12% were for real estate other than home loans, and 8% were for other miscellaneous needs. In order to see if her credit union customers had similar needs, a manager surveyed a random sample of 100 loans and found that 25 were for home mortgages, 44 for automobile purchases, 19 for credit card and unsecured loans, 8 for real estate other than home loans, and 4 for miscellaneous needs. At $\alpha = 0.05$, is the distribution the same as reported in the newspaper?

Source: USA TODAY.

12. Greenhouse Gas Emissions Statistics Canada reports national sources of greenhouse gas emissions by sector. The breakdown is business sector, 81.2%; non-business sector, 2.6%; and household sector, 16.2%. A provincial environment official wants to see if her province is the same. Her study of 300 emission sources finds business sector, 230; non-business sector, 6; and household sector, 64. At $\alpha = 0.05$, can she claim the percentages are the same?

Source: Statistics Canada.

13. Smoking Survey Health Canada reports the results of a recent survey on the smoking status of Canadians age 15 years and older as follows.

Smoking status	Daily	Nondaily	Former	Never
Percentage	13.2	4.1	27.2	55.5

A rural health authority wants to know if its region has the same smoker distribution. The results are shown. At $\alpha = 0.05$, test the claim that the health region has the same distribution of smokers as the Health Canada report.

Smoking status	Daily	Nondaily	Former	Never
Number	45	10	80	115

Source: Health Canada, Tobacco Control Directorate, Supplementary Tables, "CTUMS Wave 1, 2009."

14. Federal Prison Inmate Crimes The population distribution of Canada's federal prisons by serious offences are the following: crimes of violence, 52%; property crimes, 19%; drug offences, 14%; other offences, 15%. A warden wants to see how his prison compares so he surveys 500 prisoners and finds 275 committed crimes of violence; 88 committed property crimes; 77 committed drug offences; and 60 committed other offences. Can the warden conclude that the percentages are the same for his prison? Use $\alpha = 0.05$.

Source: Statistics Canada.

15. Provincial Prison Inmate Crimes The population of provincial prisons nationwide by serious offences are the following: crimes of violence, 15.5%; property crimes, 24.1%; impaired driving, 5.5%; drug offences, 4.7%, other Criminal Code offences, 29.8%; and other statutes, 20.4%. A provincial corrections officer wants to check how this compares to her province. She surveys 1000 inmates and finds 150 were sentenced for crimes of violence, 243 for property crimes, 57 for impaired driving, 60 for drug offences, 305 for other Criminal Code offences, and 185 for other statutes. Can she conclude that the percentages for her prison are the same as national statistics? Use $\alpha = 0.05$.

Source: Statistics Canada.

16. Performing Arts Patrons A researcher wants to know if attendance at live performing arts is equally distributed among Canada's language groups: Anglophone, Francophone, and Allophone (*spoken language other than English or French*). A sample of 188 adults was asked if they attended a live performance in the past year. The results are shown. At $\alpha = 0.05$, can it be concluded that the frequencies are equal? Use the P-value method. Interpret your answer.

Category	Anglophone	Francophone	Allophone
Frequency	65	67	56

Source: Decima Research.

17. Prescription Drug Payments A medical researcher wants to determine if the way Canadians pay for their retail medical prescriptions is distributed as follows: 24% out-of-pocket, 34.6% private insurers, and 41.4% public insurance. A sample of 50 people found that 11 paid out-of-pocket, 16 paid using private insurers, and 23 paid with public insurance. At $\alpha = 0.05$, is the assumption correct? Use the P-value method. What would be an implication of the results?

Source: Canadian Institute for Health Information.

Extending the Concepts »

18. Tossing Coins Three coins are tossed 72 times, and the number of heads is shown. At $\alpha = 0.05$, test the null hypothesis that the coins are balanced and randomly tossed. (*Hint:* Use the binomial distribution.)

No. of heads	0	1	2	3
Frequency	3	10	17	42

19. Lottery Number Occurrences Select a three-digit lottery number over a period of 50 days. Count the number of times each digit, 0 through 9, occurs. Test the claim, at $\alpha = 0.05$, that the digits occur at random.

11–2 | Tests Using Contingency Tables ›

LO2

Use chi-square to test two variables for independence and to test proportions for homogeneity.

When qualitative data are tabulated in table form in terms of frequencies, several types of hypotheses can be tested by using the chi-square test.

Two such tests are the independence of variables test and the homogeneity of proportions test. The test of independence of variables is used to determine whether two variables are independent of or related to each other when a single sample is selected. The test of homogeneity of proportions is used to determine whether the proportions for a variable are equal when several samples are selected from different populations. Both tests use the chi-square distribution and a contingency table, and the test value is found in the same way. The independence test will be explained first.

Test for Independence

The chi-square **independence test** can be used to test the independence of two variables. For example, suppose a new postoperative procedure is administered to a number of patients in a large hospital. One can ask the question, Do the doctors feel differently about this procedure from the nurses, or do they feel basically the same way? Note that the question is not whether they prefer the procedure but whether there is a difference of opinion between the two groups.

To answer this question, a researcher selects a sample of nurses and doctors and tabulates the data in table form, as shown.

Group	Prefer new procedure	Prefer old procedure	No preference
Nurses	100	80	20
Doctors	50	120	30

As the survey indicates, 100 nurses prefer the new procedure, 80 prefer the old procedure, and 20 have no preference; 50 doctors prefer the new procedure, 120 like the old procedure, and 30 have no preference. Since the main question is whether there is a difference in opinion, the null hypothesis is stated as follows:

H_0: The opinion about the procedure is *independent* of the profession.

The alternative hypothesis is stated as follows:

H_1: The opinion about the procedure is *dependent* on the profession.

If the null hypothesis is not rejected, the test means that both professions feel basically the same way about the procedure and the differences are due to chance. If the null hypothesis is rejected, the test means that one group feels differently about the procedure from the other. Remember that rejection does *not* mean that one group favours the procedure and the other does not. Perhaps both groups favour it or both dislike it, but in different proportions.

To test the null hypothesis by using the chi-square independence test, one must compute the expected frequencies, assuming that the null hypothesis is true. These frequencies are computed by using the observed frequencies given in the table.

When data are arranged in table form for the chi-square independence test, the table is called a **contingency table.** The table is made up of R rows and C columns. The table here has two rows and three columns.

Group	Prefer new procedure	Prefer old procedure	No preference
Nurses	100	80	20
Doctors	50	120	30

Note that row and column headings do not count in determining the number of rows and columns.

A contingency table is designated as an $R \times C$ (rows by columns) table. In this case, $R = 2$ and $C = 3$; hence, this table is a 2×3 contingency table. Each block in the table is called a *cell* and is designated by its row and column position. For example, the cell with a frequency of 80 is designated as $\text{cell}_{1,2}$, or row 1, column 2. The cells are shown below.

	Column 1	Column 2	Column 3
Row 1	$\text{Cell}_{1,1}$	$\text{Cell}_{1,2}$	$\text{Cell}_{1,3}$
Row 2	$\text{Cell}_{2,1}$	$\text{Cell}_{2,2}$	$\text{Cell}_{2,3}$

The degrees of freedom for any contingency table are (rows $-$ 1) times (columns $-$ 1); that is, d.f. $= (R - 1)(C - 1)$. In this case, $(2 - 1)(3 - 1) = (1)(2) = 2$. The reason for this formula for d.f. is that all the expected values except one are free to vary in each row and in each column.

Using the previous table, one can compute the expected frequencies for each block (or cell), as shown next.

1. Find the sum of each row and each column, and find the grand total, as shown.

Group	Prefer new procedure	Prefer old procedure	No preference	Total
Nurses	100	80	20	Row 1 sum → 200
Doctors	+50	+120	+30	Row 2 sum → 200
Total	150	200	50	400
	Column 1 sum	Column 2 sum	Column 3 sum	Grand total

2. For each cell, multiply the corresponding row sum by the column sum and divide by the grand total, to get the expected value (or expected frequency):

$$\text{Expected value} = \frac{\text{Row sum} \times \text{Column sum}}{\text{Grand total}}$$

The rationale for the computation of the expected frequencies for a contingency table uses proportions. For $\text{cell}_{1,1}$ a total of 150 out of 400 people prefer the new procedure. And since there are 200 nurses, one would expect, if the null hypothesis were true, $(150/400)(200)$, or 75, of the nurses to be in favour of the new procedure.

For example, for $\text{cell}_{1,2}$, the expected value, denoted by $E_{1,2}$, is (refer to the previous tables)

$$E_{1,2} = \frac{(200)(200)}{400} = 100$$

For each cell, the expected values are computed as follows:

$$E_{1,1} = \frac{(200)(150)}{400} = 75 \quad E_{1,2} = \frac{(200)(200)}{400} = 100 \quad E_{1,3} = \frac{(200)(50)}{400} = 25$$

$$E_{2,1} = \frac{(200)(150)}{400} = 75 \quad E_{2,2} = \frac{(200)(200)}{400} = 100 \quad E_{2,3} = \frac{(200)(50)}{400} = 25$$

The expected values can now be placed in the corresponding cells along with the observed values, as shown.

Group	Prefer new procedure	Prefer old procedure	No preference	Total
Nurses	100 (75)	80 (100)	20 (25)	200
Doctors	50 (75)	120 (100)	30 (25)	200
Total	150	200	50	400

The formula for the test statistic for the independence test is the same as the one used for the goodness-of-fit test. It is

$$\chi^2 = \sum \frac{(O - E)^2}{E}$$

For the previous example, compute the $(O - E)^2/E$ values for each cell, and then find the sum.

$$\chi^2 = \sum \frac{(O - E)^2}{E}$$

$$= \frac{(100 - 75)^2}{75} + \frac{(80 - 100)^2}{100} + \frac{(20 - 25)^2}{25} + \frac{(50 - 75)^2}{75}$$

$$+ \frac{(120 - 100)^2}{100} + \frac{(30 - 25)^2}{25}$$

$$\approx 26.667$$

The final steps are to make the decision and summarize the results. This test is always a right-tailed test, and the degrees of freedom are $(R - 1)(C - 1) = (2 - 1)(3 - 1) = 2$. If $\alpha = 0.05$, the critical value from Table G is 5.991. Hence, the decision is to reject the null hypothesis, since the test statistic ($\chi^2 = 26.667$) is in the critical region. See Figure 11–7. (The P-value is also shown.)

Figure 11–7

Critical Region and Test Statistic for Postoperative Procedures Example: χ^2 Distribution (d.f. = 2)

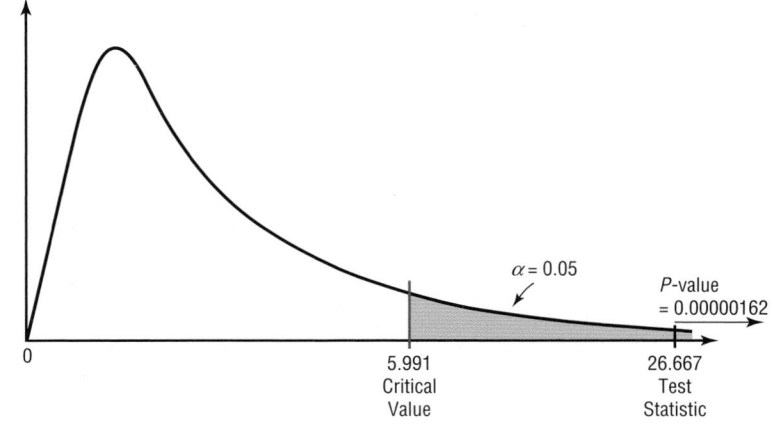

The conclusion is that there is enough evidence to support the claim that opinion is related to (dependent on) profession—that is, doctors and nurses differ in their opinions about the postoperative procedure.

P-Value Method

Using the procedures explained in Section 11–1, use Table G to determine the P-value for the doctor and nurse postoperative preference example, with d.f. $= 2$ and $\chi^2 = 21.667$. The approximate P-value obtained from Table G is to the right of $\chi^2 = 10.597$, which is less than 0.005. The exact P-value using technology is 1.620E-06 or 1.620×10^{-6}. Since the P-value (0.00000162) is less than the significance level ($\alpha = 0.05$), the decision is to reject H_0. Refer to Figure 11–7. Examples 11–4 and 11–5 illustrate the traditional and P-value methods for the chi-square test of independence.

Example 11–4

College Education and Place of Residence

A sociologist wishes to see whether the number of years of college a person has completed is related to her or his place of residence. A sample of 88 people is selected and classified as shown.

Location	No college	Four-year degree	Advanced degree	Total
Urban	15	12	8	35
Suburban	8	15	9	32
Rural	6	8	7	21
Total	29	35	24	88

At $\alpha = 0.05$, can the sociologist conclude that a person's location is dependent on the number of years of college?

Solution

Step 1 State the hypotheses and identify the claim.

H_0: The number of years of college completed is independent of a person's place of residence.

H_1: The number of years of college completed is dependent on a person's place of residence (claim).

Step 2 Find the critical value. The critical value is 9.488, since the degrees of freedom are $(3 - 1)(3 - 1) = (2)(2) = 4$.

Step 3 Compute the test statistic. To compute the test statistic, one must first compute the expected values.

$$E_{1,1} = \frac{(35)(29)}{88} = 11.53 \quad E_{1,2} = \frac{(35)(35)}{88} = 13.92 \quad E_{1,3} = \frac{(35)(24)}{88} = 9.55$$

$$E_{2,1} = \frac{(32)(29)}{88} = 10.55 \quad E_{2,2} = \frac{(32)(35)}{88} = 12.73 \quad E_{2,3} = \frac{(32)(24)}{88} = 8.73$$

$$E_{3,1} = \frac{(21)(29)}{88} = 6.92 \quad E_{3,2} = \frac{(21)(35)}{88} = 8.35 \quad E_{3,3} = \frac{(21)(24)}{88} = 5.73$$

The completed table is shown.

Location	No college	Four-year degree	Advanced degree	Total
Urban	15 (11.53)	12 (13.92)	8 (9.55)	35
Suburban	8 (10.55)	15 (12.73)	9 (8.73)	32
Rural	6 (6.92)	8 (8.35)	7 (5.73)	21
Total	29	35	24	88

Then the chi-square test statistic is

$$\chi^2 = \sum \frac{(O - E)^2}{E}$$

$$= \frac{(15 - 11.53)^2}{11.53} + \frac{(12 - 13.92)^2}{13.92} + \frac{(8 - 9.55)^2}{9.55}$$

$$+ \frac{(8 - 10.55)^2}{10.55} + \frac{(15 - 12.73)^2}{12.73} + \frac{(9 - 8.73)^2}{8.73}$$

$$+ \frac{(6 - 6.92)^2}{6.92} + \frac{(8 - 8.35)^2}{8.35} + \frac{(7 - 5.73)^2}{5.73} \approx 3.006$$

Step 4   Make the decision. At $\alpha = 0.05$, the decision is to not reject the null hypothesis, since the test statistic ($\chi^2 = 3.006$) is not in the critical region, as shown in Figure 11–8. (The P-value is also shown.)

Figure 11–8

Critical Region and Test Statistic for Example 11–4: χ^2 Distribution (d.f. = 4)

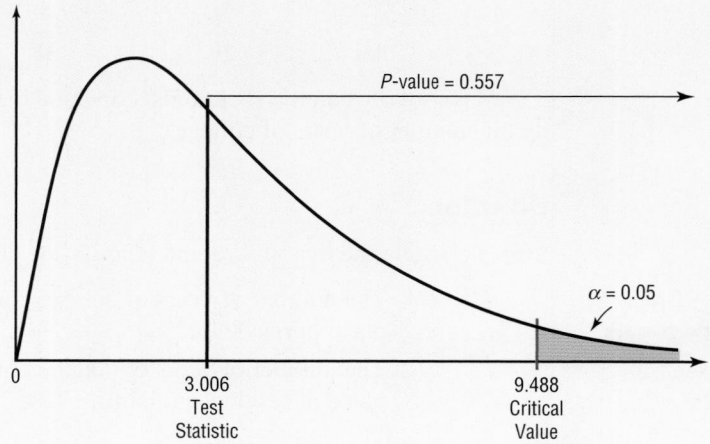

Step 5   Summarize the results. There is not enough evidence to support the claim that a person's place of residence is dependent on the number of years of college completed.

P-Value Method

Refer to Table G in Appendix C to approximate the P-value for Example 11–4, with d.f. = 4 and a test statistic $\chi^2 = 3.006$. The test statistic is between the critical values 1.064 (0.90) and 7.779 (0.10). The exact P-value using technology is 0.557. Since the P-value (0.557) > significance level ($\alpha = 0.05$), do not reject H_0.

| Example 11–5 | **Alcohol and Gender** |

A researcher wants to determine whether there is a relationship between the gender of an individual and the amount of alcohol consumed. A sample of 68 people is selected, and the following data are obtained. Use the *P*-value method.

Alcohol consumption

Gender	Low	Moderate	High	Total
Male	10	9	8	27
Female	13	16	12	41
Total	23	25	20	68

At $\alpha = 0.10$, can the researcher conclude that alcohol consumption is related to gender?

Solution

Step 1 State the hypotheses and identify the claim.

H_0: The amount of alcohol that a person consumes is independent of the individual's gender.

H_1: The amount of alcohol that a person consumes is dependent on the individual's gender (claim).

Step 2 Compute the test statistic. First, compute the expected values.

$$E_{1,1} = \frac{(27)(23)}{68} = 9.13 \quad E_{1,2} = \frac{(27)(25)}{68} = 9.93 \quad E_{1,3} = \frac{(27)(20)}{68} = 7.94$$

$$E_{2,1} = \frac{(41)(23)}{68} = 13.87 \quad E_{2,2} = \frac{(41)(25)}{68} = 15.07 \quad E_{2,3} = \frac{(41)(20)}{68} = 12.06$$

The completed table is shown.

Alcohol consumption

Gender	Low	Moderate	High	Total
Male	10 (9.13)	9 (9.93)	8 (7.94)	27
Female	13 (13.87)	16 (15.07)	12 (12.06)	41
Total	23	25	20	68

Then the test statistic is

$$\chi^2 = \sum \frac{(O - E)^2}{E}$$
$$= \frac{(10 - 9.13)^2}{9.13} + \frac{(9 - 9.93)^2}{9.93} + \frac{(8 - 7.94)^2}{7.94}$$
$$+ \frac{(13 - 13.87)^2}{13.87} + \frac{(16 - 15.07)^2}{15.07} + \frac{(12 - 12.06)^2}{12.06}$$
$$\approx 0.283$$

Step 3 Find the *P*-value.

The *P*-value, obtained from Table G in Appendix C, for the test statistic, $\chi^2 = 0.283$, with d.f. = 2 is between 0.90 and 0.10. See Figure 11–9.

Figure 11–9

Finding the P-Value

P-value is between 0.90 and 0.10

Degrees of Freedom	0.995	0.99	0.975	0.95	0.90	0.10	0.05	0.025	0.01	0.005
1	0.000	0.000	0.001	0.004	0.016	2.706	3.841	5.024	6.635	7.879
2	0.010	0.020	0.051	0.103	0.211	4.605	5.991	7.378	9.210	10.597
3	0.072	0.115	0.216	0.352	0.584	6.251	7.815	9.348	11.345	12.838
4	0.207	0.297	0.484	0.711	1.064	7.779	9.486	11.143	13.277	14.860

Test statistic is 0.283

Note: The P-value obtained from statistical software, spreadsheet, or calculator is 0.869.

Step 4   Make the decision. The decision is to fail to reject the null hypothesis, since the P-value (0.869) is greater than the significance level ($\alpha = 0.10$) as shown in Figure 11–10. (The critical value is also shown.)

Figure 11–10

Critical Region and P-Value for Example 11–5: χ^2 Distribution (d.f. = 2)

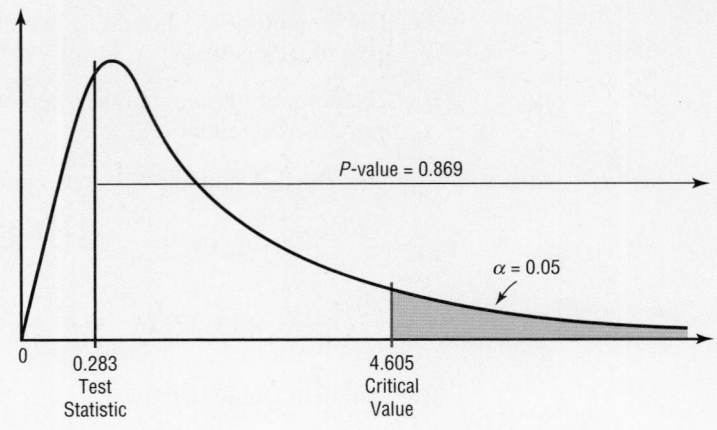

P-value = 0.869

$\alpha = 0.05$

0   0.283
Test
Statistic

4.605
Critical
Value

Step 5   Summarize the results.

There is not enough evidence to support the claim that the amount of alcohol a person consumes is dependent on the individual's gender.

Traditional Method

The critical value for $\alpha = 0.10$, d.f. $= (2 - 1)(3 - 1) = 2$, is 4.605. Fail to reject the null hypothesis, since the test statistic ($\chi^2 = 0.283$) < critical value ($\chi^2 = 4.605$), as shown in Figure 11–10.

Test for Homogeneity of Proportions

The second chi-square test that uses a contingency table is called the **homogeneity of proportions test.** In this situation, samples are selected from several different populations, and the researcher is interested in determining whether the proportions of elements that have a common characteristic are the same for each population. The sample sizes are specified in advance, making either the row totals or column totals in the contingency table known before the samples are selected. For example, a researcher may select a sample of 50 freshmen, 50 sophomores, 50 juniors, and 50 seniors and then find the proportion of students who are smokers in each level. The researcher will then compare the proportions for each group to see if they are equal. The hypotheses in this case would be

$H_0: p_1 = p_2 = p_3 = p_4$

H_1: At least one proportion is different from the others.

If one does not reject the null hypothesis, it can be assumed that the proportions are equal and the differences in them are due to chance. Hence, the proportion of students who smoke is the same for grade levels freshmen through senior. When the null hypothesis is rejected, it can be assumed that the proportions are not all equal. The computational procedure is the same as that for the test of independence shown in Example 11–6.

Example 11–6	**Lost Luggage on Airline Flights** 🛫

A researcher selected 100 passengers from each of three airlines and asked them if the airline had lost their luggage on their last flight. The data are shown in the table. At $\alpha = 0.05$, test the claim that the proportion of passengers from each airline who lost luggage on the flight is the same for each airline.

	Airline 1	Airline 2	Airline 3	Total
Yes	10	7	4	21
No	90	93	96	279
	100	100	100	300

Solution

Step 1   State the hypotheses.

$H_0: p_1 = p_2 = p_3$ (claim)

H_1: At least one proportion is different from the others.

Step 2   Find the critical value. The formula for the degrees of freedom is the same as before: (rows $-$ 1)(columns $-$ 1) $= (2 - 1)(3 - 1) = 1(2) = 2$. The critical value is 5.991.

Step 3   Compute the test statistic. First, compute the expected values.

$$E_{1,1} = \frac{(21)(100)}{300} = 7 \qquad E_{1,2} = \frac{(21)(100)}{300} = 7 \qquad E_{1,3} = \frac{(21)(100)}{300} = 7$$

$$E_{2,1} = \frac{(279)(100)}{300} = 93 \qquad E_{2,2} = \frac{(279)(100)}{300} = 93 \qquad E_{2,3} = \frac{(279)(100)}{300} = 93$$

The completed table is shown here.

	Airline 1	Airline 2	Airline 3	Total
Yes	10 (7)	7 (7)	4 (7)	21
No	90 (93)	93 (93)	96 (93)	279
	100	100	100	300

The test statistic is

$$\chi^2 = \sum \frac{(O - E)^2}{E}$$

$$= \frac{(10 - 7)^2}{7} + \frac{(7 - 7)^2}{7} + \frac{(4 - 7)^2}{7} + \frac{(90 - 93)^2}{93} + \frac{(93 - 93)^2}{93}$$

$$+ \frac{(96 - 93)^2}{93} \approx 2.765$$

Step 4   Make the decision. At $\alpha = 0.05$, the decision is to not reject the null hypothesis, since the test statistic ($\chi^2 = 2.765$) < critical value ($\chi^2 = 5.991$).

Step 5   Summarize the results. There is not enough evidence to reject the claim that the proportions of lost luggage are the same for each airline.

P-Value Method

Refer to Table G to approximate the P-value for Example 11–6 with d.f. = 2 and a test statistic $\chi^2 = 2.765$. The test statistic is between the critical values 0.211 (0.90) and 4.605 (0.10). The exact P-value using technology is 0.251. Since the P-value (0.251) > significance level ($\alpha = 0.05$), do not reject H_0.

When the degrees of freedom for a contingency table are equal to 1—that is, the table is a 2×2 table—some statisticians suggest using the *Yates correction for continuity*. The formula for the test is then

$$\chi^2 = \sum \frac{(|O - E| - 0.5)^2}{E}$$

Since the chi-square test is already conservative, most statisticians agree that the Yates correction is not necessary. (See Exercise 33 in Exercises 11–2.)

The steps for the chi-square independence and homogeneity tests are summarized in this Procedure Table.

Procedure Table

The Chi-Square Independence and Homogeneity Tests (Traditional Method)

Step 1   State the hypotheses and identify the claim.

Step 2   Find the critical value in the right tail. Use Table G.

Step 3   Compute the test statistic. To compute the test statistic, first find the expected values. For each cell of the contingency table, use the formula

$$E = \frac{(\text{Row sum})(\text{Column sum})}{\text{Grand total}}$$

to get the expected value. To find the test statistic, use the formula

$$\chi^2 = \sum \frac{(O - E)^2}{E}$$

Step 4   Make the decision.

Step 5   Summarize the results.

The assumptions for the two chi-square tests are given next.

Assumptions for the Chi-Square Independence and Homogeneity Tests

1. The data are obtained from a random sample.
2. The expected value in each cell must be 5 or more.

If the expected values are not 5 or more, combine categories.

11–2 Applying the Concepts

Satellite Dishes in Restricted Areas

Should satellite dishes be allowed in environmentally sensitive or deed-restricted areas? An opinion poll was taken to see if how a person felt about satellite dish restrictions was related to his or her age. A chi-square test was run, creating the following computer-generated information.

Degrees of freedom d.f. = 6
Test statistic χ^2 = 61.25
Critical value = 12.6
P-value = 0.00 $(2.5 \| E^{-11})$
Significance level = 0.05

	18–29	30–49	50–64	65 and up
For	96 (79.5)	96 (79.5)	90 (79.5)	36 (79.5)
Against	201 (204.75)	189 (204.75)	195 (204.75)	234 (204.75)
Don't know	3 (15.75)	15 (15.75)	15 (15.75)	30 (15.75)

1. Which number from the output is compared to the significance level to check if the null hypothesis should be rejected?
2. Which number from the output gives the probability of a type I error that is calculated from your sample data?
3. Was a right-, left-, or two-tailed test run? Why?
4. Can you tell how many rows and columns there were by looking at the degrees of freedom?
5. Does increasing the sample size change the degrees of freedom?
6. What are your conclusions? Look at the observed and expected frequencies in the table to draw some of your own specific conclusions about response and age.
7. What would your conclusions be if the level of significance was initially set at 0.10?
8. Does chi-square tell you which cell's observed and expected frequencies are significantly different?

See page 533 for the answers.

Exercises 11–2

1. How is the chi-square independence test similar to the goodness-of-fit test? How is it different?

2. How are the degrees of freedom computed for the independence test?

3. Generally, how would the null and alternative hypotheses be stated for the chi-square independence test?

4. What is the name of the table used in the independence test?

5. How are the expected values computed for each cell in the table?

6. Explain how the chi-square independence test differs from the chi-square homogeneity of proportions test.

7. How are the null and alternative hypotheses stated for the test of homogeneity of proportions?

For Exercises 8 through 31, perform the following steps.

   a. State the hypotheses and identify the claim.
   b. Find the critical value.
   c. Compute the test statistic.
   d. Make the decision.
   e. Summarize the results.

Use the traditional method of hypothesis testing unless otherwise specified.

8. **Joggers and Supplements** A study is conducted as to whether there is a relationship between joggers and the consumption of nutritional supplements. A random sample of 210 subjects is selected, and they are classified as shown. At $\alpha = 0.05$, test the claim that jogging and the consumption of supplements are not related. Why might supplement manufacturers use the results of this study?

Jogging status	Daily	Weekly	As needed
Joggers	34	52	23
Nonjoggers	18	65	18

9. **Endangered or Threatened Species** Can you conclude that a relationship exists between the class of vertebrate and whether it is endangered or threatened? Use the 0.05 level of significance. Is there a different result for the 0.01 level of significance?

	Mammal	Bird	Reptile	Amphibian	Fish
Endangered	68	76	14	13	76
Threatened	13	15	23	10	61

Source: Infoplease: www.infoplease.com.

10. **Military Status and Armed Forces Branch** This table lists the number of military personnel by status (full-time active duty or primary reserves) in each branch of the Canadian Forces. At $\alpha = 0.05$, is there sufficient evidence to conclude that a relationship exists between military personnel status and branch of the Canadian Forces?

	Active	Reserve
Army	33,000	24,000
Navy	11,200	4,200
Air Force	19,400	2,300

Source: Department of National Defence.

11. **Member of Parliament and Province** Is the composition of the House of Commons related to the province of the member of Parliament? Use $\alpha = 0.05$.

	Conservative	Liberal	New Democrat
British Columbia	18	8	10
Manitoba	8	3	3
Ontario	41	53	12
New Brunswick	3	6	1

Source: Parliament of Canada.

12. **Age Group and Residence** Is the population by age group related to the province/territory where the people reside? Use $\alpha = 0.05$. (Population values are in thousands.)

	0 to 14	15 to 64	65 and older
NL	76.0	357.7	75.2
NS	141.0	649.2	147.9
SK	195.5	682.7	151.9
NWT	9.4	31.7	2.3

Source: Statistics Canada, Summary Tables, "Population by Sex and Age Group, by Province and Territory (number, both sexes)," March 9, 2010.

13. **Occupations of Members of Parliament** It is always interesting to see what occupations elected members of the House of Commons hold in private life. Can it be concluded that the parliamentary session and the occupations of the members of Parliament are dependent? Use $\alpha = 0.05$.

	Parliamentary session		
Members' occupation fields	36th	38th	40th
Arts & Culture	16	19	13
Business & Finance	130	134	141
Health	10	9	9
Professional	125	119	123
Science & Technology	13	12	11
Trades & Related	25	26	24

Source: Parliament of Canada, Members of the House of Commons, "Comparative Table of Main Occupations by Category in the House of Commons."

14. **Information Gathering and Educational Background** An instructor wishes to see if the way people obtain information is independent of their educational background. A survey of 400 high school and college graduates yielded this information. At $\alpha = 0.05$, test the claim that the way people obtain information is independent of their educational background.

	Television	Newspapers	Other sources
High school	159	90	51
College	27	42	31

Source: USA TODAY.

15. **Gender and Legal Practice** A study was conducted to see if there was a relationship between the gender of a lawyer and the type of practice he or she is engaged in. A sample of 240 lawyers was selected, and the results are shown. At $\alpha = 0.05$, can it be assumed that gender and employment are independent?

Gender	Private practice	Law firm	Government
Male	112	16	12
Female	64	18	18

16. **Organ Transplantation** Listed below is information regarding organ transplantation in Canada for three different years. Based on these data, is there sufficient evidence at $\alpha = 0.01$ to conclude that a relationship exists between year and type of transplant?

Year	Kidney	Heart	Liver	Lung
2006	1150	178	466	171
2007	1185	163	480	187
2008	1186	164	453	165

Source: Canadian Institute for Health Information, Canadian Organ Replacement Register.

17. **Movie Rental and Age** A study is being conducted to determine whether the age of the customer is related to the type of movie he or she rents. A sample of renters gives the data shown here. At $\alpha = 0.10$, is the type of movie selected related to the customer's age?

Age	Type of movie		
	Documentary	**Comedy**	**Mystery**
12–20	14	9	8
21–29	15	14	9
30–38	9	21	39
39–47	7	22	17
48 and over	6	38	12

18. Music Sales by Genre and Year The Canadian recording industry music sales data, in thousands, for consecutive years and most popular genres is shown below. At $\alpha = 0.05$, are the sales by music genre related to the year in which the sales occurred?

Year	Alternative	Metal	Country	R & B
2008	6670	4338	2687	3014
2009	6108	3377	2990	2918

Source: Nielsen SoundScan, *Nielsen Company and Billboard 2009 Canadian Industry Report,* "Canadian Album Sales Down 2.2% in 2009."

19. Ballpark Snack and Gender A survey at a ballpark shows this selection of snacks purchased. At $\alpha = 0.10$, is the snack chosen independent of the gender of the consumer?

Gender	Snack		
	Hot dog	**Peanuts**	**Popcorn**
Male	12	21	19
Female	13	8	25

20. New Drug Effectiveness To test the effectiveness of a new drug, a researcher gives one group of individuals the new drug and another group a placebo. The results of the study are shown here. At $\alpha = 0.10$, can the researcher conclude that the drug is effective? Use the *P*-value method.

Medication	Effective	Not effective
Drug	32	9
Placebo	12	18

21. Recreational Reading and Gender A book publisher wishes to determine whether there is a difference in the type of book selected by males and females for recreational reading. A random sample provides the data given here. At $\alpha = 0.05$, test the claim that the type of book selected is independent of the gender of the individual. Use the *P*-value method.

Gender	Type of book		
	Mystery	**Romance**	**Self-help**
Male	243	201	191
Female	135	149	202

22. Signed Donor Cards and Region Environics Research Group has reported that 54% of Canadian health-care professionals have signed an organ donor card. A researcher surveys 50 randomly selected Canadian drivers in the health-care profession in each of three regions to determine the percentage who have signed an organ donor card. The results are shown here. At $\alpha = 0.01$, test the claim that the proportion of those who have signed donor cards is equal in all three regions.

Donor card	Region A	Region B	Region C
Signed	19	27	24
Not signed	31	23	26

Source: Canadian Council for Donation and Transplantation (CCDT).

23. Obesity in District Schools Statistics Canada reports that 23% of Canadians are obese. A physical educator wants to determine if the school district's students have the same percentage as the national average. Measurements for obesity (20% for males, 25% for females over ideal weight), are taken at four district schools. The results are shown here. At $\alpha = 0.05$, test the claim that the proportions who are obese in each district are equal.

	West	East	South	North
Obese	22	28	20	24
Not obese	98	92	100	96

Source: Statistics Canada.

24. Market Research Survey Participation An advertising firm has decided to ask 92 randomly selected individuals to fill out a brief survey related to their shopping experience in three shopping malls. According to previous reports, 33% of Canadians refuse to participate in surveys. The results are shown here. At $\alpha = 0.01$, test the claim that the proportion of those who are willing to participate in each mall are equal.

	Mall A	Mall B	Mall C
Will participate	52	45	36
Will not participate	40	47	56

Source: Statistics Canada.

25. Education Level and Low-Paid Workers A researcher wishes to see if the proportions of low-paid workers based on education level have changed during the last 20 years. A sample of 100 workers is selected, and the results are shown. At $\alpha = 0.05$, test the claim that the proportions have not changed.

Education level	Less than high school	High school diploma	Post-secondary certificate	University degree
20 years ago	22	17	12	6
Now	26	21	14	7

Source: Statistics Canada.

26. Mothers Working Outside the Home According to a recent survey, 59% of the population aged 8 to 17 would prefer that their mothers work outside the home, regardless of what she does now. A school district psychologist decided to select 3 samples of 60 students each in elementary, middle, and high school to see how the students in her district felt about the issue. At $\alpha = 0.10$, test the claim that the proportions of the students who prefer that their mothers have a job are equal.

	Elementary	Middle	High
Prefers mother work	29	38	51
Prefers mother not work	31	22	9

Source: Daniel Weiss, 100% American.

27. **Volunteer Practice of Students** The Bureau of Labour Statistics reported information on volunteers by selected characteristics. They found that 24.4% of the population aged 16 to 24 volunteers a median number of 36 hours per year. A survey of 75 students in each age group revealed the following data on volunteer practices. At $\alpha = 0.05$, can it be concluded that the proportions of volunteers are the same for each group?

	Age				
	18	**19**	**20**	**21**	**22**
Yes (volunteer)	19	18	23	31	13
No	56	57	52	44	62

Source: Time Almanac.

28. **Early Childhood Learning** A survey on Canadian attitudes toward learning reports that 67% of parents of young children use some form of child care on a regular basis. A researcher surveyed 300 parents in adjacent regions and asked if they used child care for their young children. The results are shown here. At $\alpha = 0.05$, is there enough evidence to reject the claim that the proportions of those who use child care are the same?

	Region			
	A	**B**	**C**	**D**
Child care	55	46	51	49
No child care	20	29	24	26

Source: Canadian Council on Learning, 2008 Survey of Canadian Attitudes toward Learning: Results for Learning throughout the Lifespan.

29. **Playground Injuries** A national Canadian survey of children's playground injuries indicated that 20% of injuries resulted in a medical visit. An insurance investigator wants to show that the proportion of playground injuries requiring a medical visit is the same across the country. Four regions are sampled with the results shown in the table below. At $\alpha = 0.05$, test the claim that the proportions are the same. Use the P-value method.

	West	Prairies	Central	Atlantic
Medical visit	7	8	4	6
No medical visit	23	22	26	24

Source: Calgary Health Region.

30. **Ban on Sunday Shopping** In 2004, 55% of Nova Scotians voted to prohibit "big stores" from opening on Sundays. In 2006, the Supreme Court of Canada sided with two grocery chains to allow Sunday shopping. Nova Scotians have strong opinions on this issue. An advocate for workers' rights wants to show that all regions of Nova Scotia are equally in favour of a ban on Sunday shopping. Four regions are selected and 125 potential shoppers are surveyed. The results are shown below. At $\alpha = 0.10$, test the claim that the proportions of Nova Scotians in favour of maintaining the ban on Sunday openings is equal in each region. Use the P-value method.

	Region 1	Region 2	Region 3	Region 4
In favour of ban	66	70	56	63
Not in favour of ban	59	55	69	62

Source: CBC.ca.

31. **Grocery Lists** The vice-president of a large supermarket chain wished to determine if her customers made a list before going grocery shopping. She surveyed 288 customers in three stores. The results are shown here. At $\alpha = 0.10$, test the claim that the proportions of the customers in the three stores who made a list before going shopping are equal.

	Store A	Store B	Store C
Made list	77	74	68
No list	19	22	28

Source: Daniel Weiss, 100% American.

Extending the Concepts »

32. For a 2 × 2 table, a, b, c, and d are the observed values for each cell, as shown.

a	b
c	d

The chi-square test value can be computed as

$$\chi^2 = \frac{n(ad - bc)^2}{(a + b)(a + c)(c + d)(b + d)}$$

where $n = a + b + c + d$. Compute the χ^2 test statistic by using the above formula and the formula $\Sigma(O - E)^2/E$, and compare the results for the following table.

12	15
9	23

33. For the contingency table shown in Exercise 32, compute the chi-square test statistic by using the Yates correction for continuity.

34. When the chi-square test value is significant and there is a relationship between the variables, the strength of this relationship can be measured by using the *contingency coefficient*. The formula for the contingency coefficient is

$$C = \sqrt{\frac{\chi^2}{\chi^2 + n}}$$

where χ^2 is the test statistic and n is the sum of frequencies of the cells. The contingency coefficient will always be less than 1. Compute the contingency coefficient for Exercises 8 and 20.

Speaking of Statistics

Does Colour Affect Your Appetite?

It has been suggested that colour is related to appetite in humans. For example, if the walls in a restaurant are painted certain colours, it is thought that the customer will eat more food. A study was done at the University of Illinois and the University of Pennsylvania. When people were given six varieties of jellybeans mixed in a bowl or separated by colour, they ate about twice as many from the bowl with the mixed jellybeans as from the bowls that were separated by colour.

It is thought that when the jellybeans were mixed, people felt that it offered a greater variety of choices, and the variety of choices increased their appetites.

In this case one variable—colour—is categorical, and the other variable—amount of jellybeans eaten—is numerical. Could a chi-square goodness-of-fit test be used here? If so, suggest how it could be set up.

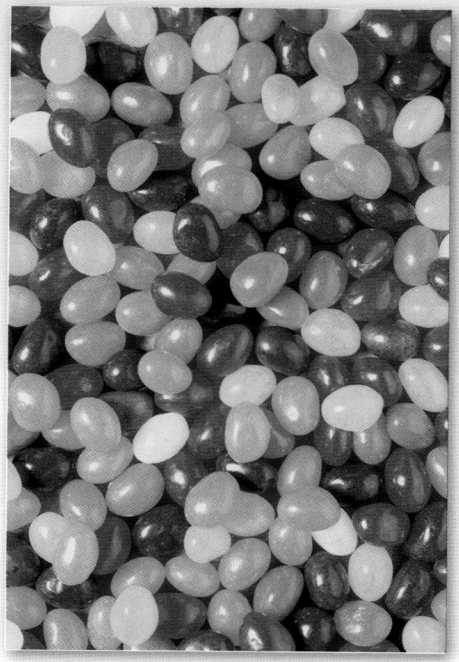

Summary >

Three uses of the chi-square distribution were explained in this chapter. It can be used as a goodness-of-fit test to determine whether the frequencies of a distribution are the same as the hypothesized frequencies. For example, is the number of defective parts produced by a factory the same each day? This test is always a right-tailed test.

The test of independence is used to determine whether two variables are related or are independent. This test uses a contingency table and is always a right-tailed test. An example of its use is a test to determine whether the attitudes of urban residents about the recycling of trash differ from the attitudes of rural residents.

Finally, the homogeneity of proportions test is used to determine if several proportions are all equal when samples are selected from different populations.

The chi-square distribution is also used for other types of statistical hypothesis tests, such as the Kruskal-Wallis test, which is explained in Chapter 13.

For step-by-step guidance on the use of Texas Instruments TI-83 Plus/TI-84 Plus programmable calculators, see Appendix E at the back of this book. For summary procedures for Minitab, SPSS, and Excel, please see the full version of Appendix E on *Connect*.

Important Terms »

contingency table 515

expected frequency 505

goodness-of-fit test 505

homogeneity
of proportions test 520

independence test 514

observed frequency 505

Important Formulas »

Formula for the chi-square test for goodness of fit:

$$\chi^2 = \sum \frac{(O - E)^2}{E}$$

with degrees of freedom equal to the number of categories minus 1 and where

O = **observed frequency**

E = **expected frequency**

Formula for the chi-square independence and homogeneity of proportions tests:

$$\chi^2 = \sum \frac{(O - E)^2}{E}$$

with degrees of freedom equal to (rows − 1) times (columns − 1). Formula for the expected value for each cell:

$$E = \frac{(\textbf{row sum})(\textbf{column sum})}{\textbf{grand total}}$$

Mc Graw Hill connect™ Practise and learn online with *Connect* with data sets and algorithmic questions related to concepts covered in this chapter. Questions and tables with online data sets are marked with 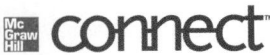.

Review Exercises »

For Exercises 1 through 10, follow these steps.

   a. State the hypotheses and identify the claim.
   b. Find the critical value(s).
   c. Compute the test statistic.
   d. Make the decision.
   e. Summarize the results.

Use the traditional method of hypothesis testing unless otherwise specified.

  1. Favourite Shopping Day A storeowner wishes to see if people have a favourite day of the week to shop. A

sample of 400 people is selected, and each is asked his or her preference. The data are shown. At $\alpha = 0.05$, test the claim that shoppers have no preference. Give one example of how retail merchants would be able to use the numbers in this study.

Day	Sun.	Mon.	Tues.	Wed.	Thurs.	Fri.	Sat.
Number	28	16	20	26	74	96	140

Source: Based on information from the International Mass Retail Association.

  2. Marital Status A researcher reads that the marital status of Canadian adults is distributed as follows: married,

48%; single, 42%; widowed 5%; divorced 5%. She selects a sample of 150 people, and the results are shown. At $\alpha = 0.01$, can it be concluded that marital status is distributed as she has read? Give one factor that might influence the results of this study.

Marital status	Married	Single	Widowed	Divorced
Number	64	79	3	4

Source: Statistics Canada.

3. **Tire Labelling** The federal government has proposed labelling tires by fuel efficiency to save fuel and cut emissions. A survey was taken to see who would use these labels. At $\alpha = 0.10$, is the gender of the individual related to whether or not a person would use these labels? The data from a sample are shown here.

Gender	Yes	No	Undecided
Men	114	30	6
Women	136	16	8

Source: USA TODAY.

4. **Gun Sale Denial** A police investigator read that the reasons why gun sales to applicants were denied were distributed as follows: criminal history of felonies, 75%; domestic violence conviction, 11%; and drug abuse, fugitive, etc., 14%. A sample of applicants in a large study who were refused sales is obtained and is distributed as follows. At $\alpha = 0.10$, can it be concluded that the distribution is as stated? Do you think the results might be different in a rural area?

Reason	Criminal history	Domestic violence	Drug abuse, etc.
Number	120	42	38

Source: Based on FBI statistics.

5. **Colour Distribution of M&M's** According to the manufacturer, M&M's are produced and distributed in the following proportions: 13% brown, 13% red, 14% yellow, 16% green, 20% orange, and 24% blue. A randomly selected 47.9-gram bag was opened and it was found to contain the following: 9 brown, 10 red, 11 yellow, 16 green, 5 orange, and 4 blue M&M's. Based on this sample, is there sufficient evidence to conclude that the proportions differ from those stated by the candy company? Use $\alpha = 0.05$.
Source: Mars, Inc.

6. **Car Type and Purchaser Gender** A car manufacturer wishes to determine whether the type of car purchased is related to the individual's gender. The data obtained from a sample are shown here. At $\alpha = 0.01$, is the gender of the purchaser related to the type of car purchased?

Gender of purchaser	Type of vehicle purchased			
	Sedan	Compact	Station wagon	SUV
Male	33	27	23	17
Female	21	34	41	18

Statistics Today

Statistics and Heredity–Revisited

Using probability, Mendel predicted the following:

	Smooth		Wrinkled	
	Yellow	Green	Yellow	Green
Expected	0.5625	0.1875	0.1875	0.0625

The observed results were these:

	Smooth		Wrinkled	
	Yellow	Green	Yellow	Green
Observed	0.5666	0.1942	0.1816	0.0556

Using chi-square tests on the data, Mendel found that his predictions were accurate in most cases (i.e., a good fit), thus supporting his theory. He reported many highly successful experiments. Mendel's genetic theory is simple but useful in predicting the results of hybridization.

A Fly in the Ointment

Although Mendel's theory is basically correct, an English statistician named R. A. Fisher examined Mendel's data some 50 years later. He found that the observed (actual) results agreed too closely with the expected (theoretical) results and concluded that the data had in some way been falsified. The results were too good to be true. Several explanations have been proposed, ranging from deliberate misinterpretation to an assistant's error, but no one can be sure how this happened.

7. **Employment of High School Females** A guidance counsellor wants to determine if the proportions of high school girls in his school district who have jobs are equal to the national average of 36%. He surveys 80 female students, ages 16 through 18, to determine if they work or not. The results are shown. At $\alpha = 0.01$, test the claim that the proportions of girls who work are equal. Use the P-value method.

	16-year-olds	17-year-olds	18-year-olds
Work	45	31	38
Don't work	35	49	42

Source: Michael D. Shook and Robert L. Shook, *The Book of Odds.*

8. **Risk of Injury** The risk of injury is higher for males compared to females (57% versus 43%). A hospital emergency room supervisor wishes to determine if the proportions of injuries to males in his hospital are the same for each of four months. He surveys 100 injuries treated in his ER for each month. The results are shown here. At $\alpha = 0.05$, can he reject the claim that the proportions of injuries for males are equal for each of the four months?

	May	June	July	August
Male	51	47	58	63
Female	49	53	42	37

Source: Michael D. Shook and Robert L. Shook, *The Book of Odds.*

9. **Anger Management** A researcher surveyed 50 randomly selected subjects in four cities and asked if they felt that their anger was the most difficult behaviour to control. The results are shown. At $\alpha = 0.10$, is there enough evidence to reject the claim that the proportion of those who felt this way in each city is the same?

	City A	City B	City C	City D
Yes	12	15	10	21
No	38	35	40	29

10. **Bill Payment** A researcher surveyed 50 randomly selected males and 50 randomly selected females to see how they paid their bills. The data are shown. At $\alpha = 0.01$, test the claim that the proportions are not equal. What might be a reason for the difference, if one exists?

	Type of payment		
	Cheques	**Online**	**In person**
Males	27	15	8
Females	22	19	9

Source: Based on information from Gallup.

Data Analysis »

The databank for these questions can be found in Appendix D at the back of the textbook and on ▓ **connect**.

1. Select a sample of 40 individuals from the databank. Use the chi-square goodness-of-fit test to see if the marital status of individuals is equally distributed.

2. Use the chi-square test of independence to test the hypothesis that smoking is independent of gender. Use a sample of at least 75 people.

3. Using the data from Data Set X in Appendix D, classify the data as 1–3, 4–6, 7–9, etc. Use the chi-square goodness-of-fit test to see if the number of times each ball is drawn is equally distributed.

Chapter Quiz »

Determine whether each statement is true or false. If the statement is false, explain why.

1. The chi-square test of independence is always two-tailed.

2. The test statistics for the chi-square goodness-of-fit test and the independence test are computed by using the same formula.

3. When the null hypothesis is rejected in the goodness-of-fit test, it means there is close agreement between the observed and expected frequencies.

Select the best answer.

4. The values of the chi-square variable cannot be

   a. Positive   c. Negative
   b. 0   d. None of the above

5. The null hypothesis for the chi-square test of independence is that the variables are

   a. Dependent   c. Related
   b. Independent   d. Always 0

6. The degrees of freedom for the goodness-of-fit test are

a. 0
b. 1
c. Sample size -1
d. Number of categories -1

Complete the following statements with the best answer.

7. The degrees of freedom for a 4×3 contingency table are _____.

8. An important assumption for the chi-square test is that the observations must be _____.

9. The chi-square goodness-of-fit test is always _____ tailed.

10. In the chi-square independence test, the expected frequency for each class must always be _____.

For Exercises 11 through 19, follow these steps.

a. State the hypotheses and identify the claim.
b. Find the critical value.
c. Compute the test statistic.
d. Make the decision.
e. Summarize the results.

Use the traditional method of hypothesis testing unless otherwise specified.

11. Job Loss Reasons A survey of why people lost their jobs produced the following results. At $\alpha = 0.05$, test the claim that the number of responses is equally distributed. Do you think the results might be different if the study was done 10 years ago?

Reason	Company closing	Position abolished	Insufficient work
Number	26	18	28

Source: Based on information from U.S. Department of Labor.

12. Consumption of Takeout Foods A food service manager read that the place where people consumed takeout food is distributed as follows: home, 53%; car, 19%; work, 14%; other, 14%. A survey of 300 individuals showed the following results. At $\alpha = 0.01$, can it be concluded that the distribution is as stated? Where would a fast-food restaurant want to target its advertisements?

Place	Home	Car	Work	Other
Number	142	57	51	50

Source: Beef Industry Council.

13. Shopping Channel Viewers A survey found that 62% of the respondents stated that they never watched the home shopping channels on cable television, 23% stated that they watched the channels rarely, 11% stated that they watched them occasionally, and 4% stated that they watched them frequently. A group of 200 college students was surveyed, and 105 stated that they never watched the home shopping channels, 72 stated that they watched them rarely, 13 stated that they watched them occasionally, and 10 stated that they watched them frequently. At $\alpha = 0.05$, can it be concluded that the college students differ in their preference for the home shopping channels?

Source: Based on information obtained from *USA TODAY* Snapshots.

14. Commuting to Work The 2006 census reported the following percentages for mode of transportation to work for Canadian workers over 15 years of age.

Motor vehicle (driver)	72.3
Motor vehicle (passenger)	7.7
Public transit	11.1
Walked	6.4
Bicycled	1.3
Other	1.2

A survey in a census metropolitan area (CMA) found that 345 drove their vehicles, 38 were vehicle passengers, 78 took public transit, 27 walked, 7 rode their bicycles and 5 used other transportation methods to commute to work. Is there sufficient evidence to conclude that the proportions of workers using each type of transportation in the CMA differ from those in the census report? Use $\alpha = 0.05$.

Source: Statistics Canada, *2006 Census: Data Products*, "Topic-Based Tabulations: Mode of Transportation."

15. Favourite Ice Cream Flavours A survey of women and men asked what their favourite ice cream flavour was. The results are shown. At $\alpha = 0.05$, can it be concluded that the favourite flavour is independent of gender?

	Flavour			
	Vanilla	Chocolate	Strawberry	Other
Women	62	36	10	2
Men	49	37	5	9

16. Types of Pizzas Purchased A pizza shop owner wishes to determine if the type of pizza a person selects is related to the age of the individual. The data obtained from a sample are shown here. At $\alpha = 0.10$, is the age of the purchaser related to the type of pizza ordered? Use the *P*-value method.

	Type of pizza			
Age	Plain	Pepperoni	Mushroom	Double cheese
10–19	12	21	39	71
20–29	18	76	52	87
30–39	24	50	40	47
40–49	52	30	12	28

17. Pennant Colours Purchased A survey at a ballpark shows the following selection of pennants sold to fans. The data are presented here. At $\alpha = 0.10$, is the colour of the pennant purchased independent of the gender of the individual?

	Blue	Yellow	Red
Men	519	659	876
Women	487	702	787

18. Tax Credit Refunds In a survey of children ages 8 through 11, these data were obtained as to what their parents should do with the money from a $400 tax credit.

	Keep it for themselves	Give it to their children	Don't know
Girls	162	132	6
Boys	147	147	6

At $\alpha = 0.10$, is there a relationship between the feelings of the children and the gender of the children?

Source: Based on information from *USA TODAY* Snapshot.

19. Employment Satisfaction A survey of 60 men and 60 women asked if they would be happy spending the rest of their careers with their present employers. The results are shown. At $\alpha = 0.10$, can it be concluded that the proportions are equal? If they are not equal, give a possible reason for the difference.

	Yes	No	Undecided
Men	40	15	5
Women	36	9	15

Source: Based on information from a Maritz Poll.

Critical Thinking Challenges ≫

1. **Random Digits** Use your calculator or the Minitab or similar technology random number generator to generate 100 two-digit random numbers. Make a grouped frequency distribution, using the chi-square goodness-of-fit test to see if the distribution is random. To do this, use an expected frequency of 10 for each class. Can it be concluded that the distribution is random? Explain.

2. **Lottery Numbers** Simulate the provincial lottery by using your calculator or Minitab or similar technology to generate 100 three-digit random numbers. Group these numbers 100–199, 200–299, etc. Use the chi-square goodness-of-fit test to see if the numbers are random. The expected frequency for each class should be 10. Explain why.

3. **M&M's Candy Colours** Purchase a bag of M&M's candy and count the number of pieces of each colour. Using the information as your sample, state a hypothesis for the distribution of colours, and compare your hypothesis to H_0: The distribution of colours of M&M's candy is 13% brown, 13% red, 14% yellow, 16% green, 20% orange, and 24% blue.

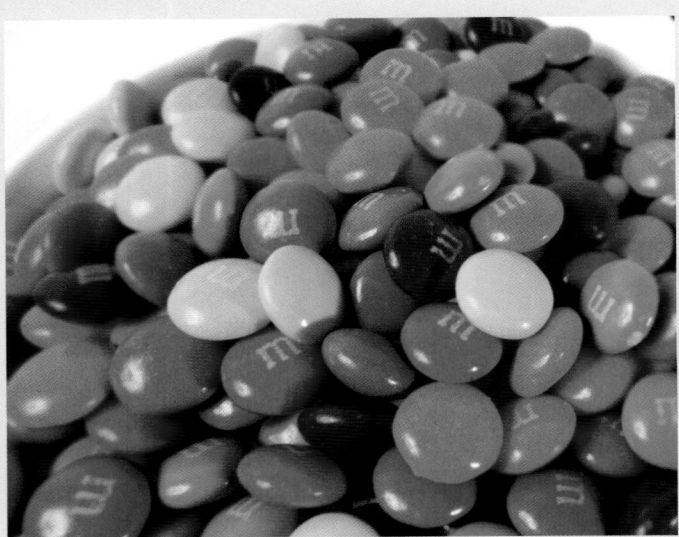

Data Projects ≫

Where appropriate, use Minitab, SPSS, TI-83 Plus, TI-84 Plus, Excel, or a computer program of your choice to complete the following exercises.

Use a significance level of 0.05 for all tests below.

1. **Business and Finance** Many of the companies that produce multicoloured candy include on their Web sites information about the production percentages for the various colours. Select a favourite multicoloured candy. Find out what percentage of each colour is produced. Open up a bag of the candy, noting how many of each colour are in the bag (be careful to count them before you eat them). Is the bag distributed as expected, based on the production percentages? If no production percentages can be found, test to see if the colours are uniformly distributed.

2. **Sports and Leisure** Select a local (or favourite) basketball, football, baseball, and hockey team as the data set. For the most recently completed season, note the teams' home record for wins and losses. Test to see whether home game advantage is independent of sport.

3. **Technology** Use the data collected in Data Project 3 of Chapter 2 regarding song genres. Do the data indicate that songs are uniformly distributed among the genres?

4. **Health and Wellness** Research the percentages of each blood type that the Canadian Blood Services states are in the population. Now use your class as a sample. For each student, note the blood type. Is the distribution of blood types in your class as expected, based on the Canadian Blood Services percentages?

5. **Politics and Economics** Research the distribution (by percentage) of Conservatives, Liberals, and a category "Other Parties" in your province or territory, based on the results of the last provincial or territorial election. Use your class as a sample. For each student, note the party affiliation. Is the distribution as expected, based on the percentages for your province or territory? What might be problematic about using your class as a sample for this exercise?

6. **Your Class** Conduct a classroom poll to determine which of the following sports each student likes best: baseball, football, basketball, hockey, tennis, or golf. Also, note the gender of the individual. Is preference for a sport independent of gender?

Answers to Applying the Concepts »

Section 11–1 Never the Same Amounts

1. The variables are quantitative.

2. We can use a chi-square goodness-of-fit test.

3. There are a total of 233 candies, so we would expect 46.6 of each colour. Our test statistic is $\chi^2 = 1.442$.

4. H_0: The colours are equally distributed.

   H_1: The colours are not equally distributed.

5. There are $5 - 1 = 4$ degrees of freedom for the test. The critical value depends on the choice of significance level. At the 0.05 significance level, the critical value is 9.488.

6. Since $1.442 < 9.488$, we fail to reject the null hypothesis. There is not enough evidence to conclude that the colours are not equally distributed.

Section 11–2 Satellite Dishes in Restricted Areas

1. We compare the P-value to the significance level of 0.05 to check if the null hypothesis should be rejected.

2. The P-value gives the probability of a type I error.

3. This is a right-tailed test, since chi-square tests of independence are always right-tailed.

4. You cannot tell how many rows and columns there were just by looking at the degrees of freedom.

5. Increasing the sample size does not increase the degrees of freedom, since the degrees of freedom are based on the number of rows and columns.

6. We will reject the null hypothesis. There are a number of cells where the observed and expected frequencies are quite different.

7. If the significance level was initially set at 0.10, we would still reject the null hypothesis.

8. No, the chi-square value does not tell us which cells have observed and expected frequencies that are very different.

Chapter 12

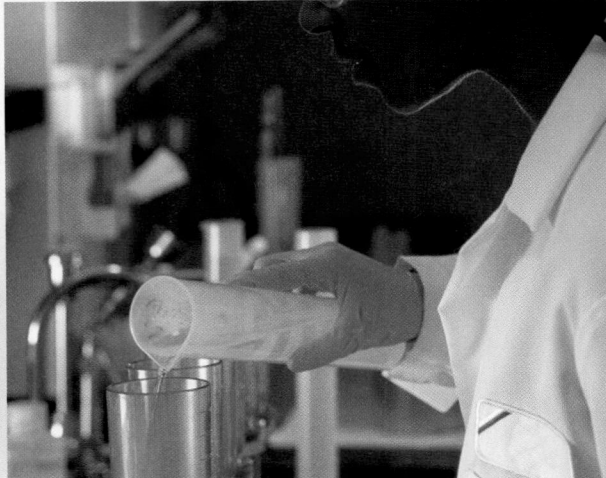

Analysis of Variance

Objectives >

After completing this chapter, you should be able to

LO1 Use the one-way ANOVA technique to determine if there is a significant difference among three or more means.

LO2 Determine which means differ, using the Scheffé or Tukey test if the null hypothesis is rejected in the ANOVA.

LO3 Use the two-way ANOVA technique to determine if there is a significant difference in the main effects or interaction.

Outline >

Mc Graw Hill connect™ Practise and learn online with *Connect* with data sets and algorithmic questions related to concepts covered in this chapter. Throughout this chapter, questions and tables with online data sets are marked with ⬈.

Statistics Today

Is Seeing Really Believing?

Many adults look on the eyewitness testimony of children with skepticism. They believe that young witnesses' testimony is less accurate than the testimony of adults in court cases. Several statistical studies have been done on this subject.

In a preliminary study, three researchers selected fourteen 8-year-olds, fourteen 12-year-olds, and fourteen adults. The researchers showed each group the same video of a crime being committed. The next day, each witness responded to direct and cross-examination questioning. Then the researchers, using statistical methods explained in this chapter, were able to determine if there were differences in the accuracy of the testimony of the three groups on direct examination and on cross-examination. The statistical methods used here differ from the ones explained in Chapter 9 because there are three

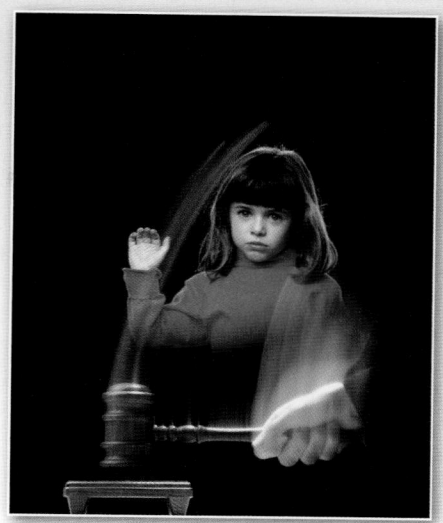

groups rather than two. See Statistics Today—Revisited, page 564.

Source: C. Luus, G. Wells, and J. Turtle, "Child Eyewitnesses: Seeing Is Believing," *Journal of Applied Psychology* 80, No. 2, pp. 317–26.

Introduction >

The *F* test, used to compare two variances as shown in Chapter 9, can also be used to compare three or more means. This technique is called *analysis of variance,* or *ANOVA.* It is used to test claims involving three or more means. (*Note:* The *F* test can also be used to test the equality of two means. But since it is equivalent to the *t* test in this case, the *t* test is usually used instead of the *F* test when there are only two means.) For example, suppose a researcher wishes to see whether the means of the time it takes three groups of students to solve a computer problem using computer languages Java, C++, and PHP are different. The researcher will use the ANOVA technique for this test. The *z* and *t* tests should not be used when three or more means are compared, for reasons given later in this chapter.

For three groups, the *F* test can show only whether a difference exists among the three means. It cannot reveal where the difference lies—that is, between $\overline{X}_1$ and $\overline{X}_2$, or $\overline{X}_1$ and $\overline{X}_3$, or $\overline{X}_2$ and $\overline{X}_3$. If the *F* test indicates that there is a difference among the means, other statistical tests are used to find where the difference exists. The most commonly used tests are the Scheffé test and the Tukey test, which are also explained in this chapter.

The analysis of variance that is used to compare three or more means is called a *one-way analysis of variance* since it contains only one variable. In the previous example, the variable is the type of computer language used. The analysis of variance can be extended to studies involving two variables, such as type of computer language used and mathematical background of the students. These studies involve a *two-way analysis of variance.* Section 12–3 explains the two-way analysis of variance.

| 12–1 | One-Way Analysis of Variance > |

Use the one-way ANOVA technique to determine if there is a significant difference among three or more means.

When an F test is used to test a hypothesis concerning the means of three or more populations, the technique is called **analysis of variance** (commonly abbreviated as **ANOVA**). At first glance, one might think that to compare the means of three or more samples, the t test can be used, comparing two means at a time. But there are several reasons why the t test should not be done.

First, when one is comparing two means at a time, the rest of the means under study are ignored. With the F test, all the means are compared simultaneously. Second, when one is comparing two means at a time and making all pairwise comparisons, the probability of rejecting the null hypothesis when it is true is increased, since the more t tests that are conducted, the greater is the likelihood of getting significant differences by chance alone. Third, the more means there are to compare, the more t tests are needed. For example, for the comparison of 3 means two at a time, 3 t tests are required. For the comparison of 5 means two at a time, 10 tests are required. And for the comparison of 10 means two at a time, 45 tests are required.

Assumptions for the F Test for Comparing Three or More Means

1. The populations from which the samples were obtained must be normally or approximately normally distributed.
2. The samples must be independent of one another.
3. The variances of the populations must be equal.

Even though one is comparing three or more means in this use of the F test, *variances* are used in order to establish whether the means differ.

With the F test, two different estimates of the population variance are made. The first estimate is called the **between-group variance,** and it involves finding the variance of the means. The second estimate, the **within-group variance,** is made by computing the variance using all the data and is not affected by differences in the means. If there is no difference in the means, the between-group variance estimate will be approximately equal to the within-group variance estimate, and the F test statistic will be approximately equal to 1. The null hypothesis will not be rejected. However, when the means differ significantly, the between-group variance will be much larger than the within-group variance; the F test statistic will be significantly greater than 1; and the null hypothesis will be rejected. Since variances are compared, this procedure is called *analysis of variance* (ANOVA).

For a test of the difference among three or more means, the following hypotheses should be used:

H_0: $\mu_1 = \mu_2 = \cdots = \mu_k$

H_1: At least one mean is different from the others.

As stated previously, a significant test statistic means that there is a high probability that this difference in means is not due to chance, but it does not indicate where the difference lies.

The degrees of freedom for this F test are d.f.N. $= k - 1$, where d.f.N. refers to degrees of freedom for the numerator and k is the number of groups, and d.f.D. $= N - k$, where d.f.D. refers to degrees of freedom for the denominator and N is the sum of the sample sizes of the groups $N = n_1 + n_2 + \cdots + n_k$. The sample sizes need not be equal.

The F test to compare means is always right-tailed. Refer to Section 9–5 which details the characteristics of the F distribution and procedures to find critical values using Table H in Appendix C.

Examples 12–1 and 12–2 illustrate the computational procedure for the ANOVA technique for comparing three or more means, and the steps are summarized in the Procedure Table shown after the examples.

Example 12–1	**Lowering Blood Pressure**

A researcher wishes to try three different techniques to lower the blood pressure of individuals diagnosed with high blood pressure. The subjects are randomly assigned to three groups; the first group takes medication, the second group exercises, and the third group follows a special diet. After four weeks, the reduction in each person's blood pressure is recorded. At $\alpha = 0.05$, test the claim that there is no difference among the means. The data are shown.

Medication	**Exercise**	**Diet**
10	6	5
12	8	9
9	3	12
15	0	8
13	2	4
$\overline{X}_1 = 11.8$	$\overline{X}_2 = 3.8$	$\overline{X}_3 = 7.6$
$s_1^2 = 5.7$	$s_2^2 = 10.2$	$s_3^2 = 10.3$

Solution

Step 1   State the hypotheses and identify the claim.

H_0: $\mu_1 = \mu_2 = \mu_3$ (claim)

H_1: At least one mean is different from the others.

Step 2   Find the critical value. Since $k = 3$ and $N = 15$,

d.f.N. $= k - 1 = 3 - 1 = 2$

d.f.D. $= N - k = 15 - 3 = 12$

The critical value is 3.89, obtained from Table H in Appendix C with $\alpha = 0.05$.

Step 3   Compute the test statistic, using the procedure outlined here.

a. Find the mean and variance of each sample (these values are shown below the data).

b. Find the grand mean. The *grand mean*, denoted by $\overline{X}_{GM}$, is the mean of all values in the samples.

$$\overline{X}_{GM} = \frac{\Sigma X}{N} = \frac{10 + 12 + 9 + \cdots + 4}{15} = \frac{116}{15} = 7.73$$

When samples are equal in size, find $\overline{X}_{GM}$ by summing the $\overline{X}$ items and dividing by k, where $k =$ the number of groups.

c. Find the between-group variance, denoted by s_B^2.

$$s_B^2 = \frac{\Sigma n_i(\overline{X}_i - \overline{X}_{GM})^2}{k - 1}$$

$$= \frac{5(11.8 - 7.73)^2 + 5(3.8 - 7.73)^2 + 5(7.6 - 7.73)^2}{3 - 1}$$

$$= \frac{160.13}{2} = 80.07$$

Note: This formula finds the variance among the means by using the sample sizes as weights and considers the differences in the means.

d. Find the within-group variance, denoted by s_W^2.

$$s_W^2 = \frac{\Sigma(n_i - 1)s_i^2}{\Sigma(n_i - 1)}$$

$$= \frac{(5 - 1)(5.7) + (5 - 1)(10.2) + (5 - 1)(10.3)}{(5 - 1) + (5 - 1) + (5 - 1)}$$

$$= \frac{104.80}{12} = 8.73$$

Note: This formula finds an overall variance by calculating a weighted average of the individual variances. It does not involve using differences of the means.

e. Find the F test statistic.

$$F = \frac{s_B^2}{s_W^2} = \frac{80.07}{8.73} = 9.17$$

Step 4 Make the decision. The decision is to reject the null hypothesis, since $9.17 > 3.89$.

Step 5 Summarize the results. There is enough evidence to reject the claim and conclude that at least one mean is different from the others.

The numerator of the fraction obtained in step 3, part c, of the computational procedure is called the **sum of squares between groups,** denoted by SS_B. The numerator of the fraction obtained in step 3, part d, of the computational procedure is called the **sum of squares within groups,** denoted by SS_W. This statistic is also called the *sum of squares for the error.* SS_B is divided by d.f.N. to obtain the between-group variance. SS_W is divided by $N - k$ to obtain the within-group or error variance. These two variances are sometimes called **mean squares,** denoted by MS_B and MS_W. These terms are used to summarize the analysis of variance and are placed in a summary table, as shown in Table 12–1.

Interesting Fact

It takes a depth of 6 centimetres of wet snow or 30 centimetres of dry, powdery snow to yield 1 centimetre of water.

Table 12–1	Analysis of Variance Summary Table			
Source	**Sum of squares**	**d.f.**	**Mean square**	**F**
Between	SS_B	$k - 1$	MS_B	
Within (error)	SS_W	$N - k$	MS_W	
Total				

In the table,

SS_B = sum of squares between groups

SS_W = sum of squares within groups

k = number of groups

$N = n_1 + n_2 + \cdots + n_k$ = sum of sample sizes for groups

$$MS_B = \frac{SS_B}{k - 1}$$

$$MS_W = \frac{SS_W}{N - k}$$

$$F = \frac{MS_B}{MS_W}$$

The totals are obtained by adding the corresponding columns. For Example 12–1, the **ANOVA summary table** is shown in Table 12–2.

Table 12–2	**Analysis of Variance Summary Table for Example 12–1**			
Source	Sum of squares	d.f.	Mean square	F
Between	160.13	2	80.07	9.17
Within (error)	104.80	12	8.73	
Total	264.93	14		

Most computer programs will print out an ANOVA summary table.

Example 12–2

Auto Thefts

A researcher wants to determine if there is a significant difference in the rate of auto thefts by census metropolitan area (CMA) in Canada. The data are shown. At $\alpha = 0.05$, can it be concluded that there is a significant difference in the average rate of auto thefts in each CMA? Rates are expressed per 10,000 population.

More than 500,000	Between 250,000–500,000	Less than 250,000
37	54	57
78	41	18
115	71	57
58	51	20
75	35	83
$\overline{X}_1 = 72.6$	$\overline{X}_2 = 50.4$	$\overline{X}_3 = 47.0$
$s_1^2 = 828.3$	$s_2^2 = 190.8$	$s_3^2 = 766.5$

Source: Adapted from Statistics Canada, *Juristat,* "Motor Vehicle Theft in Canada—2001," Catalogue 85–002, Vol. 23, No. 1.

Solution

Step 1   State the hypotheses and identify the claim.

H_0: $\mu_1 = \mu_2 = \mu_3$

H_1: At least one mean is different from the others (claim)

Step 2 Find the critical value. Since $k = 3$, $N = 15$, and $\alpha = 0.05$.

d.f.N. $= k - 1 = 3 - 1 = 2$

d.f.D. $= N - k = 15 - 3 = 12$

The critical value is 3.89.

Step 3 Compute the test statistic.

a. Find the mean and variance of each sample (these values are shown below the data columns in the example).

b. Find the grand mean.

$$\overline{X}_{\text{GM}} = \frac{\Sigma X}{N} = \frac{37 + 78 + 115 + \cdots + 83}{15} = \frac{850}{15} = 56.7.$$

c. Find the between-group variance.

$$s_B^2 = \frac{\Sigma n_i(\overline{X}_i - \overline{X}_{\text{GM}})^2}{k - 1}$$

$$= \frac{5(72.6 - 56.7)^2 + 5(50.4 - 56.7)^2 + 5(47.0 - 56.7)^2}{3 - 1}$$

$$= \frac{1932.95}{2} = 966.48$$

d. Find the within-group variance.

$$s_W^2 = \frac{\Sigma(n_i - 1)s_i^2}{\Sigma(n_i - 1)}$$

$$= \frac{(5 - 1)(828.3)^2 + (5 - 1)(190.8)^2 + (5 - 1)(766.5)^2}{(5 - 1) + (5 - 1) + (5 - 1)}$$

$$= \frac{7142.4}{12} = 595.2$$

e. Find the F test statistic.

$$F = \frac{s_B^2}{s_W^2} = \frac{966.48}{595.2} = 1.62$$

Step 4 Make the decision. Since $1.62 < 3.89$, the decision is to not reject the null hypothesis.

Step 5 Summarize the results. There is not enough evidence to support the claim that there is a difference among the means. The ANOVA summary table for this example is shown in Table 12–3.

Table 12–3	Analysis of Variance Summary Table for Example 12-2			
Source	**Sum of squares**	**d.f.**	**Mean square**	**F**
Between	1932.95	2	966.48	1.62
Within	7142.40	12	595.20	
Total	9075.35	14		

The steps for computing the F test statistic for the ANOVA are summarized in this Procedure Table.

Procedure Table

Finding the F Test Statistic for the Analysis of Variance

Step 1 Find the mean and variance of each sample:

$$(\overline{X}_1, s_1^2), (\overline{X}_2, s_2^2), \ldots, (\overline{X}_k, s_k^2)$$

Step 2 Find the grand mean.

$$\overline{X}_{GM} = \frac{\Sigma X}{N}$$

Step 3 Find the between-group variance.

$$s_B^2 = \frac{\Sigma n_i(\overline{X}_i - \overline{X}_{GM})^2}{k - 1}$$

Step 4 Find the within-group variance.

$$s_W^2 = \frac{\Sigma(n_i - 1)s_i^2}{\Sigma(n_i - 1)}$$

Step 5 Find the F test statistic.

$$F = \frac{s_B^2}{s_W^2}$$

The degrees of freedom are

d.f.N. $= k - 1$

where k is the number of groups, and

d.f.D. $= N - k$

where N is the sum of the sample sizes of the groups,

$$N = n_1 + n_2 + \cdots + n_k$$

P-Values for ANOVA

The procedure to find approximate P-values for the F distribution using Table H in Appendix C was explained in Section 9–5. For Example 12–2, find where the test statistic ($F = 1.62$) falls within Table H—F distribution using d.f.N. $= 2$ and d.f.D. $= 12$. In this case, $F = 1.62$ is less than the table value $F = 2.81$ corresponding to $\alpha = 0.10$. In other words, the P-value is greater than 0.10. The exact P-value obtained using technology is 0.238. The decision rule for the P-value method is to reject the null hypothesis if the P-value is less than α, the significance level. Since the P-value (0.238) $> \alpha = 0.05$, the decision is to not reject the null hypothesis.

In situations when the null hypothesis is rejected, it indicates that at least one of the means is different from the others. To locate the differences among the means, it is necessary to use other tests such as the Tukey or the Scheffé tests.

12–1 Applying the Concepts

Colours That Make You Look Smarter

The following set of data values was obtained from a study of people's perceptions on whether the colour of a person's clothing is related to how intelligent the person looks. The subjects rated the person's intelligence on a scale of 1 to 10. Group 1 subjects were randomly shown people with clothing in shades of blue and grey. Group 2 subjects were randomly shown people with clothing in shades of brown and yellow. Group 3 subjects were randomly shown people with clothing in shades of pink and orange. The results follow.

Group 1	Group 2	Group 3
8	7	4
7	8	9
7	7	6
7	7	7
8	5	9
8	8	8
6	5	5
8	8	8
8	7	7
7	6	5
7	6	4
8	6	5
8	6	4

1. Use ANOVA to test for any significant differences between the means.
2. What is the purpose of this study?
3. Explain why separate t tests are not accepted in this situation.

Data from this problem will be used in Applying the Concepts 12–2.

See page 568 for the answers.

Exercises 12–1

1. What test is used to compare three or more means?

2. State three reasons why multiple t tests cannot be used to compare three or more means.

3. What are the assumptions for ANOVA?

4. Define between-group variance and within-group variance.

5. What is the F test formula for comparing three or more means?

6. State the hypotheses used in the ANOVA test.

7. When there is no significant difference among three or more means, the value of F will be close to what number?

For Exercises 8 through 19, assume that all variables are normally distributed, that the samples are independent, and that the population variances are equal. Also, for each exercise, perform the following steps.

 a. State the hypotheses and identify the claim.
 b. Find the critical value.
 c. Compute the test statistic.
 d. Make the decision.
 e. Summarize the results, and explain where the differences in the means are.

Use the traditional method of hypothesis testing unless otherwise specified.

 8. **Sodium Content of Foods** The amount of sodium (in milligrams) in one serving for a random sample of three

different kinds of foods is listed here. At the 0.05 level of significance, is there sufficient evidence to conclude that a difference in mean sodium amounts exists among condiments, cereals, and desserts?

Condiment	Cereal	Dessert
270	260	100
130	220	180
230	290	250
180	290	250
80	200	300
70	320	360
200	140	300
		160

Source: The Doctor's Pocket Calorie, Fat, and Carbohydrate Counter.

9. **Hybrid Vehicles** A study was done to compare the fuel consumption, in litres, of different types of hybrid vehicles that were driven a distance of 20,000 kilometres. Based on the information given below for different models of hybrid cars, trucks, and SUVs, is there sufficient evidence to conclude a difference in the fuel consumption? Use $\alpha = 0.05$. (The information in this exercise will be used in Exercise 3 in Section 12–2.)

Hybrid car	Hybrid truck	Hybrid SUV
1000	2320	1880
900	1220	1900
1900	1380	1880
1160	1880	1900
1140	1900	
760	1880	
	1900	
	1540	

Source: Natural Resources Canada, Office of Energy Efficiency, Fuel Consumption Guide.

10. **Apprenticeship Trade Enrollments** A random sample of enrollments in selected apprenticeship trades in Atlantic Canada is shown. At $\alpha = 0.10$, test the claim that the mean apprenticeship trade enrollments are the same for the Atlantic Canada provinces. (The information in this exercise will be used in Exercise 4 in Section 12–2.)

NB	NL	NS	PEI
765	1155	755	190
770	1195	1180	140
310	1980	415	25
710	1050	940	40
840	2250	1260	185
1085	2995	1280	85

Source: Statistics Canada.

11. **Lengths of Suspension Bridges** The lengths (in metres) of a random sample of suspension bridges in North America, Europe, and Asia are shown. At $\alpha = 0.05$, is there sufficient evidence to conclude that there is a difference in mean lengths? (The information in this exercise will be used in Exercise 5 in Section 12–2.)

North America	Europe	Asia
1298	1624	1990
1067	1410	1385
701	1325	1118
564	1006	1030
668	1013	876
564	988	
472		

Source: Helsinki University of Technology, Laboratory of Bridge Engineering, World's Longest Bridge Spans, August 16, 2006.

12. **Weight Gain of Athletes** A researcher wants to see whether there is any difference in the weight gains of athletes following one of three special diets. Athletes are randomly assigned to three groups and placed on the diet for 6 weeks. The weight gains (in kilograms) are shown here. At $\alpha = 0.05$, can the researcher conclude that there is a difference in the diets?

Diet A	Diet B	Diet C
1.4	4.5	3.6
2.7	5.4	1.4
3.2	5.0	0.9
1.8	6.4	2.3
	3.6	
	2.7	

A computer printout for this problem is shown. Use the *P*-value method and the information in this printout to test the claim. (The information in this exercise will be used in Exercise 6 of Section 12–2.)

Computer Printout (Excel) for Exercise 12

```
SUMMARY
```

Groups	Count	Sum	Average	Variance
Diet A	4	9.1	2.275	0.676
Diet B	6	27.6	4.600	1.732
Diet C	4	8.2	2.050	1.403

```
ANOVA
```

Source of Variation	Sum of Squares	df	MS	F	P-value	F crit
Between Groups	20.472	2	10.236	7.558	0.00860	3.982
Within Groups	14.898	11	1.354			
Total	35.369	13				

13. University Tuition Fees Tuition fees for a selection of Canadian university undergraduate students in Arts and Sciences programs in three provinces are listed. At $\alpha = 0.05$, is there a difference in the means? If so, give a possible reason for the difference. (The information in this exercise will be used in Exercise 7 in Section 12–2.)

Alberta	Ontario	Quebec
3468	4603	2136
4767	4691	2171
5035	4647	2263
5171	4924	2842
	4982	2965
	5012	

Source: Maclean's magazine online.

14. City Populations Random samples of populations (in thousands) of Canadian cities in three regions of the country are listed. Is there evidence to conclude a difference in means at the 0.01 level of significance?

Atlantic	Great Lakes	Pacific
373	693	330
181	390	159
126	323	93
58	177	83
36	152	81
	91	55
	80	

Source: Statistics Canada, Catalogue No. 97-550-XWE2006002, Ottawa. Released March 13, 2007.

15. Farm Numbers The numbers of farms in a random selection of agricultural regions in Canada's Prairie provinces are listed. Test the claim at $\alpha = 0.05$ that the mean number of farms is the same across each Prairie province. (The information in this exercise will be used in Exercise 8 in Section 12–2.)

Manitoba	Saskatchewan	Alberta
885	1089	3123
1369	1273	3316
1556	1592	6204
1907	1968	7122
2485	2116	8655
2509	2527	
3021	2770	
	3479	
	4050	
	4438	

Source: Statistics Canada.

16. Gas Prices The price, in cents, of a litre of gasoline on the same day in three Canadian cities at a random sample of Petro-Canada gas stations is shown. Using $\alpha = 0.05$, can one conclude that there is a difference in the means? (The information in this exercise will be used in Exercise 9 in Section 12–2.)

Toronto	Calgary	Vancouver
74.2	79.9	91.4
76.5	82.9	94.5
80.2	84.9	95.3
82.9	88.4	97.9
84.4	91.9	100.8

Source: GasBuddy Organization Inc.

17. Microwave Oven Prices A research organization tested microwave ovens. At $\alpha = 0.10$, is there a significant difference in the average prices of the three types of oven?

Watts		
1000	**900**	**800**
270	240	180
245	135	155
190	160	200
215	230	120
250	250	140
230	200	180
	200	140
	210	130

A computer printout for this exercise is shown. Use the P-value method and the information in this printout to test the claim. (The information in this exercise will be used in Exercise 10 in Section 12–2.)

Computer Printout (Excel) for Exercise 17

```
SUMMARY
```

Groups	Count	Sum	Average	Variance
1000	6	1400	233.333	796.667
900	8	1625	203.125	1549.554
800	8	1245	155.625	795.982

Computer Printout (Excel) for Exercise 17 (*continued*)

```
ANOVA
```

Source of Variation	Sum of Squares	df	Mean Square	F	P-value	F crit
Between Groups	21729.735	2	10864.867	10.118	0.00102	3.522
Within Groups	20402.083	19	1073.794			
Total	42131.818	21				

18. Hotel Room Prices Three random samples of New Year's Eve hotel room prices per night in popular Canadian destinations are shown. At $\alpha = 0.05$, is there a difference in the mean prices among the three cities?

Niagara Falls	Banff	Quebec City
425	363	219
339	299	149
249	290	125
215	211	100
206	160	
194		

Source: Expedia.ca.

19. Graduate Student Enrollments The number of graduate students in universities from provinces with similar populations is shown. At a 0.10 significance level, is there a difference in the average number of graduates in the provinces?

NS	NB	MB	SK
2,890	910	2,520	2,230
320	450	90	680
170	10	50	
150			
80			

Source: Association of Universities and Colleges of Canada, *Statistics and Facts on Higher Education in Canada.*

20. Net Migration During the recession of 2008/2009, the net migration (immigrants minus emigrants) of major census metropolitan areas (CMAs) for distinct regions in Canada is shown. At $\alpha = 0.05$, is there a difference between the average net migration for these regions?

Ontario	Quebec/Atlantic	Prairies	British Columbia
58,419	30,068	27,478	38,786
13,104	5,533	19,822	4,757
4,568	3,920	8,414	3,596
3,626	2,278	5,845	2,269
3,571	1,559	3,183	
3,558	1,532		
2,481			

Source: Statistics Canada, *Annual Demographic Estimates: Subprovincial Areas Table 1.2-13, Annual Estimates of Demographic Components by Census Metropolitan Area, Canada, from July to June—Total Net Migration.*

Computer Printout (Excel) for Exercise 20

SUMMARY

Groups	Count	Sum	Average	Variance
Ontario	7	89327	12761.0	418362299.3
Quebec/Atlantic	6	44890	7481.7	124835977.1
Prairies	5	64742	12948.4	106184441.3
British Columbia	4	49408	12352.0	311591602.0

ANOVA

Source of Variation	Sum of Squares	df	Mean Square	F	P-value	F crit
Between Groups	120430124.8	3	40143374.93	0.161	0.921	3.160
Within Groups	4493866253	18	249659236.3			
Total	4614296377	21				

12–2 | The Scheffé Test and the Tukey Test ❯

LO2

Determine which means differ, using the Scheffé or Tukey test if the null hypothesis is rejected in the ANOVA.

When the null hypothesis is rejected using the *F* test, the researcher may want to know where the difference among the means is. Several procedures have been developed to determine where the significant differences in the means lie after the ANOVA procedure has been performed. Among the most commonly used tests are the *Scheffé test* and the *Tukey test.*

Scheffé Test

To conduct the **Scheffé test,** one must compare the means two at a time, using all possible combinations of means. For example, if there are three means, the following comparisons must be done:

$$\overline{X}_1 \text{ versus } \overline{X}_2 \qquad \overline{X}_1 \text{ versus } \overline{X}_3 \qquad \overline{X}_2 \text{ versus } \overline{X}_3$$

Formula for the Scheffé Test

$$F_S = \frac{(\overline{X}_i - \overline{X}_j)^2}{s_W^2[(1/n_i) + (1/n_j)]}$$

where $\overline{X}_i$ and $\overline{X}_j$ are the means of the samples being compared, n_i and n_j are the respective sample sizes, and s_W^2 is the within-group variance.

To find the critical value F' for the Scheffé test, multiply the critical value (C.V.) for the F test by $k - 1$:

$$F' = (k - 1)(\text{C.V.})$$

There is a significant difference between the two means being compared when F_S is greater than F'. Example 12–3 illustrates the use of the Scheffé test.

Example 12–3

Lowering Blood Pressure

Using the Scheffé test, test each pair of means in Example 12–1 to see whether a specific difference exists, at $\alpha = 0.05$.

Solution

    a. For $\overline{X}_1$ versus $\overline{X}_2$,

$$F_S = \frac{(\overline{X}_1 - \overline{X}_2)^2}{s_W^2[(1/n_1) + (1/n_2)]} = \frac{(11.8 - 3.8)^2}{8.73[(1/5) + (1/5)]} = 18.33.$$

    b. For $\overline{X}_2$ versus $\overline{X}_3$,

$$F_S = \frac{(\overline{X}_2 - \overline{X}_3)^2}{s_W^2[(1/n_2) + (1/n_3)]} = \frac{(3.8 - 7.6)^2}{8.73[(1/5) + (1/5)]} = 4.14.$$

    c. For $\overline{X}_1$ versus $\overline{X}_3$,

$$F_S = \frac{(\overline{X}_1 - \overline{X}_3)^2}{s_W^2[(1/n_1) + (1/n_3)]} = \frac{(11.8 - 7.6)^2}{8.73[(1/5) + (1/5)]} = 5.05.$$

    The critical value for the analysis of variance for Example 12–1 was 3.89, found by using Table H with $\alpha = 0.05$, d.f.N. $= k - 1 = 2$, and d.f.D. $= N - k = 12$. In this case, it is multiplied by $k - 1$ as shown.

    The critical value for F' at $\alpha = 0.05$, with d.f.N. $= 2$ and d.f.D. $= 12$, is

$$F' = (k - 1)(\text{C.V.}) = (3 - 1)(3.89) = 7.78$$

    Since only the F test statistic for part *a* ($\overline{X}_1$ versus $\overline{X}_2$) is greater than the critical value, 7.78, the only significant difference is between $\overline{X}_1$ and $\overline{X}_2$, that is, between medication and exercise.

Speaking of Statistics

This study involved three groups. The results showed that patients in all three groups felt better after two years. State possible null and alternative hypotheses for this study. Was the null hypothesis rejected? Explain how the statistics could have been used to arrive at the conclusion.

HEALTH

TRICKING KNEE PAIN

You sign up for a clinical trial of arthroscopic surgery used to relieve knee pain caused by arthritis. You're sedated and wake up with tiny incisions. Soon your bum knee feels better. Two years later you find out you had "placebo" surgery. In a study at the Houston VA Medical Center, researchers divided 180 patients into three groups: two groups had damaged cartilage removed, while the third got simulated surgery. Yet an equal number of patients in all groups felt better after two years. Some 650,000 people have the surgery annually, but they're wasting their money, says Dr. Nelda P. Wray, who led the study. And the patients who got fake surgery? "They aren't angry at us," she says. "They still report feeling better."

— STEPHEN P. WILLIAMS

Source: From *Newsweek* July 22, 2002 © Newsweek, Inc. All rights reserved. Reprinted by permission.

On occasion, when the F test statistic is greater than the critical value, the Scheffé test may not show any significant differences in the pairs of means. This result occurs because the difference may actually lie in the average of two or more means when compared with the other mean. The Scheffé test can be used to make these types of comparisons, but the technique is beyond the scope of this book.

Tukey Test

The **Tukey test** can also be used after the analysis of variance has been completed to make pairwise comparisons between means when the groups have the same sample size. The symbol for the test statistic in the Tukey test is q.

Formula for the Tukey Test

$$q = \frac{\overline{X}_i - \overline{X}_j}{\sqrt{s_W^2/n}}$$

where $\overline{X}_i$ and $\overline{X}_j$ are the means of the samples being compared, n is the size of the samples, and s_W^2 is the within-group variance.

When the absolute value of q is greater than the critical value for the Tukey test, there is a significant difference between the two means being compared. The procedures for finding q and the critical value from Table N in Appendix C for the Tukey test are shown in Example 12–4.

Example 12–4	**Lowering Blood Pressure**

Using the Tukey test, test each pair of means in Example 12–1 to see whether a specific difference exists, at $\alpha = 0.05$.

Solution

a. For $\overline{X}_1$ versus $\overline{X}_2$,

$$q = \frac{\overline{X}_1 - \overline{X}_2}{\sqrt{s_W^2/n}} = \frac{11.8 - 3.8}{\sqrt{8.73/5}} = \frac{8}{1.32} = 6.06$$

b. For $\overline{X}_1$ versus $\overline{X}_3$,

$$q = \frac{\overline{X}_1 - \overline{X}_3}{\sqrt{s_W^2/n}} = \frac{11.8 - 7.6}{\sqrt{8.73/5}} = \frac{4.2}{1.32} = 3.18$$

c. For $\overline{X}_2$ versus $\overline{X}_3$,

$$q = \frac{\overline{X}_2 - \overline{X}_3}{\sqrt{s_W^2/n}} = \frac{3.8 - 7.6}{\sqrt{8.73/5}} = \frac{-3.8}{1.32} = -2.88$$

To find the critical value for the Tukey test, use Table N in Appendix C. The number of means k is found in the row at the top, and the degrees of freedom for s_W^2 are found in the left column (denoted by v). Since $N = 15$, $k = 3$, d.f. $= N - k = 15 - 3 = 12$, and $\alpha = 0.05$, the critical value is 3.77. See Figure 12–1. Hence, the only q value that is greater in absolute value than the critical value is the one for the difference between $\overline{X}_1$ and $\overline{X}_2$. The conclusion, then, is that there is a significant difference in means for medication and exercise. These results agree with the Scheffé analysis.

Figure 12–1

Finding the Critical Value in Table N for the Tukey Test (Example 12–4)

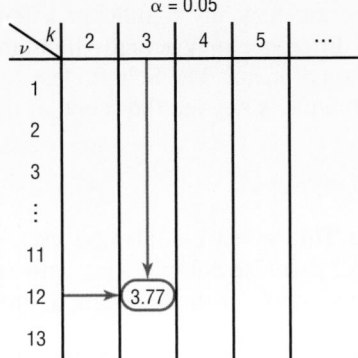

The student might wonder why there are two different tests that can be used after the ANOVA. Actually, there are several other tests that can be used in addition to the Scheffé and Tukey tests. It is up to the researcher to select the most appropriate test. The Scheffé test is the most general, and it can be used when the samples are of different sizes. Furthermore, the Scheffé test can be used to make comparisons such as the average of $\overline{X}_1$

and $\overline{X}_2$ compared with $\overline{X}_3$. However, the Tukey test is more powerful than the Scheffé test for making pairwise comparisons for the means. A rule of thumb for pairwise comparisons is to use the Tukey test when the samples are equal in size and the Scheffé test when the samples differ in size. This rule will be followed in this textbook.

12–2 Applying the Concepts

Colours That Make You Look Smarter

The following set of data values was obtained from a study of people's perceptions on whether the colour of a person's clothing is related to how intelligent the person looks. The subjects rated the person's intelligence on a scale of 1 to 10. Group 1 subjects were randomly shown people with clothing in shades of blue and grey. Group 2 subjects were randomly shown people with clothing in shades of brown and yellow. Group 3 subjects were randomly shown people with clothing in shades of pink and orange. The results follow.

Group 1	Group 2	Group 3
8	7	4
7	8	9
7	7	6
7	7	7
8	5	9
8	8	8
6	5	5
8	8	8
8	7	7
7	6	5
7	6	4
8	6	5
8	6	4

1. Use the Tukey test to test all possible pairwise comparisons.
2. Are there any contradictions in the results?
3. Explain why separate t tests are not accepted in this situation.
4. When would Tukey's test be preferred over the Scheffé method? Explain.

See page 568 for the answers.

Exercises 12–2

1. What two tests can be used to compare two means when the null hypothesis is rejected using the one-way ANOVA F test?

2. Explain the difference between the two tests used to compare two means when the null hypothesis is rejected using the one-way ANOVA F test.

For Exercises 3 through 10, the null hypothesis was rejected. Use the Scheffé test when sample sizes are unequal, or the Tukey test when sample sizes are equal, to test the differences between the pairs of means. Assume all variables are normally distributed, **samples are independent, and the population variances are equal.**

3. **Hybrid Vehicles** For the information required to complete this exercise, refer to Exercise 9 in the Section 12–1 exercises.

4. **Apprenticeship Trade Enrollments** For the information required to complete this exercise, refer to Exercise 10 in the Section 12–1 exercises.

5. **Lengths of Suspension Bridges** For the information required to complete this exercise, refer to Exercise 11 in the Section 12–1 exercises.

6. **Weight Gain of Athletes** For the information required to complete this exercise, refer to Exercise 12 in the Section 12–1 exercises.

7. **University Tuition Fees** For the information required to complete this exercise, refer to Exercise 13 in the Section 12–1 exercises.

8. **Farm Numbers** For the information required to complete this exercise, refer to Exercise 15 in the Section 12–1 exercises.

9. **Gas Prices** For the information required to complete this exercise, refer to Exercise 16 in the Section 12–1 exercises.

10. **Microwave Oven Prices** For the information required to complete this exercise, refer to Exercise 17 in the Section 12–1 exercises.

For Exercises 11 through 14, do a complete one-way ANOVA. If the null hypothesis is rejected, use either the Scheffé or Tukey test to see if there is a significant difference in the pairs of means. Assume all assumptions are met.

11. **Precipitation in Fruit-Growing Regions** Canada's primary agricultural regions for growing fruits, including grapes for wine, require ample annual precipitation. Shown below is annual precipitation, in millimetres, for select communities in each region. At $\alpha = 0.05$, is there sufficient evidence to indicate a difference in the mean precipitation for the regions?

Annapolis Valley	Niagara Region	Okanagan Valley
1201	970	381
1508	871	333
1308	910	551
1209	991	327
1477	1037	410

Source: Environment Canada, *National Climate Data and Information Archive.*

12. **Fibre Content of Food** The number of grams of fibre per serving for a random sample of three different kinds of foods is listed. Is there sufficient evidence at the 0.05 level of significance to conclude that there is a difference in mean fibre content among breakfast cereals, fruits, and vegetables?

Breakfast cereals	Fruits	Vegetables
3	5.5	10
4	2	1.5
6	4.4	3.5
4	1.6	2.7
10	3.8	2.5
5	4.5	6.5
6	2.8	4
8		3
5		

Source: *The Doctor's Pocket Calorie, Fat, and Carbohydrate Counter.*

13. **Alternative Education** The data consist of the number of students who were enrolled in alternative forms of education for schools in four different counties. At $\alpha = 0.01$, is there a difference in the means? Give a few reasons why some people would be enrolled in an alternative type of school.

County A	County B	County C	County D
2	6	4	0
0	0	0	3
8	1	2	0
1	5	3	1
0	3	2	1

14. **City Break-and-Enter Crimes** The police services in Edmonton reported the following annual break-and-enter data for a random selection of neighbourhoods in each of five city districts. At $\alpha = 0.05$, is there a difference in the city district means for break-and-enter crimes?

North	West	Southwest	Southeast	Downtown
72	25	6	36	147
37	33	24	8	112
36	14	26	16	58
47	8	5	24	5
84	22	49	4	29

Source: Edmonton Police Service, *Neighbourhood Crime Map.*

12–3	Two-Way Analysis of Variance ›

LO3

Use the two-way ANOVA technique to determine if there is a significant difference in the main effects or interaction.

The analysis of variance technique shown previously is called a **one-way ANOVA** since there is only *one independent variable*. The **two-way ANOVA** is an extension of the one-way analysis of variance; it involves *two independent variables*. The independent variables are also called **factors.**

The two-way analysis of variance is quite complicated, and many aspects of the subject should be considered when one is using a research design involving a two-way ANOVA. For the purposes of this textbook, only a brief introduction to the subject will be given.

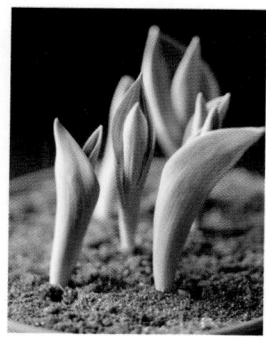

Treatment Groups for the Plant Food–Soil Type Experiment

In doing a study that involves a two-way analysis of variance, the researcher is able to test the effects of two independent variables or factors on one *dependent variable.* In addition, the interaction effect of the two variables can be tested.

For example, suppose a researcher wishes to test the effects of two different types of plant food and two different types of soil on the growth of certain plants. The two independent variables are the type of plant food and the type of soil, while the dependent variable is the plant growth. Other factors, such as water, temperature, and sunlight, are held constant.

To conduct this experiment, the researcher sets up four groups of plants. See Figure 12–2.

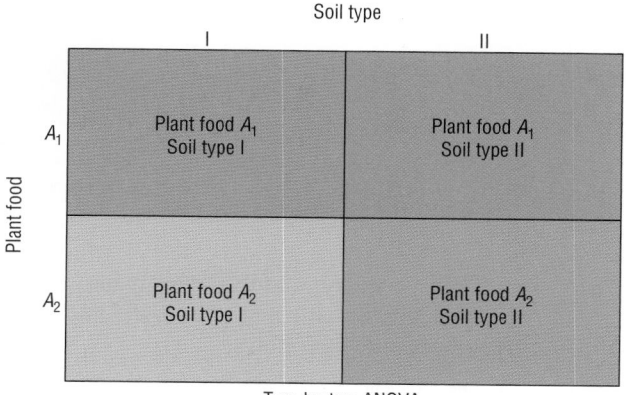

Assume that the plant food type is designated by the letters A_1 and A_2 and the soil type by the Roman numerals I and II. The groups for such a two-way ANOVA are sometimes called **treatment groups.** The four groups are

Group 1	Plant food A_1, soil type I
Group 2	Plant food A_1, soil type II
Group 3	Plant food A_2, soil type I
Group 4	Plant food A_2, soil type II

The plants are assigned to the groups at random. This design is called a 2×2 (read "two-by-two") design, since each variable consists of two **levels,** that is, two different treatments.

The two-way ANOVA enables the researcher to test the effects of the plant food and the soil type in a single experiment rather than in separate experiments involving the plant food alone and the soil type alone. Furthermore, the researcher can test an additional hypothesis about the effect of the *interaction* of the two variables—plant food and soil type—on plant growth. For example, is there a difference between the growth of plants using plant food A_1 and soil type II and the growth of plants using plant food A_2 and soil type I? When a difference of this type occurs, the experiment is said to have a significant **interaction effect.** That is, the types of plant food affect the plant growth differently in different soil types.

There are many different kinds of two-way ANOVA designs, depending on the number of levels of each variable. Figure 12–3 shows a few of these designs. As stated previously, the plant food–soil type experiment uses a 2×2 ANOVA.

The design in Figure 12–3(a) is called a 3×2 design, since the factor in the rows has three levels and the factor in the columns has two levels. Figure 12–3(b) is a 3×3 design, since each factor has three levels. Figure 12–3(c) is a 4×3 design.

Interesting Fact

As unlikely as it sounds, lightning can travel through phone wires. You should probably hold off on taking a bath or shower as well during an electrical storm. According to the *Annals of Emergency Medicine,* lightning can also travel through water pipes.

Figure 12–3

Some Types of Two-Way ANOVA Designs

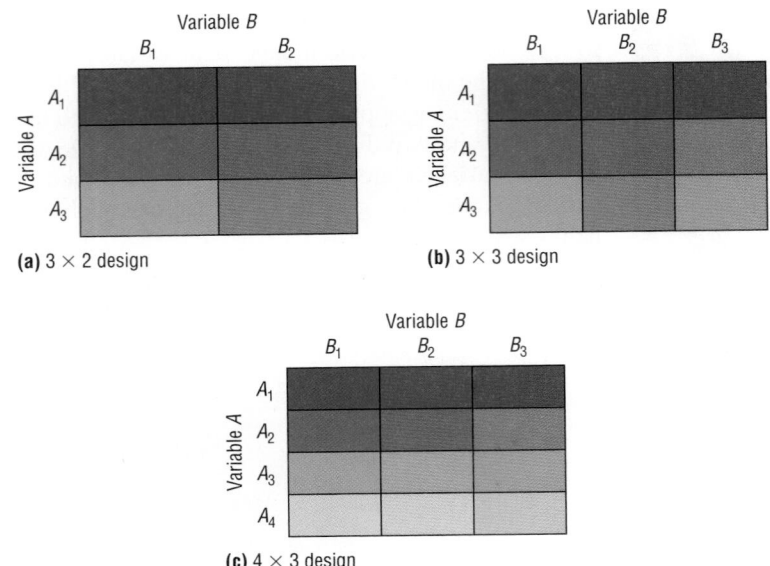

(a) 3 × 2 design

(b) 3 × 3 design

(c) 4 × 3 design

The two-way ANOVA design has several null hypotheses. There is one for each independent variable and one for the interaction. In the plant food–soil type problem, the hypotheses are as follows:

1. H_0: There is no interaction effect between type of plant food used and type of soil used on plant growth.

   H_1: There is an interaction effect between food type and soil type on plant growth.

2. H_0: There is no difference in means of heights of plants grown using different foods.

   H_1: There is a difference in means of heights of plants grown using different foods.

3. H_0: There is no difference in means of heights of plants grown in different soil types.

   H_1: There is a difference in means of heights of plants grown in different soil types.

The first set of hypotheses concerns the interaction effect; the second and third sets test the effects of the independent variables, which are sometimes called the **main effects.**

As with the one-way ANOVA, a between-group variance estimate is calculated, and a within-group variance estimate is calculated. An F test is then performed for each of the independent variables and the interaction. The results of the two-way ANOVA are summarized in a two-way table, as shown in Table 12–4 for the plant experiment.

Table 12–4	**ANOVA Summary Table for Plant Food and Soil Type**				
Source	**Sum of squares**	**d.f.**	**Mean square**	**F**
Plant food					
Soil type					
Interaction					
Within (error)					
Total					

In general, the two-way ANOVA summary table is set up as shown in Table 12–5.

Table 12–5	ANOVA Summary Table			
Source	**Sum of squares**	**d.f.**	**Mean square**	**F**
A	SS_A	$a - 1$	MS_A	F_A
B	SS_B	$b - 1$	MS_B	F_B
$A \times B$	$SS_{A \times B}$	$(a - 1)(b - 1)$	$MS_{A \times B}$	$F_{A \times B}$
Within (error)	SS_W	$ab(n - 1)$	MS_W	
Total				

In the table,

$$SS_A = \text{sum of squares for factor } A$$
$$SS_B = \text{sum of squares for factor } B$$
$$SS_{A \times B} = \text{sum of squares for interaction}$$
$$SS_W = \text{sum of squares for error term (within-group)}$$
$$a = \text{number of levels of factor } A$$
$$b = \text{number of levels of factor } B$$
$$n = \text{number of subjects in each group}$$

$$MS_A = \frac{SS_A}{a - 1}$$

$$MS_B = \frac{SS_B}{b - 1}$$

$$MS_{A \times B} = \frac{SS_{A \times B}}{(a - 1)(b - 1)}$$

$$MS_W = \frac{SS_W}{ab(n - 1)}$$

$$F_A = \frac{MS_A}{MS_W} \qquad \text{with d.f.N.} = a - 1, \text{d.f.D.} = ab(n - 1)$$

$$F_B = \frac{MS_B}{MS_W} \qquad \text{with d.f.N.} = b - 1, \text{d.f.D.} = ab(n - 1)$$

$$F_{A \times B} = \frac{MS_{A \times B}}{MS_W} \qquad \text{with d.f.N.} = (a - 1)(b - 1), \text{d.f.D.} = ab(n - 1)$$

The assumptions for the two-way analysis of variance are basically the same as those for the one-way ANOVA, except for sample size.

Assumptions for the Two-Way ANOVA

1. The populations from which the samples were obtained must be normally or approximately normally distributed.
2. The samples must be independent.
3. The variances of the populations from which the samples were selected must be equal.
4. The groups must be equal in sample size.

The computational procedure for the two-way ANOVA is quite lengthy. For this reason, it will be omitted in Example 12–5, and only the two-way ANOVA summary table will be shown. The table used in Example 12–5 is similar to the one generated by most computer programs. You should be able to interpret the table and summarize the results.

Gasoline Consumption 🏎

A researcher wishes to see whether the type of gasoline used and the type of automobile driven have any effect on gasoline consumption. Two types of gasoline, regular and high octane, will be used, and two types of automobiles, two-wheel-drive and four-wheel-drive, will be used in each group. There will be two automobiles in each group, for a total of eight automobiles used. Using a two-way analysis of variance, the researcher will perform the following steps.

Step 1 State the hypotheses.

Step 2 Find the critical value for each F test, using $\alpha = 0.05$.

Step 3 Complete the summary table to get the test statistic.

Step 4 Make the decision.

Step 5 The data (litres per 100 kilometres) are shown here, and the summary table is given in Table 12–6.

Gas	Type of automobile	
	Two-wheel-drive	**Four-wheel-drive**
Regular	8.8	8.2
	9.3	8.0
High octane	7.3	9.0
	7.2	9.7

Table 12–6 **ANOVA Summary Table for Example 12–5**

Source	Sum of squares	d.f.	Mean square	F	P-value
Gasoline A	0.151				
Automobile B	0.661				
Interaction $(A \times B)$	4.651				
Within (error)	0.395				
Total	5.858				

Solution

Step 1 State the hypotheses. The hypotheses for the interaction are

H_0: There is no interaction effect between type of gasoline used and type of automobile a person drives on gasoline consumption.

H_1: There is an interaction effect between type of gasoline used and type of automobile a person drives on gasoline consumption.

The hypotheses for the gasoline types are

H_0: There is no difference between the means of gasoline consumption for two types of gasoline.

H_1: There is a difference between the means of gasoline consumption for two types of gasoline.

The hypotheses for the types of automobile driven are

H_0: There is no difference between the means of gasoline consumption for two-wheel-drive and four-wheel-drive automobiles.

H_1: There is a difference between the means of gasoline consumption for two-wheel-drive and four-wheel-drive automobiles.

Step 2 Find the critical values for each F test. In this case, each independent variable, or factor, has two levels. Hence, a 2×2 ANOVA table is used. Factor A is designated as the gasoline type. It has two levels, regular and high octane; therefore, $a = 2$. Factor B is designated as the automobile type. It also has two levels; therefore, $b = 2$. The degrees of freedom for each factor are as follows:

$$\text{Factor } A: \quad \text{d.f.N.} = a - 1 = 2 - 1 = 1$$
$$\text{Factor } B: \quad \text{d.f.N.} = b - 1 = 2 - 1 = 1$$
$$\text{Interaction } (A \times B): \quad \text{d.f.N.} = (a - 1)(b - 1)$$
$$= (2 - 1)(2 - 1) = 1 \cdot 1 = 1$$
$$\text{Within (error):} \quad \text{d.f.D.} = ab(n - 1)$$
$$= 2 \cdot 2(2 - 1) = 4$$

where n is the number of data values in each group. In this case, $n = 2$.

The critical value for the F_A test is found by using $\alpha = 0.05$, d.f.N. = 1, and d.f.D. = 4. In this case, $F_A = 7.71$. The critical value for the F_B test is found by using $\alpha = 0.05$, d.f.N. = 1, and d.f.D. = 4; F_B is also 7.71. Finally, the critical value for the $F_{A \times B}$ test is found by using d.f.N. = 1 and d.f.D. = 4; it is also 7.71.

Note: If there are different levels of the factors, the critical values will not all be the same. For example, if factor A has three levels and factor b has four levels, and if there are two subjects in each group, then the degrees of freedom are as follows:

$$\text{d.f.N.} = a - 1 = 3 - 1 = 2 \qquad \text{factor } A$$
$$\text{d.f.N.} = b - 1 = 4 - 1 = 3 \qquad \text{factor } B$$
$$\text{d.f.N.} = (a - 1)(b - 1) = (3 - 1)(4 - 1)$$
$$= 2 \cdot 3 = 6 \qquad \text{factor } A \times B$$
$$\text{d.f.N.} = ab(n - 1) = 3 \cdot 4(2 - 1) = 12 \qquad \text{within (error) factor}$$

Step 3 Complete the ANOVA summary table to obtain the test statistics. The mean squares are calculated first.

$$\text{MS}_A = \frac{\text{SS}_A}{a - 1} = \frac{0.151}{2 - 1} = 0.151$$

$$\text{MS}_B = \frac{\text{SS}_B}{b - 1} = \frac{0.661}{2 - 1} = 0.661$$

$$\text{MS}_{A \times B} = \frac{\text{SS}_{A \times B}}{(a - 1)(b - 1)} = \frac{4.651}{(2 - 1)(2 - 1)} = 4.651$$

$$\text{MS}_W = \frac{\text{SS}_W}{ab(n - 1)} = \frac{0.395}{4} = 0.0988$$

The F test statistics are calculated next.

$$F_A = \frac{MS_A}{MS_W} = \frac{0.151}{0.0988} = 1.528 \qquad \text{d.f.N.} = a - 1 = 1 \qquad \text{d.f.D.} = ab(n-1) = 4$$

$$F_B = \frac{MS_B}{MS_W} = \frac{0.661}{0.0988} = 6.690 \qquad \text{d.f.N.} = b - 1 = 1 \qquad \text{d.f.D.} = ab(n-1) = 4$$

$$F_{A \times B} = \frac{MS_{A \times B}}{MS_W} = \frac{4.651}{0.0988} = 47.075 \quad \text{d.f.N.} = (a-1)(b-1) = 1 \quad \text{d.f.D.} = ab(n-1) = 4$$

The completed ANOVA table is shown in Table 12–7. *Note: P-values were generated using technology. Table values generated with technology may differ slightly due to rounding.*

Table 12–7	**Completed ANOVA Summary Table for Example 12–5**				
Source	Sum of squares	d.f.	Mean square	F	P-value
Gasoline A	0.151	1	0.151	1.528	0.284
Automobile B	0.661	1	0.661	6.690	0.061
Interaction $(A \times B)$	4.651	1	4.651	47.075	0.002
Within (error)	0.395	4	0.0988		
Total	5.858	7			

Step 4 Make the decision. Since $F_{A \times B} = 47.075$ is greater than the critical value 7.71, the null hypothesis concerning the interaction effect should be rejected.

Step 5 Summarize the results. Since the null hypothesis for the interaction effect was rejected, it can be concluded that the combination of type of gasoline and type of automobile does affect gasoline consumption.

In the preceding analysis, the effect of the type of gasoline used and the effect of the type of automobile driven are called the *main effects*. If there is no significant interaction effect, the main effects can be interpreted independently. However, if there is a significant interaction effect, the main effects must be interpreted cautiously.

To interpret the results of a two-way analysis of variance, researchers suggest drawing a graph, plotting the means of each group, analyzing the graph, and interpreting the results. In Example 12–5, find the means for each group or cell by adding the data values in each cell and dividing by n. The means for each cell are shown in the chart here.

	Type of automobile	
Gas	**Two-wheel-drive**	**Four-wheel-drive**
Regular	$\overline{X}_{1,1} = \dfrac{8.8 + 9.3}{2} = 9.05$	$\overline{X}_{1,2} = \dfrac{8.2 + 8.0}{2} = 8.10$
High octane	$\overline{X}_{2,1} = \dfrac{7.3 + 7.2}{2} = 7.25$	$\overline{X}_{2,2} = \dfrac{9.0 + 9.7}{2} = 9.35$

The graph of the means for each of the variables is shown in Figure 12–4. In this graph, the lines cross each other. When such an intersection occurs and the interaction is significant, the interaction is said to be a **disordinal interaction.** When there is a disordinal interaction, one should not interpret the main effects without considering the interaction effect.

Figure 12–4

Graph of the Means of the Variables in Example 12–5

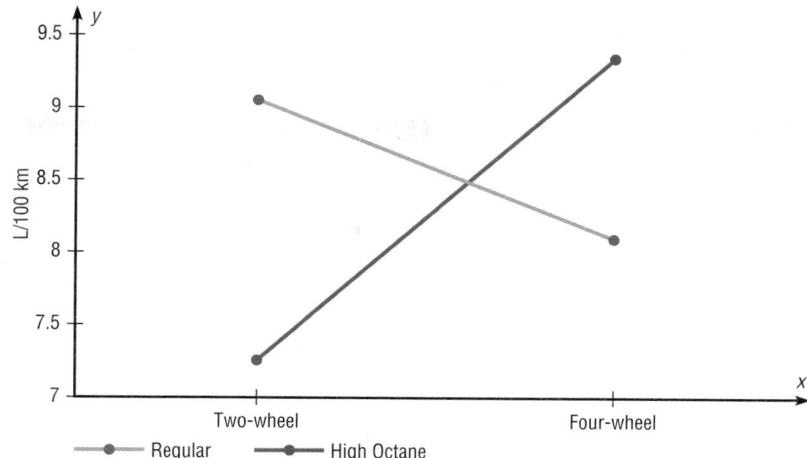

Figure 12–5

Graph of Two Variables Indicating an Ordinal Interaction

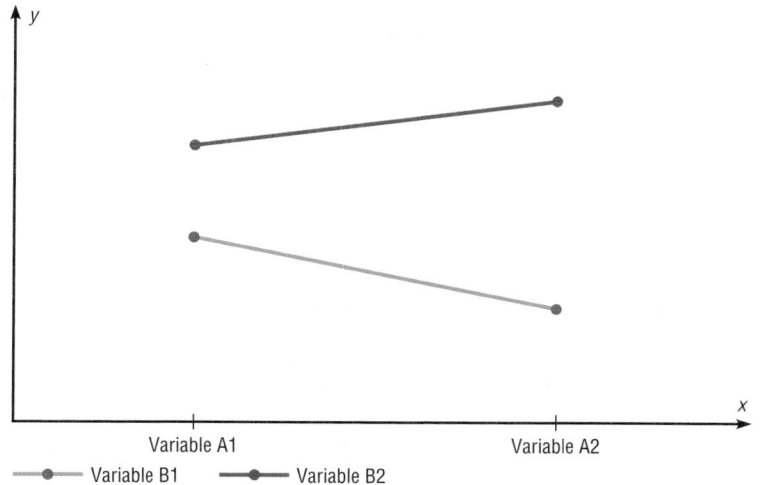

The other type of interaction that can occur is an *ordinal interaction*. Figure 12–5 shows a graph of means in which an ordinal interaction occurs between two variables. The lines do not cross each other, nor are they parallel. If the *F* test value for the interaction is significant and the lines do not cross each other, then the interaction is said to be an **ordinal interaction** and the main effects can be interpreted independently of each other.

Finally, when there is no significant interaction effect, the lines in the graph will be parallel or approximately parallel. When this situation occurs, the main effects can be interpreted independently of each other because there is no significant interaction. Figure 12–6 shows the graph of two variables when the interaction effect is not significant; the lines are parallel.

Example 12–5 was an example of a 2 × 2 two-way analysis of variance, since each independent variable had two levels. For other types of variance problems, such as a 3 × 2 or a 4 × 3 ANOVA, interpretation of the results can be quite complicated. Procedures using tests such as the Tukey and Scheffé tests for analyzing the cell means exist and are similar to the tests shown for the one-way ANOVA, but they are beyond the scope of this textbook. Many other designs for analysis of variance are available to researchers, such as three-factor designs and repeated-measure designs; they are also beyond the scope of this book.

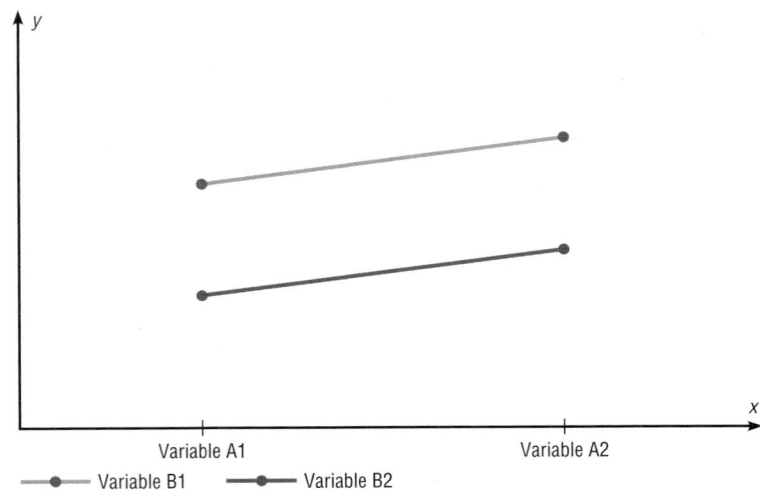

Figure 12–6

Graph of Two Variables Indicating No Interaction

In summary, the two-way ANOVA is an extension of the one-way ANOVA. The former can be used to test the effects of two independent variables and a possible interaction effect on a dependent variable.

12–3 Applying the Concepts

Automobile Sales Techniques

The following outputs are from the result of an analysis of how car sales are affected by the experience of the salesperson and the type of sales technique used. Experience was broken up into four levels, and two different sales techniques were used. Analyze the results and draw conclusions about level of experience with respect to the two different sales techniques and how they affect car sales.

Two-Way Analysis of Variance

```
Analysis of Variance for Sales
Source          DF        SS        MS
Experience       3     3414.0    1138.0
Presentation     1        6.0       6.0
Interaction      3      414.0     138.0
Error           16      838.0      52.4
Total           23     4672.0
                              Individual 95% CI
Experience     Mean    -----+---------+---------+---------+------
1              62.0     (-----*-----)
2              63.0      (-----*-----)
3              78.0                       (-----*-----)
4              91.0                                   (-----*-----)
                       -----+---------+---------+---------+------
                         60.0      70.0      80.0      90.0

                              Individual 95% CI
Presentation   Mean    ------+---------+---------+---------+-----
1              74.0       (----------------*------------------)
2              73.0     (-----------------*----------------)
                       ------+---------+---------+---------+-----
```

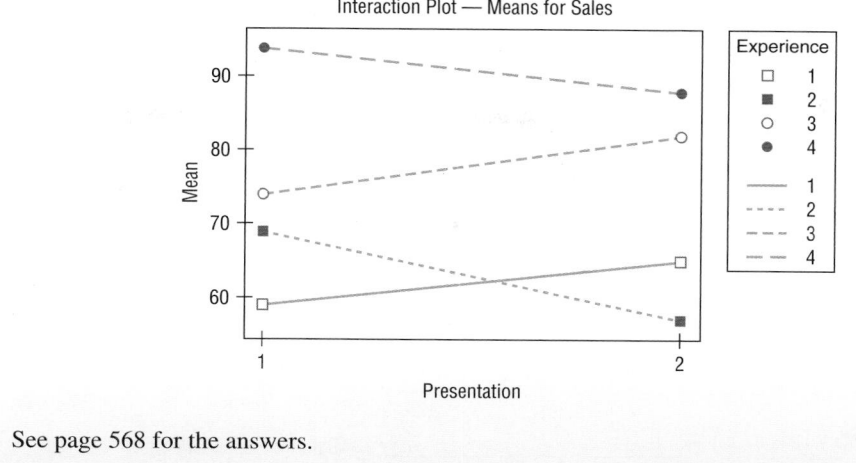

Interaction Plot — Means for Sales

See page 568 for the answers.

Exercises 12–3

1. How does the two-way ANOVA differ from the one-way ANOVA?

2. Explain what is meant by *main effects* and *interaction effect.*

3. How are the values for the mean squares computed?

4. How are the F test statistics computed?

5. In a two-way ANOVA, variable A has three levels and variable B has two levels. There are five data values in each cell. Find each degrees-of-freedom value.

  a. d.f.N. for factor A

  b. d.f.N. for factor B

  c. d.f.N. for factor $A \times B$

  d. d.f.D. for the within (error) factor

6. In a two-way ANOVA, variable A has six levels and variable B has five levels. There are seven data values in each cell. Find each degrees-of-freedom value.

  a. d.f.N. for factor A

  b. d.f.N. for factor B

  c. d.f.N. for factor $A \times B$

  d. d.f.D. for the within (error) factor

7. What are the two types of interactions that can occur in the two-way ANOVA?

8. When can the main effects for the two-way ANOVA be interpreted independently?

9. Describe what the graph of the variables would look like for each situation in a two-way ANOVA experiment.

  a. No interaction effect occurs.

  b. An ordinal interaction effect occurs.

  c. A disordinal interaction effect occurs.

For Exercises 10 through 15, perform these steps. Assume that all variables are normally or approximately normally distributed, that the samples are independent, and that the population variances are equal.

  a. State the hypotheses.

  b. Find the critical value for each F test.

  c. Complete the summary table and find the test statistic.

  d. Make the decision.

  e. Summarize the results. (Draw a graph of the cell means if necessary.)

10. Effectiveness of Advertising A company wants to test the effectiveness of its advertising. A product is selected, and two types of ads are written; one is serious and one is humorous. Also the ads are run on both television and radio. Sixteen potential customers are selected and assigned randomly to one of four groups. After seeing or listening to the ad, each customer is asked to rate its effectiveness on a scale of 1 to 20. Various points are assigned for clarity, conciseness, etc. The data are shown here. At $\alpha = 0.01$, analyze the data, using a two-way ANOVA.

Type of ad	Medium	
	Radio	**Television**
Humorous	6, 10, 11, 9	15, 18, 14, 16
Serious	8, 13, 12, 10	19, 20, 13, 17

ANOVA Summary Table for Exercise 10

Source	SS	d.f.	MS	F
Type	10.563			
Medium	175.563			
Interaction	0.063			
Within	66.250			
Total	252.439			

11. Diet Effect on Blood Sodium Levels A medical researcher wishes to test the effects of two diets and the time of day on the sodium level in a person's blood. Eight people are randomly selected, and two are randomly assigned to each of the four groups. Analyze the data shown in the tables here, using a two-way ANOVA at $\alpha = 0.05$. The sodium content is measured in milliequivalents per litre.

Time	Diet type I		Diet type II	
8:00 A.M.	135	145	138	141
8:00 P.M.	155	162	171	191

ANOVA Summary Table for Exercise 11

Source	SS	d.f.	MS	F
Time	1800.0			
Diet	242.0			
Interaction	264.5			
Within	279.0			
Total	2585.5			

13. Army Training Programs and Gender Two special training programs in outdoor survival are available for army recruits. One lasts one week and the other lasts two weeks. The officer wants to test the effectiveness of the programs to see whether there are any gender differences. Six subjects are randomly assigned to each of the programs according to gender. After completing the program, each is given a written test on his or her knowledge of survival skills. The test consists of 100 questions. The scores of the groups are shown here. Use $\alpha = 0.10$ and analyze the data, using a two-way ANOVA.

Gender	Duration One week	Duration Two weeks
Female	86, 92, 87, 88, 78, 95	78, 62, 56, 54, 65, 63
Male	52, 67, 53, 42, 68, 71	85, 94, 82, 84, 78, 91

12. Home-Building Times A contractor wishes to see whether there is a difference in the time (in days) it takes two subcontractors to build three different types of homes. At $\alpha = 0.05$, analyze the data shown here, using a two-way ANOVA. See above for raw data.

ANOVA Summary Table for Exercise 12

Source	SS	d.f.	MS	F
Subcontractor	1672.553			
Home type	444.867			
Interaction	313.267			
Within	328.800			
Total	2759.487			

Data for Exercise 12

Subcontractor	Home type I	Home type II	Home type III
A	25, 28, 26, 30, 31	30, 32, 35, 29, 31	43, 40, 42, 49, 48
B	15, 18, 22, 21, 17	21, 27, 18, 15, 19	23, 25, 24, 17, 13

ANOVA Summary Table for Exercise 13

Source	SS	d.f.	MS	F
Gender	57.042			
Duration	7.042			
Interaction	3978.375			
Within	1365.500			
Total	5407.959			

14. Types of Outdoor Paint Two types of outdoor paint, enamel and latex, were tested to see how long (in months) each lasted before it began to crack, flake, and peel. They were tested in four geographic locations in North America to study the effects of climate on the paint. At $\alpha = 0.01$, analyze the data shown, using a two-way ANOVA shown on the next page. Each group contained five test panels. See below for raw data.

Data for Exercise 14

Type of paint	Geographic location North	East	South	West
Enamel	60, 53, 58, 62, 57	54, 63, 62, 71, 76	80, 82, 62, 88, 71	62, 76, 55, 48, 61
Latex	36, 41, 54, 65, 53	62, 61, 77, 53, 64	68, 72, 71, 82, 86	63, 65, 72, 71, 63

ANOVA Summary Table for Exercise 14

Source	SS	d.f.	MS	F
Paint type	12.1			
Location	2501.0			
Interaction	268.1			
Within	2326.8			
Total	5108.0			

15. Age and Sales A company sells three items: swimming pools, spas, and saunas. The owner decides to see whether the age of the sales representative and the type of item affect monthly sales. At $\alpha = 0.05$, analyze the

data shown, using a two-way ANOVA. Sales are given in hundreds of dollars for a randomly selected month, and five salespeople were selected for each group.

ANOVA Summary Table for Exercise 15

Source	SS	d.f.	MS	F
Age	168.033			
Product	1,762.067			
Interaction	7,955.267			
Within	2,574.000			
Total	12,459.367			

Data for Exercise 15

Age of salesperson	Product		
	Pool	**Spa**	**Sauna**
Over 30	56, 23, 52, 28, 35	43, 25, 16, 27, 32	47, 43, 52, 61, 74
30 or under	16, 14, 18, 27, 31	58, 62, 68, 72, 83	15, 14, 22, 16, 27

16. Environmentally Friendly Air Freshener As a new type of environmentally friendly, natural air freshener is being developed, it is tested to see whether the effects of temperature and humidity affect the length of time that the scent is effective. The numbers of days that the air freshener had a significant level of scent are listed below for two temperature and humidity levels. Can an interaction between the two factors be concluded? Is there a difference in mean length of effectiveness with respect to humidity? With respect to temperature? Use $\alpha = 0.05$.

	Temperature 1			Temperature 2		
Humidity 1	35	25	26	35	31	37
Humidity 2	28	22	21	23	19	18

17. Sugar and Flour Doughnuts A national baking company decided to test a new recipe for its doughnuts and the glaze that it uses. Customers had the opportunity to sample the different combinations of whole wheat flour or white flour with glaze sweetened by sugar or by artificial sweetener. The sales of each type are recorded at the test site for four days. At $\alpha = 0.05$, can it be concluded that there is an interaction between the two factors? Is there a difference in mean sales with respect to flour type? With respect to sweetener type?

	Sugar				Artificial sweetener			
Wheat	62	50	78	75	60	40	50	50
White	65	60	70	70	62	38	45	52

Summary >

The F test, as shown in Chapter 9, can be used to compare two sample variances to determine whether they are equal. It can also be used to compare three or more means. When three or more means are compared, the technique is called *analysis of variance* (ANOVA). The ANOVA technique uses two estimates of the population variance. The between-group variance is the variance of the sample means; the within-group variance is the overall variance of all the values. When there is no significant difference among the means, the two estimates will be approximately equal and the F test statistic will be close to 1. If there is a significant difference among the means, the between-group variance estimate will be larger than the within-group variance estimate and a significant test statistic will result.

If there is a significant difference among means, the researcher may wish to see where this difference lies. Several statistical tests can be used to compare the sample means after the ANOVA technique has been done. The most common are the Scheffé test and the Tukey test. When the sample sizes are the same, the Tukey test can be used. The Scheffé test is more general and can be used when the sample sizes are equal or not equal.

When there is one independent variable, the analysis of variance is called a *one-way ANOVA*. When there are two independent variables, the analysis of variance is called a *two-way ANOVA*. The two-way ANOVA enables the researcher to test the effects of two independent variables and a possible interaction effect on one dependent variable.

For step-by-step guidance on the use of Texas Instruments TI-83 Plus/TI-84 Plus programmable calculators, see Appendix E at the back of this book. For summary procedures for Minitab, SPSS, and Excel, please see the full version of Appendix E on *Connect*.

Important Terms >>

analysis of variance (ANOVA) 536

ANOVA summary table 539

between-group variance 536

disordinal interaction 556

factors 550

interaction effect 551

level 551

main effect 552

mean square 538

one-way ANOVA 550

ordinal interaction 557

Scheffé test 546

sum of squares between groups 538

sum of squares within groups 538

treatment groups 551

Tukey test 547

two-way ANOVA 550

within-group variance 536

Important Formulas >>

Formulas for the ANOVA test:

$$\overline{X}_{GM} = \frac{\Sigma X}{N}$$

$$F = \frac{s_B^2}{s_W^2}$$

where

$$s_B^2 = \frac{\Sigma n_i(\overline{X}_i - \overline{X}_{GM})^2}{k - 1} \qquad s_W^2 = \frac{\Sigma(n_i - 1)s_i^2}{\Sigma(n_i - 1)}$$

$$\text{d.f.N.} = k - 1 \qquad\qquad N = n_1 + n_2 + \cdots + n_k$$

$$\text{d.f.D.} = N - k \qquad\qquad k = \text{number of groups}$$

Formulas for the Scheffé test:

$$F_s = \frac{(\overline{X}_i - \overline{X}_j)^2}{s_W^2[(1/n_i) + (1/n_j)]} \qquad \text{and} \qquad F' = (k - 1)(\text{C.V.})$$

Formula for the Tukey test:

$$q = \frac{\overline{X}_i - \overline{X}_j}{\sqrt{s_W^2/n}}$$

d.f.N. = k and **d.f.D. = degrees of freedom s_W^2**

Formulas for the two-way ANOVA:

$$MS_A = \frac{SS_A}{a-1}$$ $$F_A = \frac{MS_A}{MS_W}$$ **d.f.N. = $a - 1$**

d.f.D. = $ab(n-1)$

$$MS_B = \frac{SS_B}{b-1}$$ $$F_B = \frac{MS_B}{MS_W}$$ **d.f.N. = $b - 1$**

d.f.D. = $ab(n-1)$

$$MS_{A \times B} = \frac{SS_{A \times B}}{(a-1)(b-1)}$$ $$F_{A \times B} = \frac{MS_{A \times B}}{MS_W}$$ **d.f.N. = $(a-1)(b-1)$**

d.f.D. = $ab(n-1)$

$$MS_W = \frac{SS_W}{ab(n-1)}$$

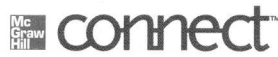 **connect**™ Practise and learn online with *Connect* with data sets and algorithmic questions related to concepts covered in this chapter. Questions and tables with online data sets are marked with .

Review Exercises »

If the null hypothesis is rejected in Exercises 1 through 9, use the Scheffé test when the sample sizes are unequal to test the differences between the means, and use the Tukey test when the sample sizes are equal. For these exercises, perform these steps.

  a. State the hypotheses and identify the claim.
  b. Find the critical value(s).
  c. Compute the test statistic.
  d. Make the decision.
  e. Summarize the results, and explain where the differences in means are.

Use the traditional method of hypothesis testing unless otherwise specified.

 1. Lengths of Various Types of Bridges The data represent the lengths (in metres) of three types of bridges in the United States. At $\alpha = 0.01$, test the claim that there is no significant difference in the means of the lengths of the types of bridges.

Simple truss	Segmented concrete	Continuous plate
227	250	192
218	229	175
213	241	160
198	205	155
197	201	146
191	195	140
185	194	137
182	189	137
168	158	137
166	137	130
163	119	128
161	113	110

Source: World Almanac and Book of Facts.

 2. Wine Prices Is there a difference in the price per bottle of three different types of wine? The data show the costs per bottle (in dollars) of three different types of wines. Use $\alpha = 0.01$ to answer the question. Why would some wines be more expensive than others?

Type 1	Type 2	Type 3
11	15	13
10	7	11
20	9	18
10	10	10
17	4	22
9	5	15

 3. Carbohydrates in Cereals The number of carbohydrates per serving in randomly selected cereals from three manufacturers is shown. At the 0.05 level of significance, is there sufficient evidence to conclude a difference in the average number of carbohydrates?

Manufacturer 1	Manufacturer 2	Manufacturer 3
25	23	24
26	44	39
24	24	28
26	24	25
26	36	23
41	27	32
26	25	
43		

Source: The Doctor's Pocket Calorie, Fat, and Carbohydrate Counter.

 4. Grams of Fat per Serving of Pizza The number of grams of fat per serving for three different kinds of pizza from several manufacturers is listed below. At the

0.01 level of significance, is there sufficient evidence that a difference exists in mean fat content?

Cheese	Pepperoni	Supreme/Deluxe
18	20	16
11	17	27
19	15	17
20	18	17
16	23	12
21	23	27
16	21	20

Source: The Doctor's Pocket Calorie, Fat, and Carbohydrate Counter.

5. Iron Content of Food The iron content in three different types of food is shown. At the 0.10 level of significance, is there sufficient evidence to conclude that a difference in mean iron content exists for meats and fish, breakfast cereals, and nutritional high-protein drinks?

Meats and fish	Breakfast cereals	Nutritional drinks
3.4	8	3.6
2.5	2	3.6
5.5	1.5	4.5
5.3	3.8	5.5
2.5	3.8	2.7
1.3	6.8	3.6
2.7	1.5	6.3
	4.5	

Source: The Doctor's Pocket Calorie, Fat, and Carbohydrate Counter.

6. Temperatures in January The average January high temperatures (in degrees Celsius) for selected tourist cities on different continents are listed below. Is there sufficient evidence to conclude a difference in mean temperatures for the three continents? Use the 0.05 level of significance.

Europe	Central/South America	Asia
5	31	32
3	24	2
2	19	28
13	29	19
10	24	9

Source: Time Almanac.

7. Violent Crimes in Metropolitan Areas A researcher wishes to see if there is a difference in the average number of violent crimes in different metropolitan areas across Canada. Random samples of cities were selected, and the violent crime rate (per 100,000 population) for a specific year was reported. At $\alpha = 0.05$, is there a difference in the means? If so, suggest a reason for the difference.

Pacific	Prairies	Central	Atlantic
1028	934	836	1343
1136	1718	489	788
	1578	910	1169
	1242	564	
		691	

Source: Statistics Canada.

8. Math Anxiety Levels and Students' Ages A teacher wants to test the math anxiety level of her students in two classes at the beginning of the semester. The classes are Calculus I and Statistics. Furthermore, she wishes to see whether there is a difference owing to the students' ages. Math anxiety is measured by the score on a 100-point anxiety test. Use $\alpha = 0.10$ and a two-way analysis of variance to see whether there is a difference. Five students are randomly assigned to each group. The data are shown here.

Age	Class	
	Calculus I	**Statistics**
Under 20	43, 52, 61, 57, 55	19, 20, 31, 36, 24
20 or over	56, 55, 42, 48, 61	63, 78, 67, 71, 75

ANOVA Summary Table for Exercise 8

Source	SS	d.f.	MS	F
Age	2376.2			
Class	105.8			
Interaction	2645.0			
Within	763.2			
Total	5890.2			

Statistics Today

Is Seeing Really Believing?—Revisited

To see if there were differences in the testimonies of the witnesses in the three age groups, the witnesses responded to 17 questions, 10 on direct examination and 7 on cross-examination. These were then scored for accuracy. An analysis of variance test with age as the independent variable was used to compare the total number of questions answered correctly by the groups. The results showed no significant differences among the age groups for the direct examination questions. However, there was a significant difference among the groups on the cross-examination questions. Further analysis showed the 8-year-olds were significantly less accurate under cross-examination compared to the other two groups. The 12-year-old and adult eyewitnesses did not differ in the accuracy of their cross-examination responses.

9. Effects of Diet and Exercise on Glucose Levels A medical researcher wishes to test the effects of two different diets and two different exercise programs on the glucose level in a person's blood. The glucose level is measured in milligrams per decilitre (mg/dL). Three subjects are randomly assigned to each group. Analyze the data shown here, using a two-way ANOVA with $\alpha = 0.05$.

Exercise program	Diet	
	A	**B**
I	62, 64, 66	58, 62, 53
II	65, 68, 72	83, 85, 91

ANOVA Summary Table for Exercise 9

Source	SS	d.f.	MS	F
Exercise	816.750			
Diet	102.083			
Interaction	444.083			
Within	108.000			
Total	1470.916			

Data Analysis »

The databank for these questions can be found in Appendix D at the back of the textbook and on ▦ connect.

1. From the databank, select a random sample of subjects, and test the hypothesis that the mean cholesterol levels of the nonsmokers, less-than-one-pack-a-day smokers, and one-pack-plus smokers are equal. Use an ANOVA test. If the null hypothesis is rejected, conduct the Scheffé test to find where the difference is. Summarize the results.

2. Repeat Exercise 2 for the mean IQs of the various educational levels of the subjects.

3. Using the databank, randomly select 12 subjects and randomly assign them to one of the four groups in the following classifications.

	Smoker	**Nonsmoker**
Male		
Female		

Use one of these variables—weight, cholesterol, or systolic pressure—as the dependent variable, and perform a two-way ANOVA on the data. Use a computer program to generate the ANOVA table.

Chapter Quiz »

Determine whether each statement is true or false. If the statement is false, explain why.

1. In analysis of variance, the null hypothesis should be rejected only when there is a significant difference among all pairs of means.

2. The F test does not use the concept of degrees of freedom.

3. When the F test statistic is close to 1, the null hypothesis should be rejected.

4. The Tukey test is generally more powerful than the Scheffé test for pairwise comparisons.

Select the best answer.

5. Analysis of variance uses the _____ test.

  a. z *c.* χ^2
  b. t *d.* F

6. The null hypothesis in ANOVA is that all the means are _____.

  a. Equal   *c.* Variable
  b. Unequal   *d.* None of the above

7. When one conducts an F test, _____ estimates of the population variance are compared.

  a. Two   *c.* Any number of
  b. Three   *d.* No

8. If the null hypothesis is rejected in ANOVA, one can use the _____ test to see where the difference in the means is found.

  a. z or t *c.* Scheffé or Tukey
  b. F or χ^2 *d.* Any of the above

Complete the following statements with the best answer.

9. When three or more means are compared, one uses the _____ technique.

10. If the null hypothesis is rejected in ANOVA, the _____ test should be used when sample sizes are equal.

11. In a two-way ANOVA, one can test _____ main hypotheses and one interactive hypothesis.

For Exercises 12 through 16 use the traditional method of hypothesis testing unless otherwise specified.

12. **Voters in Federal Elections** In a recent federal election, a sample of the percentage of voters who

voted in various regions across Canada is shown. At $\alpha = 0.05$, is there a difference in the mean percentage of voters who voted in each region.

North	West	Central	East
54.1	71.0	72.4	66.9
56.2	63.2	72.8	62.4
54.0	63.7	64.7	70.7
	48.4	64.1	

Source: Elections Canada.

13. **Ages of Late-Night TV Talk Show Viewers** A media researcher wishes to see if there is a difference in the ages of viewers of three late-night television talk shows. Three samples of viewers are selected, and the ages of the viewers are shown. At $\alpha = 0.01$, is there a difference in the means of the ages of the viewers? Why is the average age of a viewer important to a television show writer?

David Letterman	Jay Leno	Conan O'Brien
53	48	40
46	51	36
48	57	35
42	46	42
35	38	39

Source: Based on information from Nielsen Media Research.

14. **Prices of Athletic Shoes** Prices (in dollars) of men's, women's, and children's athletic shoes are shown. At the 0.05 level of significance, can it be concluded that there is a difference in mean price?

Women's	Men's	Children's
59	65	40
36	70	45
44	66	40
49	59	56
48	48	46
50	70	36

15. **Birth Weights** The birth weights (in kilograms) of randomly selected newborns at three area hospitals are shown. Using the 0.10 level of significance, test the claim that the mean weights are equal.

Hospital A	Hospital B	Hospital C
3.5	5.7	4.3
3.7	1.5	2.5
5.2	2.9	3.0
3.0	4.8	3.9
3.3	1.7	4.7
3.7	1.1	3.4

16. **Alumni Gift Solicitation** Several students volunteered for an alumni phone-a-thon to solicit alumni gifts. The number of calls made by randomly selected students from each class is listed. At $\alpha = 0.05$, is there sufficient evidence to conclude a difference in means?

Freshmen	Sophomores	Juniors	Seniors
25	17	20	20
29	25	24	25
32	20	25	26
15	26	30	32
18	30	15	19
26	28	18	20
35			

17. **Diets and Exercise Programs** A researcher conducted a study of two different diets and two different exercise programs. Three randomly selected subjects were assigned to each group for one month. The values indicate the amount of weight each lost.

Exercise program \ Diet	A	B
I	5, 6, 4	8, 10, 15
II	3, 4, 8	12, 16, 11

Answer the following questions for the information in the printout shown below.

a. What procedure is being used?
b. What are the names of the two variables?
c. How many levels does each variable contain?
d. What are the hypotheses for the study?
e. What are the F statistics for the hypotheses? State which are significant, using the P-values.
f. Based on the answers to part *e*, which hypotheses can be rejected?

Computer Printout (Minitab) for Problem 17

```
Datafile: NONAME.SST    Procedure: Two-way ANOVA

TABLE OF MEANS:

                          DIET
                 A .....          B .....      Row Mean
EX PROG I .....    5.000           11.000        8.000
      II .....     5.000           13.000        9.000
     Col Mean      5.000           12.000
     Tot Mean      8.500

SOURCE TABLE:
       Source      df     Sums of Squares   Mean Square    F Ratio     p-value
         DIET      1          147.000         147.000      21.000      0.00180
      EX PROG      1            3.000           3.000       0.429      0.53106
   DIET X EX P     1            3.000           3.000       0.429      0.53106
       Within      8           56.000           7.000
        Total     11          209.000
```

Critical Thinking Challenges »

Shown here are the abstract and two tables from a research study entitled *Adult Children of Alcoholics: Are They at Greater Risk for Negative Health Behaviors?* by Arlene E. Hall. Based on the abstract and the tables, answer these questions.

1. What was the purpose of the study?
2. How many groups were used in the study?
3. By what means were the data collected?
4. What was the sample size?
5. What type of sampling method was used?
6. How might the population be defined?
7. What may have been the hypothesis for the ANOVA part of the study?
8. Why was the one-way ANOVA procedure used, as opposed to another test, such as the *t* test?
9. What part of the ANOVA table did the conclusion "ACOAs had significantly lower wellness scores (WS) than non-ACOAs" come from?
10. What level of significance was used?
11. In the following excerpts from the article, the researcher states that

    . . . using the Tukey-HSD procedure revealed a significant difference between ACOAs and non-ACOAs, p = 0.05, but no significant difference was found between ACOAs and Unsures or between non-ACOAs and Unsures.

Using Tables 12–8 and 12–9 and the means, explain why the Tukey test would have enabled the researcher to draw this conclusion.

Abstract *The purpose of the study was to examine and compare the health behaviors of adult children of alcoholics (ACOAs) and their non-ACOA peers within a university population. Subjects were 980 undergraduate students from a major university in the East. Three groups (ACOA, non-ACOA, and Unsure) were identified from subjects' responses to three direct questions regarding parental drinking behaviors. A questionnaire was used to collect data for the study. Included were questions related to demographics, parental drinking behaviors, and the College Wellness Check (WS), a health risk appraisal designed especially for college students (Dewey & Cabral, 1986). Analysis of variance procedures revealed that ACOAs had significantly lower wellness scores (WS) than non-ACOAs. Chi-square analyses of the individual variables revealed that ACOAs and non-ACOAs were significantly different on 15 of the 50 variables of the WS. A discriminant analysis procedure revealed the similarities between Unsure subjects and ACOA subjects. The results provide valuable information regarding ACOAs in a nonclinical setting and contribute to our understanding of the influences related to their health risk behaviors.*

Table 12–8	Means and Standard Deviations for the Wellness Scores (WS) Group by ($N = 945$)		
Group	*N*	$\overline{X}$	**S.D.**
ACOAs	143	69.0	13.6
Non-ACOAs	746	73.2	14.5
Unsure	56	70.1	14.0
Total	945	212.3	42.1

Table 12–9	ANOVA of Group Means for the Wellness Scores (WS)			
Source	**d.f.**	**SS**	**MS**	*F*
Between groups	2	2,403.5	1,201.7	5.9*
Within groups	942	193,237.4	205.1	
Total	944	195,640.8		

*$p < 0.01$

Source: Arlene E. Hall, "Adult Children of Alcoholics: Are They at Greater Risk for Negative Health Behaviors?" *Journal of Health Education* 12, No. 4, pp. 232–238.

Data Projects »

Where appropriate, use Minitab, SPSS, TI-83 Plus, TI-84 Plus, Excel, or a computer program of your choice to complete these exercises.

Use a significance level of 0.05 for all tests below.

1. **Business and Finance** Select 10 stocks at random from the Dow Jones industrials, the NASDAQ, and the Toronto Stock Exchange. For each, note the gain or loss in the last quarter. Use analysis of variance to test the claim that stocks from all three groups have had equal performances.

2. **Sports and Leisure** Use total earnings data for movies that were released in the previous year. Sort them by rating (G, PG, PG 13, and R). Is the mean revenue for movies the same, regardless of rating?

3. **Technology** Use the data collected in Data Project 3 in Chapter 2 regarding song lengths. Consider only three genres. For example, use rock, alternative, and country. Conduct an analysis of variance to determine if the mean song lengths for the genres are the same.

4. **Health and Wellness** Select 10 cereals from each of the following categories: cereal targeted at children, cereal targeted at dieters, and cereal that fits neither of the previous categories. For each cereal, note its calories per cup (this may require some computation since serving sizes vary for cereals). Use analysis of variance to test the claim that the calorie content of these different types of cereals is the same.

5. **Politics and Economics** Conduct an anonymous survey to obtain your data. Ask the participants to identify which of the following federal political party platforms that they most relate to: Conservative, Liberal, New Democrat, or Other. Also ask them to give their ages. Use an analysis of variance to determine whether there is a difference in mean age between the different political designations.

6. **Your Class** Split the class into four groups, those whose favourite type of music is rock, those whose favourite is country, those whose favourite is rap or hip-hop, and those whose favourite is another type of music. Make a list of the ages of students for each of the four groups. Use analysis of variance to test the claim that the means for all four groups are equal.

Answers to Applying the Concepts »

Section 12–1 Colours That Make You Look Smarter

1. The ANOVA produces a test statistic of $F = 3.06$, with a P-value of 0.059. We would fail to reject the null hypothesis and find that there is not enough evidence to conclude that the colour of a person's clothing is related to people's perceptions of how intelligent the person looks.

2. Answers will vary. One possible answer is that the purpose of the study was to determine if the colour of a person's clothing is related to people's perceptions of how intelligent the person looks.

3. Three separate t tests would need to be performed, which would inflate the error rate.

Section 12–2 Colours That Make You Look Smarter

1. Tukey's pairwise comparisons show no significant difference in the three pairwise comparisons of the means.

2. This agrees with the nonsignificant results of the general ANOVA test conducted in Applying the Concepts 12–1.

3. The t tests should not be used since the error rate would be inflated.

4. The Tukey test is preferred over the Scheffé test when all samples are the same size.

Section 12–3 Automobile Sales Techniques

There is no significant difference between levels 1 and 2 of experience. Level 3 and level 4 salespersons did significantly better than those at levels 1 and 2, with level 4 showing the best results, on average. If type of presentation is taken into consideration, the interaction plot shows a significant difference. The best combination seems to be level 4 experience with presentation style 1.

Hypothesis-Testing Summary 2* »

7. Test of the significance of the correlation coefficient.

    Example: $H_0: \rho = 0$

    Use a t test:

    $$t = r\sqrt{\frac{n-2}{1-r^2}} \quad \text{with d.f.} = n - 2$$

8. Formula for the F test for the multiple correlation coefficient.

    Example: $H_0: \rho = 0$

    $$F = \frac{R^2/k}{(1-R^2)/(n-k-1)}$$

    d.f.N. $= n - k$ d.f.D. $= n - k - 1$

9. Comparison of a sample distribution with a specific population.

    Example: H_0: There is no difference between the two distributions.

    Use the chi-square goodness-of-fit test:

    $$\chi^2 = \sum \frac{(O-E)^2}{E}$$

    d.f. $=$ no. of categories $- 1$

10. Comparison of the independence of two variables.

    Example: H_0: Variable A is independent of variable B.

*This summary is a continuation of Hypothesis-Testing Summary 1, at the end of Chapter 9.

Use the chi-square independence test:

$$\chi^2 = \sum \frac{(O - E)^2}{E}$$

d.f. $= (R - 1)(C - 1)$

11. Test for homogeneity of proportions.

Example: $H_0: p_1 = p_2 = p_3$

Use the chi-square test:

$$\chi^2 = \sum \frac{(O - E)^2}{E}$$

d.f. $= (R - 1)(C - 1)$

12. Comparison of three or more sample means.

Example: $H_0: \mu_1 = \mu_2 = \mu_3$

Use the analysis of variance test:

$$F = \frac{s_B^2}{s_W^2}$$

where

$$s_B^2 = \frac{\sum n_i (\overline{X}_i - \overline{X}_{\mathrm{GM}})^2}{k - 1}$$

$$s_W^2 = \frac{\sum (n_i - 1)s_i^2}{\sum (n_i - 1)}$$

d.f.N. $= k - 1$ $N = n_1 + n_2 + \cdots + n_k$

d.f.D. $= N - k$ k = number of groups

13. Test when the F test statistic for the ANOVA is significant. Use the Scheffé test to find what pairs of means are significantly different.

$$F_S = \frac{(\overline{X}_i - \overline{X}_j)^2}{s_w^2[(1/n_i) + (1/n_j)]}$$

$$F' = (k - 1) \, (\text{C.V.})$$

Use the Tukey test to find which pairs of means are significantly different.

$$q = \frac{\overline{X}_j - \overline{X}_j}{\sqrt{s_W^2/n}} \quad \begin{array}{l} \text{d.f.N.} = k \\ \text{d.f.D.} = \text{degrees of freedom for } s_W^2 \end{array}$$

14. Test for the two-way ANOVA.

Example:

H_0: There is no significant difference for the main effects.

H_1: There is no significant difference for the interaction-effect.

$$\mathrm{MS}_A = \frac{\mathrm{SS}_A}{a - 1}$$

$$\mathrm{MS}_B = \frac{\mathrm{SS}_B}{b - 1}$$

$$\mathrm{MS}_{A \times B} = \frac{\mathrm{SS}_{A \times B}}{(a - 1)(b - 1)}$$

$$\mathrm{MS}_W = \frac{\mathrm{SS}_W}{ab(n - 1)}$$

$$F_A = \frac{\mathrm{MS}_A}{\mathrm{MS}_W} \quad \begin{array}{l} \text{d.f.N.} = a - 1 \\ \text{d.f.D.} = ab(n - 1) \end{array}$$

$$F_B = \frac{\mathrm{MS}_B}{\mathrm{MS}_W} \quad \begin{array}{l} \text{d.f.N.} = (b - 1) \\ \text{d.f.D.} = ab(n - 1) \end{array}$$

$$F_{A \times B} = \frac{\mathrm{MS}_{A \times B}}{\mathrm{MS}_W} \quad \begin{array}{l} \text{d.f.N.} = (a - 1)(b - 1) \\ \text{d.f.D.} = ab(n - 1) \end{array}$$

Chapter 13

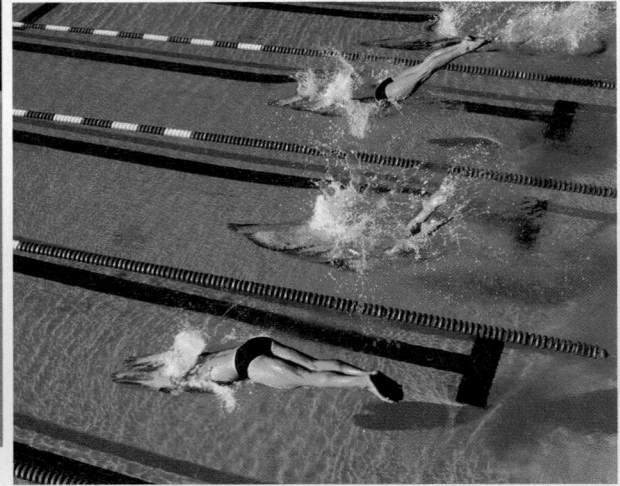

Nonparametric Statistics

Objectives >

After completing this chapter, you should be able to

LO1 State the advantages and disadvantages of nonparametric methods.

LO2 Test hypotheses, using the sign test.

LO3 Test hypotheses, using the Wilcoxon rank sum test.

LO4 Test hypotheses, using the signed-rank test.

LO5 Test hypotheses, using the Kruskal-Wallis test.

LO6 Compute the Spearman rank correlation coefficient.

LO7 Test hypotheses, using the runs test.

Outline >

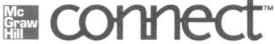 **connect**™ Practise and learn online with *Connect* with data sets and algorithmic questions related to concepts covered in this chapter. Throughout this chapter, questions and tables with online data sets are marked with ⚐.

Statistics Today

Too Much or Too Little?

Suppose a manufacturer of ketchup wants to check the bottling machines to see if they are functioning properly. That is, are they dispensing the right amount of ketchup per bottle? A 375-millilitre bottle is currently used. Because of the natural variation in the manufacturing process, the amount of ketchup in a bottle will not always be exactly 375 millilitres. Some bottles will contain less than 375 millilitres, and others will contain more than 375 millilitres. To see if the variation is due to chance or to a malfunction in the manufacturing process, a runs test can be used. The runs test is a nonparametric statistical technique. This chapter explains such techniques, which can be used to help the manufacturer determine the answer to the question. See Statistics Today—Revisited, page 609.

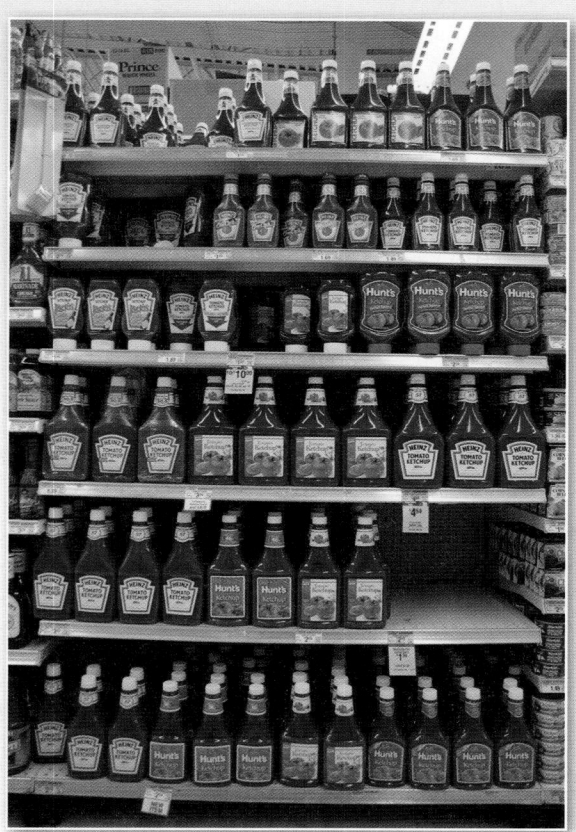

Introduction >

Statistical tests, such as the z, t, and F tests, are called *parametric tests*. **Parametric tests** are statistical tests for population parameters such as means, variances, and proportions that involve assumptions about the populations from which the samples were selected. One assumption is that these populations are normally distributed. But what if the population in a particular hypothesis-testing situation is *not* normally distributed? Statisticians have developed a branch of statistics known as **nonparametric statistics** or **distribution-free statistics** to use when the population from which the samples are selected is not normally distributed. Nonparametric statistics can also be used to test hypotheses that do not involve specific population parameters, such as μ, σ, or p.

For example, a sportswriter may want to know whether there is a relationship between the rankings of two judges on the diving abilities of ten Olympic swimmers. In another situation, a sociologist may wish to determine whether men and women enroll at random for a specific drug rehabilitation program. The statistical tests used in these situations are nonparametric or distribution-free tests. The term *nonparametric* is used for both situations.

The nonparametric tests explained in this chapter are the sign test, the Wilcoxon rank sum test, the Wilcoxon signed-rank test, the Kruskal-Wallis test, and the runs test. In addition, the Spearman rank correlation coefficient, a statistic for determining the relationship between ranks, is explained.

13–1	Advantages and Disadvantages of Nonparametric Methods >

State the advantages and disadvantages of nonparametric methods.

As stated previously, nonparametric tests and statistics can be used in place of their parametric counterparts (z, t, and F) when the assumption of normality cannot be met. However, one should not assume that these statistics are a better alternative than the parametric statistics. There are both advantages and disadvantages in the use of nonparametric methods.

Advantages

There are five advantages that nonparametric methods have over parametric methods:

1. They can be used to test population parameters when the variable is not normally distributed.
2. They can be used when the data are nominal or ordinal.
3. They can be used to test hypotheses that do not involve population parameters.
4. In most cases, the computations are easier than those for the parametric counterparts.
5. They are easy to understand.

Disadvantages

There are three disadvantages of nonparametric methods:

1. They are *less sensitive* than their parametric counterparts when the assumptions of the parametric methods are met. Therefore, larger differences are needed before the null hypothesis can be rejected.
2. They tend to use *less information* than the parametric tests. For example, the sign test requires the researcher to determine only whether the data values are above or below the median, not how much above or below the median each value is.
3. They are *less efficient* than their parametric counterparts when the assumptions of the parametric methods are met. That is, larger sample sizes are needed to overcome the loss of information. For example, the nonparametric sign test is about 60% as efficient as its parametric counterpart, the z test. Thus, a sample size of 100 is needed for use of the sign test, compared with a sample size of 60 for use of the z test to obtain the same results.

Since there are both advantages and disadvantages to the nonparametric methods, the researcher should use caution in selecting these methods. If the parametric assumptions can be met, the parametric methods are preferred. However, when parametric assumptions cannot be met, the nonparametric methods are a valuable tool for analyzing the data.

Ranking

Many nonparametric tests involve the **ranking** of data, that is, the positioning of a data value in a data array according to some rating scale. Ranking is an ordinal variable. For example, suppose a judge decides to rate five speakers on an ascending scale of 1 to 10, with 1 being the best and 10 being the worst, for categories such as voice, gestures, logical presentation, and platform personality. The ratings are shown in the chart.

Speaker	A	B	C	D	E
Rating	8	6	10	3	1

The rankings are shown next.

Speaker	E	D	B	A	C
Rating	1	3	6	8	10
Ranking	1	2	3	4	5

Interesting Fact

Older men have the biggest ears. James Heathcote, M.D., says, "On average, our ears seem to grow 0.22 millimetre a year. This is roughly a centimetre during the course of 50 years."

Since speaker E received the lowest score, 1 point, he or she is ranked first. Speaker D received the next-lower score, 3 points, so he or she is ranked second, and so on.

What happens if two or more speakers receive the same number of points? Suppose the judge awards points as follows:

Speaker	A	B	C	D	E
Rating	8	6	10	6	3

The speakers are then ranked as follows:

Speaker	E	D	B	A	C
Rating	3	6	6	8	10
Ranking	1	Tie for 2nd and 3rd		4	5

When there is a tie for two or more places, the average of the ranks must be used. In this case, each would be ranked as

$$\frac{2+3}{2} = \frac{5}{2} = 2.5$$

Hence, the rankings are as follows:

Speaker	E	D	B	A	C
Rating	3	6	6	8	10
Ranking	1	2.5	2.5	4	5

Many times, the data are already ranked, so no additional computations must be done. For example, if the judge does not have to award points but can simply select the speakers who are best, second-best, third-best, and so on, then these ranks can be used directly.

P-values can also be found for nonparametric statistical tests, and the *P*-value method can be used to test hypotheses that use nonparametric tests. For this chapter, the *P*-value method will be limited to some of the nonparametric tests that use the standard normal distribution or the chi-square distribution.

13–1 Applying the Concepts

Ranking Data

The following table lists the percentages of patients who experienced side effects from a drug used to lower a person's cholesterol level.

Side effect	Percentage
Chest pain	4.0
Rash	4.0
Nausea	7.0
Heartburn	5.4
Fatigue	3.8
Headache	7.3
Dizziness	10.0
Chills	7.0
Cough	2.6

Rank each value in the table.

See page 612 for the answer.

Exercises 13–1

1. What is meant by *nonparametric statistics?*

2. When should nonparametric statistics be used?

3. List the advantages and disadvantages of nonparametric statistics.

For Exercises 4 through 10, rank each set of data.

4. 3, 8, 6, 1, 4, 10, 7

5. 22, 66, 32, 43, 65, 43, 71, 34

6. 83, 460, 582, 177, 241

7. 9, 7, 4, 9, 8, 6, 6, 10, 13, 16, 18, 15

8. 22, 25, 28, 28, 18, 32, 37, 41, 41, 43

9. 188, 256, 197, 188, 321, 530, 763

10. 2.8, 6.8, 2.6, 3.1, 1.5, 8.9, 3.15, 2.12, 3.1

13–2   The Sign Test ❯

LO2

Test hypotheses, using the sign test.

Single-Sample Sign Test

The simplest nonparametric test, the **sign test** for single samples, is used to test the value of a median for a specific sample. When using the sign test, the researcher hypothesizes the specific value for the median of a population; then he or she selects a sample of data and compares each value with the conjectured median. If the data value is above the conjectured median, it is assigned a plus sign. If it is below the conjectured median, it is assigned a minus sign. And if it is exactly the same as the conjectured median, it is assigned a 0. Then the numbers of plus and minus signs are compared. If the null hypothesis is true, the number of plus signs should be approximately equal to the number of minus signs. If the null hypothesis is not true, there will be a disproportionate number of plus or minus signs.

Test Statistic for the Sign Test

The test statistic is the smaller number of plus or minus signs.

For example, if there are 8 positive signs and 3 negative signs, the test statistic is 3. When the sample size is 25 or less, Table J in Appendix C is used to determine the critical value. For a specific α, if the test statistic is less than or equal to the critical value obtained from the table, the null hypothesis should be rejected. The values in Table J are obtained from the binomial distribution. The derivation is omitted here.

Example 13–1

Snow Cone Sales

A convenience store owner hypothesizes that the median number of snow cones she sells per day is 40. A random sample of 20 days yields the following data for the number of snow cones sold each day.

18	43	40	16	22
30	29	32	37	36
39	34	39	45	28
36	40	34	39	52

At $\alpha = 0.05$, test the owner's hypothesis.

Solution

Step 1   State the hypotheses and identify the claim.

H_0: median = 40 (claim)   and H_1: median ≠ 40

Step 2   Find the critical value. Compare each value of the data with the median. If the value is greater than the median, replace the value with a plus sign. If it is less than the median, replace it with a minus sign. And if it is equal to the median, replace it with a 0. The completed table follows.

−	+	0	−	−
−	−	−	−	−
−	−	−	+	−
−	0	−	−	+

Refer to Table J in Appendix C, using $n = 18$ (the total number of plus and minus signs; omit the zeros) and $\alpha = 0.05$ for a two-tailed test; the critical value is 4. See Figure 13–1.

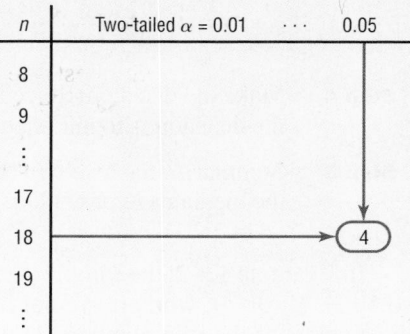

Figure 13–1

Finding the Critical Value in Table J for Example 13–1

Step 3   Compute the test statistic. Count the number of plus and minus signs obtained in step 2, and use the smaller value as the test statistic. Since there are 3 plus signs and 15 minus signs, 3 is the test statistic.

Step 4   Make the decision. Compare the test statistic 3 with the critical value 4. If the test statistic is less than or equal to the critical value, the null hypothesis is rejected. In this case, the null hypothesis is rejected since 3 < 4.

Step 5   Summarize the results. There is enough evidence to reject the claim that the median number of snow cones sold per day is 40.

When the sample size is 26 or more, the normal approximation can be used to find the test statistic. The formula is given below. The critical value is found in Table E–1 or Table E–2 in Appendix C.

Formula for the z Test Statistic in the Sign Test When $n \geq 26$

$$z = \frac{(X + 0.5) - (n/2)}{\sqrt{n}/2}$$

where

X = smaller number of + or − signs
n = sample size

Example 13–2	**Age of Workers in Region**

Based on Statistics Canada census data, the median (MD) age of Canada's labour force is 41.2 years. A researcher selects a random sample of 50 workers in his region and finds that 21 are older than 41.2 years. At $\alpha = 0.05$, test the claim that the median age of the region's workers is at least 41.2 years.

Source: Statistics Canada, *The Daily,* "2006 Census: Labour Market Activities, Industry, Occupation, Education, Language of Work, Place of Work and Mode of Transportation," March 4, 2008.

Solution

Step 1   State the hypotheses and identify the claim.

$$H_0: \text{MD} = 41.2 \text{ years (claim)} \qquad \text{and} \qquad H_1: \text{MD} < 41.2 \text{ years}$$

Step 2   Find the critical value. Since $\alpha = 0.05$ and $n = 50$, and since this is a left-tailed test, the critical value is -1.645, obtained from Table E–1.

Step 3   Compute the test statistic.

$$z = \frac{(X + 0.5) - (n/2)}{\sqrt{n}/2} = \frac{(21 + 0.5) - (50/2)}{\sqrt{50}/2} = \frac{-3.5}{3.5355} = -0.99$$

Step 4   Make the decision. Since the test statistic of -0.99 is greater than -1.645, the decision is to not reject the null hypothesis.

Step 5   Summarize the results. There is not enough evidence to reject the claim that the median age of workers in the region's labour force is at least 41.2 years.

In Example 13–2, the sample size was 50, and 21 workers were older than 41.2 years, so $50 - 21$, or 29, workers are not older than 41.2 years. The value of X corresponds to the smaller of the two numbers 21 and 29. In this case, $X = 21$ is used in the formula, since 21 is the smaller of the two numbers.

Suppose a researcher hypothesized that the median age of houses in a certain municipality was 40 years. In a random sample of 100 houses, 68 were older than 40 years. Then the value used for X in the formula would be $100 - 68$, or 32, since it is the smaller of the two numbers 68 and 32. When 40 is subtracted from the age of a house older than 40 years, the answer is positive. When 40 is subtracted from the age of a house that is less than 40 years old, the result is negative. There would be 68 positive signs and 32 negative signs (assuming that no house was exactly 40 years old). Hence, 32 would be used for X, since it is the smaller of the two values.

Paired-Sample Sign Test

The sign test can also be used to test sample means in a comparison of two dependent samples, such as a before-and-after test. Recall that when dependent samples are taken from normally distributed populations, the t test is used (Section 9–3). When the condition of normality cannot be met, the nonparametric sign test can be used, as shown in Example 13–3.

Example 13–3	**Ear Infections in Swimmers**

A medical researcher believed the number of ear infections in swimmers can be reduced if the swimmers use earplugs. A sample of 10 people was selected, and the number of infections for a four-month period was recorded. During the first two months, the swimmers did not use the earplugs; during the second two months, they did. At the beginning of the second two-month period, each swimmer was examined to make sure that no infections were present. The data are shown here. At $\alpha = 0.05$, can the researcher conclude that using earplugs reduced the number of ear infections?

Number of ear infections

Swimmer	Before, X_B	After, X_A
A	3	2
B	0	1
C	5	4
D	4	0
E	2	1
F	4	3
G	3	1
H	5	3
I	2	2
J	1	3

Solution

Step 1 State the hypotheses and identify the claim.

H_0: The number of ear infections will not be reduced.

H_1: The number of ear infections will be reduced (claim).

Step 2 Find the critical value. Subtract the *after* values X_A from the *before* values X_B and indicate the difference by a positive or negative sign or 0, according to the value, as shown in the table.

Swimmer	Before, X_B	After, X_A	Sign of difference
A	3	2	+
B	0	1	−
C	5	4	+
D	4	0	+
E	2	1	+
F	4	3	+
G	3	1	+
H	5	3	+
I	2	2	0
J	1	3	−

From Table J, with $n = 9$ (the total number of positive and negative signs; the 0 is not counted) and $\alpha = 0.05$ (one-tailed), at most 1 negative sign is needed to reject the null hypothesis because 1 is the smallest entry in the $\alpha = 0.05$ column of Table J.

Step 3 Compute the test statistic. Count the number of positive and negative signs found in step 2, and use the smaller value as the test statistic. There are 2 negative signs, so the test statistic is 2.

Step 4 Make the decision. There are 2 negative signs. The decision is to not reject the null hypothesis. The reason is that with $n = 9$, C.V. $= 1$ and $1 < 2$.

Step 5 Summarize the results. There is not enough evidence to support the claim that the use of earplugs reduced the number of ear infections.

When conducting a one-tailed sign test, the researcher must scrutinize the data to determine whether they support the null hypothesis. If the data support the null hypothesis, there is no need to conduct the test. In Example 13–3, the null hypothesis states that the number of ear infections will not be reduced. The data would support the null hypothesis if there were more negative signs than positive signs. The reason is that the *before* values X_B in most cases would be smaller than the *after* values X_A, and the $X_B - X_A$ values would be negative more often than positive. This would indicate that there is not enough evidence to reject the null hypothesis. The researcher would stop here, since there is no need to continue the procedure.

On the other hand, if the number of ear infections was reduced, the X_B values, for the most part, would be larger than the X_A values, and the $X_B - X_A$ values would most often be positive, as in Example 13–3. Hence, the researcher would continue the procedure. A word of caution is in order, and a little reasoning is required.

When the sample size is 26 or more, the normal approximation can be used in the same manner as in Example 13–2. The steps for conducting the sign test for single or paired samples are given in the Procedure Table.

Procedure Table

Sign Test for Single and Paired Samples

Step 1   State the hypotheses and identify the claim.

Step 2   Find the critical value(s). For the single-sample test, compare each value with the conjectured median. If the value is larger than the conjectured median, replace it with a positive sign. If it is smaller than the conjectured median, replace it with a negative sign.

For the paired-sample sign test, subtract the *after* values from the *before* values, and indicate the difference with a positive or negative sign or 0, according to the value. Use Table J and n = total number of positive and negative signs.

Check the data to see whether they support the null hypothesis. If they do, do not reject the null hypothesis. If not, continue with step 3.

Step 3   Compute the test statistic. Count the number of positive and negative signs found in step 2, and use the smaller value as the test statistic.

Step 4   Make the decision. Compare the test statistic with the critical value in Table J. If the test statistic is less than or equal to the critical value, reject the null hypothesis.

Step 5   Summarize the results.

Note: If the sample size n is 26 or more, use Table E–1 or Table E–2 in Appendix C and the following formula for the test statistic:

$$z = \frac{(X + 0.5) - (n/2)}{\sqrt{n}/2}$$

where

X = smaller number of $+$ or $-$ signs

n = sample size

13–2 Applying the Concepts

Clean Air

An environmentalist suggests that the median of the number of days per year that a large city failed to meet the U.S. Environmental Protection Agency (EPA) acceptable standards for clean air is 11 days per month. A random sample of 20 months shows the number of days per month that the air quality was below the EPA's standards.

15	14	1	9	0	3	3	1	10	8
6	16	21	22	3	19	16	5	23	13

1. What is the claim?
2. What test would you use to test the claim? Why?
3. What would the hypotheses be?
4. Select a value for α and find the corresponding critical value.
5. What is the test statistic?
6. What is your decision?
7. Summarize the results.
8. Could a parametric test be used?

See page 612 for the answers.

Exercises 13–2

1. Why is the sign test the simplest nonparametric test to use?

2. What population parameter can be tested with the sign test?

3. In the sign test, what is used as the test statistic when $n < 26$?

4. When $n \geq 26$, what is used in place of Table J for the sign test?

For Exercises 5 through 20, perform these steps.

   a. State the hypotheses and identify the claim.
   b. Find the critical value(s).
   c. Compute the test statistic.
   d. Make the decision.
   e. Summarize the results.

Use the traditional method of hypothesis testing unless otherwise specified.

5. **Volunteer Hours** The median number of hours spent annually in volunteer service by persons 16 to 24 years old is 36 hours. The dean of Student Activities at a particular university feels that the median number of volunteer hours for her students is 38. A sample of students had annual volunteer records as listed below. At $\alpha = 0.05$, is there enough evidence to reject her claim?

25	36	40	39	32	38	41	29	39	40
42	35	42	28	39	39	36	39	30	42

Source: Time Almanac.

6. **Game Attendance** An athletic director suggests the median number for the paid attendance at 20 local football games is 3000. The data for a sample are shown. At $\alpha = 0.05$, is there enough evidence to reject the claim? If you were printing the programs for the games, would you use this figure as a guide?

6210	3150	2700	3012	4875
3540	6127	2581	2642	2573
2792	2800	2500	3700	6030
5437	2758	3490	2851	2720

Source: Pittsburgh Post Gazette.

7. **Number of Cyber-School Students** An educator hypothesizes that the median of the number of students enrolled in cyber schools in school districts in southwestern Pennsylvania is 25. At $\alpha = 0.05$, is there enough evidence to reject the educator's claim? The data are shown here. What benefit would this information provide to the school board of a local school district?

12	41	26	14	4
38	27	27	9	11
17	11	66	5	14
8	35	16	25	17

Source: *Tribune-Review.*

8. Income of Temporary Employees A temporary employment agency advertises that its employees are placed in positions where the median weekly income is $500. A random sample of employee records revealed the following weekly earnings. At $\alpha = 0.10$, can the agency's claim be refuted?

510 490 475 495 495 520 500 480 487
500 535 500 475 482 480 495 480 498

9. Natural Gas Costs A gas marketing agency claims the median price of natural gas for a recent year was $3.82 per gigajoule (GJ). A researcher wishes to see if there is enough evidence to reject the claim. Out of 42 households, 18 paid less than $3.82 per GJ for natural gas. Test the claim at $\alpha = 0.05$. How could a prospective home buyer use this information?

Source: *Canadian Gas Association.*

10. Weight Loss and Exercise One hundred people were placed on a special exercise program. After one month, 58 lost weight, 12 gained weight, and 30 weighed the same as before. Test the hypothesis that the exercise program is effective at $\alpha = 0.10$. (*Note:* It will be effective if fewer than 50% of the people did not lose weight.)

11. Number of Faculty for Proprietary Schools An educational researcher believes that the median number of faculty for proprietary (for-profit) colleges and universities is 150. The data provided list the number of faculty at a selected number of proprietary colleges and universities. At the 0.05 level of significance, is there sufficient evidence to reject his claim?

372 111 165   95 191   83 136 149   37
142 136 137 171 122 133 133 342 126
 61 100 225 127   92 140 140   75 108
138 318 179 243 109 119   64   96

Source: *World Almanac.*

12. Television Viewers A researcher read that the median age for viewers of the Carson Daly show is 39. To test the claim, 75 viewers were surveyed, and 27 were under the age of 39. At $\alpha = 0.02$ test the claim. Give one reason why an advertiser might like to know the results of this study.

Source: *Nielsen Media Research.*

13. Students' Opinion of Longer School Year One hundred students are asked if they favour increasing the school year by 20 days. The responses are 62 no, 36 yes, and 2 undecided. At $\alpha = 0.10$, test the hypothesis that 50% of the students are against extending the school year. Use the *P*-value method.

14. Unintentional Firearm Deaths A criminologist suggests that the median number of unintentional firearms deaths per year in Canada is 56. The number of deaths for a sample of 11 years is shown. At $\alpha = 0.05$, is there enough evidence to reject the claim? If you took proper firearm safety precautions, would you feel relatively safe?

71   66   31   92   76   67
59   49   48   27   52

Source: Statistics Canada.

15. Diet Medication and Weight A study was conducted to see whether a certain diet medication had an effect on the weights (in kilograms) of eight women. Their weights were taken before and six weeks after daily administration of the medication. The data are shown here. At $\alpha = 0.05$, can one conclude that the medication had an effect (increase or decrease) on the weights of the women?

Subject	A	B	C	D	E	F	G	H
Weight before	84.8	73.9	91.2	71.7	63.0	64.9	89.8	69.9
Weight after	80.7	73.5	85.3	70.8	60.3	68.0	79.4	68.0

16. Exam Scores A statistics professor wants to investigate the relationship between a student's midterm examination score and the score on the final. Eight students were selected, and their scores on the two examinations are noted below. At the 0.10 level of significance, is there sufficient evidence to conclude that there is a difference in scores?

Student	1	2	3	4	5	6	7	8
Midterm	75	92	68	85	65	80	75	80
Final	82	90	79	95	70	83	72	79

17. Weekend Movie Attendance Is there a difference in weekend movie attendance based on the evening in question? Eight small-town movie theatres were surveyed to see how many movie patrons were in attendance on Saturday evening and on Sunday evening. Is there sufficient evidence to reject the claim that there is no difference in movie attendance for Saturday and Sunday evenings? Use $\alpha = 0.10$.

Theatre	A	B	C	D	E	F	G	H
Saturday	210	100	150	50	195	125	120	204
Sunday	165	42	92	60	172	100	108	136

18. Pill Effects on Appetite A researcher wishes to test the effects of a pill on a person's appetite. Twelve subjects are allowed to eat a meal of their choice, and their caloric intake is measured. The next day, the same subjects take the pill and eat a meal of their choice. The caloric intake of the second meal is measured. The data are shown here. At $\alpha = 0.02$, can the researcher conclude that the pill had an effect on a person's appetite?

Subject	1	2	3	4	5	6	7
Meal 1	856	732	900	1321	843	642	738
Meal 2	843	721	872	1341	805	531	740

Subject	8	9	10	11	12
Meal 1	1005	888	756	911	998
Meal 2	900	805	695	878	914

19. Television Viewers A researcher wishes to determine if the number of viewers for 10 returning television shows has not changed since last year. The data are given in millions of viewers. At $\alpha = 0.01$, test the claim that the number of viewers has not changed. Depending on your answer, would a television executive plan to air these programs for another year?

Show	1	2	3	4	5	6
Last year	28.9	26.4	20.8	25.0	21.0	19.2
This year	26.6	20.5	20.2	19.1	18.9	17.8

Show	7	8	9	10
Last year	13.7	18.8	16.8	15.3
This year	16.8	16.7	16.0	15.8

Source: Based on information from Nielson Media Research.

20. Routine Maintenance and Defective Parts A man- ufacturer believes that if routine maintenance (cleaning and oiling of machines) is increased to once a day rather than once a week, the number of defective parts produced by the machines will decrease. Nine machines are selected, and the number of defective parts produced over a 24-hour operating period is counted. Maintenance is then increased to once a day for a week, and the number of defective parts each machine produces is again counted over a 24-hour operating period. The data are shown here. At $\alpha = 0.01$, can the manufacturer conclude that increased maintenance reduces the number of defective parts manufactured by the machines?

Machine	1	2	3	4	5	6	7	8	9
Before	6	18	5	4	16	13	20	9	3
After	5	16	7	4	18	12	14	7	1

Extending the Concepts »

The confidence interval for the median of a set of values less than or equal to 25 in number can be found by ordering the data from smallest to largest, finding the median, and using Table J. For example, to find the 95% confidence interval of the true median for 17, 19, 3, 8, 10, 15, 1, 23, 2, 12, order the data:

1, 2, 3, 8, 10, 12, 15, 17, 19, 23

From Table J, select $n = 10$ and $\alpha = 0.05$, and find the critical value. Use the two-tailed row. In this case, the critical value is 1. Add 1 to this value to get 2. In the ordered list, count from the left two numbers and from the right two numbers, and use these numbers to get the confidence interval, as shown:

1, 2, 3, 8, 10, 12, 15, 17, 19, 23

$2 \leq MD \leq 19$

Always add 1 to the number obtained from the table before counting. For example, if the critical value is 3, then count 4 values from the left and right.

For Exercises 21 through 25, find the confidence interval of the median, indicated in parentheses, for each set of data.

21. 3, 12, 15, 18, 16, 15, 22, 30, 25, 4, 6, 9 (95%)

22. 101, 115, 143, 106, 100, 142, 157, 163, 155, 141, 145, 153, 152, 147, 143, 115, 164, 160, 147, 150 (90%)

23. 8.2, 7.1, 6.3, 5.2, 4.8, 9.3, 7.2, 9.3, 4.5, 9.6, 7.8, 5.6, 4.7, 4.2, 9.5, 5.1 (98%)

24. 1, 8, 2, 6, 10, 15, 24, 33, 56, 41, 58, 54, 5, 3, 42, 31, 15, 65, 21 (99%)

25. 12, 15, 18, 14, 17, 19, 25, 32, 16, 47, 14, 23, 27, 42, 33, 35, 39, 41, 21, 19 (95%)

13–3 The Wilcoxon Rank Sum Test ›

LO3

Test hypotheses, using the Wilcoxon rank sum test.

The sign test does not consider the magnitude of the data. For example, whether a value is 1 point or 100 points below the median, it will receive a negative sign. And when one compares values in the pretest/posttest situation, the magnitude of the differences is not considered. The Wilcoxon tests consider differences in magnitudes by using ranks.

The two tests considered in this section and in Section 13–4 are the **Wilcoxon rank sum test,** which is used for independent samples, and the **Wilcoxon signed-rank test,** which is used for dependent samples. Both tests are used to compare distributions. The parametric equivalents are the z and t tests for independent samples (Sections 9–1 and 9–2) and the t test for dependent samples (Section 9–3). For the parametric tests, as stated previously, the samples must be selected from approximately normally distributed populations, but the only assumption for the Wilcoxon signed-rank tests is that the population of differences has a symmetric distribution.

In the Wilcoxon tests, the values of the data for both samples are combined and then ranked. If the null hypothesis is true—meaning that there is no difference in the population distributions—then the values in each sample should be ranked approximately the same. Therefore, when the ranks are summed for each sample, the sums should be approximately equal, and the null hypothesis will not be rejected. If there is a large difference in the sums of the ranks, then the distributions are not identical, and the null hypothesis will be rejected.

The first test to be considered is the Wilcoxon rank sum test for independent samples. For this test, both sample sizes must be greater than or equal to 10. The formulas needed for the test are given next.

Formula for the Wilcoxon Rank Sum Test When Samples Are Independent

$$z = \frac{R - \mu_R}{\sigma_R}$$

where

$$\mu_R = \frac{n_1(n_1 + n_2 + 1)}{2}$$

$$\sigma_R = \sqrt{\frac{n_1 n_2(n_1 + n_2 + 1)}{12}}$$

R = sum of ranks for smaller sample size (n_1)
n_1 = smaller of sample sizes
n_2 = larger of sample sizes
$n_1 \geq 10$ and $n_2 \geq 10$

Note that if both samples are the same size, either size can be used as n_1.

Example 13–4 illustrates the Wilcoxon rank sum test for independent samples.

Example 13–4

Times to Complete an Obstacle Course

Two independent samples of army and navy recruits are selected, and the time in minutes it takes each recruit to complete an obstacle course is recorded, as shown in the table. At $\alpha = 0.05$, is there a difference in the times it takes the recruits to complete the course?

Army	15	18	16	17	13	22	24	17	19	21	26	28	Mean = 19.67
Navy	14	9	16	19	10	12	11	8	15	18	25		Mean = 14.27

Solution

Step 1 State the hypotheses and identify the claim.

H_0: There is no difference in the times it takes the recruits to complete the obstacle course.

H_1: There is a difference in the times it takes the recruits to complete the obstacle course (claim).

Step 2 Find the critical value. Since $\alpha = 0.05$ and this test is a two-tailed test, use the z values of $+1.96$ and -1.96 from Tables E–1 and E–2.

Step 3 Compute the test statistic.

a. Combine the data from the two samples, arrange the combined data in order, and rank each value. Be sure to indicate the group.

Time	8	9	10	11	12	13	14	15	15	16	16	17
Group	N	N	N	N	N	A	N	A	N	A	N	A
Rank	1	2	3	4	5	6	7	8.5	8.5	10.5	10.5	12.5

Time	17	18	18	19	19	21	22	24	25	26	28
Group	A	N	A	A	N	A	A	A	N	A	A
Rank	12.5	14.5	14.5	16.5	16.5	18	19	20	21	22	23

b. Sum the ranks of the group with the smaller sample size. (*Note:* If both groups have the same sample size, either one can be used.) In this case, the sample size for the navy is smaller.

$$R = 1 + 2 + 3 + 4 + 5 + 7 + 8.5 + 10.5 + 14.5 + 16.5 + 21$$
$$= 93$$

c. Substitute in the formulas to find the test statistic.

$$\mu_R = \frac{n_1(n_1 + n_2 + 1)}{2} = \frac{(11)(11 + 12 + 1)}{2} = 132$$

$$\sigma_R = \sqrt{\frac{n_1 n_2(n_1 + n_2 + 1)}{12}} = \sqrt{\frac{(11)(12)(11 + 12 + 1)}{12}}$$

$$= \sqrt{264} = 16.2$$

$$z = \frac{R - \mu_R}{\sigma_R} = \frac{93 - 132}{16.2} = -2.41$$

Step 4 Make the decision. The decision is to reject the null hypothesis, since $-2.41 < -1.96$.

Step 5 Summarize the results. There is enough evidence to support the claim that there is a difference in the times it takes the recruits to complete the course.

The steps for the Wilcoxon rank sum test are given in the Procedure Table.

Procedure Table

Wilcoxon Rank Sum Test

Step 1 State the hypotheses and identify the claim.

Step 2 Find the critical value(s). Use Tables E–1 and E–2.

(continued)

Procedure Table *(continued)*

Step 3   Compute the test statistic.

    a. Combine the data from the two samples, arrange the combined data in order, and rank each value.

    b. Sum the ranks of the group with the smaller sample size. (*Note:* If both groups have the same sample size, either one can be used.)

    c. Use these formulas to find the test statistic.

$$\mu_R = \frac{n_1(n_1 + n_2 + 1)}{2}$$

$$\sigma_R = \sqrt{\frac{n_1 n_2 (n_1 + n_2 + 1)}{12}}$$

$$z = \frac{R - \mu_R}{\sigma_R}$$

where R is the sum of the ranks of the data in the smaller sample and n_1 and n_2 are each greater than or equal to 10.

Step 4   Make the decision.

Step 5   Summarize the results.

13–3   Applying the Concepts

School Lunch

A nutritionist decided to see if there was a difference in the number of calories served for lunch in elementary and secondary schools. She selected a random sample of eight elementary schools and another random sample of eight secondary schools in Ontario. The data are shown.

Elementary	Secondary
648	694
589	730
625	750
595	810
789	860
727	702
702	657
564	761

1. Are the samples independent or dependent?

2. What are the hypotheses?

3. What nonparametric test would you use to test the claim?

4. What critical value would you use?

5. What is the test statistic?

6. What is your decision?

7. What is the corresponding parametric test?

8. What assumption would you need to meet to use the parametric test?

9. If this assumption was not met, would the parametric test yield the same results?

See page 612 for the answers.

Exercises 13–3

1. What are the minimum sample sizes for the Wilcoxon rank sum test?

2. What are the parametric equivalent tests for the Wilcoxon rank sum test?

3. What distribution is used for the Wilcoxon rank sum test?

For Exercises 4 through 11, use the Wilcoxon rank sum test. Assume that the samples are independent. Also perform each of these steps.

   a. State the hypotheses and identify the claim.

   b. Find the critical value(s).

   c. Compute the test statistic.

   d. Make the decision.

   e. Summarize the results.

Use the traditional method of hypothesis testing unless otherwise specified.

4. Lengths of Prison Sentences A random sample of men and women in prison was asked to give the length of sentence each received for a certain type of crime. At $\alpha = 0.05$, test the claim that there is no difference in the sentence received by each gender. The data (in months) are shown here.

Males	8	12	6	14	22	27	32	24	26
Females	7	5	2	3	21	26	30	9	4

Males	19	15	13		
Females	17	23	12	11	16

5. Calories in Deli Sandwiches Are all deli sandwiches created equal? Ten sandwiches were selected from Deli A and ten from Deli B, and the number of calories was calculated for each sandwich. At the 0.05 level of significance, is there sufficient evidence to conclude that there is a difference in the number of calories contained in sandwiches from the two delis?

Deli A	420	630	790	590	610
Deli B	680	750	430	760	450
Deli A	480	570	740	620	420
Deli B	710	430	400	860	690

6. Lifetimes of Hand-Held Video Games To test the claim that there is no difference in the lifetimes of two brands of hand-held video games, a researcher selects a sample of 11 video games of each brand. The lifetimes (in months) of each brand are shown here. At $\alpha = 0.01$, can the researcher conclude that there is a difference in the distributions of lifetimes for the two brands?

Brand A	42	34	39	42	22	47	51	34	41	39	28
Brand B	29	39	38	43	45	49	53	38	44	43	32

7. Automobile Stopping Distances A researcher wishes to see if the stopping distance (metres) for midsized automobiles is different from the stopping distance for compact automobiles at a speed of 110 kilometres per hour. The data are shown. At $\alpha = 0.10$, test the claim that the stopping distances are the same. If one of your safety concerns is stopping distance, would it make a difference which type of automobile you purchase?

Automobile	1	2	3	4	5	6	7	8	9	10
Midsized	57	58	59	59	57	59	57	57	65	62
Compact	61	64	63	91	60	62	66	65	60	59

Source: Based on information from the National Highway Traffic Safety Administration.

8. Employee Job Satisfaction Two groups of employees were given a questionnaire to ascertain their degree of job satisfaction. The scale ranged from 0 to 100. The groups were divided into those who had under 5 years of work experience and those who had 5 or more years of experience. The data are shown here. At $\alpha = 0.10$, test the claim that there is no difference in the job satisfaction of the two groups, as measured by the questionnaire. Use the *P*-value method.

Under 5	78	98	83	86	75	77	72	68
5 and over	94	79	82	85	73	66	64	59

Under 5	56	93	97	99	93
5 and over	52	58	63	68	88

9. Provincial Worker Fatalities A joint union and management safety committee wants to determine if the number of worker fatalities is different in two Canadian provinces with similar populations—Manitoba and Nova Scotia. A sample of data from the two provinces over the past several years is selected, and the numbers of worker fatalities are shown. At $\alpha = 0.05$, test the claim that there is no difference in the number of worker fatalities in the two provinces.

Manitoba	25	20	27	22	34	14	30
Nova Scotia	40	22	23	13	17	23	41

Source: Centre for Study of Living Standards.

10. Job Productivity by Marital Status Supervisors were asked to rate the productivity of employees on their jobs. A researcher wants to see whether married men receive higher ratings than single men. A rating scale of 1 to 50 yielded the data shown here. At $\alpha = 0.01$, is there evidence to support this claim?

Single men	48	46	42	50	38	36	40	31	28	24	49	34
Married men	44	35	41	37	42	43	29	31	37	32	36	

11. Product Assembly Time by Education Level A
study was conducted to see whether there is a difference in the time it takes employees of a factory to
assemble the product. Samples of high school graduates and nongraduates were timed. At $\alpha = 0.05$, is
there a difference in the distributions for the two
groups in the times needed to assemble the product?
The data (in minutes) are shown here.

Graduates	3.6	3.2	4.4	3.0	5.6	6.3	8.2
Nongraduates	2.7	3.8	5.3	1.6	1.9	2.4	2.9
Graduates	7.1	5.8	7.3	6.4	4.2	4.7	
Nongraduates	1.7	2.6	2.0	3.1	3.4	3.9	

13–4	## The Wilcoxon Signed-Rank Test >

LO4

Test hypotheses, using the signed-rank test.

When the samples are dependent, as they would be in a before-and-after test using the
same subjects, the Wilcoxon signed-rank test can be used in place of the t test for dependent samples. Again, this test does not require the condition of normality. Table K in
Appendix C is used to find the critical values.

The procedure for this test is shown in Example 13–5.

Example 13–5	**Shoplifting Incidents**

In a large department store, the owner wishes to see whether the number of
shoplifting incidents per day will change if the number of uniformed security
officers is doubled. A sample of 7 days before security is increased and 7 days
after the increase shows the number of shoplifting incidents.

	Number of shoplifting incidents	
Day	**Before**	**After**
Monday	7	5
Tuesday	2	3
Wednesday	3	4
Thursday	6	3
Friday	5	1
Saturday	8	6
Sunday	12	4

Is there enough evidence to support the claim, at $\alpha = 0.05$, that there is a
difference in the number of shoplifting incidents before and after the increase
in security?

Solution

Step 1   State the hypotheses and identify the claim.

   H_0: There is no difference in the number of shoplifting incidents before
   and after the increase in security.

   H_1: There is a difference in the number of shoplifting incidents before
   and after the increase in security (claim).

Step 2   Find the critical value from Table K. Since $n = 7$ and $\alpha = 0.05$ for this
   two-tailed test, the critical value is 2. See Figure 13–2.

Figure 13–2

Finding the Critical
Value in Table K for
Example 13–5

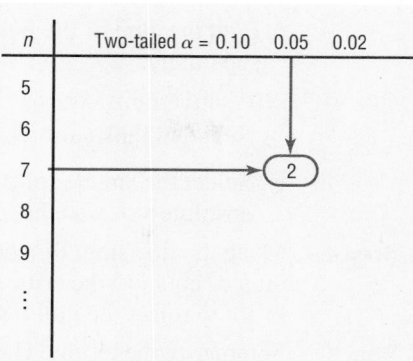

n	Two-tailed $\alpha = 0.10$	0.05	0.02
5			
6			
7			2
8			
9			
⋮			

Step 3 Find the test statistic.

a. Make a table as shown here.

Day	Before, X_B	After, X_A	Difference $D = X_B - X_A$	Absolute value $\lvert D \rvert$	Rank	Signed rank
Mon.	7	5				
Tues.	2	3				
Wed.	3	4				
Thurs.	6	3				
Fri.	5	1				
Sat.	8	6				
Sun.	12	4				

b. Find the differences (*before* minus *after*), and place the values in the Difference column.

$$7 - 5 = 2 \qquad 6 - 3 = 3 \qquad 8 - 6 = 2$$
$$2 - 3 = -1 \qquad 5 - 1 = 4 \qquad 12 - 4 = 8$$
$$3 - 4 = -1$$

c. Find the absolute value of each difference, and place the results in the Absolute value column. (*Note:* The absolute value of any number except 0 is the positive value of the number. Any differences of 0 should be ignored.)

$$\lvert 2 \rvert = 2 \qquad \lvert 3 \rvert = 3 \qquad \lvert 2 \rvert = 2$$
$$\lvert -1 \rvert = 1 \qquad \lvert 4 \rvert = 4 \qquad \lvert 8 \rvert = 8$$
$$\lvert -1 \rvert = 1$$

d. Rank each absolute value from lowest to highest, and place the rankings in the Rank column. In the case of a tie, assign the values that rank plus 0.5.

Value	2	1	1	3	4	2	8
Rank	3.5	1.5	1.5	5	6	3.5	7

e. Give each rank a plus or minus sign, according to the sign in the Difference column. The completed table is shown here.

Day	Before, X_B	After, X_A	Difference $D = X_B - X_A$	Absolute value $\lvert D \rvert$	Rank	Signed rank
Mon.	7	5	2	2	3.5	+3.5
Tues.	2	3	−1	1	1.5	−1.5
Wed.	3	4	−1	1	1.5	−1.5
Thurs.	6	3	3	3	5	+5
Fri.	5	1	4	4	6	+6
Sat.	8	6	2	2	3.5	+3.5
Sun.	12	4	8	8	7	+7

f. Find the sum of the positive ranks and the sum of the negative ranks separately.

Positive rank sum $(+3.5) + (+5) + (+6) + (+3.5) + (+7) = +25$

Negative rank sum $(-1.5) + (-1.5)$ $= -3$

g. Select the smaller of the absolute values of the sums ($|-3|$), and use this absolute value as the test statistic w_s. In this case, $w_s = |-3| = 3$.

Step 4   Make the decision. Reject the null hypothesis if the test statistic is less than or equal to the critical value. In this case, $3 > 2$; hence, the decision is not to reject the null hypothesis.

Step 5   Summarize the results. There is not enough evidence to support the claim that there is a difference in the number of shoplifting incidents. Hence, the security increase probably made no difference in the number of shoplifting incidents.

The rationale behind the signed-rank test can be explained by a diet example. If the diet is working, then the majority of the postweights will be smaller than the preweights. When the postweights are subtracted from the preweights, the majority of the signs will be positive, and the absolute value of the sum of the negative ranks will be small. This sum will probably be smaller than the critical value obtained from Table K, and the null hypothesis will be rejected. On the other hand, if the diet does not work, some people will gain weight, other people will lose weight, and still other people will remain about the same weight. In this case, the sum of the positive ranks and the absolute value of the sum of the negative ranks will be approximately equal and will be about one-half of the sum of the absolute value of all the ranks. In this case, the smaller of the absolute values of the two sums will still be larger than the critical value obtained from Table K, and the null hypothesis will not be rejected.

When $n \geq 30$, the normal distribution can be used to approximate the Wilcoxon distribution. The same critical values from Tables E–1 and E–2 used for the z test for specific α values are used. The formula is shown.

Formula for the Wilcoxon Signed-Rank Test When $n \geq 30$

$$z = \frac{w_s - \dfrac{n(n + 1)}{4}}{\sqrt{\dfrac{n(n + 1)(2n + 1)}{24}}}$$

where

n = number of pairs where difference is not 0
w_s = smaller sum in absolute value of signed ranks

The steps for the Wilcoxon signed-rank test are given in the Procedure Table.

Procedure Table

Wilcoxon Signed-Rank Test

Step 1   State the hypotheses and identify the claim.

Step 2   Find the critical value from Table K.

Step 3   Compute the test statistic.

a. Make a table, as shown.

Before, X_B	After, X_A	Difference $D = X_B - X_A$	Absolute value $|D|$	Rank	Signed rank

      b. Find the differences (before − after), and place the values in the "Difference" column.

      c. Find the absolute value of each difference, and place the results in the "Absolute" value column.

      d. Rank each absolute value from lowest to highest, and place the rankings in the "Rank" column.

      e. Give each rank a positive or negative sign, according to the sign in the "Difference" column.

      f. Find the sum of the positive ranks and the sum of the negative ranks separately.

      g. Select the smaller of the absolute values of the sums, and use this absolute value as the test statistic w_s.

Step 4 Make the decision. Reject the null hypothesis if the test statistic is less than or equal to the critical value.

Step 5 Summarize the results.

      Note: When $n \geq 30$, use Tables E–1 and E–2 and the test statistic

$$z = \frac{w_s - \dfrac{n(n+1)}{4}}{\sqrt{\dfrac{n(n+1)(2n+1)}{24}}}$$

where

      n = number of pairs where difference is not 0

      w_s = smaller sum in absolute value of signed ranks

13–4 Applying the Concepts

Pain Medication

A researcher decides to see how effective a pain medication is. Eight subjects were asked to determine the severity of their pain by using a scale of 1 to 10, with 1 being very minor and 10 being very severe. Then each was given the medication, and after 1 hour, they were asked to rate the severity of their pain, using the same scale.

Subject	1	2	3	4	5	6	7	8
Before	8	6	2	3	4	6	2	7
After	6	5	3	1	2	6	1	6

1. What is the purpose of the study?

2. Are the samples independent or dependent?

3. What are the hypotheses?

4. What nonparametric test could be used to test the claim?

5. What significance level would you use?

6. What is your decision?

7. What parametric test could you use?

8. Would the results be the same?

See page 612 for the answers.

Exercises 13–4

1. What is the parametric equivalent test for the Wilcoxon signed-rank test?

For Exercises 2 and 3, find the sum of the signed ranks. Assume that the samples are dependent. State which sum is used as the test statistic.

2. Pretest

Pretest	18	32	35	37	25	41	52	43	56	62
Posttest	20	21	26	37	29	40	31	37	51	65

3. Pretest

Pretest	108	97	115	162	156	105	153
Posttest	110	97	103	168	143	112	141

For Exercises 4 through 8, use Table K to determine whether the null hypothesis should be rejected.

4. $w_s = 62$, $n = 21$, $\alpha = 0.05$, two-tailed test

5. $w_s = 18$, $n = 15$, $\alpha = 0.02$, two-tailed test

6. $w_s = 53$, $n = 25$, $\alpha = 0.05$, one-tailed test

7. $w_s = 142$, $n = 28$, $\alpha = 0.05$, one-tailed test

8. $w_s = 109$, $n = 27$, $\alpha = 0.025$, one-tailed test

9. Human and Animal Drug Prices Eight drugs were selected, and the prices for the human doses and the animal doses for the same amounts were compared. At $\alpha = 0.05$, can it be concluded that the prices for the animal doses are significantly less than the prices for the human doses? If the null hypothesis is rejected, give one reason why animal doses might cost less than human doses.

Human dose	0.67	0.64	1.20	0.51	0.87	0.74	0.50	1.22
Animal dose	0.13	0.18	0.42	0.25	0.57	0.57	0.49	1.28

Source: U.S. House Committee on Government Reform.

10. Salary Comparison by Gender In a corporation, female and male workers were matched according to years of experience working for the company. Their salaries were then compared. The data (in thousands of dollars) are shown in the table. At $\alpha = 0.10$, is there a difference in the salaries of the males and females?

Males	18	43	32	27	15	45	21	22
Females	16	38	35	29	15	46	25	28

11. TV Viewing Hours by Language Spoken A Quebec marketing executive wanted to compare the number of hours per week that Quebec Francophones watched television programming versus Quebec Anglophones. Data are collected for the same six age categories for both groups. At $\alpha = 0.05$, can it be concluded that the Quebec Francophones watch more television per week than Quebec Anglophones? Do the results help the marketing executive focus her advertising efforts?

Francophones	22.9	12.0	17.0	20.0	25.4	37.0
Anglophones	19.8	9.5	15.7	16.5	22.0	29.7

Source: Statistics Canada.

12. Marital Compatibility Eight couples are given a questionnaire designed to measure marital compatibility. After completing a workshop, they are given a second questionnaire to see whether there is a change in their attitudes toward each other. The data are as shown here. At $\alpha = 0.10$, is there any difference in the scores of the couples?

Before	43	52	37	29	51	62	57	61
After	48	59	36	29	60	68	59	72

13. Drug Prices A researcher wished to compare the prices for prescription drugs in the United States with those in Canada. The same drugs and dosages were compared in each country. At $\alpha = 0.05$, can it be concluded that the drugs in Canada were cheaper?

Drug	1	2	3	4	5	6
United States	3.31	2.27	2.54	3.13	23.40	3.16
Canada	1.47	1.07	1.34	1.34	21.44	1.47

Drug	7	8	9	10
United States	1.98	5.27	1.96	1.11
Canada	1.07	3.39	2.22	1.13

Source: IMS Health and other sources.

13–5	The Kruskal-Wallis Test ›

LO5

Test hypotheses, using the Kruskal-Wallis test.

The analysis of variance uses the F test to compare the means of three or more populations. The assumptions for the ANOVA test are that the populations are normally distributed and that the population variances are equal. When these assumptions cannot be met, the nonparametric **Kruskal-Wallis test,** sometimes called the *H test,* can be used to compare three or more means.

In this test, each sample size must be 5 or more. In these situations, the distribution can be approximated by the chi-square distribution with $k - 1$ degrees of freedom, where k = number of groups. This test also uses ranks. The formula for the test follows.

Formula for the Kruskal-Wallis Test

$$H = \frac{12}{N(N+1)}\left(\frac{R_1^2}{n_1} + \frac{R_2^2}{n_2} + \cdots + \frac{R_k^2}{n_k}\right) - 3(N+1)$$

where

R_1 = sum of ranks of sample 1
n_1 = size of sample 1
R_2 = sum of ranks of sample 2
n_2 = size of sample 2
.
.
.
R_k = sum of ranks of sample k
n_k = size of sample k
$N = n_1 + n_2 + \cdots + n_k$
k = number of samples

In the Kruskal-Wallis test, one considers all the data values as a group and then ranks them. Next, the ranks are separated and the H formula is computed. This formula approximates the variance of the ranks. If the samples are from different populations, the sums of the ranks will be different and the H value will be large; hence, the null hypothesis will be rejected if the H value is large enough. If the samples are from the same population, the sums of the ranks will be approximately the same and the H value will be small; therefore, the null hypothesis will not be rejected. This test is always a right-tailed test. The chi-square table, Table G, with d.f. $= k - 1$, should be used for critical values.

Example 13–6 illustrates the procedure for conducting the Kruskal-Wallis test.

Example 13–6

Milliequivalents of Potassium in Breakfast Drinks

A researcher tests three different brands of breakfast drink to see how many milliequivalents of potassium per litre each contains. These data are obtained.

Brand A	Brand B	Brand C
4.7	5.3	6.3
3.2	6.4	8.2
5.1	7.3	6.2
5.2	6.8	7.1
5.0	7.2	6.6

At $\alpha = 0.05$, is there enough evidence to reject the hypothesis that all brands contain the same amount of potassium?

Solution

Step 1   State the hypotheses and identify the claim.

H_0: There is no difference in the amount of potassium contained in the brands (claim).

H_1: There is a difference in the amount of potassium contained in the brands.

Step 2 Find the critical value. Use the chi-square table, Table G, with d.f. $= k - 1$ ($k =$ number of groups). With $\alpha = 0.05$ and d.f. $= 3 - 1 = 2$, the critical value is 5.991.

Step 3 Compute the test statistic.

a. Arrange all the data from lowest to highest, and rank each value.

Amount	Brand	Rank
3.2	A	1
4.7	A	2
5.0	A	3
5.1	A	4
5.2	A	5
5.3	B	6
6.2	C	7
6.3	C	8
6.4	B	9
6.6	C	10
6.8	B	11
7.1	C	12
7.2	B	13
7.3	B	14
8.2	C	15

b. Find the sum of the ranks of each brand.

Brand A $1 + 2 + \ 3 + \ 4 + \ 5 = 15$

Brand B $6 + 9 + 11 + 13 + 14 = 53$

Brand C $7 + 8 + 10 + 12 + 15 = 52$

c. Substitute in the formula.

$$H = \frac{12}{N(N+1)}\left(\frac{R_1^2}{n_1} + \frac{R_2^2}{n_2} + \frac{R_3^2}{n_3}\right) - 3(N+1)$$

where

$$N = 15 \qquad R_1 = 15 \qquad R_2 = 53 \qquad R_3 = 52$$
$$n_1 = n_2 = n_3 = 5$$

Therefore,

$$H = \frac{12}{15(15+1)}\left(\frac{15^2}{5} + \frac{53^2}{5} + \frac{52^2}{5}\right) - 3(15+1) = 9.38$$

Step 4 Make the decision. Since the test statistic 9.38 is greater than the critical value 5.991, the decision is to reject the null hypothesis.

Step 5 Summarize the results. There is enough evidence to reject the claim that there is no difference in the amount of potassium contained in the three brands. Hence, not all brands contain the same amount of potassium.

The steps for the Kruskal-Wallis test are given in the Procedure Table.

Procedure Table

Kruskal-Wallis Test

Step 1 State the hypotheses and identify the claim.

Step 2 Find the critical value. Use the chi-square table, Table G, with d.f. $= k - 1$ (k = number of groups).

Step 3 Compute the test statistic.

    a. Arrange the data from lowest to highest and rank each value.

    b. Find the sum of the ranks of each group.

    c. Substitute in the formula.

$$H = \frac{12}{N(N+1)}\left(\frac{R_1^2}{n_1} + \frac{R_2^2}{n_2} + \cdots + \frac{R_k^2}{n_k}\right) - 3(N+1)$$

    where

$$N = n_1 + n_2 + \cdots + n_k$$
$$R_k = \text{sum of ranks for } k\text{th group}$$
$$k = \text{number of groups}$$

Step 4 Make the decision.

Step 5 Summarize the results.

13–5 Applying the Concepts

Heights of Waterfalls

You are doing research for an article on the waterfalls on our planet. You want to make a statement about the heights of waterfalls on three continents. Three samples of waterfall heights (in metres) are shown.

North America	Africa	Asia
183	124	67
366	155	253
55	192	187
189	221	335
357	146	270
135	614	101

1. What questions are you trying to answer?

2. What nonparametric test would you use to find the answer?

3. What are the hypotheses?

4. Select a significance level and run the test. What is the H value?

5. What is your conclusion?

6. What is the corresponding parametric test?

7. What assumptions would you need to make to conduct this test?

See page 612 for the answers.

Exercises 13–5

For Exercises 1 through 12, perform these steps.

 a. State the hypotheses and identify the claim.

 b. Find the critical value.

 c. Compute the test statistic.

 d. Make the decision.

 e. Summarize the results.

Use the traditional method of hypothesis testing unless otherwise specified.

 1. Calories in Cereals Samples of four different cereals show the following number of calories for the suggested servings of each brand. At $\alpha = 0.05$, is there a difference in the number of calories for the different brands?

Brand A	Brand B	Brand C	Brand D
112	110	109	106
120	118	116	122
135	123	125	130
125	128	130	117
108	102	128	116
121	101	132	114

 2. Self-Esteem and Birth Order A test to measure self-esteem is given to three different samples of individuals based on birth order. The scores range from 0 to 50. The data are shown here. At $\alpha = 0.05$, is there a difference in the scores?

Oldest child	Middle child	Youngest child
48	50	47
46	49	45
42	42	46
41	43	30
37	39	32
32	28	41

 3. Lawnmower Prices A researcher wishes to compare the prices of three types of lawnmowers. At $\alpha = 0.10$, can it be concluded that there is a difference in the prices? Based on your answer, do you feel that the cost should be a factor in determining which type of lawnmower a person would purchase?

Gas-powered self-propelled	Gas-powered push	Electric
290	320	188
325	360	245
210	200	470
300	229	395
330	160	

 4. Sodium Content of Microwave Dinners Three brands of microwave dinners were advertised as being low in sodium. Samples of the three different brands show the following milligrams of sodium. At $\alpha = 0.05$, is there a difference in the amount of sodium among the brands?

Brand A	Brand B	Brand C
810	917	893
702	912	790
853	952	603
703	958	744
892	893	623
732		743
713		609
613		

 5. Carbohydrates in Foods A nutritionist wishes to compare the number of carbohydrates in one serving of three low-carbohydrate foods. At $\alpha = 0.01$, is there a difference in the number of carbohydrates? Based on your answer, which type of food would you recommend if a person wanted to limit carbohydrates?

Pasta	Ice cream	Bread
11	5	43
22	13	62
16	10	71
29	8	49
25	12	50

 6. Job Offers for Chemical Engineers A recent study recorded the number of job offers received by newly graduated chemical engineers at three colleges. The data are shown here. At $\alpha = 0.05$, is there a difference in the average number of job offers received by the graduates at the three colleges?

College A	College B	College C
6	2	10
8	1	12
7	0	9
5	3	13
6	6	4

 7. Firearm-Related Deaths A criminologist wishes to see if there is a difference in the number of firearm-related deaths by manner/intent and age group. The data for each age group are shown here. At $\alpha = 0.10$, is there a difference in the number of firearm-related deaths for each manner/intent category?

Suicide	Homicide	Unintentional
4	7	3
87	38	3
173	59	15
247	27	7
122	6	3

Source: Statistics Canada.

8. Printer Prices An electronics store manager wishes to compare the prices (in dollars) of three types of computer printers. The data are shown. At $\alpha = 0.05$, can it be concluded that there is a difference in the prices? Based on your answer, do you think that a certain type of printer generally costs more than the other types?

Inkjet printers	Multifunction printers	Laser printers
149	98	192
199	119	159
249	149	198
239	249	198
99	99	229
79	199	

9. Number of Crimes per Week In a large city, the number of crimes per week in five precincts is recorded for five weeks. The data are shown here. At $\alpha = 0.01$, is there a difference in the number of crimes?

Precinct 1	Precinct 2	Precinct 3	Precinct 4	Precinct 5
105	87	74	56	103
108	86	83	43	98
99	91	78	52	94
97	93	74	58	89
92	82	60	62	88

10. Unemployment and Education A recent study examined the number of unemployed people in five cities who are actively seeking employment. They are listed here according to the education each received. At $\alpha = 0.05$, is there a difference in the number of unemployed based on education received? Use the P-value method.

High school diploma	College degree	Postgraduate degree
49	23	7
43	49	38
51	54	23
108	87	52
68	28	26

11. Methods of First-Aid Instruction Three different methods of first-aid instruction are given to students. The same final examination is given to each class. The data are shown here. At $\alpha = 0.10$, is there a difference in the final examination scores? Use the P-value method.

Method A	Method B	Method C
98	97	99
100	88	94
95	82	96
92	84	89
86	75	81
76	73	72
71	74	

12. Amounts of Caffeine in Beverages The amounts of caffeine in a regular (small) serving of assorted beverages are listed below. If someone wants to limit caffeine intake, does it really matter which beverage is chosen? Is there a difference in caffeine content at $\alpha = 0.05$?

Teas	Coffees	Colas
70	120	35
40	80	48
30	160	55
25	90	43
40	140	42

Source: *Doctor's Pocket Calorie, Fat & Carbohydrate Counter.*

13–6   The Spearman Rank Correlation Coefficient >

LO6

Compute the Spearman rank correlation coefficient.

The techniques of regression and correlation were explained in Chapter 10. To determine whether two variables are linearly related, one uses the Pearson product moment correlation coefficient. Its values range from $+1$ to -1. One assumption for testing the hypothesis that $\rho = 0$ for the Pearson coefficient is that the populations from which the samples are obtained are normally distributed. If this requirement cannot be met, the nonparametric equivalent, called the **Spearman rank correlation coefficient** (denoted by r_s), can be used when the data are ranked.

Rank Correlation Coefficient

The computations for the rank correlation coefficient are simpler than those for the Pearson coefficient and involve ranking each set of data. The difference in ranks is found, and r_s is computed by using these differences. If both sets of data have the same ranks, r_s will be $+1$. If the sets of data are ranked in exactly the opposite way, r_s will be -1. If there is no relationship between the rankings, r_s will be near 0.

Formula for Computing the Spearman Rank Correlation Coefficient

$$r_s = 1 - \frac{6 \, \Sigma d^2}{n(n^2 - 1)}$$

where
d = difference in ranks
n = number of data pairs

This formula is algebraically equivalent to the formula for r given in Chapter 10, except that ranks are used instead of raw data.

The computational procedure is shown in Example 13–7. For a test of the significance of r_s, Table L is used for values of n up to 30. For larger values, the normal distribution can be used. (See Exercises 15 through 19 in this section's Extending the Concepts.)

Example 13–7	**Textbook Ratings**

Two students were asked to rate 8 different textbooks for a specific course, on an ascending scale from 0 to 20 points. Points were assigned for each of several categories, such as reading level, use of illustrations, and use of colour. At $\alpha = 0.05$, test the hypothesis that there is a significant linear correlation between the two students' ratings. The data are shown in the following table.

Textbook	Student 1's rating	Student 2's rating
A	4	4
B	10	6
C	18	20
D	20	14
E	12	16
F	2	8
G	5	11
H	9	7

Solution

Step 1 State the hypotheses.

$$H_0\!: \rho = 0 \quad \text{and} \quad H_1\!: \rho \neq 0$$

Step 2 Find the critical value. Use Table L to find the value for $n = 8$ and $\alpha = 0.05$. It is 0.738. See Figure 13–3.

Figure 13–3

Finding the Critical Value in Table L for Example 13–7

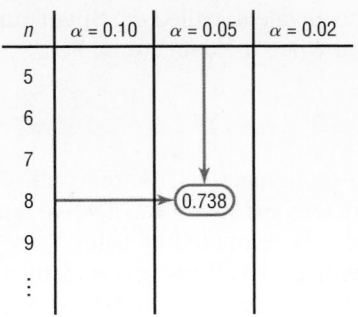

n	$\alpha = 0.10$	$\alpha = 0.05$	$\alpha = 0.02$
5			
6			
7			
8		0.738	
9			
⋮			

Step 3 Find the test statistic.

a. Rank each data set, as shown in the table.

Textbook	Student 1	Rank	Student 2	Rank
A	4	7	4	8
B	10	4	6	7
C	18	2	20	1
D	20	1	14	3
E	12	3	16	2
F	2	8	8	5
G	5	6	11	4
H	9	5	7	6

Let X_1 be the first student's rankings and X_2 be the second student's rankings.

b. Subtract the rankings $(X_1 - X_2)$.

$7 - 8 = -1 \qquad 4 - 7 = -3 \qquad$ etc.

c. Square the differences.

$(-1)^2 = 1 \qquad (-3)^2 = 9 \qquad$ etc.

d. Find the sum of the squares.

$1 + 9 + 1 + 4 + 1 + 9 + 4 + 1 = 30$

The results can be summarized in a table, as shown here.

X_1	X_2	$d = X_1 - X_2$	d^2
7	8	-1	1
4	7	-3	9
2	1	1	1
1	3	-2	4
3	2	1	1
8	5	3	9
6	4	2	4
5	6	-1	1
			$\Sigma d^2 = 30$

e. Substitute in the formula to find r_s.

$$r_s = 1 - \frac{6\Sigma d^2}{n(n^2 - 1)}$$

where $n =$ the number of data pairs. For this problem,

$$r_s = 1 - \frac{(6)(30)}{8(8^2 - 1)} = 1 - \frac{180}{504} = 0.643$$

Step 4 Make the decision. Do not reject the null hypothesis since $r_s = 0.643$, which is less than the critical value of 0.738.

Step 5 Summarize the results. There is not enough evidence to say that there is a correlation between the rankings of the two students.

Unusual Stat

You are more than 2½ times as likely to be killed walking with traffic than walking against traffic.

The steps for finding and testing the Spearman rank correlation coefficient are given in the Procedure Table. *Note:* Data sets can be ranked in ascending or descending order but the rank order must be the same for both data sets.

Procedure Table

Finding and Testing the Spearman Rank Correlation Coefficient

Step 1 State the hypotheses.

Step 2 Rank each data set.

Step 3 Subtract the rankings $(X_1 - X_2)$.

Step 4 Square the differences.

Step 5 Find the sum of the squares.

Step 6 Substitute in the formula.

$$r_s = 1 - \frac{6\Sigma d^2}{n(n^2 - 1)}$$

where
d = difference in ranks
n = number of pairs of data

Step 7 Find the critical value.

Step 8 Make the decision.

Step 9 Summarize the results.

13–6 Applying the Concepts

Tall Trees

As a biologist, you wish to see if there is a relationship between the heights of the trees and their diameters. You find the following data for the diameter (in metres) of the trees at 1.4 metres from the ground and the corresponding heights (in metres).

Diameter (m)	Height (m)
26.0	79.6
24.1	97.8
11.5	66.8
12.8	85.6
19.3	48.5
16.4	25.3
18.0	58.2
14.9	43.0
11.2	70.7
13.9	32.9

Source: The World Almanac and Book of Facts.

1. What questions are you trying to answer?
2. What type of nonparametric analysis could be used to answer the questions?
3. What would be the corresponding parametric test that could be used?
4. Which test do you think would be better?
5. Perform both tests and write a short statement comparing the results.

See page 613 for the answer.

Exercises 13–6

For Exercises 1 through 4, find the critical value from Table L for the rank correlation coefficient, given sample size n and α. Assume that the test is two-tailed.

1. $n = 14$, $\alpha = 0.01$
2. $n = 28$, $\alpha = 0.02$
3. $n = 10$, $\alpha = 0.05$
4. $n = 9$, $\alpha = 0.01$

For Exercises 5 through 14, perform these steps.

a. Find the Spearman rank correlation coefficient.
b. State the hypotheses.
c. Find the critical value. Use $\alpha = 0.05$.
d. Make the decision.
e. Summarize the results.

Use the traditional method of hypothesis testing unless otherwise specified.

5. **Forest Fire Causes** The table shows the total number of forest fires in selected Canadian provinces for a given year caused by human activity (e.g., camping, logging, construction, arson, etc.) or Mother Nature (e.g., lightning). At $\alpha = 0.10$, is there a relationship between the number of forest fires caused by human activity and Mother Nature?

Prov.	Human activity	Mother Nature
AB	336	428
BC	644	842
MB	203	105
NB	256	20
NS	398	27
ON	422	168
QC	401	74
SK	239	180

Source: Statistics Canada.

6. **Subway and Commuter Rail Passengers** Six cities are selected, and the number of daily passenger trips (in thousands) for subways and commuter rail service is obtained. At $\alpha = 0.05$, is there a relationship between the variables? Suggest one reason why the transportation authority might use the results of this study.

City	1	2	3	4	5	6
Subway	845	494	425	313	108	41
Rail	39	291	142	103	33	39

Source: American Public Transportation Association.

7. **Sentence Length and Time Served** The table shows the average maximum sentence length for certain crimes and the actual time served in months. At $\alpha = 0.05$, is there a relationship between the two?

Crime	Sentence	Time served
Murder	227	97
Rape	120	45
Robbery	106	40
Burglary	77	26
Drug offences	60	18
Weapons offences	49	21

Source: World Almanac and Book of Facts.

8. **Movie Releases and Gross Revenue** In Chapter 10, it was demonstrated that there was a significant linear relationship between the numbers of releases that a motion picture studio put out and its gross receipts for the year. Is there a relationship between the two at the 0.05 level of significance?

Number of releases	361	270	306	22	35
Receipts	2844	1967	1371	1064	667

Number of releases	10	8	12	21
Receipts	241	188	154	125

Source: ShowBIZdata: www.showbizdata.com.

9. **Music Video Rankings** Eight music videos were ranked by teenagers and their parents on style and clarity, with 1 being the highest ranking. The data are shown here. At $\alpha = 0.05$, is there a relationship between the rankings?

Music videos	1	2	3	4	5	6	7	8
Teenagers	4	6	2	8	1	7	3	5
Parents	1	7	5	4	3	8	2	6

10. **Retirees' Unused Sick Days** Eight school districts are randomly selected, and the number of employees who retired and the payment for their unused sick days are obtained. At $\alpha = 0.05$, is there a relationship between the data? How can a school board use the results of this study?

No. of employees	10	5	17	8	10	10	11	9
Amount paid in thousands of dollars	83	30	29	35	40	18	90	54

11. **Fuel and Barrel of Oil Prices** Shown are data illustrating selected Canadian monthly fuel prices (C\$/litre) and the monthly price of a barrel of oil (US\$/barrel). At $\alpha = 0.05$, is there a relationship between the prices?

Fuel price	1.02	0.92	0.87	0.95	0.89	1.12
Barrel of oil price	60.04	59.55	52.15	62.35	64.05	75.05

Source: GasBuddy.com.

12. **Motor Vehicle Thefts and Burglaries** Is there a relationship between the number of motor vehicle thefts and

the number of burglaries (per 100,000 population) for different metropolitan areas? Use $\alpha = 0.05$.

MV theft	220.5	499.4	285.6	159.2	104.3	444.0
Burglary	913.6	909.2	803.6	520.9	477.8	993.7

Source: The New York Times Almanac.

13. **Cyber-School Enrollments** Shown are the number of students enrolled in cyber-school for 5 randomly selected school districts and the per-student costs for the cyber-school education. At $\alpha = 0.10$, is there a relationship between the two variables? How might this information be useful to school administrators?

Number of students	10	6	17	8	11
Per-student cost	7200	9393	7385	4500	8203

Source: Tribune-Review.

14. **Drug Prices** Shown are the price for a human dose of several prescription drugs and the price for an equivalent dose for animals. At $\alpha = 0.10$, is there a relationship between the variables?

Humans	0.67	0.64	1.20	0.51	0.87	0.74	0.50	1.22
Animals	0.13	0.18	0.42	0.25	0.57	0.57	0.49	1.28

Source: U.S. House Committee on Government Reform.

Extending the Concepts »

When $n \geq 30$, the formula $r = \dfrac{\pm z}{\sqrt{n-1}}$ can be used to find the critical values for the rank correlation coefficient. For example, if $n = 40$ and $\alpha = 0.05$ for a two-tailed test,

$$r = \frac{\pm 1.96}{\sqrt{40-1}} = \pm 0.314$$

Hence, any r_s greater than or equal to $+0.314$ or less than or equal to -0.314 is significant.

For Exercises 15 through 19, find the critical r value for each (assume that the test is two-tailed).

15. $n = 50$, $\alpha = 0.05$

16. $n = 30$, $\alpha = 0.01$

17. $n = 35$, $\alpha = 0.02$

18. $n = 60$, $\alpha = 0.10$

19. $n = 40$, $\alpha = 0.01$

13-7   The Runs Test ›

Test hypotheses, using the runs test.

When samples are selected, one assumes that they are selected at random. How does one know if the data obtained from a sample are truly random? Before the answer to this question is given, consider the following situations for a researcher interviewing 20 people for a survey. Let their genders be denoted by M for male and F for female. Suppose the participants were chosen as follows:

Situation 1   M M M M M M M M M M F F F F F F F F F F

It does not look as if the people in this sample were selected at random, since 10 males were selected first, followed by 10 females.

Consider a different selection:

Situation 2   F M F M F M F M F M F M F M F M F M F M

In this case, it seems as if the researcher selected a female, then a male, etc. This selection is probably not random either.

Finally, consider the following selection:

Situation 3   F F F M M F M F M M F F M M M F F M M M F

This selection of data looks as if it may be random, since there is a mix of males and females and no apparent pattern to their selection.

Rather than try to guess whether the data of a sample have been selected at random, statisticians have devised a nonparametric test to determine randomness. This test is called the **runs test.**

A **run** is a succession of identical letters preceded or followed by a different letter or no letter at all, such as the beginning or end of the succession.

For example, the first situation presented has two runs:

Run 1:   M M M M M M M M M
Run 2:   F F F F F F F F F F

The second situation has 20 runs. (Each letter constitutes one run.)

The third situation has 11 runs.

Run 1:	F F F	Run 5:	F	Run 9:	F F
Run 2:	M M	Run 6:	M M	Run 10:	M M M
Run 3:	F	Run 7:	F F	Run 11:	F
Run 4:	M	Run 8:	M M		

Example 13–8

Determine the number of runs in each sequence.

a. F F F M M F F F F M

b. H H H T T T T

c. A A B B A A B B A A B B

Solution

a. There are four runs, as shown.

$$\underbrace{F\,F\,F}_{1} \quad \underbrace{M\,M}_{2} \quad \underbrace{F\,F\,F\,F}_{3} \quad \underbrace{M}_{4}$$

b. There are two runs, as shown.

$$\underbrace{H\,H\,H}_{1} \quad \underbrace{T\,T\,T\,T}_{2}$$

c. There are six runs, as shown.

$$\underbrace{A\,A}_{1} \quad \underbrace{B\,B}_{2} \quad \underbrace{A\,A}_{3} \quad \underbrace{B\,B}_{4} \quad \underbrace{A\,A}_{5} \quad \underbrace{B\,B}_{6}$$

The test for randomness considers the number of runs rather than the frequency of the letters. For example, for data to be selected at random, there should not be too few or too many runs, as in situations 1 and 2. The runs test does not consider the questions of how many males or females were selected or how many of each are in a specific run.

To determine whether the number of runs is within the random range, use Table M in Appendix C. The values are for a two-tailed test with $\alpha = 0.05$. For a sample of 12 males and 8 females, the table values shown in Figure 13–4 mean that any number of runs from 7 to 15 would be considered random. If the number of runs is 6 or less or 16 or more, the sample is probably not random, and the null hypothesis should be rejected.

Figure 13–4

**Finding the Critical
Value in Table M**

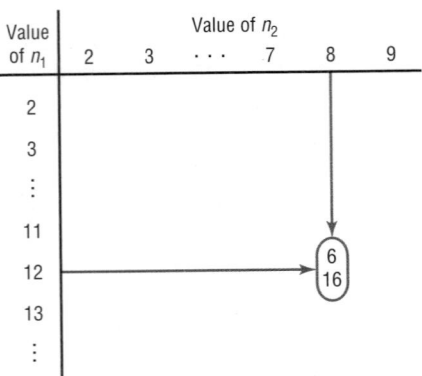

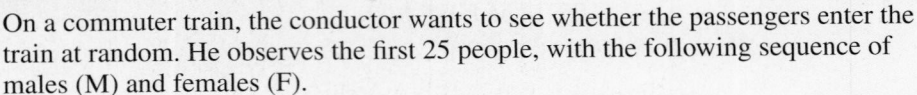

Example 13–9 shows the procedure for conducting the runs test by using letters as data. Example 13–10 shows how the runs test can be used for numerical data.

Example 13–9

Boarding of Train Passengers

On a commuter train, the conductor wants to see whether the passengers enter the train at random. He observes the first 25 people, with the following sequence of males (M) and females (F).

F F F M M F F F F M F M M M M F F F F M M F F F M M

Test for randomness at $\alpha = 0.05$.

Solution

Step 1   State the hypotheses and identify the claim.

H_0: The passengers board the train at random, according to gender (claim).

H_1: The null hypothesis is not true.

Step 2   Find the number of runs. Arrange the letters according to runs of males and females, as shown.

Run	Gender
1	F F F
2	M M
3	F F F F
4	M
5	F
6	M M M
7	F F F F
8	M M
9	F F F
10	M M

There are 15 females (n_1) and 10 males (n_2).

Step 3   Find the critical value. Find the number of runs in Table M for $n_1 = 15$, $n_2 = 10$, and $\alpha = 0.05$. The values are 7 and 18. *Note:* In this situation the critical value is found after the number of runs is determined.

Step 4 Make the decision. Compare these critical values with the number of runs. Since the number of runs is 10, and 10 is between 7 and 18, do not reject the null hypothesis.

Step 5 Summarize the results. There is not enough evidence to reject the hypothesis that the passengers board the train at random according to gender.

Quantitative data can be checked for randomization using the runs test. First find the median, a measure not affected by outliers, and then assign each numeric data value an attribute, $+/-$ or a/b, depending on whether the value is above or below the median. Omit values that are the same as the median. The decision rule for randomization is the same as the one explained for qualitative data.

Example 13–10	**Ages of Drug Program Participants** 🏹

Twenty people enrolled in a drug abuse program. Test the claim that the ages of the people, according to the order in which they enroll, occur at random, at $\alpha = 0.05$. The data are 18, 36, 19, 22, 25, 44, 23, 27, 27, 35, 19, 43, 37, 32, 28, 43, 46, 19, 20, 22.

Solution

Step 1 State the hypotheses and identify the claim.

H_0: The ages of the people, according to the order in which they enroll in a drug program, occur at random (claim).

H_1: The null hypothesis is not true.

Step 2 Find the number of runs.

a. Find the median of the data. Arrange the data in ascending order.

18 19 19 19 20 22 22 23 25 27 27

28 32 35 36 37 43 43 44 46

The median is 27.

b. Replace each number in the original sequence with an A if it is above the median and with a B if it is below the median. Eliminate any numbers that are equal to the median.

B A B B B A B A B A A A A A A B B B

c. Arrange the letters according to runs.

Run	Letters
1	B
2	A
3	B B B
4	A
5	B
6	A
7	B
8	A A A A A A
9	B B B

Step 3 Find the critical value. Table M shows that with $n_1 = 9$, $n_2 = 9$, and $\alpha = 0.05$, the number of runs should be between 5 and 15.

Step 4 Make the decision. Since there are 9 runs, and 9 falls between 5 and 15, the null hypothesis is not rejected.

Step 5 Summarize the results. There is not enough evidence to reject the hypothesis that the ages of the people who enroll occur at random.

The steps for the runs test are given in the Procedure Table.

Procedure Table

The Runs Test

Step 1 State the hypotheses and identify the claim.

Step 2 Find the number of runs.
Note: When the data are numerical, find the median. Then compare each data value with the median and classify it as above or below the median. Other methods such as odd–even can also be used. (Discard any value that is equal to the median.)

Step 3 Find the critical value. Use Table M.

Step 4 Make the decision. Compare the actual number of runs with the critical value.

Step 5 Summarize the results.

13–7 Applying the Concepts

Stock Exchange Trading Volumes

The Toronto Stock Exchange (TSX) is Canada's premier senior equity stock exchange. Millions of buy/sell orders are handled by the exchange on a daily basis. Is there a rhyme and reason to the daily market trading volumes? Listed below are TSX daily trading volumes, rounded to the nearest million, over a four-week period. Data are in rows.

54	149	199	238	142
151	131	164	158	193
355	178	166	189	165
150	177	209	231	201

Source: The Globe and Mail, Globe Investor: Stocks, "S&P/TSX Composite."

Answer the following questions.

1. Which nonparametric test would best determine whether the volume figures are random?
2. Before finding the number of runs, what needs to be determined? Calculate this value.
3. Using the $+$ sign for above and the $-$ sign for below the value in step 2, construct a table corresponding to the runs.
4. Looking at the table, does there appear to be order or randomness to the trading volumes?
5. Perform a hypothesis test of randomness on the trading volumes and interpret the results.

See page 613 for the answers.

Exercises 13–7

1. Determine the runs in each sequence.

    a. X X Y Y Y X X X X Y Y
    b. H T T T H H T H H T T T
    c. F F F M M M F F F M M M

In Exercises 2 through 10, perform these steps.

   a. State the hypotheses and identify the claim.
   b. Find the number of runs.
   c. Find the critical value. Use Table M.
   d. Make the decision.
   e. Summarize the results.

2. **Children's Dental Cavities** A school dentist wanted to test the claim, at $\alpha = 0.05$, that the number of cavities in Grade 4 students' teeth is random. Forty students were checked, and the number of cavities each had is shown here. Test for randomness of the values above or below the median.

0	4	6	0	6	2	5	3	1	5	1
2	2	1	3	7	3	6	0	2	6	0
2	3	1	5	2	1	3	0	2	3	7
3	1	5	1	1	2	2				

3. **Daily Lottery Numbers** A lottery was held each day for a month. Categorize the winning numbers as odd or even. The data follow. Test for randomness, at $\alpha = 0.05$.

409	872	235	338	472	481	318	129	229
084	291	991	356	212	457	473	834	304
361	301	051	652	405	458	094	633	809
299	712	802						

4. **Pick 3 Lottery Numbers** The winning numbers for Ontario's Pick 3 lottery for June are listed here. Classify each as odd or even and test for randomness, at $\alpha = 0.05$.

655	683	374	890	580	304
268	175	167	519	361	918
966	765	085	550	861	689
245	511	695	551	492	683
918	244	089	849	769	389

Source: Ontario Lottery and Gaming Corporation.

5. **True/False Test Answers** An irate student believes that the answers to his history professor's final true/false examination are not random. Test the claim, at $\alpha = 0.05$. The answers to the questions are shown.

    T T T F F T T T F F F F F F T
    T T F F F T T T F T F F T T F

6. **Concert Seating** As students, faculty, friends, and family arrived for the Spring Wind Ensemble Concert at Shafer Auditorium, they were asked whether they were going to sit in the balcony (B) or on the ground floor (G). Use the responses listed below and test for randomness at $\alpha = 0.05$.

    B B G G B B G B B B B B B G B B
    G G B B B B G G G G B G B B B G G

7. **Gender of Shoppers at Checkout** Twenty shoppers are in a checkout line at a grocery store. At $\alpha = 0.05$, test for randomness of their gender: male (M) or female (F). The data are shown here.

    F M M F F M F M M F
    F M M M F F F F F M

8. **Employee Absences** A supervisor records the number of employees absent over a 30-day period. Test for randomness, at $\alpha = 0.05$.

27	6	19	24	18	12	15	17	18	20
0	9	4	12	3	2	7	7	0	5
32	16	38	31	27	15	5	9	4	10

9. **Skiing Conditions** A ski lodge manager observes the weather for the month of February. If his customers are able to ski, he records S; if weather conditions do not permit skiing, he records N. Test for randomness, at $\alpha = 0.05$.

    S S S S S S N N N N N N N
    N S S S N N S S S S S S S

10. **Tossing a Coin** Toss a coin 30 times and record the outcomes (H or T). Test the results for randomness at $\alpha = 0.05$. Repeat the experiment a few times and compare your results.

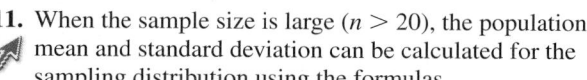

Extending the Concepts

11. When the sample size is large ($n > 20$), the population mean and standard deviation can be calculated for the sampling distribution using the formulas

$$\mu_R = \frac{2n_1 n_2}{n_1 + n_2} + 1 \qquad \sigma_R = \sqrt{\frac{(2n_1 n_2)(2n_1 n_2 - n_1 - n_2)}{(n_1 + n_2)^2 (n_1 + n_2 - 1)}}$$

where

R = observed number of runs
n_1 = frequency of the 1st attribute
n_2 = frequency of the 2nd attribute

A hypothesis test for randomness can be conducted using the test statistic $z = \dfrac{R - \mu_R}{\sigma_R}$ at an appropriate significance

level. With a large sample, the distribution is approximately normal and Tables E–1 and E–2 can be used to find the critical value. The decision rule is to reject randomness if the test statistic is in the critical region.

To test this method, a new deck of 52 playing cards is thoroughly shuffled and then each card is displayed in sequence as shown (R = red cards; B = black cards).

    R R R B B R R R R B R R B R B B B B B R R B B B R R
    B B R B B B R R R R B B R B B R R R B B R R B B B R

At a significance level of 0.05, perform a hypothesis test to determine the randomness of the shuffled playing cards.

Summary >

In many research situations, the assumptions (particularly that of normality) for the use of parametric statistics cannot be met. Also, some statistical studies do not involve parameters such as means, variances, and proportions. For both situations, statisticians have developed nonparametric statistical methods, also called *distribution-free methods.*

There are several advantages to the use of nonparametric methods. The most important one is that no knowledge of the population distributions is required. Other advantages include ease of computation and understanding. The major disadvantage is that they are less efficient than their parametric counterparts when the assumptions for the parametric methods are met. In other words, larger sample sizes are needed to get results as accurate as those given by their parametric counterparts.

This list gives the nonparametric statistical tests presented in this chapter, along with their parametric counterparts.

Nonparametric test	Parametric test	Condition
Single-sample sign test	z or t test	One sample
Paired-sample sign test	z or t test	Two dependent samples
Wilcoxon rank sum test	z or t test	Two independent samples
Wilcoxon signed-rank test	t test	Two dependent samples
Kruskal-Wallis test	ANOVA	Three or more independent samples
Spearman rank correlation coefficient	Pearson's correlation coefficient	Relationships between variables
Runs test	None	Randomness

When the assumptions of the parametric tests can be met, the parametric tests should be used instead of their nonparametric counterparts.

For step-by-step guidance on the use of Texas Instruments TI-83 Plus/TI-84 Plus programmable calculators, see Appendix E at the back of this book. For summary procedures for Minitab, SPSS, and Excel, please see the full version of Appendix E on *Connect.*

Important Terms »

Important Formulas »

Formula for the z test statistic in the sign test:

$$z = \frac{(X + 0.5) - (n/2)}{\sqrt{n}/2}$$

where

n = sample size (greater than or equal to 26)

X = smaller number of positive or negative signs

Formula for the Wilcoxon rank sum test:

$$z = \frac{R - \mu_R}{\sigma_R}$$

where

$$\mu_R = \frac{n_1(n_1 + n_2 + 1)}{2}$$

$$\sigma_R = \sqrt{\frac{n_1 n_2(n_1 + n_2 + 1)}{12}}$$

R = sum of ranks for smaller sample size (n_1)

n_1 = smaller of sample sizes

n_2 = larger of sample sizes

$n_1 \geq 10$ and $n_2 \geq 10$

Formula for the Wilcoxon signed-rank test:

$$z = \frac{w_s - \dfrac{n(n+1)}{4}}{\sqrt{\dfrac{n(n+1)(2n+1)}{24}}}$$

where

n = number of pairs where difference is not 0 and $n \geq 30$

w_s = smaller sum in absolute value of signed ranks

Formula for the Kruskal-Wallis test:

$$H = \frac{12}{N(N+1)}\left(\frac{R_1^2}{n_1} + \frac{R_2^2}{n_2} + \cdots + \frac{R_k^2}{n_k}\right) - 3(N+1)$$

where

R_1 = sum of ranks of sample 1

n_1 = size of sample 1

R_2 = sum of ranks of sample 2

n_2 = size of sample 2

$\cdot$
$\cdot$
$\cdot$

R_k = sum of ranks of sample k

n_k = size of sample k

$N = n_1 + n_2 + \cdots + n_k$

k = number of samples

Formula for the Spearman rank correlation coefficient:

$$r_s = 1 - \frac{6\Sigma d^2}{n(n^2 - 1)}$$

where

d = difference in ranks

n = number of data pairs

Mc Graw Hill Connect™ Practise and learn online with *Connect* with data sets and algorithmic questions related to concepts covered in this chapter. Questions and tables with online data sets are marked with 🏹.

Review Exercises »

For Exercises 1 through 13, follow this procedure:

　a.　State the hypotheses and identify the claim.
　b.　Find the critical value(s).
　c.　Compute the test statistic.
　d.　Make the decision.
　e.　Summarize the results.

Use the traditional method of hypothesis testing unless otherwise specified.

1. **Median Age of City Residents** The median age for the total population of Newfoundland and Labrador is 42.5 years, the highest in the nation. The mayor of a particular city believes that his population is considerably "younger" and that the median age there is 36 years. At $\alpha = 0.05$, is there sufficient evidence to reject his claim? The data here represent a random selection of persons from the household population of the city.

40	56	42	72	12	22
25	43	39	48	50	37
18	35	15	30	52	45
10	24	25	39	29	19
30	60	38	42	41	61

Source: Statistics Canada, *The Daily*, "Canada's Population by Age and Sex, Table 1: Population, Age Distribution and Median Age by Province and Territory, as of July 1, 2008," January 15, 2009.

2. **Lifetime of Truck Tires** A tire manufacturer claims that the median lifetime of a certain brand of truck tires is 65,000 kilometres. A sample of 30 tires shows that 12 lasted longer than 65,000 kilometres. Is there enough evidence to reject the claim at $\alpha = 0.05$? Use the sign test.

3. **Grocery Store Repricing** A grocery store chain has decided to help customers save money by instituting "temporary repricing" to help cut costs. The regular prices and the "temporary" new prices of 9 products in the sale flyer are shown below. Using the paired-sample sign test and $\alpha = 0.05$, is there evidence of a difference in price? Comment on your results.

Old price	2.59	0.69	1.29	3.10	1.89
New price	2.09	0.70	1.18	2.95	1.59

Old price	2.05	1.58	2.75	1.99
New price	1.75	1.32	2.19	1.99

4. **Record High Temperatures** Shown here are the record high temperatures (°C) for Dawson Creek, British Columbia, and for Whitehorse, Yukon, for 12 months. Using the Wilcoxon rank sum test at $\alpha = 0.05$, do you find a difference in the record high temperatures? Use the *P*-value method.

Dawson Creek	11 16 14 22 30 32 34 34 31 27 19 11
Whitehorse	8 10 11 21 30 32 33 30 27 19 11 8

Source: Jack Williams, *The* USA TODAY *Weather Almanac.*

5. Hours Worked by Student Employees Student employees are a major part of most college campus employment venues. Two major departments that participate in student hiring are listed below with the number of hours worked by students for a month. At the 0.10 level of significance, is there sufficient evidence to conclude a difference? Is the conclusion the same for the 0.05 level of significance?

Athletics	20 24 17 12 18 22 25 30 15 19
Library	35 28 24 20 25 18 22 26 31 21 19

6. Fuel Efficiency of Automobiles Twelve automobiles were tested to see how many litres per 100 kilometres (L/100 km) each one obtained. Under similar driving conditions, they were tested again, using a special additive. The data are shown here. At $\alpha = 0.05$, did the additive improve fuel efficiency? Use the Wilcoxon signed-rank test.

Before		After	
17.3	12.9	10.4	9.9
12.9	12.1	10.7	11.3
14.6	12.9	9.3	9.3
15.4	14.1	8.2	8.6
12.3	11.0	15.5	13.7
12.5	13.7	14.4	12.7

7. Lunch Costs Full-time employees in a large city were asked how much they spent on a typical weekday lunch and how much they spent on the weekend. The amounts are listed below. At $\alpha = 0.05$, is there sufficient evidence to conclude that there is a difference in the amounts spent?

Weekday	7.00 5.50 4.50 10.00 6.75 5.00 6.00
Weekend	6.00 10.00 7.00 12.00 8.50 7.00 8.00

8. Breaking Strength of Rope Samples of three types of ropes are tested for breaking strength. The data (in kilograms) are shown here. At $\alpha = 0.05$, is there a difference in the breaking strength of the ropes? Use the Kruskal-Wallis test.

Cotton	Nylon	Hemp
104	161	230
196	137	239
229	164	264
221	184	225
205	196	208
172	171	230
210	164	255
241	181	259
166	169	226
169	165	215
205	139	229
221	138	254
210	144	241
212	146	227

9. Rat Diet and Learning Rats were fed three different diets for one month to see whether diet has any effect on learning. Each rat was then taught to traverse a simple maze. The number of trials it took each rat to learn the correct path is shown in the table. At $\alpha = 0.05$, does diet have any effect on learning? Use the Kruskal-Wallis test.

Diet 1	8	6	12	15	9	7	5
Diet 2	2	3	6	8	7	4	
Diet 3	9	15	17	8	4	13	18	20

10. Homework Completion and Exam Scores A statistics instructor wishes to see whether there is a relationship between the number of homework exercises a student completes and her or his exam score. The data are shown here. Using the Spearman rank correlation coefficient, test the hypothesis that there is no relationship at $\alpha = 0.05$.

Homework problems	63 55 58 87 89 52 46 75 105
Exam score	85 71 75 98 93 63 72 89 100

11. TV Viewers Shown are the average number of viewers for 10 television shows for two consecutive years. At $\alpha = 0.05$, is there a relationship between the number of viewers?

Last year	28.9	26.4	20.8	25.0	21.0	19.2
This year	26.6	20.5	20.2	19.1	18.9	17.8
Last year	13.7	18.8	16.8	15.3		
This year	16.8	16.7	16.0	15.8		

12. Book Display A bookstore has a display of sale books arranged on shelves in the store window. A combination of hardbacks (H) and paperbacks (P) is arranged as follows. Test for randomness at $\alpha = 0.05$.

H H H P P P P H P H P H H H H P
P P P P H H P P P H P P P P P

13. Exam Scores An instructor wants to see whether grades of students who finish an exam occur at random. Shown here are the grades of 30 students in the order that they finished an exam. (Read from left to right across each row, and then proceed to the next row.) Test for randomness, at $\alpha = 0.05$.

87	93	82	77	64	98
100	93	88	65	72	73
56	63	85	92	95	91
88	63	72	79	55	53
65	68	54	71	73	72

Statistics Today

Too Much or Too Little?—Revisited

In this case, the manufacturer would select a sequence of bottles and see how many bottles contained more than 375 millilitres, denoted by plus, and how many bottles contained less than 375 mil- lilitres, denoted by minus. The sequence could then be analyzed according to the number of runs, as explained in Section 13–7. If the sequence was not random, then the machine would need to be checked to see if it was malfunctioning. Another method that can be used to see if machines are functioning properly is *statistical quality control*. This method is beyond the scope of this book.

Data Analysis »

The databank for these questions can be found in Appendix D at the back of the textbook and on **connect**.

1. From the databank, choose a sample and use the sign test to test one of the following hypotheses.

    a. For serum cholesterol, test H_0: median = 220 milligram percentage (mg%).

    b. For systolic pressure, test H_0: median = 120 millimetres of mercury (mm Hg).

    c. For IQ, test H_0: median = 100.

    d. For sodium level, test H_0: median = 140 mEq/L.

2. From the databank, select a sample of subjects. Use the Kruskal-Wallis test to see if the sodium levels of smokers and nonsmokers are equal.

3. From the databank select a sample of 50 subjects. Use the Wilcoxon rank sum test to see if the means of the sodium levels of the males differ from those of the females.

Chapter Quiz »

Determine whether each statement is true or false. If the statement is false, explain why.

1. Nonparametric statistics cannot be used to test the difference between two means.

2. Nonparametric statistics are more sensitive than their parametric counterparts.

3. Nonparametric statistics can be used to test hypotheses about parameters other than means, proportions, and standard deviations.

4. Parametric tests are preferred over their nonparametric counterparts, if the assumptions can be met.

Select the best answer.

5. The _____ test is used to test means when samples are dependent and the normality assumption cannot be met.

    a. Wilcoxon signed-rank
    b. Wilcoxon rank sum
    c. Sign
    d. Kruskal-Wallis

6. The Kruskal-Wallis test uses the _____ distribution.

    a. z c. χ^2
    b. t d. F

7. The nonparametric counterpart of ANOVA is the _____.

    a. Wilcoxon signed-rank test
    b. Sign test
    c. Runs test
    d. None of the above

8. To see if two rankings are related, one can use the _____.

    a. Runs test
    b. Spearman correlation coefficient
    c. Sign test
    d. Kruskal-Wallis test

Complete the following statements with the best answer.

9. When the assumption of normality cannot be met, one can use _____ tests.

10. When data are _____ or _____ in nature, non-parametric methods are used.

11. To test to see whether a median was equal to a specific value, one would use the _____ test.

12. Nonparametric tests are less _____ than their parametric counterparts.

For the following exercises, use the traditional method of hypothesis testing unless otherwise specified.

13. **Candy Bar Sales** The owner of a candy store states that she sells on average 300 candy bars per day. A random sample of 18 days shows the number of candy bars sold each day. At $\alpha = 0.10$, is the claim correct? Use the sign test.

271	297	315	282	106	297	268	215
262	305	315	256	311	375	319	297
311	299						

14. **Battery Lifetimes** A battery manufacturer claims that the median lifetime of a certain brand of heavy-duty battery is 1200 hours. A sample of 25 batteries shows that 15 lasted longer than 1200 hours. Test the claim at $\alpha = 0.05$. Use the sign test.

15. **Turkey Weights** A special diet is fed to adult turkeys to see if they will gain weight. The before and after weights (in kilograms) are given here. Use the paired-sample sign test at $\alpha = 0.05$ to see if there is weight gain.

Before	12.7	10.9	13.2	13.6	14.5	15.0	11.3	11.8	12.7
After	13.6	13.2	14.1	14.5	14.5	15.9	13.2	11.3	14.1

16. **Alcoholics' Ages for First Drink** Two groups of alcoholics, one group male and the other female, were asked at what age they first drank alcohol. The data are shown here. Using the Wilcoxon rank sum test at $\alpha = 0.05$, is there a difference in the starting ages of the females and males?

Males	6	12	14	16	17	17	13	12	10	11
Females	8	9	9	12	14	15	12	16	17	19

17. **Textbook Costs** Samples of students majoring in law and nursing are selected, and the amount each spent on textbooks for the spring semester is recorded here, in dollars. Using the Wilcoxon rank sum test at $\alpha = 0.10$, is there a difference in the amount spent by each group?

Law	167	158	162	106	98	206	112	121
Nursing	98	198	209	168	157	126	104	122

Law	133	145	151	199
Nursing	111	138	116	201

18. **Student GPAs** The grade point average of a group of students was recorded for one month. During the next nine-week grading period, the students attended a workshop on study skills. Their GPAs were recorded at the end of the grading period, and the data appear here. Using the Wilcoxon signed-rank test at $\alpha = 0.05$, can it be concluded that the GPA increased?

Before	3.0	2.9	2.7	2.5	2.1	2.6	1.9	2.0
After	3.2	3.4	2.9	2.5	3.0	3.1	2.4	2.8

19. **Breaking Strengths of Wrapping Tapes** Samples of three different types of wrapping tape are tested for breaking strength, in kilograms. The data are shown here. At $\alpha = 0.05$, is there a difference in the breaking strength of the tapes? Use the Kruskal-Wallis test.

Type A	102	151	183	176	159	127	164	195	121
Type B	116	92	118	138	105	126	118	136	123
Type C	184	194	218	180	159	186	210	214	181

Type A	160	131	164	166	123
Type B	93	93	99	101	119
Type C	184	209	196	182	170

20. **Monkey Medication and Reaction Times** Three different groups of monkeys were fed three different medications for one month to see if the medication has any effect on reaction time. Each monkey was then taught to repeat a series of steps to receive a reward. The number of trials it took each to receive the reward is shown here. At $\alpha = 0.05$, does the medication have an effect on reaction time? Use the Kruskal-Wallis test. Use the P-value method.

Med. 1	8	7	11	14	8	6	5
Med. 2	3	4	6	7	9	3	4
Med. 3	8	14	13	7	5	9	12

21. **Drug Prices** Is there a relationship between the prescription drug prices in Canada and Great Britain? Use $\alpha = 0.10$.

Canada	1.47	1.07	1.34	1.34	1.47	1.07	3.39	1.11	1.13
Great Britain	1.67	1.08	1.67	0.82	1.73	0.95	2.86	0.41	1.70

Source: USA TODAY.

22. **Funding and Enrollment for Head Start Students** Is there a relationship between the amount of money (in millions of dollars) spent on the U.S. Head Start Program by the states and the number of students enrolled (in thousands)? Use $\alpha = 0.10$.

Funding	100	50	22	88	49	219
Enrollment	16	7	3	14	8	31

Source: Gannet News Service.

23. **Birth Registry Tally** At the registry of vital statistics, the birth certificates issued for females (F) and males (M) were tallied. At $\alpha = 0.05$, test for randomness. The data are shown here.

M M F F F F F F F F M M M M F F
M F M F M M M F F F

24. Motor RPM Output The output in revolutions per minute (rpm) of 10 motors was obtained. The motors were tested again under similar conditions after they had been reconditioned. The data are shown here. At $\alpha = 0.05$, did the reconditioning improve the motors' performance? Use the Wilcoxon signed-rank test.

Before	413	701	397	602	405	512	450	487	388	351
After	433	712	406	650	450	550	450	500	402	415

25. Provincial Lottery Numbers A statistician wishes to determine if a province's lottery numbers are selected at random. The winning numbers selected for the month of February are shown here. Test for randomness at $\alpha = 0.05$.

321	909	715	700	487	808	509	606	943	761
200	123	367	012	444	576	409	128	567	908
103	407	890	193	672	867	003	578

Critical Thinking Challenges »

1. **Flipping for Bridge Toll** Two commuters ride to work together in one car. To decide who pays the toll for a bridge on the way to work, they flip a coin and the loser pays. Explain why over a period of one year, one person might have to pay the toll 5 days in a row. There is no toll on the return trip. (*Hint:* You may want to use random numbers.)

2. **Olympic Medals** Shown in the chart are the types and numbers of medals each country won in the 2010 Winter Olympic Games. You are to rank the countries from highest to lowest. Gold medals are highest, followed by silver, followed by bronze. There are many different ways to rank objects and events. Here are several suggestions.

   a. Rank the countries according to the total medals won.
   b. List some advantages and disadvantages of this method.
   c. Rank each country separately for the number of gold medals won, then for the number of silver medals won, and then for the number of bronze medals won. Then rank the countries according to the sum of the *ranks* for the categories.
   d. Are the rankings of the countries the same as those in step *a*? Explain any differences.
   e. List some advantages and disadvantages of this method of ranking.
   f. A third way to rank the countries is to assign a weight to each medal. In this case, assign 3 points for each gold medal, 2 points for each silver medal,

   and 1 point for each bronze medal the country won. Multiply the number of medals by the weights for each medal and find the sum. For example, since Canada won 14 gold medals, 7 silver medals, and 5 bronze medals, its rank sum is $(14 \times 3) + (7 \times 2) + (5 \times 1) = 61$. Rank the countries according to this method.

   g. Compare the ranks using this method with those using the other two methods. Are the rankings the same or different? Explain.
   h. List some advantages and disadvantages of this method.
   i. Select two of the rankings and run the Spearman rank correlation test to see if they differ significantly.

2010 Winter Olympic Games Final Medal Standings

Country	Gold	Silver	Bronze
Austria	4	6	6
Canada	14	7	5
China	5	2	4
France	2	3	6
Germany	10	13	7
Korea	6	6	2
Norway	9	8	6
Russian Federation	3	5	7
Sweden	5	2	4
United States	9	15	13

Source: The Vancouver Organizing Committee for the 2010 Olympic and Paralympic Winter Games.

Data Projects »

Where appropriate, use Minitab, SPSS, TI-83 Plus, TI-84 Plus, Excel, or a computer program of your choice to complete the following exercises.

Use a significance level of 0.05 for all tests below.

1. **Business and Finance** Monitor the price of a stock over a five-week period. Note the amount of gain or loss per day. Test the claim that the median is 0. Perform a runs test to see if the distribution of gains and losses is random.

2. **Sports and Leisure** Watch a basketball, baseball, football, or hockey game. For baseball, monitor an inning's pitches for balls and strikes (all fouls and balls in play also count as strikes). For football, monitor a series of plays for runs versus passing plays. For basketball, monitor one team's shots for misses versus made shots. For hockey, monitor all shots that missed the net and shots that were shots on goal. For the collected data, conduct a runs test to see if the distribution is random.

3. **Technology** Use the data collected in Data Project 3 in Chapter 2 regarding song lengths. Consider only three genres. For example, use rock, alternative, and hip-hop/rap. Conduct a Kruskal-Wallis test to determine if the mean song lengths for the genres are the same.

4. **Health and Wellness** Have everyone in class take her or his pulse during the first minute of class. Have everyone repeat this pulse-taking 30 minutes into class. Conduct a paired-sample sign test to determine if there is a difference in pulse rates.

5. **Politics and Economics** Select the ten provincial and three territorial capital cities in Canada and find the city rates for break-and-enter, homicide, and unemployment. Conduct a rank correlation analysis using break-and-enter and homicide rates, break-and-enter and unemployment rates, and homicide and unemployment rates. Which pair has the strongest relationship?

6. **Your Class** Have everyone in class take his or her temperature on a healthy day. Test the claim that the median temperature is 37°C.

Answers to Applying the Concepts »

Section 13–1 Ranking Data

Percentage	2.6	3.8	4.0	4.0	5.4	7.0	7.0	7.3	10.0
Rank	1	2	3.5	3.5	5	6.5	6.5	8	9

Section 13–2 Clean Air

1. The claim is that the median number of days that a large city failed to meet EPA standards is 11 days per month.

2. We will use the sign test, since we do not know anything about the distribution of the variable and we are testing the median.

3. H_0: median = 11 and H_1: median $\neq$ 11.

4. If $\alpha = 0.05$, then the critical value is 5.

5. The test statistic is 9.

6. Since $9 > 5$, we do not reject the null hypothesis.

7. There is enough evidence to conclude that the median is not 11 days per month.

8. We cannot use a parametric test in this situation.

Section 13–3 School Lunch

1. The samples are independent since two different random samples were selected.

2. H_0: There is no difference in the number of calories served for lunch in elementary and secondary schools.

   H_1: There is a difference in the number of calories served for lunch in elementary and secondary schools.

3. We will use the Wilcoxon rank sum test.

4. The critical value is ± 1.96 if we use $\alpha = 0.05$.

5. The test statistic is $z = -2.15$.

6. Since $-2.15 < -1.96$, we reject the null hypothesis and conclude that there is a difference in the number of calories served for lunch in elementary and secondary schools.

7. The corresponding parametric test is the two-sample t test.

8. We would need to know that the samples were normally distributed to use the parametric test.

9. Since t tests are robust against variations from normality, the parametric test would yield the same results.

Section 13–4 Pain Medication

1. The purpose of the study is to see how effective a pain medication is.

2. These are dependent samples, since we have *before* and *after* readings on the same subjects.

3. H_0: The severity of pain after is the same as the severity of pain before the medication was administered.

   H_1: The severity of pain after is less than the severity of pain before the medication was administered.

4. We will use the Wilcoxon signed-rank test.

5. We will choose to use a significance level of 0.05.

6. The test statistic is $w_s = 2.5$, since $|-2.5| < |25.5|$. The critical value is 4. Since $2.5 < 4$, we do not reject the null hypothesis. There is not enough evidence to conclude that the severity of pain after is less than the severity of pain before the medication was administered.

7. The parametric test that could be used is the t test for small dependent samples.

8. The results for the parametric test would be the same.

Section 13–5 Heights of Waterfalls

1. We are investigating the heights of waterfalls on three continents.

2. We will use the Kruskal-Wallis test.

3. H_0: There is no difference in the heights of waterfalls on the three continents.

   H_1: There is a difference in the heights of waterfalls on the three continents.

4. We will use the 0.05 significance level. The critical value is 5.991. Our test statistic is $H = 0.01$.

5. Since $0.01 < 5.991$, we fail to reject the null hypothesis. There is not enough evidence to conclude that there is a difference in the heights of waterfalls on the three continents.

6. The corresponding parametric test is analysis of variance (ANOVA).

7. To perform an ANOVA, the population must be normally distributed, the samples must be independent of each other, and the variance of the samples must be equal.

Section 13–6 Tall Trees

1. The biologist is trying to see if there is a relationship between the heights and diameters of tall trees.

2. We will use the Spearman rank correlation analysis.

3. The corresponding parametric test is the Pearson product moment correlation analysis.

4. Answers will vary.

5. The Pearson correlation coefficient is $r = 0.329$. The associated P-value is 0.353. We would fail to reject the null hypothesis that the correlation is zero. The Spearman rank correlation coefficient is $r_s = 0.115$. We would reject the null hypothesis at the 0.05 significance level, if $r_s > 0.648$. Since $0.115 < 0.648$, we do not reject the null hypothesis that the correlation is zero. Both the parametric and nonparametric tests find that the correlation is not statistically significantly different from zero. It appears that no linear relationship exists between the heights and diameters of tall trees.

Section 13–7 Stock Exchange Trading Volumes

1. The runs test is the best nonparametric test for randomness.

2. Solve for the median by sorting the data and taking the average of the two middle values, 166 and 177. The median is 171.5.

3. With the data in rows, the trading volume attributes are as follows.

Run	Attribute
1	$- -$
2	$+ +$
3	$- - - - -$
4	$+ + +$
5	$-$
6	$+$
7	$- -$
8	$+ + + +$

4. Trading volumes appear to be random.

5. H_0: The trading volumes are random (claim) and H_1: The trading volumes are not random.

   The runs are $2 -, 2 +, 5 -, 3 +, 1 -, 1 +, 2 -$, and $4 +$. The critical value at $\alpha = 0.05$ with $n_1 = 10$ and $n_2 = 10$ is 6 and 16.

   Since there are 8 runs, and 8 falls between 6 and 16, H_0 is not rejected.

   There is not sufficient evidence to reject the claim that TSX trading volumes are random.

Hypothesis-Testing Summary 3*

>>

15. Test to see whether the median of a sample is a specific value when $n \geq 26$.

    Example: H_0: median $= 100$

    Use the sign test:

    $$z = \frac{(X + 0.5) - (n/2)}{\sqrt{n}/2}$$

16. Test to see whether two independent samples are obtained from populations that have identical distributions.

    Example: H_0: There is no difference in the ages of the subjects.

    Use the Wilcoxon rank sum test:

    $$z = \frac{R - \mu_R}{\sigma_R}$$

where

$$\mu_R = \frac{n_1(n_1 + n_2 + 1)}{2}$$

$$\sigma_R = \sqrt{\frac{n_1 n_2(n_1 + n_2 + 1)}{12}}$$

17. Test to see whether two dependent samples have identical distributions.

    Example: H_0: There is no difference in the effects of a tranquilizer on the number of hours a person sleeps at night.

    Use the Wilcoxon signed-rank test:

    $$z = \frac{w_s - \frac{n(n + 1)}{4}}{\sqrt{\frac{n(n + 1)(2n + 1)}{24}}}$$

    when $n \geq 30$.

---

*This summary is a continuation of Hypothesis Testing Summary 2 at the end of Chapter 12.

18. Test to see whether three or more samples come from identical populations.

Example: H_0: There is no difference in the weights of the three groups.

Use the Kruskal-Wallis test:

$$H = \frac{12}{N(N+1)}\left(\frac{R_1^2}{n_1} + \frac{R_2^2}{n_2} + \cdots + \frac{R_k^2}{n_k}\right) - 3(N+1)$$

19. Rank correlation coefficient.

$$r_s = 1 - \frac{6\sum d^2}{n(n^2-1)}$$

20. Test for randomness: Use the runs test.

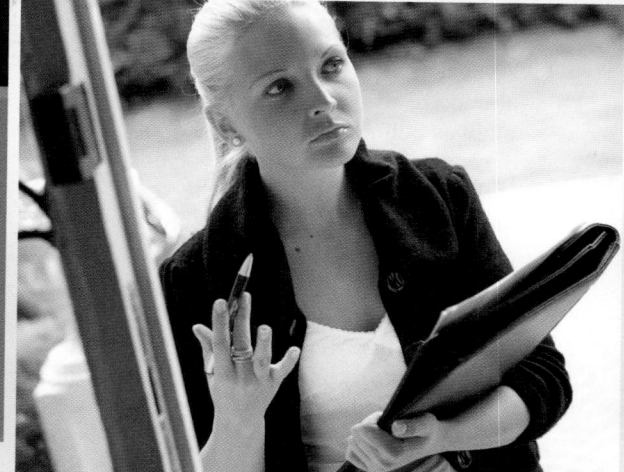

Chapter 14

Sampling and Simulation

Statistics Today

The Monty Hall Problem

On the game show *Let's Make A Deal,* Canadian-born host Monty Hall gave a contestant a choice of three doors. A valuable prize was behind one door, and nothing was behind the other two doors. When the contestant selected one door, host Monty Hall opened one of the other doors that the contestant didn't select and that had no prize behind it. (Monty Hall knew in advance which door had the prize.) Then he asked the contestant if he or she wanted to change doors or keep the one that the contestant originally selected. Now the question is, Should the contestant switch doors, or does it really matter? This chapter will show you how you can solve this problem by simulation. For the answer, see Statistics Today—Revisited, page 641.

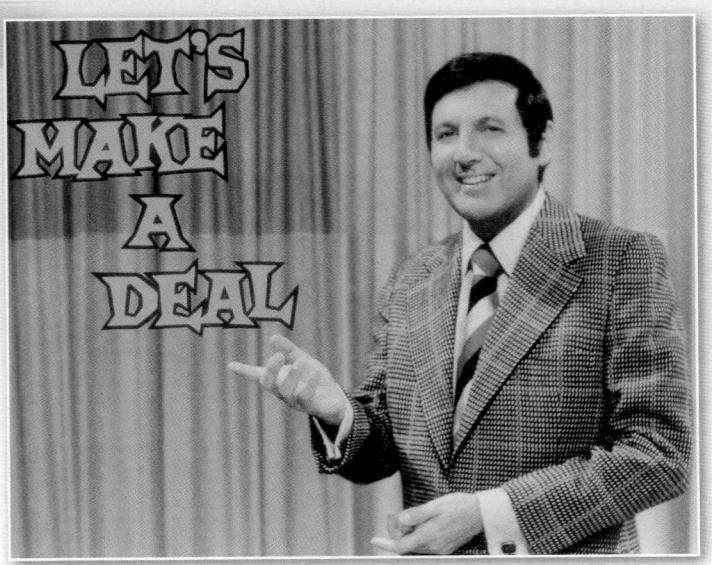

Introduction >

Most people have heard of Gallup, Ipsos Reid, and Nielsen. These and other pollsters gather information about the habits and opinions of the Canadian people. Such survey firms and Statistics Canada gather information by selecting samples from well-defined populations. Recall from Chapter 1 that the subjects in the sample should be a subgroup of the subjects in the population. Sampling methods often use what are called *random numbers* to select samples.

Since many statistical studies use surveys and questionnaires, information about these is presented in Section 14–2.

Random numbers are also used in *simulation techniques.* Instead of studying a real-life situation, which may be costly or dangerous, researchers create a similar situation in a laboratory or with a computer. Then, by studying the simulated situation, researchers can gain the necessary information about the real-life situation in a less expensive or safer manner. This chapter will explain some common methods used to obtain samples as well as the techniques used in simulations.

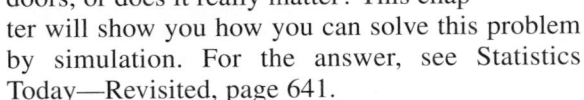

14–1 | Common Sampling Techniques >

Demonstrate a knowledge of the four basic sampling methods.

In Chapter 1, a *population* was defined as all subjects (human or otherwise) under study. Since some populations can be very large, researchers cannot use every single subject, so a sample must be selected. A *sample* is a subgroup of the population. Any subgroup of the population, technically speaking, can be called a sample. However, for researchers to make valid inferences about population characteristics, the sample must be random.

For a sample to be a **random sample,** every member of the population must have an equal chance of being selected.

When a sample is chosen at random from a population, it is said to be an **unbiased sample.** That is, the sample, for the most part, is representative of the population. Conversely, if a sample is selected incorrectly, it may be a biased sample. Samples are said to be **biased samples** when some type of systematic error has been made in the selection of the subjects.

A sample is used to get information about a population for several reasons:

1. *It saves the researcher time and money.*

2. *It enables the researcher to get information that he or she might not be able to obtain otherwise.* For example, if a person's blood is to be analyzed for cholesterol, a researcher cannot analyze every single drop of blood without killing the person. Or if the breaking strength of cables is to be determined, a researcher cannot test to destruction every cable manufactured, since the company would not have any cables left to sell.

3. *It enables the researcher to get more detailed information about a particular subject.* If only a few people are surveyed, the researcher can conduct in-depth interviews by spending more time with each person, thus getting more information about the subject. This is not to say that the smaller the sample, the better; in fact, the opposite is true. In general, larger samples—if correct sampling techniques are used—give more reliable information about the population.

It would be ideal if the sample were a perfect miniature of the population in all characteristics. This ideal, however, is impossible to achieve, because there are so many human traits (height, weight, IQ, etc.). The best that can be done is to select a sample that will be representative with respect to *some* characteristics, preferably those pertaining to the study. For example, if one-half of the population subjects are female, then approximately one-half of the sample subjects should be female. Likewise, other characteristics, such as age, socioeconomic status, and IQ, should be represented proportionately. To obtain unbiased samples, statisticians have developed several basic sampling methods. The most common methods are *random, systematic, stratified,* and *cluster sampling.* Each method will be explained in detail in this section.

In addition to the basic methods, there are other methods used to obtain samples. Some of these methods are also explained in this section.

Simple Random Sampling

A simple random sample is obtained by using methods such as random numbers, which can be generated from calculators, computers, or tables. In *simple random sampling,* the basic requirement is that for a sample of size *n,* all possible samples of this size must have an equal chance of being selected from the population. But before the correct method of obtaining a simple random sample is explained, several incorrect methods commonly used by various researchers and agencies to gain information are discussed.

One incorrect method commonly used is to ask "the person on the street." News reporters use this technique, referred to as **convenience sampling,** quite often. Selecting people haphazardly on the street does not meet the requirement for simple random sampling, since not all possible samples of a specific size have an equal chance of being selected. Many people will be at home or at work when the interview is being conducted and therefore do not have a chance of being selected.

> A **convenience sample** is a sample of subjects used because the subjects are convenient and available.

Another incorrect technique is to ask a question on either radio or television and have the listeners or viewers call the station to give their responses or opinions. Again, this sample is not random, since only those who feel strongly for or against the issue may respond and people may not have heard or seen the program. A third erroneous method is to ask people to respond by mail. Again, only those who are concerned and who have the time are likely to respond.

These methods do not meet the requirement of simple random sampling, since not all possible samples of a specific size have an equal chance of being selected. To meet this requirement, researchers can use one of two methods. The first method is to number each element of the population and then place the numbers on cards. Place the cards in a hat or fishbowl, mix them, and then select the sample by drawing the cards. When using this procedure, researchers must ensure that the numbers are well mixed. On occasion, when this procedure is used, the numbers are not mixed well, and the numbers chosen for the sample are those that were placed in the bowl last.

The second and preferred way of selecting a simple random sample is to use random numbers. Figure 14–1 shows a table of two-digit random numbers generated by a computer. A more detailed table of random numbers is found in Table D in Appendix C.

The theory behind random numbers is that each digit, 0 through 9, has an equal probability of occurring. That is, in every sequence of 10 digits, each digit has a probability of $\frac{1}{10}$ of occurring. This does not mean that in every sequence of 10 digits, one will find each digit. Rather, it means that on the average, each digit will occur once. For example, the digit 2 may occur 3 times in a sequence of 10 digits, but in later sequences, it may not occur at all, thus averaging to a probability of $\frac{1}{10}$.

To obtain a sample by using random numbers, number the elements of the population sequentially and then select each person by using random numbers. This process is shown in Example 14–1.

Simple random samples can be selected with or without replacement. If the same member of the population cannot be used more than once in the study, then the sample is selected without replacement. That is, once a random number is selected, it cannot be used later.

Figure 14–1

Table of Random Numbers

79	41	71	93	60	35	04	67	96	04	79	10	86
26	52	53	13	43	50	92	09	87	21	83	75	17
18	13	41	30	56	20	37	74	49	56	45	46	83
19	82	02	69	34	27	77	34	24	93	16	77	00
14	57	44	30	93	76	32	13	55	29	49	30	77
29	12	18	50	06	33	15	79	50	28	50	45	45
01	27	92	67	93	31	97	55	29	21	64	27	29
55	75	65	68	65	73	07	95	66	43	43	92	16
84	95	95	96	62	30	91	64	74	83	47	89	71
62	62	21	37	82	62	19	44	08	64	34	50	11
66	57	28	69	13	99	74	31	58	19	47	66	89
48	13	69	97	29	01	75	58	05	40	40	18	29
94	31	73	19	75	76	33	18	05	53	04	51	41
00	06	53	98	01	55	08	38	49	42	10	44	38
46	16	44	27	80	15	28	01	64	27	89	03	27
77	49	85	95	62	93	25	39	63	74	54	82	85
81	96	43	27	39	53	85	61	12	90	67	96	02
40	46	15	73	23	75	96	68	13	99	49	64	11

Note: In the explanations and examples of the sampling procedures, a small population will be used, and small samples will be selected from this population. Small populations are used for illustrative purposes only, because the entire population could be included with little difficulty. In real life, however, researchers must usually sample from very large populations, using the procedures shown in this chapter.

Example 14–1

Television Show Interviews

Suppose a researcher wants to produce a television show featuring in-depth interviews with Canada's city mayors on the subject of a new partnership with the federal and provincial governments. Because of time constraints, the 60-minute program will have room for only 10 mayors. The researcher wishes to select the mayors at random. Select a simple random sample of 10 cities from 50.

Solution

Step 1   Number each city from 1 to 50, as shown. In this case, they are numbered alphabetically.

01	Abbotsford	14	Hamilton	27	Oshawa	40	Sudbury
02	Barrie	15	Kamloops	28	Ottawa	41	Surrey
03	Brampton	16	Kingston	29	Quebec City	42	Thunder Bay
04	Brantford	17	Kitchener	30	Red Deer	43	Toronto
05	Burlington	18	Laval	31	Regina	44	Trois-Rivières
06	Burnaby	19	Lethbridge	32	Richmond	45	Vancouver
07	Calgary	20	Lévis	33	Saguenay	46	Victoria
08	Cambridge	21	London	34	Saint John	47	Waterloo
09	Coquitlan	22	Longueuil	35	Saskatoon	48	Whitby
10	Edmonton	23	Mississauga	36	Sault Ste. Marie	49	Windsor
11	Gatineau	24	Montreal	37	Sherbrooke	50	Winnipeg
12	Guelph	25	Niagara Falls	38	St. Catharines		
13	Halifax	26	Oakville	39	St. John's		

Step 2   Using the random numbers shown in Figure 14–1, find a starting point. To find a starting point, one generally closes one's eyes and places one's finger anywhere on the table. In this case, the first number selected was 27 in the fourth column. Going down the column and continuing on to the next column, select the first 10 numbers. They are 27, 95, 27, 73, 60, 43, 56, 34, 93, and 06. See Figure 14–2. (Note that 06 represents 6.)

Figure 14–2

Selecting a Starting Point and 10 Numbers from the Random Number Table

79	41	71	93	60 ✓	35	04	67	96	04	79	10	86
26	52	53	13	43 ✓	50	92	09	87	21	83	75	17
18	13	41	30	56 ✓	20	37	74	49	56	45	46	83
19	82	02	69	34 ✓	27	77	34	24	93	16	77	00
14	57	44	30	93 ✓	76	32	13	55	29	49	30	77
29	12	18	50	06 ✓	33	15	79	50	28	50	45	45
01	27	92	67	93	31	97	55	29	21	64	27	29
55	75	65	68	65	73	07	95	66	43	43	92	16
84	95	95	96	62	30	91	64	74	83	47	89	71
62	62	21	37	82	62	19	44	08	64	34	50	11
66	57	28	69	13	99	74	31	58	19	47	66	89
48	13	69	97	29	01	75	58	05	40	40	18	29
94	31	73	19	75	76	33	18	05	53	04	51	41
00	06	53	Start here	01	55	08	38	49	42	10	44	38
46	16	44	㉗✓	80	15	28	01	64	27	89	03	27
77	49	85	95 ✓	62	93	25	39	63	74	54	82	85
81	96	43	27 ✓	39	53	85	61	12	90	67	96	02
40	46	15	73 ✓	23	75	96	68	13	99	49	64	11

Now, refer to the list of cities and identify the city corresponding to each number. The sample consists of the following cities:

27	Oshawa	43	Toronto
95		56	
27	Oshawa	34	Saint John
73		93	
60		06	Burnaby

Step 3 Since the numbers 95, 73, 60, 56, and 93 are too large, they are disregarded. And since 27 appears twice, it is also disregarded the second time. Now, one must select six more random numbers between 1 and 50 and omit duplicates, since this sample will be selected without replacement. Make this selection by continuing down the column and moving over to the next column until a total of 10 numbers is selected. The final 10 numbers are 27, 43, 34, 06, 13, 29, 01, 39, 23, and 35. See Figure 14–3.

Figure 14–3

The Final 10 Numbers Selected

79	41	71	93	60	㉟	04	67	96	04	79	10	86
26	52	53	13	㊸	50	92	09	87	21	83	75	17
18	13	41	30	56	20	37	74	49	56	45	46	83
19	82	02	69	㉞	27	77	34	24	93	16	77	00
14	57	44	30	93	76	32	13	55	29	49	30	77
29	12	18	50	ⓞ6	33	15	79	50	28	50	45	45
01	27	92	67	93	31	97	55	29	21	64	27	29
55	75	65	68	65	73	07	95	66	43	43	92	16
84	95	95	96	62	30	91	64	74	83	47	89	71
62	62	21	37	82	62	19	44	08	64	34	50	11
66	57	28	69	⑬	99	74	31	58	19	47	66	89
48	13	69	97	㉙	01	75	58	05	40	40	18	29
94	31	73	19	75	76	33	18	05	53	04	51	41
00	06	53	98	ⓞ1	55	08	38	49	42	10	44	38
46	16	44	㉗	80	15	28	01	64	27	89	03	27
77	49	85	95	62	93	25	39	63	74	54	82	85
81	96	43	27	㊴	53	85	61	12	90	67	96	02
40	46	15	73	㉓	75	96	68	13	99	49	64	11

These numbers correspond to the following cities:

27	Oshawa	29	Quebec City
43	Toronto	01	Abbotsford
34	Saint John	39	St. John's
06	Burnaby	23	Mississauga
13	Halifax	35	Saskatoon

Thus, the mayors of these 10 cities will constitute the sample.

Simple random sampling has one limitation. If the population is extremely large, it is time-consuming to number and select the sample elements. Also, notice that the random numbers in the table are two-digit numbers. If three digits are needed, then the first digit from the next column can be used, as shown in Figure 14–4. Table D in Appendix C gives five-digit random numbers.

Speaking of Statistics

Should We Be Afraid of Lightning?

Environment Canada and the United States National Weather Service collect various types of data about the weather. North America averages 400 million lightning strikes each year, with Alberta's Rocky Mountain foothills having recorded 5000 lightning strikes in a 24-hour period. Lightning strikes kill or injure an estimated 120 to 190 people each year in Canada, with over 90% of the deaths occurring in Ontario, Quebec, and the Prairie provinces. The cause of most of these deaths is not burns, even though temperatures as high as 30,000°C are reached, but heart attacks. The lightning strike short-circuits the body's autonomic nervous system, causing the heart to stop beating. In some instances, the heart will restart on its own. In other cases, the heart victim will need emergency resuscitation.

The most dangerous places to be during a thunderstorm are open fields, golf courses, under trees,

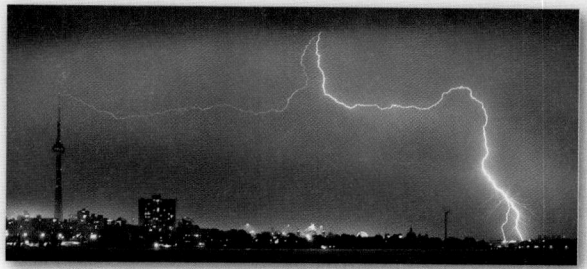

and near water, such as a lake or swimming pool. It's best to be inside a building during a thunderstorm, although there's no guarantee that the building won't be struck by lightning. Are these statistics descriptive or inferential? Why do you think more men are struck by lightning than women? Should you be afraid of lightning?

Sources: Environment Canada, *Lightning Activity,* and *Current Results: Research News and Science Facts,* "What Are the Odds You'll Get Struck by Lightening?" Liz Osborn.

79	41	71	93	60	35	04	67	96	04	79	10	86
26	52	53	13	43	50	92	09	87	21	83	75	17
18	13	41	30	56	20	37	74	49	56	45	46	83
19	82	02	69	34	27	77	34	24	93	16	77	00
14	57	44	30	93	76	32	13	55	29	49	30	77
29	12	18	50	06	33	15	79	50	28	50	45	45
01	27	92	67	93	31	97	55	29	21	64	27	29
55	75	65	68	65	73	07	95	66	43	43	92	16
84	95	95	96	62	30	91	64	74	83	47	89	71
62	62	21	37	82	62	19	44	08	64	34	50	11
66	57	28	69	13	99	74	31	58	19	47	66	89
48	13	69	97	29	01	75	58	05	40	40	18	29
94	31	73	19	75	76	33	18	05	53	04	51	41
00	06	53	98	01	55	08	38	49	42	10	44	38
46	16	44	27	80	15	28	01	64	27	89	03	27
77	49	85	95	62	93	25	39	63	74	54	82	85
81	96	43	27	39	53	85	61	12	90	67	96	02
40	46	15	73	23	75	96	68	13	99	49	64	11

Figure 14–4
Method for Selecting Three-Digit Numbers

Use one column and part of the next column for three digits, that is, 404.

Systematic Sampling

A **systematic sample** is a sample obtained by numbering each element in the population and then selecting every third or fifth or tenth, etc., number from the population to be included in the sample. This is done after the first number is selected at random.

The procedure of systematic sampling is illustrated in Example 14–2.

Example 14–2	**Television Show Interviews**

Using the population of 50 cities in Example 14–1, select a systematic sample of 10 cities.

Solution

Step 1 Number the population units as shown in Example 14–1.

Step 2 Since there are 50 cities and 10 are to be selected, the rule is to select every fifth city. This rule was determined by dividing 50 by 10, which yields 5.

Step 3 Using the table of random numbers, select the first digit (from 1 to 5) at random. In this case, 4 was selected.

Step 4 Select every fifth number on the list, starting with 4. The numbers include the following:

1 2 3 ④ 5 6 7 8 ⑨ 10 11 12 13 ⑭ . . .

The selected cities are as follows:

4	Brantford	29	Quebec City
9	Coquitlan	34	Saint John
14	Hamilton	39	St. John's
19	Lethbridge	44	Trois-Rivières
24	Montreal	49	Windsor

The advantage of systematic sampling is the ease of selecting the sample elements. Also, in many cases, a numbered list of the population units may already exist. For example, the manager of a factory may have a list of employees who work for the company, or there may be an in-house telephone directory.

When doing systematic sampling, one must be careful how the items are arranged on the list. For example, if each unit was arranged, say, as

1. Husband
2. Wife
3. Husband
4. Wife

then the selection of the starting number could produce a sample of all males or all females, depending on whether the starting number is even or odd and whether the number to be added is even or odd. As another example, if the list was arranged in order of heights of individuals, one would get a different average from two samples if the first was selected by using a small starting number and the second by using a large starting number.

Stratified Sampling

A **stratified sample** is a sample obtained by dividing the population into subgroups, called *strata*, according to various homogeneous characteristics and then selecting members from each stratum for the sample.

For example, a population may consist of males and females who are smokers or nonsmokers. The researcher will want to include in the sample people from each group—that is, males who smoke, males who do not smoke, females who smoke, and females who do not smoke. To accomplish this selection, the researcher divides the population into four subgroups and then selects a random sample from each subgroup. This method ensures that the sample is representative on the basis of the characteristics of gender and smoking. Of course, it may not be representative on the basis of other characteristics.

Example 14–3

Student Selection 🖋

Using the population of 20 students shown in Figure 14–5, select a sample of 8 students on the basis of gender (male/female) and grade level (freshman/sophomore) by stratification.

Figure 14–5

Population of Students for Example 14–3

1. Ald, Peter	M	Fr	11. Martin, Janice	F	Fr
2. Brown, Danny	M	So	12. Meloski, Gary	M	Fr
3. Bear, Theresa	F	Fr	13. Oeler, George	M	So
4. Carson, Susan	F	Fr	14. Peters, Michele	F	So
5. Collins, Carolyn	F	Fr	15. Peterson, John	M	Fr
6. Davis, William	M	Fr	16. Smith, Nancy	F	Fr
7. Hogan, Michael	M	Fr	17. Thomas, Jeff	M	So
8. Jones, Lois	F	So	18. Toms, Debbie	F	So
9. Lutz, Harry	M	So	19. Unger, Roberta	F	So
10. Lyons, Larry	M	So	20. Zibert, Mary	F	So

Solution

Step 1 Divide the population into two subgroups, consisting of males and females, as shown in Figure 14–6.

Figure 14–6

Population Divided into Subgroups by Gender

Males			**Females**		
1. Ald, Peter	M	Fr	1. Bear, Theresa	F	Fr
2. Brown, Danny	M	So	2. Carson, Susan	F	Fr
3. Davis, William	M	Fr	3. Collins, Carolyn	F	Fr
4. Hogan, Michael	M	Fr	4. Jones, Lois	F	So
5. Lutz, Harry	M	So	5. Martin, Janice	F	Fr
6. Lyons, Larry	M	So	6. Peters, Michele	F	So
7. Meloski, Gary	M	Fr	7. Smith, Nancy	F	Fr
8. Oeler, George	M	So	8. Toms, Debbie	F	So
9. Peterson, John	M	Fr	9. Unger, Roberta	F	So
10. Thomas, Jeff	M	So	10. Zibert, Mary	F	So

Step 2 Divide each subgroup further into two groups of freshmen and sophomores, as shown in Figure 14–7.

Figure 14–7

Each Subgroup Divided into Subgroups by Grade Level

Group 1			**Group 2**		
1. Ald, Peter	M	Fr	1. Bear, Theresa	F	Fr
2. Davis, William	M	Fr	2. Carson, Susan	F	Fr
3. Hogan, Michael	M	Fr	3. Collins, Carolyn	F	Fr
4. Meloski, Gary	M	Fr	4. Martin, Janice	F	Fr
5. Peterson, John	M	Fr	5. Smith, Nancy	F	Fr

Group 3			**Group 4**		
1. Brown, Danny	M	So	1. Jones, Lois	F	So
2. Lutz, Harry	M	So	2. Peters, Michele	F	So
3. Lyons, Larry	M	So	3. Toms, Debbie	F	So
4. Oeler, George	M	So	4. Unger, Roberta	F	So
5. Thomas, Jeff	M	So	5. Zibert, Mary	F	So

Step 3 Determine how many students need to be selected from each subgroup to have a proportional representation of each subgroup in the sample. There are four groups, and since a total of eight students is needed for the sample, two students must be selected from each subgroup.

Step 4 Select two students from each group by using random numbers. In this case, the random numbers are as follows:

Group 1	Students 5 and 4	Group 2	Students 5 and 2
Group 3	Students 1 and 3	Group 4	Students 3 and 4

The stratified sample then consists of the following people:

Peterson, John	M	Fr	Smith, Nancy	F	Fr
Meloski, Gary	M	Fr	Carson, Susan	F	Fr
Brown, Danny	M	So	Toms, Debbie	F	So
Lyons, Larry	M	So	Unger, Roberta	F	So

The major advantage of stratification is that it ensures representation of all population subgroups that are important to the study. There are two major drawbacks to stratification, however. First, if there are many variables of interest, dividing a large population into representative subgroups requires a great deal of effort. Second, if the variables are somewhat complex or ambiguous (such as beliefs, attitudes, or prejudices), it is difficult to separate individuals into the subgroups according to these variables.

Cluster Sampling

A **cluster sample** is a sample obtained by selecting a pre-existing or natural group, called a *cluster*, and using the members in the cluster for the sample.

For example, many studies in education use already existing classes, such as the Grade 7 class in Markham Elementary School. The voters of a certain district might be surveyed to determine their preferences for a mayoral candidate in the upcoming election. Or the residents of an entire city block might be polled to ascertain the percentage of households that have two or more incomes. In cluster sampling, researchers may use all units of a cluster if that is feasible, or they may select only part of a cluster to use as a sample. This selection is done by random methods.

There are three advantages to using a cluster sample instead of other types of samples: (1) A cluster sample can reduce costs, (2) it can simplify fieldwork, and (3) it is convenient. For example, in a dental study involving X-raying Grade 4 students' teeth to see how many cavities each child had, it would be a simple matter to select a single classroom and bring the X-ray equipment to the school to conduct the study. If other sampling methods were used, researchers might have to transport the machine to several different schools or transport the students to the dental office.

The major disadvantage of cluster sampling is that the elements in a cluster may not have the same variations in characteristics as elements selected individually from a population. The reason is that groups of people may be more homogeneous (alike) in specific clusters such as neighbourhoods or clubs. For example, the people who live in a certain neighbourhood tend to have similar incomes, drive similar cars, live in similar houses, and, for the most part, have similar habits.

Speaking of Statistics

In this study, the researchers found that subjects did better on fill-in-the-blank questions than on multiple-choice questions. Do you agree with the professor's statement, "Trusting your first impulse is your best strategy?" Explain your answer.

TESTS

Is That Your Final Answer?

Beating game shows takes more than smarts: Contestants must also overcome self-doubt and peer pressure. Two new studies suggest today's hottest game shows are particularly challenging because the very mechanisms employed to help contestants actually lead them astray.

Multiple-choice questions are one such offender, as alternative answers seem to make test-takers ignore gut instincts. To learn why, researchers at Southern Methodist University gave two identical tests: one using multiple-choice questions and the other fill-in-the-blank. The results, recently published in the *Journal of Educational Psychology*, show that test-takers were incorrect more often when given false alternatives, and that the longer they considered those alternatives, the more credible the answers looked.

"If you sit and stew, you forget that you know the right answer," says Alan Brown, Ph.D., a psychology professor at Southern Methodist University. "Trusting your first impulse is your best strategy." Audiences can also be trouble, says Jennifer Butler, Ph.D., a Wittenberg University psychology professor. Her recent study in the *Journal of Personality and Social Psychology* found that contestants who see audience participation as peer pressure slow down to avoid making embarrassing mistakes. But this strategy backfires, as more contemplation produces more wrong answers. Worse, Butler says, if perceived peer pressure grows unbearable, contestants may opt out of answering at all, "thinking that it's better to stop than to have your once supportive audience come to believe you're an idiot."

— *Sarah Smith*

Source: Reprinted with permission from *Psychology Today,* Copyright © 2000 Sussex Publishers, Inc.

Other Types of Sampling Techniques

In addition to the four basic sampling methods, other methods are sometimes used. In **sequence sampling,** which is used in quality control, successive units taken from production lines are sampled to ensure that the products meet certain standards set by the manufacturing company.

In **double sampling,** a very large population is given a questionnaire to determine those who meet the qualifications for a study. After the questionnaires are reviewed, a second, smaller population is defined. Then a sample is selected from this group.

In **multistage sampling,** the researcher uses a combination of sampling methods. For example, suppose a research organization wants to conduct a nationwide survey for a new product being manufactured. A sample can be obtained by using the following combination of methods. First, the researchers divide the 50 cities from across the country into four or five regions (or clusters). Then, several cities from each region are selected at random. Next the selected cities are divided into various areas by using districts and wards (or neighbourhoods). Samples of these areas are then selected. Finally, streets in these wards are selected at random, and the families living on these streets are given samples of the product to test and are asked to report the results. This hypothetical example illustrates a typical multistage sampling method.

The steps for conducting a sample survey are given in the Procedure Table.

Interesting Fact

Folks in extra-large aerobics classes—those with 70 to 90 participants—show up more often and are more fond of their classmates than exercisers in sessions of 18 to 26 people, report researchers at the University of Arizona.

Procedure Table

Conducting a Sample Survey

Step 1 Decide what information is needed.

Step 2 Determine how the data will be collected (phone interview, mail survey, etc.).

Step 3 Select the information-gathering instrument or design the questionnaire if one is not available.

Step 4 Set up a sampling list, if possible.

Step 5 Select the best method for obtaining the sample (random, systematic, stratified, cluster, or other).

Step 6 Conduct the survey and collect the data.

Step 7 Tabulate the data.

Step 8 Conduct the statistical analysis.

Step 9 Report the results.

14–1 Applying the Concepts

The White or Brown Bread Debate

Read the following study and answer the questions.

A baking company selected 36 women with various body weights and randomly assigned them to four different groups. The four groups were white bread only, brown bread only, low-fat white bread only, and low-fat brown bread only. Each group could eat only the type of bread assigned to the group. The study lasted for eight weeks. No other changes in any of the women's diets were allowed. A trained evaluator was used to check for any differences in the women's diets. The results showed that there were no differences in weight gain between the groups over the eight-week period.

1. Did the researchers use a population or a sample for their study?
2. Based on who conducted this study, would you consider the study to be biased?
3. Which sampling method do you think was used to obtain the original 36 women for the study (random, systematic, stratified, clustered, or convenience?
4. Which sampling method would you use? Why?
5. How would you collect a random sample for this study?
6. Does random assignment help representativeness the same as random selection does? Explain.

See page 644 for the answers.

Exercises 14–1

1. Name the four basic sampling techniques.

2. Why are samples used in statistics?

3. What is the basic requirement for a sample?

4. Why should random numbers be used when one is selecting a random sample?

5. List three incorrect methods that are often used to obtain a sample.

6. What is the principle behind random numbers?

7. List the advantages and disadvantages of random sampling.

8. List the advantages and disadvantages of systematic sampling.

9. List the advantages and disadvantages of stratified sampling.

10. List the advantages and disadvantages of cluster sampling.

Using the student survey at Utopia University, shown in Figure 14–8, as the population, complete Exercises 11 through 15.

11. Using the table of random numbers in Figure 14–1, select 10 students and find the sample mean (average) of the GPA, IQ, and distance travelled to school. Compare these sample means with the population means.

12. Select a sample of 10 students by the systematic method, and compute the sample means of the GPA, IQ, and distance travelled to school of this sample. Compare these sample means with the population means.

13. Select a cluster of 10 students, for example, students 9 through 18, and compute the sample means of their GPA, IQ, and distance travelled to school. Compare these sample means with the population means.

14. Divide the 50 students into subgroups according to class rank. Then select a sample of 2 students from each rank and compute the means of these 10 students for the GPA, IQ, and distance travelled to school each day. Compare these sample means with the population means.

15. In your opinion, which sampling method(s) provided the best sample to represent the population?

Figure 14–8

Student Survey at Utopia University (for Exercises 11 through 15)

Student number	Gender	Class rank	GPA	Kilometres travelled to school	IQ	Major field	Student number	Gender	Class rank	GPA	Kilometres travelled to school	IQ	Major field
1	M	Fr	1.4	1	104	Bio	26	M	Fr	1.1	8	100	Ed
2	M	Fr	2.3	2	95	Ed	27	F	Jr	2.1	3	101	Bus
3	M	So	2.7	6	108	Psy	28	M	Gr	3.7	5	99	Bio
4	F	So	3.2	7	119	Eng	29	M	Se	2.4	8	105	Eng
5	F	Gr	3.8	12	114	Ed	30	M	So	2.1	15	108	Bus
6	M	Jr	4.0	13	91	Psy	31	M	Gr	3.9	2	112	Ed
7	F	Jr	3.0	2	106	Eng	32	F	Jr	2.4	4	111	Psy
8	M	Jr	3.3	6	100	Bio	33	M	Se	2.7	6	107	Eng
9	F	Se	2.7	9	102	Eng	34	F	So	2.5	1	104	Bio
10	F	So	2.3	5	99	Ed	35	M	Se	3.2	3	96	Bus
11	M	Se	1.6	18	100	Bus	36	F	Fr	3.4	7	98	Bio
12	M	Gr	3.2	7	105	Psy	37	M	Gr	3.6	14	105	Ed
13	F	Gr	3.8	3	103	Bus	38	M	Jr	3.8	4	115	Psy
14	F	Se	3.1	5	97	Eng	39	F	Se	2.2	8	113	Eng
15	F	Jr	2.7	5	106	Bio	40	F	So	2.0	8	103	Psy
16	F	Fr	1.4	4	114	Bus	41	F	Fr	2.3	9	103	Eng
17	M	So	3.6	17	102	Ed	42	F	Se	2.5	10	99	Bus
18	M	Fr	2.2	1	101	Psy	43	M	Gr	3.7	13	114	Ed
19	F	Gr	4.0	7	108	Bus	44	M	Fr	3.0	11	121	Bus
20	M	Jr	2.1	4	97	Ed	45	M	Jr	2.1	10	101	Eng
21	F	Fr	2.0	3	113	Bio	46	F	Jr	3.4	2	104	Ed
22	F	So	3.6	4	104	Bio	47	M	So	3.6	9	105	Psy
23	F	Gr	3.3	16	110	Eng	48	M	Se	2.1	1	97	Psy
24	F	Se	2.5	4	99	Psy	49	F	Gr	3.3	12	111	Bio
25	M	So	3.0	5	96	Psy	50	F	Fr	2.2	11	102	Bio

Use Figure 14–9 as the population to complete Exercises 16 through 19. The data show the top 50 municipalities in Canada, by population, based on the *2006 Census*. Precipitation and frost-free days are yearly averages. House prices are 2009 averages in $1000s.

16. Municipal Population Find the population mean (all 50 municipalities) for the population data. Use the table of random numbers in Figure 14–1 to select 10 municipalities. Find the mean of the sample from the population data. Compare these sample means with the population means.

Figure 14–9

Top 50 Municipalities in Canada (by population, based on the *2006 Census*)

	Municipality	Province	Population	Precipitation (mm/year)	Frost-free days	House prices ($1000s)
1	Abbotsford	BC	123,864	1573	303	330
2	Barrie	ON	128,430	700	205	274
3	Brampton	ON	433,806	793	219	314
4	Burlington	ON	164,415	879	236	324
5	Burnaby	BC	202,799	2020	317	561
6	Calgary	AB	988,193	413	169	363
7	Cambridge	ON	120,371	958	209	245
8	Cape Breton	NS	102,250	1505	197	101
9	Chatham-Kent	ON	108,177	887	244	135
10	Coquitlam	BC	114,565	2253	296	561
11	Delta	BC	96,723	1008	330	313
12	Edmonton	AB	730,372	477	186	311
13	Gatineau	QC	242,124	943	212	150
14	Greater Sudbury	ON	157,857	899	183	197
15	Guelph	ON	114,943	923	204	272
16	Halifax	NS	372,679	1452	208	234
17	Hamilton	ON	504,559	910	223	235
18	Kelowna	BC	106,707	381	207	545
19	Kingston	ON	117,207	960	228	228
20	Kitchener	ON	204,668	908	205	263
21	Laval	QC	368,709	987	211	242
22	Lévis	QC	130,006	1230	189	200
23	London	ON	352,395	987	217	193
24	Longueuil	QC	229,330	1053	225	231
25	Markham	ON	261,573	892	217	441
26	Mississauga	ON	668,549	793	219	326
27	Montreal	QC	1,620,693	793	215	326
28	Oakville	ON	165,613	1056	222	315
29	Oshawa	ON	141,590	878	212	204
30	Ottawa	ON	812,129	914	212	273
31	Quebec City	QC	491,142	1230	189	200
32	Regina	SK	179,246	388	165	228
33	Richmond	BC	174,461	1199	319	561
34	Richmond Hill	BC	162,704	892	217	379
35	Saanich	BC	108,265	608	312	537
36	Saguenay	QC	143,692	920	172	149
37	Saskatoon	SK	202,340	350	166	266
38	Sherbrooke	QC	147,427	1144	176	194
39	St. Catharines	ON	131,989	874	236	193
40	St. John's	NL	100,646	1514	191	177

Figure 14–9 *(Continued)*

41	Surrey	BC	394,976	1370	315	379
42	Thunder Bay	ON	109,140	712	162	135
43	Toronto	ON	2,503,281	836	218	387
44	Trois-Rivières	QC	126,323	859	193	114
45	Vancouver	BC	578,041	1276	330	561
46	Vaughan	ON	238,866	798	207	439
47	Waterloo	ON	97,475	908	205	263
48	Whitby	ON	111,184	878	212	270
49	Windsor	ON	216,473	918	242	151
50	Winnipeg	MB	633,451	514	171	183

Source: Statistics Canada, 2006 Census.

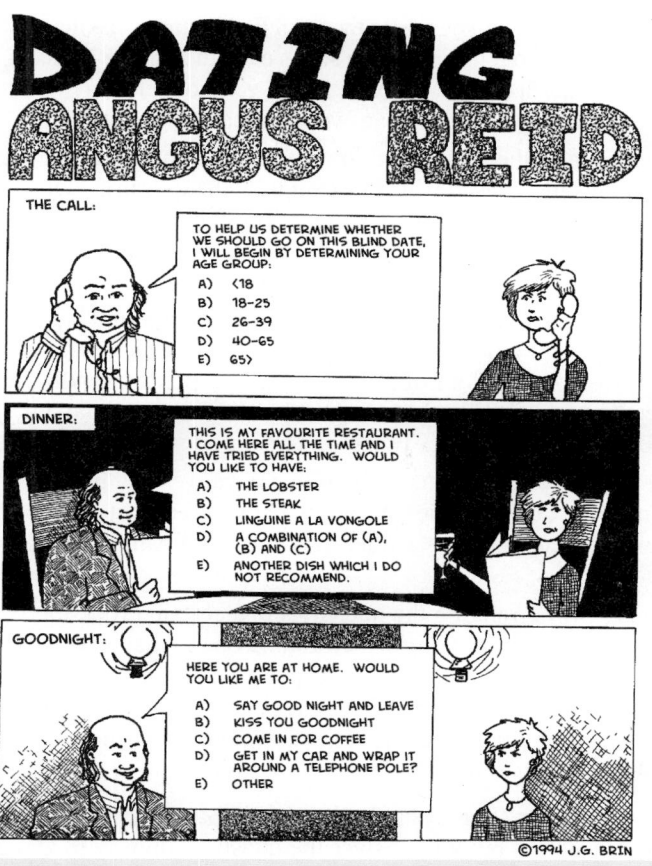

Source: "Dating Angus Reid" by J.G. Brin, Bubonic Press, www.bubonicpress.com.

17. Municipal Precipitation Find the population mean (all 50 municipalities) for precipitation data. Use the table of random numbers in Figure 14–1 to select 10 municipalities. Find the sample mean of the annual precipitation, in millimetres. Repeat the random selection and compare the sample means with the population mean.

18. Municipal Frost-Free Days Find the population mean (all 50 municipalities) for the frost-free days data. Use the systematic method to select 10 municipalities and find the sample mean of the frost-free days. Compare the sample mean with the population mean.

19. Municipal House Prices Find the population mean (all 50 municipalities) for the house price data. Perform a stratified sample by dividing the municipalities into three regions (West: BC, AB, SK, and MB; Central: ON; East: QC, NS, and NL) and select 12 municipalities (4 from each region) using the table of random numbers in Figure 14–1. Find the sample mean of the house prices and compare with the population mean.

20. Many research studies described in newspapers and magazines do not report the sample size or the sampling method used. Try to find a research article that gives this information; state the sampling method that was used and the sample size.

14–2 Surveys and Questionnaire Design ›

LO2

Recognize faulty questions on a survey and other factors that can bias responses.

Many statistical studies obtain information from *surveys*. A survey is conducted when a sample of individuals is asked to respond to questions about a particular subject. There are two types of surveys: interviewer-administered and self-administered. Interviewer-administered surveys require a person to ask the questions. The interview can be conducted face to face in an office, on a street, or in a mall, or via telephone.

Self-administered surveys can be done by mail or in a group setting such as a classroom.

When analyzing the results of surveys, you should be very careful about the interpretations. The way a question is phrased can influence the way people respond. For example, when a group of people were asked if they favoured a waiting period and background check before guns could be sold, 91% of the respondents were in favour of it and 7% were against it. However, when asked if there should be a national gun registration program costing about 20% of all dollars spent on crime control, only 33% of the respondents were in favour of it and 61% were against it.

As you can see, by phrasing questions in different ways, different responses can be obtained, since the purpose of a national gun registry would include a waiting period and a background check.

When you are writing questions for a questionnaire, it is important to avoid these common mistakes.

1. *Asking biased questions.* By asking questions in a certain way, the researcher can lead the respondents to answer in the way he or she wants them to. For example, asking a question such as "Are you going to vote for candidate Jones even though the latest survey indicates that he will lose the election?" instead of "Are you going to vote for candidate Jones?" may dissuade some people from answering in the affirmative.

2. *Using confusing words.* In this case, the participant misinterprets the meaning of the words and answers the questions in a biased way. For example, the question "Do you think people would live longer if they were on a diet?" could be misinterpreted since there are many different types of diets—weight-loss diets, low-salt diets, medically prescribed diets, etc.

3. *Asking double-barrelled questions.* Sometimes questions contain compound sentences that require the participant to respond to two questions at the same time. For example, the question "Are you in favour of a special tax to support Canada's commitment to reduce greenhouse gases?" asks two questions: "Are you in favour of greenhouse gas reduction?" and "Do you favour a tax to support it?"

4. *Using double negatives in questions.* Questions with double negatives can be confusing to the respondents. For example, the question " Do you feel that it is not appropriate to have areas where people cannot smoke?" is very confusing since *not* is used twice in the sentence.

5. *Ordering questions improperly.* By arranging the questions in a certain order, the researcher can lead the participant to respond in a way that he or she may otherwise not have done. For example, a question might ask the respondent, "At what age should an elderly person not be permitted to drive?" A later question might ask the respondent to list some problems of elderly people. The respondent may indicate that transportation is a problem based on reading the previous question.

Other factors can also bias a survey. For example, the participant may not know anything about the subject of the question but will answer the question anyway to avoid being considered uninformed. For example, many people might respond yes or no to the following question: "Would you be in favour of giving pensions to the widows of unknown soldiers?" In this case, the question makes no sense since if the soldiers were unknown, their widows would also be unknown.

Many people will make responses on the basis of what they think the person asking the questions wants to hear. For example, if a question asks, "How often do you lie?" people may *understate* the incidences of their lying.

Participants will, in some cases, respond differently to questions depending on whether their identity is known. This is especially true if the questions concern sensitive issues such as income, sexuality, and abortion. Researchers try to ensure confidentiality (i.e., keeping the respondent's identity secret) rather than anonymity (soliciting unsigned responses); however, many people will be suspicious in either case.

Still other factors that could bias a survey include the time and place of the survey and whether the questions are open-ended or closed-ended. The time and place where a survey is conducted can influence the results. For example, if a survey on airline safety is conducted immediately after a major airline crash, the results may differ from those obtained in a year in which no major airline disasters occurred.

Finally, the type of questions asked influences the responses. In this case, the concern is whether the question is open-ended or closed-ended.

An *open-ended question* would be one such as "List three activities that you plan to spend more time on when you retire." A *closed-ended question* would be one such as "Select three activities that you plan to spend more time on after you retire: travelling; eating out; fishing, hunting; exercising; visiting relatives."

One problem with a closed-ended question is that the respondent is forced to choose the answers that the researcher gives and cannot supply his or her own. But there is also a problem with open-ended questions in that the results may be so varied that attempting to summarize them might be difficult, if not impossible. Hence, you should be aware of what types of questions are being asked before you draw any conclusions from the survey.

There are several other things to consider when you are conducting a study that uses questionnaires. For example, a pilot study should be done to test the design and usage of the questionnaire (i.e., the *validity* of the questionnaire). The pilot study helps the researcher to pretest the questionnaire to determine if it meets the objectives of the study. It also helps the researcher to rewrite any questions that may be misleading, ambiguous, etc.

If the questions are being asked by an interviewer, some training should be given to that person. If the survey is being done by mail, a cover letter and clear directions should accompany the questionnaire.

Questionnaires help researchers to gather needed statistical information for their studies; however, much care must be given to proper questionnaire design and usage; otherwise, the results will be unreliable.

Unusual Stat

Of people who are struck by lightning, 85% are men.

14–2 Applying the Concepts

Smoking Bans and Profits

Assume you are a tavern owner and are concerned about the recent bans on smoking in public places. Will your business lose money if you do not allow smoking in your tavern? You decide to research this question and find two related articles published on the Internet. The first article states that bar and pub sales were reduced by 23.5% in Ottawa after the smoking ban was enforced. In that study, a telephone survey was used and owners were asked how much business that they thought they lost. The survey was conducted by a special interest group, PUBCO (Pub and Bar Coalition of Canada). It was reported in the second article that there had been a modest increase in business at various taverns that banned smoking in that same area. Sales receipts were collected and analyzed against last year's profits. The second survey was conducted by chartered accountants KPMG for the City of Ottawa.

1. How did the public smoking ban affect tavern business in Ottawa?
2. Why do you think the surveys reported conflicting results?
3. Should surveys based on anecdotal responses be allowed to be published?
4. Can the results of a sample be representative of a population and still offer misleading information?
5. How critical is measurement error in survey sampling?

See page 644 for the answers.

Exercises 14–2

Exercises 1 through 8 include questions that contain a flaw. Identify the flaw and rewrite the question, following the guidelines presented in this section.

1. Will you vote for John Doe for class president or will you vote for Bill Jones, the football star?

2. Would you buy an ABC car even if you knew the manufacturer used imported parts?

3. Should banks charge their chequing account customers a fee to balance their chequebooks when customers are not able to do so?

4. Do you think that students who did not attend Friday's class should not be allowed to take the retest?

5. How long have you studied for this examination?

6. Which artificial sweetener do you prefer?

7. If a plane was to crash on the border of Ontario and Quebec, where should the survivors be buried?

8. Are you in favour of imposing a tax on tobacco to pay for health care related to diseases caused by smoking?

9. Find a study that uses a questionnaire. Select any questions that you feel are improperly written.

10. Many television and radio stations have a phone vote poll. If there is one in your area, select a specific day and write a brief paragraph stating the question of the day and if it could be misleading in any way.

14–3 | Simulation Techniques >

LO3

Solve problems using simulation techniques.

Many real-life problems can be solved by employing simulation techniques.

> A **simulation technique** uses a probability experiment to mimic a real-life situation.

Instead of studying the actual situation, which might be too costly, too dangerous, or too time-consuming, scientists and researchers create a similar situation but one that is less expensive, less dangerous, or less time-consuming. For example, NASA uses space shuttle flight simulators so that its astronauts can practise flying the shuttle. Most video games use the computer to simulate real-life sports such as boxing, wrestling, baseball, and hockey.

Simulation techniques go back to ancient times when the game of chess was invented to simulate warfare. Modern techniques date to the mid-1940s when two mathematicians, John Von Neumann and Stanislaw Ulam, developed simulation techniques to study the behaviour of neutrons in the design of atomic reactors.

Mathematical simulation techniques use probability and random numbers to create conditions similar to those of real-life problems. Computers have played an important role in simulation techniques, since they can generate random numbers, perform experiments, tally the outcomes, and compute the probabilities much faster than human beings. The basic simulation technique is called the *Monte Carlo method*. This topic is discussed next.

The Monte Carlo Method

The **Monte Carlo method** is a simulation technique using random numbers. Monte Carlo simulation techniques are used in business and industry to solve problems that are extremely difficult or involve a large number of variables. The steps for simulating real-life experiments in the Monte Carlo method are as follows:

1. List all possible outcomes of the experiment.
2. Determine the probability of each outcome.
3. Set up a correspondence between the outcomes of the experiment and the random numbers.
4. Select random numbers from a table and conduct the experiment.

5. Repeat the experiment and tally the outcomes.

6. Compute any statistics and state the conclusions.

Before examples of the complete simulation technique are given, an illustration is needed for step 3 (set up a correspondence between the outcomes of the experiment and the random numbers). Tossing a coin, for instance, can be simulated by using random numbers as follows: Since there are only two outcomes, heads and tails, and since each outcome has a probability of $\frac{1}{2}$, the odd digits (1, 3, 5, 7, and 9) can be used to represent a head, and the even digits (0, 2, 4, 6, and 8) can represent a tail.

Suppose a random number 8631 is selected. This number represents four tosses of a single coin and the results T, T, H, H. Or this number could represent one toss of four coins with the same results.

An experiment of rolling a single die can also be simulated by using random numbers. In this case, the digits 1, 2, 3, 4, 5, and 6 can represent the number of spots that appear on the face of the die. The digits 7, 8, 9, and 0 are ignored, since they cannot be rolled.

When two dice are rolled, two random digits are needed. For example, the number 26 represents a 2 on the first die and a 6 on the second die. The random number 37 represents a 3 on the first die, but the 7 cannot be used, so another digit must be selected. As another example, a three-digit daily lotto number can be simulated by using three-digit random numbers. Finally, a spinner with four numbers, as shown in Figure 14–10, can be simulated by letting the random numbers 1 and 2 represent 1 on the spinner, 3 and 4 represent 2 on the spinner, 5 and 6 represent 3 on the spinner, and 7 and 8 represent 4 on the spinner, since each number has a probability of $\frac{1}{4}$ of being selected. The random numbers 9 and 0 are ignored in this situation.

Many real-life games, such as bowling and baseball, can be simulated by using random numbers, as shown in Figure 14–11.

Figure 14–10

Spinner with Four Numbers

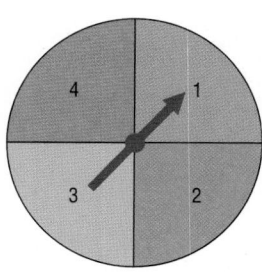

Example 14–4	**Gender of Children**

Using random numbers, simulate the gender of children born.

Solution

There are only two possibilities, female and male. Since the probability of each outcome is 0.5, the odd digits can be used to represent male births and the even digits to represent female births.

Example 14–5	**Outcomes of a Tennis Game**

Using random numbers, simulate the outcomes of a tennis game between Bill and Mike, with the additional condition that Bill is twice as good, winning two games for every one game that Mike wins.

Solution

Since Bill is twice as good as Mike, he will win at a two-to-one ratio by winning two out of every three games; hence, the probability that Bill wins will be $\frac{2}{3}$, and the probability that Mike wins will be $\frac{1}{3}$. The random digits 1 through 6 can be used to represent a game Bill wins; the random digits 7, 8, and 9 can be used to represent Mike's wins. The digit 0 is disregarded. Suppose they play five games, and the random number 86314 is selected. This number means that Bill won games 2, 3, 4, and 5 and Mike won the first game. The sequence is

8	6	3	1	4
M	B	B	B	B

Unusual Stat

The average 6-year-old laughs 300 times a day; the average adult, just 17.

Figure 14–11

Example of Simulation of a Game

Source: Albert Shuylte, "Simulated Bowling Game," *Student Math Notes,* March 1986. Published by the National Council of Teachers of Mathematics. Reprinted with permission.

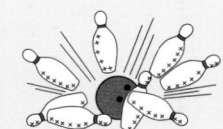

Simulated Bowling Game

Let's use the random digit table to simulate a bowling game. Our game is much simpler than commercial simulation games.

		Second Ball			
First Ball		2-Pin Split		No split	
Digit	Results	Digit	Results	Digit	Results
1–3	Strike	1	Spare	1–3	Spare
4–5	2-pin split	2–8	Leave one pin	4–6	Leave 1 pin
6–7	9 pins down	9–0	Miss both pins	7–8	*Leave 2 pins
8	8 pins down			9	+Leave 3 pins
9	7 pins down			0	Leave all pins
0	6 pins down				

*If there are fewer than 2 pins, result is a spare.
+If there are fewer than 3 pins, those pins are left.

Here's how to score bowling:
1. There are 10 frames to a **game** or **line**.
2. You roll two balls for each frame, unless you knock all the pins down with the first ball (a **strike**).
3. Your score for a frame is the sum of the pins knocked down by the two balls, if you don't knock down all 10.
4. If you knock all 10 pins down with two balls (a **spare**, shown as ⟋), your score is 10 pins plus the number knocked down with the next ball.
5. If you knock all 10 pins down with the first ball (a **strike**, shown as ⊠), your score is 10 pins plus the number knocked down by the next **two** balls.
6. A **split** (shown as 0) is when there is a big space between the remaining pins. Place in the circle the number of pins remaining after the second ball.
7. A **miss** is shown as —.

Here is how one person simulated a bowling game using the random digits 7 2 7 4 8 2 2 3 6 1 6 0 4 6 1 5 5, chosen in that order from the table.

Frame

	1	2	3	4	5	6	7	8	9	10	
Digit(s)	7/2	7/4	8/2	2	3	6/1	6/0	4/6	1	5/5	
Bowling result	9⟋ 19	9— 28	8⟋ 48	⊠ 77	⊠ 97	9⟋ 116	9— 125	8① 134	⊠ 153	8① 162	162

Now you try several.

Frame

	1	2	3	4	5	6	7	8	9	10	
Digit(s)											
Bowling result											

	1	2	3	4	5	6	7	8	9	10	
Digit(s)											
Bowling result											

If you wish to, you can change the probabilities in the simulation to better reflect *your* actual bowling ability.

More complex problems can be solved by using random numbers, as shown in Examples 14–6 through 14–8.

Example 14–6

Rolling a Die

A die is rolled until a 6 appears. Using simulation, find the average number of rolls needed. Try the experiment 20 times.

Solution

Step 1 List all possible outcomes. They are 1, 2, 3, 4, 5, 6.

Step 2 Assign the probabilities. Each outcome has a probability of $\frac{1}{6}$.

Step 3 Set up a correspondence between the random numbers and the outcome. Use random numbers 1 through 6. Omit the numbers 7, 8, 9, and 0.

Step 4   Select a block of random numbers, and count each digit 1 through 6 until the first 6 is obtained. For example, the block 857236 means that it takes 4 rolls to get a 6.

$$
\begin{array}{cccccc}
8 & 5 & 7 & 2 & 3 & 6 \\
 & \uparrow & & \uparrow & \uparrow & \uparrow \\
 & 5 & & 2 & 3 & 6
\end{array}
$$

Step 5   Repeat the experiment 19 more times and tally the data as shown.

Trial	Random number	Number of rolls
1	8 5 7 2 3 6	4
2	2 1 0 4 8 0 1 5 1 1 0 1 5 3 6	11
3	2 3 3 6	4
4	2 4 1 3 0 4 8 3 6	7
5	4 2 1 6	4
6	3 7 5 2 0 3 9 8 7 5 8 1 8 3 7 1 6	9
7	7 7 9 2 1 0 6	3
8	9 9 5 6	2
9	9 6	1
10	8 9 5 7 9 1 4 3 4 2 6	7
11	8 5 4 7 5 3 6	5
12	2 8 9 1 8 6	3
13	6	1
14	0 9 4 2 9 9 3 9 6	4
15	1 0 3 6	3
16	0 7 1 1 9 9 7 3 3 6	5
17	5 1 0 8 5 1 2 7 6	6
18	0 2 3 6	3
19	0 1 0 1 1 5 4 0 9 2 3 3 3 6	10
20	5 2 1 6	4
		Total 96

Step 6   Compute the results and draw a conclusion. In this case, one must find the average.

$$\overline{X} = \frac{\Sigma X}{n} = \frac{96}{20} = 4.8$$

Hence, the average is about 5 rolls.

Note: The theoretical average obtained from the expected value formula is 6. If this experiment is done many times, say 1000 times, the results should be closer to the theoretical results.

Example 14–7

Selecting a Key

A person selects a key at random from four keys to open a lock. Only one key fits. If the first key does not fit, she tries other keys until one fits. Find the average of the number of keys a person will have to try to open the lock. Try the experiment 25 times.

Solution

Assume that each key is numbered from 1 through 4 and that key 2 fits the lock. Naturally, the person doesn't know this, so she selects the keys at random. For the simulation, select a sequence of random digits, using only 1 through 4, until the digit 2 is reached. The trials are shown here.

Trial	Random digit (key)	Number	Trial	Random digit (key)	Number
1	2	1	14	2	1
2	2	1	15	4 2	2
3	1 2	2	16	1 3 2	3
4	1 4 3 2	4	17	1 2	2
5	3 2	2	18	2	1
6	3 1 4 2	4	19	3 4 2	3
7	4 2	2	20	2	1
8	4 3 2	3	21	2	1
9	4 2	2	22	2	1
10	2	1	23	4 2	2
11	4 2	2	24	4 3 1 2	4
12	3 1 2	3	25	3 1 2	3
13	3 1 2	3		Total	54

Next, find the average:

$$\overline{X} = \frac{\Sigma X}{n} = \frac{1 + 1 + \cdots + 3}{25} = \frac{54}{25} = 2.16$$

The theoretical average is 2.2. Again, only 25 repetitions were used; more repetitions should give a result closer to the theoretical average.

Example 14–8

Selecting a Monetary Bill

A box contains five $5 bills, three $10 bills, and two $20 bills. A person selects a bill at random. What is the expected value of the bill? Perform the experiment 25 times.

Solution

Step 1 List all possible outcomes. They are $5, $10, and $20.

Step 2 Assign the probabilities to each outcome.

$$P(\$5) = \frac{5}{10} \quad P(\$10) = \frac{3}{10} \quad P(\$20) = \frac{2}{10}$$

Step 3 Set up a correspondence between the random numbers, and the outcomes. Use random numbers 1 through 5 to represent the $5 bill being selected, 6 through 8 to represent the $10 bill being selected, and 9 and 0 to represent the $20 bill being selected.

Steps 4 and 5 Select the random numbers and tally the results.

Number	Results ($)
4 5 8 2 9	5, 5, 10, 5, 20
2 5 6 4 6	5, 5, 10, 5, 10
9 1 8 0 3	20, 5, 10, 20, 5
8 4 0 6 0	10, 5, 20, 10, 20
9 6 9 4 3	20, 10, 20, 5, 5

Step 6   Compute the average:

$$\overline{X} = \frac{\Sigma X}{n} = \frac{\$5 + \$5 + \$10 + \cdots + \$5}{25} = \frac{\$265}{25} = \$10.60$$

Hence, the average (expected value) is \$10.60.

Recall that using the expected value formula $E(X) = \Sigma X \cdot P(X)$ gives a theoretical average of

$$E(X) = \Sigma[X \cdot P(X)] = (0.5)(\$5) + (0.3)(\$10) + (0.2)(\$20) = \$9.50$$

Remember that simulation techniques do not give exact results. The more times the experiment is performed, though, the closer the actual results should be to the theoretical results. (Recall the law of large numbers.)

The steps for solving problems using the Monte Carlo method are summarized in the Procedure Table.

Procedure Table

Simulating Experiments Using the Monte Carlo Method

Step 1   List all possible outcomes of the experiment.

Step 2   Determine the probability of each outcome.

Step 3   Set up a correspondence between the outcomes of the experiment and the random numbers.

Step 4   Select random numbers from a table and conduct the experiment.

Step 5   Repeat the experiment and tally the outcomes.

Step 6   Compute any statistics and state the conclusions.

14–3   Applying the Concepts

Simulations

Answer the following questions:

1. Define *simulation techniques*.
2. Have simulation techniques been used for very many years?
3. Is it cost-effective to do simulation testing on some things such as airplanes or automobiles?
4. Why might simulation testing be better than real-life testing? Give examples.
5. When did mathematicians develop computer simulation techniques to study neutrons?
6. When could simulations be misleading or harmful? Give examples.
7. Could simulations have prevented the Hindenburg or space shuttle disasters?
8. What discipline is simulation theory based in?

See page 644 for the answers.

Exercises 14–3

1. What is the purpose of simulations?

2. Give three examples of simulation techniques.

3. Who was responsible for the development of modern simulation techniques?

4. What role does the computer play in simulation?

5. What are the steps in the simulation of an experiment?

6. What purpose do random numbers play in simulation?

7. What happens when the number of repetitions is increased?

For Exercises 8 through 13, explain how each experiment can be simulated by using random numbers.

8. **Octahedral Die** A game is played using an octahedral die.

9. **Computer Use** Approximately 75% of Canadians use a computer on the job.

10. **Defective DVDs** A certain brand of DVD player has a 10% defective rate.

11. **Batting Average** A baseball player is batting 0.300; another is batting 0.271.

12. **Matching Pennies** Two players match pennies.

13. **Odd Man Out** Three players play odd man out. (Three coins are tossed; if all three match, the game is repeated and no one wins. If two players match, the third person wins all three coins.)

For Exercises 14 through 21, use random numbers to simulate the experiments. The number in parentheses is the number of times the experiment should be repeated.

14. **Tossing a Coin** A coin is tossed until four heads are obtained. Find the average number of tosses necessary. (50)

15. **Rolling a Die** A die is rolled until all faces appear at least once. Find the average number of tosses. (30)

16. **Prizes in Caramel Corn Boxes** A caramel corn company gives four different prizes, one in each box. They are placed in the boxes at random. Find the average number of boxes a person needs to buy to get all four prizes. (40)

17. **Keys to a Door** The probability that a door is locked is 0.6, and there are five keys, one of which will unlock the door. The experiment consists of choosing one key at random and seeing if you can open the door. Calculate the empirical probability of opening the door. Compare your result to the theoretical probability for this experiment (50).

18. **Lottery Winner** To win a certain lottery, a person must spell the word *big,* using tickets with letters printed on them. Sixty percent of the tickets contain the letter *b,* 30% contain the letter *i,* and 10% contain the letter *g.* Find the average number of tickets a person must buy to win the prize. (30)

19. **Clay Pigeon Shooting** Two shooters shoot clay pigeons. Gail has an 80% accuracy rate and Paul has a 60% accuracy rate. Paul shoots first. The first person who hits the target wins. Find each shooter's probability of winning. (30).

20. **Clay Pigeon Shooting** In Exercise 19, find the average number of shots fired. (30)

21. **Basketball Foul Shots** A basketball player has a 60% success rate for shooting foul shots. If she gets two shots, find the probability that she will make one or both shots. (50).

22. **Baseball or Soccer Games** Which would be easier to simulate with random numbers, baseball or soccer? Explain.

23. **Dealing Cards** Explain how cards can be used to generate random numbers.

24. **Rolling Dice** Explain how a pair of dice can be used to generate random numbers.

Summary >

To obtain information and make inferences about a large population, researchers select a sample. A sample is a subgroup of the population. Using a sample rather than a population, researchers can save time and money, get more detailed information, and get information that otherwise would be impossible to obtain.

The four most common methods researchers use to obtain samples are random, systematic, stratified, and cluster sampling methods. In random sampling, some type of random method (usually random numbers) is used to obtain the sample. In systematic sampling, the researcher selects every *k*th person or item after selecting the *first* one at random. In stratified sampling, the population is divided into subgroups according to various characteristics, and elements are then selected at random from the subgroups. In cluster sampling, the researcher selects an intact group to use as a sample. When the population is large, multistage sampling (a combination of methods) is used to obtain a subgroup of the population.

Researchers must use caution when conducting surveys and designing questionnaires; otherwise, conclusions obtained from these will be inaccurate. Guidelines were presented in Section 14–2.

Most sampling methods use random numbers, which can also be used to simulate many real-life problems or situations. The basic method of simulation is known as the *Monte Carlo method*. The purpose of simulation is to duplicate situations that are too dangerous, too costly, or too time-consuming to study in real life. Most simulation techniques can be done on the computer or calculator, since they can rapidly generate random numbers, count the outcomes, and perform the necessary computations.

Sampling and simulation are two techniques that enable researchers to gain information that might otherwise be unobtainable.

For step-by-step guidance on the use of Texas Instruments TI-83 Plus/TI-84 Plus programmable calculators, see Appendix E at the back of this book. For summary procedures for Minitab, SPSS, and Excel, please see the full version of Appendix E on *Connect*.

Important Terms >>

biased sample 617	double sampling 625	random sample 617	stratified sample 622
convenience sample 618	Monte Carlo method 632	sequence sampling 625	systematic sample 621
cluster sample 624	multistage sampling 625	simulation technique 632	unbiased sample 617

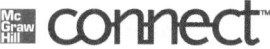 Practise and learn online with *Connect* with data sets and algorithmic questions related to concepts covered in this chapter. Questions and tables with online data sets are marked with .

Review Exercises >>

Use Figure 14–12 (next page) for Exercises 1 through 8.

1. **Weights of Individuals** Select a random sample of 10 people and find the mean of the weights of the individuals. Compare this mean with the population mean.

2. **Weights of Individuals** Select a systematic sample of 10 people, and compute the mean of their weights. Compare this mean with the population mean.

3. **Weights by Gender** Divide the individuals into subgroups of males and females. Select 5 individuals from each group, and find the mean of their weights. Compare these means with the population mean.

4. **Weights of Groups** Select a cluster of 10 people, and find the mean of their weights. Compare this mean with the population mean.

5. **Blood Pressure of Individuals** Repeat Exercise 1 for blood pressure.

6. **Blood Pressure of Individuals** Repeat Exercise 2 for blood pressure.

7. **Blood Pressure by Gender** Repeat Exercise 3 for blood pressure.

8. **Blood Pressure of Groups** Repeat Exercise 4 for blood pressure.

Figure 14–12

Population for Exercises 1 through 8

Individual	Gender	Weight	Systolic blood pressure	Individual	Gender	Weight	Systolic blood pressure	Individual	Gender	Weight	Systolic blood pressure
1	F	122	132	18	F	118	125	35	M	172	116
2	F	128	116	19	F	107	138	36	M	175	123
3	M	183	140	20	M	214	121	37	F	101	114
4	M	165	136	21	F	114	127	38	F	123	113
5	M	192	120	22	M	119	125	39	M	186	145
6	F	116	118	23	F	125	114	40	F	100	119
7	M	206	116	24	M	182	137	41	M	202	135
8	F	131	120	25	F	127	127	42	F	117	121
9	M	155	118	26	F	132	130	43	F	120	130
10	F	106	122	27	M	198	114	44	M	193	125
11	F	103	119	28	F	135	119	45	M	200	115
12	M	169	136	29	M	183	137	46	F	118	132
13	M	173	134	30	F	140	123	47	F	121	143
14	M	195	145	31	M	189	135	48	M	189	128
15	F	107	113	32	M	165	121	49	M	114	118
16	M	201	111	33	M	211	117	50	M	174	138
17	F	114	141	34	F	111	127				

For Exercises 9 through 13, explain how to simulate each experiment by using random numbers.

9. **Baseball Strikeouts** A baseball player strikes out 40% of the time.

10. **Airline Overbooking** An airline overbooks 15% of the time.

11. **Rolling a Die** Two players roll a die. The higher number wins.

12. **Rolling Dice** Player 1 rolls two dice. Player 2 rolls one die. If the number on the single die matches one number of the player who rolled the two dice, player 2 wins. Otherwise, player 1 wins.

13. **Rock, Paper, Scissors** Two players play rock, paper, scissors. The rules are as follows: Since paper covers rock, paper wins. Since rock breaks scissors, rock wins. Since scissors cut paper, scissors win. Each person selects rock, paper, or scissors by random numbers and then compares results.

For Exercises 14 through 18, use random numbers to simulate the experiments. The number in parentheses is the number of times the experiment should be repeated.

14. **Football Game** A football is placed on the 10-yard line, and a team has four downs to score a touchdown. The team can move the ball only 0 to 5 yards per play. Find the average number of times the team will score a touchdown. (30)

15. **Football Game** In Exercise 14, find the average number of plays it will take to score a touchdown. Ignore the four-downs rule and keep playing until a touchdown is scored. (30)

16. **Rolling Dice** Four dice are rolled 50 times. Find the average of the sum of the number of spots that will appear. (50)

17. **Field Goals** A field goal kicker is successful in 60% of his kicks inside the 35-yard line. Find the probability of kicking three field goals in a row. (50)

18. **Making a Sale** A sales representative finds that there is a 30% probability of making a sale by visiting the potential customer personally. For every 20 calls, find the probability of making three sales in a row. (50)

For Exercises 19 through 22, explain what is wrong with each question. Rewrite each one following the guidelines in this chapter.

19. **Running Red Lights** How often do you run red lights?

20. **Student and Tutors** Do you think students who are not failing should not be tutored?

21. **Automobile Bumpers and Car Prices** Do you think all automobiles should have heavy-duty bumpers, even though it will raise the price of the cars by $500?

22. **Question Types** Explain the difference between an open-ended question and a closed-ended question.

Data Analysis >>

The databank for these questions can be found in Appendix D at the back of the textbook and on ▓ **connect**.

1. From the databank, choose a variable. Select a random sample of 20 individuals, and find the mean of the data.

2. Select a systematic sample of 20 individuals, and using the same variable as in Exercise 1, find the mean.

3. Select a cluster sample of 20 individuals, and using the same variable as in Exercise 1, find the mean.

4. Stratify the data according to marital status and gender, and sample 20 individuals. Compute the mean of the sample variable selected in Exercise 1 (use four groups of five individuals).

5. Compare all four means and decide which one is most appropriate. (*Hint:* Find the population mean.)

Chapter Quiz >>

Determine whether each statement is true or false. If the statement is false, explain why.

1. When researchers are sampling from large populations, such as adult citizens living in Canada, they may use a combination of sampling techniques to ensure representativeness.

2. Simulation techniques using random numbers are a substitute for performing the actual statistical experiment.

3. When researchers perform simulation experiments, they do not need to use random numbers since they can make up random numbers.

4. Random samples are said to be unbiased.

 Statistics Today

The Monty Hall Problem–Revisited

It appears that it does not matter whether the contestant switches doors because he or she is given a choice of two doors, and the chance of winning the prize is 1 out of 2, or $\frac{1}{2}$. This reasoning, however, is incorrect. Consider the three possibilities for the prize. It could be behind door A, B, or C. Also consider the fact that the contestant has selected door A. Now the three situations look like this:

	Door		
Case	**A**	**B**	**C**
1	Prize	Empty	Empty
2	Empty	Prize	Empty
3	Empty	Empty	Prize

In case 1, the contestant selected door A, and if the contestant switched after being shown that there was no prize behind either door B or door C, he'd lose. In case 2, the contestant selected door A, and Monty will open door C, so if the contestant would switch, he would win the prize. In case 3, the contestant selected door A, and Monty will open door B, so if the contestant would switch, he would win the prize. Hence, by switching, the probability of winning is $\frac{2}{3}$ and the probability of losing is $\frac{1}{3}$. The same reasoning can be used no matter which door you select.

You can simulate this problem by using three cards, say, an ace (prize) and two other cards. Have a person arrange the cards in a row and let you select a card. After the person turns over one of the cards (not an ace), then switch. Keep track of the number of times you win. You can also play this game on the Internet by going to the website www.stat.sc.edu/~west/javahtml/LetsMakeaDeal.html.

Select the best answer.

5. When all subjects under study are used, the group is called a _____.

   a. Population
   b. Large group
   c. Sample
   d. Study group

6. When a population is divided into subgroups with similar characteristics and then a sample is obtained, this method is called _____ sampling.

   a. Random
   b. Systematic
   c. Stratified
   d. Cluster

7. Interviewing selected people at a local supermarket can be considered an example of _____ sampling.

   a. Random *c.* Convenience
   b. Systematic *d.* Stratified

Complete the following statements with the best answer.

8. In general, when one conducts sampling, the _____ the sample, the more representative it will be.

9. When samples are not representative, they are said to be _____ .

10. When all residents of a street are interviewed for a survey, the sampling method used is _____ .

Use Figure 14–13 for Exercises 11 through 14.

Figure 14–13

World's 50 Richest Cities by Gross Domestic Product (GDP)

City/Urban area	Country	GDP ($US billions)	City/Urban area	Country	GDP ($US billions)
Atlanta	USA	$236	Montreal	Canada	$120
Baltimore	USA	110	Moscow	Russia	181
Barcelona	Spain	140	Mumbai	India	126
Beijing	China	99	New York	USA	1133
Boston	USA	290	Osaka/Kobe	Japan	341
Buenos Aires	Argentina	245	Paris	France	460
Cairo	Egypt	98	Philadelphia	USA	312
Chicago	USA	460	Phoenix	USA	156
Dallas/Fort Worth	USA	268	Pusan	South Korea	95
Denver	USA	130	Rio de Janeiro	Brazil	141
Detroit	USA	203	Rome	Italy	123
Hong Kong	China	244	San Diego	USA	153
Houston	USA	235	San Francisco/Oakland	USA	242
Istanbul	Turkey	133	Sao Paulo	Brazil	225
Jakarta	Indonesia	98	Seattle	USA	186
Kolkata	India	94	Seoul	South Korea	218
London	UK	452	Shanghai	China	139
Los Angeles	USA	639	Singapore	Singapore	129
Madrid	Spain	188	St Louis	USA	101
Melbourne	Australia	135	Sydney	Australia	172
Metro Manila	Philippines	108	Tampa/St Petersburg	USA	97
Mexico City	Mexico	315	Tokyo	Japan	1191
Miami	USA	231	Toronto	Canada	209
Milan	Italy	115	Vienna	Austria	93
Minneapolis	USA	155	Washington DC	USA	299

Source: City Mayors Statistics, *Tokyo Is Number One among the Richest Cities in the World (A Report by PricewaterhouseCoopers)*, March 11, 2007.

11. **GDP of Cities** Find the population mean (all 50 cities) for the gross domestic product (GDP) data. Use the table of random numbers in Figure 14–1 to select 10 cities. Find the cities' GDP sample mean, in $US billions. Repeat the random selection and compare the sample means with the population mean.

12. **GDP of Cities** Find the population mean (all 50 cities) for the gross domestic product (GDP) data. Use the systematic method to select 10 cities and find the cities' GDP sample mean, in $US billions. Repeat the random selection and compare the sample means with the population mean.

13. **GDP of Cities by Region** Find the population mean (all 50 cities) for the gross domestic product (GDP) data. Perform a stratified sample by dividing the cities into two regions Americas (Canada, United States, Mexico, Argentina, and Brazil) and the Rest of the World. Select 7 cities from each region using the table of random numbers in Figure 14–1. Find the cities' GDP sample mean, in $US billions, and compare with the population mean.

14. **GDP of Cities by Continent** Find the population mean (all 50 cities) for the gross domestic product (GDP) data. Perform a cluster sample by organizing the cities

by continent (North America, South America, Asia, Europe, Africa, and Australia). Use the table of random numbers in Figure 14–1 to select a continent. Find the GDP sample mean, in \$US billions, for all cities in that continent and compare with the population mean.

For Exercises 15 through 19, explain how each could be simulated by using random numbers.

15. **Winning at Chess** A chess player wins 45% of his games.

16. **Travel Cancellations** A travel agency has a 5% cancellation rate.

17. **Card Selection** Two players select a card from a deck with no face cards. The player who gets the higher card wins.

18. **Dice Roll and Card Selection** One player rolls two dice. The other player selects a card from a deck. Face cards count as 11 for a jack, 12 for a queen, and 13 for a king. The player with the higher total points wins.

19. **Tossing Coins** Two players toss two coins. If they match, player 1 wins; otherwise, player 2 wins.

For Exercises 20 through 24, use random numbers to simulate the experiments. The number in parentheses is the number of times the experiment should be done.

20. **Phone Sales** A telephone solicitor finds that there is a 15% probability of selling her product over the phone. For every 20 calls, find the probability of making two sales in a row. (100)

21. **Field Goals** A field goal kicker is successful in 65% of his kicks inside the 40-yard line. Find the probability of his kicking four field goals in a row. (40)

22. **Tossing Coins** Two coins are tossed. Find the average number of times two tails will appear. (40)

23. **Drawing Cards** A single card is drawn from a deck. Find the average number of times it takes to draw an ace. (30)

24. **Bowling** A bowler finds that there is a 30% probability that he will make a strike. For every 15 frames he bowls, find the probability of making two strikes. (30)

Critical Thinking Challenges ≫

1. **Opinion Polls** Explain why two different opinion polls might yield different results on a survey. Also, give an example of an opinion poll and explain how the data may have been collected.

2. **Blood Donors** Use a computer to generate random numbers to simulate the following real-life problem.

In a certain geographic region, 40% of the people have type O blood. On a certain day, the blood centre needs 1.8 litres of type O blood. On average, how many donors are needed to obtain 1.8 litres of type O blood? Approximately 450 millilitres (1 pint) of blood is collected during a blood donation.

Data Projects ≫

Where appropriate, use Minitab, SPSS, TI-83 Plus, TI-84 Plus, Excel, or a computer program of your choice to complete the following exercises.

1. **Business and Finance** A car salesperson has six automobiles on the car lot. Roll a die, using the numbers 1 through 6 to represent each car. If only one car can be sold on each day, how long will it take him to sell all the automobiles? In other words, see how many tosses of the die it will take to get the numbers 1 through 6.

2. **Sports and Leisure** Using the rules given in Figure 14–11 on page 634, play the simulated bowling game. Each game consists of 10 frames.

3. **Technology** In a carton of 12 iPods, three are defective. If four are sold on Saturday, find the probability that at least one will be defective. Use random numbers to simulate this exercise 50 times.

4. **Health and Wellness** Of people who go on a special diet, 25% will lose at least 5 kilograms in 10 weeks. A drug manufacturer says that if people take its special herbal pill, the number of people who lose at least 5 kilograms in 10 weeks will increase. The company conducts an experiment, giving its pill to 20 people. Seven people lost at least 5 kilograms in 10 weeks. The drug manufacturer claims that the study "proves" the success of the herbal pill. Using random numbers, simulate the experiment 30 times, assuming the pill is ineffective. What can you conclude about the result that 7 out of 20 people lost at least 5 kilograms?

5. **Politics and Economics** Research the home provinces of all prime ministers of Canada since Confederation. Select two of the prime ministers at random. What is the probability that both prime ministers will be from the same province? Use random numbers to simulate the experiment and perform the experiment 50 times.

6. **Your Class** Simulate the classical birthday problem given in Critical Thinking Challenge 3 in Chapter 4. Select a sample size of 25 and generate random numbers between 1 and 365. Are any two random numbers the same? Select a sample of 50. Are any two random numbers the same? Repeat the experiments 10 times each and explain your answers.

Answers to Applying the Concepts »

Section 14–1 The White or Brown Bread Debate

1. The researchers used a sample for their study.

2. Answers will vary. One possible answer is that we might have doubts about the validity of the study, since the baking company that conducted the experiment has an interest in the outcome of the experiment.

3. The sample was probably a convenience sample.

4. Answers will vary. One possible answer would be to use a simple random sample.

5. Answers will vary. One possible answer is that a list of women's names could be obtained from the city in which the women live. Then a simple random sample could be selected from this list.

6. The random assignment helps to spread variation among the groups. The random selection helps to generalize from the sample back to the population. These are two different issues.

Section 14–2 Smoking Bans and Profits

1. It is uncertain how public smoking bans affected tavern business in Ottawa, since the survey results were conflicting.

2. Since the data were collected in different ways, the survey results were bound to have different answers. Perceptions of the owners will definitely be different from an analysis of actual sales receipts, particularly if the owners assumed that the public smoking bans would hurt business.

3. Answers will vary. One possible answer is that it would be difficult to not allow publication of surveys based on anecdotal responses. At the same time, it would be good for those publishing such results to comment on the limitations of these surveys.

4. We can get results from a representative sample that offers misleading information about the population.

5. Answers will vary. One possible answer is that measurement error is important in survey sampling in order to give ranges for the population parameters that are being investigated.

Section 14–3 Simulations

1. A simulation uses a probability experiment to mimic a real-life situation.

2. Simulation techniques date back to ancient times.

3. It is definitely cost-effective to run simulations for expensive items such as airplanes and automobiles.

4. Simulation testing is safer, faster, and less expensive than many real-life testing situations.

5. Computer simulation techniques were developed in the mid-1940s.

6. Answers will vary. One possible answer is that some simulations are far less harmful than conducting an actual study on the real-life situation of interest.

7. Answers will vary. Simulations could have possibly prevented the Hindenburg or the space shuttle disasters. For example, data analysis after the space shuttle disaster showed that there was a "likelihood . . . closer to 1 in 100" that something would go wrong on that flight according to the *Rogers Commission Report,* produced for a U.S. Presidential Commission.

8. Simulation theory is based on probability theory.

Appendix A

Algebra Review

A–1 Factorials

Definition and Properties of Factorials

The notation called factorial notation is used in probability. *Factorial notation* uses the exclamation point and involves multiplication. For example,

$$5! = 5 \cdot 4 \cdot 3 \cdot 2 \cdot 1 = 120$$
$$4! = 4 \cdot 3 \cdot 2 \cdot 1 = 24$$
$$3! = 3 \cdot 2 \cdot 1 = 6$$
$$2! = 2 \cdot 1 = 2$$
$$1! = 1$$

In general, a factorial is evaluated as follows:

$$n! = n(n-1)(n-2) \cdots 3 \cdot 2 \cdot 1$$

Note that the factorial is the product of n factors, with the number decreased by 1 for each factor.

One property of factorial notation is that it can be stopped at any point by using the exclamation point. For example,

$5! = 5 \cdot 4!$	since	$4! = 4 \cdot 3 \cdot 2 \cdot 1$
$\quad = 5 \cdot 4 \cdot 3!$	since	$3! = 3 \cdot 2 \cdot 1$
$\quad = 5 \cdot 4 \cdot 3 \cdot 2!$	since	$2! = 2 \cdot 1$
$\quad = 5 \cdot 4 \cdot 3 \cdot 2 \cdot 1$		

Thus,
$$n! = n(n-1)!$$
$$\quad = n(n-1)(n-2)!$$
$$\quad = n(n-1)(n-2)(n-3)! \quad \text{etc.}$$

Another property of factorials is

$$0! = 1$$

This fact is needed for formulas.

Operations with Factorials

Factorials cannot be added or subtracted directly. They must be multiplied out. Then the products can be added or subtracted.

Example A–1

Evaluate $3! + 4!$.

Solution

$$3! + 4! = (3 \cdot 2 \cdot 1) + (4 \cdot 3 \cdot 2 \cdot 1)$$
$$= 6 + 24 = 30$$

Note: $3! + 4! \neq 7!$, since $7! = 5040$.

Example A–2

Evaluate $5! - 3!$.

Solution

$$5! - 3! = (5 \cdot 4 \cdot 3 \cdot 2 \cdot 1) - (3 \cdot 2 \cdot 1)$$
$$= 120 - 6 = 114$$

Note: $5! - 3! \neq 2!$, since $2! = 2$.

Factorials cannot be multiplied directly. Again, one must multiply them out and then multiply the products.

Example A–3

Evaluate $3! \cdot 2!$.

Solution

$$3! \cdot 2! = (3 \cdot 2 \cdot 1) \cdot (2 \cdot 1) = 6 \cdot 2 = 12$$

Note: $3! \cdot 2! \neq 6!$, since $6! = 720$.

Finally, factorials cannot be divided directly unless they are equal.

Example A–4

Evaluate $6! \div 3!$.

Solution

$$\frac{6!}{3!} = \frac{6 \cdot 5 \cdot 4 \cdot 3 \cdot 2 \cdot 1}{3 \cdot 2 \cdot 1} = \frac{720}{6} = 120$$

Note: $\dfrac{6!}{3!} \neq 2!$ since $2! = 2$

But $\dfrac{3!}{3!} = \dfrac{3 \cdot 2 \cdot 1}{3 \cdot 2 \cdot 1} = \dfrac{6}{6} = 1$

In division, one can take some shortcuts, as shown:

$$\dfrac{6!}{3!} = \dfrac{6 \cdot 5 \cdot 4 \cdot 3!}{3!} \quad \text{and} \quad \dfrac{3!}{3!} = 1$$

$$= 6 \cdot 5 \cdot 4 = 120$$

$$\dfrac{8!}{6!} = \dfrac{8 \cdot 7 \cdot 6!}{6!} \quad \text{and} \quad \dfrac{6!}{6!} = 1$$

$$= 8 \cdot 7 = 56$$

Another shortcut that can be used with factorials is cancellation, after factors have been expanded. For example,

$$\dfrac{7!}{(4!)(3!)} = \dfrac{7 \cdot 6 \cdot 5 \cdot 4!}{3 \cdot 2 \cdot 1 \cdot 4!}$$

Now cancel both instances of 4!. Then cancel the $3 \cdot 2$ in the denominator with the 6 in the numerator.

$$\dfrac{7 \cdot \overset{1}{6} \cdot 5 \cdot \overset{1}{4!}}{\underset{1}{3} \cdot \underset{1}{2} \cdot 1 \cdot \underset{1}{4!}} = 7 \cdot 5 = 35$$

Example A–5

Evaluate $10! \div (6!)(4!)$.

Solution

$$\dfrac{10!}{(6!)(4!)} = \dfrac{10 \cdot \overset{3}{9} \cdot \overset{1}{8} \cdot 7 \cdot \overset{1}{6!}}{\underset{1}{4} \cdot \underset{1}{3} \cdot \underset{1}{2} \cdot 1 \cdot \underset{1}{6!}} = 10 \cdot 3 \cdot 7 = 210$$

Exercises

Evaluate each expression.

A–1. $9!$

A–2. $7!$

A–3. $5!$

A–4. $0!$

A–5. $1!$

A–6. $3!$

A–7. $\dfrac{12!}{9!}$

A–8. $\dfrac{10!}{2!}$

A–9. $\dfrac{5!}{3!}$

A–10. $\dfrac{11!}{7!}$

A–11. $\dfrac{9!}{(4!)(5!)}$

A–12. $\dfrac{10!}{(7!)(3!)}$

A–13. $\dfrac{8!}{(4!)(4!)}$

A–14. $\dfrac{15!}{(12!)(3!)}$

A–15. $\dfrac{10!}{(10!)(0!)}$

A–16. $\dfrac{5!}{(3!)(2!)(1!)}$

A–17. $\dfrac{8!}{(3!)(3!)(2!)}$

A–18. $\dfrac{11!}{(7!)(2!)(2!)}$

A–19. $\dfrac{10!}{(3!)(2!)(5!)}$

A–20. $\dfrac{6!}{(2!)(2!)(2!)}$

A–2   Summation Notation

In mathematics, the symbol Σ (Greek capital letter sigma) means to add or find the sum. For example, ΣX means to add the numbers represented by the variable X. Thus, when X represents 5, 8, 2, 4, and 6, then ΣX means $5 + 8 + 2 + 4 + 6 = 25$.

Sometimes, a subscript notation is used, such as

$$\sum_{i=1}^{5} X_i$$

This notation means to find the sum of five numbers represented by X, as shown:

$$\sum_{i=1}^{5} X_i = X_1 + X_2 + X_3 + X_4 + X_5$$

When the number of values is not known, the unknown number can be represented by n, such as

$$\sum_{i=1}^{n} X_i = X_1 + X_2 + X_3 + \cdots + X_n$$

There are several important types of summation used in statistics. The notation ΣX^2 means to square each value before summing. For example, if the values of the X's are 2, 8, 6, 1, and 4, then

$$\Sigma X^2 = 2^2 + 8^2 + 6^2 + 1^2 + 4^2$$
$$= 4 + 64 + 36 + 1 + 16 = 121$$

The notation $(\Sigma X)^2$ means to find the sum of X's and then square the answer. For instance, if the values for X are 2, 8, 6, 1, and 4, then

$$(\Sigma X)^2 = (2 + 8 + 6 + 1 + 4)^2$$
$$= (21)^2 = 441$$

Another important use of summation notation is in finding the mean (shown in Section 3–2). The mean $\overline{X}$ is defined as

$$\overline{X} = \dfrac{\Sigma X}{n}$$

For example, to find the mean of 12, 8, 7, 3, and 10, use the formula and substitute the values, as shown:

$$\overline{X} = \dfrac{\Sigma X}{n} = \dfrac{12 + 8 + 7 + 3 + 10}{5} = \dfrac{40}{5} = 8$$

The notation $\Sigma(X - \overline{X})^2$ means to perform the following steps.

STEP 1 Find the mean.

STEP 2 Subtract the mean from each value.

STEP 3 Square the answers.

STEP 4 Find the sum.

Example A–6

Find the value of $\Sigma(X - \overline{X})^2$ for the values 12, 8, 7, 3, and 10 of X.

Solution

STEP 1 Find the mean.

$$\overline{X} = \frac{12 + 8 + 7 + 3 + 10}{5} = \frac{40}{5} = 8$$

STEP 2 Subtract the mean from each value.

$$12 - 8 = 4 \qquad 7 - 8 = -1 \qquad 10 - 8 = 2$$
$$8 - 8 = 0 \qquad 3 - 8 = -5$$

STEP 3 Square the answers.

$$4^2 = 16 \qquad (-1)^2 = 1 \qquad 2^2 = 4$$
$$0^2 = 0 \qquad (-5)^2 = 25$$

STEP 4 Find the sum.

$$16 + 0 + 1 + 25 + 4 = 46$$

Example A–7

Find $\Sigma(X - \overline{X})^2$ for the following values of X: 5, 7, 2, 1, 3, 6.

Solution

Find the mean:

$$\overline{X} = \frac{5 + 7 + 2 + 1 + 3 + 6}{6} = \frac{24}{6} = 4$$

Then the steps in Example A–6 can be shortened as follows:

$$\Sigma(X - \overline{X})^2 = (5 - 4)^2 + (7 - 4)^2 + (2 - 4)^2$$
$$+ (1 - 4)^2 + (3 - 4)^2 + (6 - 4)^2$$
$$= 1^2 + 3^2 + (-2)^2 + (-3)^2$$
$$+ (-1)^2 + 2^2$$
$$= 1 + 9 + 4 + 9 + 1 + 4 = 28$$

Exercises

For each set of values, find ΣX, ΣX^2, $(\Sigma X)^2$, and $\Sigma(X - \overline{X})^2$.

A–21. 9, 17, 32, 16, 8, 2, 9, 7, 3, 18

A–22. 4, 12, 9, 13, 0, 6, 2, 10

A–23. 5, 12, 8, 3, 4

A–24. 6, 2, 18, 30, 31, 42, 16, 5

A–25. 80, 76, 42, 53, 77

A–26. 123, 132, 216, 98, 146, 114

A–27. 53, 72, 81, 42, 63, 71, 73, 85, 98, 55

A–28. 43, 32, 116, 98, 120

A–29. 12, 52, 36, 81, 63, 74

A–30. −9, −12, 18, 0, −2, −15

A–3 The Line

The following figure shows the *rectangular coordinate system* or *Cartesian plane*. This figure consists of two axes: the horizontal axis, called the x axis, and the vertical axis, called the y axis. Each axis has numerical scales. The point of intersection of the axes is called the *origin*.

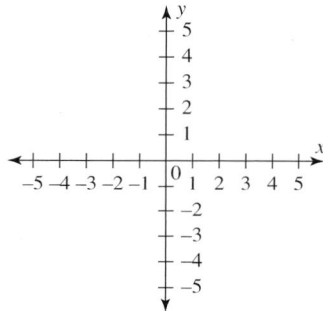

Points can be graphed by using coordinates. For example, the notation for point $P(3, 2)$ means that the x coordinate is 3 and the y coordinate is 2. Hence, P is located at the intersection of $x = 3$ and $y = 2$, as shown.

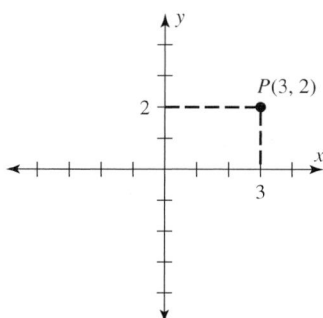

Other points, such as $Q(-5, 2)$, $R(4, 1)$, and $S(-3, -4)$, can be plotted, as shown in the next figure.

When a point lies on the y axis, the x coordinate is 0, as in $(0, 6)(0, -3)$, etc. When a point lies on the x axis, the y coordinate is 0, as in $(6, 0)(-8, 0)$, etc., as shown at the top of the next page.

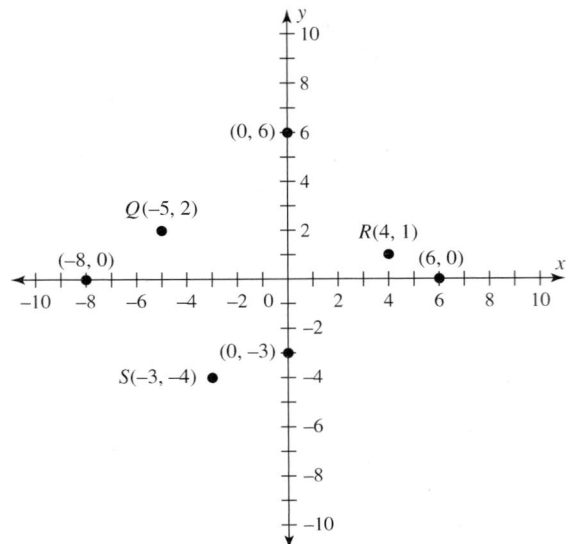

Two points determine a line. There are two properties of a line: its slope and its equation. The *slope m* of a line is determined by the ratio of the rise (called Δy) to the run (Δx).

$$m = \frac{\text{rise}}{\text{run}} = \frac{\Delta y}{\Delta x}$$

For example, the slope of the line shown below is $\frac{3}{2}$, or 1.5, since the height Δy is 3 units and the run Δx is 2 units.

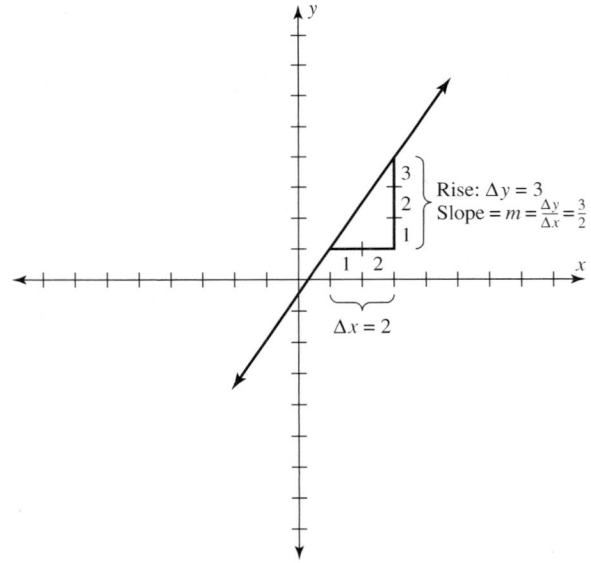

The slopes of lines can be positive, negative, or zero. A line going uphill from left to right has a positive slope. A line going downhill from left to right has a negative slope. And a line that is horizontal has a slope of zero.

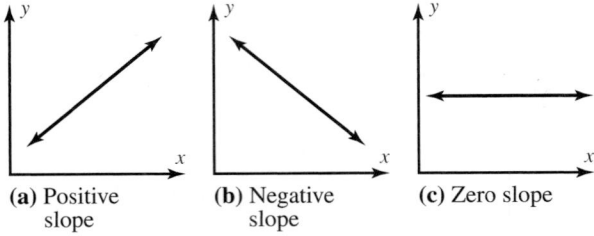

A point *b* where the line crosses the *x* axis is called the *x intercept* and has the coordinates (*b*, 0). A point *a* where the line crosses the *y* axis is called the *y intercept* and has the coordinates (0, *a*).

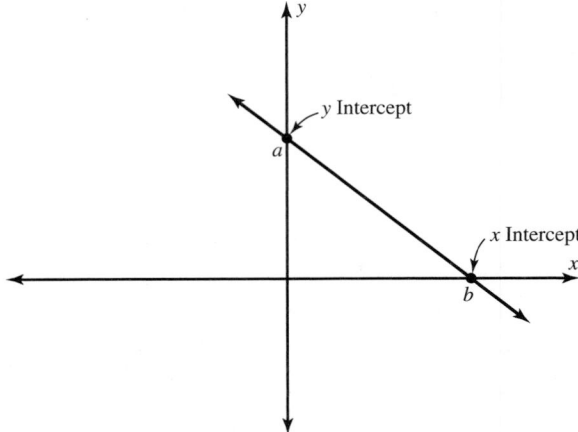

Every line has a unique equation of the form $y = a + bx$. For example, the equations

$$y = 5 + 3x$$
$$y = 8.6 + 3.2x$$
$$y = 5.2 - 6.1x$$

all represent different, unique lines. The number represented by *a* is the *y* intercept point; the number represented by *b* is the slope. The line whose equation is $y = 3 + 2x$ has a *y* intercept at 3 and a slope of 2, or $\frac{2}{1}$. This line can be shown as in the following graph.

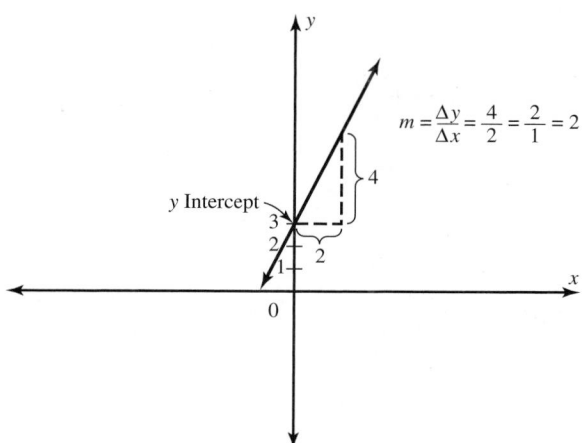

If two points are known, then the graph of the line can be plotted. For example, to find the graph of a line passing through the points $P(2, 1)$ and $Q(3, 5)$, plot the points and connect them as shown below.

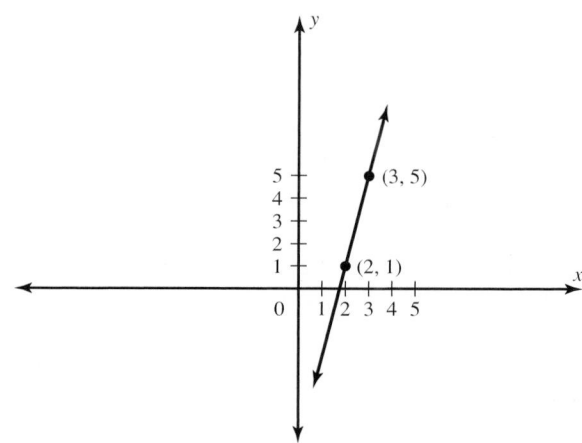

Given the equation of a line, one can graph the line by finding two points and then plotting them.

Example A–8

Plot the graph of the line whose equation is $y = 3 + 2x$.

Solution

Select any number as an x value, and substitute it in the equation to get the corresponding y value. Let $x = 0$.

Then

$$y = 3 + 2x = 3 + 2(0) = 3$$

Hence, when $x = 0$, then $y = 3$, and the line passes through the point $(0, 3)$.

Now select any other value of x, say, $x = 2$.

$$y = 3 + 2x = 3 + 2(2) = 7$$

Hence, a second point is $(2, 7)$. Then plot the points and graph the line.

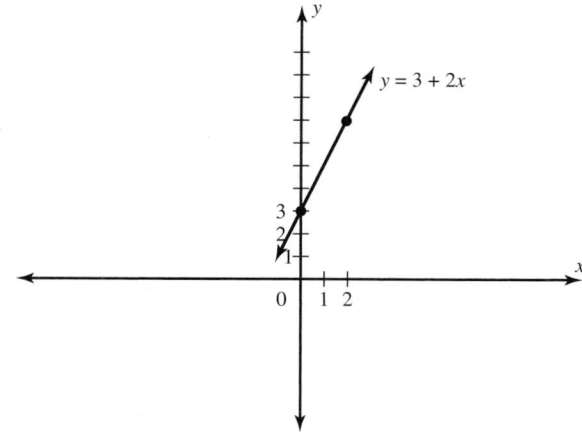

Exercises

Plot the line passing through each set of points.

A–31. $P(3, 2)$, $Q(1, 6)$ **A–34.** $P(-1, -2)$, $Q(-7, 8)$

A–32. $P(0, 5)$, $Q(8, 0)$ **A–35.** $P(6, 3)$, $Q(10, 3)$

A–33. $P(-2, 4)$, $Q(3, 6)$

Find at least two points on each line, and then graph the line containing these points.

A–36. $y = 5 + 2x$ **A–39.** $y = -2 - 2x$

A–37. $y = -1 + x$ **A–40.** $y = 4 - 3x$

A–38. $y = 3 + 4x$

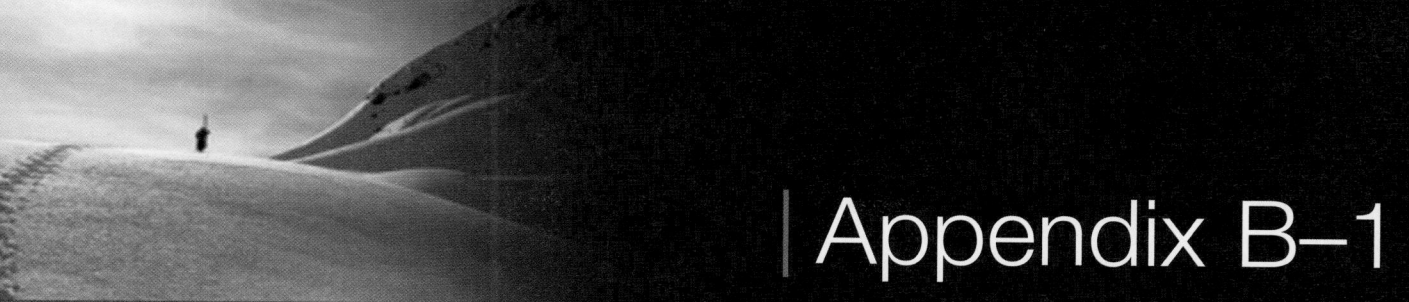

Appendix B–1

Writing the Research Report

After conducting a statistical study, a researcher must write a final report explaining how the study was conducted and giving the results. The formats of research reports, theses, and dissertations vary from school to school; however, they tend to follow the general format explained here.

Front Materials

The front materials typically include the following items:

> Title page
> Copyright page
> Acknowledgements
> Table of contents
> Table of appendices
> List of tables
> List of figures

Chapter 1: Nature and Background of the Study

This chapter should introduce the reader to the nature of the study and present some discussion on the background. It should contain the following information:

> Introduction
> Statement of the problem
> Background of the problem
> Rationale for the study
> Research questions and/or hypotheses
> Assumptions, limitations, and delimitations
> Definitions of terms

Chapter 2: Review of Literature

This chapter should explain what has been done in previous research related to the study. It should contain the following information:

> Prior research
> Related literature

Chapter 3: Methodology

This chapter should explain how the study was conducted. It should contain the following information:

> Development of questionnaires, tests, survey instruments, etc.
> Definition of the population
> Sampling methods used
> How the data were collected
> Research design used
> Statistical tests that will be used to analyze the data

Chapter 4: Analysis of Data

This chapter should explain the results of the statistical analysis of the data. It should state whether the null hypothesis should be rejected. Any statistical tables used to analyze the data should be included here.

Chapter 5: Summary, Conclusions, and Recommendations

This chapter summarizes the results of the study and explains any conclusions that have resulted from the statistical analysis of the data. The researchers should cite and explain any shortcomings of the study. Recommendations obtained from the study should be included here, and further studies should be suggested.

Bayes' Theorem

Objective B-1

Find the probability of an event, using Bayes' theorem.

Historical Note

Thomas Bayes was born around 1701 and lived in London. He was an ordained minister who dabbled in mathematics and statistics. All his findings and writings were published after his death in 1761.

Given two dependent events A and B, the previous formulas for conditional probability allow one to find $P(A$ and $B)$, or $P(B|A)$. Related to these formulas is a rule developed by the English Presbyterian minister Thomas Bayes (1702–61). The rule is known as **Bayes' theorem.**

It is possible, given the outcome of the second event in a sequence of two events, to determine the probability of various possibilities for the first event. In Example 4–31, there were two boxes, each containing red balls and blue balls. A box was selected and a ball was drawn. The example asked for the probability that the ball selected was red. Now, a different question can be asked: If the ball is red, what is the probability it came from box 1? In this case, the outcome is known, a red ball was selected, and one is asked to find the probability that it is a result of a previous event, that it came from box 1. Bayes' theorem can enable one to compute this probability and can be explained by using tree diagrams.

The tree diagram for the solution of Example 4–31 is shown in Figure B–1, along with the appropriate notation and the corresponding probabilities. In this case, A_1 is the event of selecting box 1, A_2 is the event of selecting box 2, R is the event of selecting a red ball, and B is the event of selecting a blue ball.

To answer the question "If the ball selected is red, what is the probability that it came from box 1?" the two formulas

$$P(B|A) = \frac{P(A \text{ and } B)}{P(A)} \tag{1}$$

$$P(A \text{ and } B) = P(A) \cdot P(B|A) \tag{2}$$

can be used. The notation that will be used is that of Example 4–31, shown in Figure B–1. Finding the probability that box 1 was selected given that the ball selected was red can be written symbolically as $P(A_1|R)$. By formula 1,

$$P(A_1|R) = \frac{P(R \text{ and } A_1)}{P(R_1)}$$

Note: $P(R \text{ and } A_1) = P(A_1 \text{ and } R)$.

Figure B–1

Tree Diagram for Example 4–31

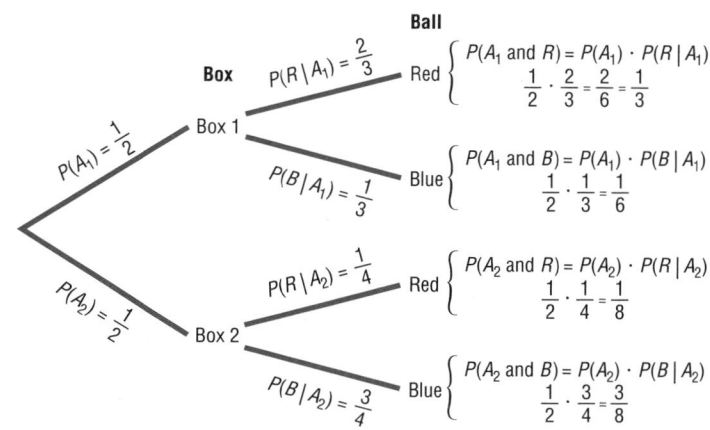

By formula 2,

$$P(A_1 \text{ and } R) = P(A_1) \cdot P(R|A_1)$$

and

$$P(R) = P(A_1 \text{ and } R) + P(A_2 \text{ and } R)$$

as shown in Figure B–1; $P(R)$ was found by adding the products of the probabilities of the branches in which a red ball was selected. Now,

$$P(A_1 \text{ and } R) = P(A_1) \cdot P(R|A_1)$$

$$P(A_2 \text{ and } R) = P(A_2) \cdot P(R|A_2)$$

Substituting these values in the original formula for $P(A_1|R)$, one gets

$$P(A_1|R) = \frac{P(A_1) \cdot P(R|A_1)}{P(A_1) \cdot P(R|A_1) + P(A_2) \cdot P(R|A_2)}$$

Refer to Figure B–1. The numerator of the fraction is the product of the top branch of the tree diagram, which consists of selecting a red ball and selecting box 1. And the denominator is the sum of the products of the two branches of the tree where the red ball was selected.

Using this formula and the probability values shown in Figure B–1, one can find the probability that box 1 was selected given that the ball was red, as shown.

$$P(A_1|R) = \frac{P(A_1) \cdot P(R|A_1)}{P(A_1) \cdot P(R|A_1) + P(A_2) \cdot P(R|A_2)}$$

$$= \frac{\frac{1}{2} \cdot \frac{2}{3}}{\frac{1}{2} \cdot \frac{2}{3} + \frac{1}{2} \cdot \frac{1}{4}} = \frac{\frac{1}{3}}{\frac{1}{3} + \frac{1}{8}} = \frac{\frac{1}{3}}{\frac{8}{24} + \frac{3}{24}} = \frac{\frac{1}{3}}{\frac{11}{24}}$$

$$= \frac{1}{3} \div \frac{11}{24} = \frac{1}{\overset{1}{\cancel{3}}} \cdot \frac{\overset{8}{\cancel{24}}}{11} = \frac{8}{11}$$

This formula is a simplified version of Bayes' theorem.

Before Bayes' theorem is stated, another example is shown.

Example B–1 Defective Phones

A shipment of two boxes, each containing six telephones, is received by a store. Box 1 contains one defective phone, and box 2 contains two defective phones. After the boxes are unpacked, a phone is selected and found to be defective. Find the probability that it came from box 2.

Solution

STEP 1   Select the proper notation. Let A_1 represent box 1 and A_2 represent box 2. Let D represent a defective phone and ND represent a phone that is not defective.

STEP 2   Draw a tree diagram and find the corresponding probabilities for each branch. The probability of selecting box 1 is $\frac{1}{2}$, and the probability of selecting box 2 is $\frac{1}{2}$. Since there is one defective phone in box 1, the probability of selecting it is $\frac{1}{6}$. The probability of selecting a nondefective phone from box 1 is $\frac{5}{6}$.

   Since there are two defective phones in box 2, the probability of selecting a defective phone from box 2 is $\frac{2}{6}$, or $\frac{1}{3}$; and the probability of selecting a nondefective phone is $\frac{4}{6}$, or $\frac{2}{3}$. The tree diagram is shown in Figure B–2.

STEP 3   Write the corresponding formula. Since the example is asking for the probability that, given a defective phone, it came from box 2, the corresponding formula is as shown.

$$P(A_2|D) = \frac{P(A_2) \cdot P(D|A_2)}{P(A_1) \cdot P(D|A_1) + P(A_2) \cdot P(D|A_2)}$$

$$= \frac{\frac{1}{2} \cdot \frac{2}{6}}{\frac{1}{2} \cdot \frac{1}{6} + \frac{1}{2} \cdot \frac{2}{6}} = \frac{\frac{1}{6}}{\frac{1}{12} + \frac{2}{12}} = \frac{\frac{1}{6}}{\frac{3}{12}}$$

$$= \frac{1}{6} \div \frac{3}{12} = \frac{1}{\overset{1}{\cancel{6}}} \cdot \frac{\overset{2}{\cancel{12}}}{3} = \frac{2}{3}$$

Figure B–2

Tree Diagram for Example B–1

Bayes' theorem can be generalized to events with three or more outcomes and formally stated as in the next box.

> **Bayes' theorem** For two events A and B, where event B follows event A, event A can occur in $A_1, A_2, \ldots, A_n$ mutually exclusive ways, and event B can occur in $B_1, B_2, \ldots, B_m$ mutually exclusive ways,
>
> $$P(A_1|B_1) = \frac{P(A_1) \cdot P(B_1|A_1)}{[P(A_1) \cdot P(B_1|A_1) + P(A_2) \cdot P(B_1|A_2) + \cdots + P(A_n) \cdot P(B_1|A_n)]}$$
>
> for any specific events A_1 and B_1.

The numerator is the product of the probabilities on the branch of the tree that consists of outcomes A_1 and B_1. The denominator is the sum of the products of the probabilities of the branches containing B_1 and A_1, B_1 and A_2, ..., B_1 and A_n.

Example B–2 Coin Boxes

On a game show, a contestant can select one of four boxes. Box 1 contains one $100 coin and nine $1 coins. Box 2 contains two $100 coins and eight $1 coins. Box 3 contains three $100 coins and seven $1 coins. Box 4 contains five $100 coins and five $1 coins. The contestant selects a box at random and selects a coin from the box at random. If a $100 coin is selected, find the probability that it came from box 4.

Solution

STEP 1   Select the proper notation. Let B_1, B_2, B_3, and B_4 represent the boxes and 100 and 1 represent the values of the coins in the boxes.

STEP 2   Draw a tree diagram and find the corresponding probabilities. The probability of selecting each box is $\frac{1}{4}$, or 0.25. The probabilities of selecting the $100 coin from each box, respectively, are $\frac{1}{10} = 0.1$, $\frac{2}{10} = 0.2$, $\frac{3}{10} = 0.3$, and $\frac{5}{10} = 0.5$. The tree diagram is shown in Figure B–3.

STEP 3   Using Bayes' theorem, write the corresponding formula. Since the example asks for the probability that box 4 was selected, given that $100 was obtained, the corresponding formula is as follows:

$$P(B_4|100) = \frac{P(B_4) \cdot P(100|B_4)}{[P(B_1) \cdot P(100|B_1) + P(B_2) \cdot P(100|B_2) + P(B_3) \cdot P(100|B_3) + P(B_4) \cdot P(100|B_4)]}$$

$$= \frac{0.125}{0.025 + 0.05 + 0.075 + 0.125}$$

$$= \frac{0.125}{0.275} = 0.455$$

Figure B–3

Tree Diagram for
Example B–2

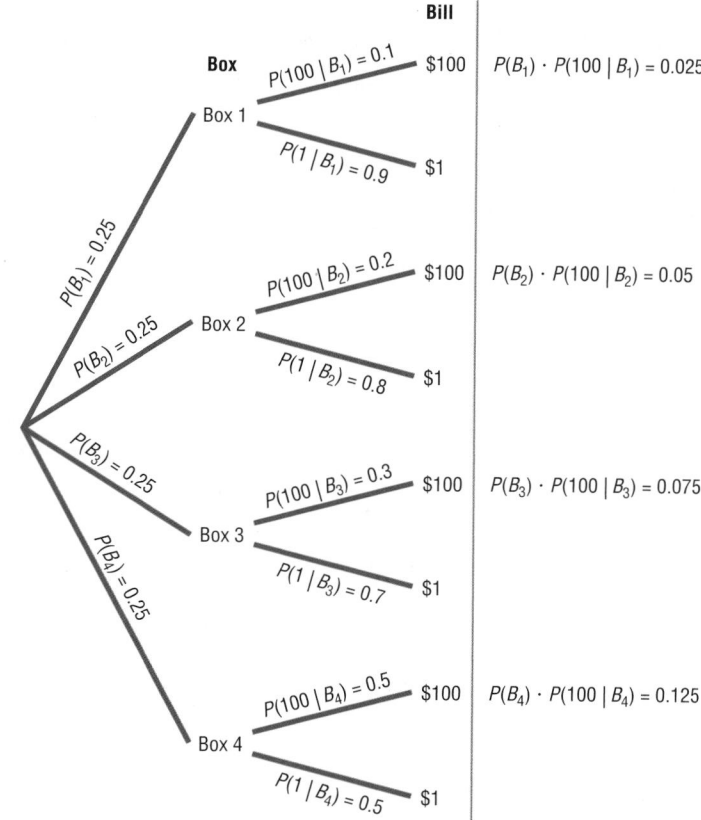

In Example B–2, the original probability of selecting box 4 was 0.25. However, once additional information was obtained—and the condition was considered, that a $100 coin was selected—the revised probability of selecting box 4 became 0.455.

Bayes' theorem can be used to revise probabilities of events once additional information becomes known. Bayes' theorem is used as the basis for a branch of statistics called *Bayesian decision making*, which includes the use of subjective probabilities in making statistical inferences.

Exercises

B–1. Defective Ranges An appliance store purchases electric ranges from two companies. From company A, 500 ranges are purchased and 2% are defective. From company B, 850 ranges are purchased and 2% are defective. Given that a range is defective, find the probability that it came from company B.

B–2. Irregular Blankets Two manufacturers supply blankets to emergency relief organizations. Manufacturer A supplies 3000 blankets, and 4% are irregular in workmanship. Manufacturer B supplies 2400 blankets, and 7% are found to be irregular. Given that a blanket is irregular, find the probability that it came from manufacturer B.

B–3. Disease Test A test for a certain disease is found to be 95% accurate, meaning that it will correctly diagnose the disease in 95 out of 100 people who have the ailment. For a certain segment of the population, the incidence of the disease is 9%. If a person tests positive, find the probability that the person actually has the disease. The test is also 95% accurate for a negative result.

B–4. Disease Test Using the test in Exercise B–3, if a person tests negative for the disease, find the probability that the person actually has the disease. Remember, 9% of the population has the disease.

B–5. Employee Training A corporation has three methods of training employees. Because of time, space, and location, it sends 20% of its employees to location A, 35% to location B, and 45% to location C. Location A has an 80% success rate. That is, 80% of the employees who complete the course will pass the licensing exam. Location B has a 75% success rate, and location C has a 60% success rate. If a person has passed the exam, find the probability that the person went to location B.

B–6. Employee Training In Exercise B–5, if a person failed the exam, find the probability that the person went to location C.

B–7. Selecting Hats A store purchases baseball hats from three different manufacturers. In manufacturer A's box, there are 12 blue hats, 6 red hats, and 6 green hats. In manufacturer B's box, there are 10 blue hats, 10 red hats, and 4 green hats. In manufacturer C's box, there are 8 blue hats, 8 red hats, and 8 green hats. A box is selected at random, and a hat is selected at random from that box. If the hat is red, find the probability that it came from manufacturer A's box.

B–8. Selecting Hats In Exercise B–7, if the hat selected is green, find the probability that it came from manufacturer B's box.

B–9. Driving Routes A driver has three ways to get from one city to another. There is an 80% probability of encountering a traffic jam on route 1, a 60% probability on route 2, and a 30% probability on route 3. Because of other factors, such as distance and speed limits, the driver uses route 1 just 50% of the time and routes 2 and 3 each 25% of the time. If the driver calls the dispatcher to inform him that she is in a traffic jam, find the probability that she has selected route 1.

B–10. Driving Routes In Exercise B–9, if the driver did not encounter a traffic jam, find the probability that she selected route 3.

B–11. Defective Phones A store owner purchases telephones from two companies. From company A, 350 telephones are purchased and 2% are defective. From company B, 1050 telephones are purchased and 4% are defective. Given that a phone is defective, find the probability that it came from company B.

B–12. Dented Cans Two manufacturers supply food to a large cafeteria. Manufacturer A supplies 2400 cans of soup, and 3% are found to be dented. Manufacturer B supplies 3600 cans, and 1% are found to be dented. Given that a can of soup is dented, find the probability that it came from manufacturer B.

Appendix C

Tables

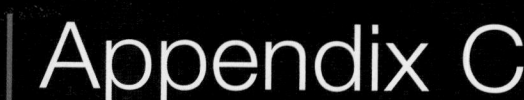

Table A	Factorials
n	$n!$
0	1
1	1
2	2
3	6
4	24
5	120
6	720
7	5,040
8	40,320
9	362,880
10	3,628,800
11	39,916,800
12	479,001,600
13	6,227,020,800
14	87,178,291,200
15	1,307,674,368,000
16	20,922,789,888,000
17	355,687,428,096,000
18	6,402,373,705,728,000
19	121,645,100,408,832,000
20	2,432,902,008,176,640,000

Table B		Binomial Distribution										
							p					
n	x	0.05	0.1	0.2	0.3	0.4	0.5	0.6	0.7	0.8	0.9	0.95
2	0	0.902	0.810	0.640	0.490	0.360	0.250	0.160	0.090	0.040	0.010	0.002
	1	0.095	0.180	0.320	0.420	0.480	0.500	0.480	0.420	0.320	0.180	0.095
	2	0.002	0.010	0.040	0.090	0.160	0.250	0.360	0.490	0.640	0.810	0.902
3	0	0.857	0.729	0.512	0.343	0.216	0.125	0.064	0.027	0.008	0.001	
	1	0.135	0.243	0.384	0.441	0.432	0.375	0.288	0.189	0.096	0.027	0.007
	2	0.007	0.027	0.096	0.189	0.288	0.375	0.432	0.441	0.384	0.243	0.135
	3		0.001	0.008	0.027	0.064	0.125	0.216	0.343	0.512	0.729	0.857
4	0	0.815	0.656	0.410	0.240	0.130	0.062	0.026	0.008	0.002		
	1	0.171	0.292	0.410	0.412	0.346	0.250	0.154	0.076	0.026	0.004	
	2	0.014	0.049	0.154	0.265	0.346	0.375	0.346	0.265	0.154	0.049	0.014
	3		0.004	0.026	0.076	0.154	0.250	0.346	0.412	0.410	0.292	0.171
	4			0.002	0.008	0.026	0.062	0.130	0.240	0.410	0.656	0.815
5	0	0.774	0.590	0.328	0.168	0.078	0.031	0.010	0.002			
	1	0.204	0.328	0.410	0.360	0.259	0.156	0.077	0.028	0.006		
	2	0.021	0.073	0.205	0.309	0.346	0.312	0.230	0.132	0.051	0.008	0.001
	3	0.001	0.008	0.051	0.132	0.230	0.312	0.346	0.309	0.205	0.073	0.021
	4			0.006	0.028	0.077	0.156	0.259	0.360	0.410	0.328	0.204
	5				0.002	0.010	0.031	0.078	0.168	0.328	0.590	0.774
6	0	0.735	0.531	0.262	0.118	0.047	0.016	0.004	0.001			
	1	0.232	0.354	0.393	0.303	0.187	0.094	0.037	0.010	0.002		
	2	0.031	0.098	0.246	0.324	0.311	0.234	0.138	0.060	0.015	0.001	
	3	0.002	0.015	0.082	0.185	0.276	0.312	0.276	0.185	0.082	0.015	0.002
	4		0.001	0.015	0.060	0.138	0.234	0.311	0.324	0.246	0.098	0.031
	5			0.002	0.010	0.037	0.094	0.187	0.303	0.393	0.354	0.232
	6				0.001	0.004	0.016	0.047	0.118	0.262	0.531	0.735
7	0	0.698	0.478	0.210	0.082	0.028	0.008	0.002				
	1	0.257	0.372	0.367	0.247	0.131	0.055	0.017	0.004			
	2	0.041	0.124	0.275	0.318	0.261	0.164	0.077	0.025	0.004		
	3	0.004	0.023	0.115	0.227	0.290	0.273	0.194	0.097	0.029	0.003	
	4		0.003	0.029	0.097	0.194	0.273	0.290	0.227	0.115	0.023	0.004
	5			0.004	0.025	0.077	0.164	0.261	0.318	0.275	0.124	0.041
	6				0.004	0.017	0.055	0.131	0.247	0.367	0.372	0.257
	7					0.002	0.008	0.028	0.082	0.210	0.478	0.698
8	0	0.663	0.430	0.168	0.058	0.017	0.004	0.001				
	1	0.279	0.383	0.336	0.198	0.090	0.031	0.008	0.001			
	2	0.051	0.149	0.294	0.296	0.209	0.109	0.041	0.010	0.001		
	3	0.005	0.033	0.147	0.254	0.279	0.219	0.124	0.047	0.009		
	4		0.005	0.046	0.136	0.232	0.273	0.232	0.136	0.046	0.005	
	5			0.009	0.047	0.124	0.219	0.279	0.254	0.147	0.033	0.005
	6			0.001	0.010	0.041	0.109	0.209	0.296	0.294	0.149	0.051
	7				0.001	0.008	0.031	0.090	0.198	0.336	0.383	0.279
	8					0.001	0.004	0.017	0.058	0.168	0.430	0.663

Table B		(continued)									
						p					
n	*x*	0.05	0.1	0.2	0.3	0.4	0.5	0.6	0.7	0.8	0.9	0.95
9	0	0.630	0.387	0.134	0.040	0.010	0.002					
	1	0.299	0.387	0.302	0.156	0.060	0.018	0.004				
	2	0.063	0.172	0.302	0.267	0.161	0.070	0.021	0.004			
	3	0.008	0.045	0.176	0.267	0.251	0.164	0.074	0.021	0.003		
	4	0.001	0.007	0.066	0.172	0.251	0.246	0.167	0.074	0.017	0.001	
	5		0.001	0.017	0.074	0.167	0.246	0.251	0.172	0.066	0.007	0.001
	6			0.003	0.021	0.074	0.164	0.251	0.267	0.176	0.045	0.008
	7				0.004	0.021	0.070	0.161	0.267	0.302	0.172	0.063
	8					0.004	0.018	0.060	0.156	0.302	0.387	0.299
	9						0.002	0.010	0.040	0.134	0.387	0.630
10	0	0.599	0.349	0.107	0.028	0.006	0.001					
	1	0.315	0.387	0.268	0.121	0.040	0.010	0.002				
	2	0.075	0.194	0.302	0.233	0.121	0.044	0.011	0.001			
	3	0.010	0.057	0.201	0.267	0.215	0.117	0.042	0.009	0.001		
	4	0.001	0.011	0.088	0.200	0.251	0.205	0.111	0.037	0.006		
	5		0.001	0.026	0.103	0.201	0.246	0.201	0.103	0.026	0.001	
	6			0.006	0.037	0.111	0.205	0.251	0.200	0.088	0.011	0.001
	7			0.001	0.009	0.042	0.117	0.215	0.267	0.201	0.057	0.010
	8				0.001	0.011	0.044	0.121	0.233	0.302	0.194	0.075
	9					0.002	0.010	0.040	0.121	0.268	0.387	0.315
	10						0.001	0.006	0.028	0.107	0.349	0.599
11	0	0.569	0.314	0.086	0.020	0.004						
	1	0.329	0.384	0.236	0.093	0.027	0.005	0.001				
	2	0.087	0.213	0.295	0.200	0.089	0.027	0.005	0.001			
	3	0.014	0.071	0.221	0.257	0.177	0.081	0.023	0.004			
	4	0.001	0.016	0.111	0.220	0.236	0.161	0.070	0.017	0.002		
	5		0.002	0.039	0.132	0.221	0.226	0.147	0.057	0.010		
	6			0.010	0.057	0.147	0.226	0.221	0.132	0.039	0.002	
	7			0.002	0.017	0.070	0.161	0.236	0.220	0.111	0.016	0.001
	8				0.004	0.023	0.081	0.177	0.257	0.221	0.071	0.014
	9				0.001	0.005	0.027	0.089	0.200	0.295	0.213	0.087
	10					0.001	0.005	0.027	0.093	0.236	0.384	0.329
	11							0.004	0.020	0.086	0.314	0.569
12	0	0.540	0.282	0.069	0.014	0.002						
	1	0.341	0.377	0.206	0.071	0.017	0.003					
	2	0.099	0.230	0.283	0.168	0.064	0.016	0.002				
	3	0.017	0.085	0.236	0.240	0.142	0.054	0.012	0.001			
	4	0.002	0.021	0.133	0.231	0.213	0.121	0.042	0.008	0.001		
	5		0.004	0.053	0.158	0.227	0.193	0.101	0.029	0.003		
	6			0.016	0.079	0.177	0.226	0.177	0.079	0.016		
	7			0.003	0.029	0.101	0.193	0.227	0.158	0.053	0.004	
	8			0.001	0.008	0.042	0.121	0.213	0.231	0.133	0.021	0.002
	9				0.001	0.012	0.054	0.142	0.240	0.236	0.085	0.017
	10					0.002	0.016	0.064	0.168	0.283	0.230	0.099
	11						0.003	0.017	0.071	0.206	0.377	0.341
	12						0.002	0.014	0.069	0.282	0.540

Table B		(continued)										
							p					
n	*x*	0.05	0.1	0.2	0.3	0.4	0.5	0.6	0.7	0.8	0.9	0.95
13	0	0.513	0.254	0.055	0.010	0.001						
	1	0.351	0.367	0.179	0.054	0.011	0.002					
	2	0.111	0.245	0.268	0.139	0.045	0.010	0.001				
	3	0.021	0.100	0.246	0.218	0.111	0.035	0.006	0.001			
	4	0.003	0.028	0.154	0.234	0.184	0.087	0.024	0.003			
	5		0.006	0.069	0.180	0.221	0.157	0.066	0.014	0.001		
	6		0.001	0.023	0.103	0.197	0.209	0.131	0.044	0.006		
	7			0.006	0.044	0.131	0.209	0.197	0.103	0.023	0.001	
	8			0.001	0.014	0.066	0.157	0.221	0.180	0.069	0.006	
	9				0.003	0.024	0.087	0.184	0.234	0.154	0.028	0.003
	10				0.001	0.006	0.035	0.111	0.218	0.246	0.100	0.021
	11					0.001	0.010	0.045	0.139	0.268	0.245	0.111
	12						0.002	0.011	0.054	0.179	0.367	0.351
	13							0.001	0.010	0.055	0.254	0.513
14	0	0.488	0.229	0.044	0.007	0.001						
	1	0.359	0.356	0.154	0.041	0.007	0.001					
	2	0.123	0.257	0.250	0.113	0.032	0.006	0.001				
	3	0.026	0.114	0.250	0.194	0.085	0.022	0.003				
	4	0.004	0.035	0.172	0.229	0.155	0.061	0.014	0.001			
	5		0.008	0.086	0.196	0.207	0.122	0.041	0.007			
	6		0.001	0.032	0.126	0.207	0.183	0.092	0.023	0.002		
	7			0.009	0.062	0.157	0.209	0.157	0.062	0.009		
	8			0.002	0.023	0.092	0.183	0.207	0.126	0.032	0.001	
	9				0.007	0.041	0.122	0.207	0.196	0.086	0.008	
	10				0.001	0.014	0.061	0.155	0.229	0.172	0.035	0.004
	11					0.003	0.022	0.085	0.194	0.250	0.114	0.026
	12					0.001	0.006	0.032	0.113	0.250	0.257	0.123
	13						0.001	0.007	0.041	0.154	0.356	0.359
	14							0.001	0.007	0.044	0.229	0.488
15	0	0.463	0.206	0.035	0.005							
	1	0.366	0.343	0.132	0.031	0.005						
	2	0.135	0.267	0.231	0.092	0.022	0.003					
	3	0.031	0.129	0.250	0.170	0.063	0.014	0.002				
	4	0.005	0.043	0.188	0.219	0.127	0.042	0.007	0.001			
	5	0.001	0.010	0.103	0.206	0.186	0.092	0.024	0.003			
	6		0.002	0.043	0.147	0.207	0.153	0.061	0.012	0.001		
	7			0.014	0.081	0.177	0.196	0.118	0.035	0.003		
	8			0.003	0.035	0.118	0.196	0.177	0.081	0.014		
	9			0.001	0.012	0.061	0.153	0.207	0.147	0.043	0.002	
	10				0.003	0.024	0.092	0.186	0.206	0.103	0.010	0.001
	11				0.001	0.007	0.042	0.127	0.219	0.188	0.043	0.005
	12					0.002	0.014	0.063	0.170	0.250	0.129	0.031
	13						0.003	0.022	0.092	0.231	0.267	0.135
	14							0.005	0.031	0.132	0.343	0.366
	15								0.005	0.035	0.206	0.463

Table B		(continued)									
						p					
n	x	0.05	0.1	0.2	0.3	0.4	0.5	0.6	0.7	0.8	0.9	0.95
16	0	0.440	0.185	0.028	0.003							
	1	0.371	0.329	0.113	0.023	0.003						
	2	0.146	0.275	0.211	0.073	0.015	0.002					
	3	0.036	0.142	0.246	0.146	0.047	0.009	0.001				
	4	0.006	0.051	0.200	0.204	0.101	0.028	0.004				
	5	0.001	0.014	0.120	0.210	0.162	0.067	0.014	0.001			
	6		0.003	0.055	0.165	0.198	0.122	0.039	0.006			
	7			0.020	0.101	0.189	0.175	0.084	0.019	0.001		
	8			0.006	0.049	0.142	0.196	0.142	0.049	0.006		
	9			0.001	0.019	0.084	0.175	0.189	0.101	0.020		
	10				0.006	0.039	0.122	0.198	0.165	0.055	0.003	
	11				0.001	0.014	0.067	0.162	0.210	0.120	0.014	0.001
	12					0.004	0.028	0.101	0.204	0.200	0.051	0.006
	13					0.001	0.009	0.047	0.146	0.246	0.142	0.036
	14						0.002	0.015	0.073	0.211	0.275	0.146
	15							0.003	0.023	0.113	0.329	0.371
	16								0.003	0.028	0.185	0.440
17	0	0.418	0.167	0.023	0.002							
	1	0.374	0.315	0.096	0.017	0.002						
	2	0.158	0.280	0.191	0.058	0.010	0.001					
	3	0.041	0.156	0.239	0.125	0.034	0.005					
	4	0.008	0.060	0.209	0.187	0.080	0.018	0.002				
	5	0.001	0.017	0.136	0.208	0.138	0.047	0.008	0.001			
	6		0.004	0.068	0.178	0.184	0.094	0.024	0.003			
	7		0.001	0.027	0.120	0.193	0.148	0.057	0.009			
	8			0.008	0.064	0.161	0.185	0.107	0.028	0.002		
	9			0.002	0.028	0.107	0.185	0.161	0.064	0.008		
	10				0.009	0.057	0.148	0.193	0.120	0.027	0.001	
	11				0.003	0.024	0.094	0.184	0.178	0.068	0.004	
	12				0.001	0.008	0.047	0.138	0.208	0.136	0.017	0.001
	13					0.002	0.018	0.080	0.187	0.209	0.060	0.008
	14						0.005	0.034	0.125	0.239	0.156	0.041
	15						0.001	0.010	0.058	0.191	0.280	0.158
	16							0.002	0.017	0.096	0.315	0.374
	17								0.002	0.023	0.167	0.418

Table B												
(continued)												
							p					
n	x	0.05	0.1	0.2	0.3	0.4	0.5	0.6	0.7	0.8	0.9	0.95
18	0	0.397	0.150	0.018	0.002							
	1	0.376	0.300	0.081	0.013	0.001						
	2	0.168	0.284	0.172	0.046	0.007	0.001					
	3	0.047	0.168	0.230	0.105	0.025	0.003					
	4	0.009	0.070	0.215	0.168	0.061	0.012	0.001				
	5	0.001	0.022	0.151	0.202	0.115	0.033	0.004				
	6		0.005	0.082	0.187	0.166	0.071	0.015	0.001			
	7		0.001	0.035	0.138	0.189	0.121	0.037	0.005			
	8			0.012	0.081	0.173	0.167	0.077	0.015	0.001		
	9			0.003	0.039	0.128	0.185	0.128	0.039	0.003		
	10			0.001	0.015	0.077	0.167	0.173	0.081	0.012		
	11				0.005	0.037	0.121	0.189	0.138	0.035	0.001	
	12				0.001	0.015	0.071	0.166	0.187	0.082	0.005	
	13					0.004	0.033	0.115	0.202	0.151	0.022	0.001
	14					0.001	0.012	0.061	0.168	0.215	0.070	0.009
	15						0.003	0.025	0.105	0.230	0.168	0.047
	16						0.001	0.007	0.046	0.172	0.284	0.168
	17							0.001	0.013	0.081	0.300	0.376
	18								0.002	0.018	0.150	0.397
19	0	0.377	0.135	0.014	0.001							
	1	0.377	0.285	0.068	0.009	0.001						
	2	0.179	0.285	0.154	0.036	0.005						
	3	0.053	0.180	0.218	0.087	0.017	0.002					
	4	0.011	0.080	0.218	0.149	0.047	0.007	0.001				
	5	0.002	0.027	0.164	0.192	0.093	0.022	0.002				
	6		0.007	0.095	0.192	0.145	0.052	0.008	0.001			
	7		0.001	0.044	0.153	0.180	0.096	0.024	0.002			
	8			0.017	0.098	0.180	0.144	0.053	0.008			
	9			0.005	0.051	0.146	0.176	0.098	0.022	0.001		
	10			0.001	0.022	0.098	0.176	0.146	0.051	0.005		
	11				0.008	0.053	0.144	0.180	0.098	0.071		
	12				0.002	0.024	0.096	0.180	0.153	0.044	0.001	
	13				0.001	0.008	0.052	0.145	0.192	0.095	0.007	
	14					0.002	0.022	0.093	0.192	0.164	0.027	0.002
	15					0.001	0.007	0.047	0.149	0.218	0.080	0.011
	16						0.002	0.017	0.087	0.218	0.180	0.053
	17							0.005	0.036	0.154	0.285	0.179
	18							0.001	0.009	0.068	0.285	0.377
	19								0.001	0.014	0.135	0.377

Table B		(concluded)										
							p					
n	*x*	0.05	0.1	0.2	0.3	0.4	0.5	0.6	0.7	0.8	0.9	0.95
20	0	0.358	0.122	0.012	0.001							
	1	0.377	0.270	0.058	0.007							
	2	0.189	0.285	0.137	0.028	0.003						
	3	0.060	0.190	0.205	0.072	0.012	0.001					
	4	0.013	0.090	0.218	0.130	0.035	0.005					
	5	0.002	0.032	0.175	0.179	0.075	0.015	0.001				
	6		0.009	0.109	0.192	0.124	0.037	0.005				
	7		0.002	0.055	0.164	0.166	0.074	0.015	0.001			
	8			0.022	0.114	0.180	0.120	0.035	0.004			
	9			0.007	0.065	0.160	0.160	0.071	0.012			
	10			0.002	0.031	0.117	0.176	0.117	0.031	0.002		
	11				0.012	0.071	0.160	0.160	0.065	0.007		
	12				0.004	0.035	0.120	0.180	0.114	0.022		
	13				0.001	0.015	0.074	0.166	0.164	0.055	0.002	
	14					0.005	0.037	0.124	0.192	0.109	0.009	
	15					0.001	0.015	0.075	0.179	0.175	0.032	0.002
	16						0.005	0.035	0.130	0.218	0.090	0.013
	17						0.001	0.012	0.072	0.205	0.190	0.060
	18							0.003	0.028	0.137	0.285	0.189
	19								0.007	0.058	0.270	0.377
	20								0.001	0.012	0.122	0.358

Note: All values of 0.0005 or less are omitted.

Source: John E. Freund, *Modern Elementary Statistics,* 8th ed., © 1992. Reprinted by permission of Prentice-Hall, Inc., Upper Saddle River, N.J.

| Table C | | Poisson Distribution | | | | | | | |

λ

x	0.1	0.2	0.3	0.4	0.5	0.6	0.7	0.8	0.9	1.0
0	.9048	.8187	.7408	.6703	.6065	.5488	.4966	.4493	.4066	.3679
1	.0905	.1637	.2222	.2681	.3033	.3293	.3476	.3595	.3659	.3679
2	.0045	.0164	.0333	.0536	.0758	.0988	.1217	.1438	.1647	.1839
3	.0002	.0011	.0033	.0072	.0126	.0198	.0284	.0383	.0494	.0613
4	.0000	.0001	.0003	.0007	.0016	.0030	.0050	.0077	.0111	.0153
5	.0000	.0000	.0000	.0001	.0002	.0004	.0007	.0012	.0020	.0031
6	.0000	.0000	.0000	.0000	.0000	.0000	.0001	.0002	.0003	.0005
7	.0000	.0000	.0000	.0000	.0000	.0000	.0000	.0000	.0000	.0001

λ

x	1.1	1.2	1.3	1.4	1.5	1.6	1.7	1.8	1.9	2.0
0	.3329	.3012	.2725	.2466	.2231	.2019	.1827	.1653	.1496	.1353
1	.3662	.3614	.3543	.3452	.3347	.3230	.3106	.2975	.2842	.2707
2	.2014	.2169	.2303	.2417	.2510	.2584	.2640	.2678	.2700	.2707
3	.0738	.0867	.0998	.1128	.1255	.1378	.1496	.1607	.1710	.1804
4	.0203	.0260	.0324	.0395	.0471	.0551	.0636	.0723	.0812	.0902
5	.0045	.0062	.0084	.0111	.0141	.0176	.0216	.0260	.0309	.0361
6	.0008	.0012	.0018	.0026	.0035	.0047	.0061	.0078	.0098	.0120
7	.0001	.0002	.0003	.0005	.0008	.0011	.0015	.0020	.0027	.0034
8	.0000	.0000	.0001	.0001	.0001	.0002	.0003	.0005	.0006	.0009
9	.0000	.0000	.0000	.0000	.0000	.0000	.0001	.0001	.0001	.0002

λ

x	2.1	2.2	2.3	2.4	2.5	2.6	2.7	2.8	2.9	3.0
0	.1225	.1108	.1003	.0907	.0821	.0743	.0672	.0608	.0550	.0498
1	.2572	.2438	.2306	.2177	.2052	.1931	.1815	.1703	.1596	.1494
2	.2700	.2681	.2652	.2613	.2565	.2510	.2450	.2384	.2314	.2240
3	.1890	.1966	.2033	.2090	.2138	.2176	.2205	.2225	.2237	.2240
4	.0992	.1082	.1169	.1254	.1336	.1414	.1488	.1557	.1622	.1680
5	.0417	.0476	.0538	.0602	.0668	.0735	.0804	.0872	.0940	.1008
6	.0146	.0174	.0206	.0241	.0278	.0319	.0362	.0407	.0455	.0504
7	.0044	.0055	.0068	.0083	.0099	.0118	.0139	.0163	.0188	.0216
8	.0011	.0015	.0019	.0025	.0031	.0038	.0047	.0057	.0068	.0081
9	.0003	.0004	.0005	.0007	.0009	.0011	.0014	.0018	.0022	.0027
10	.0001	.0001	.0001	.0002	.0002	.0003	.0004	.0005	.0006	.0008
11	.0000	.0000	.0000	.0000	.0000	.0001	.0001	.0001	.0002	.0002
12	.0000	.0000	.0000	.0000	.0000	.0000	.0000	.0000	.0000	.0001

λ

x	3.1	3.2	3.3	3.4	3.5	3.6	3.7	3.8	3.9	4.0
0	.0450	.0408	.0369	.0334	.0302	.0273	.0247	.0224	.0202	.0183
1	.1397	.1304	.1217	.1135	.1057	.0984	.0915	.0850	.0789	.0733
2	.2165	.2087	.2008	.1929	.1850	.1771	.1692	.1615	.1539	.1465
3	.2237	.2226	.2209	.2186	.2158	.2125	.2087	.2046	.2001	.1954
4	.1734	.1781	.1823	.1858	.1888	.1912	.1931	.1944	.1951	.1954

| Table C | (continued) |

					λ					
x	3.1	3.2	3.3	3.4	3.5	3.6	3.7	3.8	3.9	4.0
5	.1075	.1140	.1203	.1264	.1322	.1377	.1429	.1477	.1522	.1563
6	.0555	.0608	.0662	.0716	.0771	.0826	.0881	.0936	.0989	.1042
7	.0246	.0278	.0312	.0348	.0385	.0425	.0466	.0508	.0551	.0595
8	.0095	.0111	.0129	.0148	.0169	.0191	.0215	.0241	.0269	.0298
9	.0033	.0040	.0047	.0056	.0066	.0076	.0089	.0102	.0116	.0132
10	.0010	.0013	.0016	.0019	.0023	.0028	.0033	.0039	.0045	.0053
11	.0003	.0004	.0005	.0006	.0007	.0009	.0011	.0013	.0016	.0019
12	.0001	.0001	.0001	.0002	.0002	.0003	.0003	.0004	.0005	.0006
13	.0000	.0000	.0000	.0000	.0001	.0001	.0001	.0001	.0002	.0002
14	.0000	.0000	.0000	.0000	.0000	.0000	.0000	.0000	.0000	.0001

					λ					
x	4.1	4.2	4.3	4.4	4.5	4.6	4.7	4.8	4.9	5.0
0	.0166	.0150	.0136	.0123	.0111	.0101	.0091	.0082	.0074	.0067
1	.0679	.0630	.0583	.0540	.0500	.0462	.0427	.0395	.0365	.0337
2	.1393	.1323	.1254	.1188	.1125	.1063	.1005	.0948	.0894	.0842
3	.1904	.1852	.1798	.1743	.1687	.1631	.1574	.1517	.1460	.1404
4	.1951	.1944	.1933	.1917	.1898	.1875	.1849	.1820	.1789	.1755
5	.1600	.1633	.1662	.1687	.1708	.1725	.1738	.1747	.1753	.1755
6	.1093	.1143	.1191	.1237	.1281	.1323	.1362	.1398	.1432	.1462
7	.0640	.0686	.0732	.0778	.0824	.0869	.0914	.0959	.1002	.1044
8	.0328	.0360	.0393	.0428	.0463	.0500	.0537	.0575	.0614	.0653
9	.0150	.0168	.0188	.0209	.0232	.0255	.0280	.0307	.0334	.0363
10	.0061	.0071	.0081	.0092	.0104	.0118	.0132	.0147	.0164	.0181
11	.0023	.0027	.0032	.0037	.0043	.0049	.0056	.0064	.0073	.0082
12	.0008	.0009	.0011	.0014	.0016	.0019	.0022	.0026	.0030	.0034
13	.0002	.0003	.0004	.0005	.0006	.0007	.0008	.0009	.0011	.0013
14	.0001	.0001	.0001	.0001	.0002	.0002	.0003	.0003	.0004	.0005
15	.0000	.0000	.0000	.0000	.0001	.0001	.0001	.0001	.0001	.0002

					λ					
x	5.1	5.2	5.3	5.4	5.5	5.6	5.7	5.8	5.9	6.0
0	.0061	.0055	.0050	.0045	.0041	.0037	.0033	.0030	.0027	.0025
1	.0311	.0287	.0265	.0244	.0225	.0207	.0191	.0176	.0162	.0149
2	.0793	.0746	.0701	.0659	.0618	.0580	.0544	.0509	.0477	.0446
3	.1348	.1293	.1239	.1185	.1133	.1082	.1033	.0985	.0938	.0892
4	.1719	.1681	.1641	.1600	.1558	.1515	.1472	.1428	.1383	.1339

Table C	(continued)								
					λ				
x	5.1	5.2	5.3	5.4	5.5	5.6	5.7	5.8	5.9	6.0
5	.1753	.1748	.1740	.1728	.1714	.1697	.1678	.1656	.1632	.1606
6	.1490	.1515	.1537	.1555	.1571	.1584	.1594	.1601	.1605	.1606
7	.1086	.1125	.1163	.1200	.1234	.1267	.1298	.1326	.1353	.1377
8	.0692	.0731	.0771	.0810	.0849	.0887	.0925	.0962	.0998	.1033
9	.0392	.0423	.0454	.0486	.0519	.0552	.0586	.0620	.0654	.0688
10	.0200	.0220	.0241	.0262	.0285	.0309	.0334	.0359	.0386	.0413
11	.0093	.0104	.0116	.0129	.0143	.0157	.0173	.0190	.0207	.0225
12	.0039	.0045	.0051	.0058	.0065	.0073	.0082	.0092	.0102	.0113
13	.0015	.0018	.0021	.0024	.0028	.0032	.0036	.0041	.0046	.0052
14	.0006	.0007	.0008	.0009	.0011	.0013	.0015	.0017	.0019	.0022
15	.0002	.0002	.0003	.0003	.0004	.0005	.0006	.0007	.0008	.0009
16	.0001	.0001	.0001	.0001	.0001	.0002	.0002	.0002	.0003	.0003
17	.0000	.0000	.0000	.0000	.0000	.0000	.0001	.0001	.0001	.0001

					λ				
x	6.1	6.2	6.3	6.4	6.5	6.6	6.7	6.8	6.9	7.0
0	.0022	.0020	.0018	.0017	.0015	.0014	.0012	.0011	.0010	.0009
1	.0137	.0126	.0116	.0106	.0098	.0090	.0082	.0076	.0070	.0064
2	.0417	.0390	.0364	.0340	.0318	.0296	.0276	.0258	.0240	.0223
3	.0848	.0806	.0765	.0726	.0688	.0652	.0617	.0584	.0552	.0521
4	.1294	.1249	.1205	.1162	.1118	.1076	.1034	.0992	.0952	.0912
5	.1579	.1549	.1519	.1487	.1454	.1420	.1385	.1349	.1314	.1277
6	.1605	.1601	.1595	.1586	.1575	.1562	.1546	.1529	.1511	.1490
7	.1399	.1418	.1435	.1450	.1462	.1472	.1480	.1486	.1489	.1490
8	.1066	.1099	.1130	.1160	.1188	.1215	.1240	.1263	.1284	.1304
9	.0723	.0757	.0791	.0825	.0858	.0891	.0923	.0954	.0985	.1014
10	.0441	.0469	.0498	.0528	.0558	.0588	.0618	.0649	.0679	.0710
11	.0245	.0265	.0285	.0307	.0330	.0353	.0377	.0401	.0426	.0452
12	.0124	.0137	.0150	.0164	.0179	.0194	.0210	.0227	.0245	.0264
13	.0058	.0065	.0073	.0081	.0089	.0098	.0108	.0119	.0130	.0142
14	.0025	.0029	.0033	.0037	.0041	.0046	.0052	.0058	.0064	.0071
15	.0010	.0012	.0014	.0016	.0018	.0020	.0023	.0026	.0029	.0033
16	.0004	.0005	.0005	.0006	.0007	.0008	.0010	.0011	.0013	.0014
17	.0001	.0002	.0002	.0002	.0003	.0003	.0004	.0004	.0005	.0006
18	.0000	.0001	.0001	.0001	.0001	.0001	.0001	.0002	.0002	.0002
19	.0000	.0000	.0000	.0000	.0000	.0000	.0000	.0001	.0001	.0001

Table C	(continued)								
					λ				
x	7.1	7.2	7.3	7.4	7.5	7.6	7.7	7.8	7.9	8.0
0	.0008	.0007	.0007	.0006	.0006	.0005	.0005	.0004	.0004	.0003
1	.0059	.0054	.0049	.0045	.0041	.0038	.0035	.0032	.0029	.0027
2	.0208	.0194	.0180	.0167	.0156	.0145	.0134	.0125	.0116	.0107
3	.0492	.0464	.0438	.0413	.0389	.0366	.0345	.0324	.0305	.0286
4	.0874	.0836	.0799	.0764	.0729	.0696	.0663	.0632	.0602	.0573
5	.1241	.1204	.1167	.1130	.1094	.1057	.1021	.0986	.0951	.0916
6	.1468	.1445	.1420	.1394	.1367	.1339	.1311	.1282	.1252	.1221
7	.1489	.1486	.1481	.1474	.1465	.1454	.1442	.1428	.1413	.1396
8	.1321	.1337	.1351	.1363	.1373	.1382	.1388	.1392	.1395	.1396
9	.1042	.1070	.1096	.1121	.1144	.1167	.1187	.1207	.1224	.1241
10	.0740	.0770	.0800	.0829	.0858	.0887	.0914	.0941	.0967	.0993
11	.0478	.0504	.0531	.0558	.0585	.0613	.0640	.0667	.0695	.0722
12	.0283	.0303	.0323	.0344	.0366	.0388	.0411	.0434	.0457	.0481
13	.0154	.0168	.0181	.0196	.0211	.0227	.0243	.0260	.0278	.0296
14	.0078	.0086	.0095	.0104	.0113	.0123	.0134	.0145	.0157	.0169
15	.0037	.0041	.0046	.0051	.0057	.0062	.0069	.0075	.0083	.0090
16	.0016	.0019	.0021	.0024	.0026	.0030	.0033	.0037	.0041	.0045
17	.0007	.0008	.0009	.0010	.0012	.0013	.0015	.0017	.0019	.0021
18	.0003	.0003	.0004	.0004	.0005	.0006	.0006	.0007	.0008	.0009
19	.0001	.0001	.0001	.0002	.0002	.0002	.0003	.0003	.0003	.0004
20	.0000	.0000	.0001	.0001	.0001	.0001	.0001	.0001	.0001	.0002
21	.0000	.0000	.0000	.0000	.0000	.0000	.0000	.0000	.0001	.0001

					λ				
x	8.1	8.2	8.3	8.4	8.5	8.6	8.7	8.8	8.9	9.0
0	.0003	.0003	.0002	.0002	.0002	.0002	.0002	.0002	.0001	.0001
1	.0025	.0023	.0021	.0019	.0017	.0016	.0014	.0013	.0012	.0011
2	.0100	.0092	.0086	.0079	.0074	.0068	.0063	.0058	.0054	.0050
3	.0269	.0252	.0237	.0222	.0208	.0195	.0183	.0171	.0160	.0150
4	.0544	.0517	.0491	.0466	.0443	.0420	.0398	.0377	.0357	.0337
5	.0882	.0849	.0816	.0784	.0752	.0722	.0692	.0663	.0635	.0607
6	.1191	.1160	.1128	.1097	.1066	.1034	.1003	.0972	.0941	.0911
7	.1378	.1358	.1338	.1317	.1294	.1271	.1247	.1222	.1197	.1171
8	.1395	.1392	.1388	.1382	.1375	.1366	.1356	.1344	.1332	.1318
9	.1256	.1269	.1280	.1290	.1299	.1306	.1311	.1315	.1317	.1318

Table C	(continued)								
					λ				
x	8.1	8.2	8.3	8.4	8.5	8.6	8.7	8.8	8.9	9.0
10	.1017	.1040	.1063	.1084	.1104	.1123	.1140	.1157	.1172	.1186
11	.0749	.0776	.0802	.0828	.0853	.0878	.0902	.0925	.0948	.0970
12	.0505	.0530	.0555	.0579	.0604	.0629	.0654	.0679	.0703	.0728
13	.0315	.0334	.0354	.0374	.0395	.0416	.0438	.0459	.0481	.0504
14	.0182	.0196	.0210	.0225	.0240	.0256	.0272	.0289	.0306	.0324
15	.0098	.0107	.0116	.0126	.0136	.0147	.0158	.0169	.0182	.0194
16	.0050	.0055	.0060	.0066	.0072	.0079	.0086	.0093	.0101	.0109
17	.0024	.0026	.0029	.0033	.0036	.0040	.0044	.0048	.0053	.0058
18	.0011	.0012	.0014	.0015	.0017	.0019	.0021	.0024	.0026	.0029
19	.0005	.0005	.0006	.0007	.0008	.0009	.0010	.0011	.0012	.0014
20	.0002	.0002	.0002	.0003	.0003	.0004	.0004	.0005	.0005	.0006
21	.0001	.0001	.0001	.0001	.0001	.0002	.0002	.0002	.0002	.0003
22	.0000	.0000	.0000	.0000	.0001	.0001	.0001	.0001	.0001	.0001

					λ				
x	9.1	9.2	9.3	9.4	9.5	9.6	9.7	9.8	9.9	10.0
0	.0001	.0001	.0001	.0001	.0001	.0001	.0001	.0001	.0001	.0000
1	.0010	.0009	.0009	.0008	.0007	.0007	.0006	.0005	.0005	.0005
2	.0046	.0043	.0040	.0037	.0034	.0031	.0029	.0027	.0025	.0023
3	.0140	.0131	.0123	.0115	.0107	.0100	.0093	.0087	.0081	.0076
4	.0319	.0302	.0285	.0269	.0254	.0240	.0226	.0213	.0201	.0189
5	.0581	.0555	.0530	.0506	.0483	.0460	.0439	.0418	.0398	.0378
6	.0881	.0851	.0822	.0793	.0764	.0736	.0709	.0682	.0656	.0631
7	.1145	.1118	.1091	.1064	.1037	.1010	.0982	.0955	.0928	.0901
8	.1302	.1286	.1269	.1251	.1232	.1212	.1191	.1170	.1148	.1126
9	.1317	.1315	.1311	.1306	.1300	.1293	.1284	.1274	.1263	.1251
10	.1198	.1210	.1219	.1228	.1235	.1241	.1245	.1249	.1250	.1251
11	.0991	.1012	.1031	.1049	.1067	.1083	.1098	.1112	.1125	.1137
12	.0752	.0776	.0799	.0822	.0844	.0866	.0888	.0908	.0928	.0948
13	.0526	.0549	.0572	.0594	.0617	.0640	.0662	.0685	.0707	.0729
14	.0342	.0361	.0380	.0399	.0419	.0439	.0459	.0479	.0500	.0521
15	.0208	.0221	.0235	.0250	.0265	.0281	.0297	.0313	.0330	.0347
16	.0118	.0127	.0137	.0147	.0157	.0168	.0180	.0192	.0204	.0217
17	.0063	.0069	.0075	.0081	.0088	.0095	.0103	.0111	.0119	.0128
18	.0032	.0035	.0039	.0042	.0046	.0051	.0055	.0060	.0065	.0071
19	.0015	.0017	.0019	.0021	.0023	.0026	.0028	.0031	.0034	.0037

Table C	(continued)								

	λ									
x	**9.1**	**9.2**	**9.3**	**9.4**	**9.5**	**9.6**	**9.7**	**9.8**	**9.9**	**10.0**
20	.0007	.0008	.0009	.0010	.0011	.0012	.0014	.0015	.0017	.0019
21	.0003	.0003	.0004	.0004	.0005	.0006	.0006	.0007	.0008	.0009
22	.0001	.0001	.0002	.0002	.0002	.0002	.0003	.0003	.0004	.0004
23	.0000	.0001	.0001	.0001	.0001	.0001	.0001	.0001	.0002	.0002
24	.0000	.0000	.0000	.0000	.0000	.0000	.0000	.0001	.0001	.0001

	λ									
x	**11**	**12**	**13**	**14**	**15**	**16**	**17**	**18**	**19**	**20**
0	.0000	.0000	.0000	.0000	.0000	.0000	.0000	.0000	.0000	.0000
1	.0002	.0001	.0000	.0000	.0000	.0000	.0000	.0000	.0000	.0000
2	.0010	.0004	.0002	.0001	.0000	.0000	.0000	.0000	.0000	.0000
3	.0037	.0018	.0008	.0004	.0002	.0001	.0000	.0000	.0000	.0000
4	.0102	.0053	.0027	.0013	.0006	.0003	.0001	.0001	.0000	.0000
5	.0224	.0127	.0070	.0037	.0019	.0010	.0005	.0002	.0001	.0001
6	.0411	.0255	.0152	.0087	.0048	.0026	.0014	.0007	.0004	.0002
7	.0646	.0437	.0281	.0174	.0104	.0060	.0034	.0018	.0010	.0005
8	.0888	.0655	.0457	.0304	.0194	.0120	.0072	.0042	.0024	.0013
9	.1085	.0874	.0661	.0473	.0324	.0213	.0135	.0083	.0050	.0029
10	.1194	.1048	.0859	.0663	.0486	.0341	.0230	.0150	.0095	.0058
11	.1194	.1144	.1015	.0844	.0663	.0496	.0355	.0245	.0164	.0106
12	.1094	.1144	.1099	.0984	.0829	.0661	.0504	.0368	.0259	.0176
13	.0926	.1056	.1099	.1060	.0956	.0814	.0658	.0509	.0378	.0271
14	.0728	.0905	.1021	.1060	.1024	.0930	.0800	.0655	.0514	.0387
15	.0534	.0724	.0885	.0989	.1024	.0992	.0906	.0786	.0650	.0516
16	.0367	.0543	.0719	.0866	.0960	.0992	.0963	.0884	.0772	.0646
17	.0237	.0383	.0550	.0713	.0847	.0934	.0963	.0936	.0863	.0760
18	.0145	.0256	.0397	.0554	.0706	.0830	.0909	.0936	.0911	.0844
19	.0084	.0161	.0272	.0409	.0557	.0699	.0814	.0887	.0911	.0888
20	.0046	.0097	.0177	.0286	.0418	.0559	.0692	.0798	.0866	.0888
21	.0024	.0055	.0109	.0191	.0299	.0426	.0560	.0684	.0783	.0846
22	.0012	.0030	.0065	.0121	.0204	.0310	.0433	.0560	.0676	.0769
23	.0006	.0016	.0037	.0074	.0133	.0216	.0320	.0438	.0559	.0669
24	.0003	.0008	.0020	.0043	.0083	.0144	.0226	.0328	.0442	.0557
25	.0001	.0004	.0010	.0024	.0050	.0092	.0154	.0237	.0336	.0446
26	.0000	.0002	.0005	.0013	.0029	.0057	.0101	.0164	.0246	.0343
27	.0000	.0001	.0002	.0007	.0016	.0034	.0063	.0109	.0173	.0254
28	.0000	.0000	.0001	.0003	.0009	.0019	.0038	.0070	.0117	.0181
29	.0000	.0000	.0001	.0002	.0004	.0011	.0023	.0044	.0077	.0125

Table C	(concluded)								
					λ				
x	11	12	13	14	15	16	17	18	19	20
30	.0000	.0000	.0000	.0001	.0002	.0006	.0013	.0026	.0049	.0083
31	.0000	.0000	.0000	.0000	.0001	.0003	.0007	.0015	.0030	.0054
32	.0000	.0000	.0000	.0000	.0001	.0001	.0004	.0009	.0018	.0034
33	.0000	.0000	.0000	.0000	.0000	.0001	.0002	.0005	.0010	.0020
34	.0000	.0000	.0000	.0000	.0000	.0000	.0001	.0002	.0006	.0012
35	.0000	.0000	.0000	.0000	.0000	.0000	.0000	.0001	.0003	.0007
36	.0000	.0000	.0000	.0000	.0000	.0000	.0000	.0001	.0002	.0004
37	.0000	.0000	.0000	.0000	.0000	.0000	.0000	.0000	.0001	.0002
38	.0000	.0000	.0000	.0000	.0000	.0000	.0000	.0000	.0000	.0001
39	.0000	.0000	.0000	.0000	.0000	.0000	.0000	.0000	.0000	.0001

Reprinted with permission from W. H. Beyer, *Handbook of Tables for Probability and Statistics,* 2nd ed. Copyright CRC Press, Boca Raton, Fla., 1986.

Table D		Random Numbers											
10480	15011	01536	02011	81647	91646	67179	14194	62590	36207	20969	99570	91291	90700
22368	46573	25595	85393	30995	89198	27982	53402	93965	34095	52666	19174	39615	99505
24130	48360	22527	97265	76393	64809	15179	24830	49340	32081	30680	19655	63348	58629
42167	93093	06243	61680	07856	16376	39440	53537	71341	57004	00849	74917	97758	16379
37570	39975	81837	16656	06121	91782	60468	81305	49684	60672	14110	06927	01263	54613
77921	06907	11008	42751	27756	53498	18602	70659	90655	15053	21916	81825	44394	42880
99562	72905	56420	69994	98872	31016	71194	18738	44013	48840	63213	21069	10634	12952
96301	91977	05463	07972	18876	20922	94595	56869	69014	60045	18425	84903	42508	32307
89579	14342	63661	10281	17453	18103	57740	84378	25331	12566	58678	44947	05584	56941
85475	36857	43342	53988	53060	59533	38867	62300	08158	17983	16439	11458	18593	64952
28918	69578	88231	33276	70997	79936	56865	05859	90106	31595	01547	85590	91610	78188
63553	40961	48235	03427	49626	69445	18663	72695	52180	20847	12234	90511	33703	90322
09429	93969	52636	92737	88974	33488	36320	17617	30015	08272	84115	27156	30613	74952
10365	61129	87529	85689	48237	52267	67689	93394	01511	26358	85104	20285	29975	89868
07119	97336	71048	08178	77233	13916	47564	81056	97735	85977	29372	74461	28551	90707
51085	12765	51821	51259	77452	16308	60756	92144	49442	53900	70960	63990	75601	40719
02368	21382	52404	60268	89368	19885	55322	44819	01188	65255	64835	44919	05944	55157
01011	54092	33362	94904	31273	04146	18594	29852	71585	85030	51132	01915	92747	64951
52162	53916	46369	58586	23216	14513	83149	98736	23495	64350	94738	17752	35156	35749
07056	97628	33787	09998	42698	06691	76988	13602	51851	46104	88916	19509	25625	58104
48663	91245	85828	14346	09172	30168	90229	04734	59193	22178	30421	61666	99904	32812
54164	58492	22421	74103	47070	25306	76468	26384	58151	06646	21524	15227	96909	44592
32639	32363	05597	24200	13363	38005	94342	28728	35806	06912	17012	64161	18296	22851
29334	27001	87637	87308	58731	00256	45834	15398	46557	41135	10367	07684	36188	18510
02488	33062	28834	07351	19731	92420	60952	61280	50001	67658	32586	86679	50720	94953
81525	72295	04839	96423	24878	82651	66566	14778	76797	14780	13300	87074	79666	95725
29676	20591	68086	26432	46901	20849	89768	81536	86645	12659	92259	57102	80428	25280
00742	57392	39064	66432	84673	40027	32832	61362	98947	96067	64760	64584	96096	98253
05366	04213	25669	26422	44407	44048	37937	63904	45766	66134	75470	66520	34693	90449
91921	26418	64117	94305	26766	25940	39972	22209	71500	64568	91402	42416	07844	69618
00582	04711	87917	77341	42206	35126	74087	99547	81817	42607	43808	76655	62028	76630
00725	69884	62797	56170	86324	88072	76222	36086	84637	93161	76038	65855	77919	88006
69011	65797	95876	55293	18988	27354	26575	08625	40801	59920	29841	80150	12777	48501
25976	57948	29888	88604	67917	48708	18912	82271	65424	69774	33611	54262	85963	03547
09763	83473	73577	12908	30883	18317	28290	35797	05998	41688	34952	37888	38917	88050
91567	42595	27958	30134	04024	86385	29880	99730	55536	84855	29080	09250	79656	73211
17955	56349	90999	49127	20044	59931	06115	20542	18059	02008	73708	83517	36103	42791
46503	18584	18845	49618	02304	51038	20655	58727	28168	15475	56942	53389	20562	87338
92157	89634	94824	78171	84610	82834	09922	25417	44137	48413	25555	21246	35509	20468
14577	62765	35605	81263	39667	47358	56873	56307	61607	49518	89656	20103	77490	18062
98427	07523	33362	64270	01638	92477	66969	98420	04880	45585	46565	04102	46880	45709
34914	63976	88720	82765	34476	17032	87589	40836	32427	70002	70663	88863	77775	69348
70060	28277	39475	46473	23219	53416	94970	25832	69975	94884	19661	72828	00102	66794
53976	54914	06990	67245	68350	82948	11398	42878	80287	88267	47363	46634	06541	97809
76072	29515	40980	07391	58745	25774	22987	80059	39911	96189	41151	14222	60697	59583
90725	52210	83974	29992	65831	38857	50490	83765	55657	14361	31720	57375	56228	41546
64364	67412	33339	31926	14883	24413	59744	92351	97473	89286	35931	04110	23726	51900
08962	00358	31662	25388	61642	34072	81249	35648	56891	69352	48373	45578	78547	81788
95012	68379	93526	70765	10593	04542	76463	54328	02349	17247	28865	14777	62730	92277
15664	10493	20492	38391	91132	21999	59516	81652	27195	48223	46751	22923	32261	85653

Reprinted with permission from W. H. Beyer, *Handbook of Tables for Probability and Statistics,* 2nd ed. Copyright CRC Press, Boca Raton, Fla., 1986.

NEGATIVE *z* Scores

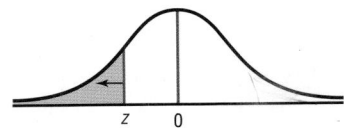

Table E-1	Standard Normal Distribution								

Cumulative Area to the Left of z score

z	0.00	0.01	0.02	0.03	0.04	0.05	0.06	0.07	0.08	0.09
−3.7	0.0001									
−3.6	0.0002	0.0002	0.0001	0.0001	0.0001	0.0001	0.0001	0.0001	0.0001	0.0001
−3.5	0.0002	0.0002	0.0002	0.0002	0.0002	0.0002	0.0002	0.0002	0.0002	0.0002
−3.4	0.0003	0.0003	0.0003	0.0003	0.0003	0.0003	0.0003	0.0003	0.0003	0.0002
−3.3	0.0005	0.0005	0.0005	0.0004	0.0004	0.0004	0.0004	0.0004	0.0004	0.0003
−3.2	0.0007	0.0007	0.0006	0.0006	0.0006	0.0006	0.0006	0.0005	0.0005	0.0005
−3.1	0.0010	0.0009	0.0009	0.0009	0.0008	0.0008	0.0008	0.0008	0.0007	0.0007
−3.0	0.0013	0.0013	0.0013	0.0012	0.0012	0.0011	0.0011	0.0011	0.0010	0.0010
−2.9	0.0019	0.0018	0.0018	0.0017	0.0016	0.0016	0.0015	0.0015	0.0014	0.0014
−2.8	0.0026	0.0025	0.0024	0.0023	0.0023	0.0022	0.0021	0.0021	0.0020	0.0019
−2.7	0.0035	0.0034	0.0033	0.0032	0.0031	0.0030	0.0029	0.0028	0.0027	0.0026
−2.6	0.0047	0.0045	0.0044	0.0043	0.0041	0.0040	0.0039	0.0038	0.0037	0.0036
−2.5	0.0062	0.0060	0.0059	0.0057	0.0055	0.0054	0.0052	0.0051 *	0.0049	0.0048
−2.4	0.0082	0.0080	0.0078	0.0075	0.0073	0.0071	0.0069	0.0068	0.0066	0.0064
−2.3	0.0107	0.0104	0.0102	0.0099	0.0096	0.0094	0.0091	0.0089	0.0087	0.0084
−2.2	0.0139	0.0136	0.0132	0.0129	0.0125	0.0122	0.0119	0.0116	0.0113	0.0110
−2.1	0.0179	0.0174	0.0170	0.0166	0.0162	0.0158	0.0154	0.0150	0.0146	0.0143
−2.0	0.0228	0.0222	0.0217	0.0212	0.0207	0.0202	0.0197	0.0192	0.0188	0.0183
−1.9	0.0287	0.0281	0.0274	0.0268	0.0262	0.0256	0.0250	0.0244	0.0239	0.0233
−1.8	0.0359	0.0351	0.0344	0.0336	0.0329	0.0322	0.0314	0.0307	0.0301	0.0294
−1.7	0.0446	0.0436	0.0427	0.0418	0.0409	0.0401	0.0392	0.0384	0.0375	0.0367
−1.6	0.0548	0.0537	0.0526	0.0516	0.0505 *	0.0495	0.0485	0.0475	0.0465	0.0455
−1.5	0.0668	0.0655	0.0643	0.0630	0.0618	0.0606	0.0594	0.0582	0.0571	0.0559
−1.4	0.0808	0.0793	0.0778	0.0764	0.0749	0.0735	0.0721	0.0708	0.0694	0.0681
−1.3	0.0968	0.0951	0.0934	0.0918	0.0901	0.0885	0.0869	0.0853	0.0838	0.0823
−1.2	0.1151	0.1131	0.1112	0.1093	0.1075	0.1056	0.1038	0.1020	0.1003	0.0985
−1.1	0.1357	0.1335	0.1314	0.1292	0.1271	0.1251	0.1230	0.1210	0.1190	0.1170
−1.0	0.1587	0.1562	0.1539	0.1515	0.1492	0.1469	0.1446	0.1423	0.1401	0.1379
−0.9	0.1841	0.1814	0.1788	0.1762	0.1736	0.1711	0.1685	0.1660	0.1635	0.1611
−0.8	0.2119	0.2090	0.2061	0.2033	0.2005	0.1977	0.1949	0.1922	0.1894	0.1867
−0.7	0.2420	0.2389	0.2358	0.2327	0.2296	0.2266	0.2236	0.2206	0.2177	0.2148
−0.6	0.2743	0.2709	0.2676	0.2643	0.2611	0.2578	0.2546	0.2514	0.2483	0.2451
−0.5	0.3085	0.3050	0.3015	0.2981	0.2946	0.2912	0.2877	0.2843	0.2810	0.2776
−0.4	0.3446	0.3409	0.3372	0.3336	0.3300	0.3264	0.3228	0.3192	0.3156	0.3121
−0.3	0.3821	0.3783	0.3745	0.3707	0.3669	0.3632	0.3594	0.3557	0.3520	0.3483
−0.2	0.4207	0.4168	0.4129	0.4090	0.4052	0.4013	0.3974	0.3936	0.3897	0.3859
−0.1	0.4602	0.4562	0.4522	0.4483	0.4443	0.4404	0.4364	0.4325	0.4286	0.4247
0.0	0.5000	0.4960	0.4920	0.4880	0.4840	0.4801	0.4761	0.4721	0.4681	0.4641

Note: For all values less than −3.70, use 0.0001 for the area.

z score	Area
−1.645	0.0500
−2.575	0.0050

POSITIVE z Scores

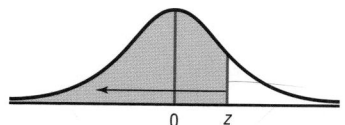

Table E-2	Standard Normal Distribution								
	Cumulative Area to the Left of z score								
z	0.00	0.01	0.02	0.03	0.04	0.05	0.06	0.07	0.08	0.09
0.0	0.5000	0.5040	0.5080	0.5120	0.5160	0.5199	0.5239	0.5279	0.5319	0.5359
0.1	0.5398	0.5438	0.5478	0.5517	0.5557	0.5596	0.5636	0.5675	0.5714	0.5753
0.2	0.5793	0.5832	0.5871	0.5910	0.5948	0.5987	0.6026	0.6064	0.6103	0.6141
0.3	0.6179	0.6217	0.6255	0.6293	0.6331	0.6368	0.6406	0.6443	0.6480	0.6517
0.4	0.6554	0.6591	0.6628	0.6664	0.6700	0.6736	0.6772	0.6808	0.6844	0.6879
0.5	0.6915	0.6950	0.6985	0.7019	0.7054	0.7088	0.7123	0.7157	0.7190	0.7224
0.6	0.7257	0.7291	0.7324	0.7357	0.7389	0.7422	0.7454	0.7486	0.7517	0.7549
0.7	0.7580	0.7611	0.7642	0.7673	0.7704	0.7734	0.7764	0.7794	0.7823	0.7852
0.8	0.7881	0.7910	0.7939	0.7967	0.7995	0.8023	0.8051	0.8078	0.8106	0.8133
0.9	0.8159	0.8186	0.8212	0.8238	0.8264	0.8289	0.8315	0.8340	0.8365	0.8389
1.0	0.8413	0.8438	0.8461	0.8485	0.8508	0.8531	0.8554	0.8577	0.8599	0.8621
1.1	0.8643	0.8665	0.8686	0.8708	0.8729	0.8749	0.8770	0.8790	0.8810	0.8830
1.2	0.8849	0.8869	0.8888	0.8907	0.8925	0.8944	0.8962	0.8980	0.8997	0.9015
1.3	0.9032	0.9049	0.9066	0.9082	0.9099	0.9115	0.9131	0.9147	0.9162	0.9177
1.4	0.9192	0.9207	0.9222	0.9236	0.9251	0.9265	0.9279	0.9292	0.9306	0.9319
1.5	0.9332	0.9345	0.9357	0.9370	0.9382	0.9394	0.9406	0.9418	0.9429	0.9441
1.6	0.9452	0.9463	0.9474	0.9484	0.9495 *	0.9505	0.9515	0.9525	0.9535	0.9545
1.7	0.9554	0.9564	0.9573	0.9582	0.9591	0.9599	0.9608	0.9616	0.9625	0.9633
1.8	0.9641	0.9649	0.9656	0.9664	0.9671	0.9678	0.9686	0.9693	0.9699	0.9706
1.9	0.9713	0.9719	0.9726	0.9732	0.9738	0.9744	0.9750	0.9756	0.9761	0.9767
2.0	0.9772	0.9778	0.9783	0.9788	0.9793	0.9798	0.9803	0.9808	0.9812	0.9817
2.1	0.9821	0.9826	0.9830	0.9834	0.9838	0.9842	0.9846	0.9850	0.9854	0.9857
2.2	0.9861	0.9864	0.9868	0.9871	0.9875	0.9878	0.9881	0.9884	0.9887	0.9890
2.3	0.9893	0.9896	0.9898	0.9901	0.9904	0.9906	0.9909	0.9911	0.9913	0.9916
2.4	0.9918	0.9920	0.9922	0.9925	0.9927	0.9929	0.9931	0.9932	0.9934	0.9936
2.5	0.9938	0.9940	0.9941	0.9943	0.9945	0.9946	0.9948	0.9949 *	0.9951	0.9952
2.6	0.9953	0.9955	0.9956	0.9957	0.9959	0.9960	0.9961	0.9962	0.9963	0.9964
2.7	0.9965	0.9966	0.9967	0.9968	0.9969	0.9970	0.9971	0.9972	0.9973	0.9974
2.8	0.9974	0.9975	0.9976	0.9977	0.9977	0.9978	0.9979	0.9979	0.9980	0.9981
2.9	0.9981	0.9982	0.9982	0.9983	0.9984	0.9984	0.9985	0.9985	0.9986	0.9986
3.0	0.9987	0.9987	0.9987	0.9988	0.9988	0.9989	0.9989	0.9989	0.9990	0.9990
3.1	0.9990	0.9991	0.9991	0.9991	0.9992	0.9992	0.9992	0.9992	0.9993	0.9993
3.2	0.9993	0.9993	0.9994	0.9994	0.9994	0.9994	0.9994	0.9995	0.9995	0.9995
3.3	0.9995	0.9995	0.9995	0.9996	0.9996	0.9996	0.9996	0.9996	0.9996	0.9997
3.4	0.9997	0.9997	0.9997	0.9997	0.9997	0.9997	0.9997	0.9997	0.9997	0.9998
3.5	0.9998	0.9998	0.9998	0.9998	0.9998	0.9998	0.9998	0.9998	0.9998	0.9998
3.6	0.9998	0.9998	0.9999	0.9999	0.9999	0.9999	0.9999	0.9999	0.9999	0.9999
3.7	0.9999									

Note: For all values greater than 3.70, use 0.9999 for the area.

z score	Area
1.645	0.9500
2.575	0.9950

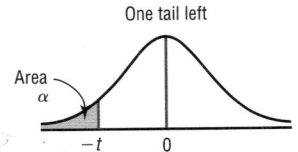

One tail left

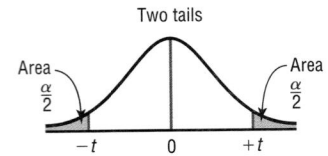

Two tails

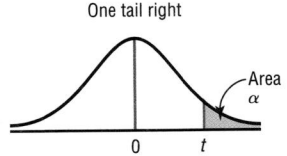

One tail right

Table F	*t* Distribution						
Degrees of freedom d.f.	**Confidence Intervals**	**50%**	**80%**	**90%**	**95%**	**98%**	**99%**
	One tail, α	**0.25**	**0.10**	**0.05**	**0.025**	**0.01**	**0.005**
	Two tails, α	**0.50**	**0.20**	**0.10**	**0.05**	**0.02**	**0.01**
1		1.000	3.078	6.314	12.706	31.821	63.657
2		0.816	1.886	2.920	4.303	6.965	9.925
3		0.765	1.638	2.353	3.182	4.541	5.841
4		0.741	1.533	2.132	2.776	3.747	4.604
5		0.727	1.476	2.015	2.571	3.365	4.032
6		0.718	1.440	1.943	2.447	3.143	3.707
7		0.711	1.415	1.895	2.365	2.998	3.499
8		0.706	1.397	1.860	2.306	2.896	3.355
9		0.703	1.383	1.833	2.262	2.821	3.250
10		0.700	1.372	1.812	2.228	2.764	3.169
11		0.697	1.363	1.796	2.201	2.718	3.106
12		0.695	1.356	1.782	2.179	2.681	3.055
13		0.694	1.350	1.771	2.160	2.650	3.012
14		0.692	1.345	1.761	2.145	2.624	2.977
15		0.691	1.341	1.753	2.131	2.602	2.947
16		0.690	1.337	1.746	2.120	2.583	2.921
17		0.689	1.333	1.740	2.110	2.567	2.898
18		0.688	1.330	1.734	2.101	2.552	2.878
19		0.688	1.328	1.729	2.093	2.539	2.861
20		0.687	1.325	1.725	2.086	2.528	2.845
21		0.686	1.323	1.721	2.080	2.518	2.831
22		0.686	1.321	1.717	2.074	2.508	2.819
23		0.685	1.319	1.714	2.069	2.500	2.807
24		0.685	1.318	1.711	2.064	2.492	2.797
25		0.684	1.316	1.708	2.060	2.485	2.787
26		0.684	1.315	1.706	2.056	2.479	2.779
27		0.684	1.314	1.703	2.052	2.473	2.771
28		0.683	1.313	1.701	2.048	2.467	2.763
29		0.683	1.311	1.699	2.045	2.462	2.756
30		0.683	1.310	1.697	2.042	2.457	2.750
35		0.682	1.306	1.690	2.030	2.438	2.724
40		0.681	1.303	1.684	2.021	2.423	2.704
50		0.679	1.299	1.676	2.009	2.403	2.678
75		0.678	1.293	1.665	1.992	2.377	2.643
100		0.677	1.290	1.660	1.984	2.364	2.626
200		0.676	1.286	1.653	1.972	2.345	2.601
500		0.675	1.283	1.648	1.965	2.334	2.586
1000		0.675	1.282	1.646	1.962	2.330	2.581
(*z*)∞		0.674	1.282	1.645	1.960	2.326	2.576

✈ **Please visit *Connect* for an expanded version of the *t* Distribution table.**

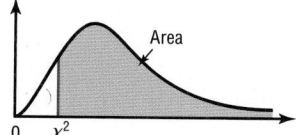

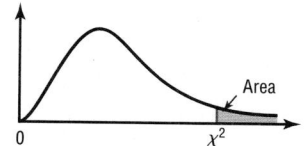

Table G	Chi-Square Distribution									
Degrees of freedom	**Area to the Right of Critical Value**									
	0.995	**0.99**	**0.975**	**0.95**	**0.90**	**0.10**	**0.05**	**0.025**	**0.01**	**0.005**
1	0.000	0.000	0.001	0.004	0.016	2.706	3.841	5.024	6.635	7.879
2	0.010	0.020	0.051	0.103	0.211	4.605	5.991	7.378	9.210	10.597
3	0.072	0.115	0.216	0.352	0.584	6.251	7.815	9.348	11.345	12.838
4	0.207	0.297	0.484	0.711	1.064	7.779	9.488	11.143	13.277	14.860
5	0.412	0.554	0.831	1.145	1.610	9.236	11.070	12.833	15.086	16.750
6	0.676	0.872	1.237	1.635	2.204	10.645	12.592	14.449	16.812	18.548
7	0.989	1.239	1.690	2.167	2.833	12.017	14.067	16.013	18.475	20.278
8	1.344	1.646	2.180	2.733	3.490	13.362	15.507	17.535	20.090	21.955
9	1.735	2.088	2.700	3.325	4.168	14.684	16.919	19.023	21.666	23.589
10	2.156	2.558	3.247	3.940	4.865	15.987	18.307	20.483	23.209	25.188
11	2.603	3.053	3.816	4.575	5.578	17.275	19.675	21.920	24.725	26.757
12	3.074	3.571	4.404	5.226	6.304	18.549	21.026	23.337	26.217	28.300
13	3.565	4.107	5.009	5.892	7.042	19.812	22.362	24.736	27.688	29.819
14	4.075	4.660	5.629	6.571	7.790	21.064	23.685	26.119	29.141	31.319
15	4.601	5.229	6.262	7.261	8.547	22.307	24.996	27.488	30.578	32.801
16	5.142	5.812	6.908	7.962	9.312	23.542	26.296	28.845	32.000	34.267
17	5.697	6.408	7.564	8.672	10.085	24.769	27.587	30.191	33.409	35.718
18	6.265	7.015	8.231	9.390	10.865	25.989	28.869	31.526	34.805	37.156
19	6.844	7.633	8.907	10.117	11.651	27.204	30.144	32.852	36.191	38.582
20	7.434	8.260	9.591	10.851	12.443	28.412	31.410	34.170	37.566	39.997
21	8.034	8.897	10.283	11.591	13.240	29.615	32.671	35.479	38.932	41.401
22	8.643	9.542	10.982	12.338	14.041	30.813	33.924	36.781	40.289	42.796
23	9.260	10.196	11.689	13.091	14.848	32.007	35.172	38.076	41.638	44.181
24	9.886	10.856	12.401	13.848	15.659	33.196	36.415	39.364	42.980	45.559
25	10.520	11.524	13.120	14.611	16.473	34.382	37.652	40.646	44.314	46.928
26	11.160	12.198	13.844	15.379	17.292	35.563	38.885	41.923	45.642	48.290
27	11.808	12.879	14.573	16.151	18.114	36.741	40.113	43.195	46.963	49.645
28	12.461	13.565	15.308	16.928	18.939	37.916	41.337	44.461	48.278	50.993
29	13.121	14.256	16.047	17.708	19.768	39.087	42.557	45.722	49.588	52.336
30	13.787	14.953	16.791	18.493	20.599	40.256	43.773	46.979	50.892	53.672
40	20.707	22.164	24.433	26.509	29.051	51.805	55.758	59.342	63.691	66.766
50	27.991	29.707	32.357	34.764	37.689	63.167	67.505	71.420	76.154	79.490
60	35.534	37.485	40.482	43.188	46.459	74.397	79.082	83.298	88.379	91.952
70	43.275	45.442	48.758	51.739	55.329	85.527	90.531	95.023	100.425	104.215
80	51.172	53.540	57.153	60.391	64.278	96.578	101.879	106.629	112.329	116.321
90	59.196	61.754	65.647	69.126	73.291	107.565	113.145	118.136	124.116	128.299
100	67.328	70.065	74.222	77.929	82.358	118.498	124.342	129.561	135.807	140.169

Source: Donald B. Owen, *Handbook of Statistics Tables,* The Chi-Square Distribution Table, © 1962 by Addison-Wesley Publishing Company, Inc. Copyright renewal © 1990. Reprinted by permission of Pearson Education, Inc.

Table H   **F Distribution**

α = 0.005

d.f.N.: degrees of freedom, numerator

d.f.D.: degrees of freedom, denominator	1	2	3	4	5	6	7	8	9	10	12	15	20	24	30	40	60	120	∞
1	16,211	20,000	21,615	22,500	23,056	23,437	23,715	23,925	24,091	24,224	24,426	24,630	24,836	24,940	25,044	25,148	25,253	25,359	25,465
2	198.5	199.0	199.2	199.2	199.3	199.3	199.4	199.4	199.4	199.4	199.4	199.4	199.4	199.5	199.5	199.5	199.5	199.5	199.5
3	55.55	49.80	47.47	46.19	45.39	44.84	44.43	44.13	43.88	43.69	43.39	43.08	42.78	42.62	42.47	42.31	42.15	41.99	41.83
4	31.33	26.28	24.26	23.15	22.46	21.97	21.62	21.35	21.14	20.97	20.70	20.44	20.17	20.03	19.89	19.75	19.61	19.47	19.32
5	22.78	18.31	16.53	15.56	14.94	14.51	14.20	13.96	13.77	13.62	13.38	13.15	12.90	12.78	12.66	12.53	12.40	12.27	12.14
6	18.63	14.54	12.92	12.03	11.46	11.07	10.79	10.57	10.39	10.25	10.03	9.81	9.59	9.47	9.36	9.24	9.12	9.00	8.88
7	16.24	12.40	10.88	10.05	9.52	9.16	8.89	8.68	8.51	8.38	8.18	7.97	7.75	7.65	7.53	7.42	7.31	7.19	7.08
8	14.69	11.04	9.60	8.81	8.30	7.95	7.69	7.50	7.34	7.21	7.01	6.81	6.61	6.50	6.40	6.29	6.18	6.06	5.95
9	13.61	10.11	8.72	7.96	7.47	7.13	6.88	6.69	6.54	6.42	6.23	6.03	5.83	5.73	5.62	5.52	5.41	5.30	5.19
10	12.83	9.43	8.08	7.34	6.87	6.54	6.30	6.12	5.97	5.85	5.66	5.47	5.27	5.17	5.07	4.97	4.86	4.75	4.64
11	12.23	8.91	7.60	6.88	6.42	6.10	5.86	5.68	5.54	5.42	5.24	5.05	4.86	4.76	4.65	4.55	4.44	4.34	4.23
12	11.75	8.51	7.23	6.52	6.07	5.76	5.52	5.35	5.20	5.09	4.91	4.72	4.53	4.43	4.33	4.23	4.12	4.01	3.90
13	11.37	8.19	6.93	6.23	5.79	5.48	5.25	5.08	4.94	4.82	4.64	4.46	4.27	4.17	4.07	3.97	3.87	3.76	3.65
14	11.06	7.92	6.68	6.00	5.56	5.26	5.03	4.86	4.72	4.60	4.43	4.25	4.06	3.96	3.86	3.76	3.66	3.55	3.44
15	10.80	7.70	6.48	5.80	5.37	5.07	4.85	4.67	4.54	4.42	4.25	4.07	3.88	3.79	3.69	3.58	3.48	3.37	3.26
16	10.58	7.51	6.30	5.64	5.21	4.91	4.69	4.52	4.38	4.27	4.10	3.92	3.73	3.64	3.54	3.44	3.33	3.22	3.11
17	10.38	7.35	6.16	5.50	5.07	4.78	4.56	4.39	4.25	4.14	3.97	3.79	3.61	3.51	3.41	3.31	3.21	3.10	2.98
18	10.22	7.21	6.03	5.37	4.96	4.66	4.44	4.28	4.14	4.03	3.86	3.68	3.50	3.40	3.30	3.20	3.10	2.99	2.87
19	10.07	7.09	5.92	5.27	4.85	4.56	4.34	4.18	4.04	3.93	3.76	3.59	3.40	3.31	3.21	3.11	3.00	2.89	2.78
20	9.94	6.99	5.82	5.17	4.76	4.47	4.26	4.09	3.96	3.85	3.68	3.50	3.32	3.22	3.12	3.02	2.92	2.81	2.69
21	9.83	6.89	5.73	5.09	4.68	4.39	4.18	4.01	3.88	3.77	3.60	3.43	3.24	3.15	3.05	2.95	2.84	2.73	2.61
22	9.73	6.81	5.65	5.02	4.61	4.32	4.11	3.94	3.81	3.70	3.54	3.36	3.18	3.08	2.98	2.88	2.77	2.66	2.55
23	9.63	6.73	5.58	4.95	4.54	4.26	4.05	3.88	3.75	3.64	3.47	3.30	3.12	3.02	2.92	2.82	2.71	2.60	2.48
24	9.55	6.66	5.52	4.89	4.49	4.20	3.99	3.83	3.69	3.59	3.42	3.25	3.06	2.97	2.87	2.77	2.66	2.55	2.43
25	9.48	6.60	5.46	4.84	4.43	4.15	3.94	3.78	3.64	3.54	3.37	3.20	3.01	2.92	2.82	2.72	2.61	2.50	2.38
26	9.41	6.54	5.41	4.79	4.38	4.10	3.89	3.73	3.60	3.49	3.33	3.15	2.97	2.87	2.77	2.67	2.56	2.45	2.33
27	9.34	6.49	5.36	4.74	4.34	4.06	3.85	3.69	3.56	3.45	3.28	3.11	2.93	2.83	2.73	2.63	2.52	2.41	2.25
28	9.28	6.44	5.32	4.70	4.30	4.02	3.81	3.65	3.52	3.41	3.25	3.07	2.89	2.79	2.69	2.59	2.48	2.37	2.29
29	9.23	6.40	5.28	4.66	4.26	3.98	3.77	3.61	3.48	3.38	3.21	3.04	2.86	2.76	2.66	2.56	2.45	2.33	2.24
30	9.18	6.35	5.24	4.62	4.23	3.95	3.74	3.58	3.45	3.34	3.18	3.01	2.82	2.73	2.63	2.52	2.42	2.30	2.18
40	8.83	6.07	4.98	4.37	3.99	3.71	3.51	3.35	3.22	3.12	2.95	2.78	2.60	2.50	2.40	2.30	2.18	2.06	1.93
60	8.49	5.79	4.73	4.14	3.76	3.49	3.29	3.13	3.01	2.90	2.74	2.57	2.39	2.29	2.19	2.08	1.96	1.83	1.69
120	8.18	5.54	4.50	3.92	3.55	3.28	3.09	2.93	2.81	2.71	2.54	2.37	2.19	2.09	1.98	1.87	1.75	1.61	1.43
∞	7.88	5.30	4.28	3.72	3.35	3.09	2.90	2.74	2.62	2.52	2.36	2.19	2.00	1.90	1.79	1.67	1.53	1.36	1.00

Table H (continued)

$\alpha = 0.01$

d.f.D: degrees of freedom, denominator	\multicolumn{19}{c}{d.f.N.: degrees of freedom, numerator}
	1	2	3	4	5	6	7	8	9	10	12	15	20	24	30	40	60	120	∞
---	---	---	---	---	---	---	---	---	---	---	---	---	---	---	---	---	---	---	---
1	4052	4999.5	5403	5625	5764	5859	5928	5982	6022	6056	6106	6157	6209	6235	6261	6287	6313	6339	6366
2	98.50	99.00	99.17	99.25	99.30	99.33	99.36	99.37	99.39	99.40	99.42	99.43	99.45	99.46	99.47	99.47	99.48	99.49	99.50
3	34.12	30.82	29.46	28.71	28.24	27.91	27.67	27.49	27.35	27.23	27.05	26.87	26.69	26.60	26.50	26.41	26.32	26.22	26.13
4	21.20	18.00	16.69	15.98	15.52	15.21	14.98	14.80	14.66	14.55	14.37	14.20	14.02	13.93	13.84	13.75	13.65	13.56	13.46
5	16.26	13.27	12.06	11.39	10.97	10.67	10.46	10.29	10.16	10.05	9.89	9.72	9.55	9.47	9.38	9.29	9.20	9.11	9.02
6	13.75	10.92	9.78	9.15	8.75	8.47	8.26	8.10	7.98	7.87	7.72	7.56	7.40	7.31	7.23	7.14	7.06	6.97	6.88
7	12.25	9.55	8.45	7.85	7.46	7.19	6.99	6.84	6.72	6.62	6.47	6.31	6.16	6.07	5.99	5.91	5.82	5.74	5.65
8	11.26	8.65	7.59	7.01	6.63	6.37	6.18	6.03	5.91	5.81	5.67	5.52	5.36	5.28	5.20	5.12	5.03	4.95	4.86
9	10.56	8.02	6.99	6.42	6.06	5.80	5.61	5.47	5.35	5.26	5.11	4.96	4.81	4.73	4.65	4.57	4.48	4.40	4.31
10	10.04	7.56	6.55	5.99	5.64	5.39	5.20	5.06	4.94	4.85	4.71	4.56	4.41	4.33	4.25	4.17	4.08	4.00	3.91
11	9.65	7.21	6.22	5.67	5.32	5.07	4.89	4.74	4.63	4.54	4.40	4.25	4.10	4.02	3.94	3.86	3.78	3.69	3.60
12	9.33	6.93	5.95	5.41	5.06	4.82	4.64	4.50	4.39	4.30	4.16	4.01	3.86	3.78	3.70	3.62	3.54	3.45	3.36
13	9.07	6.70	5.74	5.21	4.86	4.62	4.44	4.30	4.19	4.10	3.96	3.82	3.66	3.59	3.51	3.43	3.34	3.25	3.17
14	8.86	6.51	5.56	5.04	4.69	4.46	4.28	4.14	4.03	3.94	3.80	3.66	3.51	3.43	3.35	3.27	3.18	3.09	3.00
15	8.68	6.36	5.42	4.89	4.56	4.32	4.14	4.00	3.89	3.80	3.67	3.52	3.37	3.29	3.21	3.13	3.05	2.96	2.87
16	8.53	6.23	5.29	4.77	4.44	4.20	4.03	3.89	3.78	3.69	3.55	3.41	3.26	3.18	3.10	3.02	2.93	2.84	2.75
17	8.40	6.11	5.18	4.67	4.34	4.10	3.93	3.79	3.68	3.59	3.46	3.31	3.16	3.08	3.00	2.92	2.83	2.75	2.65
18	8.29	6.01	5.09	4.58	4.25	4.01	3.84	3.71	3.60	3.51	3.37	3.23	3.08	3.00	2.92	2.84	2.75	2.66	2.57
19	8.18	5.93	5.01	4.50	4.17	3.94	3.77	3.63	3.52	3.43	3.30	3.15	3.00	2.92	2.84	2.76	2.67	2.58	2.49
20	8.10	5.85	4.94	4.43	4.10	3.87	3.70	3.56	3.46	3.37	3.23	3.09	2.94	2.86	2.78	2.69	2.61	2.52	2.42
21	8.02	5.78	4.87	4.37	4.04	3.81	3.64	3.51	3.40	3.31	3.17	3.03	2.88	2.80	2.72	2.64	2.55	2.46	2.36
22	7.95	5.72	4.82	4.31	3.99	3.76	3.59	3.45	3.35	3.26	3.12	2.98	2.83	2.75	2.67	2.58	2.50	2.40	2.31
23	7.88	5.66	4.76	4.26	3.94	3.71	3.54	3.41	3.30	3.21	3.07	2.93	2.78	2.70	2.62	2.54	2.45	2.35	2.26
24	7.82	5.61	4.72	4.22	3.90	3.67	3.50	3.36	3.26	3.17	3.03	2.89	2.74	2.66	2.58	2.49	2.40	2.31	2.21
25	7.77	5.57	4.68	4.18	3.85	3.63	3.46	3.32	3.22	3.13	2.99	2.85	2.70	2.62	2.54	2.45	2.36	2.27	2.17
26	7.72	5.53	4.64	4.14	3.82	3.59	3.42	3.29	3.18	3.09	2.96	2.81	2.66	2.58	2.50	2.42	2.33	2.23	2.13
27	7.68	5.49	4.60	4.11	3.78	3.56	3.39	3.26	3.15	3.06	2.93	2.78	2.63	2.55	2.47	2.38	2.29	2.20	2.10
28	7.64	5.45	4.57	4.07	3.75	3.53	3.36	3.23	3.12	3.03	2.90	2.75	2.60	2.52	2.44	2.35	2.26	2.17	2.06
29	7.60	5.42	4.54	4.04	3.73	3.50	3.33	3.20	3.09	3.00	2.87	2.73	2.57	2.49	2.41	2.33	2.23	2.14	2.03
30	7.56	5.39	4.51	4.02	3.70	3.47	3.30	3.17	3.07	2.98	2.84	2.70	2.55	2.47	2.39	2.30	2.21	2.11	2.01
40	7.31	5.18	4.31	3.83	3.51	3.29	3.12	2.99	2.89	2.80	2.66	2.52	2.37	2.29	2.20	2.11	2.02	1.92	1.80
60	7.08	4.98	4.13	3.65	3.34	3.12	2.95	2.82	2.72	2.63	2.50	2.35	2.20	2.12	2.03	1.94	1.84	1.73	1.60
120	6.85	4.79	3.95	3.48	3.17	2.96	2.79	2.66	2.56	2.47	2.34	2.19	2.03	1.95	1.86	1.76	1.66	1.53	1.38
∞	6.63	4.61	3.78	3.32	3.02	2.80	2.64	2.51	2.41	2.32	2.18	2.04	1.88	1.79	1.70	1.59	1.47	1.32	1.00

Table H (continued)

α = 0.025

d.f.N.: degrees of freedom, numerator

d.f.D.: degrees of freedom, denominator	1	2	3	4	5	6	7	8	9	10	12	15	20	24	30	40	60	120	∞
1	647.8	799.5	864.2	899.6	921.8	937.1	948.2	956.7	963.3	968.6	976.7	984.9	993.1	997.2	1001	1006	1010	1014	1018
2	38.51	39.00	39.17	39.25	39.30	39.33	39.36	39.37	39.39	39.40	39.41	39.43	39.45	39.46	39.46	39.47	39.48	39.49	39.50
3	17.44	16.04	15.44	15.10	14.88	14.73	14.62	14.54	14.47	14.42	14.34	14.25	14.17	14.12	14.08	14.04	13.99	13.95	13.90
4	12.22	10.65	9.98	9.60	9.36	9.20	9.07	8.98	8.90	8.84	8.75	8.66	8.56	8.51	8.46	8.41	8.36	8.31	8.26
5	10.01	8.43	7.76	7.39	7.15	6.98	6.85	6.76	6.68	6.62	6.52	6.43	6.33	6.28	6.23	6.18	6.12	6.07	6.02
6	8.81	7.26	6.60	6.23	5.99	5.82	5.70	5.60	5.52	5.46	5.37	5.27	5.17	5.12	5.07	5.01	4.96	4.90	4.85
7	8.07	6.54	5.89	5.52	5.29	5.12	4.99	4.90	4.82	4.76	4.67	4.57	4.47	4.42	4.36	4.31	4.25	4.20	4.14
8	7.57	6.06	5.42	5.05	4.82	4.65	4.53	4.43	4.36	4.30	4.20	4.10	4.00	3.95	3.89	3.84	3.78	3.73	3.67
9	7.21	5.71	5.08	4.72	4.48	4.32	4.20	4.10	4.03	3.96	3.87	3.77	3.67	3.61	3.56	3.51	3.45	3.39	3.33
10	6.94	5.46	4.83	4.47	4.24	4.07	3.95	3.85	3.78	3.72	3.62	3.52	3.42	3.37	3.31	3.26	3.20	3.14	3.08
11	6.72	5.26	4.63	4.28	4.04	3.88	3.76	3.66	3.59	3.53	3.43	3.33	3.23	3.17	3.12	3.06	3.00	2.94	2.88
12	6.55	5.10	4.47	4.12	3.89	3.73	3.61	3.51	3.44	3.37	3.28	3.18	3.07	3.02	2.96	2.91	2.85	2.79	2.72
13	6.41	4.97	4.35	4.00	3.77	3.60	3.48	3.39	3.31	3.25	3.15	3.05	2.95	2.89	2.84	2.78	2.72	2.66	2.60
14	6.30	4.86	4.24	3.89	3.66	3.50	3.38	3.29	3.21	3.15	3.05	2.95	2.84	2.79	2.73	2.67	2.61	2.55	2.49
15	6.20	4.77	4.15	3.80	3.58	3.41	3.29	3.20	3.12	3.06	2.96	2.86	2.76	2.70	2.64	2.59	2.52	2.46	2.40
16	6.12	4.69	4.08	3.73	3.50	3.34	3.22	3.12	3.05	2.99	2.89	2.79	2.68	2.63	2.57	2.51	2.45	2.38	2.32
17	6.04	4.62	4.01	3.66	3.44	3.28	3.16	3.06	2.98	2.92	2.82	2.72	2.62	2.56	2.50	2.44	2.38	2.32	2.25
18	5.98	4.56	3.95	3.61	3.38	3.22	3.10	3.01	2.93	2.87	2.77	2.67	2.56	2.50	2.44	2.38	2.32	2.26	2.19
19	5.92	4.51	3.90	3.56	3.33	3.17	3.05	2.96	2.88	2.82	2.72	2.62	2.51	2.45	2.39	2.33	2.27	2.20	2.13
20	5.87	4.46	3.86	3.51	3.29	3.13	3.01	2.91	2.84	2.77	2.68	2.57	2.46	2.41	2.35	2.29	2.22	2.16	2.09
21	5.83	4.42	3.82	3.48	3.25	3.09	2.97	2.87	2.80	2.73	2.64	2.53	2.42	2.37	2.31	2.25	2.18	2.11	2.04
22	5.79	4.38	3.78	3.44	3.22	3.05	2.93	2.84	2.76	2.70	2.60	2.50	2.39	2.33	2.27	2.21	2.14	2.08	2.00
23	5.75	4.35	3.75	3.41	3.18	3.02	2.90	2.81	2.73	2.67	2.57	2.47	2.36	2.30	2.24	2.18	2.11	2.04	1.97
24	5.72	4.32	3.72	3.38	3.15	2.99	2.87	2.78	2.70	2.64	2.54	2.44	2.33	2.27	2.21	2.15	2.08	2.01	1.94
25	5.69	4.29	3.69	3.35	3.13	2.97	2.85	2.75	2.68	2.61	2.51	2.41	2.30	2.24	2.18	2.12	2.05	1.98	1.91
26	5.66	4.27	3.67	3.33	3.10	2.94	2.82	2.73	2.65	2.59	2.49	2.39	2.28	2.22	2.16	2.09	2.03	1.95	1.88
27	5.63	4.24	3.65	3.31	3.08	2.92	2.80	2.71	2.63	2.57	2.47	2.36	2.25	2.19	2.13	2.07	2.00	1.93	1.85
28	5.61	4.22	3.63	3.29	3.06	2.90	2.78	2.69	2.61	2.55	2.45	2.34	2.23	2.17	2.11	2.05	1.98	1.91	1.83
29	5.59	4.20	3.61	3.27	3.04	2.88	2.76	2.67	2.59	2.53	2.43	2.32	2.21	2.15	2.09	2.03	1.96	1.89	1.81
30	5.57	4.18	3.59	3.25	3.03	2.87	2.75	2.65	2.57	2.51	2.41	2.31	2.20	2.14	2.07	2.01	1.94	1.87	1.79
40	5.42	4.05	3.46	3.13	2.90	2.74	2.62	2.53	2.45	2.39	2.29	2.18	2.07	2.01	1.94	1.88	1.80	1.72	1.64
60	5.29	3.93	3.34	3.01	2.79	2.63	2.51	2.41	2.33	2.27	2.17	2.06	1.94	1.88	1.82	1.74	1.67	1.58	1.48
120	5.15	3.80	3.23	2.89	2.67	2.52	2.39	2.30	2.22	2.16	2.05	1.94	1.82	1.76	1.69	1.61	1.53	1.43	1.31
∞	5.02	3.69	3.12	2.79	2.57	2.41	2.29	2.19	2.11	2.05	1.94	1.83	1.71	1.64	1.57	1.48	1.39	1.27	1.00

Table H (continued)

α = 0.05

d.f.D.: degrees of freedom, denominator	d.f.N.: degrees of freedom, numerator																		
	1	2	3	4	5	6	7	8	9	10	12	15	20	24	30	40	60	120	∞
1	161.4	199.5	215.7	224.6	230.2	234.0	236.8	238.9	240.5	241.9	243.9	245.9	248.0	249.1	250.1	251.1	252.2	253.3	254.3
2	18.51	19.00	19.16	19.25	19.30	19.33	19.35	19.37	19.38	19.40	19.41	19.43	19.45	19.45	19.46	19.47	19.48	19.49	19.50
3	10.13	9.55	9.28	9.12	9.01	8.94	8.89	8.85	8.81	8.79	8.74	8.70	8.66	8.64	8.62	8.59	8.57	8.55	8.53
4	7.71	6.94	6.59	6.39	6.26	6.16	6.09	6.04	6.00	5.96	5.91	5.86	5.80	5.77	5.75	5.72	5.69	5.66	5.63
5	6.61	5.79	5.41	5.19	5.05	4.95	4.88	4.82	4.77	4.74	4.68	4.62	4.56	4.53	4.50	4.46	4.43	4.40	4.36
6	5.99	5.14	4.76	4.53	4.39	4.28	4.21	4.15	4.10	4.06	4.00	3.94	3.87	3.84	3.81	3.77	3.74	3.70	3.67
7	5.59	4.74	4.35	4.12	3.97	3.87	3.79	3.73	3.68	3.64	3.57	3.51	3.44	3.41	3.38	3.34	3.30	3.27	3.23
8	5.32	4.46	4.07	3.84	3.69	3.58	3.50	3.44	3.39	3.35	3.28	3.22	3.15	3.12	3.08	3.04	3.01	2.97	2.93
9	5.12	4.26	3.86	3.63	3.48	3.37	3.29	3.23	3.18	3.14	3.07	3.01	2.94	2.90	2.86	2.83	2.79	2.75	2.71
10	4.96	4.10	3.71	3.48	3.33	3.22	3.14	3.07	3.02	2.98	2.91	2.85	2.77	2.74	2.70	2.66	2.62	2.58	2.54
11	4.84	3.98	3.59	3.36	3.20	3.09	3.01	2.95	2.90	2.85	2.79	2.72	2.65	2.61	2.57	2.53	2.49	2.45	2.40
12	4.75	3.89	3.49	3.26	3.11	3.00	2.91	2.85	2.80	2.75	2.69	2.62	2.54	2.51	2.47	2.43	2.38	2.34	2.30
13	4.67	3.81	3.41	3.18	3.03	2.92	2.83	2.77	2.71	2.67	2.60	2.53	2.46	2.42	2.38	2.34	2.30	2.25	2.21
14	4.60	3.74	3.34	3.11	2.96	2.85	2.76	2.70	2.65	2.60	2.53	2.46	2.39	2.35	2.31	2.27	2.22	2.18	2.13
15	4.54	3.68	3.29	3.06	2.90	2.79	2.71	2.64	2.59	2.54	2.48	2.40	2.33	2.29	2.25	2.20	2.16	2.11	2.07
16	4.49	3.63	3.24	3.01	2.85	2.74	2.66	2.59	2.54	2.49	2.42	2.35	2.28	2.24	2.19	2.15	2.11	2.06	2.01
17	4.45	3.59	3.20	2.96	2.81	2.70	2.61	2.55	2.49	2.45	2.38	2.31	2.23	2.19	2.15	2.10	2.06	2.01	1.96
18	4.41	3.55	3.16	2.93	2.77	2.66	2.58	2.51	2.46	2.41	2.34	2.27	2.19	2.15	2.11	2.06	2.02	1.97	1.92
19	4.38	3.52	3.13	2.90	2.74	2.63	2.54	2.48	2.42	2.38	2.31	2.23	2.16	2.11	2.07	2.03	1.98	1.93	1.88
20	4.35	3.49	3.10	2.87	2.71	2.60	2.51	2.45	2.39	2.35	2.28	2.20	2.12	2.08	2.04	1.99	1.95	1.90	1.84
21	4.32	3.47	3.07	2.84	2.68	2.57	2.49	2.42	2.37	2.32	2.25	2.18	2.10	2.05	2.01	1.96	1.92	1.87	1.81
22	4.30	3.44	3.05	2.82	2.66	2.55	2.46	2.40	2.34	2.30	2.23	2.15	2.07	2.03	1.98	1.94	1.89	1.84	1.78
23	4.28	3.42	3.03	2.80	2.64	2.53	2.44	2.37	2.32	2.27	2.20	2.13	2.05	2.01	1.96	1.91	1.86	1.81	1.76
24	4.26	3.40	3.01	2.78	2.62	2.51	2.42	2.36	2.30	2.25	2.18	2.11	2.03	1.98	1.94	1.89	1.84	1.79	1.73
25	4.24	3.39	2.99	2.76	2.60	2.49	2.40	2.34	2.28	2.24	2.16	2.09	2.01	1.96	1.92	1.87	1.82	1.77	1.71
26	4.23	3.37	2.98	2.74	2.59	2.47	2.39	2.32	2.27	2.22	2.15	2.07	1.99	1.95	1.90	1.85	1.80	1.75	1.69
27	4.21	3.35	2.96	2.73	2.57	2.46	2.37	2.31	2.25	2.20	2.13	2.06	1.97	1.93	1.88	1.84	1.79	1.73	1.67
28	4.20	3.34	2.95	2.71	2.56	2.45	2.36	2.29	2.24	2.19	2.12	2.04	1.96	1.91	1.87	1.82	1.77	1.71	1.65
29	4.18	3.33	2.93	2.70	2.55	2.43	2.35	2.28	2.22	2.18	2.10	2.03	1.94	1.90	1.85	1.81	1.75	1.70	1.64
30	4.17	3.32	2.92	2.69	2.53	2.42	2.33	2.27	2.21	2.16	2.09	2.01	1.93	1.89	1.84	1.79	1.74	1.68	1.62
40	4.08	3.23	2.84	2.61	2.45	2.34	2.25	2.18	2.12	2.08	2.00	1.92	1.84	1.79	1.74	1.69	1.64	1.58	1.51
60	4.00	3.15	2.76	2.53	2.37	2.25	2.17	2.10	2.04	1.99	1.92	1.84	1.75	1.70	1.65	1.59	1.53	1.47	1.39
120	3.92	3.07	2.68	2.45	2.29	2.17	2.09	2.02	1.96	1.91	1.83	1.75	1.66	1.61	1.55	1.50	1.43	1.35	1.25
∞	3.84	3.00	2.60	2.37	2.21	2.10	2.01	1.94	1.88	1.83	1.75	1.67	1.57	1.52	1.46	1.39	1.32	1.22	1.00

Table H (concluded)

$\alpha = 0.10$

	d.f.N: degrees of freedom, numerator																		
d.f.D.: degrees of freedom, denominator	1	2	3	4	5	6	7	8	9	10	12	15	20	24	30	40	60	120	∞
1	39.86	49.50	53.59	55.83	57.24	58.20	58.91	59.44	59.86	60.19	60.71	61.22	61.74	62.00	62.26	62.53	62.79	63.06	63.33
2	8.53	9.00	9.16	9.24	9.29	9.33	9.35	9.37	9.38	9.39	9.41	9.42	9.44	9.45	9.46	9.47	9.47	9.48	9.49
3	5.54	5.46	5.39	5.34	5.31	5.28	5.27	5.25	5.24	5.23	5.22	5.20	5.18	5.18	5.17	5.16	5.15	5.14	5.13
4	4.54	4.32	4.19	4.11	4.05	4.01	3.98	3.95	3.94	3.92	3.90	3.87	3.84	3.83	3.82	3.80	3.79	3.78	3.76
5	4.06	3.78	3.62	3.52	3.45	3.40	3.37	3.34	3.32	3.30	3.27	3.24	3.21	3.19	3.17	3.16	3.14	3.12	3.10
6	3.78	3.46	3.29	3.18	3.11	3.05	3.01	2.98	2.96	2.94	2.90	2.87	2.84	2.82	2.80	2.78	2.76	2.74	2.72
7	3.59	3.26	3.07	2.96	2.88	2.83	2.78	2.75	2.72	2.70	2.67	2.63	2.59	2.58	2.56	2.54	2.51	2.49	2.47
8	3.46	3.11	2.92	2.81	2.73	2.67	2.62	2.59	2.56	2.54	2.50	2.46	2.42	2.40	2.38	2.36	2.34	2.32	2.29
9	3.36	3.01	2.81	2.69	2.61	2.55	2.51	2.47	2.44	2.42	2.38	2.34	2.30	2.28	2.25	2.23	2.21	2.18	2.16
10	3.29	2.92	2.73	2.61	2.52	2.46	2.41	2.38	2.35	2.32	2.28	2.24	2.20	2.18	2.16	2.13	2.11	2.08	2.06
11	3.23	2.86	2.66	2.54	2.45	2.39	2.34	2.30	2.27	2.25	2.21	2.17	2.12	2.10	2.08	2.05	2.03	2.00	1.97
12	3.18	2.81	2.61	2.48	2.39	2.33	2.28	2.24	2.21	2.19	2.15	2.10	2.06	2.04	2.01	1.99	1.96	1.93	1.90
13	3.14	2.76	2.56	2.43	2.35	2.28	2.23	2.20	2.16	2.14	2.10	2.05	2.01	1.98	1.96	1.93	1.90	1.88	1.85
14	3.10	2.73	2.52	2.39	2.31	2.24	2.19	2.15	2.12	2.10	2.05	2.01	1.96	1.94	1.91	1.89	1.86	1.83	1.80
15	3.07	2.70	2.49	2.36	2.27	2.21	2.16	2.12	2.09	2.06	2.02	1.97	1.92	1.90	1.87	1.85	1.82	1.79	1.76
16	3.05	2.67	2.46	2.33	2.24	2.18	2.13	2.09	2.06	2.03	1.99	1.94	1.89	1.87	1.84	1.81	1.78	1.75	1.72
17	3.03	2.64	2.44	2.31	2.22	2.15	2.10	2.06	2.03	2.00	1.96	1.91	1.86	1.84	1.81	1.78	1.75	1.72	1.69
18	3.01	2.62	2.42	2.29	2.20	2.13	2.08	2.04	2.00	1.98	1.93	1.89	1.84	1.81	1.78	1.75	1.72	1.69	1.66
19	2.99	2.61	2.40	2.27	2.18	2.11	2.06	2.02	1.98	1.96	1.91	1.86	1.81	1.79	1.76	1.73	1.70	1.67	1.63
20	2.97	2.59	2.38	2.25	2.16	2.09	2.04	2.00	1.96	1.94	1.89	1.84	1.79	1.77	1.74	1.71	1.68	1.64	1.61
21	2.96	2.57	2.36	2.23	2.14	2.08	2.02	1.98	1.95	1.92	1.87	1.83	1.78	1.75	1.72	1.69	1.66	1.62	1.59
22	2.95	2.56	2.35	2.22	2.13	2.06	2.01	1.97	1.93	1.90	1.86	1.81	1.76	1.73	1.70	1.67	1.64	1.60	1.57
23	2.94	2.55	2.34	2.21	2.11	2.05	1.99	1.95	1.92	1.89	1.84	1.80	1.74	1.72	1.69	1.66	1.62	1.59	1.55
24	2.93	2.54	2.33	2.19	2.10	2.04	1.98	1.94	1.91	1.88	1.83	1.78	1.73	1.70	1.67	1.64	1.61	1.57	1.53
25	2.92	2.53	2.32	2.18	2.09	2.02	1.97	1.93	1.89	1.87	1.82	1.77	1.72	1.69	1.66	1.63	1.59	1.56	1.52
26	2.91	2.52	2.31	2.17	2.08	2.01	1.96	1.92	1.88	1.86	1.81	1.76	1.71	1.68	1.65	1.61	1.58	1.54	1.50
27	2.90	2.51	2.30	2.17	2.07	2.00	1.95	1.91	1.87	1.85	1.80	1.75	1.70	1.67	1.64	1.60	1.57	1.53	1.49
28	2.89	2.50	2.29	2.16	2.06	2.00	1.94	1.90	1.87	1.84	1.79	1.74	1.69	1.66	1.63	1.59	1.56	1.52	1.48
29	2.89	2.50	2.28	2.15	2.06	1.99	1.93	1.89	1.86	1.83	1.78	1.73	1.68	1.65	1.62	1.58	1.55	1.51	1.47
30	2.88	2.49	2.28	2.14	2.05	1.98	1.93	1.88	1.85	1.82	1.77	1.72	1.67	1.64	1.61	1.57	1.54	1.50	1.46
40	2.84	2.44	2.23	2.09	2.00	1.93	1.87	1.83	1.79	1.76	1.71	1.66	1.61	1.57	1.54	1.51	1.47	1.42	1.38
60	2.79	2.39	2.18	2.04	1.95	1.87	1.82	1.77	1.74	1.71	1.66	1.60	1.54	1.51	1.48	1.44	1.40	1.35	1.29
120	2.75	2.35	2.13	1.99	1.90	1.82	1.77	1.72	1.68	1.65	1.60	1.55	1.48	1.45	1.41	1.37	1.32	1.26	1.19
∞	2.71	2.30	2.08	1.94	1.85	1.77	1.72	1.67	1.63	1.60	1.55	1.49	1.42	1.38	1.34	1.30	1.24	1.17	1.00

From M. Merrington and C. M. Thompson (1943). Table of Percentage Points of the Inverted Beta (F) Distribution. *Biometrika 33*, pp. 74–87. Reprinted with permission from Biometrika.

Table I	Critical Values for PPMC

Reject H_0: $\rho = 0$ if the absolute value of r is greater than the value given in the table. The values are for a two-tailed test; d.f. $= n - 2$.

d.f	$\alpha = 0.05$	$\alpha = 0.01$
1	0.999	0.999
2	0.950	0.999
3	0.878	0.959
4	0.811	0.917
5	0.754	0.875
6	0.707	0.834
7	0.666	0.798
8	0.632	0.765
9	0.602	0.735
10	0.576	0.708
11	0.553	0.684
12	0.532	0.661
13	0.514	0.641
14	0.497	0.623
15	0.482	0.606
16	0.468	0.590
17	0.456	0.575
18	0.444	0.561
19	0.433	0.549
20	0.423	0.537
25	0.381	0.487
30	0.349	0.449
35	0.325	0.418
40	0.304	0.393
45	0.288	0.372
50	0.273	0.354
60	0.250	0.325
70	0.232	0.302
80	0.217	0.283
90	0.205	0.267
100	0.195	0.254

Source: From *Biometrika Tables for Statisticians,* vol. 1 (1962), p. 138. Reprinted with permission.

Table J	Critical Values for the Sign Test

Reject the null hypothesis if the smaller number of positive or negative signs is less than or equal to the value in the table.

	One-tailed, $\alpha = 0.005$	$\alpha = 0.01$	$\alpha = 0.025$	$\alpha = 0.05$
n	Two-tailed, $\alpha = 0.01$	$\alpha = 0.02$	$\alpha = 0.05$	$\alpha = 0.10$
8	0	0	0	1
9	0	0	1	1
10	0	0	1	1
11	0	1	1	2
12	1	1	2	2
13	1	1	2	3
14	1	2	3	3
15	2	2	3	3
16	2	2	3	4
17	2	3	4	4
18	3	3	4	5
19	3	4	4	5
20	3	4	5	5
21	4	4	5	6
22	4	5	5	6
23	4	5	6	7
24	5	5	6	7
25	5	6	6	7

Note: Table J is for one-tailed or two-tailed tests. The term n represents the total number of positive and negative signs. The test value is the number of less frequent signs.

Source: From *Journal of American Statistical Association,* vol. 41 (1946), pp. 557–66. W. J. Dixon and A. M. Mood.

Table K	Critical Values for the Wilcoxon Signed-Rank Test

Reject the null hypothesis if the test value is less than or equal to the value given in the table.

	One-tailed, $\alpha = 0.05$	$\alpha = 0.025$	$\alpha = 0.01$	$\alpha = 0.005$
n	Two-tailed, $\alpha = 0.10$	$\alpha = 0.05$	$\alpha = 0.02$	$\alpha = 0.01$
5	1			
6	2	1		
7	4	2	0	
8	6	4	2	0
9	8	6	3	2
10	11	8	5	3
11	14	11	7	5
12	17	14	10	7
13	21	17	13	10
14	26	21	16	13
15	30	25	20	16
16	36	30	24	19
17	41	35	28	23
18	47	40	33	28
19	54	46	38	32
20	60	52	43	37
21	68	59	49	43
22	75	66	56	49
23	83	73	62	55
24	92	81	69	61
25	101	90	77	68
26	110	98	85	76
27	120	107	93	84
28	130	117	102	92
29	141	127	111	100
30	152	137	120	109

Source: From *Some Rapid Approximate Statistical Procedures,* Copyright 1949, 1964 Lerderle Laboratories, American Cyanamid Co., Wayne, N.J. Reprinted with permission.

Table L	Critical Values for the Rank Correlation Coefficient

Reject H_0: $\rho = 0$ if the absolute value of r_S is greater than the value given in the table.

n	$\alpha = 0.10$	$\alpha = 0.05$	$\alpha = 0.02$	$\alpha = 0.01$
5	0.900	—	—	—
6	0.829	0.886	0.943	—
7	0.714	0.786	0.893	0.929
8	0.643	0.738	0.833	0.881
9	0.600	0.700	0.783	0.833
10	0.564	0.648	0.745	0.794
11	0.536	0.618	0.709	0.818
12	0.497	0.591	0.703	0.780
13	0.475	0.566	0.673	0.745
14	0.457	0.545	0.646	0.716
15	0.441	0.525	0.623	0.689
16	0.425	0.507	0.601	0.666
17	0.412	0.490	0.582	0.645
18	0.399	0.476	0.564	0.625
19	0.388	0.462	0.549	0.608
20	0.377	0.450	0.534	0.591
21	0.368	0.438	0.521	0.576
22	0.359	0.428	0.508	0.562
23	0.351	0.418	0.496	0.549
24	0.343	0.409	0.485	0.537
25	0.336	0.400	0.475	0.526
26	0.329	0.392	0.465	0.515
27	0.323	0.385	0.456	0.505
28	0.317	0.377	0.488	0.496
29	0.311	0.370	0.440	0.487
30	0.305	0.364	0.432	0.478

Source: From N. L. Johnson and F. C. Leone, *Statistical and Experimental Design,* vol. I (1964), p. 412. Reprinted with permission from the Institute of Mathematical Statistics.

Table M	Critical Values for the Number of Runs

This table gives the critical values at $\alpha = 0.05$ for a two-tailed test. Reject the null hypothesis if the number of runs is less than or equal to the smaller value or greater than or equal to the larger value.

Value of n_1	Value of n_2 2	3	4	5	6	7	8	9	10	11	12	13	14	15	16	17	18	19	20
2	1	1	1	1	1	1	1	1	1	1	2	2	2	2	2	2	2	2	2
	6	6	6	6	6	6	6	6	6	6	6	6	6	6	6	6	6	6	6
3	1	1	1	1	2	2	2	2	2	2	2	2	2	3	3	3	3	3	3
	6	8	8	8	8	8	8	8	8	8	8	8	8	8	8	8	8	8	8
4	1	1	1	2	2	2	3	3	3	3	3	3	3	3	4	4	4	4	4
	6	8	9	9	9	10	10	10	10	10	10	10	10	10	10	10	10	10	10
5	1	1	2	2	3	3	3	3	3	4	4	4	4	4	4	4	5	5	5
	6	8	9	10	10	11	11	12	12	12	12	12	12	12	12	12	12	12	12
6	1	2	2	3	3	3	3	4	4	4	4	5	5	5	5	5	5	6	6
	6	8	9	10	11	12	12	13	13	13	13	14	14	14	14	14	14	14	14
7	1	2	2	3	3	3	4	4	5	5	5	5	5	6	6	6	6	6	6
	6	8	10	11	12	13	13	14	14	14	14	15	15	15	16	16	16	16	16
8	1	2	3	3	3	4	4	5	5	5	6	6	6	6	6	7	7	7	7
	6	8	10	11	12	13	14	14	15	15	16	16	16	16	17	17	17	17	17
9	1	2	3	3	4	4	5	5	5	6	6	6	7	7	7	7	8	8	8
	6	8	10	12	13	14	14	15	16	16	16	17	17	18	18	18	18	18	18
10	1	2	3	3	4	5	5	5	6	6	7	7	7	7	8	8	8	8	9
	6	8	10	12	13	14	15	16	16	17	17	18	18	18	19	19	19	20	20
11	1	2	3	4	4	5	5	6	6	7	7	7	8	8	8	9	9	9	9
	6	8	10	12	13	14	15	16	17	17	18	19	19	19	20	20	20	21	21
12	2	2	3	4	4	5	6	6	7	7	7	8	8	8	9	9	9	10	10
	6	8	10	12	13	14	16	16	17	18	19	19	20	20	21	21	21	22	22
13	2	2	3	4	5	5	6	6	7	7	8	8	9	9	9	10	10	10	10
	6	8	10	12	14	15	16	17	18	19	19	20	20	21	21	22	22	23	23
14	2	2	3	4	5	5	6	7	7	8	8	9	9	9	10	10	10	11	11
	6	8	10	12	14	15	16	17	18	19	20	20	21	22	22	23	23	23	24
15	2	3	3	4	5	6	6	7	7	8	8	9	9	10	10	11	11	11	12
	6	8	10	12	14	15	16	18	18	19	20	21	22	22	23	23	24	24	25
16	2	3	4	4	5	6	6	7	8	8	9	9	10	10	11	11	11	12	12
	6	8	10	12	14	16	17	18	19	20	21	21	22	23	23	24	25	25	25
17	2	3	4	4	5	6	7	7	8	9	9	10	10	11	11	11	12	12	13
	6	8	10	12	14	16	17	18	19	20	21	22	23	23	24	25	25	26	26
18	2	3	4	5	5	6	7	8	8	9	9	10	10	11	11	12	12	13	13
	6	8	10	12	14	16	17	18	19	20	21	22	23	24	25	25	26	26	27
19	2	3	4	5	6	6	7	8	8	9	10	10	11	11	12	12	13	13	13
	6	8	10	12	14	16	17	18	20	21	22	23	23	24	25	26	26	27	27
20	2	3	4	5	6	6	7	8	9	9	10	10	11	12	12	13	13	13	14
	6	8	10	12	14	16	17	18	20	21	22	23	24	25	25	26	27	27	28

Source: Adapted from C. Eisenhart and F. Swed, "Tables for Testing Randomness of Grouping in a Sequence of Alternatives," *The Annals of Statistics,* vol. 14 (1943), pp. 83–86. Reprinted with permission of the Institute of Mathematical Statistics and of the Benjamin/Cummings Publishing Company, in whose publication, *Elementary Statistics,* 3rd ed. (1989), by Mario F. Triola, this table appears.

Table N — Critical Values for the Tukey Test

α = 0.01

k / v	2	3	4	5	6	7	8	9	10	11	12	13	14	15	16	17	18	19	20
1	90.03	135.0	164.3	185.6	202.2	215.8	227.2	237.0	245.6	253.2	260.0	266.2	271.8	277.0	281.8	286.3	290.4	294.3	298.0
2	14.04	19.02	22.29	24.72	26.63	28.20	29.53	30.68	31.69	32.59	33.40	34.13	34.81	35.43	36.00	36.53	37.03	37.50	37.95
3	8.26	10.62	12.17	13.33	14.24	15.00	15.64	16.20	16.69	17.13	17.53	17.89	18.22	18.52	18.81	19.07	19.32	19.55	19.77
4	6.51	8.12	9.17	9.96	10.58	11.10	11.55	11.93	12.27	12.57	12.84	13.09	13.32	13.53	13.73	13.91	14.08	14.24	14.40
5	5.70	6.98	7.80	8.42	8.91	9.32	9.67	9.97	10.24	10.48	10.70	10.89	11.08	11.24	11.40	11.55	11.68	11.81	11.93
6	5.24	6.33	7.03	7.56	7.97	8.32	8.61	8.87	9.10	9.30	9.48	9.65	9.81	9.95	10.08	10.21	10.32	10.43	10.54
7	4.95	5.92	6.54	7.01	7.37	7.68	7.94	8.17	8.37	8.55	8.71	8.86	9.00	9.12	9.24	9.35	9.46	9.55	9.65
8	4.75	5.64	6.20	6.62	6.96	7.24	7.47	7.68	7.86	8.03	8.18	8.31	8.44	8.55	8.66	8.76	8.85	8.94	9.03
9	4.60	5.43	5.96	6.35	6.66	6.91	7.13	7.33	7.49	7.65	7.78	7.91	8.03	8.13	8.23	8.33	8.41	8.49	8.57
10	4.48	5.27	5.77	6.14	6.43	6.67	6.87	7.05	7.21	7.36	7.49	7.60	7.71	7.81	7.91	7.99	8.08	8.15	8.23
11	4.39	5.15	5.62	5.97	6.25	6.48	6.67	6.84	6.99	7.13	7.25	7.36	7.46	7.56	7.65	7.73	7.81	7.88	7.95
12	4.32	5.05	5.50	5.84	6.10	6.32	6.51	6.67	6.81	6.94	7.06	7.17	7.26	7.36	7.44	7.52	7.59	7.66	7.73
13	4.26	4.96	5.40	5.73	5.98	6.19	6.37	6.53	6.67	6.79	6.90	7.01	7.10	7.19	7.27	7.35	7.42	7.48	7.55
14	4.21	4.89	5.32	5.63	5.88	6.08	6.26	6.41	6.54	6.66	6.77	6.87	6.96	7.05	7.13	7.20	7.27	7.33	7.39
15	4.17	4.84	5.25	5.56	5.80	5.99	6.16	6.31	6.44	6.55	6.66	6.76	6.84	6.93	7.00	7.07	7.14	7.20	7.26
16	4.13	4.79	5.19	5.49	5.72	5.92	6.08	6.22	6.35	6.46	6.56	6.66	6.74	6.82	6.90	6.97	7.03	7.09	7.15
17	4.10	4.74	5.14	5.43	5.66	5.85	6.01	6.15	6.27	6.38	6.48	6.57	6.66	6.73	6.81	6.87	6.94	7.00	7.05
18	4.07	4.70	5.09	5.38	5.60	5.79	5.94	6.08	6.20	6.31	6.41	6.50	6.58	6.65	6.73	6.79	6.85	6.91	6.97
19	4.05	4.67	5.05	5.33	5.55	5.73	5.89	6.02	6.14	6.25	6.34	6.43	6.51	6.58	6.65	6.72	6.78	6.84	6.89
20	4.02	4.64	5.02	5.29	5.51	5.69	5.84	5.97	6.09	6.19	6.28	6.37	6.45	6.52	6.59	6.65	6.71	6.77	6.82
24	3.96	4.55	4.91	5.17	5.37	5.54	5.69	5.81	5.92	6.02	6.11	6.19	6.26	6.33	6.39	6.45	6.51	6.56	6.61
30	3.89	4.45	4.80	5.05	5.24	5.40	5.54	5.65	5.76	5.85	5.93	6.01	6.08	6.14	6.20	6.26	6.31	6.36	6.41
40	3.82	4.37	4.70	4.93	5.11	5.26	5.39	5.50	5.60	5.69	5.76	5.83	5.90	5.96	6.02	6.07	6.12	6.16	6.21
60	3.76	4.28	4.59	4.82	4.99	5.13	5.25	5.36	5.45	5.53	5.60	5.67	5.73	5.78	5.84	5.89	5.93	5.97	6.01
120	3.70	4.20	4.50	4.71	4.87	5.01	5.12	5.21	5.30	5.37	5.44	5.50	5.56	5.61	5.66	5.71	5.75	5.79	5.83
∞	3.64	4.12	4.40	4.60	4.76	4.88	4.99	5.08	5.16	5.23	5.29	5.35	5.40	5.45	5.49	5.54	5.57	5.61	5.65

Table N (continued)

$\alpha = 0.05$

v \ k	2	3	4	5	6	7	8	9	10	11	12	13	14	15	16	17	18	19	20
1	17.97	26.98	32.82	37.08	40.41	43.12	45.40	47.36	49.07	50.59	51.96	53.20	54.33	55.36	56.32	57.22	58.04	58.83	59.56
2	6.08	8.33	9.80	10.88	11.74	12.44	13.03	13.54	13.99	14.39	14.75	15.08	15.38	15.65	15.91	16.14	16.37	16.57	16.77
3	4.50	5.91	6.82	7.50	8.04	8.48	8.85	9.18	9.46	9.72	9.95	10.15	10.35	10.53	10.69	10.84	10.98	11.11	11.24
4	3.93	5.04	5.76	6.29	6.71	7.05	7.35	7.60	7.83	8.03	8.21	8.37	8.52	8.66	8.79	8.91	9.03	9.13	9.23
5	3.64	4.60	5.22	5.67	6.03	6.33	6.58	6.80	6.99	7.17	7.32	7.47	7.60	7.72	7.83	7.93	8.03	8.12	8.21
6	3.46	4.34	4.90	5.30	5.63	5.90	6.12	6.32	6.49	6.65	6.79	6.92	7.03	7.14	7.24	7.34	7.43	7.51	7.59
7	3.34	4.16	4.68	5.06	5.36	5.61	5.82	6.00	6.16	6.30	6.43	6.55	6.66	6.76	6.85	6.94	7.02	7.10	7.17
8	3.26	4.04	4.53	4.89	5.17	5.40	5.60	5.77	5.92	6.05	6.18	6.29	6.39	6.48	6.57	6.65	6.73	6.80	6.87
9	3.20	3.95	4.41	4.76	5.02	5.24	5.43	5.59	5.74	5.87	5.98	6.09	6.19	6.28	6.36	6.44	6.51	6.58	6.64
10	3.15	3.88	4.33	4.65	4.91	5.12	5.30	5.46	5.60	5.72	5.83	5.93	6.03	6.11	6.19	6.27	6.34	6.40	6.47
11	3.11	3.82	4.26	4.57	4.82	5.03	5.20	5.35	5.49	5.61	5.71	5.81	5.90	5.98	6.06	6.13	6.20	6.27	6.33
12	3.08	3.77	4.20	4.51	4.75	4.95	5.12	5.27	5.39	5.51	5.61	5.71	5.80	5.88	5.95	6.02	6.09	6.15	6.21
13	3.06	3.73	4.15	4.45	4.69	4.88	5.05	5.19	5.32	5.43	5.53	5.63	5.71	5.79	5.86	5.93	5.99	6.05	6.11
14	3.03	3.70	4.11	4.41	4.64	4.83	4.99	5.13	5.25	5.36	5.46	5.55	5.64	5.71	5.79	5.85	5.91	5.97	6.03
15	3.01	3.67	4.08	4.37	4.59	4.78	4.94	5.08	5.20	5.31	5.40	5.49	5.57	5.65	5.72	5.78	5.85	5.90	5.96
16	3.00	3.65	4.05	4.33	4.56	4.74	4.90	5.03	5.15	5.26	5.35	5.44	5.52	5.59	5.66	5.73	5.79	5.84	5.90
17	2.98	3.63	4.02	4.30	4.52	4.70	4.86	4.99	5.11	5.21	5.31	5.39	5.47	5.54	5.61	5.67	5.73	5.79	5.84
18	2.97	3.61	4.00	4.28	4.49	4.67	4.82	4.96	5.07	5.17	5.27	5.35	5.43	5.50	5.57	5.63	5.69	5.74	5.79
19	2.96	3.59	3.98	4.25	4.47	4.65	4.79	4.92	5.04	5.14	5.23	5.31	5.39	5.46	5.53	5.59	5.65	5.70	5.75
20	2.95	3.58	3.96	4.23	4.45	4.62	4.77	4.90	5.01	5.11	5.20	5.28	5.36	5.43	5.49	5.55	5.61	5.66	5.71
24	2.92	3.53	3.90	4.17	4.37	4.54	4.68	4.81	4.92	5.01	5.10	5.18	5.25	5.32	5.38	5.44	5.49	5.55	5.59
30	2.89	3.49	3.85	4.10	4.30	4.46	4.60	4.72	4.82	4.92	5.00	5.08	5.15	5.21	5.27	5.33	5.38	5.43	5.47
40	2.86	3.44	3.79	4.04	4.23	4.39	4.52	4.63	4.73	4.82	4.90	4.98	5.04	5.11	5.16	5.22	5.27	5.31	5.36
60	2.83	3.40	3.74	3.98	4.16	4.31	4.44	4.55	4.65	4.73	4.81	4.88	4.94	5.00	5.06	5.11	5.15	5.20	5.24
120	2.80	3.36	3.68	3.92	4.10	4.24	4.36	4.47	4.56	4.64	4.71	4.78	4.84	4.90	4.95	5.00	5.04	5.09	5.13
∞	2.77	3.31	3.63	3.86	4.03	4.17	4.29	4.39	4.47	4.55	4.62	4.68	4.74	4.80	4.85	4.89	4.93	4.97	5.01

Table N *(concluded)*

$\alpha = 0.10$

k / v	2	3	4	5	6	7	8	9	10	11	12	13	14	15	16	17	18	19	20
1	8.93	13.44	16.36	18.49	20.15	21.51	22.64	23.62	24.48	25.24	25.92	26.54	27.10	27.62	28.10	28.54	28.96	29.35	29.71
2	4.13	5.73	6.77	7.54	8.14	8.63	9.05	9.41	9.72	10.01	10.26	10.49	10.70	10.89	11.07	11.24	11.39	11.54	11.68
3	3.33	4.47	5.20	5.74	6.16	6.51	6.81	7.06	7.29	7.49	7.67	7.83	7.98	8.12	8.25	8.37	8.48	8.58	8.68
4	3.01	3.98	4.59	5.03	5.39	5.68	5.93	6.14	6.33	6.49	6.65	6.78	6.91	7.02	7.13	7.23	7.33	7.41	7.50
5	2.85	3.72	4.26	4.66	4.98	5.24	5.46	5.65	5.82	5.97	6.10	6.22	6.34	6.44	6.54	6.63	6.71	6.79	6.86
6	2.75	3.56	4.07	4.44	4.73	4.97	5.17	5.34	5.50	5.64	5.76	5.87	5.98	6.07	6.16	6.25	6.32	6.40	6.47
7	2.68	3.45	3.93	4.28	4.55	4.78	4.97	5.14	5.28	5.41	5.53	5.64	5.74	5.83	5.91	5.99	6.06	6.13	6.19
8	2.63	3.37	3.83	4.17	4.43	4.65	4.83	4.99	5.13	5.25	5.36	5.46	5.56	5.64	5.72	5.80	5.87	5.93	6.00
9	2.59	3.32	3.76	4.08	4.34	4.54	4.72	4.87	5.01	5.13	5.23	5.33	5.42	5.51	5.58	5.66	5.72	5.79	5.85
10	2.56	3.27	3.70	4.02	4.26	4.47	4.64	4.78	4.91	5.03	5.13	5.23	5.32	5.40	5.47	5.54	5.61	5.67	5.73
11	2.54	3.23	3.66	3.96	4.20	4.40	4.57	4.71	4.84	4.95	5.05	5.15	5.23	5.31	5.38	5.45	5.51	5.57	5.63
12	2.52	3.20	3.62	3.92	4.16	4.35	4.51	4.65	4.78	4.89	4.99	5.08	5.16	5.24	5.31	5.37	5.44	5.49	5.55
13	2.50	3.18	3.59	3.88	4.12	4.30	4.46	4.60	4.72	4.83	4.93	5.02	5.10	5.18	5.25	5.31	5.37	5.43	5.48
14	2.49	3.16	3.56	3.85	4.08	4.27	4.42	4.56	4.68	4.79	4.88	4.97	5.05	5.12	5.19	5.26	5.32	5.37	5.43
15	2.48	3.14	3.54	3.83	4.05	4.23	4.39	4.52	4.64	4.75	4.84	4.93	5.01	5.08	5.15	5.21	5.27	5.32	5.38
16	2.47	3.12	3.52	3.80	4.03	4.21	4.36	4.49	4.61	4.71	4.81	4.89	4.97	5.04	5.11	5.17	5.23	5.28	5.33
17	2.46	3.11	3.50	3.78	4.00	4.18	4.33	4.46	4.58	4.68	4.77	4.86	4.93	5.01	5.07	5.13	5.19	5.24	5.30
18	2.45	3.10	3.49	3.77	3.98	4.16	4.31	4.44	4.55	4.65	4.75	4.83	4.90	4.98	5.04	5.10	5.16	5.21	5.26
19	2.45	3.09	3.47	3.75	3.97	4.14	4.29	4.42	4.53	4.63	4.72	4.80	4.88	4.95	5.01	5.07	5.13	5.18	5.23
20	2.44	3.08	3.46	3.74	3.95	4.12	4.27	4.40	4.51	4.61	4.70	4.78	4.85	4.92	4.99	5.05	5.10	5.16	5.20
24	2.42	3.05	3.42	3.69	3.90	4.07	4.21	4.34	4.44	4.54	4.63	4.71	4.78	4.85	4.91	4.97	5.02	5.07	5.12
30	2.40	3.02	3.39	3.65	3.85	4.02	4.16	4.28	4.38	4.47	4.56	4.64	4.71	4.77	4.83	4.89	4.94	4.99	5.03
40	2.38	2.99	3.35	3.60	3.80	3.96	4.10	4.21	4.32	4.41	4.49	4.56	4.63	4.69	4.75	4.81	4.86	4.90	4.95
60	2.36	2.96	3.31	3.56	3.75	3.91	4.04	4.16	4.25	4.34	4.42	4.49	4.56	4.62	4.67	4.73	4.78	4.82	4.86
120	2.34	2.93	3.28	3.52	3.71	3.86	3.99	4.10	4.19	4.28	4.35	4.42	4.48	4.54	4.60	4.65	4.69	4.74	4.78
∞	2.33	2.90	3.24	3.48	3.66	3.81	3.93	4.04	4.13	4.21	4.28	4.35	4.41	4.47	4.52	4.57	4.61	4.65	4.69

Source: "Tables of Range and Studentized Range," *Annals of Mathematical Statistics*, vol. 31, no. 4. Reprinted with permission of the Institute of Mathematical Sciences.

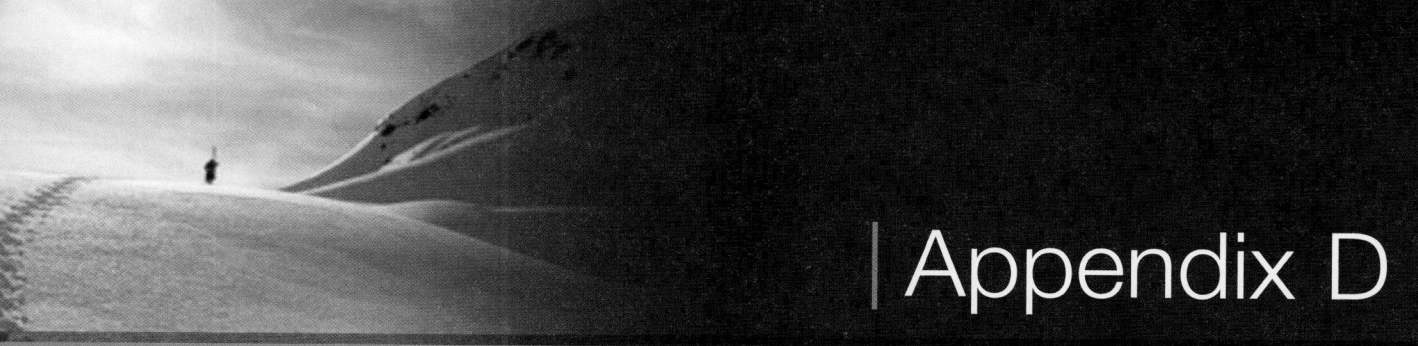

Databank

Databank Values

This list explains the values given for the categories in the databank.

1. "Age" is given in years.
2. "Educational level" values are defined as follows:
   0 = no high school degree   2 = college graduate
   1 = high school graduate   3 = graduate degree
3. "Smoking status" values are defined as follows:
   0 = does not smoke
   1 = smokes less than one pack per day
   2 = smokes one or more than one pack per day
4. "Exercise" values are defined as follows:
   0 = none   2 = moderate
   1 = light   3 = heavy

5. "Weight" is given in kilograms.
6. "Serum cholesterol" is given in millimoles per litre (mmol/L).
7. "Systolic pressure" is given in millimetres of mercury (mm Hg).
8. "IQ" is given in standard IQ test score values.
9. "Sodium" is given in milliequivalents per litre (mEq/L).
10. "Gender" is listed as male (M) or female (F).
11. "Marital status" values are defined as follows:
    M = married   S = single
    W = widowed   D = divorced

Data Bank

ID number	Age	Educational level	Smoking status	Exercise	Weight	Serum cholesterol	Systolic pressure	IQ	Sodium	Gender	Marital status
1	27	2	1	1	54.4	5.0	126	118	136	F	M
2	18	1	0	1	65.8	5.4	120	105	137	M	S
3	32	2	0	0	53.5	5.1	128	115	135	F	M
4	24	2	0	1	73.5	5.4	129	108	142	M	M
5	19	1	2	0	48.1	4.9	119	106	133	F	S
6	56	1	0	0	64.9	5.3	136	111	138	F	W
7	65	1	2	0	72.6	6.2	131	99	140	M	W
8	36	2	1	0	97.5	5.6	163	106	151	M	D
9	43	1	0	1	57.6	5.2	132	111	134	F	M
10	47	1	1	1	59.9	5.6	138	109	135	F	D

Data Bank

ID number	Age	Educational level	Smoking status	Exercise	Weight	Serum cholesterol	Systolic pressure	IQ	Sodium	Gender	Marital status
11	48	3	1	2	88.9	5.2	148	115	146	M	D
12	25	2	2	3	49.4	5.4	115	114	141	F	S
13	63	0	1	0	77.1	6.3	149	101	152	F	D
14	37	2	0	3	84.8	5.0	142	109	144	M	M
15	40	0	1	1	106.1	5.4	156	98	147	M	M
16	25	1	2	1	90.3	6.6	135	103	148	M	S
17	72	0	0	0	64.9	7.5	156	103	145	F	M
18	56	1	1	0	70.8	4.2	153	99	144	F	D
19	37	2	0	2	64.4	5.5	122	110	135	M	M
20	41	1	1	1	55.8	5.7	142	108	134	F	M
21	33	2	1	1	74.8	5.0	122	112	137	M	S
22	52	1	0	1	71.2	5.3	119	106	134	M	D
23	44	2	0	1	54.9	5.8	135	116	133	F	M
24	53	1	0	0	59.4	5.2	133	121	136	F	M
25	19	1	0	3	58.1	5.3	118	122	132	M	S
26	25	1	0	0	64.9	5.2	118	103	135	M	M
27	31	2	1	1	68.9	5.3	120	119	136	M	M
28	28	2	0	0	54.0	5.3	118	116	138	F	M
29	23	1	0	0	50.3	6.2	120	105	135	F	S
30	47	2	1	0	67.6	5.2	132	123	136	F	M
31	47	2	1	0	81.2	6.1	131	113	139	M	W
32	59	1	2	0	93.4	6.7	151	99	143	M	D
33	36	2	1	0	86.6	5.2	148	118	145	M	D
34	59	0	1	1	70.8	6.1	142	100	132	F	W
35	35	1	0	0	55.3	6.0	131	106	135	F	M
36	29	2	0	2	79.4	5.1	129	121	148	M	M
37	43	3	0	3	88.0	5.5	138	129	146	M	M
38	44	1	2	0	59.9	6.2	130	109	132	F	S
39	63	2	2	1	85.3	6.6	156	121	145	M	M
40	36	2	1	1	56.7	5.7	126	117	140	F	S
41	21	1	0	1	49.4	5.3	114	102	136	F	M
42	31	2	0	2	50.8	5.2	116	123	133	F	M
43	57	1	1	1	75.7	5.5	141	103	143	M	W
44	20	1	2	3	45.8	5.0	110	111	125	F	S
45	24	2	1	3	48.1	4.9	113	114	127	F	D
46	42	1	0	1	67.1	5.3	136	107	140	M	S
47	55	1	0	0	77.1	6.7	152	106	130	F	M
48	23	0	0	1	68.9	5.3	116	95	142	M	M
49	32	2	0	0	86.6	5.4	132	115	147	M	M
50	28	1	0	1	67.1	5.8	135	100	135	M	M
51	67	0	0	0	72.6	6.5	141	116	146	F	W
52	22	1	1	1	49.4	5.7	121	103	144	F	M
53	19	1	1	1	59.4	6.0	117	112	133	M	S
54	25	2	0	2	69.4	5.5	121	119	149	M	D
55	41	3	2	2	74.8	6.1	130	131	152	M	M

Data Bank

ID number	Age	Educational level	Smoking status	Exercise	Weight	Serum cholesterol	Systolic pressure	IQ	Sodium	Gender	Marital status
56	24	2	0	3	50.8	5.3	118	100	132	F	S
57	32	2	0	1	52.2	4.8	115	109	136	F	S
58	50	3	0	1	78.5	5.3	136	126	146	M	M
59	32	2	1	0	84.4	6.4	119	122	149	M	M
60	26	2	0	1	82.1	5.4	123	121	142	M	S
61	36	1	1	0	50.8	4.9	117	98	135	F	D
62	40	1	1	0	59.0	5.2	121	105	136	F	D
63	19	1	1	1	59.9	6.1	115	111	137	M	S
64	37	2	0	2	81.2	5.9	141	127	141	F	M
65	65	3	2	1	96.2	5.7	158	129	148	M	M
66	21	1	2	2	44.9	4.9	117	103	131	F	S
67	25	2	2	1	58.1	5.1	120	121	131	F	S
68	68	0	0	0	75.7	5.4	142	98	140	M	W
69	18	1	1	2	54.9	5.1	123	113	136	F	S
70	26	0	1	1	73.9	6.1	128	99	140	M	M
71	45	1	1	1	83.9	5.9	125	101	143	M	M
72	44	3	0	0	59.0	5.6	128	128	137	F	M
73	50	1	0	0	64.4	6.0	135	104	138	F	M
74	63	0	0	0	75.3	7.0	143	103	147	F	W
75	48	1	0	3	73.9	5.3	131	103	144	M	M
76	27	2	0	3	66.7	4.8	118	114	134	M	M
77	31	3	1	1	68.9	5.9	116	126	138	M	D
78	28	2	0	2	50.8	5.1	120	123	133	F	M
79	36	2	1	2	86.2	5.9	123	121	147	M	M
80	43	3	2	0	81.2	6.5	127	131	145	M	D
81	21	1	0	1	53.1	4.8	116	105	137	F	S
82	32	2	1	0	56.7	5.0	123	119	135	F	M
83	29	2	1	0	55.8	5.0	131	116	131	F	D
84	49	2	2	1	83.9	4.9	129	127	144	M	M
85	24	1	1	1	60.3	6.1	121	114	129	M	M
86	36	2	0	2	73.9	5.1	115	119	139	M	M
87	34	1	2	0	61.2	5.2	133	117	135	F	M
88	36	0	0	1	64.4	5.6	138	88	137	F	M
89	29	1	1	1	70.3	5.5	120	98	135	M	S
90	42	0	0	2	76.7	5.2	123	96	137	M	D
91	41	1	1	1	61.7	5.5	133	102	141	F	D
92	29	1	1	0	50.8	5.3	120	102	130	F	M
93	43	1	1	0	83.9	5.4	127	100	143	M	M
94	61	1	2	0	78.5	6.4	142	101	141	M	M
95	21	1	1	3	48.1	5.4	111	105	131	F	S
96	56	0	0	0	67.6	6.0	142	103	141	F	M
97	63	0	1	0	87.1	5.0	163	95	147	M	M
98	74	1	0	0	73.5	6.4	151	99	151	F	W
99	35	2	0	1	68.5	6.5	147	113	145	F	M
100	28	2	0	3	73.0	5.2	129	116	138	M	M

Data Set I North American Record Temperatures

Record high temperatures for Canadian provinces/territories (in °C)

43.3	44.4	44.4	39.4	41.7
38.3	33.9	39.4	42.2	36.7
40.0	45.0	36.1		

Record low temperatures for Canadian provinces/territories (in °C)

−61.1	−58.9	−52.8	−47.2	−51.1
−41.1	−57.8	−57.2	−58.3	−37.2
−54.4	−56.7	−63.0		

Record high temperatures for the United States (in °C)

44.4	37.8	53.3	48.9	56.7
47.8	41.1	43.3	42.8	44.4
37.8	47.8	47.2	46.7	47.8
49.4	45.6	45.6	40.6	42.8
41.7	44.4	45.6	46.1	47.8
47.2	47.8	51.7	41.1	43.3
50.0	42.2	43.3	49.4	45.0
48.9	48.3	43.9	40.0	43.9
48.9	45.0	48.9	47.2	40.6
43.3	47.8	44.4	45.6	46.1

Record low temperatures for the United States (in °C)

−32.8	−62.2	−40.0	−33.9	−42.8
−51.7	−35.6	−27.2	−18.9	−27.2
−11.1	−51.1	−37.8	−37.8	−43.9
−40.0	−38.3	−26.7	−44.4	−40.0
−37.2	−46.1	−51.1	−28.3	−40.0
−56.7	−43.9	−45.6	−43.9	−36.7
−45.6	−46.7	−36.7	−51.1	−39.4
−32.8	−47.8	−41.1	−31.7	−28.3
−50.0	−35.6	−30.6	−56.1	−45.6
−34.4	−44.4	−38.3	−48.3	−54.4

Sources: Canadian data–Current Results, *Weather Extremes,* "Hottest Places in Canada" and "Coldest Places in Canada," Liz Osborn; U.S. data–*The World Almanac and Book of Facts 2010,* p. 305 (U.S. data converted from °Fahrenheit to °Celsius).

Data Set II Identity Theft Complaints

The data values show the number of complaints of identity theft for 50 selected cities in the year 2009.

1,016	709	989	151	199
1,758	251	5,444	5,315	159
457	570	1,169	1,619	6,728
10,457	176	16,588	289	418
265	247	862	2,539	483
189	263	130	6,589	298
424	201	144	499	136
710	564	361	631	151
413	272	1,066	139	675
1,330	8,377	196	2,428	2,892

Source: Federal Trade Commission, *Consumer Sentinel Network Data Book for January–December 2009,* February 1010.

Data Set III Length of Major North American Rivers (kilometres)

1173	982	523	631	843
2348	724	748	974	531
1529	1458	529	467	1609
966	2334	1387	856	1432
655	845	1159	2000	1368
1044	1175	566	628	676
1143	547	1115	492	402
756	1165	534	417	3766
901	1706	1246	534	5971
3726	4088	995	1885	740
694	1287	974	660	2108
805	1271	855	1579	740
1490	604	2076	1947	2108
616	612	483	499	661
3058	698	676	877	916
684	1287	1392	612	716
866	1670	682	563	607
869	1061	1049	505	579
484	824	805	504	982
579	692	1098	1426	719
544	781	1006	1162	845
1287	497	700		

Source: Reprinted with permission from *The World Almanac and Book of Facts 2004.* Copyright © 2004 K-III Reference Corporation. All rights reserved.

Data Set IV Heights (in Metres) of 80 Tallest Buildings in New York City

381.0	262.4	318.8	290.2	168.2
278.9	237.1	260.9	259.1	282.5
222.2	227.1	230.7	229.2	248.1
228.6	212.4	226.5	225.2	228.6
213.4	204.2	218.2	215.5	222.5
207.9	197.5	209.4	209.4	214.9
198.1	193.2	202.4	205.4	208.8
195.1	191.4	192.0	199.0	205.1
190.5	189.0	191.4	196.6	198.1
187.5	180.4	189.0	192.0	192.0
181.4	176.8	187.1	188.4	191.7
178.9	175.3	179.8	185.6	187.5
175.3	174.3	176.8	179.2	183.8
175.0	171.6	175.3	175.9	178.9
172.2	169.2	171.3	173.7	175.6
169.8	173.7	169.2	171.0	175.0

Heights (in Metres) of 25 Tallest Buildings in Calgary, Alberta

210.0	161.5	140.2	125.0
196.6	160.0	136.9	125.0
196.6	154.5	134.4	124.4
190.8	152.4	132.6	124.1
185.3	143.0	132.6	
176.8	142.6	131.7	
161.5	141.1	128.0	

Source: Reprinted with permission from *The World Almanac and Book of Facts 2004.* Copyright © 2004 K-III Reference Corporation. All rights reserved.

Data Set V   School Suspensions

The data values show the number of students suspended and student enrollment for 72 district school boards in Ontario.

Suspensions	Enrollment	Suspensions	Enrollment
1,158	11,875	48	1,352
407	12,613	782	11,356
843	18,567	1,905	25,885
821	20,169	1,750	22,775
649	11,441	960	12,106
71	3,832	1,290	24,744
810	14,759	157	3,364
661	17,710	286	2,723
107	11,005	43	1,311
206	7,261	1,465	40,696
133	2,413	3,268	72,359
150	1,634	5,286	148,890
247	12,687	855	15,338
493	11,717	1,282	15,926
19	708	226	3,232
217	7,638	141	5,147
409	7,473	670	10,723
213	7,369	3,827	56,212
183	3,263	1,145	22,432
370	41,792	391	10,712
1,005	8,817	611	6,781
2,892	88,109	33	764
1,302	25,350	103	2,182
4,704	71,055	4,920	79,684
1,018	22,494	409	8,677
3,019	29,087	3,059	92,051
2,816	37,988	8,814	264,783
252	28,748	1,249	19,713
1,564	52,299	2,145	33,696
1,677	29,944	1,698	35,285
3,369	54,095	1,502	23,937
1,295	18,487	2,457	61,020
167	5,003	288	8,772
215	6,110	2,447	26,396
2,162	38,214	1,351	54,989
332	6,078	1,828	111,643

Source: Government of Ontario, Ministry of Education, *Number of Students Suspended, Enrollment, and Rate of Suspension by District School Boards during School Years 2000–2001 to 2007–2008.*

Data Set VI   Area of Canada's National Parks and National Park Reserves (in km²)

12,200	26	404	16	400
21,417	1,349	22,013	3,874	9,600
6,641	907	1,406	22	16,340
154	1,942	239	1,878	20,500
949	33	544	39,500	4,345
194	1,495	151	2,973	11,475
112	3,050	260	439	505
240	10,168	4,766	22,200	44,807
206	10,878	500	9	1,313

Source: Natural Resources Canada, *The Atlas of Canada,* "National Parks."

Data Set VII   Area of Canada's 30 Most Populated Cities (in km²)

630	545	97	366	450
366	465	146	446	1166
115	1117	20	77	289
2779	422	57	212	87
727	139	144	359	141
684	383	119	3200	75

Source: Wikipedia, "List of the 100 Largest Cities and Towns in Canada by Area."

Data Set VIII   Oceans of the World

Ocean	Area (thousands of square kilometres)	Maximum depth (metres)
Arctic	13,986	5,450
Caribbean Sea	2,753	7,680
Mediterranean Sea	2,505	5,020
Norwegian Sea	1,546	4,020
Gulf of Mexico	1,544	4,380
Hudson Bay	1,230	259
Greenland Sea	1,204	4,846
North Sea	575	661
Black Sea	461	2,243
Baltic Sea	422	439
Atlantic Ocean	82,439	9,219
South China Sea	3,447	5,560
Sea of Okhotsk	1,580	3,372
Bering Sea	2,269	4,191
Sea of Japan	1,008	3,743
East China Sea	751	2,782
Yellow Sea	417	91
Pacific Ocean	165,241	11,034
Arabian Sea	3,864	5,800
Bay of Bengal	2,173	5,258
Red Sea	438	2,246
Indian Ocean	73,452	7,450

Source: The Universal Almanac 1995, p. 330.

Data Set IX Commuter and Rapid Rail Systems in the United States

System	Stations	Kilometres	Vehicles Operated
Long Island RR	134	1027	947
NY Metro-North	108	862	702
New Jersey Transit	158	1490	582
Chicago RTA	117	671	358
Chicago & NW Transit	62	498	277
Boston Amtrak/MBTA	101	853	291
Chicago, Burlington, Northern	27	121	139
NW Indiana CTD	18	217	39
New York City TA	469	793	4923
Washington Metro Area TA	70	261	534
Metro Boston TA	53	123	368
Chicago TA	137	307	924
Philadelphia SEPTA	76	122	300
San Francisco BART	34	229	415
Metro Atlantic RTA	29	108	136
New York PATH	13	46	282
Miami/Dade Co TA	21	68	82
Baltimore MTA	12	43	48
Philadelphia PATCO	13	51	102
Cleveland RTA	18	61	30
New York, Staten Island RT	22	46	36

Source: The Universal Almanac 1995, p. 287.

Data Set X Lotto 649 Jackpot Analysis*

Ball	Times Drawn	Ball	Times Drawn	Ball	Times Drawn
1	354	17	353	33	352
2	349	18	342	34	411
3	352	19	368	35	345
4	362	20	386	36	361
5	350	21	353	37	359
6	346	22	344	38	363
7	373	23	356	39	358
8	348	24	333	40	393
9	357	25	345	41	355
10	335	26	362	42	361
11	335	27	382	43	392
12	355	28	331	44	349
13	349	29	364	45	380
14	334	30	370	46	387
15	325	31	400	47	387
16	345	32	377	48	345
				49	359

* Times each number has been selected, excluding bonus numbers, in the regular drawings by the Interprovincial Lottery Corporation since June 12, 1982.

Source: Ontario Lottery and Gaming Corporation, *Lotteries,* "Most Frequent Winning Numbers."

Data Set XI Pages in Statistics Books

The data values represent the number of pages found in statistics textbooks.

616	578	569	511	468
493	564	801	483	847
525	881	757	272	703
741	556	500	668	967
608	465	739	669	651
495	613	774	274	542
739	488	601	727	556
589	724	731	662	680
589	435	742	567	574
733	576	526	443	478
586	282			

Source: Allan G. Bluman.

Data Set XII Fifty Top Grossing Movies–2008

The data values represent the gross income in millions of dollars for the 50 top movies for the year 2008.

530.9	152.6	102.5	82.4	70.2
318.3	144.1	101.7	81.2	69.4
317.0	141.6	101.3	80.2	66.5
227.9	134.8	100.5	80.2	65.6
223.8	134.5	100.0	80.0	65.3
215.4	130.3	94.8	77.0	65.0
176.1	115.4	93.5	76.8	64.5
172.3	112.0	92.6	76.0	63.7
165.7	110.5	90.0	72.3	63.2
154.5	106.6	87.3	71.2	60.6

Source: The World Almanac and Book of Facts 2010.

Data Set XIII   Hospital Data*

Data Set XIII   Hospital Data (continued)

Number	Number of beds	Admissions	Payroll ($000)	Personnel	Number	Number of beds	Admissions	Payroll ($000)	Personnel
1	235	6,559	18,190	722	45	85	2,114	4,522	221
2	205	6,237	17,603	692	46	120	3,435	11,479	417
3	371	8,915	27,278	1,187	47	84	1,768	4,360	184
4	342	8,659	26,722	1,156	48	667	22,375	74,810	2,461
5	61	1,779	5,187	237	49	36	1,008	2,311	131
6	55	2,261	7,519	247	50	598	21,259	113,972	4,010
7	109	2,102	5,817	245	51	1,021	40,879	165,917	6,264
8	74	2,065	5,418	223	52	233	4,467	22,572	558
9	74	3,204	7,614	326	53	205	4,162	21,766	527
10	137	2,638	7,862	362	54	80	469	8,254	280
11	428	18,168	70,518	2,461	55	350	7,676	58,341	1,525
12	260	12,821	40,780	1,422	56	290	7,499	57,298	1,502
13	159	4,176	11,376	465	57	890	31,812	134,752	3,933
14	142	3,952	11,057	450	58	880	31,703	133,836	3,914
15	45	1,179	3,370	145	59	67	2,020	8,533	280
16	42	1,402	4,119	211	60	317	14,595	68,264	2,772
17	92	1,539	3,520	158	61	123	4,225	12,161	504
18	28	503	1,172	72	62	285	7,562	25,930	952
19	56	1,780	4,892	195	63	51	1,932	6,412	472
20	68	2,072	6,161	243	64	34	1,591	4,393	205
21	206	9,868	30,995	1,142	65	194	5,111	19,367	753
22	93	3,642	7,912	305	66	191	6,729	21,889	946
23	68	1,558	3,929	180	67	227	5,862	18,285	731
24	330	7,611	33,377	1,116	68	172	5,509	17,222	680
25	127	4,716	13,966	498	69	285	9,855	27,848	1,180
26	87	2,432	6,322	240	70	230	7,619	29,147	1,216
27	577	19,973	60,934	1,822	71	206	7,368	28,592	1,185
28	310	11,055	31,362	981	72	102	3,255	9,214	359
29	49	1,775	3,987	180	73	76	1,409	3,302	198
30	449	17,929	53,240	1,899	74	540	396	22,327	788
31	530	15,423	50,127	1,669	75	110	3,170	9,756	409
32	498	15,176	49,375	1,549	76	142	4,984	13,550	552
33	60	565	5,527	251	77	380	335	11,675	543
34	350	11,793	34,133	1,207	78	256	8,749	23,132	907
35	381	13,133	49,641	1,731	79	235	8,676	22,849	883
36	585	22,762	71,232	2,608	80	580	1,967	33,004	1,059
37	286	8,749	28,645	1,194	81	86	2,477	7,507	309
38	151	2,607	12,737	377	82	102	2,200	6,894	225
39	98	2,518	10,731	352	83	190	6,375	17,283	618
40	53	1,848	4,791	185	84	85	3,506	8,854	380
41	142	3,658	11,051	421	85	42	1,516	3,525	166
42	73	3,393	9,712	385	86	60	1,573	15,608	236
43	624	20,410	72,630	2,326	87	485	16,676	51,348	1,559
44	78	1,107	4,946	139	88	455	16,285	50,786	1,537

*This information was obtained from a sample of hospitals in a selected U.S. state. The hospitals are identified by number instead of name.

(continued)

Data Set XIII   Hospital Data *(continued)*

Number	Number of beds	Admissions	Payroll ($000)	Personnel
92	36	519	1,526	80
93	34	615	1,342	74
94	37	1,123	2,712	123
95	100	2,478	6,448	265
96	65	2,252	5,955	237
97	58	1,649	4,144	203
98	55	2,049	3,515	152
99	109	1,816	4,163	194
100	64	1,719	3,696	167
101	73	1,682	5,581	240
102	52	1,644	5,291	222
103	326	10,207	29,031	1,074
104	268	10,182	28,108	1,030
105	49	1,365	4,461	215
106	52	763	2,615	125
107	106	4,629	10,549	456
108	73	2,579	6,533	240
109	163	201	5,015	260
110	32	34	2,880	124
111	385	14,553	52,572	1,724
112	95	3,267	9,928	366
113	339	12,021	54,163	1,607
114	50	1,548	3,278	156
115	55	1,274	2,822	162
116	278	6,323	15,697	722
117	298	11,736	40,610	1,606
118	136	2,099	7,136	255
119	97	1,831	6,448	222
120	369	12,378	35,879	1,312
121	288	10,807	29,972	1,263
122	262	10,394	29,408	1,237
123	94	2,143	7,593	323
124	98	3,465	9,376	371
125	136	2,768	7,412	390
126	70	824	4,741	208
127	35	883	2,505	142
128	52	1,279	3,212	158

Technology Step by Step (in brief)

The following technologies will assist the learner through common statistical procedures for describing and analyzing data.

- Minitab Statistical Software
- IBM SPSS Statistics
- Microsoft Excel spreadsheet application
- Texas Instruments TI-83 Plus or TI-84 Plus programmable calculators

This brief version of Appendix E contains only the Texas Instruments TI-83 Plus/TI-84 Plus programmable calculator step-by-step instructions. For Minitab, SPSS, and Excel, please see the full version of Appendix E on *Connect*.

TI-83 Plus/TI-84 Plus

The TI-83 Plus and TI-84 Plus are multifunction programmable calculators that include capabilities to edit, describe, graph, and analyze data.

Restore Default Settings

Press ON > 2nd [MEM] > 7 : Reset > 2 : Defaults > 2 : Reset

Clear All Lists

2nd [MEM] > 4 : ClrAllLists > Enter

Input Data

Press STAT > EDIT 1: Edit > {type data in L_1}. Press 2nd [QUIT] when completed.

Histogram (ungrouped data)

Input data in L_1. Press WINDOW. Change Xmin and Xmax (data range), Ymin and Ymax (data frequency) values appropriate to input data. Press 2nd [QUIT]. Press 2nd [STAT PLOT] ENTER twice to turn plot on. Select Histogram symbol, press ENTER. Xlist is L_1 and Freq is 1. Press GRAPH. Press TRACE and ▶ or ◀ keys to display number of data values for each class.

Histogram (grouped data)

Input data midpoints in L_1 and class frequencies in L_2. Press WINDOW and change values appropriate to input data. Press 2nd [QUIT]. Press 2nd [STAT PLOT] ENTER twice to turn plot on. Select Histogram symbol, press ENTER. Xlist is L_1 and Freq is L_2. Press GRAPH. Press TRACE and ▶ or ◀ keys to display number of data values for each class.

Note: A similar procedure for confidence intervals for the difference between two means (z distribution) is available using the STATS > TESTS > 9:2-SampZInt . . . option. Input appropriate values and calculate.

t Distribution → Repeat z Distribution procedure except select STATS > TESTS > 9:2-SampTTest . . . standard deviations are calculated from L_1 and L_2 lists. In Pooled: select No (standard deviations are assumed not equal) or Yes (standard deviations are assumed equal).

Note: A similar procedure for confidence intervals for the difference between two means (t distribution) is available using the STATS > TESTS > 0:2-SampTInt . . . option. Input appropriate values and calculate.

Dependent Samples → Input 2 sets of data in L_1 and L_2. Move to L_3 heading. Type L_1 - L_2. Press ENTER. Select STATS > TESTS > 2:T-Test . . . Input $\mu_0 = 0$, List: L_3, Freq: 1. Check List: L_1 and Freq: 1. Select required alternative, $\mu: \neq \mu_0 < \mu_0 > \mu_0$. Select Calculate to display results.

Note: A similar procedure for confidence intervals for the difference between two means (dependent samples) is available using the STATS > TESTS > 8:TInterval . . . option. Input appropriate values using L_3 and calculate.

Hypothesis Test: Difference Between Two Variances

Input 2 sets of data in L_1 and L_2. Select STATS > TESTS > D:2-SampFTest . . . Select Data. Check List1: L_1, List2: L_2, Freq1:1, and Freq2: 1. Select required alternative, $\sigma 1: \neq \sigma 2 < \sigma 2 > \sigma 2$. Calculate to display results including F (test statistic) and p (P-value). *Note:* If summary statistics mean and standard deviation are known for each data set, select Stats instead of Data and input appropriate values.

Hypothesis Test: Difference Between Two Proportions

No data is required. Select STAT > TESTS > 6:2-PropZTest . . . Type appropriate values for x1:, n1:, x2:, n2:. Select p1:$\neq$2. Press Calculate to display results.

Note: A similar procedure for confidence intervals for the difference between two proportions is available. Select STAT > TESTS > B:2-PropZInt . . . Input appropriate values and calculate.

Scatter Plot

Input x values in L_1 and y values in L_2. Select WINDOW and adjust Xmin, Xmax, Ymin, and Ymax to match data set. Press 2nd [STAT PLOT] > Plot 1 > On. Select: Type: first chart, XList: L_1, Ylist: L_2. Press GRAPH to display scatter plot.

Correlation and Regression

Turn on correlation display. Press 2nd [CATALOG]. Scroll to DiagnosticON. Press ENTER twice. Feature will remain on unless calculator's memory is reset.

Input x values in L_1 and y values in L_2. Press STAT > CALC > LinReg($a + bx$). Press ENTER to display values for a (y-intercept) and b (slope) and r (correlation coefficient).

Plot Regression Equation on Scatter Plot

Follow procedure for Scatter Plot and Correlation and Regression. Press Y= > CLEAR to clear previous equations. Press VARS > 5:Statistics > EQ > 1:RegEQ to display regression equation. Press GRAPH to display resulting graph.

Multiple Regression

No built-in functions for multiple regression. Downloadable MULREG program is available on *Connect.* Follow included instructions.

Chi-Square Hypothesis Test

X^2 Goodness-of-Fit Test → Input observed frequencies in L_1 and expected L_2. Press 2nd [QUIT] to exit to home screen. To calculate test statistic, press 2nd [LIST] > MATH 5:sum(> input $(L_1\text{-}L_2)^2/L_2$) > ENTER. To calculate P-value, press 2nd [DIST] > 7:X^2cdf(> command format X^2cdf (test statistic, ∞, degrees of freedom). *Note:* Use 2nd [EE], type 99 for ∞.

　X^2 Independence Test → Press 2nd [MATRX] > EDIT. Input number of rows and columns in contingency table over 1 × 1 (i.e., 2 × 3, for 2 rows, 3 columns). Input observed frequencies in displayed matrix (table) pressing ENTER after each data entry. Press STAT > TESTS > C:X^2-Test . . . Check the Observed: [A] and Expected [B]. Select Calculate to display results including X^2 (test statistic) and p (P-value).

One-Way Analysis of Variance (ANOVA)

Input data into L_1, L_2, L_3, etc. Press STAT > TESTS > F:ANOVA(. Type each list followed by a comma (i.e., F:ANOVA(L_1, L_2, L_3). Press ENTER to display F (test statistic) and p (P-value).

Two-Way Analysis of Variance

No built-in functions for two-way analysis of variance. Downloadable TWOWAY program is available on *Connect.* Follow included instructions.

Random Numbers

To generate a random number from 0 to 1, press MATH > PRB > 1:rand > ENTER to display results. Continue to press ENTER to display more random numbers.

　To generate a list of random numbers between specified values, press MATH > PRB > 5:randInt(. Type a desired minimum value, comma, maximum value, comma, number of desired values. (i.e., randInt(1,99,10) will generate 10 random number between 1 and 99.) *Note:* Use arrow ▶ keys to scroll right to see numbers.

Glossary

adjusted R^2 used in multiple regression when n and k are approximately equal, to provide a more realistic value of R^2

alpha the probability of a type I error, represented by the Greek letter α

alternative hypothesis a statistical hypothesis that states a parameter is either less than, not equal to, or greater than a specific value, or states that there is a difference between two parameters; also known as a *research hypothesis*

analysis of variance (ANOVA) a statistical technique used to test a hypothesis concerning the means of three or more populations

ANOVA summary table the table used to summarize the results of an ANOVA test

Bayes' theorem a theorem that allows one to compute the revised probability of an event that occurred before another event when the events are dependent

beta the probability of a type II error, represented by the Greek letter β

between-group variance a variance estimate using the means of the groups or between the groups in an F test

biased sample a sample for which some type of systematic error has been made in the selection of subjects for the sample

bimodal a data set with two modes

binomial distribution a discrete probability distribution of the number of successes in a series of n independent trials, with each trial having two possible outcomes and a constant probability of success

binomial experiment a probability experiment in which each trial has only two outcomes, there are a fixed number of trials, the outcomes of the trials are independent, and the probability of success remains the same for each trial

boxplot a graph used to represent a data set when the data set contains a small number of values

categorical frequency distribution a frequency distribution used when the data are categorical (nominal)

central limit theorem a theorem that states that as the sample size increases, the shape of the distribution of the sample means taken from the population with mean μ and standard deviation σ will approach a normal distribution; the distribution will have a mean μ and a standard deviation $\sigma/\sqrt{n}$

Chebyshev's theorem a theorem that states that the proportion of values from a data set that fall within k standard deviations of the mean will be at least $1 - 1/k^2$, where k is a number greater than 1

chi-square distribution a probability distribution obtained from the values of $(n - 1)s^2/\sigma^2$ when random samples are selected from a normally distributed population whose variance is σ^2

class a quantitative or qualitative category

class boundaries the upper and lower values of a class for a grouped frequency distribution whose values have one additional decimal place more than the data and end in the digit 5

class midpoint a value for a class in a frequency distribution obtained by adding the lower and upper class boundaries (or the lower and upper class limits) and dividing by 2

class width the difference between the upper class boundary and the lower class boundary for a class in a frequency distribution

classical probability the type of probability that uses sample spaces to determine the numerical probability that an event will happen

cluster sample a sample obtained by selecting a pre-existing or natural group, called a *cluster,* and using the members in the cluster for the sample

coefficient of determination a measure of the percentage of variation of the dependent variable that is explained by the regression line and the independent variable; the ratio of the explained variation to the total variation

coefficient of variation the standard deviation divided by the mean; the result is expressed as a percentage

combination a selection of objects without regard to order

complement of an event the set of outcomes in the sample space that are not among the outcomes of the event itself

compound event an event that consists of two or more outcomes or simple events

conditional probability the probability that an event B occurs after an event A has already occurred

confidence interval a specific interval estimate of a parameter determined by using data obtained from a sample and the specific confidence level of the estimate

confidence level the probability that a parameter lies within the specified interval estimate of the parameter

confounded variables two variables confounded when their effects on a response variable cannot be distinguished from each other

consistent estimator an estimator whose value approaches the value of the parameter estimated as the sample size increases

contingency table data arranged in table form for the chi-square independence test, with R rows and C columns

continuous variable a variable that can assume all values between any two specific values; a variable obtained by measuring

control group a group in an experimental study that is not given any special treatment

convenience sample sample of subjects used because they are convenient and available

correction for continuity a correction employed when a continuous distribution is used to approximate a discrete distribution

correlation a statistical method used to determine whether a linear relationship exists between variables

correlation coefficient a statistic or parameter that measures the strength and direction of a linear relationship between two variables

critical or **rejection region** the range of values of the test value that indicates that there is a significant difference and the null hypothesis should be rejected in a hypothesis test

critical value a value that separates the critical region from the noncritical region in a hypothesis test

cumulative frequency the sum of the frequencies accumulated up to the upper boundary of a class in a frequency distribution

data measurements or observations for a variable

data array a data set that has been ordered

data set a collection of data values

data value or **datum** a value in a data set

decile a location measure of a data value; it divides the distribution into ten groups

degrees of freedom the number of values that are free to vary after a sample statistic has been computed; used when a distribution (such as the t distribution) consists of a family of curves

dependent events events for which the outcome or occurrence of the first event affects the outcome or occurrence of the second event in such a way that the probability is changed

dependent samples samples in which the subjects are paired or matched in some way; i.e., the samples are related

dependent variable a variable in correlation and regression analysis that cannot be controlled or manipulated

descriptive statistics a branch of statistics that consists of the collection, organization, summarization, and presentation of data

discrete probability distribution a distribution that consists of the values a random variable can assume and the corresponding probabilities of the values

discrete variable a variable that assumes values that can be counted

disordinal interaction an interaction between variables in ANOVA, indicated when the graphs of the lines connecting the mean intersect

distribution-free statistics *see* **nonparametric statistics**

double-blind study a common experimental procedure in which neither the subjects of the experiment nor the persons administering the experiment know the critical aspects of the experiment; for example, neither the doctor nor the patient knows whether a drug or a placebo is administered

double sampling a sampling method in which a very large population is given a questionnaire to determine those who meet the qualifications for a study; the questionnaire is reviewed, a second smaller population is defined, and a sample is selected from this group

element an object contained in a set of data

empirical probability the type of probability that uses frequency distributions based on observations to determine numerical probabilities of events

empirical rule a rule that states that when a distribution is bell-shaped (normal), approximately 68% of the data values will fall within 1 standard deviation of the mean; approximately 95% of the data values will fall within 2 standard deviations of the mean; and approximately 99.7% of the data values will fall within 3 standard deviations of the mean

equally likely events the events in the sample space that have the same probability of occurring

estimation the process of estimating the value of a parameter from information obtained from a sample

estimator a statistic used to estimate a parameter

event outcome of a probability experiment

expected frequency the frequency obtained by calculation (as if there were no preference) and used in the chi-square test

expected value the theoretical average of a variable that has a probability distribution

experimental study a study in which the researcher manipulates one of the variables and tries to determine how the manipulation influences other variables

explanatory variable a variable that is being manipulated by the researcher to see if it affects the outcome variable

exploratory data analysis the act of analyzing data to determine what information can be obtained by using stem and leaf plots, medians, interquartile ranges, and boxplots

extrapolation use of the equation for the regression line to predict y' for a value of x that is beyond the range of the data values of x

F distribution the sampling distribution of the variances when two independent samples are selected from two normally distributed populations in which the variances are equal ($\sigma_1^2 = \sigma_2^2$) and the variances s_1^2 and s_2^2 are compared as s_1^2 / s_2^2

F test a statistical test used to compare two variances or three or more means

factors the independent variables in ANOVA tests

finite population correction factor a correction factor used to correct the standard error of the mean when the sample size is greater than 5% of the population size

five-number summary five specific values for a data set that consist of the lowest and highest values, Q_1 and Q_3, and the median

frequency the number of values in a specific class of a frequency distribution

frequency distribution an organization of raw data in table form, using classes and frequencies

frequency polygon a graph that displays the data by using lines that connect points plotted for the frequencies at the midpoints of the classes

fundamental counting rule in a sequence of n events in which the first event has k_1 possibilities, the second event has k_2 possibilities, the third has k_3 possibilities, etc.; the total number of possibilities of the sequence will be $k_1 \cdot k_2 \cdot k_3 \cdots k_n$

goodness-of-fit test a chi-square test used to see whether a frequency distribution fits a specific pattern

grouped frequency distribution a distribution used when the range is large and classes of several units in width are needed

Hawthorne effect an effect on an outcome variable caused by the fact that subjects of the study know that they are participating in the study

histogram a bar chart in which vertical bars represent class frequencies

homogeneity of proportions test a test used to determine the equality of three or more proportions

hypergeometric distribution the distribution of a variable that has two outcomes when sampling is done without replacement

hypothesis testing a decision-making process for evaluating claims about a population

independence test a chi-square test used to test the independence of two variables when data are tabulated in table form in terms of frequencies

independent events events for which the probability of the first occurring does not affect the probability of the second occurring

independent samples the measurements in one sample are not related to the measurements in the other sample

independent variable a variable in correlation and regression analysis that can be controlled or manipulated

inferential statistics a branch of statistics that consists of generalizing from samples to populations, performing hypothesis testing, determining relationships among variables, and making predictions

influential observation an observation that, when removed from the data values, would markedly change the position of the regression line

interaction effect the effect of two or more variables on each other in a two-way ANOVA study

interquartile range $Q_3 - Q_1$

interval estimate a range of values used to estimate a parameter

interval level of measurement a measurement level that ranks data and in which precise differences between units of measure exist; *see also* **nominal, ordinal,** and **ratio levels of measurement**

Kruskal-Wallis test a nonparametric test used to compare three or more means

law of large numbers when a probability experiment is repeated a large number of times, the relative frequency probability of an outcome will approach its theoretical probability

least-squares line another name for the regression line

left-tailed test a test used on a hypothesis when the critical region is on the left side of the distribution

level a treatment in ANOVA for a variable

level of significance the maximum probability of committing a type I error in hypothesis testing

lower class limit the lower value of a class in a frequency distribution that has the same decimal place value as the data

lurking variable a variable that influences the relationship between x and y, but was not considered in the study

main effect the effect of the factors or independent variables when there is a nonsignificant interaction effect in a two-way ANOVA study

marginal change the magnitude of the change in the dependent variable when the independent variable changes one unit

margin of error the maximum likely difference between the point estimate of a parameter and the actual value of the parameter

mean the sum of the values, divided by the total number of values

mean square the variance found by dividing the sum of the squares of a variable by the corresponding degrees of freedom; used in ANOVA

measurement scales a type of classification that tells how variables are categorized, counted, or measured; the four types of scales are nominal, ordinal, interval, and ratio

median the midpoint of a data array

midrange the sum of the lowest and highest data values, divided by 2

modal class the class with the largest frequency

mode the value that occurs most often in a data set

Monte Carlo method a simulation technique using random numbers

multimodal a data set with three or more modes

multinomial distribution a probability distribution for an experiment in which each trial has more than two outcomes

multiple correlation coefficient a measure of the strength of the relationship between the independent variables and the dependent variable in a multiple regression study

multiple regression a study that seeks to determine if several independent variables are related to a dependent variable

multiple relationship a relationship in which many variables are under study

multistage sampling a sampling technique that uses a combination of sampling methods

mutually exclusive events probability events that cannot occur at the same time

negative relationship a relationship between variables such that as one variable increases, the other variable decreases, and vice versa

negatively skewed or left-skewed distribution a distribution in which the majority of the data values fall to the right of the mean

nominal level of measurement a measurement level that classifies data into mutually exclusive (nonoverlapping) exhaustive categories in which no order or ranking can be imposed on them; *see also* **interval, ordinal**, and **ratio levels of measurement**

noncritical or nonrejection region the range of values of the test value that indicates that the difference was probably due to chance and the null hypothesis should not be rejected

nonparametric statistics a branch of statistics for use when the population from which the samples are selected is not normally distributed and for use in testing hypotheses that do not involve specific population parameters

nonrejection region *see* **noncritical region**

normal distribution a continuous, symmetric, bell-shaped distribution of a variable

normal quantile plot a graphical plot used to determine whether a variable is approximately normally distributed

null hypothesis a statistical hypothesis that states that a parameter is equal to a specific value, or that there is no difference between two parameters

observational study a study in which the researcher merely observes what is happening or what has happened in the past and draws conclusions based on these observations

observed frequency the actual frequency value obtained from a sample and used in the chi-square test

ogive a graph that represents the cumulative frequencies for the classes in a frequency distribution

one-tailed test a test that indicates that the null hypothesis should be rejected when the test statistic value is in the critical region on one side of the mean

one-way ANOVA a study used to test for differences among means for a single independent variable when there are three or more groups

open-ended distribution a frequency distribution that has no specific beginning value or no specific ending value

ordinal interaction an interaction between variables in ANOVA, indicated when the graphs of the lines connecting the means do not intersect

ordinal level of measurement a measurement level that classifies data into categories that can be ranked; however, precise differences between the ranks do not exist; *see also* **interval, nominal,** and **ratio levels of measurement**

outcome the result of a single trial of a probability experiment

outcome variable a variable that is studied to see if it has changed significantly due to the manipulation of the explanatory variable

outlier an extreme value in a data set; it is omitted from a boxplot

parameter a characteristic or measure obtained by using all the data values for a specific population

parametric tests statistical tests for population parameters such as means, variances, and proportions that involve assumptions about the populations from which the samples were selected

Pareto chart a chart that uses vertical bars to represent frequencies for a categorical variable

Pearson product moment correlation coefficient (PPMCC) a statistic used to determine the strength of a relationship when the variables are normally distributed

percentile a location measure of a data value; it divides a data set into 100 equal parts in which the pth percentile is a value that at most $p\%$ of the observations in the data set are less than this value and the remainder are greater

permutation an arrangement of n objects in a specific order

pie graph a circle that is divided into sections or wedges according to the percentage of frequencies in each category of the distribution

point estimate a specific numerical value estimate of a parameter

Poisson distribution a probability distribution used when n is large and p is small and when the independent variables occur over a period of time

pooled estimate of the variance a weighted average of the variance using the two sample variances and their respective degrees of freedom as the weights

population the totality of all subjects possessing certain common characteristics that are being studied

population correlation coefficient the value of the correlation coefficient computed by using all possible pairs of data values (x, y) taken from a population

positive relationship a relationship between two variables such that as one variable increases, the other variable increases, or as one variable decreases, the other decreases

positively skewed or right-skewed distribution a distribution in which the majority of the data values fall to the left of the mean

power of a test the probability of rejecting the null hypothesis when it is false

prediction interval a confidence interval for a predicted value y

probability the chance of an event occurring

probability distribution the values a random variable can assume and the corresponding probabilities of the values

probability experiment a chance process that leads to well-defined results called *outcomes*

proportion a part of a whole, represented by a fraction, a decimal, or a percentage

***P*-value (or probability value)** the probability that a sample statistic (such as the sample mean) could have been selected from the population(s) being tested (or that a more improbable sample could be selected in the direction of the alternative hypothesis), given the assumption that the null hypothesis is true

qualitative variable a variable that can be placed into distinct categories, according to some characteristic or attribute

quantiles values that separate the data into approximately equal groups

quantitative variable a variable that is numerical in nature and that can be ordered or ranked

quartile a location measure of a data value; it divides the distribution into four groups

quasi-experimental study a study that uses intact groups rather than random assignment of subjects to groups

random sample a sample obtained by using random or chance methods; a sample for which every member of the population has an equal chance of being selected

random variable a variable whose values are determined by chance; a function that assigns a unique numerical value, determined by chance, to each outcome of an experiment

range the highest data value minus the lowest data value

range rule of thumb dividing the range by 4, given an approximation of the standard deviation

ranking the positioning of a data value in a data array according to some rating scale

ratio level of measurement a measurement level that possesses all the characteristics of interval measurement and a true zero; it also has true ratios between different units of measure; *see also* **interval, nominal,** and **ordinal levels of measurement**

raw data data collected in original form

regression a statistical method used to describe the nature of the relationship between variables; that is, a positive or negative, linear or nonlinear relationship

regression line the line of best fit of the data

rejection region *see* **critical region**

relative frequency graph a graph using proportions instead of raw data as frequencies

relatively efficient estimator an estimator that has the smallest variance from among all the statistics that can be used to estimate a parameter

research hypothesis an unverified claim about a population parameter that is opposite the null hypothesis; also known as the *alternative hypothesis*

residual the difference between the actual value of y and the predicted value $y9$ for a specific value of x

resistant statistic a statistic that is not affected by an extremely skewed distribution

right-tailed test a test used on a hypothesis when the critical region is on the right side of the distribution

run a succession of identical letters preceded by or followed by a different letter or no letter at all, such as the beginning or end of the succession

runs test a nonparametric test used to determine whether data are random

sample a group of subjects selected from the population

sample space the set of all possible outcomes of a probability experiment

sampling distribution of means a distribution obtained by using the means computed from random samples taken from a population

sampling error the difference between the sample measure and the corresponding population measure due to the fact that the sample is not a perfect representation of the population

scatter plot a graph of the independent and dependent variables in regression and correlation analysis

Scheffé test a test used after ANOVA if the null hypothesis is rejected, to locate significant differences in the means

sequence sampling a sampling technique used in quality control in which successive units are taken from production lines and tested to see whether they meet the standards set by the manufacturing company

sign test a nonparametric test used to test the value of the median for a specific sample or to test sample means in a comparison of two dependent samples

simple event an outcome that results from a single trial of a probability experiment

simulation techniques techniques that use probability experiments to mimic real-life situations

Spearman rank correlation coefficient the nonparametric equivalent to the correlation coefficient, used when the data are ranked

standard deviation the square root of the variance

standard error of the estimate the standard deviation of the observed y values about the predicted y' values in regression and correlation analysis

standard error of the mean the standard deviation of the sample means for samples taken from the same population

standard normal distribution a normal distribution for which the mean is equal to 0 and the standard deviation is equal to 1

standard score the difference between a data value and the mean, divided by the standard deviation

statistic a characteristic or measure obtained by using the data values from a sample

statistical hypothesis a conjecture about a population parameter, which may or may not be true

statistical test a test that uses data obtained from a sample to make a decision about whether the null hypothesis should be rejected

statistics the science of conducting studies to collect, organize, summarize, analyze, and draw conclusions from data

stem and leaf plot a data plot that uses the stem as the leading part of the data value, with the leaf as the remaining part of the data value to form groups or classes

stratified sample a sample obtained by dividing the population into subgroups, called *strata,* according to various homogeneous characteristics and then selecting members from each stratum

subjective probability the type of probability that uses a probability value based on an educated guess or estimate, employing opinions and inexact information

sum of squares between groups a statistic computed in the numerator of the fraction used to find the between-group variance in ANOVA

sum of squares within groups a statistic computed in the numerator of the fraction used to find the within-group variance in ANOVA

symmetric distribution a distribution in which the data values are uniformly distributed about the mean

systematic sample a sample obtained by numbering each element in the population and then selecting every kth number from the population to be included in the sample

t **distribution** a family of bell-shaped curves based on degrees of freedom, similar to the standard normal distribution with the exception that the variance is greater than 1; used when one is testing small samples and when the population standard deviation is unknown

t **test** a statistical test for the mean of a population, used when the population is normally distributed, the population standard deviation is unknown, and the sample size is less than 30

test statistic the numerical value calculated from the sample data in a statistical test

time series graph a graph that represents data that occur over a specific time

treatment group a group in an experimental study that has received some type of treatment

treatment groups the groups used in an ANOVA study

tree diagram a schematic with branches emanating from a starting point, showing all possible outcomes of a probability experiment

Tukey test a test used to make pairwise comparisons of means in an ANOVA study when samples are the same size

two-tailed test a test that indicates that the null hypothesis should be rejected when the test value is in either of the two critical regions

two-way ANOVA a study used to test the effects of two or more independent variables and the possible interaction between them

type I error the error that occurs if one rejects the null hypothesis when it is true

type II error the error that occurs if one does not reject the null hypothesis when it is false

unbiased estimator an estimator whose value approximates the expected value of a population parameter, used for the variance or standard deviation when the sample size is less than 30; an estimator whose expected value or mean must be equal to the mean of the parameter being estimated

unbiased sample a sample chosen at random from the population that is, for the most part, representative of the population

ungrouped frequency distribution a distribution that uses individual data and has a small range of data

uniform distribution a distribution whose values are evenly distributed over its range

unimodal a data set that has only one value that occurs with the greatest frequency

upper class limit the upper value of a class in a frequency distribution that has the same decimal place value as the data

variable a characteristic or attribute capable of assuming any value within the data set

variance the average of the squares of the distance that each value is from the mean

Venn diagram a diagram used as a pictorial representative for a probability concept or rule

weighted mean the mean found by multiplying each value by its corresponding weight and dividing by the sum of the weights

Wilcoxon rank sum test a nonparametric test used to test independent samples and compare distributions

Wilcoxon signed-rank test a nonparametric test used to test dependent samples and compare distributions

within-group variance a variance estimate using all the sample data for an F test; it is not affected by differences in the means

z **distribution** *see* **standard normal distribution**

z **score** *see* **standard score**

z **test** a statistical test for means and proportions of a population, used when the population is normally distributed and the population standard deviation is known or the sample size is 30 or more

Glossary of Symbols

a	y intercept of a line	GM	Geometric mean
α	Probability of a type I error	H	Kruskal-Wallis test statistic
b	Slope of a line	H_0	Null hypothesis
β	Probability of a type II error	H_1	Alternative hypothesis
C	Column frequency	HM	Harmonic mean
cf	Cumulative frequency	k	Number of samples
$_nC_r$	Number of combinations of n objects taking r objects at a time	λ	Expected number of occurrences for the Poisson distribution
C.V.	Critical value	s_D	Standard deviation of the differences
CVar	Coefficient of variation	s_{est}	Standard error of estimate
D	Difference; decile	SS_B	Sum of squares between groups
$\overline{D}$	Mean of the differences	SS_W	Sum of squares within groups
d.f.	Degrees of freedom	s_B^2	Between-group variance
d.f.N.	Degrees of freedom, numerator	s_W^2	Within-group variance
d.f.D.	Degrees of freedom, denominator	t	t test statistic
E	Event; expected frequency; maximum error of estimate	$t_{\alpha/2}$	Two-tailed t critical value
$\overline{E}$	Complement of an event	μ	Population mean
e	Euler's constant ≈ 2.7183	μ_D	Mean of the population differences
$E(X)$	Expected value	$\mu_{\overline{X}}$	Mean of the sample means
f	Frequency	w	Class width; weight
F	F test value; failure	r	Sample correlation coefficient
F'	Critical value for the Scheffé test	R	Multiple correlation coefficient
MD	Median	r^2	Coefficient of determination
MR	Midrange	ρ	Population correlation coefficient
MS_B	Mean square between groups	r_S	Spearman rank correlation coefficient
MS_W	Mean square within groups (error)	S	Sample space; success
n	Sample size	s	Sample standard deviation
N	Population size	s^2	Sample variance
$n(E)$	Number of ways E can occur	σ	Population standard deviation
$n(S)$	Number of outcomes in the sample space	σ^2	Population variance
O	Observed frequency	$\sigma_{\overline{X}}$	Standard error of the mean
P	Percentile; probability	$\sum$	Summation notation
p	Probability; population proportion	w_s	Smaller sum of signed ranks, Wilcoxon signed-rank test
$\hat{p}$	Sample proportion		
$\overline{p}$	Weighted estimate of p	X	Data value; number of successes for a binomial distribution
$P(B|A)$	Conditional probability		
$P(E)$	Probability of an event E	$\overline{X}$	Sample mean
$P(\overline{E})$	Probability of the complement of E	x	Independent variable in regression
$_nP_r$	Number of permutations of n objects taking r objects at a time	$\overline{X}_{GM}$	Grand mean
π	Pi ≈ 3.14	X_m	Midpoint of a class
Q	Quartile	χ^2	Chi-square
q	$1 - p$; test value for Tukey test	y	Dependent variable in regression
$\hat{q}$	$1 - \hat{p}$	y'	Predicted y value
$\overline{q}$	$1 - \overline{p}$	z	z test value or z score
R	Range; rank sum	$z_{\alpha/2}$	Two-tailed critical z value
F_S	Scheffé test statistic	!	Factorial

Bibliography

Aczel, Amir D. *Complete Business Statistics,* 3rd ed. Chicago: Irwin, 1996.

Beyer, William H. *CRC Handbook of Tables for Probability and Statistics,* 2nd ed. Boca Raton, Fla.: CRC Press, 1986.

Brase, Charles, and Corrinne P. Brase. *Understanding Statistics,* 5th ed. Lexington, Mass.: D.C. Heath, 1995.

Chao, Lincoln L. *Introduction to Statistics.* Monterey, Calif.: Brooks/Cole, 1980.

Daniel, Wayne W., and James C. Terrell. *Business Statistics,* 4th ed. Boston: Houghton Mifflin, 1986.

Edwards, Allan L. *An Introduction to Linear Regression and Correlation,* 2nd ed. New York: Freeman, 1984.

Eves, Howard. *An Introduction to the History of Mathematics,* 3rd ed. New York: Holt, Rinehart and Winston, 1969.

Famighetti, Robert, ed. *The World Almanac and Book of Facts 1996.* New York: Pharos Books, 1995.

Freund, John E., and Gary Simon. *Statistics—A First Course,* 6th ed. Englewood Cliffs, N.J.: Prentice-Hall, 1995.

Gibson, Henry R. *Elementary Statistics.* Dubuque, Iowa: Wm. C. Brown Publishers, 1994.

Glass, Gene V., and Kenneth D. Hopkins. *Statistical Methods in Education and Psychology,* 2nd ed. Englewood Cliffs, N.J.: Prentice-Hall, 1984.

Guilford, J. P. *Fundamental Statistics in Psychology and Education,* 4th ed. New York: McGraw-Hill, 1965.

Haack, Dennis G. *Statistical Literacy:* A Guide to *Interpretation.* Boston: Duxbury Press, 1979.

Hartwig, Frederick, with Brian Dearing. *Exploratory Data Analysis.* Newbury Park, Calif.: Sage Publications, 1979.

Henry, Gary T. *Graphing Data: Techniques for Display and Analysis.* Thousand Oaks, Calif.: Sage Publications, 1995.

Isaac, Stephen, and William B. Michael. *Handbook in Research and Evaluation,* 2nd ed. San Diego: EdITS, 1990.

Johnson, Robert. *Elementary Statistics,* 6th ed. Boston: PWS-Kent, 1992.

Kachigan, Sam Kash. *Statistical Analysis.* New York: Radius Press, 1986.

Khazanie, Ramakant. *Elementary Statistics in a World of Applications,* 3rd ed. Glenview, Ill.: Scott, Foresman, 1990.

Kuzma, Jan W. *Basic Statistics for the Health Sciences.* Mountain View, Calif.: Mayfield, 1984.

Lapham, Lewis H., Michael Pollan, and Eric Ethridge. *The Harper's Index Book.* New York: Henry Holt, 1987.

Lipschultz, Seymour. *Schaum's Outline of Theory and Problems of Probability.* New York: McGraw-Hill, 1968.

Marascuilo, Leonard A., and Maryellen McSweeney. *Nonparametric and Distribution-Free Methods for the Social Sciences.* Monterey, Calif.: Brooks/Cole, 1977.

Marzillier, Leon F. *Elementary Statistics.* Dubuque, Iowa: Wm. C. Brown Publishers, 1990.

Mason, Robert D., Douglas A. Lind, and William G. Marchal. *Statistics: An Introduction.* New York: Harcourt Brace Jovanovich, 1988.

Minitab. *Minitab Reference Manual.* State College, Pa.: Minitab, Inc., 1994.

Minium, Edward W. *Statistical Reasoning in Psychology and Education.* New York: Wiley, 1970.

Moore, David S. *The Basic Practice of Statistics.* New York: W. H. Freeman and Co., 1995.

Moore, Davis S., and George P. McCabe. *Introduction to the Practice of Statistics,* 3rd ed. New York: W. H. Freeman, *1999.*

Newmark, Joseph. *Statistics and Probability in Modern Life.* New York: Saunders, 1988.

Pagano, Robert R. *Understanding Statistics,* 3rd ed. New York: West, 1990.

Phillips, John L., Jr. *How to Think about Statistics.* New York: Freeman, 1988.

Reinhardt, Howard E., and Don O. Loftsgaarden. *Elementary Probability and Statistical Reasoning.* Lexington, Mass.: Heath, 1977.

Roscoe, John T. *Fundamental Research Statistics for the Behavioral Sciences,* 2nd ed. New York: Holt, Rinehart and Winston, 1975.

Rossman, Allan J. *Workshop Statistics, Discovery with Data.* New York: Springer, 1996.

Runyon, Richard P., and Audrey Haber. *Fundamentals of Behavioral Statistics,* 6th ed. New York: Random House, 1988.

Shulte, Albert P., 1981 yearbook editor, and James R. Smart, general yearbook editor. *Teaching Statistics and Probability, 1981 Yearbook.* Reston, Va.: National Council of Teachers of Mathematics, 1981.

Smith, Gary. *Statistical Reasoning.* Boston: Allyn and Bacon, 1985.

Spiegel, Murray R. *Schaum's Outline of Theory and Problems of Statistics.* New York: McGraw-Hill, 1961.

Texas Instruments. *TI-83 Graphing Calculator Guidebook.* Temple, Tex.: Texas Instruments, 1996.

Triola, Mario G. *Elementary Statistics,* 7th ed. Reading, Mass.: Addison-Wesley, 1998.

Wardrop, Robert L. *Statistics: Learning in the Presence of Variation.* Dubuque, Iowa: Wm. C. Brown Publishers, 1995.

Warwick, Donald P., and Charles A. Lininger. *The Sample Survey: Theory and Practice.* New York: McGraw-Hill, 1975.

Weiss, Daniel Evan. *100% American.* New York: Poseidon Press, 1988.

Williams, Jack. *The USA Today Weather Almanac 1995.* New York: Vintage Books, 1994.

Wright, John W., ed. *The Universal Almanac 1995.* Kansas City, Mo.: Andrews & McMeel, 1994.

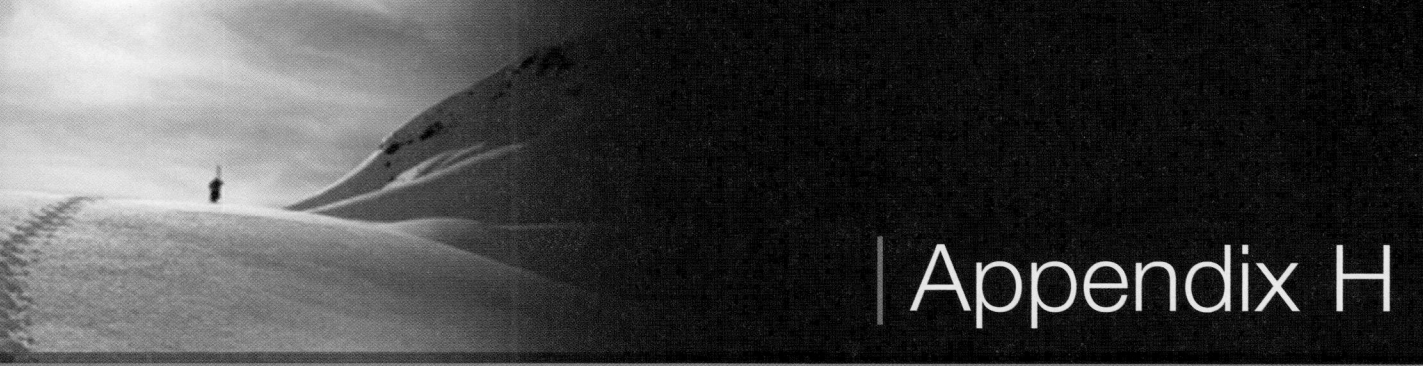

Photo Credits

Chapter 1

Opener: Reproduced with the permission of the Minister of Public Works and Government Services Canada, 2006, and courtesy of Natural Resources Canada, *Geological Survey of Canada;* p. 2: © Vol. 102/Corbis; p. 5: NASA; p. 10: © Banana Stock Ltd. RF; p. 12 (Table 1–4): iStockphoto; p. 17: Ryan McVay/Getty Images; pp. 19 and 20: © John Mayer.

Chapter 2

Opener: The Canadian Press/Larry MacDougal; p. 31: Image Source—Joseph Turp/The Canadian Press; p. 61: Roger Bamber/Almay; p. 64: © Bank of Canada/Banque du Canada; photo Gord Carter; used and altered with permission from the Bank of Canada.

Chapter 3

Opener: © Comstock/Jupiter Images; p. 81: Royalty-free/CORBIS; p. 82: © Brand X Pictures/PunchStock; p. 86: CREA—Canadian Real Estate Association (May 2007); p. 143: Janis Christie/Getty Images; p. 144: © Sherburne/PhotoLink/Getty Images.

Chapter 4

Opener: Steve Cole/Getty Images; p. 148: © Getty RF; p. 190: Uppercut RF/Getty Images; p. 195: Royalty-free/CORBIS; p. 198: Royalty-free/CORBIS.

Chapter 5

Opener: Image Source/Alamy; p. 210: © Vol. 41/Corbis; p. 214: CFL—Peter McCabe/The Canadian Press; p. 227: Richard Lautens/GetStock.com.

Chapter 6

Opener: Library of Congress; p. 253: © Vol. 106/Corbis; p. 268: © Digital Vision/PunchStock.

Chapter 7

Opener: USDA; p. 303: © Brand X Pictures/PunchStock; p. 325: © Brand X Pictures/Getty Images; p. 329: © Corbis RF.

Chapter 8

Opener: Geostock/Getty Images; p. 342: BananaStock/JupiterImages; p. 373: © Digital Vision/SuperStock; p. 393: © Vol. 48/PhotoDisc.

Chapter 9

Opener (both): © Bob Shirtz/SuperStock; p. 407: The McGraw-Hill Companies, Inc./Jill Braaten, photographer; p. 428: © Antonio Reeve/Photo Researchers.

Chapter 10

Opener: © PhotoDisc; p. 456: © Digital Vision/PunchStock; p. 468: © Getty RF; p. 470: PhotoLink/Getty Images; p. 489: © Frederick Bass/Getty Images.

Chapter 11

Opener: Tony Bock/GetStock.com; p. 504: © Vol. 130/Corbis; p. 527: © Vol. 56/PhotoDisc; p. 532: © The McGraw-Hill Companies, Inc./Jill Braaten, photographer.

Chapter 12

Opener: © Brand X Pictures/PunchStock; p. 535: © Al Francekevich/CORBIS; p. 551: Ingram Publishing/SuperStock.

Chapter 13

Opener: © Getty RF; p. 571: © The McGraw-Hill Companies, Inc./Andrew Resek, Photographer.

Chapter 14

Opener: Chris Rout/GetStock.com; p. 616: Courtesy of Hastos-Hall Productions; p. 621: Lucas Oleniuk/GetStock.com.

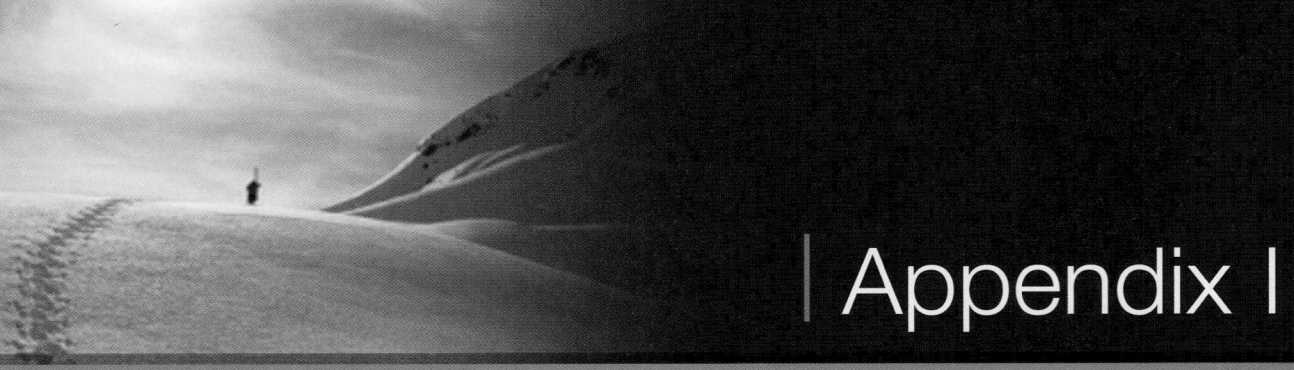

Credits for Unusual Stats, Interesting Facts, Historical Notes, and Exercises

Chapter 1

p. 2: Unusual Stat: SPCA.com; p. 3: Interesting Fact: *Time* magazine, Apr. 3, 2006; p. 4: Unusual Stat: Reuters; p. 5: Unusual Stat: Statistics Canada, *Criminal Victimization in Canada, 2004;* p. 7: Unusual Stat: *Canada World View,* Issue 24; p. 10: Interesting Fact: Canadian Radio-television and Telecommunications Commission, *Key Facts for Exempt Telemarketers,* modified May 1, 2009; p.13: Interesting Fact: Statistics Canada, *The Daily,* "Study: Work Injuries," July 10, 2007; p. 15: Interesting Fact: 50PLUS.com; p. 17: Interesting Fact: ccnmatthews.com, Jan. 25, 2006; p. 17: Unusual Stat: craigmarlatt.com; p. 23: Unusual Stat: *What Canadians Think . . . About Almost Everything,* Darrell Bricker and John Wright of Ipsos-Reid; p. 24, 6a: Adapted from Futron Corporation: www.futron.com; 6b: Adapted from Canadian Wireless Telecommunications Association: *Wireless Facts and Figures;* 6c: Adapted from Statistics Canada, *The Daily,* "Building Permits, Mar. 6, 2006; 6d: Adapted from Statistics Canada, *The Daily,* "Homicide in Canada," Oct. 28, 2009; 6f: Adapted from Statistics Canada, CANSIM Table 052-0004 and Catalogue 91-520-X, Feb. 28, 2007; 6g: Adapted from Canadian Institute for Health Information, *Health Care Spending in Canada to Exceed $180 Billion This Year,* Nov. 19, 2009; 6h: Adapted from canada.com, *Canada's Deficit to Balloon to $55.9 B: Flaherty,* Sept. 10, 2009; p. 25, 16a: Adapted from Top-Law-Schools.com, *Canada: University of Toronto Faculty of Law,* Matthew G. Scott; 16b: Adapted from *blogTO,* "Cat City," Sept. 23, 2010; p. 27, 22b: Adapted from United Nations, Department of Economic and Social Affairs, Population Division, *World Population to 2300,* 2004; 22c: Adapted from Hill Strategies Research Inc., *Statistical Insights on the Arts,* Vol. 7, No. 4, Feb. 2009; 22e: Adapted from Health Canada, *Healthy Canadians: A Federal Report on Comparable Health Indicators 2008.*

Chapter 2

p. 33: Interesting Fact: *Forbes.com,* "The World's Billionaires," edited by Luisa Kroll, Matthew Miller, and Tatiana Serafin, Mar. 11, 2009; p. 35: Unusual Stat: *Softpedia,* "32 Things You Did Not Know about Mosquitoes"; p. 38: Interesting Fact: Statistics Canada, CANSIM Table 502-0004 and Catalogue

87F0006XIE, Feb. 28, 2007; p. 42, 14: Adapted from Transport Canada, *Collisions and Casualties, 1985–2004,* reprinted with the permission of the Minister of Public Works and Government Services Canada, 2007; p. 43, 16: Adapted from Parks Canada, reproduced with permission of the Minister of Public Works and Government Services Canada, 2007; p. 48: Unusual Stat: *National Post,* Aug. 30, 2005; p. 53, 10: Adapted from Transport Canada, *Percentage of Driver and Passenger Fatalities and Serious Injuries by Age Group,* 2004, reprinted with the permission of the Minister of Public Works and Government Services Canada, 2007; p. 61: Interesting Fact: University of Guelph, Dairy Science and Technology, *Ice Cream Flavours,* 2006; p. 73, 13: Adapted from Statistics Canada, *Juristat,* "Homicide in Canada, 2004," Vol. 26, No. 6, p. 17, Catalogue 85-002; p. 74, 17: Adapted from *Canadian Insolvency Statistics—Up to 2004: Consumer Insolvencies by Major Region, Canada (2003–2009),* reproduced with the permission of the Minister of Public Works and Government Services, 2006.

Chapter 3

p. 81: Interesting Fact: FunFactz, www.funfactz.com; p. 93: Interesting Fact *and* Unusual Stat: Statistics Canada, *Excerpts from Canadian Agriculture at a Glance 1999,* Feb. 28, 2007; p. 108: Unusual Stat: *MenStuff,* "Male Privilege: A Different Perspective"; p. 116, 41: Adapted from Statistics Canada, *Food Statistics,* Catalogue 21-020, Feb, 28, 2007; p. 119: Interesting Fact: Goddard Space Flight Center, NASA; 126, Unusual Stat: *Science News Magazine,* "Drugged Money," Janet Raloff, Sept. 12, 2009; p. 135, 11: Adapted from Statistics Canada, *The Daily,* "Police Personnel and Expenditures," Dec. 15, 2005; p. 136, 15: Adapted from Environment Canada, *Canadian Climate Normals & Averages, 1971–2000,* reproduced with the permission of the Minister of Public Works and Government Services Canada, 2007; p. 138, 1: Adapted from Statistics Canada, *The Daily,* "Radio Listening," July 8, 2005; p. 142, 25: Adapted from Environment Canada, *Canadian Climate Normals & Averages, 1971–2000,* reproduced with the permission of the Minister of Public Works and Government Services Canada, 2007.

Chapter 4

p. 159: Interesting Fact: Chess.com, *How Many Possible Games Are There?* posted June 24, 2010; p. 163, 26: © Correctional Service of Canada, 2004, reproduced with the permission of the Minister of Public Works and Government Services Canada, 2007; 30: Adapted from Finance Canada, *Where Your Tax Dollar Goes,* 2005, reproduced with the permission of the Minister of Public Works and Government Services, 2007; p. 182, 4: Adapted from Transport Canada, *Road Safety,* reprinted with the permission of the Minister of Public Works and Government Services Canada, 2007; 5: Adapted from Statistics Canada, *Women in Canada: Work Chapter Updates,* 2003, Catalogue 89X0133XIE, Mar. 2004; 6: Adapted from Statistics Canada, *Adult Correctional Services in Canada, 2003–2004,* Catalogue 85-211, Dec. 2005, p. 13; p. 184, 35: Adapted from Canadian Intellectual Patents Office, *Annual Report 2004–2005—Data on Trademarks, Copyrights and Patents,* reprinted with the permission of the Minister of Public Works and Government Services, 2006; 37: Adapted from Statistics Canada, *The Daily,* "Marriages," Dec. 21, 2004; 38: Adapted from Transport Canada, *Canadian Motor Vehicle Traffic Collision Statistics: 2004,* "Fatalities by Road User Class—2000–2004," reprinted with the permission of the Minister of Public Works and Government Services Canada, 2007; 41: Adapted from Statistics Canada, *Canada at a Glance, 2005,* Catalogue 12-581, Mar. 10, 2006; p. 191, Interesting Fact: Statistics Canada, *The Daily,* "Police-Reported Crime Statistics: Table 1—Selected Violations, by Most Serious Offences, Canada," July 21, 2009; p. 202, 26: Adapted from Health Canada, *It's Your Health: Asthma,* May 2006, reproduced with the permission of the Minister of Public Works and Government Services Canada, 2007.

Chapter 5

p. 235, 10: Adapted from Statistics Canada, *Juristat,* "Criminal Victimization in Canada, 2004," Catalogue 85-002, Vol. 25, No. 7; p. 235, 11: Adapted from Fisheries and Oceans Canada, *Canadian Attitudes toward the Seal Hunt,* reproduced with the permission of Her Majesty the Queen in Right of Canada, 2007; p. 235, 19: Adapted from Statistics Canada, *Viewing Habits of the Average Canadian Family,* Feb. 28, 2007; p. 236, 22: Adapted from Statistics Canada, *The Daily,* "Residential Telephone Service Survey," Apr. 5, 2006; p. 236, 27: Adapted from Statistics Canada, *Juristat,* "Crime Statistics in Canada, 2004," Catalogue 85-002, Vol. 25, No. 5; p. 242: Interesting Fact: CNet news.com; p. 247, 20: Adapted from Statistics Canada, *Canadian Social Trends,* Catalogue 11-008, No. 80, Spring 2006; p. 247, 21: Adapted from Health Canada, *Canadian Tobacco Use Monitoring Survey* (CTUMS), 2005, reproduced with the permission of the Minister of Public Works and Government Services Canada, 2007.

Chapter 6

p. 270: Interesting Fact: Canadian Centre for Policy Alternatives; p. 271, 3: © Correctional Service of Canada, 2004, adapted and reproduced with the permission of the Minister of Public Works and Government Services Canada, 2007; p. 279: Interesting

Fact: www.bbc.co.uk/news and www.wikipedia.org; p. 283: Interesting Fact: TheMiddleAges.net, *The Black Death: Bubonic Plague;* p. 284, 8: Adapted from Statistics Canada, *Waste Management Industry Survey: Business and Government Sectors, 2002,* Catalogue 16F0023X, Sept. 24, 2004; p. 285, 13: Adapted from Statistics Canada publication *Food Expenditure in Canada, 2001,* Catalogue 62-554, Feb. 2003; p. 285, 17: Adapted from Health Canada, adapted and reproduced with the permission of the Minister of Public Works and Government Services Canada, 2007; p. 286, 25: Adapted from Statistics Canada, *Summary Tables,* "Food and Nutrition: Food Available, by Major Food Groups (Animal Products)," Catalogue no. 21-020-X; p. 288: Interesting Fact: abcNews.com, *Summertime Mystery: More Born, Fewer Die in August,* Aug. 16, 2005; p. 293, 7: Adapted from Statistics Canada, *Summary Tables,* "Educational Achievement: Population 15 Years and Over by Highest Degree, Certificate or Diploma (1986 to 2006 Census)"; p. 293, 9: Adapted from Statistics Canada, *Update in Education, Canadian Social Trends,* Catalogue 11-008, Winter 2003, No. 71, p. 20; p. 293, 12: Adapted from Statistics Canada, *Summary Tables,* "Employment and Unemployment: Experienced Labour Force 15 Years and over by Class of Worker, by Sex, by Province and Territory (2006 Census) (Newfoundland and Labrador, Prince Edward Island, Nova Scotia, New Brunswick)"; p. 295, 3: Adapted from Statistics Canada, *Earnings of Canadians, 2001 Census,* Catalogue 97F0019XIE2001002, Mar. 11, 2003; p. 295, 7: Adapted from Environment Canada, *Canadian Climate Normals & Averages 1971–2000,* reproduced with the permission of the Minister of Public Works and Government Services Canada, 2007; p. 296, 13: Adapted from Statistics Canada, *Summary Tables,* "Employment and Unemployment: Experienced Labour Force 15 Years and over by Occupation (Census 1991 to 2006); p. 297, 20: Adapted from Environment Canada, *Canadian Climate Normals & Averages 1971–2000,* reproduced with the permission of the Minister of Public Works and Government Services Canada, 2007; p. 297, 22: Adapted from Statistics Canada, *Food Consumption in Canada (2002),* Catalogue 32-229; p. 291, 29: Adapted from Statistics Canada, *The Daily,* Catalogue 11-001, Nov. 16, 2005; p. 298, 32: Adapted from Statistics Canada, *Summary Tables,* "Employment and Unemployment: Experienced Labour Force 15 Years and over by Occupation (Census 1991 to 2006).

Chapter 7

p. 305: Interesting Fact: *Prevention* magazine; p. 311: Interesting Fact: Adapted from Statistics Canada, *Family Expenditure Survey* (1982, 1986, 1992) and *Survey of Household Spending* (1997, 2002); p. 336, 16: Adapted from Health Canada, *Fish and Seafood Survey, 2002,* reproduced with the permission of the Minister of Public Works and Government Services Canada, 2007.

Chapter 8

p. 347, Unusual Stat: Digital Home Canada, *Average Canadian Watches over 25,000 TV Commercials Annually,* Oct. 13, 2009; p. 364, 6: Adapted from Statistics Canada, *Canadian Potato Production,* Catalogue 22-008, Vol. 4, No. 3; p. 365, 11: Adapted from Statistics Canada, *The Daily,* "Television Viewing—Fall 2004," Catalogue 11-001, Mar. 31, 2006; p. 365, 16: Adapted from Statistics Canada, *Food Consumption in Canada: Part 1,* Catalogue 32-229-XIB, 2002, June 27, 2003, p. 13; p. 365, 17: Adapted from Government of Ontario, © Queen's Printer for Ontario, 2004; p. 366, 21: Adapted from Statistics Canada, *Farming Facts, 2002,* Catalogue 21-522-XPE, Apr. 2003; p. 366, 22: Adapted from Statistics Canada, *Farming Facts, 2002,* Catalogue 21-522-XPE Apr. 2003; p. 371: Interesting Fact: *National Post,* Sept. 2006; p. 374, 5: Adapted from Environment Canada, *Climate Data,* reproduced with the permission of the Minister of Public Works and Government Services Canada, 2007; p. 374, 8: Adapted from Statistics Canada, *Canadian Social Trends,* "Traffic Report: Weekday Commuting Patterns," Catalogue 11-008, Spring 2000, No. 56, p. 19; p. 375, 14: Adapted from Health Canada, *Healthy Living: Canada's Guide to Healthy Eating and Physical Activity,* 2004, reproduced with the permission of the Minister of Public Works and Government Services Canada, 2007; p. 375, 18: Adapted from Statistics Canada, *Changes in Job Tenure and Job Stability in Canada,* Table 2, p. 9, Catalogue 11F0019MPE; p. 379: Interesting Fact: *National Geographic,* "Key to Lightning Deaths: Location, Location, Location," June 22, 2004; p. 381, 11: Adapted from Transport Canada, *Canadian Motor Vehicle Traffic Collision Statistics: 2004,* "Fatalities by Road User Class: 2000–2004," reproduced with the permission of the Minister of Public Works and Government Services Canada, 2007; p. 382, 14: Adapted from Statistics Canada, *The Daily,* "Spending Patterns in Canada, 2003," Catalogue 62-202; p. 382, 18: Adapted from Statistics Canada, "Survey of Earned Doctorates: A Profile of Doctoral Degree Recipients," Catalogue 11-001, July 5, 2005; p. 385: Interesting Fact: Adapted from Statistics Canada, *Farming Facts, 2002,* Catalogue 21-522-XIE2002001, p. 15; p. 391, 5: Adapted from Statistics Canada, *Juristat,* "Motor Vehicle Theft in Canada, 2001," Catalogue 85-002, Vol. 23, No. 1; p. 392, 10: Adapted from Environment Canada, *Climate Data,* reproduced with the permission of the Minister of Public Works and Government Services Canada, 2007; p. 399, 1: Adapted from Environment Canada, *Climate Data,* reproduced with the permission of the Minister of Public Works and Government Services Canada, 2007; p. 399, 5: Adapted from Environment Canada, *Climate Data,* reproduced with the permission of the Minister of Public Works and Government Services Canada, 2007.

Chapter 9

p. 418: Unusual Stat: *A Study on the Simulation of Proxemic Behavior,* William J. Ickinger, Tulane University, and Marjorie Fox Utsey, Tulane University, 2001; p. 423: Unusual Stat: Statistics Canada, *Food Consumption in Canada: Part 1,* Catalogue 32-229-XIB, 2002, p. 13; p. 422: Unusual Stat: Statistics Canada, *Food Consumption in Canada: Part 1,* Catalogue 32-229-XIB, 2002, p. 13; p. 427: Unusual Stat: Statistics Canada, *Canadian Social Trends,* "Across the Generations: Grandparents and Grandchildren," Winter 2003, Catalogue 11-008; p. 445, 16: Adapted from Statistics Canada, *Farm Data for the 2001 Census of Agriculture* (initial release), Catalogue 95F0301XIE; p. 445, 24: Adapted from Statistics

Canada, *Employment, Earnings and Hours,* Catalogue 72-002; p. 447, 4: Adapted from Environment Canada, *Canadian Climate Normals & Averages, 1971–2000,* reproduced with the permission of the Minister of Public Works and Government Services Canada, 2007.

Chapter 10

p. 457: Interesting Fact: Natural Resources Canada, Canadian Forest Service; p. 458: Interesting Fact: Public Safety Canada, *Earthquakes,* reproduced with the permission of the Minister of Public Works and Government Services Canada, 2007; p. 471, 17: Adapted from Statistics Canada, *Juristat,* "Crime Statistics in Canada, 2004," Catalogue 85-002, Vol. 25, No. 5; p. 471, 21: Adapted from Statistics Canada, *The Visible Minority Population, by Census Metropolitan Areas (2001 Census);* p. 472, 23: Adapted from Environment Canada, *Canadian Climate Normals & Averages, 1971–2000,* reproduced with the permission of the Minister of Public Works and Government Services Canada, 2007; p. 477: Interesting Fact: Cochrane Collaboration, *Helmets for Preventing Injury In Motorcycle Riders,* B. C. Liu, R. Ivers, R. Norton, S. Boufous, S. Blows, S. K. Lo; p. 480, 23: Adapted from Environment Canada, *Canadian Climate Normals & Averages, 1971–2000,* reproduced with the permission of the Minister of Public Works and Government Services Canada, 2007; p. 481, 31: Adapted from Statistics Canada, *Canadian Economic Observer,* "Head Office Employment in Canada, 1999 to 2005," Catalogue 11-010-XIB2006007; p. 483: Unusual Stat: Random Anything, *Rubik's Cube Colour Combinations;* p. 497, 2: Adapted from Statistics Canada, *Summary Tables,* "Sports Involvement by Sex.".

Chapter 11

p. 513, 12: Adapted from Statistics Canada, CANSIM database, Table 153-0034, "Greenhouse Gas Emissions (Carbon Dioxide Equivalents), by Sector, Annual (kilotonnes)"; p. 513, 14: Adapted from Statistics Canada, *Juristat,* "Adult Correctional Services in Canada, 2003/04," Table 3, Vol. 25 No. 8, Catalogue 85-002; p. 513, 15: Adapted from Statistics Canada, *Juristat,* "Adult Correctional Services in Canada, 2003/04," Table 3, Vol. 25 No. 8, Catalogue 85-002; p. 515: Interesting Fact: Adapted from *This Thing Called Age: You're Never Too Old to Be at Your Best,* Judd Biasiotto, Ph.D.; p. 517: Interesting Fact: U.S. Environmental Protection Agency; p. 520: Interesting Fact: U.S. Center for Health & Athletic Performance, Inc.; p. 524, 10: Government of Canada, *Canadian Ally 2007,* reproduced with the permission of the Minister of Public Works and Government Services, courtesy of the Department of National Defence, 2007; p. 525, 23: Adapted from Statistics Canada, *The Daily,* "Health Reports: Regional Differences in Obesity," Aug. 22, 2006, Catalogue 11-001; p. 525, 25: Adapted from Statistics Canada, *Perspectives on Labour and Income,* Catalogue 75-001, October 2004; p. 528, 2: Adapted from Statistics Canada, *Summary Tables,* "Population by Marital Status and Sex, 2003–2007."

Chapter 12

p. 538: Interesting Fact: *The Weather Network;* p. 539: Unusual Stat: Nedic, *Understanding Statistics on Eating Disorders;* p. 554:

Unusual Stat: World Health Organization; p. 556: Interesting Fact: *Audubon* magazine; p. 564, 7: Adapted from Statistics Canada, *Exploring Crime Patterns in Canada,* Catalogue 85-561-MIE2005005, 2005.

Chapter 13

p. 572: Interesting Fact: James A. Heathcote, *BMJ,* December 23, 1995, 311:1668; p. 570: Unusual Stat: Environment Canada, www.climate.weatheroffice.ec.gc.ca/climate_normals/index_e.html, reproduced with the permission of the Minister of Public Works and Government Services Canada, 2007; p. 580, 14: Adapted from Statistics Canada, *Health Reports,* "Deaths Involving Firearms," Catalogue 82-003-XPE2004004, Vol. 16, No. 4, released June 28, 2005; p. 587: Interesting Fact: Transport Canada: www.tc.gc.ca/roadsafety/tp2436/rs200104/menu.htm, reproduced with the permission of the Minister of Public Works and Government Services Canada, 2007; p. 590, 11: Adapted

from Statistics Canada, *The Daily,* "Television Viewing," March 31, 2006; 592: Interesting Fact: Home of Beliefs, *Pi Day Is Albert Einstein's Birthday;* p. 594, 7: Statistics Canada, *Health Reports,* "Deaths Involving Firearms," Catalogue 82-003-XPE2004004, Vol. 16, No. 4, released June 28, 2005; p. 597: Unusual Stat: Transport Canada, www.tc.gc.ca/roadsafety/tp2436/rs200104/page8.htm, reproduced with the permission of the Minister of Public Works and Government Services Canada, 2007; p. 599, 5: Statistics Canada, *Summary Tables,* "Forest Fires and Forest Land Burned, by Province and Territory."

Chapter 14

p. 631: Unusual Stat: *Sky-Fire.tv*: http://www.sky-fire.tv/index.cgi/lightning.html#sexist; p. 635: Interesting Fact: Adapted from Statistics Canada, *2003 General Social Survey on Social Engagement,* "Cycle 17: *An Overview of Findings, Table 4,*" Catalogue 89-598.

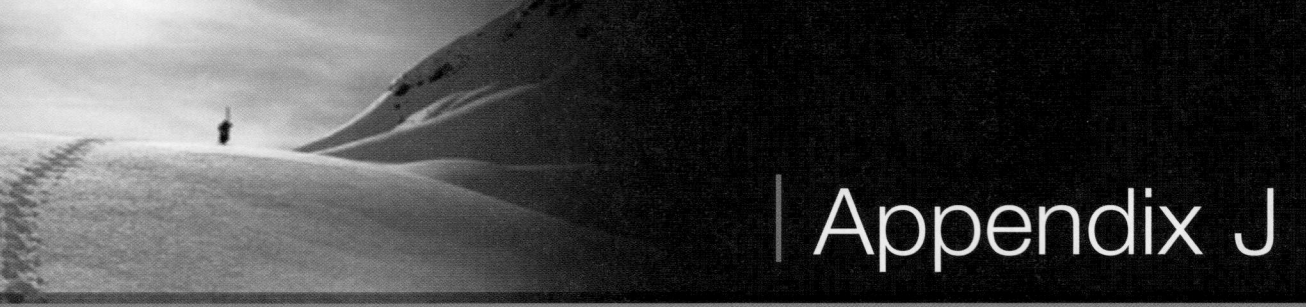

Selected Answers*

Chapter 1

Review Exercises

1. Descriptive statistics describes a set of data. Inferential statistics uses a set of data to make predictions about a population.

3. Answers will vary.

5. When the population is large, the researcher saves time and money using samples. Samples are used when the units must be destroyed.

7. *a.* ratio *e.* ratio *i.* nominal
 b. ordinal *f.* ordinal *j.* ratio
 c. ratio *g.* ratio
 d. interval *h.* ratio

8. *a.* quantitative *d.* quantitative *g.* qualitative
 b. qualitative *e.* qualitative
 c. quantitative *f.* quantitative

9. *a.* discrete *c.* continuous *e.* discrete
 b. continuous *d.* continuous *f.* continuous

11. Random samples are selected by using chance methods or random numbers. Systematic samples are selected by numbering each subject and selecting every *k*th number. Stratified samples are selected by dividing the population into groups and selecting from each group. Cluster samples are selected by using intact groups called *clusters*.

12. *a.* cluster *c.* random *e.* stratified
 b. systematic *d.* systematic

13. Answers will vary.

15. Answers will vary.

17. *a.* experimental *c.* observational
 b. observational *d.* experimental

19. Answers will vary. Possible answers include:
 a. overall health of participants, amount of exposure to infected individuals through the workplace or home

 b. gender and/or age of driver, time of day
 c. diet, general health, heredity factors
 d. amount of exercise, heredity factors

21. Claims can be proven only if the entire population is used.

23. Since the results are not typical, the advertisers selected only a few people for whom the product worked extremely well.

25. "74% more calories" than what? No comparison group is stated.

27. What is meant by "24 hours of acid control"?

29. Possible reasons for conflicting results: The amount of caffeine in the coffee or tea or the brewing method.

31. Answers will vary.

Chapter Quiz

1. True   2. False
3. False   4. False
5. False   6. True
7. False   8. *c*
9. *b*   10. *d*
11. *a*   12. *c*
13. *a*   14. descriptive, inferential
15. gambling, insurance 16. population
17. sample
18. *a.* saves time *c.* use when population is infinite
 b. saves money
19. *a.* random *c.* cluster
 b. systematic *d.* stratified
20. quasi-experimental 21. random
22. *a.* descriptive *d.* inferential
 b. inferential *e.* inferential
 c. descriptive

*Answers may vary due to rounding or use of technology.

Note: These answers to odd-numbered and selected even-numbered exercises include all quiz answers.

23. *a.* nominal   *d.* interval
    b. ratio   *e.* ratio
    c. ordinal

24. *a.* continuous   *d.* continuous
    b. discrete   *e.* discrete
    c. continuous

25. *a.* 47.5–48.5 seconds
    b. 0.555–0.565 centimetres
    c. 9.05–9.15 litres
    d. 13.65–13.75 kilograms
    e. 6.5–7.5 metres

Chapter 2

Exercises 2–1

1. Frequency distributions are used to organize data in a meaningful way, to facilitate computational procedures for statistics, to make it easier to draw charts and graphs, and to make comparisons among different sets of data.

3. *a.* $11.5 - 18.5$, $\frac{12 + 18}{2} = \frac{30}{2} = 15$, $18.5 - 11.5 = 7$
    b. $55.5 - 74.5$, $\frac{56 + 74}{2} = \frac{130}{2} = 65$, $74.5 - 55.5 = 19$
    c. $694.5 - 705.5$, $\frac{695 + 705}{2} = \frac{1400}{2} = 700$, $705.5 - 694.5 = 11$
    d. $13.55 - 14.75$, $\frac{13.6 + 14.7}{2} = \frac{28.3}{2} = 14.15$, $14.75 - 13.75 = 1.2$
    e. $2.145 - 3.935$, $\frac{2.15 + 3.93}{2} = \frac{6.08}{2} = 3.04$, $3.935 - 2.145 = 1.79$

5. *a.* Class width is not uniform.
    b. Class limits overlap, and class width is not uniform.
    c. A class has been omitted.
    d. Class width is not uniform.

7.

Class	Tally	*f*	Percent
A	////	4	10%
M	⊬⊬ ⊬⊬ ⊬⊬ ⊬⊬ ⊬⊬ ///	28	70%
H	⊬⊬ /	6	15%
S	//	2	5%
		40	100%

9. Max: 215; Min: 70; Range: 145; Classes: 8; Width: 18.1 (use 20). First class: 70–89.

Class limits	Class boundaries	*f*	cf
70–89	69.5–89.5	2	2
90–109	89.5–109.5	6	8
110–129	109.5–129.5	7	15
130–149	129.5–149.5	11	26
150–169	149.5–169.5	6	32
170–189	169.5–189.5	1	33
190–209	189.5–209.5	4	37
210–229	209.5–229.5	2	39

11. Max: 780; Min: 746; Range: 34; Classes: 6; Width: 5.7 (use 6). First class: 746–751.

Class limits	Class boundaries	*f*	cf
746–751	745.5–751.5	4	4
752–757	751.5–757.5	4	89
758–763	757.5–763.5	7	15
764–769	763.5–769.5	6	21
770–775	769.5–775.5	6	27
776–781	775.5–781.5	3	30

13. Max: 183; Min: 3; Range: 180; Classes: 8; Width: 22.5. For convenience use class width: 24 and first class: 1–24.

Class limits	Class boundaries	*f*	cf
1–24	0.5–24.5	9	9
25–48	24.5–48.5	3	12
49–72	48.5–72.5	7	19
73–96	72.5–96.5	1	20
97–120	96.5–120.5	2	22
121–144	120.5–144.5	2	24
145–168	144.5–168.5	2	26
169–192	168.5–192.5	1	27

15. Max: 90; Min: 63; Range: 27; Classes: 7; Width: 3.9 (use 4). First class: 63–66.

Class limits	Class boundaries	*f*	cf
63–66	62.5–66.5	11	11
67–70	66.5–70.5	9	20
71–74	70.5–74.5	10	30
75–78	74.5–78.5	3	33
79–82	78.5–82.5	3	36
83–86	82.5–86.5	3	39
87–90	86.5–90.5	1	40

17. Max: 8848; Min: 7129; Range: 1719; Classes: 7; Class width: 245.6 (use 300); Convenient first class: 7000–7299.

Class limits	Class boundaries	*f*	cf
7000–7299	7699.5–7299.5	9	9
7300–7599	7299.5–7599.5	10	19
7600–7899	7599.5–7899.5	17	36
7900–8199	7899.5–8199.5	8	44
8200–8499	8199.5–8499.5	2	46
8500–8799	8499.5–8799.5	3	49
8800–9099	8799.5–9099.5	1	50

19. The percentages add up to 101%. They should total 100% unless rounding was used.

Exercises 2–2

1.

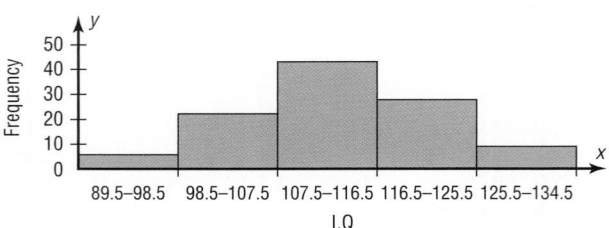

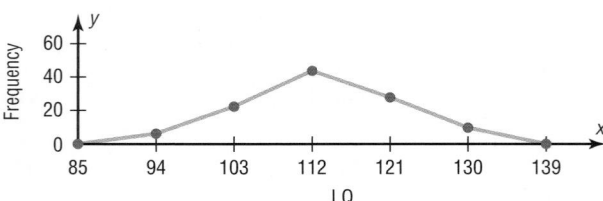

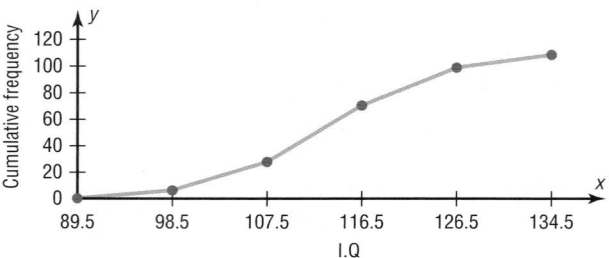

Eighty applicants do not need to enroll in the summer programs.

3.

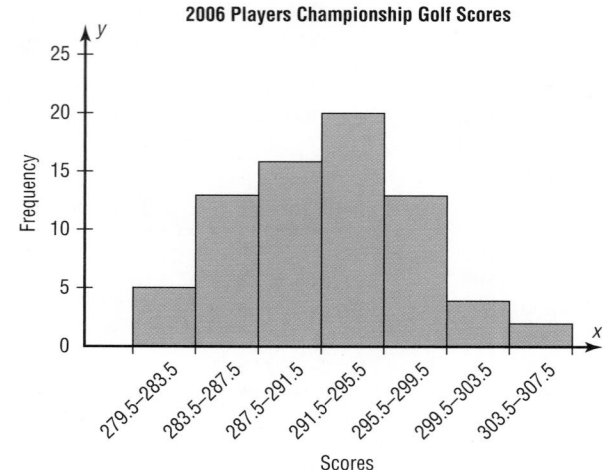

2006 Players Championship Golf Scores

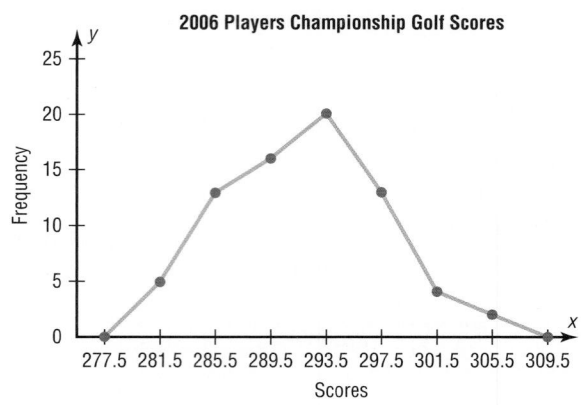

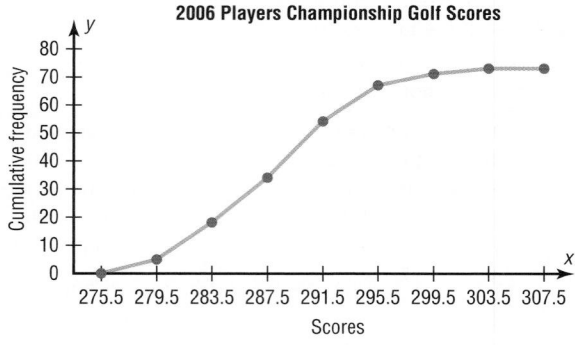

5.

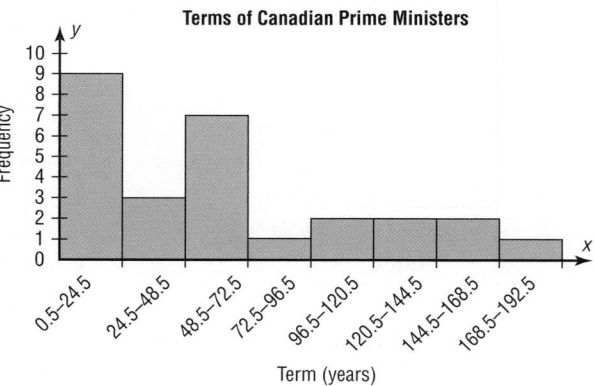

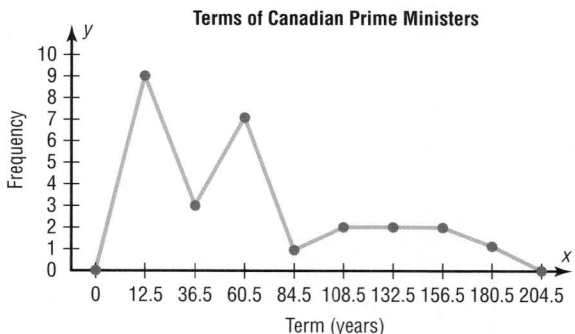

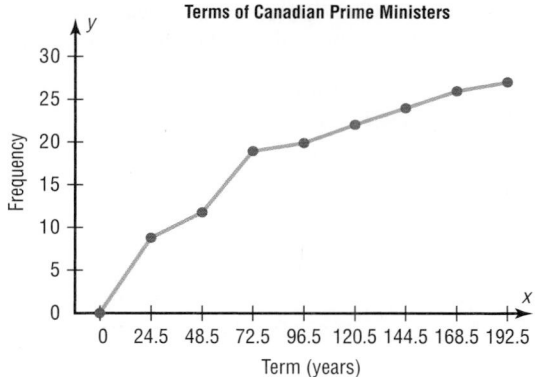

Terms of Canadian Prime Ministers

7. Max: 49; Min: 8; Range: 41;
Classes: 7; Class width: 5.9 (use 6). First class: 8–13.

Class limits	Class boundaries	Class midpoints	f	cf
8–13	7.5–13.5	10.5	5	5
14–19	13.5–19.5	16.5	12	17
20–25	19.5–25.5	22.5	10	27
26–31	25.5–31.5	28.5	4	31
32–37	31.5–37.5	34.5	3	34
38–43	37.5–43.5	40.5	1	35
44–49	43.5–49.5	46.5	1	36

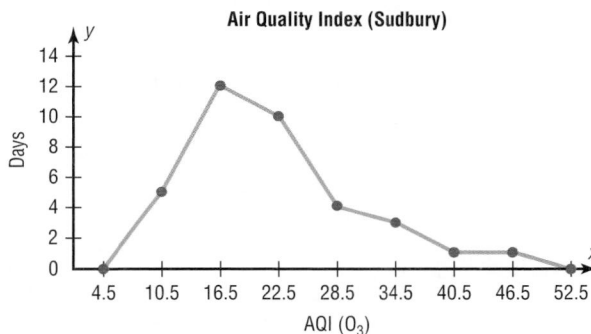

Air Quality Index (Sudbury)

9.

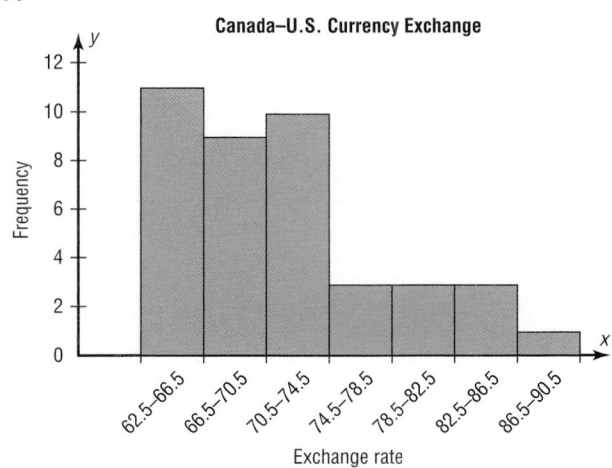

Canada–U.S. Currency Exchange

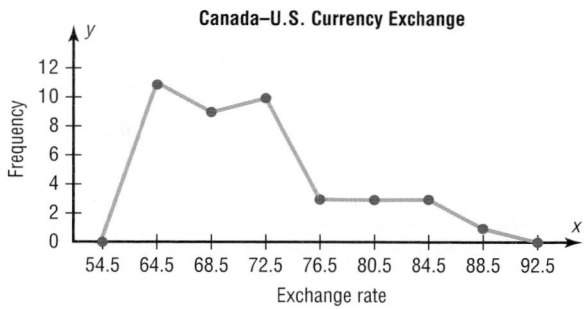

Canada–U.S. Currency Exchange

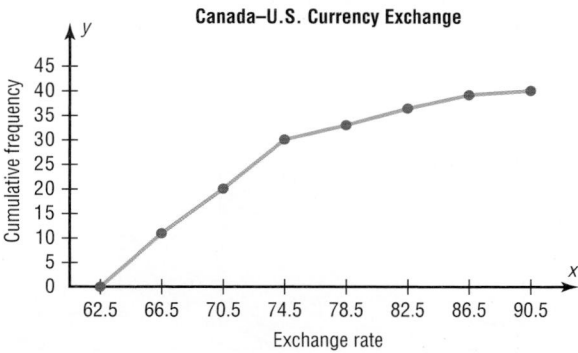

Canada–U.S. Currency Exchange

11.

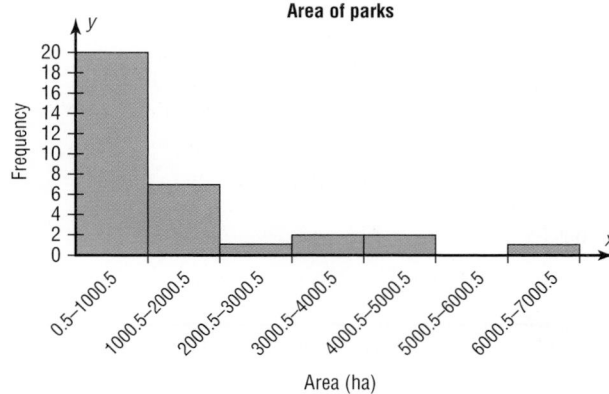

Area of parks

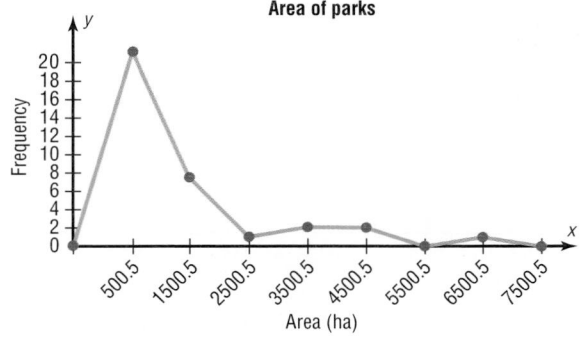

Area of parks

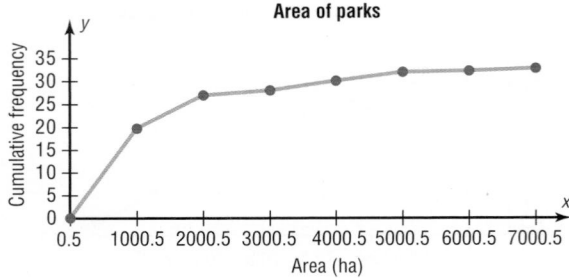

Area of parks

The peak is in the first class, followed by a smaller peak in the second class, and then the histogram is rather uniform after the second class. Most of the parks have less than 2000 hectares as compared with any other class of values.

13.

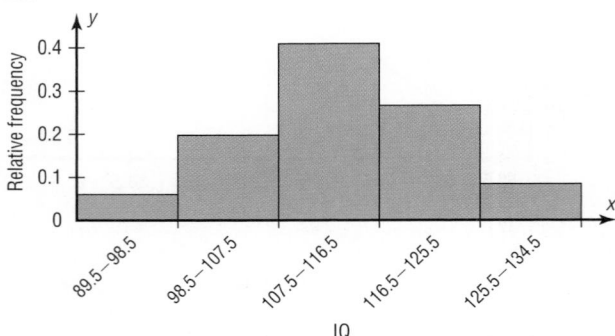

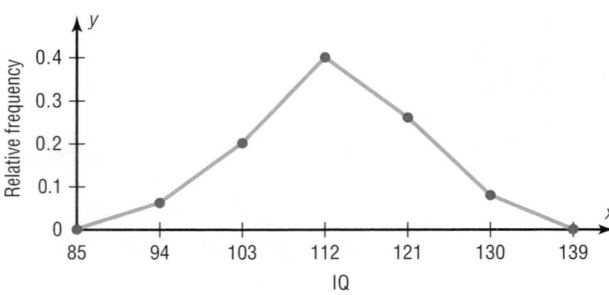

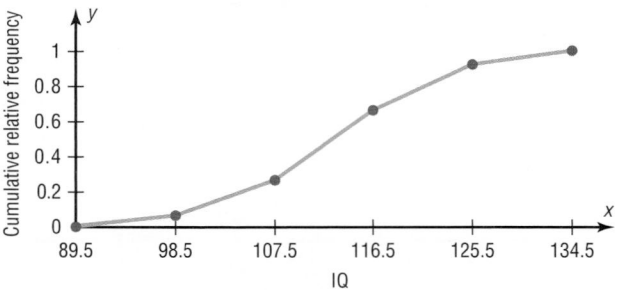

The proportion of applicants who need to enroll in a summer program is 0.26 or 26%.

15. Max: 270; Min: 80; Range: 190; Classes: 7; Width: 27.1 (use 29—rule 2 odd-numbered width)

Class limits	Class boundaries	f	rf	crf
80–108	79.5–108.5	8	0.17	0.17
109–137	108.5–137.5	13	0.28	0.45
138–166	137.5–166.5	2	0.04	0.49
167–195	166.5–195.5	9	0.20	0.69
196–224	195.5–224.5	10	0.22	0.91
225–253	224.5–253.5	2	0.04	0.95
254–282	253.5–282.5	2	0.04	0.99*
			0.99	

*Due to rounding

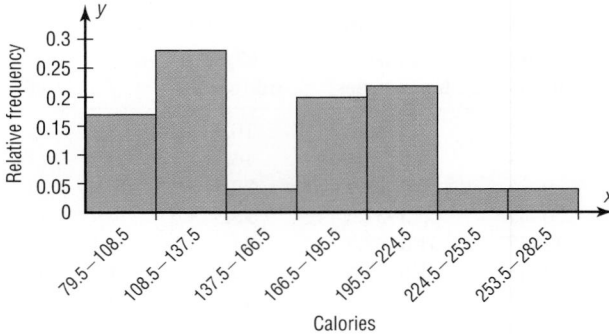

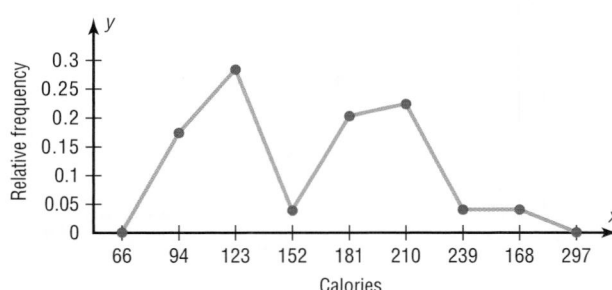

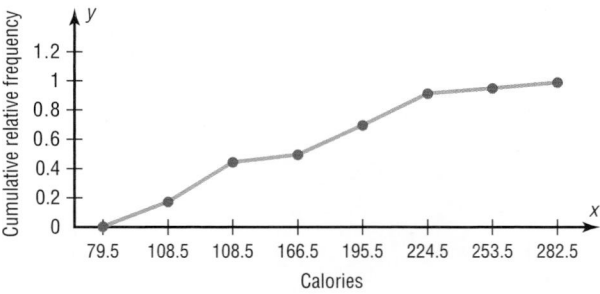

The histogram has two peaks.

17.

Class boundaries	Class midpoints	f	rf
7.5–13.5	10.5	5	0.14
13.5–19.5	16.5	12	0.33
19.5–25.5	22.5	10	0.28
25.5–31.5	28.5	4	0.11
31.5–37.5	34.5	3	0.08
37.5–43.5	40.5	1	0.03
43.5–49.5	46.5	1	0.03

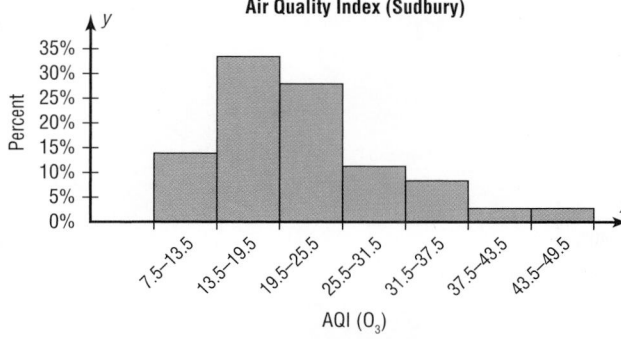

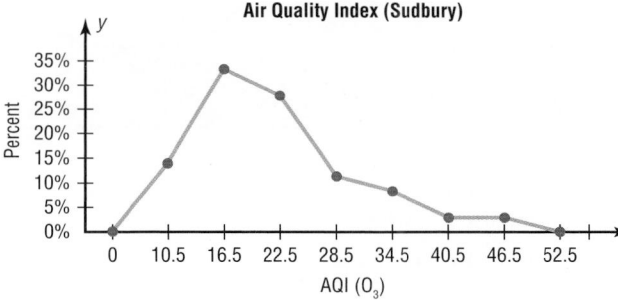

The distribution is positively or right-skewed, with the greatest proportion of days having a fair air quality reading in the range 13.5 to 25.5.

19.

Class limits	Class boundaries	Class midpoints	f	cf
22–24	21.5–24.5	23	1	1
25–27	24.5–27.5	26	3	4
28–30	27.5–30.5	29	0	4
31–33	30.5–33.5	32	6	10
34–36	33.5–36.5	35	5	15
37–39	36.5–39.5	38	3	18
40–42	39.5–42.5	41	2	20
			20	

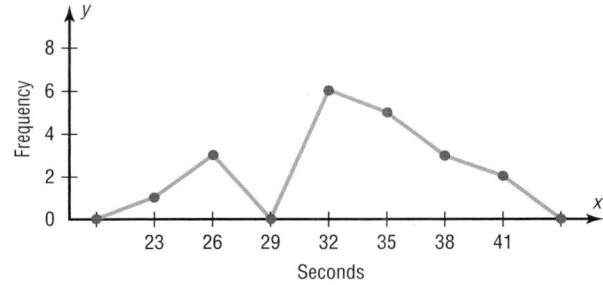

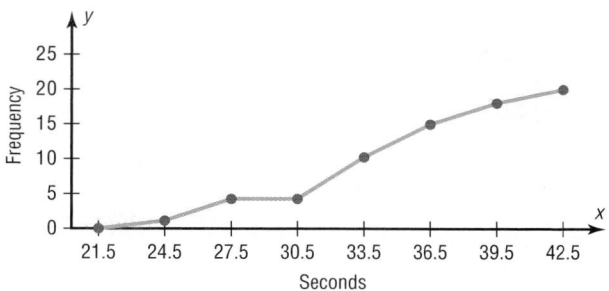

Exercises 2–3

1.

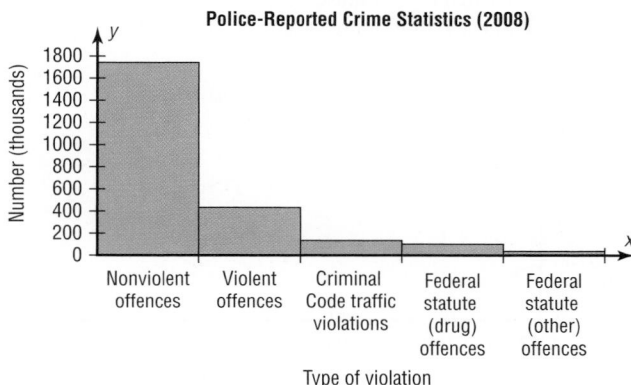

Police activity and public education should address the problem of nonviolent offences, followed by allocation of resources to address the problem of violent offences.

3.

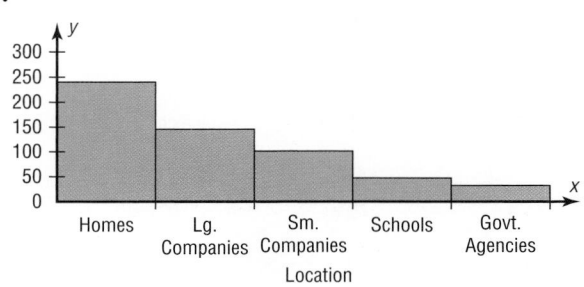

The best place to market products would be to residential users.

5.

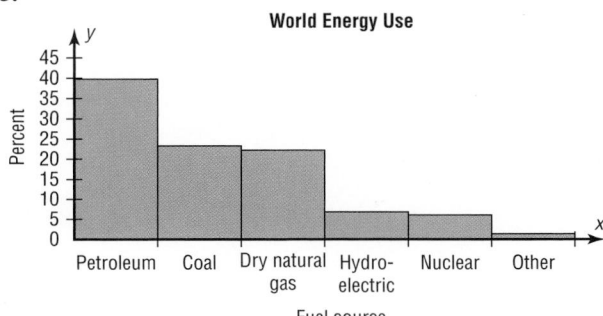

7.

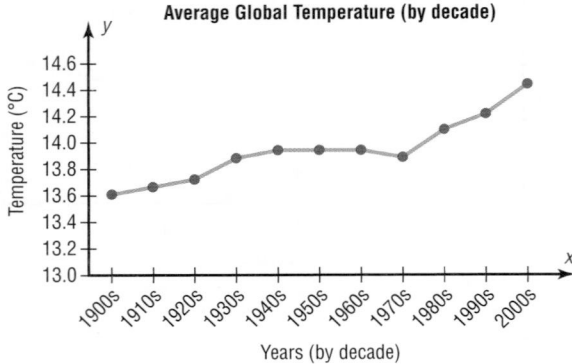

Temperatures steadily increased throughout the twentieth century, with escalating increases after the 1970s.

9.

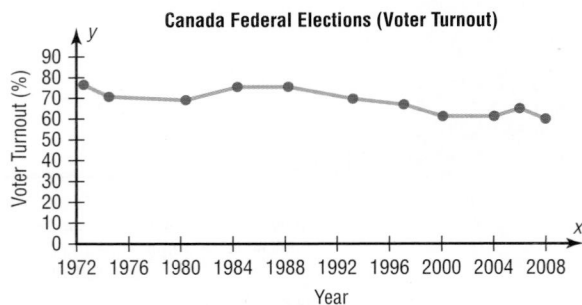

Canadian voter turnout dropped slightly from 1972 to 1980, returned to the 1972 levels in the 1984 and 1988 elections, but then declined in the 2008 election to the lowest level in the 1972–2008 period.

11.

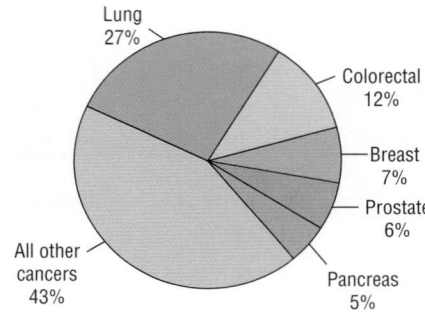

13.

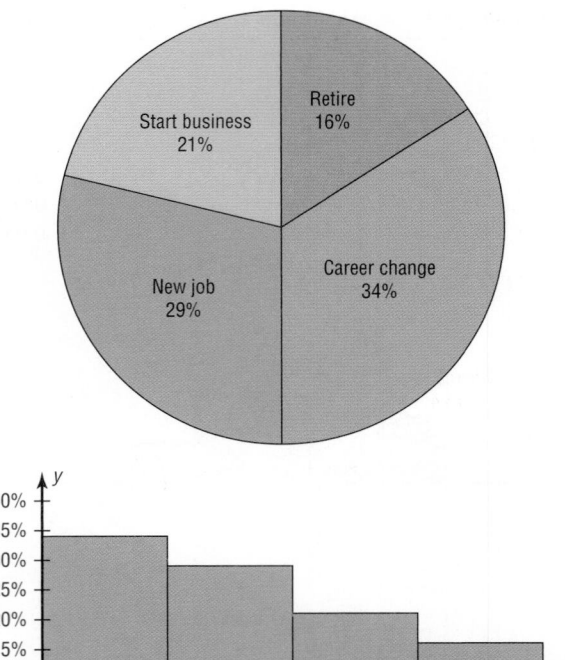

The pie graph better represents the data since we are looking at parts of a whole.

15.

Stem	Leaves
3	9
4	5 6 6 6 7 7 8
5	1 2 4 5 7 9
6	0 1 5 6 6 9
7	0 4

17.

	Variety 1			Variety 2		
	2	1	3 8			
	3	0	2	5		
9 8 8 5	2	3	6 8			
3 3 1	4	1 2 5 5				
9 9 8 5 3 3 2 1 0	5	0 3 5 5 6 7 9				
	6	2 2				

The distributions are similar but variety 2 seems to be more variable than variety 1.

19. Answers will vary. Two possible solutions are a pie chart and a Pareto chart.

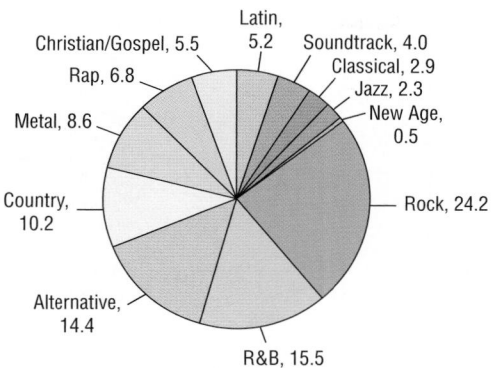

2007 Music Sales (by genre)

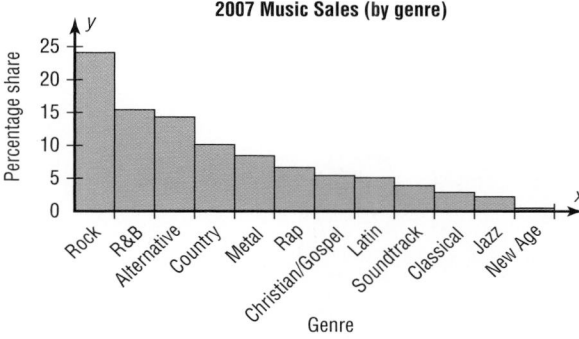

2007 Music Sales (by genre)

Both the pie chart and Pareto chart clearly illustrate that rock is the most popular genre.

21.

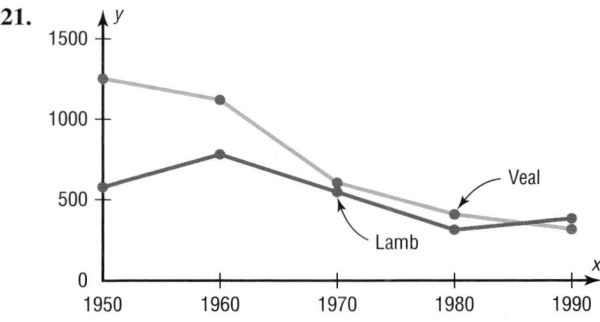

In 1950, veal production was considerably higher than lamb. By 1970, production was approximately the same for both.

23.

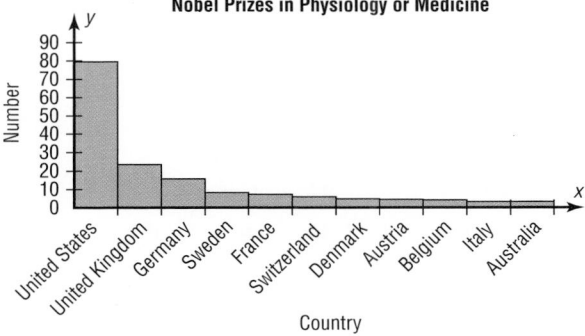

Nobel Prizes in Physiology or Medicine

25. The values on the y axis start at 3.5. Also there are no data values shown for the years 2004 through 2011.

Review Exercises

1.

Class	f
Newspaper	10
Television	16
Radio	12
Internet	12
	50

3.

Class	f
baseball	4
golf ball	5
tennis ball	6
soccer ball	5
football	5
	25

5.

Class	f	cf
11	1	1
12	2	3
13	2	5
14	2	7
15	1	8
16	2	10
17	4	14
18	2	16
19	2	18
20	1	19
21	0	19
22	1	20
	20	

7.

Class limits	Class boundaries	f	cf
85–105	84.5–105.5	4	4
106–126	105.5–126.5	7	11
127–147	126.5–147.5	9	20
148–168	147.5–168.5	10	30
169–189	168.5–189.5	9	39
190–210	189.5–210.5	1	40
		40	

9.

Class limits	Class boundaries	f	cf
170–188	169.5–188.5	11	11
189–207	188.5–207.5	9	20
208–226	207.5–226.5	4	24
227–245	226.5–245.5	5	29
246–264	245.5–264.5	0	29
265–283	264.5–283.5	0	29
284–302	283.5–302.5	0	29
303–321	302.5–321.5	1	30
		30	

11.

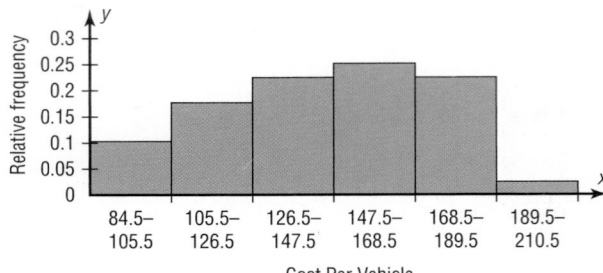

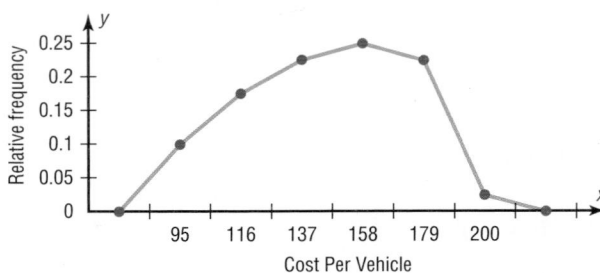

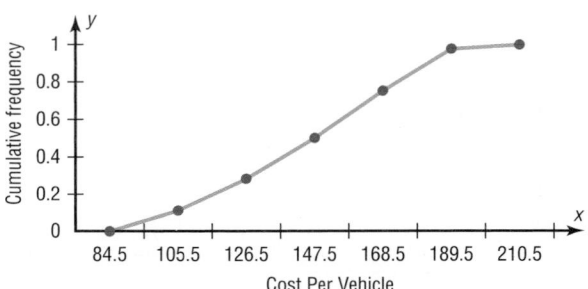

13.

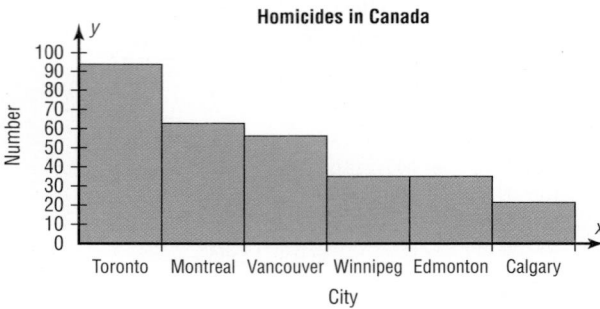

Toronto leads Canadian cities in number of homicides.

15.

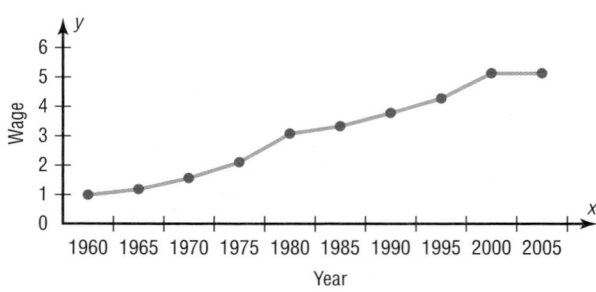

The minimum wage has increased over the years with the largest increase occurring between 1975 and 1980.

17.

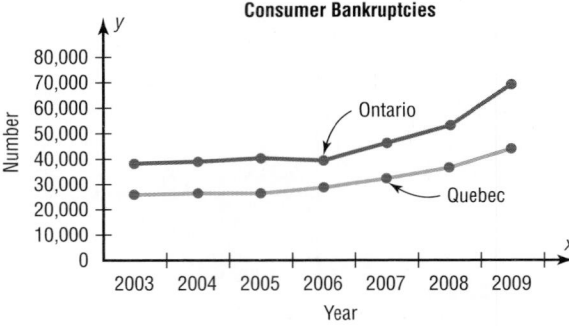

Consumer bankruptcies are on the increase but more so in Ontario than Quebec.

19.

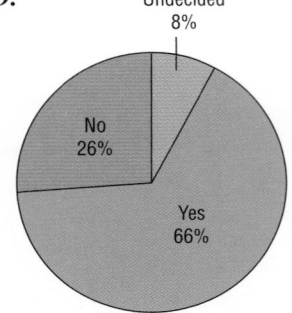

The majority of people surveyed would like to spend the rest of their careers with their present employer.

21.
```
1 | 2  4
1 | 6  7  8  8  9
2 | 0  2  3  4
2 | 5  5  5  6  6  9  9
3 | 2  3
3 | 5  7  8  8  9
```
The peak of the distribution is in the range of 25–29.

Chapter Quiz

1. False   **2.** False

3. False   **4.** True

5. True   **6.** False

7. False   **8.** *c*

9. *c*   **10.** *b*

11. *b*

12. Categorical, ungrouped, grouped

13. 5, 20   **14.** categorical

15. time series   **16.** stem and leaf plot

17. vertical or *y*

18.

Class	f	cf
H	6	6
A	5	11
M	6	17
C	8	25
	25	

19.

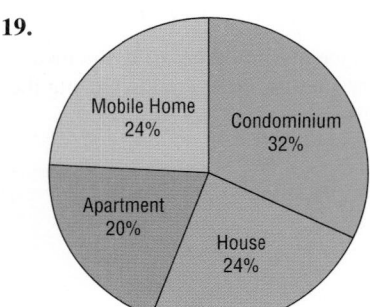

20.

Class	f	cf
0.5–1.5	1	1
1.5–2.5	5	6
2.5–3.5	3	9
3.5–4.5	4	13
4.5–5.5	2	15
5.5–6.5	6	21
6.5–7.5	2	23
7.5–8.5	3	26
8.5–9.5	4	30
	30	

21.

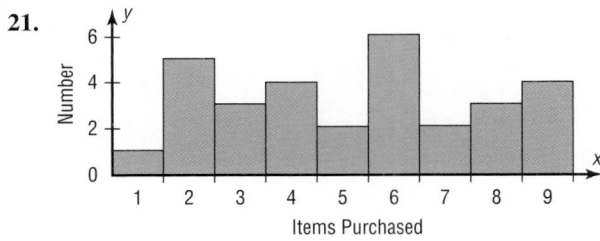

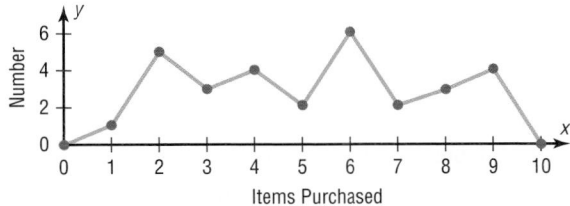

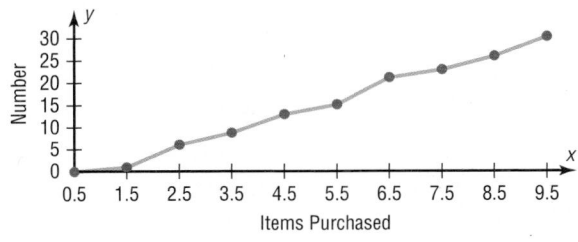

22.

Class limits	Class boundaries	f	cf
27–90	26.5–90.5	13	13
91–154	90.5–154.5	2	15
155–218	154.5–218.5	0	15
219–282	218.5–282.5	5	20
283–346	282.5–346.5	0	20
347–410	346.5–410.5	2	22
411–474	410.5–474.5	0	22
475–538	474.5–538.5	1	23
539–602	538.5–602.5	2	25
		25	

23. The distribution is positively skewed with one more than half of the data values in the lowest class.

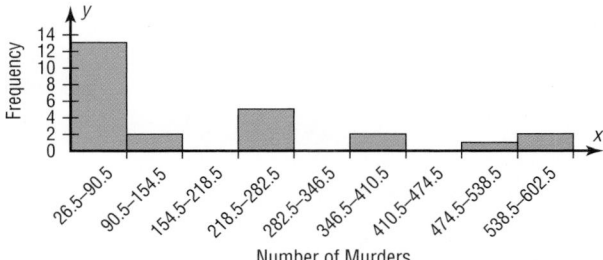

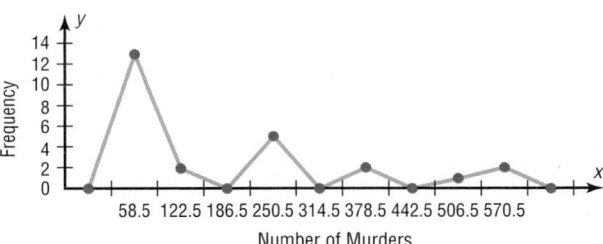

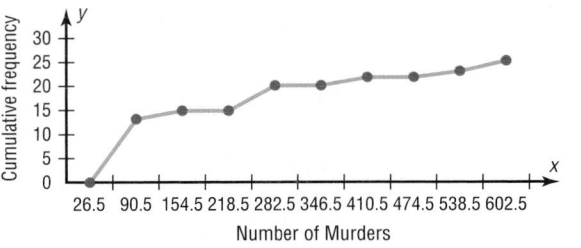

24.

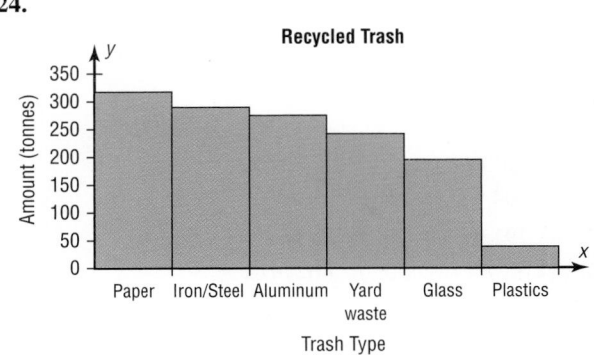

25.

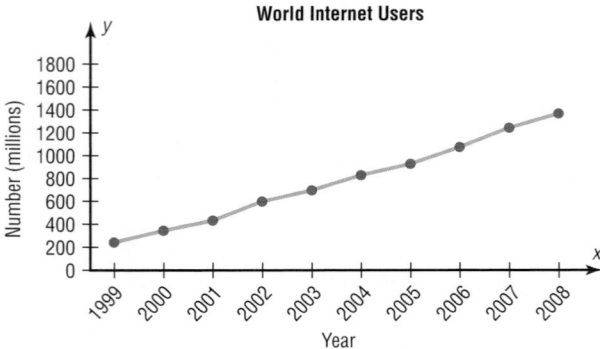

World Internet Users

World Internet use is growing at a steady pace.

26.

1	5	9			
2	6	8			
3	1	5	8	8	9
4	1	7	8		
5	3	3	4		
6	2	3	7	8	
7	6	9			
8	6	8	9		
9	8				

Chapter 3

Note: Answers may vary due to rounding or use of a calculator or computer program.

Exercises 3–1

1. *a.* 3.724   *b.* 3.73   *c.* 3.74 and 3.70   *d.* 3.715

3. *a.* 16.6   *b.* 8.5   *c.* 13.0   *d.* 37.5

5. *a.* 270.75   *c.* No mode
 b. 209   *d.* 369
 It would seem that the average number of identity thefts is not higher than 300.

7. *a.* 6.63   *c.* Mode: 5.4, 6.2, 6.4, 7.2
 b. 6.45   *d.* 6.7
 For the best measure of average, answers will vary.

9. *a.* 7746.9   *c.* 7756
 b. 7732.5   *d.* 7988.5
 The distribution is positively (right) skewed.

11. For 2001:
 a. 658.8   *b.* 302   *c.* 148   *d.* 2400
 For 2006:
 a. 704.9   *b.* 326.5   *c.* 330   *d.* 2619

13. *a.* 291.9   *b.* 292–295

15. *a.* 90.7   *b.* 60–79

17. *a.* 85.1   *b.* 74.5–85.5

19. *a.* 33.8   *b.* 27–33

21. *a.* 23.7   *b.* 21.5–24.5

23. 63.17; 1–14

25. 66.6; 63–66   **27.** 10.35 g/100 g

29. $545,666.67   **31.** 82.7

33. *a.* Median   *c.* Mode   *e.* Mode
 b. Mean   *d.* Mode   *f.* Mean

35. Both could be true since one could be using the mean for the average salary, and the other could be using the mode for the average.

37. 6

39. *a.* 54.55 km/h   *b.* 94.74 km/h   *c.* $8.33

41. 5.48

Exercises 3–2

1. The square root of the variance is equal to the standard deviation.

3. σ^2, σ

5. When the sample size is less than 30, the formula for the true standard deviation of the sample will underestimate the population standard deviation.

7. 3.6, 1.43, 1.20. Data vary based on large range and standard deviation.

9. High life expectancy:
 $R = 3.5$
 $s^2 = 1.114$
 $s = 1.55$
 Low life expectancy:
 $R = 3.5$
 $s^2 = 11.463$
 $s = 3.386$
 Low life expectancy data are more variable.

11. Hong Kong buildings:
 $R = 36$
 $s^2 = 104.4$
 $s = 10.2$
 New York buildings:
 $R = 42$
 $s^2 = 190.4$
 $s = 13.8$
 New York building data are more variable.

13. Using the range rule of thumb,
 $s = \frac{range}{4} = \frac{17.5 - 11.5}{4} = \frac{6}{4} = 1.5$; therefore, approximately 1.5 students are within 1 standard deviation from the mean of 15.9 students.

15. For Year 1:   For Year 2:
 $R = 4123$ $R = 3970$
 $s^2 = 1,030,817.63$ $s^2 = 1,019,853.85$
 $s = 1015.3$ $s = 1009.9$
 The fatalities in Year 1 are more variable.

17. $R = 11{,}263$; 7,436,475.0; 2727.0

19. 133.6; 11.6   **21.** 45.93; 6.78

23. 211.2; 14.5   **25.** 211.2; 14.5;

No, the variability of the lifetimes of the batteries is quite large.

27. 11.7; 3.4

29. For West, CVar $= 46.4\%$. For East, CVar $= 48.3\%$. The data for East are more variable.

31. 23.1%; 12.9%.

The age is more variable.

33. *a.* 96%   *b.* 93.75%

35. $7.60–$8.92   **37.** 89–101

39. 86%   **41.** 2.5%

43. $n = 30$ $\overline{X} = 214.97$ $s = 20.76$.   At least 75% of the data values will fall between $\overline{X} \pm 2s$.
$\overline{X} - 2(20.76) = 214.97 - 41.52 = 173.45$ and
$\overline{X} + 2(20.76) = 214.97 + 41.52 = 256.49$

In this case all 30 values fall within this range; hence Chebyshev's theorem is correct for this example.

45. 56%; 75%; 84%; 88.89%; 92%

47. 4.36

49. It must be an incorrect data value, since it is beyond the range using the formula $s\sqrt{n-1}$.

Exercises 3–3

1. A z score tells how many standard deviations the data value is above or below the mean.

3. A percentile is a relative measure while a percent is an absolute measure of the part to the total.

5. $Q_1 = P_{25}, Q_2 = P_{50}, Q_3 = P_{75}$

7. $D_1 = P_{10}, D_2 = P_{20}, D_3 = P_{30}$, etc.

9. Canada: $z = -0.40$
Italy: $z = 1.47$
United States: $z = -1.91$

11. *a.* 0.75   *b.* −1.25   *c.* 2.25   *d.* −2   *e.* −0.5

13. Chemistry: $z = 2.0$
Biology: $z = 2.4$
The biology exam score is relatively better.

15. Verbal reasoning: $z = 1.1$
Quantitative reasoning: $z = 1.5$
Analytical writing: $z = 1.33$
The quantitative reasoning score is relatively best.

17. *a.* 22nd   *b.* 67th   *c.* 48th   *d.* 88th

19. *a.* 234   *b.* 251   *c.* 263   *d.* 274   *e.* 284

21. a. 611 km/h ≈ 14th percentile
b. 684 km/h ≈ 41st percentile
c. 732 km/h ≈ 56th percentile

d. 813 km/h ≈ 79th percentile
e. 845 km/h ≈ 93rd percentile

23. *a.* $P_{60} = 411$ *c.* $D_4 = P_{40} = 381$
b. $Q_3 = P_{75} = 415$ *d.* $P_{85} = 427$

25. $P_{70} = 1155$

27. $P_{40} = 2.15$ **29.** $P_{33} = 31$

31. *a.* $Q_1 = 12, Q_2 = 20.5, Q_3 = 32$
Midquartile $= \frac{12 + 32}{2} = 22$ Interquartile range: $32 - 12 = 20$

b. $Q_1 = 62, Q_2 = 94, Q_3 = 99$
Midquartile $= \frac{62 + 99}{2} = 80.5$ Interquartile range: $99 - 62 = 37$

Exercises 3–4

1. 6, 8, 19, 32, 54; 24

3. 188, 192, 339, 437, 589; 245

5. 14.6, 15.5, 16.3, 18.2, 19.8; 2.7

7. 11, 3, 8, 5, 9, 4

9. 95, 55, 70, 65, 90, 25

11.

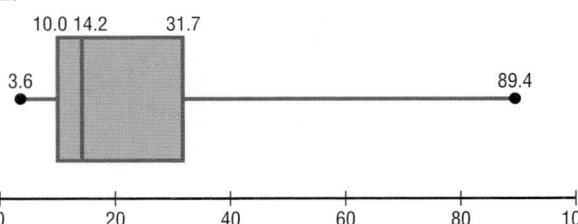

Since the median is to the left of the box centre and the line to the right of the box is longer than the line to the left of the box, the distribution is positively skewed.

13.

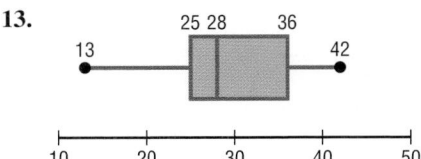

15.

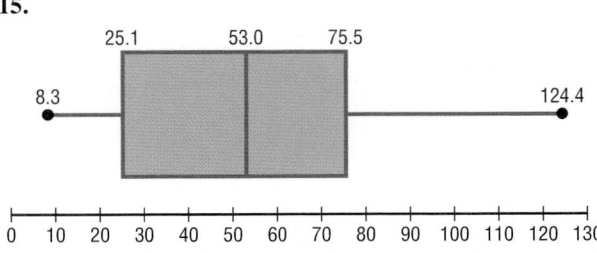

The median is slightly to the right of the box centre and the line to the right of the box is longer than the line to the left of the box, which indicates a moderate negative skew.

17. *a.* May

b. 2008

c. The five-number summaries for each year are as follows.

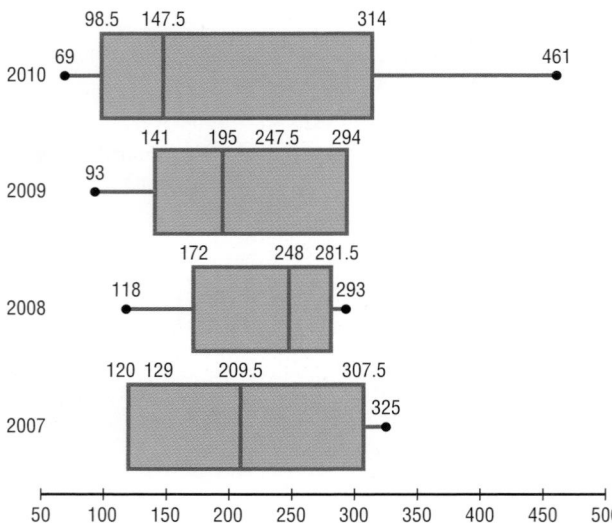

The distribution for 2008 is approximately symmetric with median near centre. The distributions for 2009 and 2010 are positively skewed. The distribution for 2008 is negatively skewed.

Review Exercises

1. *a.* 15.75   *c.* No mode.   *e.* 6.5   *g.* 2.56

b. 15.15   *d.* 16.15   *f.* 6.57

3. *a.* 7.25   *b.* 7–9   *c.* 10.0   *d.* 3.2

5. *Note:* Technically the first class should read −0.05, which is redundant. The class limits are 0–2.9, 3–5.9, 6–8.9, etc.

a. 6.034

b. 2.95–5.95 (frequency = 7)

c. 16.318

d. 4.040

7. 1.1   **9.** 6

11. Magazines: 21.4%

Year: 41.7%

The magazine data are more variable.

13. *a.*

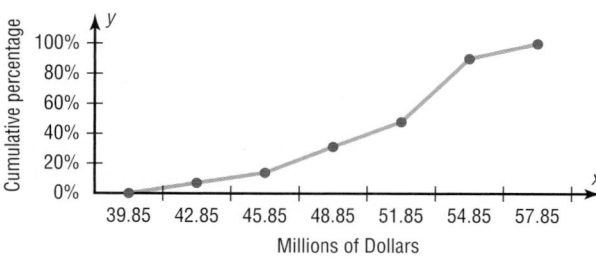

b. 49, 52, 53 (answers are approximate)

c. 15th; 33rd; 91st (answers are approximate)

15. $0.26–$0.38   **17.** 56%

19. 88.89%

21.

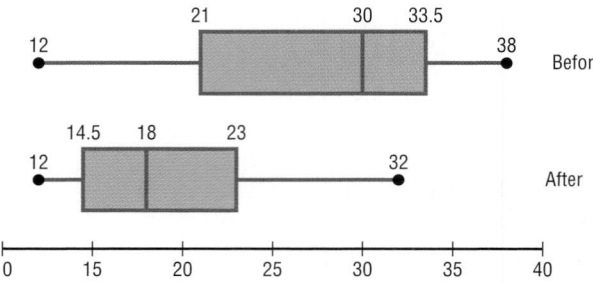

The employees worked more hours before Christmas than after Christmas. Also, the range and variability of the distribution of hours worked before Christmas are greater than those of hours worked after Christmas.

Chapter Quiz

1. True   **2.** True

3. False   **4.** False

5. False   **6.** False

7. False   **8.** False

9. False   **10.** *c*

11. *c*   **12.** *a* and *b*

13. *b*   **14.** *d*

15. *b*   **16.** statistic

17. parameters, statistics **18.** standard deviation

19. σ **20.** midrange

21. positively   **22.** outlier

23. *a.* 22.7   *c.* 22.9   *e.* 3.9   *g.* 0.994

b. 22.8   *d.* 22.75   *f.* 0.989

24. *a.* 6.4   *b.* 6–8   *c.* 11.6   *d.* 3.4

25. *a.* 64.4   *b.* 0.5–25.5   *c.* 2167.1   *d.* 46.6

26. *a.* 8.2   *b.* 7–9   *c.* 21.6   *d.* 4.6

27. 1.6

28. 4.46 or 4.5

29. 33.3%; 16.2%; newspapers

30. 31.3%; 22.9%; brands

31. −0.75; −1.67; science

32. Verbal reasoning: −0.50

Quantitative reasoning: −0.75

Science: −0.33

Science is relatively better.

33. *a.* 95, 85, 75, 65, 55, 45, 35, 25, 15, 5

  b. 269.75

  c.

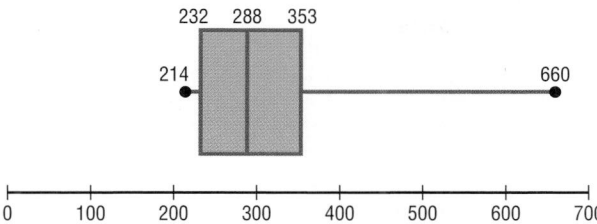

The median is to the left of the box centre and the right tail is longer than the left tail, which infers a positively skewed distribution.

34. *a.*

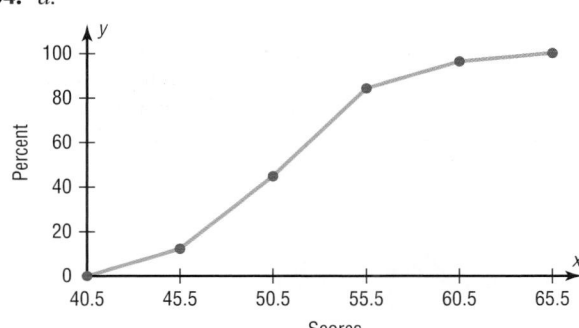

  b. 47; 54; 65

  c. 60th percentile; 6th percentile; 98th percentile

35.

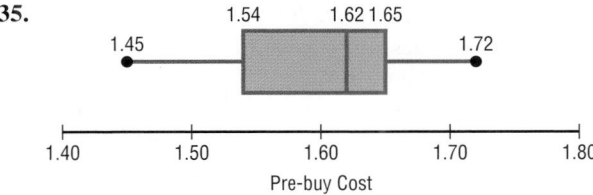

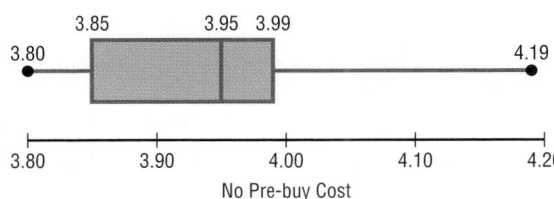

The cost of pre-buy gas is much less than to return the car without filling it with gas. The variability of the return without filling with gas is larger than the variability of the pre-buy gas.

36. *a.* 31.2 *b.* 36.3 *c.* 38.8

Chapter 4

Note: Answers may vary due to rounding or use of a calculator or computer program.

Exercises 4–1

1. A probability experiment is a chance process that leads to well-defined outcomes.

3. An outcome is the result of a single trial of a probability experiment, whereas an event can consist of one or more outcomes.

5. The range of values is $0 \leq P(E) \leq 1$.

7. 0

9. 0.80. Since the probability that it won't rain is 80%, you could leave your umbrella at home and be fairly safe.

11. *a.* empirical *d.* classical *f.* empirical

  b. classical *e.* empirical *g.* subjective

  c. empirical

12. *a.* $\frac{1}{6}$ *c.* $\frac{1}{3}$ *e.* 1 *g.* $\frac{1}{6}$

  b. $\frac{1}{2}$ *d.* 1 *f.* $\frac{5}{6}$

13. There are 6^2 or 36 outcomes.

  a. $\frac{5}{36}$ *b.* $\frac{1}{6}$ *c.* $\frac{2}{9}$ *d.* $\frac{1}{6}$ *e.* $\frac{1}{6}$

14. *a.* $\frac{1}{13}$ *c.* $\frac{1}{52}$ *e.* $\frac{4}{13}$ *g.* $\frac{1}{2}$ *i.* $\frac{7}{13}$

  b. $\frac{1}{4}$ *d.* $\frac{2}{13}$ *f.* $\frac{4}{13}$ *h.* $\frac{1}{26}$ *j.* $\frac{1}{26}$

15. There are 20 possible outcomes.

  a. $\frac{1}{6}$ *b.* $\frac{1}{2}$ *c.* $\frac{1}{2}$

17. *a.* 0.46 *b.* 0.51 *c.* 0.12

19. *a.* 0.512 or 51.2% *b.* 0.342 or 34.2%

  c. 0.897 or 89.7%

  d. Probability of fewer than 3 children, $P(E) = 89\%$, is most likely to occur.

21. *a.* $\frac{1}{8}$ *b.* $\frac{1}{4}$ *c.* $\frac{3}{4}$ *d.* $\frac{3}{4}$

23. $\frac{1}{9}$

25. *a.* $\frac{9}{19}$ *b.* $\frac{9}{38}$ *c.* $\frac{5}{38}$.

  d. The event in part *a* is most likely to occur since it has the highest probability of occurring.

27. *a.* 0.736 or 73.6% *b.* 0.264 or 26.4%

  c. 0.838 or 83.8%

29. *a.*

	1	2	3	4	5	6
1	1	2	3	4	5	6
2	2	4	6	8	10	12
3	3	6	9	12	15	18
4	4	8	12	16	20	24
5	5	10	15	20	25	30
6	6	12	18	24	30	36

  b. $\frac{5}{12}$ *c.* $\frac{17}{36}$

31. Tree Diagram—Outcomes represent the sample space ($n = 16$)

	1st child	2nd child	Outcomes

```
1st child
  1¢ ──┬── 1¢      1¢   1¢
       ├── 5¢      1¢   5¢
       ├── 10¢     1¢   10¢
       └── 25¢     1¢   25¢

  5¢ ──┬── 1¢      5¢   1¢
       ├── 5¢      5¢   5¢
       ├── 10¢     5¢   10¢
       └── 25¢     5¢   25¢

  10¢ ─┬── 1¢      10¢  1¢
       ├── 5¢      10¢  5¢
       ├── 10¢     10¢  10¢
       └── 25¢     10¢  25¢

  25¢ ─┬── 1¢      25¢  1¢
       ├── 5¢      25¢  5¢
       ├── 10¢     25¢  10¢
       └── 25¢     25¢  25¢
```

33.

```
1 ──┬── 1    1,1
    ├── 2    1,2
    ├── 3    1,3
    └── 4    1,4

2 ──┬── 1    2,1
    ├── 2    2,2
    ├── 3    2,3
    └── 4    2,4

3 ──┬── 1    3,1
    ├── 2    3,2
    ├── 3    3,3
    └── 4    3,4

4 ──┬── 1    4,1
    ├── 2    4,2
    ├── 3    4,3
    └── 4    4,4
```

35.

```
1 ──┬── 1 ──┬── 1    1,1,1
    │       ├── 2    1,1,2
    │       ├── 3    1,1,3
    │       ├── 4    1,1,4
    │       └── 5    1,1,5
    │
    ├── 2 ──┬── 1    1,2,1
    │       ├── 2    1,2,2
    │       ├── 3    1,2,3
    │       ├── 4    1,2,4
    │       └── 5    1,2,5
    │
    └── 3 ──┬── 1    1,3,1
            ├── 2    1,3,2
            ├── 3    1,3,3
            ├── 4    1,3,4
            └── 5    1,3,5

2 ──┬── 1 ──┬── 1    2,1,1
    │       ├── 2    2,1,2
    │       ├── 3    2,1,3
    │       ├── 4    2,1,4
    │       └── 5    2,1,5
    │
    ├── 2 ──┬── 1    2,2,1
    │       ├── 2    2,2,2
    │       ├── 3    2,2,3
    │       ├── 4    2,2,4
    │       └── 5    2,2,5
    │
    └── 3 ──┬── 1    2,3,1
            ├── 2    2,3,2
            ├── 3    2,3,3
            ├── 4    2,3,4
            └── 5    2,3,5
```

37. *a.* 0.08   *b.* 0.01   *c.* 0.35   *d.* 0.36

39. The statement is probably not based on empirical probability and probably not true.

41. Actual outcomes will vary, however each number should occur approximately $\frac{1}{6}$ of the time.

43. *a.* 1:5, 5:1   *d.* 1:1, 1:1   *g.* 1:1, 1:1
b. 1:1, 1:1   *e.* 1:12, 12:1
c. 1:3, 3:1   *f.* 1:3, 3:1

Exercises 4–2

1. Two events are mutually exclusive if they cannot occur at the same time. Examples will vary.

3. *a.* 0.797 or 79.7%   *c.* 0.012 or 1.2%
b. 0.623 or 62.3%   *d.* 0.819 or 81.9%

5. $\frac{11}{19}$ or 0.579

7. *a.* $\frac{7}{25}$ or 0.28   *b.* $\frac{3}{8}$ or 0.375   *c.* $\frac{17}{100}$ or 0.17
d. Event *b* has the highest probability so it is most likely to occur.

9. 0.55

11. *a.* $\frac{6}{7}$ *b.* $\frac{4}{7}$ *c.* 1

13. *a.* 0.150   *b.* 0.649   *c.* 0.705

15. *a.* 0.434   *b.* 0.390   *c.* 0.279   *d.* 0.651

17. *a.* $\frac{14}{31}$ *b.* $\frac{23}{31}$ *c.* $\frac{19}{31}$

19. *a.* $\frac{1}{15}$ *b.* $\frac{1}{3}$ *c.* $\frac{5}{6}$ *d.* $\frac{5}{6}$ *e.* $\frac{1}{3}$

21. *a.* $\frac{5}{12}$ *b.* $\frac{1}{8}$ *c.* $\frac{2}{3}$ *d.* $\frac{23}{24}$

23. *a.* $\frac{3}{13}$ *b.* $\frac{3}{4}$ *c.* $\frac{19}{52}$ *d.* $\frac{7}{13}$ *e.* $\frac{15}{26}$

25. $\frac{7}{10}$ **27.** 0.06

29. 0.30

Exercises 4–3

1. *a.* independent   *e.* independent
    b. dependent   *f.* dependent
    c. dependent   *g.* dependent
    d. dependent   *h.* independent

3. 0.706 or 70.6%; the event is somewhat but not highly likely to occur since the probability is greater than 0.5.

5. 0.437 or 43.7%; the event is unlikely because the probability is less than 0.5.

7. *a.* 0.2   *b.* 0.8   *c.* 0.512

9. 0.154 or 15.4%   **11.** 0.0298 or 2.98%

13. 0.498 or 49.8%   **15.** $\frac{243}{1024}$

17. $\frac{5}{28}$

19. 0.210; the event is unlikely to occur since the probability is less than 0.5.

21. 0.116   **23.** 0.03

25. $\frac{49}{72}$ **27.** 0.116

29. 89%   **31.** 70%

33. *a.* 0.714   *b.* 0.435   *c.* 0.156

35. *a.* 0.108 or 10.8%   *b.* 0.0278

37. *a.* 0.002 or 0.2%   *b.* 0.998

39. 0.999936   **41.** 0.000151

43. $\frac{14,498}{20,825}$ **45.** 26.6%

47. $\frac{31}{32}$

49. 0.721; the event is likely to occur since the probability is about 72%.

51. $\frac{7}{8}$

53. No, because $P(A \cap B) = 0$ therefore $P(A \cap B) \neq P(A) \cdot P(B)$

55. Yes.
    $P(\text{enroll}) = 0.55$
    $P(\text{enroll} \mid DW) > P(\text{enroll})$, which indicates that DW has a positive effect on enrollment.
    $P(\text{enroll} \mid LP) = P(\text{enroll})$, which indicates that LP has no effect on enrollment.
    $P(\text{enroll} \mid MH) < P(\text{enroll})$, which indicates that MH has a low effect on enrollment.
    Thus, all students should meet with DW.

Exercises 4–4

1. 100,000; 30,240   **3.** 5040

5. 40,320   **7.** 5040

9. 1000;72   **11.** 600

13. *a.* 40,320   *e.* 2520   *i.* 120
    b. 3,628,800   *f.* 11,880   *j.* 30
    c. 1   *g.* 60
    d. 1   *h.* 1

15. 24   **17.** 7315

19. 840   **21.** 151,200

23. 5,527,200   **25.** 495; 11,880

27. *a.* 10   *c.* 35   *e.* 15   *g.* 1   *i.* 66
    b. 56   *d.* 15   *f.* 1   *h.* 36   *j.* 4

29. 120   **31.** 210

33. 15,504   **35.** 43,758; 12,870

37. 495; 210; 420   **39.** 340; 475

41. 2970   **43.** 28

45. 330   **47.** 190,040

49. 15

51. *a.* 48   *b.* 60   *c.* 72

Exercises 4–5

1. $\frac{11}{221}$

3. *a.* $\frac{4}{35}$ *b.* $\frac{1}{35}$ *c.* $\frac{12}{35}$ *d.* $\frac{18}{35}$

5. *a.* 0.000269 or 0.0269%
    b. 0.00000439 or 0.000439%

7. $\frac{1}{1225}$

9. *a.* $\frac{10}{143}$ *c.* $\frac{15}{1001}$ *e.* $\frac{48}{143}$
    b. $\frac{60}{143}$ *d.* $\frac{160}{1001}$

11. *a.* 0.3216   *b.* 0.1637   *c.* 0.5146
    d. It probably got lost in the wash!

13. $\frac{5}{72}$ **15.** $\frac{1}{60}$

Review Exercises

1. *a.* $\frac{1}{6}$ *b.* $\frac{1}{6}$ *c.* $\frac{2}{3}$

3. *a.* 0.7   *b.* 0.5

5. $\frac{17}{30}$ **7.** 0.19

9. 0.98   **11.** 0.289 or 28.9%

13. *a.* $\frac{2}{17}$ *b.* $\frac{11}{850}$ *c.* $\frac{1}{5525}$

15. *a.* 0.603   *b.* 0.340   *c.* 0.324   *d.* 0.379

17. 0.4

19. 0.51   **21.** 57.3%

23. *a.* $\frac{19}{44}$ *b.* $\frac{1}{4}$

25. $\frac{31}{32}$

27. 17,576,000; 11,232,000; 12,654,720

29. 350   **31.** 45

33. 26,000   **35.** 495

37. 15,504

39. 1/258,336,000

41. 0.097

Chapter Quiz

1. False   **2.** False

3. True   **4.** False

5. False   **6.** False

7. True   **8.** False

9. *b*   **10.** *b* and *d*

11. *d*   **12.** *b*

13. *c*   **14.** *b*

15. *d*   **16.** *b*

17. *b*   **18.** sample space

19. zero and one **20.** zero

21. one   **22.** mutually exclusive

23. *a.* $\frac{1}{13}$ *b.* $\frac{1}{13}$ *c.* $\frac{4}{13}$

24. *a.* $\frac{1}{4}$ *b.* $\frac{4}{13}$ *c.* $\frac{1}{52}$ *d.* $\frac{1}{13}$ *e.* $\frac{1}{2}$

25. *a.* $\frac{12}{31}$ *b.* $\frac{12}{31}$ *c.* $\frac{27}{31}$ *d.* $\frac{24}{31}$

26. *a.* $\frac{11}{36}$ *c.* $\frac{11}{36}$ *e.* 0
     b. $\frac{5}{18}$ *d.* $\frac{1}{3}$ *f.* $\frac{11}{12}$

27. 0.84   **28.** 0.002

29. *a.* $\frac{253}{9996}$ *b.* $\frac{33}{66,640}$ *c.* 0

30. 0.54   **31.** 0.53

32. 0.81   **33.** 0.056

34. *a.* $\frac{1}{2}$ *b.* $\frac{3}{7}$

35. 0.99   **36.** 0.518

37. 0.9999886   **38.** 2,646

39. 40,320   **40.** 1,365

41. 1,188,137,600; 710,424,000

42. 720   **43.** 33,554,432

44. 56   **45.** $\frac{1}{4}$

46. $\frac{3}{14}$ **47.** $\frac{12}{55}$

48.

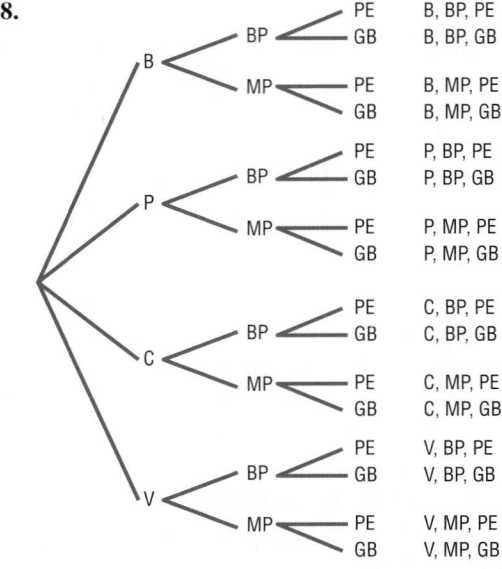

Chapter 5

Exercises 5–1

1. A random variable is a variable whose values are determined by chance. Examples will vary.

3. The number of commercials a radio station plays during each hour. The number of times a student uses his or her calculator during a mathematics exam. The number of leaves on a specific type of tree.

5. A probability distribution is a distribution that consists of the values a random variable can assume, along with the corresponding probabilities of these values.

7. No; probabilities cannot be negative and the sum of the probabilities is not one.

9. Yes

11. No, probability values cannot be greater than 1.

13. Discrete   **15.** Continuous

17. Discrete

19.

X	0	1	2	3
$P(X)$	$\frac{6}{15}$	$\frac{5}{15}$	$\frac{3}{15}$	$\frac{1}{15}$

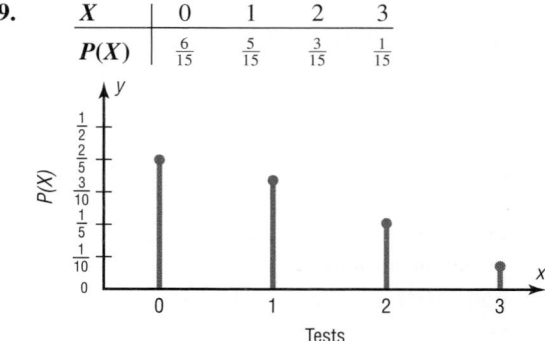

21.

X	0	1	2	3	4	5
P(X)	0.75	0.17	0.04	0.025	0.01	0.005

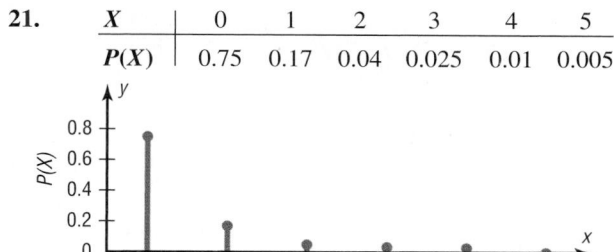

23.

X	1	2	3	4	5	6
P(X)	$\frac{1}{2}$	$\frac{1}{6}$	$\frac{1}{12}$	$\frac{1}{12}$	$\frac{1}{12}$	$\frac{1}{12}$

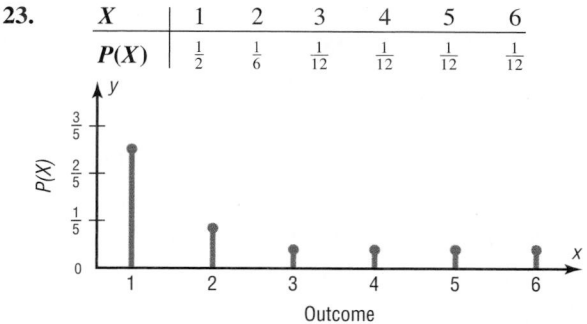

25.

X	3	4	5	6	7
P(X)	0.15	0.20	0.25	0.2	0.2

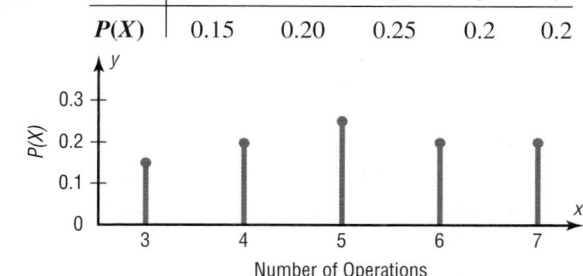

27. Let X = Canadian currency ($bills)

X	f	P(X)
$5	2	0.222
$10	3	0.333
$20	1	0.111
$50	3	0.333
	9	1.000

29.

X	1	2	3	4
P(X)	$\frac{1}{4}$	$\frac{1}{4}$	$\frac{3}{8}$	$\frac{1}{8}$

31.

X	1	2	3
P(X)	$\frac{1}{6}$	$\frac{1}{3}$	$\frac{1}{2}$

Yes.

33.

X	3	4	7
P(X)	$\frac{3}{6}$	$\frac{4}{6}$	$\frac{7}{6}$

No, the sum of the probabilities is greater than one and $P(7) = \frac{7}{6}$, which is also greater than one.

35.

X	1	2	3
P(X)	$\frac{1}{7}$	$\frac{2}{7}$	$\frac{4}{7}$

Yes.

Exercises 5–2

1. 0.15; 0.3075; 0.55; 2

3. 1.3; 0.9; 1. No, on average each person has about one credit card.

5. 5.4; 2.94; 2.71   **7.** 6.6; 1.3; 1.1

9. 13.9; 1.3; 1.1   **11.** $260

13. $0.83   **15.** −$1.00

17. −$0.50; − $0.52   **19.** $4

21. 10.5   **23.** Answers will vary.

25. Answers will vary.

Exercises 5–3

1. *a.* Yes   *c.* Yes   *e.* No   *g.* Yes   *i.* No
  b. Yes   *d.* No   *f.* Yes   *h.* Yes   *j.* Yes

2. *a.* 0.420   *c.* 0.590   *e.* 0.000   *g.* 0.418   *i.* 0.246
  b. 0.346   *d.* 0.251   *f.* 0.250   *h.* 0.176

3. *a.* 0.0005   *c.* 0.342   *e.* 0.173
  b. 0.131   *d.* 0.007

5. 0.021; no, it's only about a 2% chance.

7. *a.* 0.275   *b.* 0.423   *c.* 0.852   *d.* 0.757

9. 0.071

11. *a.* 0.292   *b.* 0.773   *c.* 0.556   *d.* 0.0444

13. *a.* 0.281   *b.* 0.723   *c.* 0.574   *d.* 0.707

15. 3.5; 3.476; 1.864   **17.** 9; 8.73; 2.95

19. 80; 8.579; 73.6   **21.** 0.199

23. 0.514   **25.** 0.409

27. 0.172

29.

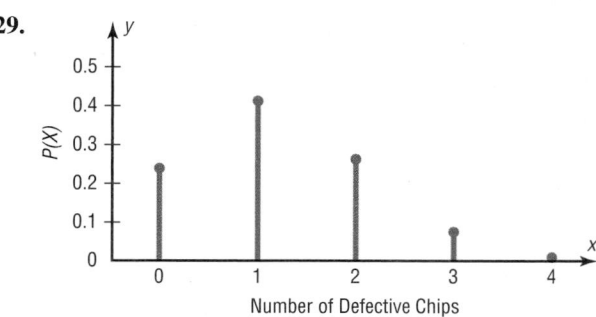

Exercises 5–4

1. *a.* 0.135   *c.* 0.0096   *e.* 0.0112
  b. 0.0324   *d.* 0.18

3. 0.063   **5.** $\frac{1}{108}$

7. *a.* 0.1563   *c.* 0.0504   *e.* 0.1241
  b. 0.1465   *d.* 0.071

9. *a.* 0.0183   *c.* 0.1465
    b. 0.0733   *d.* 0.7619

11. 0.3554   **13.** 0.0498

15. 0.1563   **17.** 0.117

19. 0.13   **21.** 0.597

Review Exercises

1. Yes.

3. No, the sum of the probabilities is greater than one.

5. *a.* 0.35   *b.* 1.55; 1.808; 1.345

7.

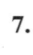

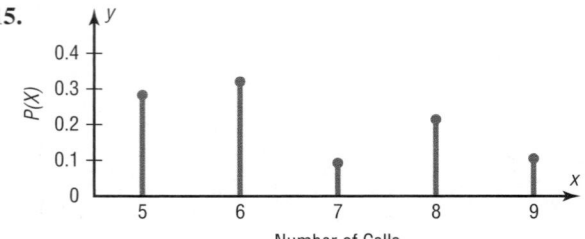

9. 15.2; 1.6; 1.3   **11.** 24.2; 1.5; 1.2

13. $2.15

15. *a.* 0.122   *b.* 0.989   *c.* 0.043

17. 135; 33.8; 5.8   **19.** 0.967

21. 0.175   **23.** 0.008

25. 0.050

27. *a.* 0.5543   *b.* 0.8488   *c.* 0.4457

29. 0.27   **31.** 0.0862

Chapter Quiz

1. True   **2.** False

3. False   **4.** True

5. chance   **6.** $\mu = n \cdot p$

7. one   **8.** *c*

9. *c*   **10.** *d*

11. No, the sum of the probabilities is greater than one.

12. Yes   **13.** Yes

14. Yes

15.

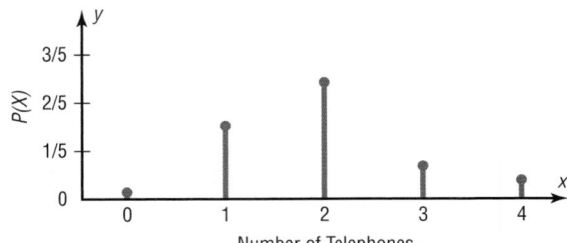

16.

X	0	1	2	3	4
$P(X)$	0.02	0.30	0.48	0.13	0.07

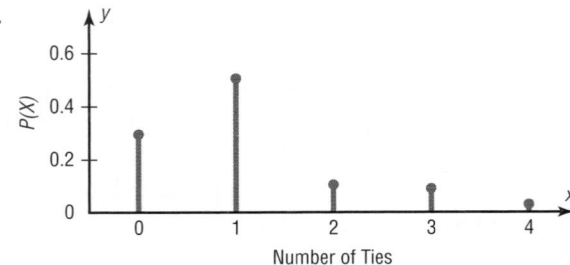

17. 2.0; 1.3; 1.1   **18.** 32.2; 1.1; 1.0

19. 5.2   **20.** $9.65

21. 0.124

22. *a.* 0.075   *b.* 0.872   *c.* 0.126

23. 240; 48; 6.9   **24.** 9; 7.9; 2.8

25. 0.00797   **26.** 0.000332

27. 0.0614   **28.** 0.122

29. *a.* 0.5471   *b.* 0.9863   *c.* 0.4529

30. 0.128

31. *a.* 0.16   *b.* 0.42   *c.* 0.0699

Chapter 6

Exercises 6–1

1. The properties of the normal distribution are:
    a. It is bell-shaped.
    b. It is symmetric about the mean.
    c. The mean, median, and mode are equal.
    d. It is continuous.
    e. It never touches the *x* axis.
    f. The area under the curve is equal to one.
    g. It is unimodal.

3. One or 100%.   **5.** 68%, 95%, 99.7%

7. 0.2734   **9.** 0.4808

11. 0.4090   **13.** 0.0764

15. 0.1145   **17.** 0.0258

19. 0.8417   **21.** 0.9826

23. 0.5596   **25.** 0.3574

27. 0.2486   **29.** 0.4418

31. 0.0023   **33.** 0.1131

35. 0.9522   **37.** 0.0706

39. 0.9222   **41.** −1.94

43. −2.13   **45.** −1.26

47. *a.* −2.28   *b.* −0.92   *c.* −0.27

49. *a.* $z = \pm 1.96$
  b. $z = \pm 1.645$
  c. $z = \pm 2.575$

51. 0.6826; 0.9544; 0.9974; they are very close.

53. 2.10   **55.** -1.45 and 0.11

57.

x	−2	−2	−1	−1	0	0.5	1	1.5	2
y	0.1	0.1	0.2	0.4	0.4	0.4	0.2	0.1	0.1

58.

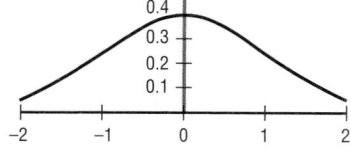

Exercises 6–2

1. 0.1401 or 14.01%

3. *a.* 0.2776   *b.* 0.1518

5. *a.* 0.3023 or 30.23%
  b. 0.0062 or 0.62%

7. *a.* 0.6628 or 66.28%
  b. 0.0436 or 4.36%

9. *a.* 0.1251 or 12.51%
  b. 0.2317 or 23.17%
  c. 0.2451 or 24.51%

11. *a.* 0.2776 or 27.76%
  b. 0.2702 or 27.02%
  c. 0.4522 or 45.22%

13. *a.* 0.3281 or 32.81%
  b. 0.4002 or 40.02%
  c. 0.0091 or 0.91%

15. 15.7; 18.9

17. The prices are between $5518.25 and $7465.75. Yes, a boat priced at $5550 would be sold in this store.

19. 139.8; 158.2   **21.** $21,718

23. $7290; $9222

25. *a.* 8.56 or approximately 9 days
  b. 5.95 or approximately 6 days

27. $18,840.48

29. 18.6 months.

31. *a.* $\mu = 120, \sigma = 20$ *b.* $\mu = 15, \sigma = 2.5$ *c.* $\mu = 30, \sigma = 5$

33. There are several mathematical tests that can be used including drawing a histogram and calculating Pearson's index of skewness.

35. 1.05

37. $\mu = 0.45$ and $\sigma = 1.34$

39.

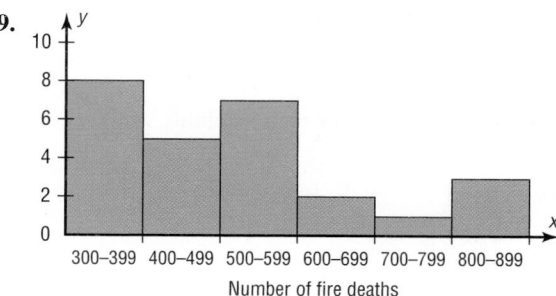

Histogram is positive or right-skewed.
Not skewed, since Pearson's index of skewness of 0.27 is within ±1 range.
There are no outliers.
Inconclusive, check for normality using normal probability plot.

41.

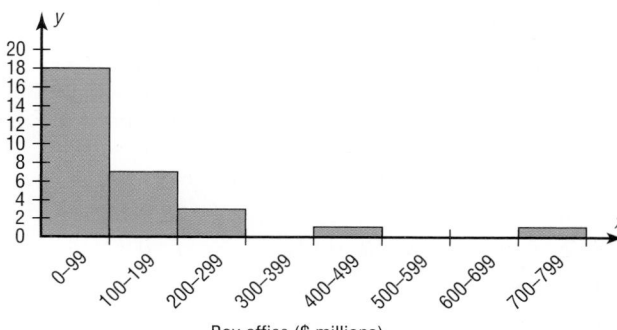

Histogram is positive or right-skewed.
Skewed, since Pearson's index of skewness of 1.16 is outside the ±1 range.
There are outliers.
The distribution is not normal.

Exercises 6–3

1. The distribution is called the sampling distribution of sample means.

3. The mean of the sample means is equal to the population mean.

5. The distribution will be approximately normal when the sample size is large.

7. $z = \frac{\bar{x} - \mu}{\sigma / \sqrt{n}}$ **9.** 0.0045 or 0.45%

11. 0.1190 or 11.90%. If overweight is considered to be the top 15%, or above the 85th percentile of weights, then the group is overweight.

13. 0.0107

15. *a.* 0.3859   *b.* 0.1841
  c. Individual values are more variable than means.

17. 0.8966   **19.** 0.9153

21. *a.* 0.3446   *b.* 0.0023
   c. Yes, since it is within one standard deviation of the mean.
   d. Very unlikely, since the probability would be less than 1%.

23. *a.* 0.6406   *b.* 0.0392

25. *a.* 0.2164   *b.* 0.8805

27. 0.9778

29. $\sigma_x = \frac{\sigma}{\sqrt{n}} = \frac{15}{\sqrt{100}} = 1.5$
   $2(1.5) = \frac{15}{\sqrt{n}}$
   $3 \cdot \sqrt{n} = 5$
   $n = 25$

Exercises 6–4

1. When *p* is approximately 0.5, and as *n* increases, the shape of the binomial distribution becomes similar to the normal distribution. The normal approximation should be used only when *n p* and *n q* are both greater than or equal to 5. The correction for continuity is necessary because the normal distribution is continuous and the binomial is discrete.

2. *a.* 0.811   *c.* 0.1052   *e.* 0.2327
   b. 0.0516   *d.* 0.1711   *f.* 0.9988

3. *a.* Yes   *c.* No   *e.* Yes
   b. No   *d.* Yes   *f.* No

5. 0.1660   **7.** 0.4960

9. 0.3483   **11.** 0.4761

13. 0.9951; yes

Review Exercises

1. *a.* 0.4744   *e.* 0.2139   *i.* 0.0183
   b. 0.1443   *f.* 0.8284   *j.* 0.9535
   c. 0.0590   *g.* 0.0233
   d. 0.8329   *h.* 0.9131

3. *a.* 0.500   *b.* 0.2358
   c. A salary of $18,000 is the cutoff for the bottom 23.58% of salaries or 76.42% of 15- to 24-year-olds earns a higher salary.

5. 0.9686; 0.9099

7. *a.* 0.6915   *b.* 0.8686

9. *a.* 0.6628   *b.* 0.0014

11. 0.0655   **13.** 0.8389

15. 0.9686

17.

School FTEs

Histogram is positive or right-skewed.
Pearson's index of skewness of 0.7 is within ±1 range; indicates no skew.
There are outliers.
The distribution is not normal.

Chapter Quiz

1. False   **2.** True

3. True   **4.** True

5. False   **6.** False

7. *a*   **8.** *a*

9. *b*   **10.** *b*

11. *c*   **12.** 0.5

13. Sampling error.   **14.** The population mean.

15. The standard error of the mean.

16. 5   **17.** 5%

18. *a.* 0.4332   *d.* 0.1029   *g.* 0.0401   *j.* 0.9131
   b. 0.3944   *e.* 0.2912   *h.* 0.8997
   c. 0.0344   *f.* 0.8284   *i.* 0.017

19. *a.* 0.4846   *d.* 0.0188   *g.* 0.0089   *j.* 0.8461
   b. 0.4693   *e.* 0.7461   *h.* 0.9582
   c. 0.9334   *f.* 0.0384   *i.* 0.9788

20. *a.* 0.4207   *b.* 0.3409   *c.* 0.2347
   d. If we use the 90th percentile or top 10% of rainfalls as extremely wet, the top 10% of rainfalls would exceed 101.5 mm.

21. *a.* 0.1335   *b.* 0.3156   *c.* 0.5733
   d. 152.6; 173.4

22. *a.* 0.3090   *b.* 0.1711   *c.* 0.9686   *d.* 0.8051

23. *a.* 0.0013   *b.* 0.0668   *c.* 0.2144   *d.* 0.8664

24. *a.* 0.0037   *b.* 0.0228   *c.* 0.5   *d.* 0.3232

25. 8.804 cm

26. The lowest acceptable score is 121.24.

27. 0.015   **28.** 0.9738

29. 0.5793 **30.** 0.0630

31. 0.2177 **32.** 0.7123

33.

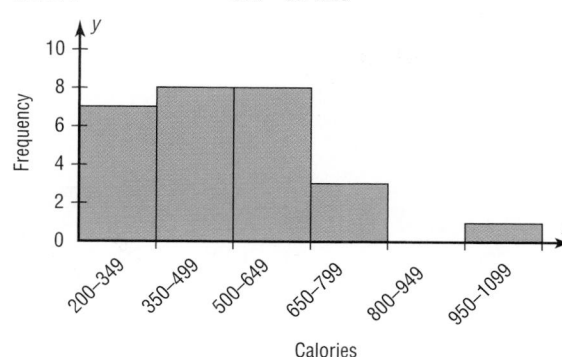

Calories

Histogram is positive or right-skewed.
Pearson's index of skewness of 0.4 is within ±1 range; indicates not skewed.
There are outliers.
Distribution is not normal.

34.

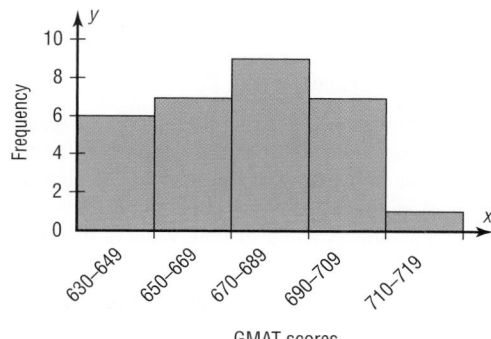

GMAT scores

Histogram is approximately normal.
Pearson's index of skewness of –0.4 is within ±1 range; indicates not skewed.
There are no outliers.
Distribution is approximately normal.

Chapter 7

Exercises 7–1

1. A point estimate of a parameter specifies a specific value such as $\mu = 87$, whereas an interval estimate specifies a range of values for the parameter such as $84 < \mu < 90$. The advantage of an interval estimate is that a specific confidence level (say 95%) can be selected, and one can be 95% confident that the parameter being estimated lies in the interval.

3. The margin of error, also known as the *maximum error of estimate*, is a range of values to the right or left of the statistic, point estimate, which is likely to contain the population parameter.

5. A good estimator should be unbiased, consistent, and relatively efficient.

7. To determine sample size, the margin of error and the degree of confidence must be specified and the population standard deviation must be known.

9. *a.* 2.575   *c.* 1.96   *e.* 1.88
  b. 2.33   *d.* 1.645

11. *a.* 82   *b.* $77 < \mu < 87$ *c.* $75.5 < \mu < 88.5$
  d. The 99% confidence interval is larger because the confidence level is larger.

13. *a.* 12.6   *b.* $11.9 < \mu < 13.3$
  c. It would be highly unlikely since this is far larger than 13.3 minutes.

15. $\$145,030 < \mu < \$154,970$

17. $1.72 < \mu < 1.88$

19. $127.1 < \mu < 134.9$ **21.** 114

23. 25   **25.** 239

Exercises 7–2

1. The characteristics of the t distribution are: It is bell-shaped, symmetrical about the mean, and never touches the x axis. The mean, median, and mode are equal to 0 and are located at the centre of the distribution. The variance is greater than 1. The t distribution is a family of curves based on degrees of freedom. As sample size increases the t distribution approaches the normal distribution.

3. The t distribution should be used when σ is unknown and $n < 30$.

4. *a.* 2.898   *c.* 2.624   *e.* 2.093
  b. 2.074   *d.* 1.833

5. $14.72 < \mu < 17.3$

7. $\$3,585.93 < \mu < \$5,093.27$

9. $120.5 < \mu < 129.5$ **11.** $21.84 < \mu < 24.16$

13. $\$17.29 < \mu < \$19.77$ **15.** $108.7 < \mu < 121.3$

17. $38.8 < \mu < 44.4$ **19.** Answers will vary.

21. $\overline{X} = 2.175$; $s = 0.585$; $\mu > \$1.95$ means that one can be 95% confident that the mean revenue is greater than $\$1.95$; $\mu < \$2.40$ means that one can be 95% confident that the mean revenue is less than $\$2.40$.

Exercises 7–3

1. *a.* 0.5, 0.5   *c.* 0.46, 0.54   *e.* 0.45, 0.55
  b. 0.45, 0.55   *d.* 0.58, 0.42

2. *a.* $\hat{p} = 0.15$; $\hat{q} = 0.85$ *d.* $\hat{p} = 0.51$; $\hat{q} = 0.49$
  b. $\hat{p} = 0.37$; $\hat{q} = 0.63$ *e.* $\hat{p} = 0.79$; $\hat{q} = 0.21$
  c. $\hat{p} = 0.71$; $\hat{q} = 0.29$

3. $0.370 < p < 0.410$ **5.** $0.023 < p < 0.031$

7. $0.524 < p < 0.576$

9. $0.075 < p < 0.185$.

The Health Canada proportion of 10% is within the confidence interval range for the proportion of 15- to 17-year-olds who are current smokers.

11. $0.048 < p < 0.132$ **13.** $0.419 < p < 0.481$

15. *a.* 3108.1 or 3109
    b. 4144.1 or 4145

17. *a.* 556.97 or 557
    b. 663.06 or 664

19. *a.* 1082.4 or 1083
    b. 463.7 or 464

21. 1.96 corresponds to a 95% degree of confidence.

Exercises 7–4

1. χ^2

3.

	χ^2 **left**	χ^2 **right**
a.	3.816	21.920
b.	10.117	30.144
c.	13.844	41.923
d.	0.412	16.750
e.	26.509	55.758

5. $8.64 < \sigma^2 < 28.93$
  $2.94 < \sigma^2 < 5.38$
  Yes. The times deviate between 3 and 5 minutes.

7. $0.40 < \sigma^2 < 2.25$
  $0.63 < \sigma < 1.50$

9. $232.1 < \sigma^2 < 691.6$
  $15.2 < \sigma^2 < 26.3$

11. $4.03 < \sigma^2 < 6.95$

13. $16.2 < \sigma < 19.8$

Review Exercises

1. 12.6; $12.35 < \mu < 12.85$

3. 13; $12.92 < \mu < 13.08$

5. $25.1 < \mu < 30.9$ **7.** 27.71 or 28

9. $0.434 < p < 0.660$; yes; it seems that as many as 66% were dissatisfied.

11. 833.02 or 834

13. $0.217 < \sigma < 0.435$; yes; it seems that there is a large standard deviation.

15. $5.1 < \sigma^2 < 18.3$

Chapter Quiz

1. True **2.** True

3. False **4.** True

5. *b* **6.** *a*

7. *b*

8. unbiased, consistent, relatively efficient

9. margin of error

10. point **11.** 90, 95, 99

12. $23.45; $22.78 < \mu < 24.12

13. $364.40; $341.01 < \mu < 387.79

14. 1882; $1793.2 < \mu < 1970.8$

15. $45.7 < \mu < 51.5$ **16.** $418 < \mu < 458$

17. $26.3 < \mu < 35.7$ **18.** 179.3 or 180

19. 24.4 or 25 **20.** $0.604 < p < 0.810$

21. $0.296 < p < 0.424$ **22.** $0.342 < p < 0.547$

23. 544.2 or 545 **24.** $7.1 < \sigma < 12.5$

25. $30.9 < \sigma^2 < 78.2$ **26.** $1.8 < \sigma < 3.2$
  $5.6 < \sigma < 8.9$

Chapter 8

Exercises 8–1

Note: For Chapters 8–13, specific *P*-values are given in parentheses after the *P*-value intervals. When the specific *P*-value is extremely small, it is not given.

1. The null hypothesis states that there is no difference between a parameter and a specific value or that there is no difference between two parameters. The alternative hypothesis states that there is a specific difference between a parameter and a specific value or that there is a difference between two parameters. Examples will vary.

3. A statistical test uses the data obtained from a sample to make a decision about whether the null hypothesis should be rejected.

5. The critical region is the range of values of the test statistic that indicates that there is a significant difference and the null hypothesis should be rejected. The noncritical region is the range of values of the test statistic that indicates that the difference was probably due to chance and the null hypothesis should not be rejected.

7. α, β

9. A one-tailed test should be used when a specific direction, such as greater than or less than, is being hypothesized; when no direction is specified, a two-tailed test should be used.

11. Hypotheses can be proved true only when the entire population is used to compute the test statistic. In most cases, this is impossible.

12. *a.* ± 1.96 *d.* $+2.33$ *g.* $+1.65$ *i.* -1.75
    b. -2.33 *e.* -1.65 *h.* ± 2.58 *j.* $+2.05$
    c. $+2.58$ *f.* -2.05

13. *a.* H_0: $\mu = 24.6$
      H_1: $\mu \neq 24.6$
    b. H_0: $\mu = $51,497$
      H_1: $\mu \neq $51,497$

c. H_0: $\mu = 25.4$
  H_1: $\mu > 25.4$
d. H_0: $\mu = 88$
  H_1: $\mu < 88$
e. H_0: $\mu = 70$
  H_1: $\mu < 70$
f. H_0: $\mu = \$10,000$
  H_1: $\mu \neq \$10,000$
g. H_0: $\mu = 3.7$
  H_1: $\mu \neq 3.7$

Exercises 8–2

1. H_0: $\mu = 5000$ and H_1: $\mu > 5000$ (claim); C.V. $= +1.96$; $z = 4.53$. Reject the null hypothesis. There is enough evidence at $\alpha = 0.05$ to conclude that the mean is greater than 5000 steps.

3. H_0: $\mu = \$15$ billion and H_1: $\mu < \$15$ billion (claim); C.V. $= -1.645$; $z = -1.97$; reject. There is not enough evidence to reject the claim that the average revenue of the top 1000 Canadian companies is less than $15 billion.

5. H_0: $\mu = 9.8$ and H_1: $\mu < 9.8$ (claim); C.V. $= -2.33$; $z = -5.67$; reject. There is not enough evidence to reject the claim that the average age of Air Canada's commercial fleet is less than 9.8 years.

7. H_0: $\mu = 73.7$ and H_1: $\mu \neq 73.7$ (claim); C.V. $= \pm 1.96$; $z = 0.93$; do not reject. There is enough evidence to reject the claim that the average length of 1-year-old toddlers in northern communities is not equal to 73.7 cm.

9. H_0: $\mu = \$19,410$ and H_1: $\mu > \$19,410$ (claim); C.V. $= 2.33$; $z = 2.81$; reject. There is not enough evidence to reject the claim that the average tuition cost has increased.

11. H_0: $\mu = 21.4$ and H_1: $\mu \neq 21.4$ (claim); C.V. $= \pm 2.575$; $z = 3.51$; reject. There is not enough evidence to reject the claim that the average Quebec TV viewing hours per week differ from the Canadian national average.

13. H_0: $\mu = \$850$ and H_1: $\mu \neq \$850$ (claim); at $\alpha = 0.01$, C.V. $= \pm 2.575$; $z = -2.19$. Do not reject. There is enough evidence to reject the claim that the average out-of-pocket health service costs are not equal to $850. At $\alpha = 0.05$, C.V. $= \pm 1.96$. Reject. There is not enough evidence to reject the claim that the average out-of-pocket health service costs are not equal to $850.

15. a. Do not reject. d. Reject.
   b. Do not reject. e. Reject.
   c. Do not reject.

17. H_0: $\mu = 213$ and H_1: $\mu < 213$ (claim); $z = -2.61$; P-value (0.0045) is $\leq \alpha$ (0.01); reject the null hypothesis. There is not enough evidence to reject the tire manufacturer's claim that the average stopping distance is less than 213 metres.

19. H_0: $\mu = 546$ and H_1: $\mu < 546$ (claim); $z = -2.4$; P-value (0.0082) is $\leq \alpha$ (0.01); reject the null hypothesis. There is not enough evidence to reject the claim that the number of calories burned is less than 546.

21. H_0: $\mu = 246$ and H_1: $\mu > 246$ (claim); $z = 5.99$; P-value (0.0001) $\leq \alpha$ (0.05); reject the null hypothesis. There is not enough evidence to reject the claim that the average farm size is larger than 246 hectares.

23. H_0: $\mu = 48,000$ (claim) and H_1: $\mu \neq 48,000$; $z = 1.71$; P-value (0.0872) $\leq \alpha$ (0.10); reject the null hypothesis. There is enough evidence to reject the claim that the average vehicle transmission is serviced at 48,000 kilometres.

25. H_0: $\mu = 10$ and H_1: $\mu < 10$ (claim); $z = -8.67$; P-value (0.0001) is $\leq \alpha$ (0.05); reject the null hypothesis. There is not enough evidence to reject the claim that the average number of days missed per year is less than 10.

27. H_0: $\mu = 8.65$ (claim) and H_1: $\mu \neq 8.65$; C.V. $= \pm 1.96$; $z = -1.35$; do not reject. Yes; there is not enough evidence to reject the claim that the average hourly wage of the employees is $8.65.

Exercises 8–3

1. It is bell-shaped, it is symmetric about the mean, and it never touches the x axis. The mean, median, and mode are all equal to 0, and they are located at the centre of the distribution. The t distribution differs from the standard normal distribution in that it is a family of curves and the variance is greater than 1; and as the degrees of freedom increase, the t distribution approaches the standard normal distribution.

3. a. $+1.833$ c. -3.365 e. ± 2.145 g. $+2.438$
   b. ± 1.740 d. $+2.306$ f. -2.819 h. ± 2.021

4. Specific P-values are in parentheses.
   a. $0.01 <$ P-value < 0.025 (0.018)
   b. $0.05 <$ P-value < 0.10 (0.062)
   c. $0.10 <$ P-value < 0.25 (0.123)
   d. $0.10 <$ P-value < 0.20 (0.138)
   e. P-value < 0.005 (0.003)
   f. $0.10 <$ P-value < 0.25 (0.158)
   g. P-value $= 0.05$ (0.05)
   h. P-value > 0.25 (0.261)

5. H_0: $\mu = 281.5$ and H_1: $\mu < 281.5$ (claim); C.V. $= -1.833$; $t = -2.962$; reject. There is not enough evidence to reject the claim that the average Maritime summer rainfall differs from 281.5 millimetres.

7. H_0: $\mu = \$120,000$ and H_1: $\mu \neq \$120,000$ (claim); C.V. $= \pm 2.776$; $t = 2.286$. Do not reject. There is enough evidence to reject the claim that the average Canadian mayor's salary is $120,000 is not correct.

9. $H_0: \mu = 200$ and $H_1: \mu < 200$ (claim); C.V. $= -2.262$
$t = -0.711$; do not reject. There is not enough
evidence to reject the claim that the average height of
Canada's tallest buildings is at least 200 metres.

11. $H_0: \mu = \$13,252$ and $H_1: \mu > \$13,252$ (claim);
C.V. $= 2.539$; d.f. $= 19$; $t = 2.949$; reject. There is not
enough evidence to reject the claim that the average
tuition cost has increased.

13. $H_0: \mu = \$54.8$ million and $H_1: \mu > \$54.8$ million
(claim); C.V. $= 1.761$; d.f. $= 14$; $t = 3.058$; reject.
There is not enough evidence to reject the claim
that the cost to produce an action movie is more
than \$54.8 million.

15. $H_0: \mu = 132$ (claim) and $H_1: \mu \neq 132$; C.V. $= \pm 2.365$;
d.f. $= 7$; $t = -1.800$; do not reject. Yes; there is not
enough evidence to reject the claim that the average
time is 132 minutes.

17. $H_0: \mu = 5.8$ and $H_1: \mu \neq 5.8$ (claim); d.f. $= 19$;
$t = -3.462$; P-value $(0.00262) \leq \alpha$ (0.05); reject the
null hypothesis. There is not enough evidence to reject
the claim that, on average, a woman visits her
physician 5.8 times per year.

19. $H_0: \mu = \$15,000$ and $H_1: \mu \neq \$15,000$ (claim);
C.V. $= \pm 2.201$; d.f. $= 11$; $t = -1.103$; do not reject.
There is enough evidence to reject the claim that the
average stipend differs from \$15,000.

Exercises 8–4

1. Answers will vary.

3. $np \geq 5$ and $nq \geq 5$

5. $H_0: p = 0.684$ (claim) and $H_1: p \neq 0.684$.
C.V. $= \pm 2.33$; $z = -1.87$; do not reject. There
is not enough evidence to reject the claim that the
proportion of homeowners is equal to 68.4%.

7. $H_0: p = 0.40$ and $H_1: p \neq 0.40$ (claim); C.V. $= \pm 2.575$;
$z = -1.07$; do not reject. No. There is not enough
evidence to support the claim that the proportion is
different from 0.40.

9. $H_0: p = 0.71$ (claim) and $H_1: p \neq 0.71$;
C.V. $= \pm 1.96$; $z = 1.60$; do not reject. There is
not enough evidence to reject the claim that the new
city has the same proportion as the Industry Canada
report.

11. $H_0: p = 0.073$ (claim) and $H_1: p \neq 0.073$;
C.V. $= \pm 1.96$; $z = 0.19$; do not reject. There is not
enough evidence to reject the claim that 7.3% of
vehicle fatalities involve motorcyclists.

13. $H_0: p = 0.133$ (claim) and $H_1: p \neq 0.133$;
$z = 0.78$; P-value $(0.2542) > \alpha$ (0.10); do not reject.
There is not enough evidence to reject the claim that
13.3% of food bank users have jobs.

15. $H_0: p = 0.18$ (claim) and $H_1: p \neq 0.18$; $z = -0.59$; the
P-value $(0.5552) > \alpha$ (0.05); do not reject. There is not

enough evidence to reject the claim that 18% of all
high school students smoke at least a pack of cigarettes
a day.

17. $H_0: p = 0.44$ (claim) and $H_1: p \neq 0.44$;
C.V. $= \pm 1.96$; $z = 3.02$; reject. There is sufficient
evidence to reject the claim that 44% of Canadians
using library services borrow books.

19. $H_0: p = 0.10$ and $H_1: p < 0.10$ (claim);
C.V. $= -1.645$; $z = -0.38$; do not reject. There is
enough evidence to reject the claim that fewer than
10% of injury deaths are firearm-related fatalities.

21. Binomial distribution with $p = 0.50$ and $n = 9$. The
P-value is $2 \cdot P(X \leq 3) = 2(0.254) = 0.508$. Since the
P-value > 0.10, do not reject. The conclusion is that
the coin is balanced.

23. $\mu = np$ and $\sigma = \sqrt{npq}$ and $\hat{p} = \dfrac{X}{n}$

$$z = \frac{X - \mu}{\sigma} \qquad z = \frac{\hat{p} - p}{\dfrac{\sqrt{npq}}{n}}$$

$$z = \frac{X - np}{\sqrt{npq}} \times \frac{\dfrac{1}{n}}{\dfrac{1}{n}} \qquad z = \frac{\hat{p} - p}{\sqrt{\dfrac{npq}{n^2}}}$$

$$z = \frac{\dfrac{X}{n} - \dfrac{np}{n}}{\dfrac{\sqrt{npq}}{n}} \qquad z = \frac{\hat{p} - p}{\sqrt{\dfrac{pq}{n}}}$$

Exercises 8–5

1. a. $H_0: \sigma^2 = 225$ and $H_1: \sigma^2 > 225$; C.V. $= 27.587$;
d.f. $= 17$

b. $H_0: \sigma^2 = 225$ and $H_1: \sigma^2 < 225$; C.V. $= 14.042$;
d.f. $= 22$

c. $H_0: \sigma^2 = 225$ and $H_1: \sigma^2 \neq 225$; C.V. $= 5.629$;
26.119; d.f. $= 14$

d. $H_0: \sigma^2 = 225$ and $H_1: \sigma^2 \neq 225$; C.V. $= 2.167$;
14.067; d.f. $= 7$

e. $H_0: \sigma^2 = 225$ and $H_1: \sigma^2 > 225$; C.V. $= 32.000$;
d.f. $= 16$

f. $H_0: \sigma^2 = 225$ and $H_1: \sigma^2 < 225$; C.V. $= 8.907$;
d.f. $= 19$

g. $H_0: \sigma^2 = 225$ and $H_1: \sigma^2 \neq 225$; C.V. $= 3.074$;
28.299; d.f. $= 12$

h. $H_0: \sigma^2 = 225$ and $H_1: \sigma^2 < 225$; C.V. $= 15.308$;
d.f. $= 28$

3. $H_0: \sigma = 60$ (claim) and $H_1: \sigma \neq 60$; C.V. $= 8.672$;
27.587; d.f. $= 17$; $\chi^2 = 19.707$; do not reject. There is
not enough evidence to reject the claim that the
standard deviation is 60.

5. H_0: $\sigma = 500$ and H_1: $\sigma < 500$ (claim); C.V. $= 10.851$; d.f. $= 20$; $\chi^2 = 16.121$; do not reject. There is enough evidence to reject the claim that the standard deviation of motor vehicle theft rate per year in Canada is less than 500.

7. H_0: $\sigma = 1.2$ (claim) and H_1: $\sigma > 1.2$; $\alpha = 0.01$; d.f. $= 14$; $\chi^2 = 31.5$; P-value < 0.005 (0.0047); since P-value < 0.01, reject. There is enough evidence to reject the claim that the standard deviation is less than or equal to 1.2 minutes.

9. H_0: $\sigma = 20$ and H_1: $\sigma > 20$ (claim); C.V. $= 36.191$; d.f. $= 19$; $\chi^2 = 58.55$; reject. There is not enough evidence to reject the claim that the standard deviation is greater than 20 calories.

11. H_0: $\sigma = 150$ and H_1: $\sigma < 150$ (claim); C.V. $= 3.940$; d.f. $= 10$; $\chi^2 = 9.669$; do not reject. There is enough evidence to reject the claim that the standard deviation of annual deaths from fires in Canada is less than 150.

13. H_0: $\sigma^2 = 25$ and H_1: $\sigma^2 > 25$ (claim); C.V. $= 22.362$; d.f. $= 13$; $\chi^2 = 23.622$; reject. There is not enough evidence to reject the claim that the variance is greater than 25.

Exercises 8–6

1. H_0: $\mu = 1800$ (claim) and H_1: $\mu \neq 1800$; C.V. $= \pm 1.96$; $z = 0.47$; $1706.04 < \mu < 1953.96$; do not reject. There is not enough evidence to reject the claim that the average of the sales is $1800.

3. H_0: $\mu = 86$ (claim) and H_1: $\mu \neq 86$; C.V. $= \pm 2.575$; $z = -1.29$; $80.01 < \mu < 87.99$; do not reject. There is not enough evidence to reject the claim that the average monthly maintenance is $86.

5. H_0: $\mu = 22$ and H_1: $\mu \neq 22$ (claim); C.V. $= \pm 2.575$; $z = -2.32$; $19.47 < \mu < 22.13$; do not reject. There is enough evidence to reject the claim that the average study time has changed.

7. The power of a statistical test is the probability of rejecting the null hypothesis when it is false.

9. The power of a test can be increased by increasing α or selecting a larger sample size.

Review Exercises

1. H_0: $\mu = 37°C$ (claim) and H_1: $\mu \neq 37°C$; C.V. $= \pm 1.96$; $z = -2.61$; reject. There is enough evidence to reject the claim that the average eastern Canada high temperature is equal to 37°C.

3. H_0: $\mu = \$40,000$ and H_1: $\mu > \$40,000$ (claim); C.V. $= 1.645$; $z = 2.00$; reject. There is not enough evidence to reject the claim that the average salary is more than $40,000.

5. H_0: $\mu = 26.8°C$ and H_1: $\mu > 26.8°C$ (claim); C.V. $= 1.833$; d.f. $= 9$; $t = 1.626$; do not reject.

There is enough evidence to reject the claim that the July 2006 was hotter than normal.

7. H_0: $\mu = 18,000$ and H_1: $\mu < 18,000$ (claim); C.V. $= -2.462$; $t = -3.578$; reject. There is not enough evidence to reject the claim that average debt is less than $18,000.

9. H_0: $p = 0.256$ and H_1: $p \neq 0.256$ (claim); C.V. $= \pm 1.96$; $z = 1.072$; do not reject. There is enough evidence to reject the claim that the union's membership differs from 25.6%.

11. H_0: $p = 0.67$ and H_1: $p > 0.67$ (claim); $z = 1.27$; P-value (0.0102) $\leq \alpha$ (0.05); reject. There is enough evidence to reject the theological researcher's claim that more than 67% of constituents attend yearly religious services.

13. H_0: $\mu = 10$ and H_1: $\mu < 10$ (claim); $z = -2.22$; P-value (0.0132) $\leq \alpha$ (0.05); reject. There is not enough evidence to reject the claim that the average digestion relief time is less than 10 minutes.

15. H_0: $\sigma = 1.6$ L/100 km and H_1: $\sigma < 1.6$ L/100 (claim); d.f. $= 19$; $\chi^2 = 6.012$; P-value < 0.05 (0.002); reject. There is not enough evidence to reject the claim that the standard deviation of automobile fuel consumption is less than 1.6 L/100.

17. H_0: $\sigma^2 = 40$ and H_1: $\sigma^2 \neq 40$ (claim); C.V. $= 2.700$, 19.023 (d.f. $= 9$, two tails); $\chi^2 = 9.68$; do not reject. There is enough evidence to reject the claim that the variance in NBA games played is not equal to 40.

19. H_0: $\mu = 241.3$ and H_1: $\mu \neq 241.3$ (claim): C.V. $= \pm 1.690$; $z = -3.014$; reject. $225.07 < \mu < 236.75$. There is not enough evidence to reject the claim that people are not keeping their tires inflated to the correct pressure of 241.3 kPa.

Chapter Quiz

1. True
2. True
3. False
4. True
5. False
6. b
7. d
8. c
9. b
10. Type I
11. β
12. Statistical hypothesis.
13. Right.
14. $n - 1$

15. H_0: $\mu = 28.6$ (claim) and H_1: $\mu \neq 28.6$; $z = 2.10$; C.V. $= \pm 1.96$; reject. There is enough evidence to reject the claim that the average age of the mothers is 28.6 years.

16. H_0: $\mu = \$6500$ (claim) and H_1: $\mu \neq \$6500$; $z = 5.27$; C.V. $= \pm 1.96$; reject. There is enough evidence to reject the agent's claim.

17. H_0: $\mu = 80$ and H_1: $\mu \neq 80$ (claim); C.V. $= \pm 2.33$; $z = 2.14$; reject. There is not enough evidence to reject the Nielsen report claim.

18. H_0: $\mu = 500$ (claim) and H_1: $\mu \neq 500$; d.f. = 6; $t = -0.571$; C.V. = ± 3.707; do not reject. There is not enough evidence to reject the claim that the mean is 500.

19. H_0: $\mu = 170$ and H_1: $\mu < 170$ (claim); $t = -3.016$; P-value < 0.01 (0.00355); since P-value < 0.05; reject. There is not enough evidence to reject the claim that the average height of female models is less than 170 cm.

20. H_0: $\mu = 12.4$ and H_1: $\mu < 12.4$ (claim); $t = -2.324$; C.V. = -1.345; reject. There is not enough evidence to reject the claim that the average taxi driver's experience is less than the company claimed.

21. H_0: $\mu = 63.5$ and H_1: $\mu > 63.5$ (claim); $t = 0.47075$; P-value > 0.25 (0.322); since P-value > 0.05; do not reject. There is enough evidence to reject the claim that the average age of robbery victims is greater than 63.5.

22. H_0: $\mu = 26$ (claim) and H_1: $\mu \neq 26$; $t = -1.5$; C.V. = ± 2.492; do not reject. There is not enough evidence to reject the claim that the average is 26.

23. H_0: $p = 0.39$ (claim) and H_1: $p \neq 0.39$; C.V. = ± 1.96; $z = -0.62$; do not reject. There is not enough evidence to reject the claim that 39% took supplements. The study supports the results of the previous study.

24. H_0: $p = 0.55$ (claim) and H_1: $p < 0.55$; $z = -0.899$; C.V. = -1.28; do not reject. There is not enough evidence to reject the dietician's claim.

25. H_0: $p = 0.35$ (claim) and H_1: $p \neq 0.35$; C.V. = ± 2.33; $z = 0.666$; do not reject. There is not enough evidence to reject the claim that the proportion is 35%.

26. H_0: $p = 0.27$ (claim) and H_1: $p \neq 0.27$; C.V. = ± 2.575; $z = 1.87$; do not reject. There is not enough evidence to reject the claim.

27. P-value = 0.0324

28. P-value = 0.0001

29. H_0: $\sigma = 6$ and H_1: $\sigma > 6$ (claim); $\chi^2 = 54$; C.V. = 36.415; reject. There is not enough evidence to reject the claim that the standard deviation is more than 6 pages.

30. H_0: $\sigma = 8$ (claim) and H_1: $\sigma \neq 8$; $\chi^2 = 33.189$; C.V. = 27.991, 79.490; do not reject. There is not enough evidence to reject the claim that $\sigma = 8$.

31. H_0: $\sigma = 18$ and H_1: $\sigma < 18$ (claim); C.V. = 10.117; $\chi^2 = 13.194$; do not reject. There is enough evidence to reject the claim that the standard deviation of the pollution by-products for automobiles is less than previously indicated.

32. H_0: $\sigma = 4.1$ (claim) and H_1: $\sigma \neq 4.1$; d.f. = 9; $\chi^2 = 13.385$; $0.10 < P$-value < 0.90 (0.146); do not reject. There is not enough evidence to reject the claim that the standard deviation of wrapping cord strength is equal to 4.1 kg.

33. $28.7 < \mu < 31.4$; no.

34. $\$6562.81 < \mu < \$6637.19$; no.

Chapter 9

Exercises 9–1

1. Testing a single mean involves comparing a sample mean to a specific value such as $\mu = 100$; testing the difference between two means involves comparing the means of two samples, such as $\mu_1 = \mu_2$.

3. The populations must be independent of each other, and they must be normally distributed; s_1 and s_2 can be used in place of σ_1 and σ_2 when σ_1 and σ_2 are unknown and both samples are each greater than or equal to 30.

5. H_0: $\mu_1 = \mu_2$ (claim) and H_1: $\mu_1 \neq \mu_2$; C.V. = ± 2.575; $z = -0.857$; do not reject. There is not enough evidence to reject the claim that the average lengths of the rivers are the same.

7. H_0: $\mu_1 = \mu_2$ and H_1: $\mu_1 > \mu_2$ (claim); C.V. = $+1.645$; $z = 2.561$; reject. There is not enough evidence to reject the claim that pulse rates of smokers are higher than pulse rates of nonsmokers.

9. H_0: $\mu_1 = \mu_2$ and H_1: $\mu_1 > \mu_2$ (claim); C.V. = 2.33; $z = 3.75$; reject. There is not enough evidence to reject the claim that the average stay is longer for men than for women.

11. H_0: $\mu_1 = \mu_2$ and H_1: $\mu_1 < \mu_2$ (claim); C.V. = -1.645; $z = -2.01$; reject. There is not enough evidence to reject the claim that leavers have a lower GPA than stayers.

13. H_0: $\mu_1 = \mu_2$ and H_1: $\mu_1 > \mu_2$ (claim); C.V. = $+2.33$; $z = +1.09$; do not reject. There is enough evidence to reject the claim that colleges spend more money on male sports than they spend on female sports.

15. H_0: $\mu_1 = \mu_2$ and H_1: $\mu_1 \neq \mu_2$ (claim); $z = 1.01$; P-value = 0.3124; do not reject. There is not enough evidence to support the claim that there is a difference in self-esteem scores.

17. $2.83 < \mu_1 - \mu_2 < 5.97$

19. $-7.29 < \mu_1 - \mu_2 < -1.31$

21. H_0: $\mu_1 - \mu_2 = 8$ (claim) and H_1: $\mu_1 - \mu_2 > 8$; C.V. = $+1.645$; $z = -0.73$; do not reject. There is not enough evidence to reject the claim that private school students have exam scores that are at most 8 points higher than those of students in public schools.

Exercises 9–2

1. H_0: $\mu_1 = \mu_2$ and H_1: $\mu_1 \neq \mu_2$ (claim); C.V. = ± 2.262; $t = -4.02$; reject. There is not enough evidence to reject the claim that there is a significant difference in the values of the homes based on the appraisers' values. $-7966.65 < \mu_1 - \mu_2 < -2229.35$.

3. H_0: $\mu_1 = \mu_2$ and H_1: $\mu_1 \neq \mu_2$ (claim); C.V. = ± 2.145; $t = -1.07$; do not reject. There is enough evidence to reject the claim that there is no difference between the salaries.

5. H_0: $\mu_1 = \mu_2$ and H_1: $\mu_1 \neq \mu_2$ (claim); C.V. $= \pm 2.365$; $t = 1.057$; do not reject. There is enough evidence to reject the claim that there is a difference between the scoring means.

7. H_0: $\mu_1 = \mu_2$ and H_1: $\mu_1 \neq \mu_2$ (claim); C.V. $= \pm 2.821$; $t = -2.84$; reject. There is not enough evidence to reject the claim that there is a difference in the average times of the two groups. $-11.955 < \mu_1 - \mu_2 < -0.045$. (TI: $-11.45 < \mu_1 - \mu_2 < -0.55$)

9. H_0: $\mu_1 = \mu_2$ and H_1: $\mu_1 \neq \mu_2$ (claim); C.V. $= \pm 2.365$; $t = -3.21$; reject. There is not enough evidence to reject the claim that fruits and vegetables differ in moisture content.

11. H_0: $\mu_1 = \mu_2$ and H_1: $\mu_1 \neq \mu_2$ (claim); C.V. $= \pm 2.571$; $t = 0.119$; do not reject. There is enough evidence to reject the claim that the colour of the mice made a difference. $-6.812 < \mu_1 - \mu_2 < 7.472$. (TI: $-5.863 < \mu_1 - \mu_2 < 6.529$)

13. $-10097.1 < \mu_1 - \mu_2 < -5982.5$. (TI: $-12154 < \mu_1 - \mu_2 < -3925$)

Exercises 9–3

1. *a.* Dependent   *d.* Dependent
   b. Dependent   *e.* Independent
   c. Independent

3. H_0: $\mu_D = 0$ and H_1: $\mu_D < 0$ (claim); C.V. $= -1.397$; d.f. $= 8$; $t = -2.80$; reject. There is not enough evidence to reject the claim that the seminar increased the number of hours students studied.

5. H_0: $\mu_D = 0$ and H_1: $\mu_D \neq 0$ (claim); C.V. $= \pm 2.365$; d.f. $= 7$; $t = 1.659$; do not reject. There is enough evidence to reject the claim that there is a difference in the mean number of hours slept.

7. H_0: $\mu_D \leq 0$ and H_1: $\mu_D > 0$ (claim); C.V. $= 2.571$; d.f. $= 5$; $t = 2.24$; do not reject. There is enough evidence to reject the claim that the errors have been reduced.

9. H_0: $\mu_D = 0$ and H_1: $\mu_D \neq 0$ (claim); d.f. $= 7$; $t = 0.978$; $0.20 < P$-value < 0.50 (0.361). Do not reject since P-value > 0.01. There is enough evidence to reject the claim that there is a difference in the pulse rates. $-3.23 < \mu_D < 5.73$

11. Using the previous problem, $\overline{D} = 2.286$, whereas the mean of the 2005 values is 35.5714 and the mean of the 2009 values is 33.2857; hence, $\overline{D} = 35.5714 - 33.2857 = 2.286$ (rounded)

Exercises 9–4

1a. *a.* $\hat{p} = \frac{34}{48}, \hat{q} = \frac{14}{48}$
   b. $\hat{p} = \frac{28}{75}, \hat{q} = \frac{47}{75}$
   c. $\hat{p} = \frac{50}{100}, \hat{q} = \frac{50}{100}$
   d. $\hat{p} = \frac{6}{24}, \hat{q} = \frac{18}{24}$
   e. $\hat{p} = \frac{12}{144}, \hat{q} = \frac{132}{144}$

1b. *a.* 16   *c.* 48   *e.* 30
   b. 4   *d.* 104

3. $\hat{p}_1 = 0.533$; $\hat{p}_2 = 0.3$; $\overline{p} = 0.44$; $\overline{q} = 0.56$; H_0: $p_1 = p_2$ and H_1: $p_1 \neq p_2$ (claim); C.V. $= \pm 1.96$; $z = 3.64$; reject. There is not enough evidence to reject the claim that there is a significant difference in the proportions.

5. $\hat{p}_1 = 0.747$; $\hat{p}_2 = 0.75$; $\overline{p} = 0.749$; $\overline{q} = 0.251$; H_0: $p_1 = p_2$ and H_1: $p_1 \neq p_2$ (claim); C.V. $= \pm 1.96$; $z = -0.07$; do not reject. There is not enough evidence to support the claim that the proportions are different.

7. $\hat{p}_1 = 0.83$; $\hat{p}_2 = 0.75$; $\overline{p} = 0.79$; $\overline{q} = 0.21$; H_0: $p_1 = p_2$ (claim) and H_1: $p_1 \neq p_2$; C.V. $= \pm 1.96$; $z = 1.39$; do not reject. There is not enough evidence to reject the claim that the proportions are equal. $-0.032 < p_1 - p_2 < 0.192$

9. $\hat{p}_1 = 0.55$; $\hat{p}_2 = 0.45$; $\overline{p} = 0.497$; $\overline{q} = 0.503$; H_0: $p_1 = p_2$ and H_1: $p_1 \neq p_2$ (claim); C.V. $= \pm 2.575$; $z = 1.302$; do not reject. There is not enough evidence to support the claim that the proportions are different. $-0.097 < p_1 - p_2 < 0.297$

11. $\hat{p}_1 = 0.347$; $\hat{p}_2 = 0.433$; $\overline{p} = 0.385$; $\overline{q} = 0.615$; H_0: $p_1 = p_2$ and H_1: $p_1 \neq p_2$ (claim); C.V. $= \pm 1.96$; $z = -1.027$; do not reject. There is not enough evidence to say that the proportion of dog owners has changed ($-0.252 < p_1 - p_2 < 0.079$). Yes, the confidence interval contains 0. This is another way to conclude that there is no difference in the proportions.

13. $\hat{p}_1 = 0.25$; $\hat{p}_2 = 0.31$; $\overline{p} = 0.3575$; $\overline{q} = 0.6425$; H_0: $p_1 = p_2$ and H_1: $p_1 \neq p_2$ (claim); C.V. $= \pm 2.575$; $z = -1.252$; do not reject. There is not enough evidence to support the claim that the proportions are different. $-0.165 < p_1 - p_2 < 0.045$

15. $-0.294 < p_1 - p_2 < 0.014$

17. $\hat{p}_1 = 0.43$; $\hat{p}_2 = 0.58$; $\overline{p} = 0.505$; $\overline{q} = 0.495$; H_0: $p_1 = p_2$ and H_1: $p_1 \neq p_2$ (claim); C.V. $= \pm 1.96$; $z = -2.12$; reject; there is not enough evidence to reject the claim that the proportions are different.

19. $-0.0631 < p_1 - p_2 < 0.0667$. It does agree with the *Almanac* statistics stating a difference of -0.042 since -0.042 is contained in the interval.

Exercises 9–5

1. The variance in the numerator should be the larger of the two variances.

3. One degree of freedom is used for the variance associated with the numerator, and one is used for the variance associated with the denominator.

5. *a.* d.f.N. $= 15$, d.f.D. $= 22$; C.V. $= 3.36$
   b. d.f.N. $= 24$, d.f.D. $= 13$; C.V. $= 3.59$
   c. d.f.N. $= 45$, d.f.D. $= 29$; C.V. $= 2.03$
   d. d.f.N. $= 20$, d.f.D. $= 16$; C.V. $= 2.28$
   e. d.f.N. $= 10$, d.f.D. $= 10$; C.V. $= 2.98$

6. Specific *P*-values are in parentheses.

   a. $0.025 < P\text{-value} < 0.05\ (0.033)$

   b. $0.05 < P\text{-value} < 0.10\ (0.072)$

   c. $P\text{-value} = 0.05$

   d. $0.005 < P\text{-value} < 0.01\ (0.006)$

   e. $P\text{-value} = 0.05$

   f. $P\text{-value} > 0.10\ (0.112)$

   g. $0.05 < P\text{-value} < 0.10\ (0.068)$

   h. $0.01 < P\text{-value} < 0.02\ (0.015)$

7. $H_0: \sigma_1^2 = \sigma_2^2$ and $H_1: \sigma_1^2 \neq \sigma_2^2$ (claim); C.V. = 2.53; d.f.N. = 14; d.f.D. = 14; F = 4.52; reject. There is enough evidence to support the claim that there is a difference in the variances.

9. $H_0: \sigma_1^2 = \sigma_2^2$ and $H_1: \sigma_1^2 \neq \sigma_2^2$ (claim); C.V. = 2.86; d.f.N. = 15; d.f.D. = 15; F = 7.85; reject. There is enough evidence to support the claim that the variances are different. Since both data sets vary greatly from normality, the results are suspect.

11. $H_0: \sigma_1^2 = \sigma_2^2$ and $H_1: \sigma_1^2 \neq \sigma_2^2$ (claim); C.V. = 4.99; d.f.N. = 7; d.f.D. = 7; F = 1; do not reject. There is not enough evidence to support the claim that there is a difference in the variances.

13. $H_0: \sigma_1 = \sigma_2$ and $H_1: \sigma_1 \neq \sigma_2$ (claim); C.V. = 2.27; F = 4.52; reject. There is enough evidence to support the claim that the standard deviations of the ages are different. One reason is that there are many more people who play the slot machines than people who play roulette. This could possibly account for the larger standard deviation in the ages of the players.

15. $H_0: \sigma_1^2 = \sigma_2^2$ and $H_1: \sigma_1^2 \neq \sigma_2^2$ (claim); C.V. = 4.03; d.f.N. = 9; d.f.D. = 9; F = 1.103; do not reject. There is not enough evidence to support the claim that the variances are not equal.

17. $H_0: \sigma_1^2 = \sigma_2^2$ (claim) and $H_1: \sigma_1^2 \neq \sigma_2^2$; C.V. = 3.44; d.f.N. = 8; d.f.D. = 8; F = 3.980; reject. There is enough evidence to reject the claim that the variance in Montreal and Calgary building heights is different.

19. $H_0: \sigma_1^2 = \sigma_2^2$ (claim) and $H_1: \sigma_1^2 \neq \sigma_2^2$; F = 5.319; d.f.N. = 14; d.f.D. = 14; $P\text{-value} < 0.005\ (0.0035)$; reject. There is enough evidence to reject the claim that the variances in the shoe weights are equal.

Review Exercises

1. $H_0: \mu_1 = \mu_2$ and $H_1: \mu_1 > \mu_2$ (claim); C.V. = 2.33; z = 0.586; do not reject. There is enough evidence to reject the claim that single people do more pleasure driving than married people.

3. $H_0: \mu_1 = \mu_2$ and $H_1: \mu_1 > \mu_2$ (claim); C.V. = 1.729; t = 4.595; reject. There is not enough evidence to reject the claim that single people spend more time each day communicating.

5. $H_0: \mu_1 = \mu_2$ and $H_1: \mu_1 \neq \mu_2$ (claim); C.V. = ±2.624; t = 3.315; reject. There is not enough evidence to reject the claim that there is a significant difference in teachers' salaries between the two provinces. $767.92 < \mu_1 - \mu_2 < 6604.08$ (TI: 836.86, 6535.1)

7. $H_0: \mu_D = 0$ and $H_1: \mu_D < 0$ (claim); C.V. = −2.821; t = −4.17; reject. There is not enough evidence to reject the claim that the tutoring sessions helped to improve the students' vocabulary.

9. $H_0: p_1 = p_2$ and $H_1: p_1 \neq p_2$ (claim); C.V. = ±2.33; z = 3.03; reject. There is not enough evidence to reject the claim that the proportions are different.

11. $H_0: \sigma_1 = \sigma_2$ and $H_1: \sigma_1 \neq \sigma_2$ (claim); C.V. = 2.77; F = 10.365; reject. There is not enough evidence to reject the claim that there is a difference in the standard deviations.

Chapter Quiz

1. False

2. False

3. True

4. False

5. *d*

6. *a*

7. *c*

8. *a*

9. $\mu_1 = \mu_2$

10. *t*

11. Normal

12. Negative

13. $\dfrac{s_1^2}{s_2^2}$

14. $H_0: \mu_1 = \mu_2$ and $H_1: \mu \neq \mu_2$ (claim); C.V. = ±2.575; z = −3.693; reject. There is enough evidence to support the claim that there is a difference in the cholesterol levels of the two groups. $-10.184 < \mu_1 - \mu_2 < -1.816$

15. $H_0: \mu_1 = \mu_2$ and $H_1: \mu > \mu_2$ (claim); C.V. = 1.303; t = 1.601; reject. There is not enough evidence to reject the claim that the average rental fees for the apartments in the east are greater than the average rental fees for the apartments in the west.

16. $H_0: \mu_1 = \mu_2$ and $H_1: \mu_1 \neq \mu_2$ (claim); C.V. = ±3.106; t = 11.094; reject. There is not enough evidence to reject the claim that the average prices are different. $0.288 < \mu_1 - \mu_2 < 0.512$ (TI: 0.2995, 0.5005)

17. $H_0: \mu_1 = \mu_2$ and $H_1: \mu_1 > \mu_2$ (claim); C.V. = 1.303; t = 3.250; reject. There is not enough evidence to reject the claim that the average number of accidents has decreased.

18. $H_0: \mu_1 = \mu_2$ and $H_1: \mu_1 > \mu_2$ (claim); C.V. = ±2.718; t = 9.807; reject. There is not enough evidence to reject the claim that there is a difference in salaries. $6653.91 < \mu_1 - \mu_2 < 11756.09$ (TI: 6919, 11491)

19. $H_0: \mu_1 = \mu_2$ and $H_1: \mu_1 > \mu_2$ (claim); t = 0.875. Since the $P\text{-value}\ (0.198) > \alpha\ (0.05)$, do not reject. There is enough evidence to reject the claim that incomes of city residents are greater than incomes of rural residents.

20. H_0: $\mu_D = 0$ and H_1: $\mu_D < 0$ (claim); C.V. $= -2.821$; $\overline{D} = -6.5$; $s_D = 4.927$; $t = -4.172$; reject. There is not enough evidence to reject the claim that the tutoring sessions helped to improve the students' vocabulary.

21. H_0: $\mu_D = 0$ and H_1: $\mu_D < 0$ (claim); C.V. $= -1.833$; $\overline{D} = -0.8$; $s_D = 1.476$; $t = -1.714$; do not reject. There is enough evidence to reject the claim that the lengthened light time increases hen egg production.

22. H_0: $p_1 = p_2$ and H_1: $p_1 \neq p_2$ (claim); C.V. $= \pm 1.645$; $z = -0.693$; do not reject. There is enough evidence to reject the claim that there is a difference in the proportions. $-0.1047 < p_1 - p_2 < 0.0447$

23. H_0: $p_1 = p_2$ and H_1: $p_1 \neq p_2$ (claim); C.V. $= \pm 1.96$; $z = -0.306$; do not reject. There is enough evidence to reject the claim that there is a difference in the proportions. $-0.037 < p_1 - p_2 < 0.027$. Yes, the confidence interval contains 0; hence, the null hypothesis is not rejected.

24. H_0: $\sigma_1^2 = \sigma_2^2$ and H_1: $\sigma_1^2 \neq \sigma_2^2$ (claim); $F = 1.637$; P-value $> 0.20 \cdot (0.357) > \alpha$ (0.05); do not reject. There is enough evidence to reject the claim that the variances are different.

25. H_0: $\sigma_1^2 = \sigma_2^2$ and H_1: $\sigma_1^2 \neq \sigma_2^2$ (claim); C.V. $= 1.90$; $F = 1.292$; do not reject. There is enough evidence to reject the claim that the variances are different.

Chapter 10

Exercises 10–1

Note: Critical values use Table I: Critical Values for PPMC. Answers do not show t test and P values.

1. Two variables are related when a discernible pattern exists between them.

3. r, ρ (rho)

5. A positive relationship means that as x increases, y increases. A negative relationship means that as x increases, y decreases.

7. Answers will vary.

9. Pearson product moment correlation coefficient.

11. There are many other possibilities, such as chance, or relationship to a third variable.

13. H_0: $\rho = 0$ and H_1: $\rho \neq 0$; $r = -0.832$; C.V. $= \pm 0.811$; reject. There is a significant relationship between a person's age and the number of hours he or she exercises.

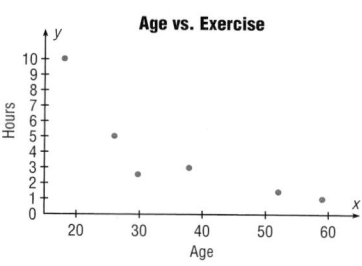
Age vs. Exercise

15. H_0: $\rho = 0$ and H_1: $\rho \neq 0$; $r = -0.883$; C.V. $= \pm 0.811$; reject. There is a significant relationship between the number of years a person has been out of school and his or her contribution.

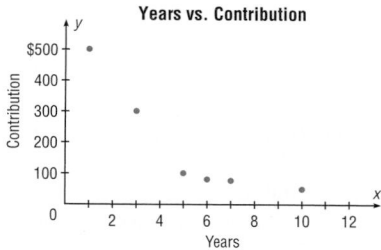
Years vs. Contribution

17. H_0: $\rho = 0$ and H_1: $\rho \neq 0$; $r = 0.893$; C.V. $= \pm 0.754$; reject. There is a significant linear correlation between the robbery and homicide crime rates.

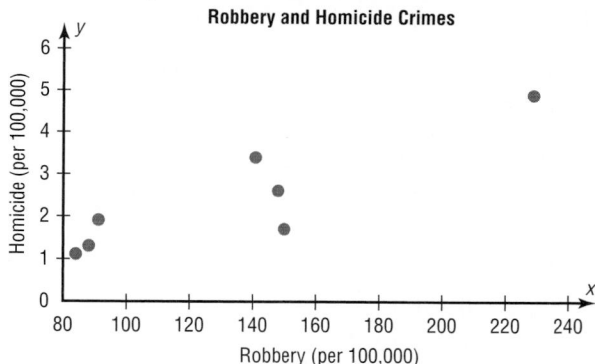
Robbery and Homicide Crimes

19. H_0: $\rho = 0$ and H_1: $\rho \neq 0$; $r = -0.833$; C.V. $= \pm 0.811$; reject. There is a significant linear relationship between the number of eggs produced and the price per dozen.

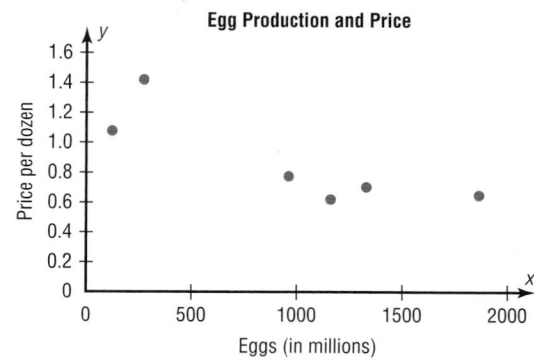
Egg Production and Price

21. $H_0: \rho = 0$ and $H_1: \rho \neq 0$; $r = 0.963$; C.V. $= \pm 0.878$; reject. There is a significant linear correlation between the Black and Asian visible minorities.

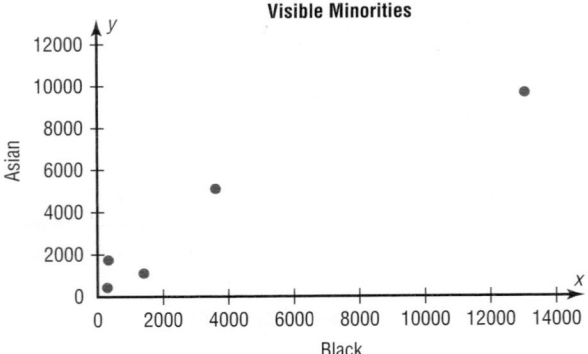

Visible Minorities

23. $H_0: \rho = 0$ and $H_1: \rho \neq 0$; $r = 0.560$; C.V. $= \pm 0.754$; do not reject. There is no significant linear correlation between Canadian city temperatures and average monthly precipitation.

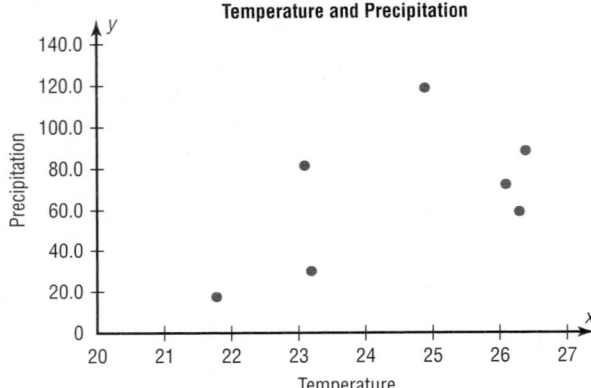

Temperature and Precipitation

25. $H_0: \rho = 0$ and $H_1: \rho \neq 0$; $r = 0.725$; C.V. $= \pm 0.754$; do not reject. There is no significant linear relationship between the number of calories and the cholesterol content of fast-food chicken sandwiches.

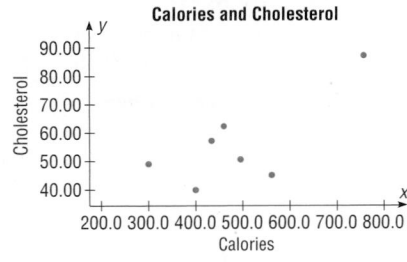

Calories and Cholesterol

27. $H_0: \rho = 0$ and $H_1: \rho \neq 0$; $r = 0.831$; C.V. $= \pm 0.754$; reject. There is a significant linear relationship between the number of licensed beds in a hospital and the number of staffed beds.

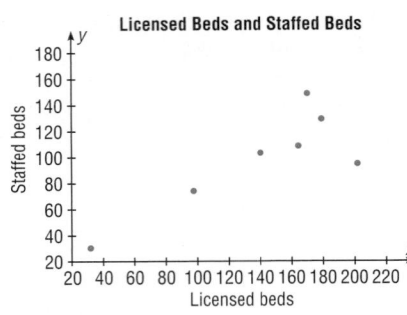

Licensed Beds and Staffed Beds

29. $r = 1.00$: All values fall in a straight line. $r = 1.00$: The value of r between x and y is the same when x and y are interchanged.

Exercises 10–2

1. A scatter plot should be drawn, and the value of the correlation coefficient should be tested to see whether it is significant.

3. $y' = a + bx$

5. It is the line that is drawn through the points on the scatter plot such that the sum of the squares of the vertical distances from each point to the line is a minimum.

7. When r is positive, b will be positive. When r is negative, b will be negative.

9. The closer r is to $+1$ or -1, the more accurate the predicted value will be.

11. When r is not significant, the mean of the y values should be used to predict y.

13. $y' = 10.499 - 0.18x$; 4.2

15. $y' = 453.176 - 50.439x$; 251.42

17. $y' = -0.69 + 0.02x$; 1.64

19. $y' = 1.252 - 0.000398x$; 0.614

21. $y' = 1015.2 + 0.7x$; 2730.2

23. Since r is not significant, no regression should be done.

25. Since r is not significant, no regression should be done.

27. $y' = 22.659 + 0.582x$; 48.267

29. $H_0: \rho = 0$ and $H_1: \rho \neq 0$; $r = +0.956$; C.V. $= \pm 0.754$; reject; d.f. $= 5$; $y' = -10.944 + 1.969x$; when $x = 30$, $y' = 48.13$. There is a significant relationship between the amount of lung damage and the number of years a person has been smoking.

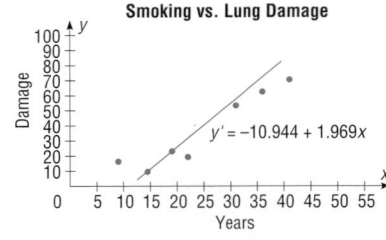

Smoking vs. Lung Damage

31. $H_0: \rho = 0$ and $H_1: \rho \neq 0$; $r = 0.987$; C.V. $= \pm 0.754$; reject. $y' = -2.679 + 1.042x$; when $x = 200$, $y' = 205.72$. There is a significant linear correlation between the number of business head offices in 1999 and 2005.

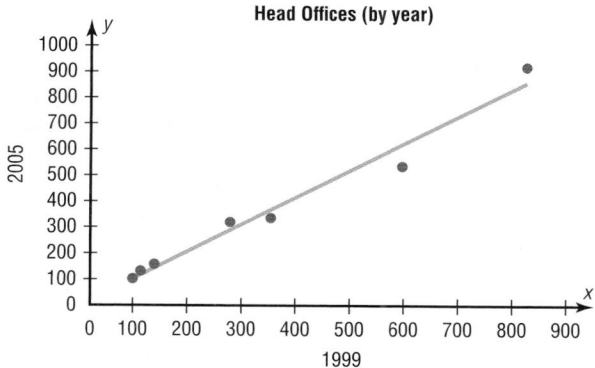

Head Offices (by year)

33. $H_0: \rho = 0$ and $H_1: \rho \neq 0$; $r = -0.981$; C.V. $= \pm 0.811$; reject. There is a significant relationship between the number of absences and the final grade; $y' = 96.784 - 2.668x$.

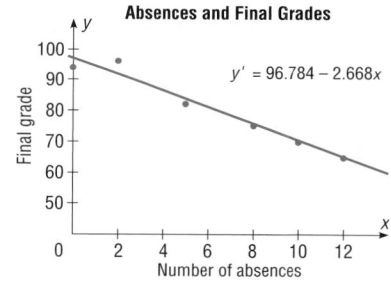

Absences and Final Grades

35. $H_0: \rho = 0$ and $H_1: \rho \neq 0$; $r = -0.265$; $t = -0.777$; $0.2 < P\text{-value} > 0.5$ (0.459); do not reject. There is no significant linear relationship between the ages of billionaires and their net worth. No regression should be done.

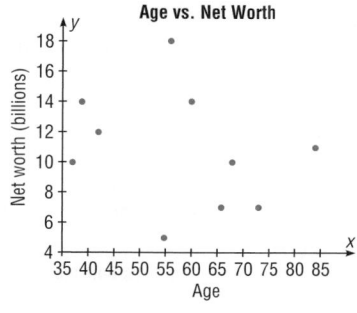

Age vs. Net Worth

37. 453.173; 21.1

Exercises 10–3

1. Explained variation is the variation due to the relationship. It is computed by $\Sigma(y' - \bar{y})^2$.

3. Total variation is the sum of the squares of the vertical distances of the points from the mean. It is computed by $\Sigma(y - \bar{y})^2$.

5. The coefficient of determination is found by squaring the value of the correlation coefficient.

7. $r^2 = 0.49$; 49% of the variation of y is due to the variation of x; 51% of the variation of y is due to chance.

9. $r^2 = 0.1369$; 13.69% of the variation of y is due to the variation of x; 86.31% of the variation of y is due to chance.

11. $r^2 = 0.0025$; 0.25% of the variation of y is due to the variation of x; 99.75% of the variation of y is due to chance.

13. 2.092*   **15.** 94.221*

17. $1.587 < y < 12.211$*   **19.** $31.273 < y < 471.527$*

*Answers may vary due to rounding.

Exercises 10–4

1. Simple regression has one dependent variable and one independent variable. Multiple regression has one dependent variable and two or more independent variables.

3. The relationship would include all variables in one equation.

5. They will all be smaller.

7. 3.48 or 3   **9.** 85.75

11. R is the strength of the relationship between the dependent variable and all the independent variables.

13. R^2 is the coefficient of multiple determination. R^2_{adj} is adjusted for sample size and number of predictors.

15. The F test.

Review Exercises

1. $H_0: \rho = 0$ and $H_1: \rho \neq 0$; $r = 0.479$; C.V. $= \pm 0.765$; do not reject. There is no significant linear relationship between the number of shots on goal and goals scored. Since r is not significant, no regression should be done.

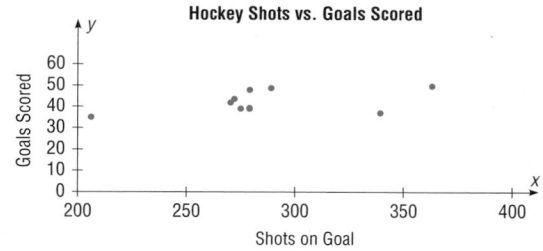

Hockey Shots vs. Goals Scored

3. H_0: $\rho = 0$ and H_1: $\rho \neq 0$; $r = 0.891$; C.V. $= \pm 0.875$; reject. There is a significant linear relationship between gasoline and diesel fuel prices. $y' = -7.485 + 1.042x$; $y' = 96.715$.

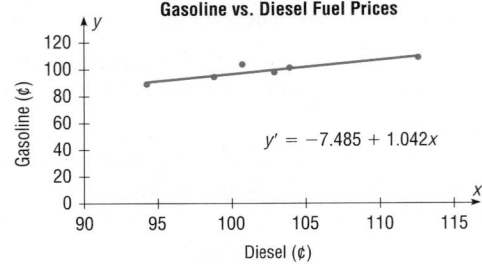

Gasoline vs. Diesel Fuel Prices

$y' = -7.485 + 1.042x$

5. H_0: $\rho = 0$ and H_1: $\rho \neq 0$; $r = -0.974$; C.V. $= \pm 0.708$; reject. There is a significant relationship between speed and time; $y' = 14.086 - 0.137x$; $y' = 4.222$.

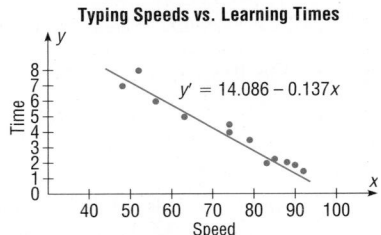

Typing Speeds vs. Learning Times

$y' = 14.086 - 0.137x$

7. H_0: $\rho = 0$ and H_1: $\rho \neq 0$; $r = 0.889$; C.V. $= \pm 0.834$; reject. There is a significant relationship between vehicle's age and repair costs. $y' = 297.603 + 84.621x$; $y' = \$889.95$.

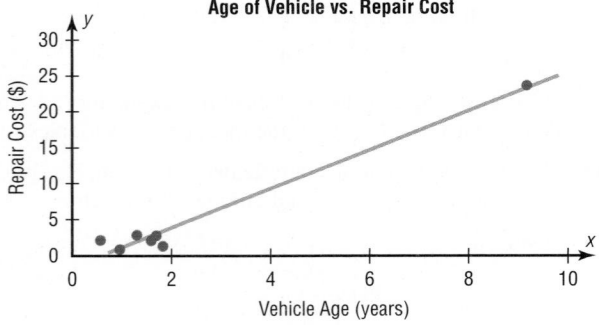

Age of Vehicle vs. Repair Cost

9. 0.468* (TI: 0.513)

11. $3.331 < y < 5.113$*

13. 22.01*

15. $R^2_{adj} = 0.643$*

*Answers may vary due to rounding.

Chapter Quiz

1. False   **2.** True

3. True   **4.** False

5. False   **6.** False

7. *a*   **8.** *a*

9. *d*   **10.** *c*

11. *b*   **12.** Scatter plot

13. Independent   **14.** $-1, +1$

15. *b*   **16.** Line of best fit

17. $+1, -1$

18. H_0: $\rho = 0$ and H_1: $\rho \neq 0$; $r = 0.988$; C.V. $= \pm 0.754$; reject. There is a significant linear relationship between Canada and U.S. drug prices; $y' = -1.44 + 2.70x$; $y' = \$8.68$.

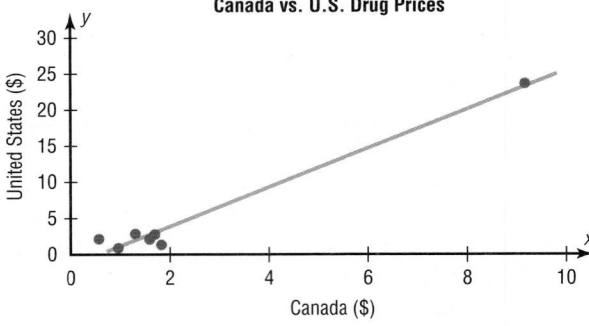

Canada vs. U.S. Drug Prices

19. H_0: $\rho = 0$ and H_1: $\rho \neq 0$; $r = -0.078$; C.V. $= \pm 0.754$; do not reject. No regression should be done.

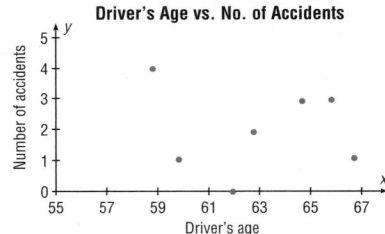

Driver's Age vs. No. of Accidents

20. H_0: $\rho = 0$ and H_1: $\rho \neq 0$; $r = 0.842$; C.V. $= \pm 0.811$; reject. $y' = -1.918 + 0.551x$; 4.14 or 4.

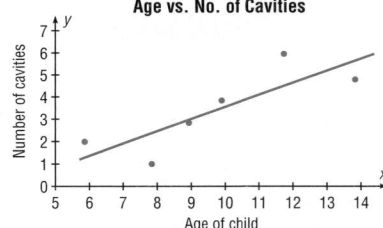

Age vs. No. of Cavities

21. H_0: $\rho = 0$ and H_1: $\rho \neq 0$; $r = 0.602$; C.V. $= \pm 0.707$; do not reject. No regression should be done.

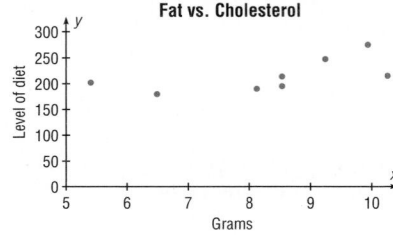

Fat vs. Cholesterol

22. 1.129*

23. 29.5* For calculation purposes only. No regression should be done.

24. $0 < y < 5$*

25. 217.5 (average of y' values is used since there is no significant relationship)

26. 119.9*   27. $R = 0.729$*

28. $R^2_{adj} = 0.439$*

*These answers may vary due to the method of calculation or rounding.

Chapter 11

Exercises 11–1

1. The variance test compares a sample variance with a hypothesized population variance; the goodness-of-fit test compares a distribution obtained from a sample with a hypothesized distribution.

3. The expected values are computed on the basis of what the null hypothesis states about the distribution.

5. H_0: The ages of automobiles are equally distributed over the three categories (claim). H_1: The ages of automobiles are not equally distributed over the three categories. C.V. = 5.991; d.f. = 2; $\chi^2 = 0.8$; do not reject. There is not enough evidence to reject the claim that the average age of automobiles is equally distributed over the three categories. Tire manufacturers need to make enough tires to fit automobiles of all ages.

7. H_0: New vehicle market share in Canada is General Motors, 29.0%; Chrysler, 14.3%; Ford, 14.1%; Toyota, 10.2%; Other Manufacturers, 32.4%. H_1: The distribution is different then stated in the null hypothesis (claim). C.V. = 9.488; d.f. = 4; $\chi^2 = 1.3423$; do not reject. There is not enough evidence to support the claim that the distribution is not the same.

9. H_0: 35% feel that genetically modified food is safe to eat, 52% feel that genetically modified food is not safe to eat, and 13% have no opinion. H_1: The distribution is not the same as stated in the null hypothesis (claim). C.V. = 9.210; d.f. = 2; $\chi^2 = 1.4286$; do not reject. There is not enough evidence to support the claim that the proportions are different from those reported in the survey.

11. H_0: The types of loans are distributed as follows: 21% for home mortgages, 39% for automobile purchases, 20% for credit card, 12% for real estate, and 8% for miscellaneous (claim). H_1: The distribution is different from that stated in the null hypothesis. C.V. = 9.488; d.f. = 4; $\chi^2 = 4.786$; do not reject. There is not enough evidence to reject the claim that the distribution is the same as reported in the newspaper.

13. H_0: Smoking status of Canadians 15 years and older is daily, 13.2%; nondaily, 4.1%; former, 27.2%; and never, 55.5% (claim). H_1: At least one proportion is different than stated in the null hypothesis. C.V. = 7.815. $\chi^2 = 10.5527$; reject. There is no significant evidence to reject the claim that the rural health authority smoking distribution is the same as the Health Canada report.

15. H_0: Canada's provincial prison population is distributed as crimes of violence, 15.5%; property crimes, 24.1%; impaired driving, 5.5%; drug offences, 4.7%; other Criminal Code offences, 29.8%; and other statutes, 20.4% (claim). H_1: The distribution is different then stated in the null hypothesis. C.V. = 11.071; d.f. = 5; $\chi^2 = 5.7804$; do not reject. There is not enough evidence to reject the claim that the proportions are the same as stated in the null hypothesis.

17. H_0: Distribution of Canadian retail medical prescription payments is 24% out-of-pocket, 34.6% private insurers, and 41.4% public insurance (claim). H_1: The distribution is not the same as stated in the null hypothesis. The d.f. = 2; $\chi^2 = 0.4366$; do not reject at $\alpha = 0.05$ since $0.90 < P$-value < 0.10 (0.8039). There is not enough evidence to reject the claim that the proportions are the same as stated in the null hypothesis.

19. Answers will vary.

Exercises 11–2

1. The independence test and the goodness-of-fit test both use the same formula for computing the test value. However, the independence test uses a contingency table, whereas the goodness-of-fit test does not.

3. H_0: The variables are independent (or not related). H_1: The variables are dependent (or related).

5. The expected values are computed as (row total $\times$ column total) $\div$ grand total.

7. H_0: $p_1 = p_2 = p_3 = p_4 = \cdots = p_n$. H_1: At least one proportion is different from the others.

9. H_0: The class of vertebrate is independent of whether the species is endangered or threatened. H_1: The class of vertebrate is dependent on whether the species is endangered or threatened (claim); C.V. = 9.488; $\chi^2 = 45.3145$; reject. There is significant evidence that a relationship exists between the class of vertebrate and whether it is an endangered or threatened species.

11. H_0: The composition of the House of Commons is independent of the province of the Member of Parliament. H_1: The composition of the House of Commons is dependent of the province of the Member of Parliament (claim). C.V. = 12.592; $\chi^2 = 14.083$; reject. There is significant evidence to support the claim that the composition of the House of Commons is dependent of the province of the Member of Parliament.

13. H_0: A member of Parliament's occupation is independent of the session of Parliament. H_1: A member of Parliament's occupation is dependent on the session of Parliament (claim); C.V. = 18.307; χ^2 = 2.05; do not reject. There is not enough evidence to support the claim that a member of Parliament's occupation is dependent on the session of Parliament.

15. H_0: The type of practice of an attorney is independent of the gender of the attorney (claim). H_1: The type of practice of an attorney is dependent on the gender of the attorney. C.V. = 5.991; χ^2 = 7.963; reject. There is enough evidence to reject the claim that the type of practice is independent of the gender of the attorney.

17. H_0: The type of video rented is independent of the person's age. H_1: The type of video rented is dependent on the person's age (claim). C.V. = 13.362; χ^2 = 46.733; reject. Yes, there is enough evidence to support the claim that the type of movie selected is related to the age of the customer.

19. H_0: The type of snack purchased is independent of the gender of the consumer (claim). H_1: The type of snack purchased is dependent on the gender of the consumer. C.V. = 4.605; χ^2 = 6.342; reject. There is enough evidence to reject the claim that the type of snack is independent of the gender of the consumer.

21. H_0: The type of book purchased by an individual is independent of the gender of the individual (claim). H_1: The type of book purchased by an individual is dependent on the gender of the individual. P-value (0.00006) $< \alpha$ (0.05); reject. There is enough evidence to reject the claim that the type of book purchased by an individual is independent of the gender of the individual.

23. H_0: $p_1 = p_2 = p_3 = p_4$ (claim). H_1: At least one proportion is different from the others. C.V. = 7.815; χ^2 = 1.852; do not reject. There is not enough evidence to reject the claim that the proportions for obesity are equal for each district.

25. H_0: $p_1 = p_2 = p_3 = p_4$ (claim). H_1: At least one proportion is different from the others. C.V. = 7.815; χ^2 = 0.017; do not reject. There is not enough evidence to reject the null hypothesis that the proportions are the same as they were 20 years ago.

27. H_0: $p_1 = p_2 = p_3 = p_4 = p_5$ (claim). H_1: At least one proportion is different from the others. C.V. = 9.488; χ^2 = 12.028; reject. There is significant evidence to reject the claim that the proportions of volunteers are the same for each group.

29. H_0: $p_1 = p_2 = p_3 = p_4$ (claim). H_1: At least one proportion is different. χ^2 = 1.768; α = 0.05; 0.90 $< P$-value < 0.10 (0.622); do not reject. There is not sufficient evidence to reject the claim that the proportions are the same.

31. H_0: $p_1 = p_2 = p_3$ (claim). H_1: At least one proportion is different. C.V. = 4.605; χ^2 = 2.401; do not reject. There is not enough evidence to reject the claim that the proportions are equal.

33. χ^2 = 1.075

Review Exercises

1. H_0: People show no preference for the day of the week that they do their shopping (claim). H_1: People show a preference for the day of the week that they do their shopping. C.V. = 12.592; χ^2 = 237.15; reject. There is enough evidence to reject the claim that shoppers have no preference for the day of the week that they do their shopping. Retail merchants should probably plan for more shoppers on Fridays and Saturdays than they will have on the other days of the week.

3. H_0: Opinion is independent of gender. H_1: Opinion is dependent on gender (claim). C.V. = 4.605; χ^2 = 6.166; reject. There is enough evidence to support the claim that opinion is dependent on gender.

5. H_0: The distribution of M&Ms is 13% brown, 13% red, 14% yellow, 16% green, 20% orange, and 24% blue. H_1: The distribution is not the same as stated in the null hypothesis (claim); C.V. = 11.070; χ^2 = 18.6047; reject. There is significant evidence to support the claim that the proportion of M&M colours differs from those stated by the candy company.

7. H_0: $p_1 = p_2 = p_3$ (claim). H_1: At least one proportion is different. χ^2 = 4.912; α = 0.01; 0.05 $< P$-value < 0.10 (0.086); do not reject since P-value > 0.01. There is not enough evidence to reject the claim that the proportions are equal.

9. H_0: $p_1 = p_2 = p_3 = p_4$ (claim). H_1: At least one proportion is different. C.V. = 6.251; χ^2 = 6.702; reject. There is enough evidence to reject the claim that the proportions are equal.

Chapter Quiz

1. False

2. True

3. False

4. *c*

5. *b*

6. *d*

7. 6

8. Independent

9. Right

10. At least five

11. H_0: The reasons why people lost their jobs are equally distributed (claim). H_1: The reasons why people lost their jobs are not equally distributed. C.V. = 5.991; χ^2 = 2.333; do not reject. There is not enough evidence to reject the claim that the reasons why people lost their jobs are equally distributed. The results could have been different 10 years ago since different factors of the economy existed then.

12. H_0: Takeout food is consumed according to the following distribution: 53% at home, 19% in the car, 14% at work, and 14% at other places (claim). H_1: The distribution is different from that stated in the null hypothesis. C.V. = 11.345; χ^2 = 5.270; do not reject. There is not enough evidence to reject the claim that the distribution is as stated. Fast-food restaurants may want to make their advertisements appeal to those who like to take their food home to eat.

13. H_0: College students show the same preference for shopping channels as those surveyed. H_1: College students show a different preference for shopping channels (claim). C.V. = 7.815; α = 0.05; χ^2 = 21.789; reject. There is enough evidence to support the claim that college students show a different preference for shopping channels.

14. H_0: The mode of transportation to work is distributed as motor vehicle (driver), 72.3%; motor vehicle (passenger), 7.7%; public transit, 11.0%; walk, 6.4%; bicycle, 1.3%; and other, 1.2%. H_1: At least one proportion is different than stated in the null hypothesis (claim); C.V. = 11.070; χ^2 = 10.8676; do not reject. There is not enough evidence to support the claim that the proportion of workers using each type of transportation is different for the CMA than stated in the census.

15. H_0: Ice cream flavour is independent of the gender of the purchaser (claim). H_1: Ice cream flavour is dependent on the gender of the purchaser. C.V. = 7.815; χ^2 = 7.198; do not reject. There is not enough evidence to reject the claim that ice cream flavour is independent of the gender of the purchaser.

16. H_0: The type of pizza ordered is independent of the age of the individual who purchases it. H_1: The type of pizza ordered is dependent on the age of the individual who purchases it (claim). χ^2 = 107.3; P-value < 0.005 (0.000) < α (0.10); reject. There is enough evidence to support the claim that the pizza purchased is related to the age of the purchaser.

17. H_0: The colour of the pennant purchased is independent of the gender of the purchaser (claim). H_1: The colour of the pennant purchased is dependent on the gender of the purchaser. χ^2 = 5.632; C.V. = 4.605; reject. There is enough evidence to reject the claim that the colour of the pennant purchased is independent of the gender of the purchaser.

18. H_0: The opinion of the children on the use of the tax credit is independent of the gender of the children. H_1: The opinion of the children on the use of the tax credit is dependent on the gender of the children (claim). C.V. = 4.605; χ^2 = 1.535; do not reject. There is not enough evidence to support the claim that the opinion of the children on the use of the tax is dependent on their gender.

19. H_0: $p_1 = p_2 = p_3$ (claim). H_1: At least one proportion is different from the others. C.V. = 4.605; χ^2 = 6.711;

reject. There is enough evidence to reject the claim that the proportions are equal. It seems that more women are undecided about their jobs. Perhaps they want better income or greater chances of advancement.

Chapter 12

Exercises 12–1

1. The analysis of variance using the F test can be employed to compare three or more means.

3. The populations from which the samples were obtained must be normally distributed. The samples must be independent of each other. The variances of the populations must be equal.

5. $F = \dfrac{S_B^2}{S_W^2}$

7. If the F test indicates that there is a difference among the means, use the Scheffé test. Use the Tukey test to determine where the difference among the means lies.

9. H_0: $\mu_1 = \mu_2 = \mu_3$. H_1: At least one mean is different from the others (claim). C.V. = 3.68; α = 0.05; d.f.N. = 2; d.f.D. = 15; F = 7.955; reject. There is not enough evidence to reject the claim that at least one mean is different.

11. H_0: $\mu_1 = \mu_2 = \mu_3$. H_1: At least one mean is different from the others (claim). C.V. = 3.68; d.f.N. = 2; d.f.D. = 15; F = 4.620; reject. There is not enough evidence to reject the claim that at least one mean bridge length is different.

13. H_0: $\mu_1 = \mu_2 = \mu_3$. H_1: At least one mean is different from the others (claim). C.V. = 3.89; d.f.N. = 2; d.f.D. = 12; F = 39.409; reject There is sufficient evidence to support the claim that the tuition fees are different. One possible reason for the difference is that provinces may provide different levels of subsidies that support lower tuition fees.

15. H_0: $\mu_1 = \mu_2 = \mu_3$ (claim). H_1: At least one mean is different from the others. C.V. = 3.52; α = 0.05; d.f.N. = 2; d.f.D. = 19; F = 11.231; reject. There is enough evidence to reject the claim that the mean number of farms in the Prairie provinces is the same.

17. H_0: $\mu_1 = \mu_2 = \mu_3$. H_1: At least one mean is different from the others (claim). F = 10.118; since P-value (0.00102) < α (0.10), reject. There is not enough evidence to reject the claim that a not enough difference exists in the average price of the microwave ovens.

19. H_0: $\mu_1 = \mu_2 = \mu_3 = \mu_4$. H_1: At least one mean is different from the others (claim). C.V. = 2.81, d.f.N. = 3, d.f.D. = 9, α = 0.10; F = 0.3290; do not reject. There is enough evidence to reject the claim that the average number of graduate students in each province is different.

Exercises 12–2

1. Scheffé test—unequal sample sizes; Tukey test—equal sample sizes.

3. Scheffé test: C.V. = 3.67; $F' = 7.34$; $\overline{X}_1$ vs $\overline{X}_2$; $F_S = 11.46$; $\overline{X}_1$ vs $\overline{X}_3$; $F_S = 12.05$; $\overline{X}_2$ vs $\overline{X}_3$; $F_S = 0.45$. There is a significant difference between $\overline{X}_1$ and $\overline{X}_2$ and between $\overline{X}_1$ and $\overline{X}_3$.

5. Scheffé test: C.V. = 3.68; $F' = 7.36$; $\overline{X}_1$ vs $\overline{X}_2$; $F_S = 6.27$; $\overline{X}_1$ vs $\overline{X}_3$; $F_S = 7.00$; $\overline{X}_2$ vs $\overline{X}_3$; $F_S = 0.07$. There is no significant difference between pairs.

7. Scheffé test: C.V. = 3.89; $F' = 7.78$; $\overline{X}_1$ vs $\overline{X}_2$; $F_S = 0.51$; $\overline{X}_1$ vs $\overline{X}_3$; $F_S = 54.57$; $\overline{X}_2$ vs $\overline{X}_3$; $F_S = 77.30$. There is a significant difference between $\overline{X}_1$ and $\overline{X}_3$ and between $\overline{X}_2$ and $\overline{X}_3$.

9. Tukey test: C.V. 3.77; $\overline{X}_1$ vs $\overline{X}_2$; $q = -3.04$; $\overline{X}_1$ vs $\overline{X}_3$; $q = -8.33$; $\overline{X}_2$ vs $\overline{X}_3$; $q = -5.29$. There is a significant difference between $\overline{X}_1$ and $\overline{X}_3$ and between $\overline{X}_2$ and $\overline{X}_3$.

11. H_0: $\mu_1 = \mu_2 = \mu_3$. H_1: At least one mean is different (claim). C.V. = 3.89; $\alpha = 0.05$, d.f.N. = 2, d.f.D. = 12; $F = 99.372$; reject. There is significant evidence to indicate a difference in the mean precipitation for the region. Tukey test: C.V. = 3.77; $\overline{X}_1$ vs $\overline{X}_2$; $q = 8.12$; $\overline{X}_1$ vs $\overline{X}_3$; $q = 19.83$; $\overline{X}_2$ vs $\overline{X}_3$; $q = 11.71$. There is a significant difference between $\overline{X}_1$ and $\overline{X}_2$ and between $\overline{X}_1$ and $\overline{X}_3$ and between $\overline{X}_2$ and $\overline{X}_3$.

13. H_0: $\mu_1 = \mu_2 = \mu_3 = \mu_4$. H_1: At least one mean is different (claim). C.V. = 5.29; $\alpha = 0.01$, d.f.N. = 3, d.f.D. = 16; $F = 0.636$; do not reject. There is not enough evidence to support the claim that at least one mean is different. Students might have had discipline problems. Parents might not like the regular school district, etc.

Exercises 12–3

1. The two-way ANOVA allows the researcher to test the effects of two independent variables and a possible interaction effect. The one-way ANOVA can test the effects of only one independent variable.

3. The mean square values are computed by dividing the sum of squares by the corresponding degrees of freedom.

5. *a.* For factor A, d.f.$_A$ = 2
   b. For factor B, d.f.$_B$ = 1
   c. d.f.$_{A \times B}$ = 2
   d. d.f.$_{within}$ = 24

7. The two types of interactions that can occur are ordinal and disordinal.

9. *a.* The lines will be parallel or approximately parallel. They may also coincide.
   b. The lines will not intersect and they will not be parallel.
   c. The lines will intersect.

11. H_0: There is no interaction effect between the time of day and the type of diet on a person's sodium level. H_1: There is an interaction effect between the time of day and the type of diet on a person's sodium level.

   H_0: There is no difference between the means for the sodium level for the times of day. H_1: There is a difference between the means for the sodium level for the times of day.

   H_0: There is no difference between the means for the sodium level for the type of diet. H_1: There is a difference between the means for the sodium level for the type of diet.

ANOVA Summary Table

Source	SS	d.f.	MS	F
Time	1800.0	1	1800.000	25.806
Diet	242.0	1	242.000	3.470
Interaction	264.5	1	264.500	3.792
Within	279.0	4	69.750	
Total	2585.5	7		

The critical value at $\alpha = 0.05$ with d.f.N. = 1 and d.f.D. = 4 is 7.71 for F_A, F_B, and $F_{A \times B}$. Since the only F test statistic that exceeds 7.71 is the one for the time, 25.806, it can be concluded that there is a difference in the means for the sodium level taken at two different times.

13. H_0: There is no interaction effect between the gender of the individual and the duration of the training on the test scores. H_1: There is an interaction effect between the gender of the individual and the duration of the training on the test scores.

   H_0: There is no difference between the means of the test scores for the males and females. H_1: There is a difference between the means of the test scores for the males and females.

   H_0: There is no difference between the means of the test scores for the two different durations. H_1: There is a difference between the means of the test scores for the two different durations.

ANOVA Summary Table

Source	SS	d.f.	MS	F
Gender	57.042	1	57.042	0.835
Duration	7.042	1	7.042	0.103
Interaction	3978.375	1	3978.375	58.270
Within	1365.500	20	68.275	
Total	5407.959	23		

The critical value at $\alpha = 0.10$ with d.f.N. = 1 and d.f.D. = 20 is 2.97. Since the F test value for the interaction is greater than the critical value, it can be concluded that gender affects test scores differently for the duration levels.

15. H_0: There is no interaction effect between the ages of the salespeople and the products they sell on the monthly sales. H_1: There is an interaction effect between the ages of the salespeople and the products they sell on the monthly sales.

H_0: There is no difference in the means of the monthly sales of the two age groups. H_1: There is a difference in the means of the monthly sales of the two age groups.

H_0: There is no difference among the means of the sales for the different products. H_1: There is a difference among the means of the sales for the different products.

ANOVA Summary Table

Source	SS	d.f.	MS	F
Age	168.033	1	168.033	1.567
Product	1,762.067	2	881.034	8.215
Interaction	7,955.267	2	3,977.634	37.087
Error	2,574.000	24	107.250	
Total	12,459.367	29		

At $\alpha = 0.05$, the critical values are: for age, d.f.N. = 1, d.f.D. = 24, C.V. = 4.26; for product and interaction, d.f.N. = 2 and d.f.D. = 24; C.V. = 3.40. The null hypotheses for the interaction effect and for the type of product sold are rejected since the F test statistic is greater than the critical value 3.40. The cell means are as follows:

Product / Age	Pools	Spas	Saunas
Over 30	38.8	28.6	55.4
30 and under	21.2	68.6	18.8

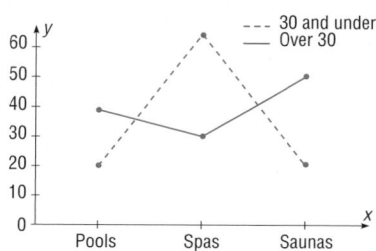

Since the lines cross, there is a disordinal interaction; hence, there is an interaction effect between the ages of salespeople and the type of products sold.

17. H_0: There is no interaction effect between the type of flour and the sweetening agent in the glaze.
H_1: There is an interaction effect between the type of flour and the sweetening agent in the glaze.

H_0: There is no difference in mean sales based on the type of flour used.
H_1: There is a difference in mean sales based on the type of flour used.

H_0: There is no difference in mean sales based on the type of sweetener used in the glaze.
H_1: There is a difference in mean sales based on the type of sweetener used in the glaze.

ANOVA Summary Table

Source	SS	d.f.	MS	F
Flour	0.5625	1	0.5625	0.0062
Sweetener	1105.563	1	1105.563	12.2812
Interaction	0.5625	1	0.5625	0.0062
Error	1080.25	12	90.0208	
Total	470.6667	15		

The critical value at $\alpha = 0.05$ with d.f.N. = 1 and d.f.D. = 12 is 4.747. Since the F test statistic for the sweetener is greater than the critical value, it can be concluded that there is a difference in mean sales based on the type of sweetener used in the glaze.

Review Exercises

1. H_0: $\mu_1 = \mu_2 = \mu_3$ (claim). H_1: At least one mean is different from the others. C.V. = 5.39; $\alpha = 0.01$; d.f.N. = 2, d.f.D. = 33 (use 30); $F = 6.931$; reject. Tukey test; C.V. = 5.05; $\overline{X}_1$ versus $\overline{X}_2$; $q = 0.344$; $\overline{X}_1$ versus $\overline{X}_3$; $q = 4.722$; $\overline{X}_2$ versus $\overline{X}_3$; $q = 4.378$. There is no significant difference between the paired means.

3. H_0: $\mu_1 = \mu_2 = \mu_3$. H_1: At least one mean is different from the others (claim). C.V. = 3.59; $\alpha = 0.05$; d.f.N. = 2; d.f.D. = 17; $F = 0.0155$; do not reject. There is not enough evidence to support the claim that at least one mean is different from the others.

5. H_0: $\mu_1 = \mu_2 = \mu_3$. H_1: At least one mean is different from the others (claim). C.V. = 2.61; $\alpha = 0.10$; d.f.N. = 2; d.f.D. = 19; $F = 0.4876$; do not reject. There is not enough evidence to support the claim that at least one mean is different from the others.

7. H_0: $\mu_1 = \mu_2 = \mu_3 = \mu_4$. H_1: At least one mean is different from the others (claim). C.V. = 3.710; $\alpha = 0.05$, d.f.N. = 3, d.f.D. = 10; $F = 5.1656$; reject. Scheffé test: C.V. = 12.30; $F' = 7.78$. $\overline{X}_1$ vs $\overline{X}_2$; $F_s = 1.74$; $\overline{X}_1$ vs $\overline{X}_3$; $F_s = 3.35$; $\overline{X}_1$ vs $\overline{X}_3$; $F_s = 3.35$; $\overline{X}_1$ vs $\overline{X}_4$; $F_s = 0.01$; $\overline{X}_2$ vs $\overline{X}_3$; $F_s = 15.887$; $\overline{X}_2$ vs $\overline{X}_4$; $F_s = 1.96$; $\overline{X}_3$ vs $\overline{X}_4$; $F_s = 4.83$. There is a significant difference between $\overline{X}_2$ and $\overline{X}_3$.

9. H_0: There is no interaction effect between the type of exercise program and the type of diet on a person's glucose level. H_1: There is an interaction effect between type of exercise program and the type of diet on a person's glucose level.

H_0: There is no difference in the means for the glucose levels of the people in the two exercise programs. H_1: There is a difference in the means for the glucose levels of the people in the two exercise programs.

H_0: There is no difference in the means for the glucose levels of the people in the two diet programs. H_1: There is a difference in the means for the glucose levels of the people in the two diet programs.

ANOVA Summary Table

Source	SS	d.f.	MS	F
Exercise	816.750	1	816.750	60.50
Diet	102.083	1	102.083	7.56
Interaction	444.083	1	444.083	32.90
Within	108.000	8	13.500	
Total	1470.916	11		

At $\alpha = 0.05$, d.f.N. $= 1$, d.f.D. $= 8$, and the critical value is 5.32 for each F_A, F_B, and $F_{A \times B}$. Hence, all three null hypotheses are rejected. The cell means should be calculated.

Exercise \ Diet	A	B
I	64.000	57.667
II	68.333	86.333

Since the means for exercise program I are both smaller than those for exercise program II and the vertical differences are not the same, the interaction is ordinal. Hence one can say that there is a difference for exercise and diet, and that an interaction effect is present.

Chapter Quiz

1. False
2. False
3. False
4. True
5. *d*
6. *a*
7. *a*
8. *c*
9. ANOVA
10. Tukey
11. Two
12. H_0: $\mu_1 = \mu_2 = \mu_3 = \mu_4$. H_1: At least one mean is different from the others (claim). C.V. $= 3.71$; $\alpha = 0.05$; d.f.N. $= 3$; d.f.D. $= 10$; $F = 3.312$; do not reject. There is enough evidence to reject the claim that at least one mean is different from the others.
13. H_0: $\mu_1 = \mu_2 = \mu_3$. H_1: At least one mean is different from the others (claim). C.V. $= 6.93$; $\alpha = 0.01$; d.f.N. $= 2$; d.f.D. $= 12$; $F = 3.497$. Do not reject. There is enough evidence reject the claim that at least one mean is different from the others. Writers would want to target their material to the age group of the viewers.

14. H_0: $\mu_1 = \mu_2 = \mu_3$. H_1: At least one mean is different from the others (claim). C.V. $= 3.68$; $\alpha = 0.05$; d.f.N. $= 2$; d.f.D. $= 15$; $F = 10.494$; reject. There is not enough evidence to reject the claim that at least one mean is different from the others.

15. H_0: $\mu_1 = \mu_2 = \mu_3$ (claim). H_1: At least one mean is different from the others. C.V. $= 2.70$; $\alpha = 0.10$; d.f.N. $= 2$; d.f.D. $= 15$; $F = 0.670$; do not reject. There is not enough evidence to reject the claim that the means are equal.

16. H_0: $\mu_1 = \mu_2 = \mu_3 = \mu_4$. H_1: At least one mean is different from the others (claim). C.V. $= 3.07$; $\alpha = 0.05$; d.f.N. $= 3$; d.f.D. $= 21$; $F = 0.4564$; do not reject. There is enough evidence to reject the claim that at least one mean is different from the others.

17. *a.* Two-way ANOVA.
   b. Diet and exercise program.
   c. 2
   d. H_0: There is no interaction effect between the type of exercise program and the type of diet on a person's weight loss. H_1: There is an interaction effect between the type of exercise program and the type of diet on a person's weight loss.

   H_0: There is no difference in the means of the weight losses of people in the exercise programs. H_1: There is a difference in the means of the weight losses of people in the exercise programs.

   H_0: There is no difference in the means of the weight losses of people in the diet programs. H_1: There is a difference in the means of the weight losses of people in the diet programs.

   e. Diet: $F = 21.0$, significant; exercise program: $F = 0.429$, not significant; interaction: $F = 0.429$, not significant.
   f. Reject the null hypothesis for the diets.

Chapter 13

Exercises 13–1

1. *Nonparametric* means hypotheses other than those using population parameters can be tested; *distribution-free* means no assumptions about the population distributions have to be satisfied.

3. Nonparametric methods have the following advantages:
   a. They can be used to test population parameters when the variable is not normally distributed.
   b. They can be used when data are nominal or ordinal.
   c. They can be used to test hypotheses other than those involving population parameters.
   d. The computations are easier in some cases than the computations of the parametric counterparts.
   e. They are easier to understand.

The disadvantages are as follows:

   a. They are less sensitive than their parametric counterparts.

   b. They tend to use less information than their parametric counterparts.

   c. They are less efficient than their parametric counterparts.

5.

Data	22	32	34	43	43	65	66	71
Rank	1	2	3	4.5	4.5	6	7	8

7.

Data	4	6	6	7	8	9	9	10	13	15	16	18
Rank	1	2.5	2.5	4	5	6.5	6.5	8	9	10	11	12

9.

Data	188	188	197	256	321	530	763
Rank	1.5	1.5	3	4	5	6	7

Exercises 13–2

1. The sign test uses only positive or negative signs.

3. The smaller number of positive or negative signs.

5. H_0: median = 38 (claim) and H_1: median $\neq$ 38; C.V. = 5; test statistic = 5; do not reject. There is not enough evidence to reject the claim that the median is 38.

7. H_0: median = 25 (claim) and H_1: median $\neq$ 25; test statistic = 7; C.V. = 4; T.S. (7) > C.V. (4); do not reject. There is not enough evidence to reject the claim that the median is 25. School boards could use the median to plan for the costs of cyber school enrollments.

9. H_0: median = \$3.82 (claim) and H_1: median $\neq$ \$3.82; C.V. = +1.96; z = −0.77; do not reject. There is not enough evidence to reject the claim that the median is \$3.82. Home buyers could estimate the yearly cost of their gas bills.

11. H_0: Median = 150 (claim). H_1: Median $\neq$ 150. C.V. = ±1.96; z = −2.70; reject. There is enough evidence to reject the claim that the median number of faculty members is 150.

13. H_0: median = 50 (claim) and H_1: median $\neq$ 50; z = −2.3; P-value (0.0214) $< \alpha$ (0.10); reject. There is enough evidence to reject the claim that 50% of the students are against extending the school year.

15. H_0: The medication has no effect on weight loss. H_1: The medication affects weight loss (claim). C.V. = 0; test statistic = 1; T.S. (1) > C.V. (0); do not reject. There is enough evidence to reject the claim that the medication affects weight loss.

17. H_0: There is no difference in attendance (claim). H_1: There is a difference in attendance. C.V. = 1. Test statistic: T.S. = 1; T.S. (1) = C.V. (1); reject. There is enough evidence to reject the claim that there is no difference in attendance.

19. H_0: The number of viewers is the same as last year (claim); H_1: The number of viewers is not the same as last year; C.V. = 0; test statistic = 2; T.S. (2) > C.V. (1); do not reject. There is not enough evidence to reject the claim that the number of viewers is the same as last year.

21. 6 $\leq$ median $\leq$ 22   **23.** 4.7 $\leq$ median $\leq$ 9.3

25. 4.7 $\leq$ median $\leq$ 9.3

Exercises 13–3

1. n_1 and n_2 are each greater than or equal to 10.

3. The standard normal distribution.

5. H_0: There is no difference in calories between the two delis. H_1: There is a difference in calories between the two delis (claim). C.V. = ±1.96; z = −0.60; do not reject. There is not enough evidence to support the claim that there is a difference in calories.

7. H_0: There is no difference in the stopping distances of the two types of automobiles (claim). H_1: There is a difference between the stopping distances of the two types of automobiles. C.V. = ±1.645; z = 2.797; reject. There is enough evidence to reject the claim that there is no difference in the stopping distances of the two types of automobiles.

9. *Note:* Data do not meet the recommended sample size requirements of $n \geq 10$. Answer would apply only if conditions are met (i.e., more data). H_0: There is no difference in the number of worker fatalities in the two regions (claim). H_1: There is a difference in the number of worker fatalities in the two regions. C.V. = ±1.96; z = 0.128; do not reject. There is not enough evidence to reject the claim that there is no difference in the number of worker fatalities in the two regions.

11. H_0: There is no difference in the times needed to assemble the product. H_1: There is a difference in the times needed to assemble the product (claim). C.V. = ±1.96; z = +3.56; reject. There is enough evidence to support the claim that there is a difference in the productivity of the two groups.

Exercises 13–4

1. The t test for dependent samples.

3. Sum of minus ranks is −6; sum of plus ranks is +15. The test statistic is 6.

5. C.V. = 20; w_s = 18; 18 $\leq$ 20; reject.

7. C.V. = 130; w_s = 142; 142 > 130; do not reject.

9. H_0: The human dose is less than or equal to the animal dose. H_1: The human dose is more than the animal dose (claim). C.V. = 6; w_s = 2; 2 < 6; reject. There is not enough evidence to reject the claim that the human dose costs more than the equivalent animal dose. One reason is that some people might not be inclined to pay a lot of money for their pets' medication.

11. H_0: Quebec Francophones watch the same or less TV then Quebec Anglophones. H_1: Quebec Francophones watch more TV then Quebec Anglophones (claim). C.V. = 2; $w_x = 0$; $0 < 2$; reject. There is not enough evidence to reject the claim that Quebec Francophones watch more TV than Quebec Angolophones.

13. H_0: The prices of prescription drugs in the United States are greater than or equal to the prices in Canada. H_1: The drugs sold in Canada are cheaper (claim). C.V. = 11; $w_s = 3$; $3 < 11$; reject. There is not enough evidence to reject the claim that the drugs are less expensive in Canada.

Exercises 13–5

1. H_0: There is no difference in the number of calories. H_1: There is a difference in the number of calories (claim). C.V. = 7.815; $H = 2.842$; do reject. There is enough evidence to reject the claim that there is a difference in the number of calories.

3. H_0: There is no difference in the prices of the three types of lawnmowers. H_1: There is a difference in the prices of the three types of lawnmowers (claim). C.V. = 4.605; $H = 1.07$; do not reject. There is enough evidence to reject the claim that the prices are different. No, price is not a factor. Results are suspect since one sample is less than 5.

5. H_0: There is no difference in the number of carbohydrates in one serving of each of the three types of food. H_1: There is a difference in the number of carbohydrates in each of the three types of food (claim). C.V. = 9.210; $H = 11.58$; reject. There is not enough evidence to reject the claim that there is a difference in the number of carbohydrates in the three foods. You should recommend the ice cream.

7. H_0: There is no difference in the number of firearm-related deaths by manner/intent for each age group. H_1: There is a difference in the number of firearm-related deaths by manner/intent for each age group (claim). C.V. = 4.605; $H = 8.385$; reject. There is not enough evidence to reject the claim that there is a difference in the number of firearm-related deaths by manner/intent for each age group.

9. H_0: There is no difference in the number of crimes in the five precincts. H_1: There is a difference in the number of crimes in the five precincts (claim). C.V. = 13.277; $H = 20.753$; reject. There is not enough evidence to reject the claim that there is a difference in the number of crimes in the five precincts.

11. H_0: There is no difference in the final exam scores of the three groups. H_1: There is a difference in the final exam scores of the three groups (claim). $H = 1.710$; P-value > 0.10 (0.425); do not reject. There is enough evidence to reject the claim that there is a difference in the final exam scores of the three groups.

Exercises 13–6

1. 0.716   **3.** 0.648

5. $r_s = 0.286$; H_0: $\rho = 0$ and H_1: $\rho \neq 0$; C.V. = ± 0.643; do not reject. There is not enough evidence to indicate that there is a correlation between the number of forest fires caused by human activity and lightning.

7. $r_s = 0.943$; H_0: $\rho = 0$ and H_1: $\rho \neq 0$; C.V. = ± 0.886; reject. There is a significant relationship between the sentence and the time period.

9. $r_s = 0.5$; H_0: $\rho = 0$ and H_1: $\rho \neq 0$; C.V. = ± 0.738; do not reject. There is not enough evidence to say that a significant correlation exists.

11. $r_s = 0.6$; H_0: $\rho = 0$ and H_1: $\rho \neq 0$; C.V. = ± 0.886; do not reject. There is not enough evidence to indicate that a correlation exists between monthly fuel prices and monthly prices of a barrel of oil.

13. $r_s = -0.10$; H_0: $\rho = 0$ and H_1: $\rho \neq 0$; C.V. = ± 0.900; do not reject. There is no significant relationship between the number of cyber school students and the cost per pupil. In this case, the cost per pupil is different in each district.

15. $r = \pm 0.28$ **17.** $r = \pm 0.400$

19. $r = \pm 0.413$

Exercises 13–7

1. *a.* 4 runs   *b.* 6 runs   *c.* 4 runs

3. H_0: The numbers occur at random (claim). H_1: The null hypothesis is not true. For $n_1 = O = 17$, $n_2 = E = 13$; C.V.: 9 and 21; since 18 runs is between 9 and 21, do not reject. There is not enough evidence to reject the claim of randomness.

5. H_0: The answers to the test questions are random (claim). H_1: The null hypothesis is not true. For $n_1 = T = 15$, $n_2 = E = 15$; C.V.: 10 and 22; since 12 runs is between 10 and 22, do not reject. The answers are random.

7. H_0: The gender of the shoppers occurs at random (claim). H_1: The null hypothesis is not true. For $n_1 = M = 9$, $n_2 = F = 11$; C.V.: 6 and 16; since 10 runs is between 6 and 16, do not reject. There is not enough evidence to reject the claim that the gender of the shoppers in line is random.

9. H_0: The days on which customers are able to ski occur at random (claim). H_1: The null hypothesis is false. For $n_1 = S = 17$, $n_2 = N = 11$; C.V.: 9 and 20; since 5 runs is not between 9 and 20, reject. There is enough evidence to reject the claim that the days that customers are able to ski occur at random.

11. H_0: The shuffled card colours occur randomly (claim). H_1: The null hypothesis is false. C.V. = ± 1.96; $z = -1.142$; do not reject. There is enough evidence to conclude that the shuffled card colours occur randomly.

Review Exercises

1. H_0: Median = 42.5 (claim). H_1: Median $\neq$ 42.5. C.V. = ± 0.05; $z = -2.008$; reject. There is enough evidence to reject the claim that the median is 42.5.

3. H_0: There is no difference in prices. H_1: There is a difference in prices (claim). C.V. = 0; test statistic = 1; since $0 < 1$, do not reject. There is not enough evidence to support the claim that the prices are different.

5. H_0: There is no difference in the number of hours worked. H_1: There is a difference in the number of hours worked (claim). C.V. = ± 1.645; $z = -1.760$; reject. There is enough evidence to support the claim that there is a difference in the hours worked.

7. H_0: There is no difference in the amount spent. H_1: There is a difference in the amount spent (claim). C.V. = 2; $w_s = 1$; reject. There is enough evidence to conclude that there is a difference in the amount spent.

9. H_0: The diet has no effect on learning. H_1: The diet affects learning (claim). C.V. = 5.991; $H = 8.5$. Reject; there is enough evidence to support the claim that the diets do affect learning.

11. $r_s = 0.891$; H_0: $\rho = 0$ and H_1: $\rho \neq 0$; C.V. = ± 0.648; reject. There is a significant relationship in the average number of people who are watching the television shows for both years.

13. H_0: The grades of students who finish the exam occur at random. H_1: The null hypothesis is not true. Since there are 8 runs and this value does not fall in the 9-to-21 interval, the null hypothesis is rejected. The grades do not occur at random.

Chapter Quiz

1. False
2. False
3. True
4. True
5. a
6. c
7. d
8. b
9. Nonparametric
10. Nominal, ordinal
11. Sign
12. Sensitive

13. H_0: median = 300 (claim) and H_1: median $\neq$ 300. There are 7 plus signs. Do not reject since 7 is greater than the critical value of 5. There is not enough evidence to reject the claim that the median is 300.

14. H_0: median = 1200 (claim) and H_1: median $\neq$ 1200. There are 10 minus signs. Do not reject since the 10 is greater than the critical value 6. There is not enough evidence to reject the claim that the median is 1200.

15. H_0: There will be no change in the weight of the turkeys after the special diet. H_1: The turkeys will weigh more after the special diet (claim). C.V. = 1; + signs = 1, test statistic = 1; reject. There is enough evidence to support the claim that the turkeys gained weight after the special diet.

16. H_0: The distributions are the same. H_1: The distributions are different (claim). $z = 0.076$; C.V. = ± 1.96; do not reject the null hypothesis. There is not enough evidence to reject the claim that the distributions are the same.

17. H_0: The distributions are the same. H_1: The distributions are different (claim). $z = 0.144$; C.V. = ± 1.645; do not reject the null hypothesis. There is not enough evidence to support the claim that the distributions are different.

18. H_0: There is no difference in the GPA of the students before and after the workshop. H_1: There is a difference in the GPA of the students before and after the workshop (claim). C.V. = 4; $w_s = 1$; reject the null hypothesis. There is enough evidence to support the claim that there is a difference in the GPAs of the students.

19. H_0: There is no difference in the breaking strengths of the tapes. H_1: There is a difference in the breaking strengths of the tapes (claim); $\chi^2 = 5.991$; $H = 29.236$; reject. There is sufficient evidence to support the claim that there is a difference in the breaking strengths of the tapes.

20. H_0: There is no difference in the reaction times of the monkeys. H_1: There is a difference in the reaction times of the monkeys (claim). $H = 6.852$; $0.025 < P$-value < 0.05 (0.032); reject the null hypothesis. There is enough evidence to support the claim that there is a difference in the reaction times of the monkeys.

21. $r_s = 0.683$; H_0: $\rho = 0$ and H_1: $\rho \neq 0$; C.V. = ± 0.600; reject. There is enough evidence to say that there is a significant relationship between the drug prices.

22. $r_s = 0.943$; H_0: $\rho = 0$ and H_1: $\rho \neq 0$; C.V. = ± 0.829; reject. There is a significant relationship between the amount of money spent on Head Start and the number of students enrolled in the program.

23. H_0: The births of babies occur at random according to gender. H_1: The null hypothesis is not true. There are 10 runs, and since this is between 8 and 19, the null hypothesis is not rejected. There is not enough evidence to reject the null hypothesis that the gender occurs at random.

24. H_0: There is no difference in the rpm of the motors before and after the reconditioning. H_1: There is a difference in the rpm of the motors before and after the reconditioning (claim). Reject the null hypothesis since $w_s (0) \leq$ C.V. (6). There is not enough evidence to reject the claim that there is a difference in the rpm of the motors before and after reconditioning.

25. H_0: The numbers occur at random. H_1: The null hypothesis is not true. There are 16 runs, and since this is between 9 and 21, the null hypothesis is not rejected. There is not enough evidence to reject the null hypothesis that the numbers occur at random.

Chapter 14

Exercises 14–1

1. Random, systematic, stratified, cluster

3. A sample must be randomly selected.

5. Talking to people on the street, calling people on the phone, and asking one's friends are three incorrect ways of obtaining a sample.

7. Random sampling has the advantage that each unit of the population has an equal chance of being selected. One disadvantage is that the units of the population must be numbered; if the population is large, this could be somewhat time-consuming.

9. An advantage of stratified sampling is that it ensures representation for the groups used in stratification; however, it is virtually impossible to stratify the population so that all groups are represented.

11. Answers will vary.   13. Answers will vary.

15. Answers will vary.   17. Answers will vary.

19. Answers will vary.

Exercises 14–2

1. Flaw—asking a biased question. Change question to "Will you vote for John Doe or Bill Jones for class president?"

3. Flaw—asking a biased question. Change question to "Should banks charge a fee to balance their customers' chequebooks?"

5. Flaw—confusing words. Change question to "How many hours did you study for this exam?"

7. Flaw—confusing words. Change question to "If a plane was to crash on the border of Ontario and Quebec where should the victims be buried?"

9. Answers will vary.

Exercises 14–3

1. Simulation involves setting up probability experiments that mimic the behaviour of real-life events.

3. John Von Neumann and Stanislaw Ulam.

5. The steps are as follows:
   a. List all possible outcomes.
   b. Determine the probability of each outcome.
   c. Set up a correspondence between the outcomes and the random numbers.
   d. Conduct the experiment by using random numbers.
   e. Repeat the experiment and tally the outcomes.
   f. Compute any statistics and state the conclusions.

7. When the repetitions increase, there is a higher probability that the simulation will yield more precise answers.

9. Use two-digit random numbers, 00 to 99, where digits 00 through 74 will represent the users and digits 75 through 99 will represent non-users.

11. Use two-digit random numbers, 00 through 03, to represent a hit. Use three digits, 000 through 270, to represent a miss.

13. Let an odd number represent heads and an even number represent tails. Then each person selects a digit at random.

15. Answers will vary.   17. Answers will vary.

19. Answers will vary.   21. Answers will vary.

23. Answers will vary.

Review Exercises

1. Answers will vary.   3. Answers will vary.

5. Answers will vary.   7. Answers will vary.

9. Use one-digit random numbers 1 through 4 for a strikeout and 5 through 9 and 0 to represent anything other than a strikeout.

11. In this case, a one-digit random number is selected. Numbers 1 through 6 represent the numbers on the face. Ignore 7, 8, 9, and 0 and select another number.

13. Let the digits 1–3 represent rock, let 4–6 represent paper, let 7–9 represent scissors, and omit 0.

15. Answers will vary.   17. Answers will vary.

19. Flaw—asking a biased question. Change question to "Have you ever driven through a red light?"

21. Flaw—asking a double-barreled question. Change question to "Do you think all automobiles should have heavy-duty bumpers?"

Chapter Quiz

1. True   2. True   3. False

4. True   5. a   6. c

7. c   8. Larger   9. Biased

10. Cluster

11.–14. Answers will vary.

15. Use two-digit random numbers: 01 through 45 means the player wins. Any other two-digit random number means the player loses.

16. Use two-digit random numbers: 01 through 05 means a cancellation. Any other two-digit random number means the person shows up.

17. The random numbers 01 through 13 represent the 13 cards in hearts. The random numbers 14 through 26 represent the 13 cards in diamonds. The random numbers 27 through 39 represent the 13 spades, and 40 through 52 represent the 13 clubs. Any number over 52 is ignored.

18. Use two-digit random numbers to represent the spots on the face of the dice. Ignore any two-digit random numbers with 7, 8, 9, or 0. For cards, use two-digit random numbers between 01 and 13.

19. Use two-digit random numbers. The first digit represents the first player, and the second digit represents the second player. If both numbers are odd or even, player 1 wins. If a digit is odd and the other digit is even, player 2 wins.

20.–24. Answers will vary.

Appendix A

A–1. 362,880

A–3. 120

A–5. 1

A–7. 1320

A–9. 20

A–11. 126

A–13. 70

A–15. 1

A–17. 560

A–19. 2520

A–21. 121; 2181; 14,641; 716.9

A–23. 32; 258; 1024; 53.2

A–25. 328; 22,678; 107,584; 1161.2

A–27. 693; 50,511; 480,249; 2486.1

A–29. 318; 20,150; 101,124; 3296

A–31.

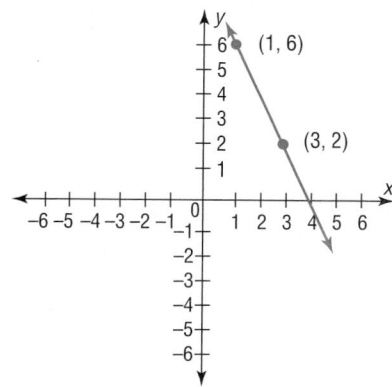

A–33.

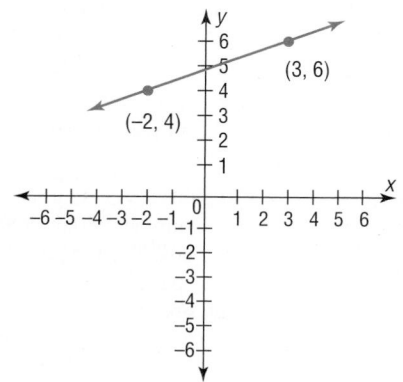

A–35.

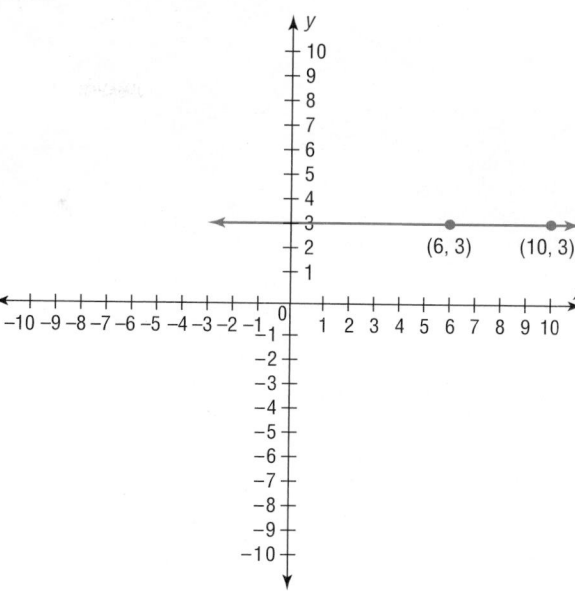

A–37.

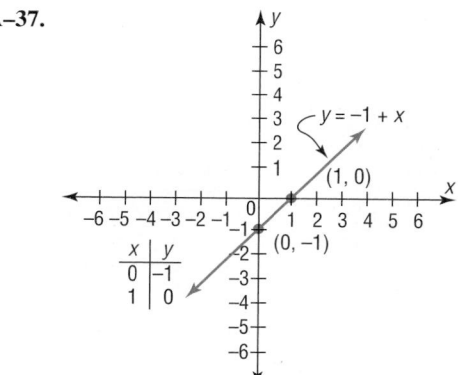

A–39.

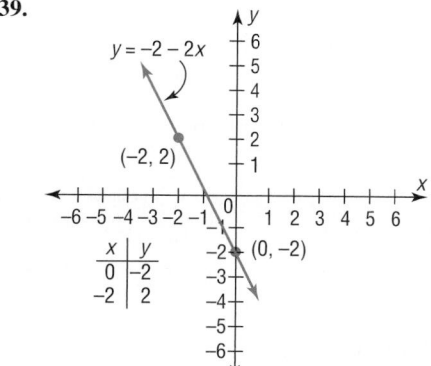

Appendix B–2

B–1. 0.65

B–3. 0.653

B–5. 0.379

B–7. $\frac{1}{4}$

B–9. 0.64

B–11. 0.857

Index